D1707979

SCVIR SYLLABUS

Thoracic and Visceral Nonvascular Interventions

~

Genitourinary Interventions

Jeet Sandhu, M.D., *Editor*
Assistant Professor of Radiology
University of North Carolina
Chapel Hill, North Carolina

Allen J. Meglin, M.D., *Editor*
Assistant Professor of Radiology
Uniformed Services University of the Health Sciences
Director, Interventional Radiology
Walter Reed Army Medical Center
Washington, D.C.

Scott O. Trerotola, M.D., *Editor in Chief*
Associate Professor of Radiology
Indiana University School of Medicine
Indianapolis, Indiana

Published by

The Society of Cardiovascular & Interventional Radiology

Notice

The usage of supply items and indications and dosages of drugs in this book have been recommended in the medical literature. Products mentioned may or may not be approved by the United States Food and Drug Administration for use in the diseases and dosages for which they are recommended by their manufacturers. Please consult package inserts and other product information for current approved standards.

Library of Congress Catalog Card Number 97-67421

The Society of Cardiovascular & Interventional Radiology is accredited by the Accreditation Council for Continuing Medical Education to sponsor continuing medical education for physicians.

The Society of Cardiovascular & Interventional Radiology designates this continuing medical education activity for 20 credit hours in Category 1 of the Physicians Recognition Award of the American Medical Association. This activity has been approved for AMA/PRA 1 CME credit for the period from July 1997 through June 2000.

FOREWORD

I feel privileged to have witnessed the early labor pains of angiography and interventional radiology during the sixties and seventies before this field became the healthy, kicking, independent specialty that we know today. When it was first realized that the Seldinger vascular technique for exchanging a small needle for a much larger catheter became equally applicable to drainage procedures, it became quite obvious that many surgical procedures in the abdomen and pelvis might be replaced or complemented by percutaneous techniques with less patient discomfort and shorter hospital stay. Progress in this regard was initially slow because many were concerned about the safety of needling retroperitoneal structures, especially so when our surgical colleagues asserted that puncture of the bowel or biopsy of the pancreas, accidental or otherwise, would lead inexorably to life-threatening complications. With increasing experience with fine needle puncture and aspiration biopsy within the abdomen under fluoroscopic, angiographic, and ultrasound control, it became quite obvious that almost any abdominal structure could be punctured safely with the "skinny" needle. The advent of CT imaging provided our specialty with a wonderful tool for percutaneously accessing and draining abscesses and postoperative collections without disturbing tissue planes. One can only appreciate the value of this interventional technique if we remember how hazardous surgical drainage was in the past, with mortality rates in the 10%–40% range.

The fear of severe complicating hemorrhage and laceration initially slowed down the wide acceptance of nephrostomy and biliary drainage; the development of fine needle "one-stick" catheter systems did much to facilitate the safe insertion of catheters while the introduction of soft locking-loop drain catheters served to increase patient comfort and markedly decrease the incidence of accidental withdrawals.

The reason for the success and safety of percutaneous gastrostomy and jejunostomy has always puzzled me when it is realized that the equivalent surgical procedures performed with various complex maneuvers to prevent pericatheter leakage have a higher incidence of complications. It would seem that gradual dilatation of tissues following needling of hollow viscous tamponades the track more effectively than surgical incision followed by a purse-string suture around the drain.

The growing impact and sophistication of nonvascular interventions began by radiologists has been noticed by gastroenterologists and laparoscopists. In the future we must anticipate that further progress and ideas in our field will spring not only from interventional radiologists but also from other interested specialties. This cross-fertilization will certainly be beneficial to our specialty and hopefully will lead to constructive cooperation among the interested players! The editors and authors of this book are to be congratulated for providing us with tutorials and interesting cases for a thorough overview of genitourinary, thoracic, and visceral nonvascular interventions. This kind of work should provide our younger members with a tool to confirm their understanding of the present but also with a challenge for the future.

Constantin Cope, M.D.
Professor of Radiology
Hospital of the University of Pennsylvania

PREFACE

The mission of the SCVIR Educational Materials Committee is to provide high-quality educational materials to our membership, and Volume VII of the SCVIR Syllabus/Videodisc series is no exception. The Committee is proud to introduce the current volume, which covers a broad variety of interventions in the thorax, abdomen and pelvis. The material covered in this Syllabus ranges from the tried and true "bread and butter" techniques of nephrostomy and abscess drainage, to recent developments such as tracheal and esophageal stent placement. The split cover design reflects the diversity of content and serves to remind the reader that this is in effect a two-in-one volume. As with prior Syllabi, the content is divided into didactic tutorials and quiz-type teaching file cases. The SCVIR offers Category 1 CME credit for those wishing to complete the CME quizzes at the end of the volume.

Jeet Sandhu and Allen Meglin are to be commended for assembling an outstanding group of contributors. The result is a truly comprehensive review of thoracoabdominal nonvascular and genitourinary interventions. On behalf of the SCVIR Educational Materials Committee, I would like to congratulate the authors and editors on their fine effort, and thank them for their generous contribution of time and expertise. In addition, Belinda Byrne and her production staff deserve thanks for their excellent work.

The SCVIR Syllabus series is the result of hard work and careful planning by a great many individuals. The continued success of the series is due in part to these individuals, but also to the strong support and interest among the SCVIR membership. Undoubtedly, however, the series would not have generated such momentum without the vision and energy of Jeanne LaBerge, who laid so much of the initial groundwork. Thanks, Jeanne!

The next volume of the Syllabi, Vascular Diagnosis, is already underway. In addition to the Syllabus series, the Educational Materials Committee is developing ideas for other enduring materials, both electronic (such as Internet projects) and conventional. Stay tuned.

Scott O. Trerotola, M.D.
Editor in Chief
Chairman, SCVIR Educational Materials Committee

ACKNOWLEDGMENTS

The production of any manuscript or text requires the effort of many individuals. I would like to thank Belinda Byrne and her production staff for their ceaseless efforts in transforming numerous images and text into a highly professional production while maintaining an incredibly good disposition. I would like to thank all of the contributors of tutorials and teaching files for their efforts in making such a superb syllabus a reality. Volunteering their time and effort exemplifies the dedication, enthusiasm, and commitment typical of the SCVIR membership. I would like to thank my partners Paul Jaques and Matt Mauro for their suggestions and support during production of the syllabus. I would like to thank Scott Trerotola for his guidance, advice, and superb editorial skills. His unflagging dedication and attention to detail contributed mightily to the syllabus. My secretary, Angela Lyght, deserves extraordinary thanks for the magnificent job she did in organizing, typing, reminding, calling, cajoling, and all of the little things it took to finish the project. Although not directly involved in the syllabus, I would like to acknowledge my parents, Jind and Shingara Sandhu, for their never ending love and for everything that they have done as great parents. Thanks Mom and Dad. Most of all, I would like to thank my wife Maury for her love, support, patience, understanding, and encouragement. Without her, it wouldn't have been possible.

Jeet Sandhu, M.D.

I am deeply indebted to many coworkers without whom this project would have been impossible. I would like to thank Faith Smit for her tireless and meticulous participation in each and every manuscript draft. Without her I would have been lost. Doug LeFevre and Jill Duhan, the office managers, were invaluable for their organizational skills and follow-up. Ellen Chung and Mark Lukens contributed heavily to the text, to my morale, and to the overall forward movement of the project. God has truly blessed me with two superb partners. I would also like to thank my immediate supervisors Curt Stoldt, Theodore Raia, and Mike Brazaitis who taught me leadership through their example. I would also like to acknowledge Scott Trerotola whose guidance and support has taken me through fellowship and beyond. A special mention of gratitude to the copy editor, Paula Sinclair, whose superlative editing skills have once again contributed to the high caliber of this book. And finally, I will forever be indebted to the SCVIR production team—Belinda Byrne, Koreen Piazza, Kevin Havener, and Martha Borelli. Thank you for all your help, guidance, support, professionalism, and ability to deliver during crunch time.

Anyone who has worked on a project such as this knows that it is a significant undertaking similar to parenting. It is both painful and rewarding and requires the inspiration of others. I would like to dedicate this project to Anthony C. Venbrux, the most decent and honorable person I know, to the residents and faculty at Walter Reed who taught me more than I can ever teach them, to my wife, Nancy, whom I love with all my heart, and to my children, Michelle, Mathew, Melissa, and Michael, who make life worth living.

Allen J. Meglin, M.D.

CME INFORMATION

CME Essentials

The SCVIR Syllabus, *Thoracic and Visceral Nonvascular Interventions/Genitourinary Interventions*, is part of a series of enduring materials planned and produced in accordance with the Accreditation Council for Continuing Medical Education Essentials. It has been developed for interventional radiologists, both practicing and in training, in two formats: instructional textbook and computer-assisted videodisc.

Thoracic and Visceral Nonvascular Interventions/Genitourinary Interventions constitutes a planned activity of continuing medical education with an estimated completion time of 20 hours. This activity has been approved for AMA/PRA 1 CME credit for the period from July 1997 through June 2000. Topics covered for this CME activity are represented by the Table of Contents, Part One: Tutorials, on pages xv and xvi of this volume, and principal faculty and their credentials can be found on pages ix–xiii. An evaluation survey is provided as part of this CME activity to assess the value of these materials in meeting the educational needs of the end user.

After completing *Thoracic and Visceral Nonvascular Interventions/Genitourinary Interventions*, the reader should be able to:

1) Discuss indications and techniques for percutaneous biopsy of the thorax, liver, pancreas, and adrenal gland.
2) Describe the appearance of abscesses in the liver, peritoneum, pelvis, and within the thorax, and define the fundamental principles of their percutaneous management.
3) Discuss indications for and techniques of percutaneous nephrostomy for decompression, as well as access for stone removal.
4) Discuss indications for and techniques of percutaneous enterostomy, including gastrostomy and gastrojejunostomy, as well as direct percutaneous jejunostomy.
5) Describe complications of percutaneous biopsy, abscess drainage, nephrostomy, and enterostomy, and discuss management options.

To become eligible for 20 hours of Category 1 CME credit, the user must submit the enclosed application form, an evaluation survey, and a completed quiz answer sheet, along with a $20 administrative fee, to:

SCVIR
Attention: CME Administrator
10201 Lee Highway, Suite 500
Fairfax, VA 22030

Financial Disclosure

The Society of Cardiovascular & Interventional Radiology has a policy requiring disclosure of the existence of any significant financial interest or other relationship that authors have to the manufacturer(s) of any commercial product(s) discussed in any SCVIR-sponsored educational activity.

The following authors have disclosed a financial relationship with companies about whose products or services they have reported:

Amy Thurmond, M.D. (Conceptus, Inc.; Cook, Inc.)
Rendon C. Nelson, M.D. (Bracco Diagnostics; GE CT Medical Advisory Board)

Each of the remaining authors have indicated that he or she has no financial relationship with companies or organizations about whose products or services they are reporting.

SCVIR Syllabus Volume VII
Thoracic and Visceral Nonvascular Interventions/Genitourinary Interventions

Date of next CME review: June 2000

CONTRIBUTORS

Lance Arnder, M.D.
Radiology Resident
University of North Carolina
Chapel Hill, North Carolina

Robert T. Andrews, M.D.
Clinical Instructor in Interventional Radiology
The Johns Hopkins Medical Institutions
Baltimore, Maryland

Dean E. Baird, M.D.
Staff Radiologist
Tripler Army Medical Center
Honolulu, Hawaii

Mark Berger, M.D.
Clinical Associate
Duke University Medical Center
Durham, North Carolina

Robert D. Bloch, Ph.D., M.D.
Instructor in Interventional Radiology
Dotter Institute of Interventional Therapy
Oregon Health Sciences University
Portland, Oregon

Daniel Boyle, M.D.
Staff Radiologist
Walter Reed Army Medical Center
Washington, D.C.

Stephen J. Brown, M.D.
Staff Radiologist
Walter Reed Army Medical Center
Washington, D.C.

John F. Cardella, M.D.
Professor of Radiology
Pennsylvania State University School of Medicine
Chief, Interventional Radiology
Hershey Medical Center
Hershey, Pennsylvania

C. Humberto Carrasco, M.D.
Professor of Radiology
Chief, Angiography and Interventional Radiology
M.D. Anderson Cancer Center
University of Texas
Houston, Texas

Paul R. Cazier, M.D.
Neuroradiology Fellow
University of California, San Francisco
San Francisco, California

Shailendra Chopra, M.D., M.R.C.P., F.R.C.R.
Assistant Professor of Radiology
University of Texas Health Science Center
San Antonio, Texas

Ellen M. Chung, M.D.
Staff Radiologist
Walter Reed Army Medical Center
Washington, D.C.

William Clark, M.D.
Fellow Associate
University of Iowa Hospital and Clinics
Iowa City, Iowa

Dewey J. Conces, Jr., M.D.
Professor of Radiology
Indiana University School of Medicine
Indianapolis, Indiana

Allen A. Currier, Jr., M.D.
Radiology Resident
Hartford Hospital
Hartford, Connecticut

Gerald D. Dodd III, M.D.
Professor of Radiology
Chief, Abdominal Imaging
University of Texas Health Science Center
San Antonio, Texas

CONTRIBUTORS

Siobhan Dumbleton, M.D.
Clinical Instructor in Interventional Radiology
University of North Carolina
Chapel Hill, North Carolina

Georges Y. El-Khoury, M.D.
Professor of Radiology and Orthopaedics
Director, Diagnostic Division
University of Iowa Hospital and Clinics
Iowa City, Iowa

Christine C. Esola, M.D.
Assistant Professor of Radiology
University of Texas Health Science Center
San Antonio, Texas

Vickie A. Feldstein, M.D.
Assistant Professor of Radiology
University of California, San Francisco
San Francisco, California

Hector Ferral, M.D.
Interventional Radiologist
School of Medicine in New Orleans
Louisiana State University Medical Center
New Orleans, Louisiana

Jeffrey A. Golden, M.D.
Professor of Medicine
University of California, San Francisco
San Francisco, California

Roy L. Gordon, M.D.
Professor of Radiology
Chief, Interventional Radiology
University of California, San Francisco
San Francisco, California

James F. Gruden, M.D.
Assistant Professor of Radiology
New York University School of Medicine
New York, New York

John R. Haaga, M.D.
Professor of Radiology
Chairman and Director, Department of Radiology
University Hospitals of Cleveland
Cleveland, Ohio

Michael J. Hallisey, M.D.
Assistant Clinical Professor of Radiology
University of Connecticut School of Medicine
Staff Physician
Hartford Hospital
Hartford, Connecticut

Joseph L. Higgins, Ph.D., M.D.
Assistant Professor of Radiology
Chief, Computed Tomography
School of Medicine in New Orleans
Louisiana State University Medical Center
New Orleans, Louisiana

Jeffrey P. Houston, M.D.
Assistant Professor of Radiology
Yale University School of Medicine
New Haven, Connecticut

Pierce B. Irby, M.D.
Director, Urology Stone Center
Walter Reed Army Medical Center
Washington, D.C.

Philip J. Kenney, M.D.
Professor of Radiology
University of Alabama at Birmingham
Birmingham, Alabama
Armed Forces Institute of Pathology
Washington, D.C.

Robert K. Kerlan, Jr., M.D.
Clinical Professor of Radiology
University of California, San Francisco
San Francisco, California

CONTRIBUTORS

Jeffrey S. Klein, M.D.
Chief, Thoracic Radiology
Medical Center Hospital of Vermont
Burlington, Vermont

Phillip Kohanski, M.D.
Chief, Interventional Radiology
D.D. Eisenhower Army Medical Center
Fort Gordon, Georgia

David D. Lawrence, M.D.
Associate Professor of Radiology
M.D. Anderson Cancer Center
University of Texas
Houston, Texas

Ricardo Lencioni, M.D.
Instituto di Radiologia
Universita degli Studi di Pisa
Pisa, Italy

David L. Levin, Ph.D., M.D.
Assistant Professor of Radiology
Chief, Chest Radiology
Beth Israel Deaconess Medical Center
Boston, Massachussetts

Curtis A. Lewis, M.D.
Assistant Professor of Radiology
Emory University School of Medicine
Atlanta, Georgia

Mark L. Lukens, M.D.
Assistant Director, Interventional Radiology
Walter Reed Army Medical Center
Washington, D.C.

Robert D. Lyon, M.D.
Staff Radiologist
Brooke Army Medical Center
Fort Sam Houston, Texas

Shelley R. Marder, M.D.
Assistant Clinical Professor of Radiology
University of California, San Francisco
Chief, Interventional Radiology
San Francisco General Hospital
San Francisco, California

William H. Marshall, M.D.
Staff Radiologist
Walter Reed Army Medical Center
Washington, D.C.

Vincent D. McCormick, M.D.
Associate Clinical Professor of Radiology
University of California, San Francisco
San Francisco General Hospital
San Francisco, California

J. Mark McKinney, M.D.
Senior Associate Consultant
Diagnostic Radiology
Mayo Clinic Jacksonville
Jacksonville, Florida

Allen J. Meglin, M.D.
Assistant Professor of Radiology
Uniformed Services University of the Health Sciences
Bethesda, Maryland
Director, Interventional Radiology
Walter Reed Army Medical Center
Washington, D.C.

Rendon C. Nelson, M.D.
Professor of Radiology
Director, Abdominal Imaging
Duke University Medical Center
Durham, North Carolina

Albert A. Nemcek, Jr., M.D.
Associate Professor of Radiology
Northwestern University Medical School
Northwestern Memorial Hospital
Chicago, Illinois

CONTRIBUTORS

Michelle Neuder, M.D.
Radiology Resident
Bowman-Gray School of Medicine
North Carolina Baptist Hospital
Winston-Salem, North Carolina

Dennis S. Orwig, M.D.
Assistant Clinical Professor of Radiology
University of California, San Francisco
Marin Radiology Medical Group
Novato, California

David E. Panzer, M.D.
Associate Consultant
Diagnostic Radiology
Mayo Clinic Jacksonville
Jacksonville, Florida

L. Alden Parker, M.D.
Associate Professor of Radiology
Chief, Thoracic Radiology
University of North Carolina Hospitals
Chapel Hill, North Carolina

Nilesh H. Patel, M.D.
Director, Angiography and
Interventional Radiology
Harborview Medical Center
University of Washington
Seattle, Washington

Dennis S. Peppas, M.D.
Director, Pediatric Urology
Walter Reed Army Medical Center
Washington, D.C.

Bryan Peterson, M.D.
Assistant Professor of Diagnostic Radiology
Dotter Institute of Interventional Therapy
Oregon Health Sciences University
Director, Angiography
Veterans Administration Medical Center
Portland, Oregon

Jeffrey S. Pollak, M.D.
Associate Professor of Radiology
Yale University School of Medicine
New Haven, Connecticut

Kevin L. Quinn, M.D.
Interventional Radiologist
William W. Backus Hospital
Norwich, Connecticut

Richard D. Redvanly, M.D.
Assistant Professor of Radiology
Emory University School of Medicine
Atlanta, Georgia

William R. Richili, M.D.
Associate Professor of Radiology
M.D. Anderson Cancer Center
University of Texas
Houston, Texas

Ernest J. Ring, M.D.
Professor of Radiology
Associate Dean of Clinical Affairs
University of California, San Francisco
San Francisco, California

Joseph A. Ronsivalle, D.O.
Staff Radiologist
Walter Reed Army Medical Center
Washington, D.C.

Ana M. Salazar, M.D.
Assistant Professor of Radiology
Jefferson Medical College
Thomas Jefferson University Hospital
Philadelphia, Pennsylvania

Jeet Sandhu, M.D.
Assistant Professor of Radiology
University of North Carolina
Chapel Hill, North Carolina

CONTRIBUTORS

Rajiv Sawhney, M.D.
Assistant Professor of Radiology
University of California, San Francisco
Veterans Administration Medical Center
San Francisco, California

Richard R. Saxon, M.D.
Assistant Professor
Dotter Institute of Interventional Therapy
Oregon Health Sciences University
Portland, Oregon

Scott R. Schultz, M.D.
Chief, Interventional Radiology
Minneapolis Radiology Associates, Ltd.
Robbinsdale, Minnesota

Rosita M. Shah, M.D.
Assistant Professor of Radiology
Allegheny University Hospital
Philadelphia, Pennsylvania

Steven Souza, M.D.
Interventional Radiologist
Radiology Associates of Santa Rosa
Santa Rosa, California

Aaron L. Stack, M.D.
Resident, Diagnostic Radiology
Walter Reed Army Medical Center
Washington, D.C.

John D. Statler, M.D.
Staff Radiologist
Walter Reed Army Medical Center
Washington, D.C.

Steven D. Stowell, M.D.
Staff Radiologist
Walter Reed Army Medical Center
Washington, D.C.

Charles E. Swallow, M.D.
Neuroradiology Fellow
University of Utah
Salt Lake City, Utah

Amy Thurmond, M.D.
Associate Professor of Obstetrics
and Gynecology
Oregon Health Sciences University
Portland, Oregon
Staff Radiologist
Legacy Meridian Park Hospital
Tualatin, Oregon

Anthony C. Venbrux, M.D.
Associate Professor of Radiology
and Surgery
The Johns Hopkins Medical Institutions
Baltimore, Maryland

Robert L. Vogelzang, M.D.
Professor of Radiology
Northwestern University Medical School
Northwestern Memorial Hospital
Chicago, Illinois

Kimberly A. Waugh, M.D.
Assistant Professor of Radiology
M.D. Anderson Cancer Center
University of Texas
Houston, Texas

Michael Wholey, M.D.
Interventional Radiologist
School of Medicine in New Orleans
Louisiana State University Medical Center
New Orleans, Louisiana

Mark W. Wilson, M.D.
Assistant Professor of Radiology
University of Michigan School of Medicine
Ann Arbor, Michigan

Adam B. Winick, M.D.
Assistant Professor of Radiology
George Washington University Medical Center
Washington, D.C.

CONTENTS

PART ONE: TUTORIALS

VISCERAL NONVASCULAR INTERVENTIONS

PART TWO: TEACHING FILE CASES

VISCERAL NONVASCULAR INTERVENTIONS

THORACIC NONVASCULAR INTERVENTIONS

GENITOURINARY INTERVENTIONS

OTHER TOPICS

PART THREE: CME QUIZZES

TUTORIALS

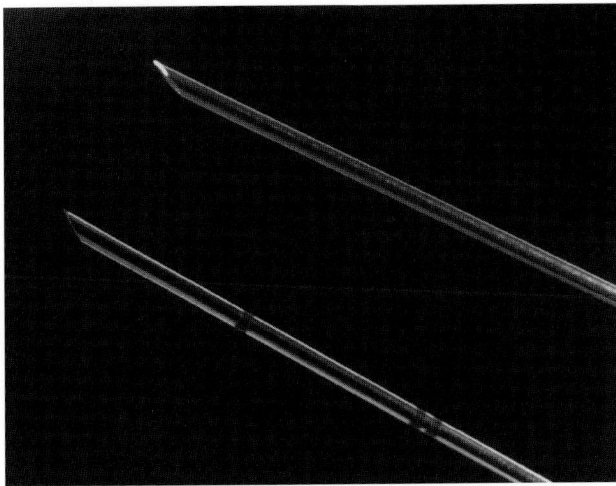

Figure 1. Chiba needles.

TUTORIAL 1
OVERVIEW OF BIOPSY TECHNIQUE AND BIOPSY NEEDLES

John R. Haaga, M.D.

Introduction

The subjects addressed in this tutorial include:

1. Aspiration technique
2. Cutting needle technique
3. Bleeding risks after needle biopsy
4. Needle selection for lung biopsy
5. Needle selection for liver biopsy
6. Needle selection for kidney and retroperitoneal biopsy.

The choice of biopsy needle varies according to the type of tissue required to answer the clinical question, the risk of complications, the target organ, the coagulation status of the patient, the vascularity of the target area, and the anatomic trajectory being chosen.[1]

For cases where a confirmatory diagnosis of malignancy is sought and a high level of safety is desired, an aspiration needle **(Fig. 1)** is appropriate. Although a variety of needles is available differing in size and tip configuration, published data clearly show that larger-caliber needles provide a better cytologic sample.[2] Furthermore, the best tip angle is approximately that of the Chiba needle, which measures 25–30 degrees.

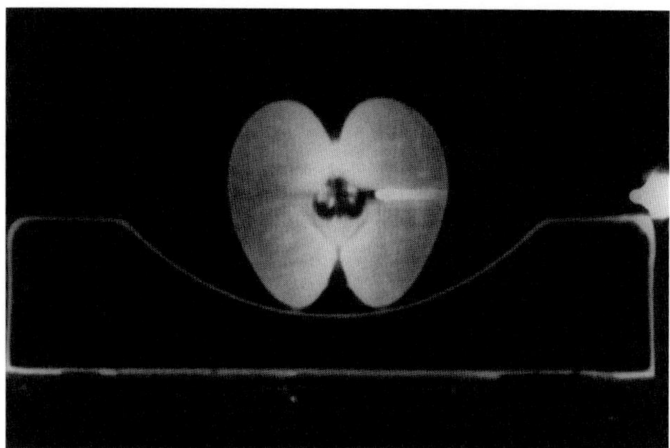

Figure 2. Aspiration needle advanced to the edge of the target (apple core).

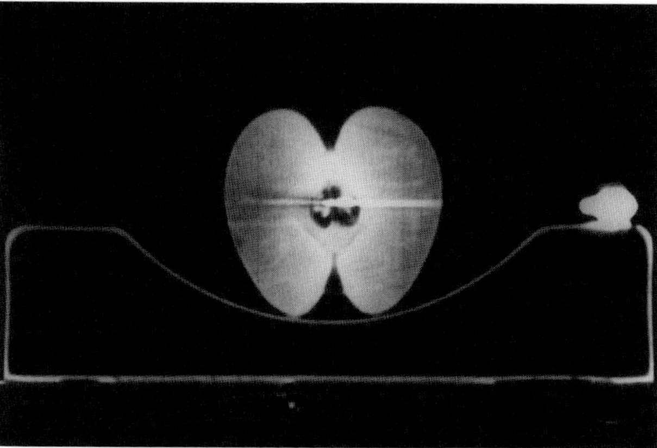

Figure 3. The needle is then advanced with suction and small reciprocating movements to obtain tissue.

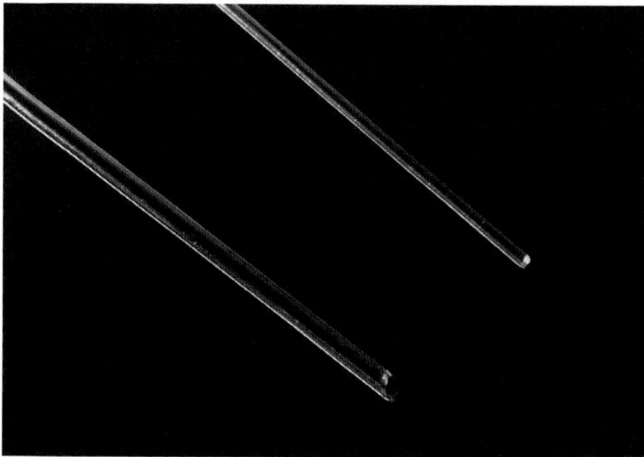

Figure 4. Menghini needles.

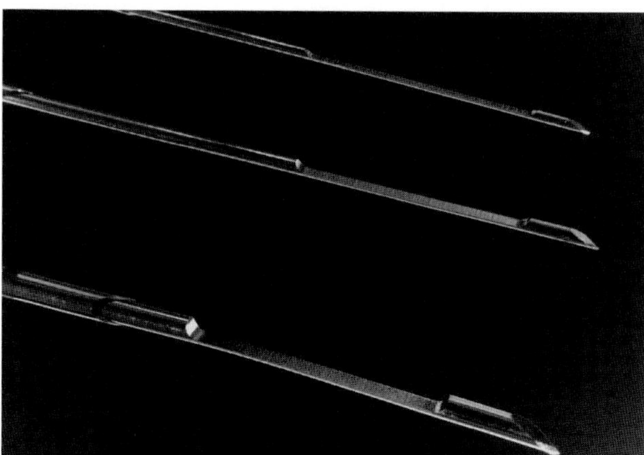

Figure 5. Tru-Cut needles.

Aspiration Technique

To perform an aspiration biopsy, the needle is first positioned adjacent to the target (core of an apple in this case) **(Fig. 2)**. Suction is then applied and the needle is inserted through the lesion with numerous short, rapid, up-and-down reciprocating movements **(Fig. 3)**. Suction with approximately 5–10 mL of syringe displacement should be maintained to obtain adequate tissue and prevent tissue from being left behind out of the needle.

Cutting Needle Techniques

The two types of devices used for cutting needles are the “Menghini” type **(Fig. 4)** and the “Tru-Cut” type (Travenol Laboratories, Deerfield, IL) **(Fig. 5)**. These vary according to the needle caliber and cutting design variation. Both types are designed to obtain core samples, although a more reliable core sample is obtained with the Tru-Cut type. The Menghini-type needle differs from aspiration (Chiba) needles in that the edge of the cylinder is sharpened. The Menghini method, as with the aspiration method, consists of placing the needle next to the target and applying suction as the needle is thrust through the target. The difference between the Menghini and aspiration methods is that numerous reciprocations are made with the aspiration and only a single thrust forward is made with the Menghini.

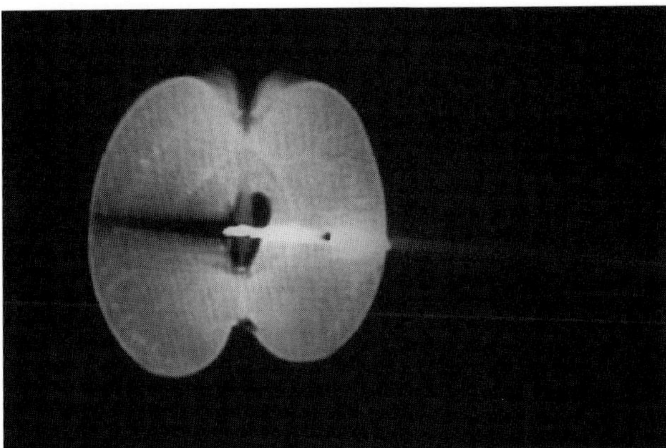

Figure 6. Technique of Tru-Cut biopsy. A Tru-Cut needle with its inner stylet withdrawn is advanced to the edge of or immediately within the lesion (apple core).

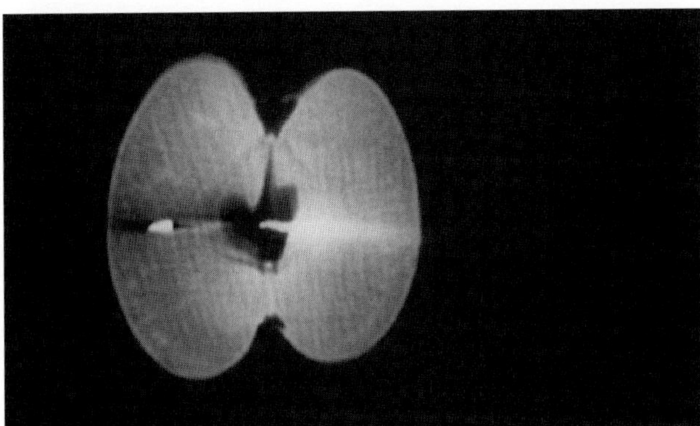

Figure 7. Inner cutting stylet advanced through the lesion.

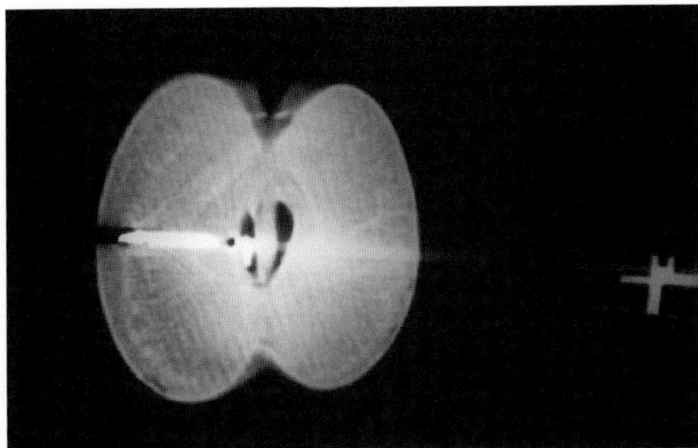

Figure 8. Outer cannula advanced while the inner stylet is held stable.

Tru-Cut Method

The method of obtaining tissue with the Tru-Cut type is the same whether a manual needle or automated needle is used. The needle tip is first placed immediately proximal to the lesion **(Fig. 6)**. The tissue stylet is then advanced into the lesion **(Fig. 7)** and the outer cutting cannula is moved over the stylet **(Fig. 8)**. The "throw" of the inner stylet—the distance the stylet and eventually the entire needle will move from the initial point of insertion—must be taken into consideration. If a critical structure lies immediately behind the targeted lesion, the stylet may advance into that structure. Best samples are taken when the inner stylet is kept absolutely still while the cutting cannula is moved forward. With manual needles, this requires practice and concentration. With automated needles, the device must be held firmly as it is "fired" to prevent recoil which will push back and compromise the correct cutting action.

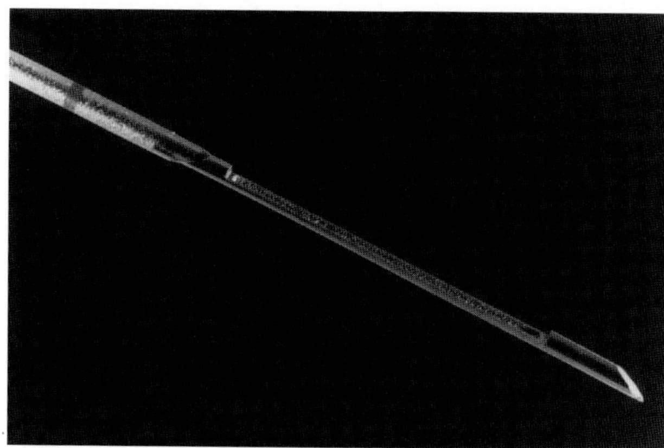

Figure 9. Channel cut Tru-Cut device.

Variations in Tru-Cut Design

A variety of Tru-Cut needle configurations and calibers is available. Recent studies in live anesthetized animals that used quantification of deoxyribonucleic acid (DNA) in recovered samples have revealed valuable information about these devices.[2,3] Modifications such as the channel cut **(Fig. 9)** have improved the recovery of tissue samples by about 40%. Various needle gauges were evaluated relative to blood loss and sample recovery. Animals with normal coagulation studies showed no difference in the amount of bleeding per microgram of DNA recovered. Larger needles were also more efficient because fewer samples were required by large needle passes to obtain a particular amount of tissue. For example, one pass with a 14-gauge needle was equivalent to three 18-gauge or six 20-gauge passes.

Bleeding Risks

The overall bleeding risks of the different needles have not varied sufficiently in clinical studies to be definitive, but controlled animal studies by Gazelle et al have clearly stratified the risks of biopsy in patients with normal coagulation and some anticoagulated states.[3] Clear differences are seen in the absolute amount of bleeding from the kidney and liver in subjects with normal and abnormal prothrombin times.

For liver biopsies, little difference in bleeding was noted between the 18-, 20-, and 22-gauge Chiba needles in normal and anticoagulated subjects (treated with either aspirin or warfarin). However, 14- and 16-gauge needles do produce significantly more bleeding. For kidney biopsies in subjects with normal coagulation, no difference in bleeding was noted with 18-, 20-, or 22-gauge needles. For kidney biopsies in anticoagulated subjects, 18- and 20-gauge needles caused equivalent bleeding, but both caused more bleeding than did 22-gauge needles.

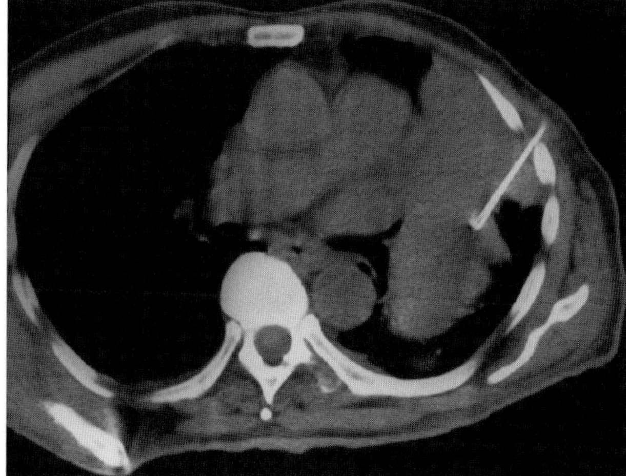

Figure 10. Aspiration lung biopsy. Note the path chosen to avoid the lung and decrease the risk of pneumothorax.

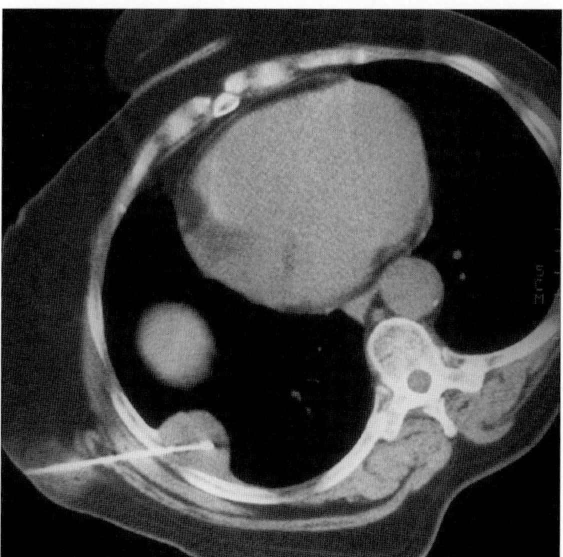

Figure 11. Tru-Cut core needle lung biopsy.

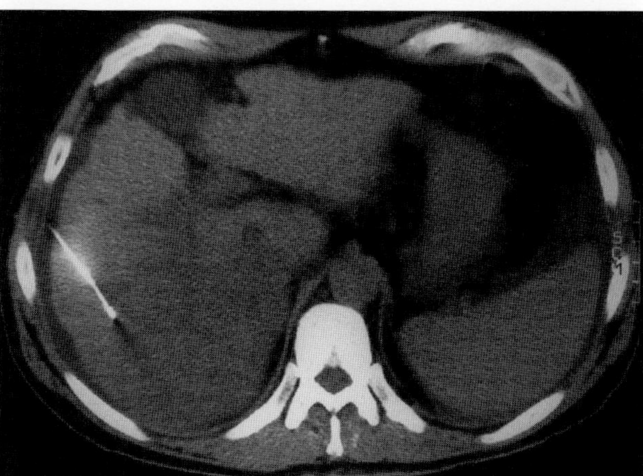

Figure 12. Tru-Cut core needle liver biopsy.

No matter which needle is used, alteration of platelet function increases bleeding.[4] This animal model correlates well with clinical experience, and patients treated with aspirin or anti-inflammatory agents should discontinue the medication for 7 days before any biopsy procedure.

To summarize, biopsies with 18–22-gauge needles carry equivalent risks of bleeding in patients with normal coagulation parameters, and the larger needle size may provide better tissue samples. In patients with uncorrectable coagulopathy, smaller needles are better. Embolization of the biopsy track with Gelfoam (Upjohn, Kalamazoo, MI) should be considered in patients with severe underlying coagulation abnormalities.

Needle Selection for Lung Biopsy

For sampling the lung, both aspiration and cutting needles can be used in selected cases. For routine lung masses, typically adenocarcinoma, small cell, or squamous cell tumors, an aspiration needle biopsy is satisfactory. Methods to minimize possible pneumothorax include planning the trajectory to have a short pathway through the lung, traversing consolidation or fibrous attachments **(Fig. 10)**, avoiding obvious blebs, minimizing the number of needle passes, placing the punctured side dependent after the procedure, and selecting patients appropriately. When attempts at aspiration fail and a mass is adjacent to the pleura, the mass can be biopsied safely with a cutting needle if the cutting chamber is confined to the lesion **(Fig. 11)**.

Needle Selection for Liver Biopsy

For liver lesions, either aspiration or cutting needles can be selected **(Fig. 12)**, depending on the following factors. A 20-gauge Chiba aspiration needle should be used for "known" malignancy, precariously located lesions (adjacent to vessels, gallbladder, etc), questionable vascular lesions, or uncooperative patients. The trajectory chosen for either needle should include a cuff of normal liver parenchyma. Cutting needles should be reserved for lesions which are "avascular" by contrast bolus (computed tomography or magnetic resonance imaging) or Doppler ultrasound. Although angled approaches are more difficult, they are preferable to penetrating uninvolved organs.

See Tutorial 3 for a more detailed discussion of liver biopsy.

Needle Selection For Kidney and Retroperitoneal Biopsy

The method for biopsy of the kidney depends on the tissue being sought. For indeterminate renal masses, aspiration biopsy is usually adequate, but cutting needles may occasionally be required **(Fig. 13)**, especially if special stains for hormonal products are needed. When renal parenchyma is needed for histologic evaluation of the kidney, a cutting needle of 14 to 18 gauge must be used. The target area of parenchyma should be superficial, to avoid the medullary region where larger vessels reside **(Fig. 14)**. The lower pole or lateral cortex should be targeted. Despite the best technique and trajectory selection, bleeding is more common with renal parenchymal biopsies and can easily be visualized around the organ **(Fig. 15)**.

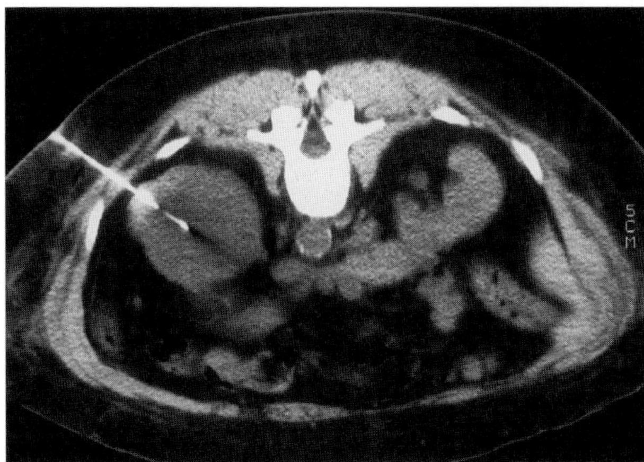

Figure 13. Core needle biopsy of a renal tumor.

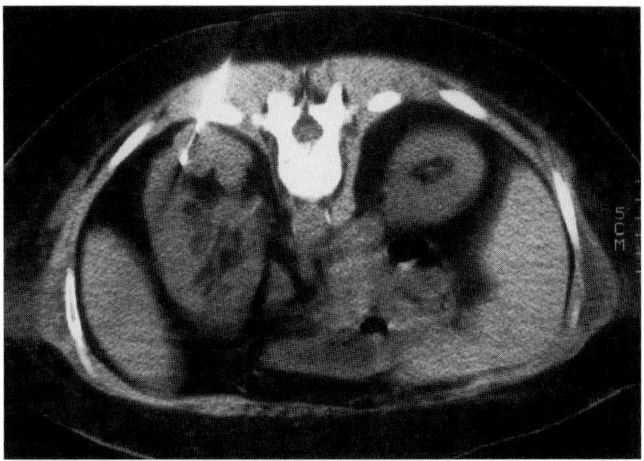

Figure 14. Cutting biopsy of renal parenchyma. Note the superficial needle trajectory which avoids large vessels.

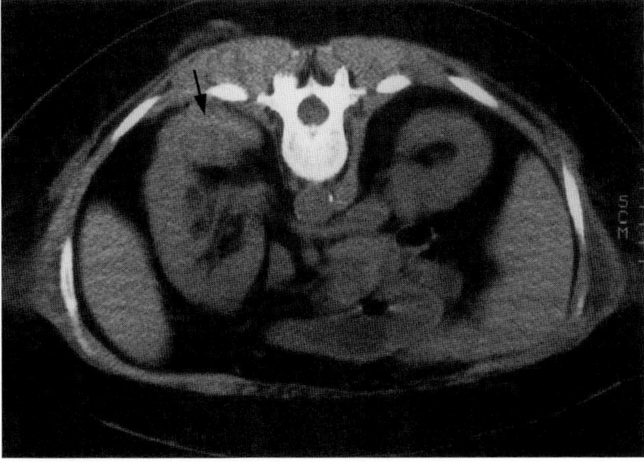

Figure 15. Small post-biopsy hematoma (arrow).

Summary

Percutaneous biopsy is a safe and effective technique of obtaining adequate material for cytologic or histologic diagnosis. If proper attention is given to the patient's coagulation status, any use of antiplatelet agents, and appropriate needle gauge, this procedure can be performed with a minimum of complications. The choice of needle design and technique will be determined by several factors that must be considered in each individual case.

References

1. Haaga JR. Interventional CT-guided procedures. In: Haaga JR, Lanzieri CF, Sartoris DJ, Zerhouni EA, eds. Computed tomography and magnetic resonance imaging of the whole body. 3rd edition. St. Louis: C.V. Mosby Company, 1994.

2. Andriole JG, Haaga JR, Adams RB, Nunez C. Biopsy needle characteristics assessed in the laboratory. Radiology 1983; 148(3):659–662.

3. Gazelle GS, Haaga JR, Rowland DY. Effect of needle gauge, level of anticoagulation, and target organ on bleeding associated with aspiration biopsy. Work in progress. Radiology 1992; 183:509–513.

4. Gazelle GS, Haaga JR, Halpern EF. Hemostatic protein-polymer sheath: improvement in hemostasis at percutaneous biopsy in the setting of platelet dysfunction. Radiology 1993; 187:269–272.

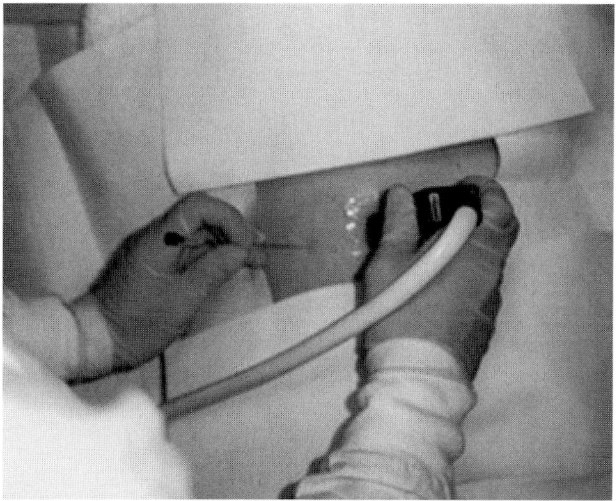

Figure 1. Demonstration of percutaneous US-guided fine needle aspiration procedure. Note the position of the needle and transducer held by a single operator.

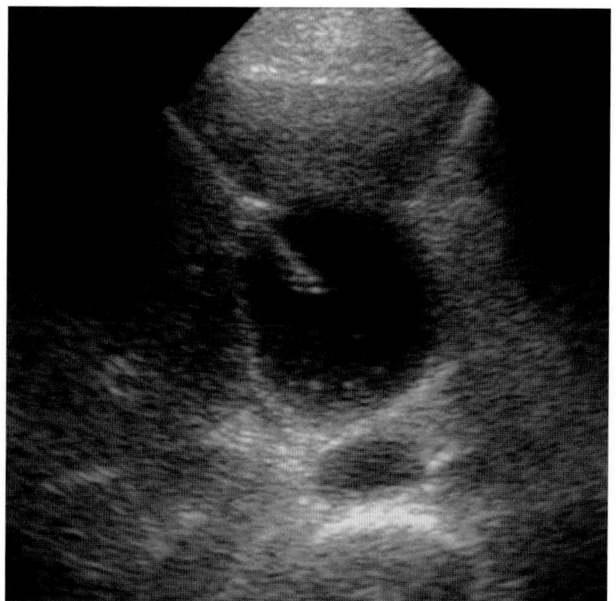

Figure 2. Transhepatic insertion of a needle into the gallbladder under ultrasound guidance.

Ultrasound-Guided Interventional Procedures

Biopsies	*Interventions*
Abdomen	Chest
Liver	Pleural tube placement
Kidney	Abscess drainage
Pancreas	Abdomen
Spleen	Peritoneal catheter placement
Retroperitoneum	Percutaneous transhepatic cholangiography
Lymph nodes	Biliary drainage
	Percutaneous cholecystostomy
Pelvis	Percutaneous nephrostomy
Uterus	Percutaneous gastrostomy
Ovaries	Abscess drainage
Lymph nodes	Pelvis
Scrotum	Abscess drainage
	Ovum retrieval
Breast	Foreign body removal
Chest	Obstetrical
Peripheral lung lesions	Chorionic villus sampling
Pleural lesions	Umbilical cord
Mediastinal masses	Blood sampling
	Transfusion
Head and Neck	Aspirations
Thyroid	Breast cysts
Parathyroid	Thoracentesis
Lymph nodes	Paracentesis
Central nervous system (intraoperative)	Renal cysts
	Joint spaces
	Vascular access
	Venous
	Arterial

Figure 3.

TUTORIAL 2 ULTRASOUND IN INTERVENTIONAL RADIOLOGY: APPLICATIONS AND TECHNIQUES

Vickie A. Feldstein, M.D., and Dennis S. Orwig, M.D.

Introduction

The subjects addressed in this tutorial include:

1. Role of ultrasound in guiding procedures
2. Advantages of ultrasound guidance
3. Technique of ultrasound guidance
4. Transducers appropriate for various procedures
5. Needle selection
6. Technical considerations.

Advances in imaging and the introduction of specially designed needles and catheters have revolutionized the radiologist's role in diagnostic medicine and patient management. Percutaneous biopsies and drainage procedures are now performed routinely in hospital-based and free-standing radiology departments **(Fig. 1)**.

All interventional procedures begin with needle placement. Imaging guidance is used during such procedures to select appropriate pathways and to direct needles and catheters into lesions, vessels, and fluid collections **(Fig. 2)**. Advances in ultrasound (US) have improved its ability to guide many procedures, often providing unique advantages over other imaging modalities **(Fig. 3)**.[1–3]

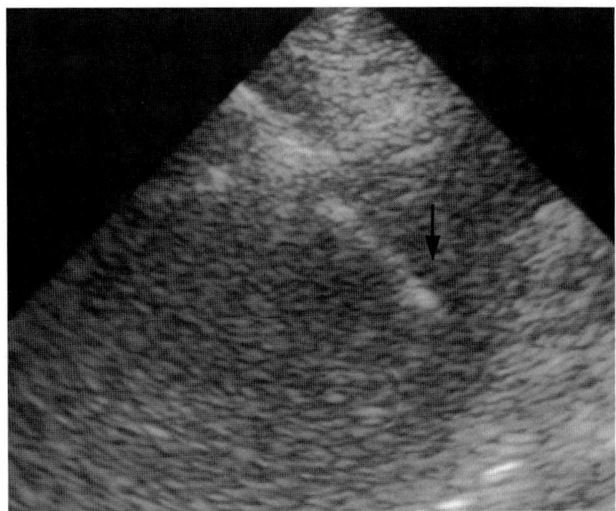

Figure 4. US-guided biopsy of a kidney with the needle (arrow) in the renal parenchyma.

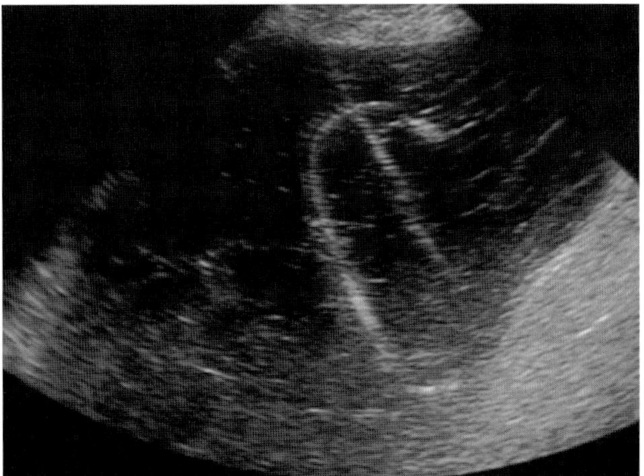

Figure 5. Initial wire placement for drainage of a subphrenic abscess.

Procedures Amenable to US Guidance

US was first introduced for guidance of percutaneous procedures in the early 1970s. With a few notable exceptions, US guidance may be used whenever percutaneous biopsy of almost any organ or region of the body is performed **(Fig. 4)**.[4] Fluid collections in pleural, peritoneal, and synovial spaces are readily identified with US. An extension of these simple needle-guidance and diagnostic techniques is the insertion of catheters into the thorax, abdomen, and pelvis for drainage of fluid collections **(Fig. 5)**.[5] Specialty transducers have been designed to allow for transrectal and transvaginal guided biopsies and aspirations.[6,7]

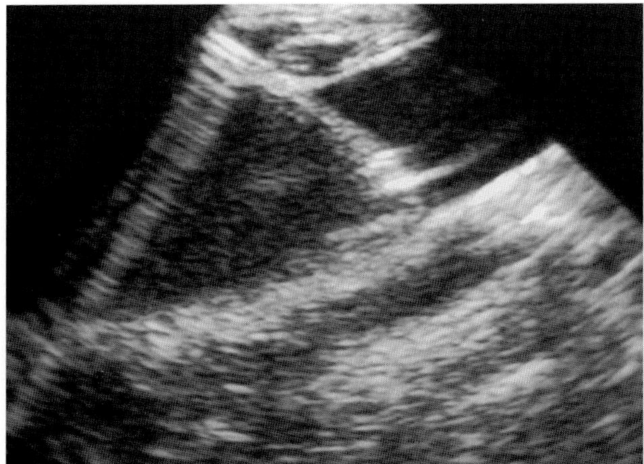

Figure 6. US guidance of a jugular vein puncture prior to placement of a central venous catheter. The needle shaft appears as a linear, brightly echogenic structure seen coursing into the dilated vein.

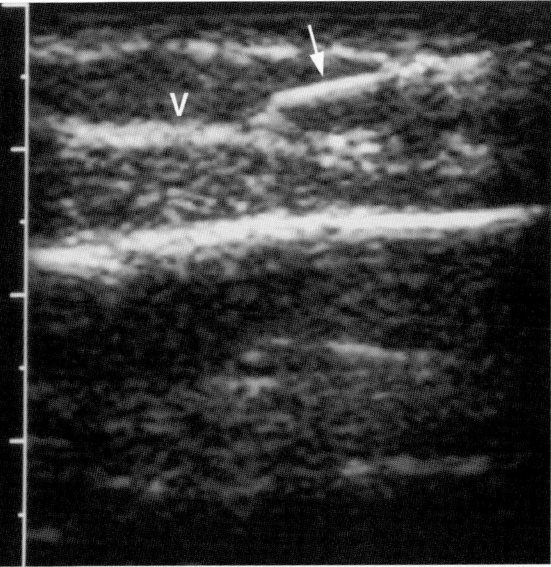

Figure 7. Puncture of the basilic vein (V) for placement of a peripherally inserted central catheter (arrow).

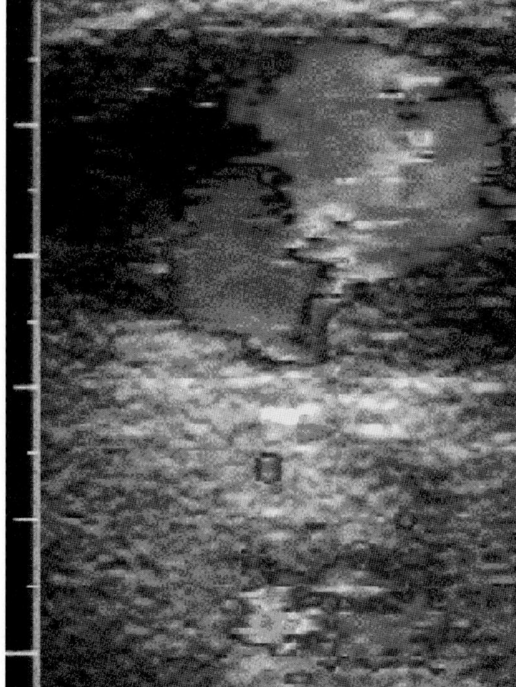

Figure 8. Pseudoaneurysm of the superficial femoral artery demonstrated on this color Doppler US image.

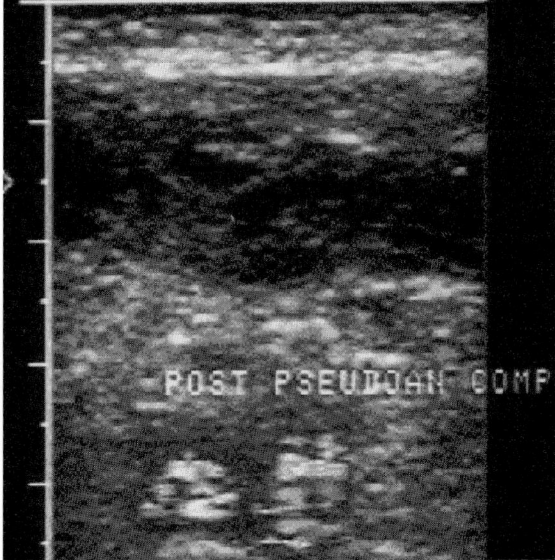

Figure 9. Following US-guided manual compression repair, the pseudoaneurysm has thrombosed and no residual intraluminal flow is seen by color Doppler US.

US may be used to guide initial venous puncture for vascular access **(Fig. 6)**. Indeed, the placement of long-term central venous access devices is a rapidly developing area for radiologists, and US greatly facilitates safe vascular access, especially when compared to "blind" techniques that rely on surface landmarks **(Fig. 7)**.[8] US also greatly facilitates the puncture of "pulseless" but patent arteries. The US transducer itself can serve as a therapeutic device in patients with iatrogenic arterial injuries by enabling US-guided compression repair of pseudoaneurysms **(Figs. 8, 9)**.[9]

US localization of foreign bodies is useful, particularly when the material is not radiopaque. Shrapnel, glass, wood, plastic, and broken needles can be identified readily, even when quite small, and their percutaneous removal can be guided with use of US.[10]

Advantages and Disadvantages of Ultrasound Guidance	
Advantages	*Disadvantages*
Real time	Dependent upon operator experience
Multiplanar	Limited by overlying bone, gas, lung
Portable	
Readily available	
Low cost	
Lack of radiation	
Time-saving	

Figure 10.

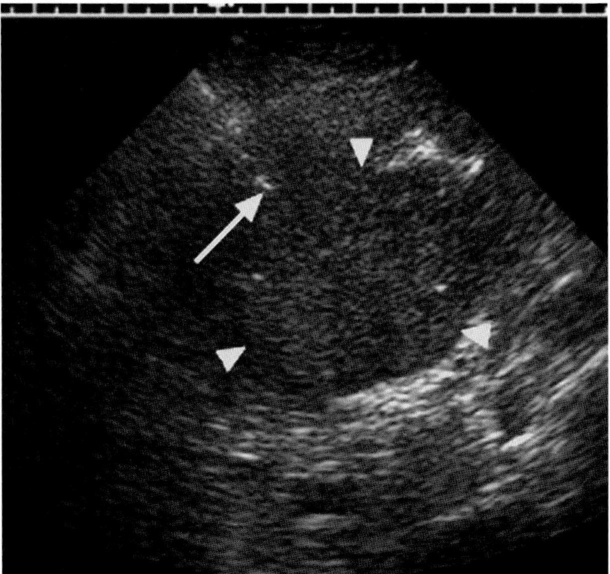

Figure 11. US-guided fine needle aspiration of a focal solid liver mass (metastasis). The needle tip appears as an echogenic focus (arrow) shown approaching the margin of the target lesion (arrowheads).

Advantages of US Guidance

US is now readily available in most radiology departments and offers several advantages over other imaging guidance modalities **(Fig. 10)**. Portable equipment allows for US guidance in the Interventional Radiology suite or at the patient's bedside. US-guided procedures are often less time-consuming and less expensive than those performed under fluoroscopic or computed tomography (CT) guidance. Furthermore, neither the patient nor the radiologist is exposed to ionizing radiation. Unlike CT, US offers rapid imaging in multiple planes merely by repositioning the transducer. Most importantly, real-time US permits constant monitoring of the course of the needle so that any necessary adjustments in needle position can be made quickly and precisely **(Fig. 11)**. Respiratory misregistration, due to variability in the depth of respiration from image to image, is a source of difficulty with CT-guided biopsies; this problem is eliminated when real-time US imaging is used.

One of the unique features of US guidance is the dynamic interaction which occurs during real-time imaging. As with fluoroscopy, US provides a moving two-dimensional image of a three-dimensional structure. Yet, with US, an operator-needle-machine feedback loop is formed in which control of the transducer and of the needle occur simultaneously.[2] To improve this dynamic interaction, US-guided needle localization and guidance techniques can be practiced with use of simple homemade or commercially available phantoms.[11] Such practice can improve operator skills dramatically, thus instilling confidence in physicians performing US-guided procedures.

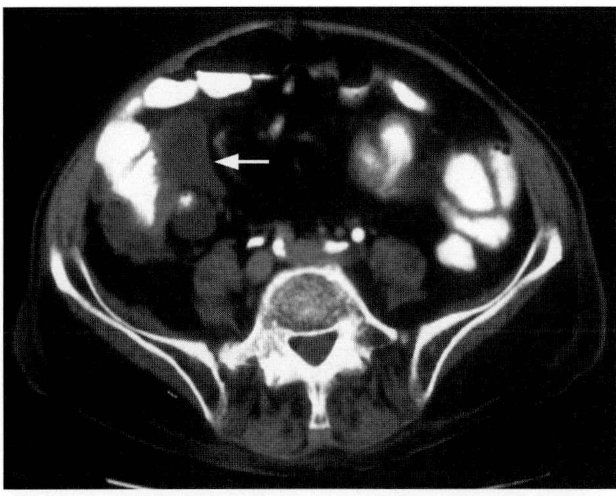

Figure 12. CT scan demonstrates an interloop abscess (arrow) with surrounding bowel loops. Air in the surrounding bowel loops precludes adequate US visualization of the abscess.

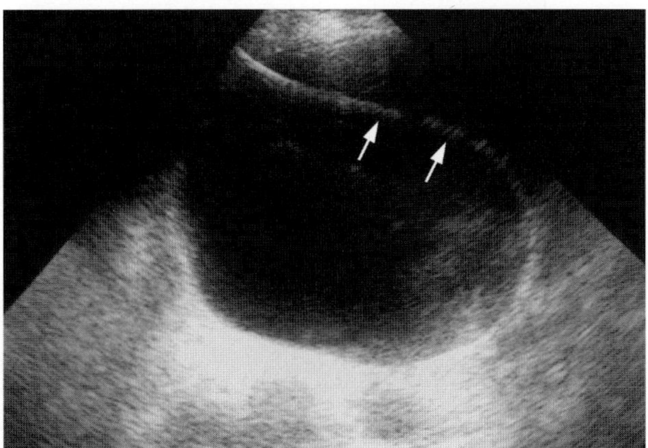

Figure 13. US-guided drainage of loculated pleural empyema with a wire (arrows) in the collection.

Despite its tremendous advantages, US guidance is limited to cases in which the lesion is well seen and a safe pathway for needle or catheter insertion can be identified by US. When adequate visualization is not possible, such as when the target is obscured by overlying gas or superficial bony structures, other modalities are used. For example, CT scanning is preferred for the assessment and guided drainage of intraabdominal interloop abscesses **(Fig. 12)**. Most intraparenchymal pulmonary lesions are better suited to fluoroscopic or CT guidance. However, drainage of pleural fluid collections is greatly facilitated with US guidance **(Fig. 13)**.

Given the many advantages of US guidance for interventional procedures, we advocate its use during any percutaneous procedure where guidance is required and where the target can be adequately visualized and accessed with the use of US.

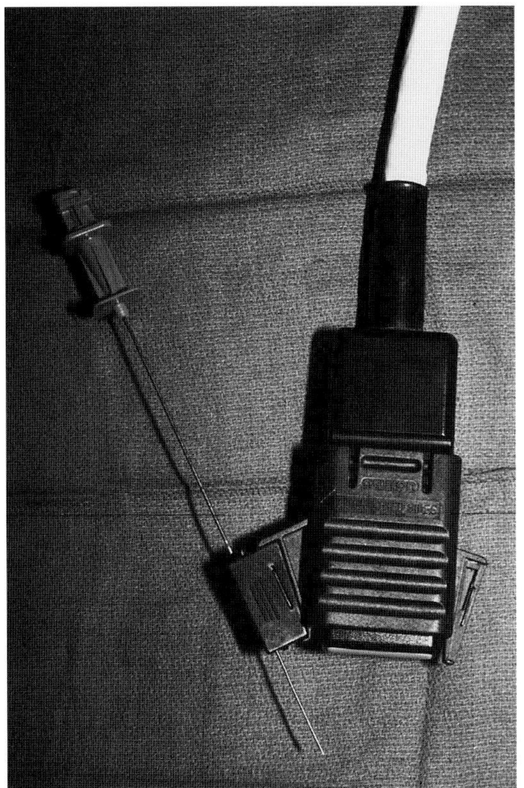

Figure 14. Transducer with needle guide device attached.

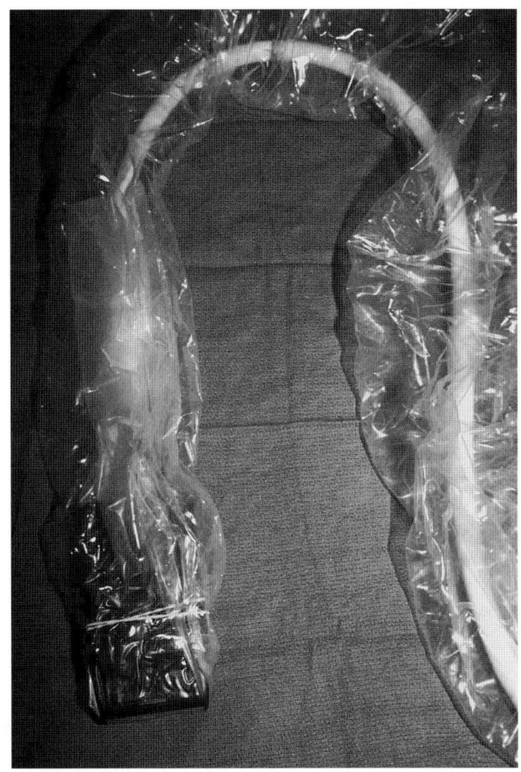

Figure 15. US transducer covered with sterile sleeve.

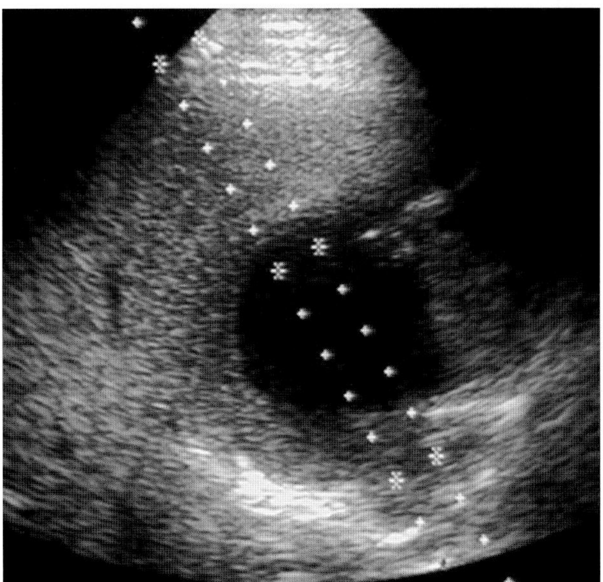

Figure 16. US transducer with a biopsy guide showing the predetermined needle path (dotted lines) entering the gallbladder in a patient with acalculous cholecystitis.

Freehand versus Needle-Guide Technique

US-guided real-time procedures can be performed with use of the freehand method or with transducers fitted with needle guide attachments. The needle guide technique is particularly helpful when operators are first becoming familiar with the use of US guidance **(Fig. 14)**. When a biopsy transducer or an attached needle guide system is used, the transducer is placed directly over the target. The transducer is sterilized or draped with sterile coverings **(Fig. 15)**. The needle guide system permits the introduction of the needle in a predetermined pathway **(Fig. 16)**.

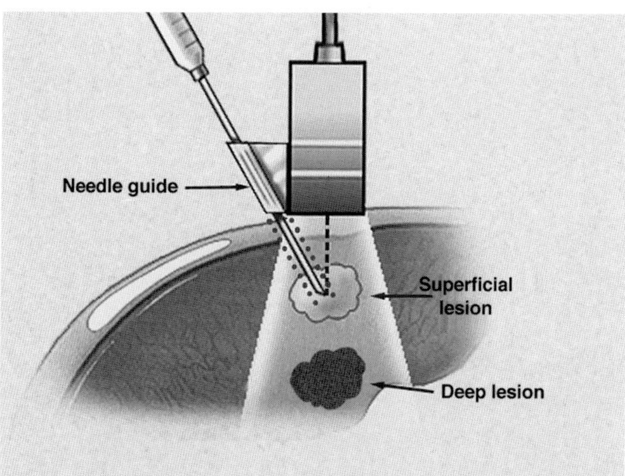

Figure 17. Diagram illustrating the use of the needle guide attachment to access a superficial hepatic lesion for fine needle aspiration. The deep lesion could not be accessed with this device.

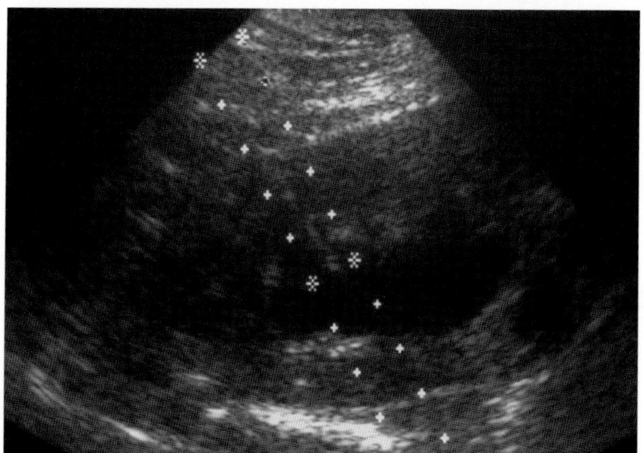

Figure 18. US-guided nephrostomy with use of a needle guide attachment. The needle shaft appears as an echogenic line between the dotted lines showing the expected needle path.

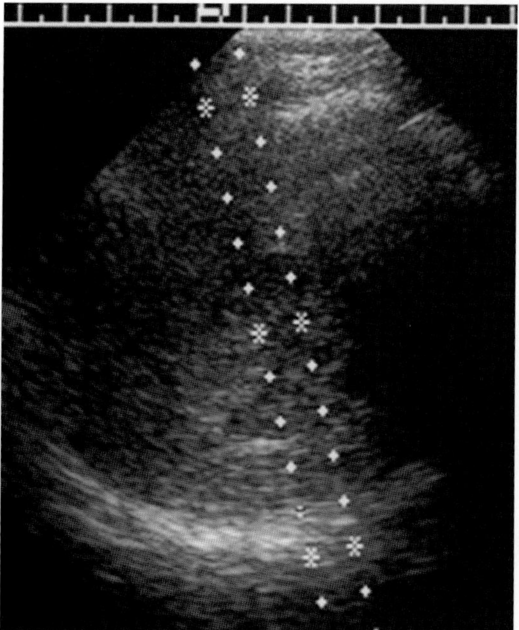

Figure 19. Needle guide attachment used to perform US-guided fine needle aspiration of a hypoechoic solid mass (hepatoma) near the dome of the liver. From this location, the prescribed needle path is seen to traverse the center of the lesion.

The prescribed angle of the needle path with a needle guide may limit its flexibility in certain applications. In particular, lesions which are very superficial or very deep to the skin surface can be extremely difficult to access with use of the needle guide technique **(Fig. 17)**. The transducer must be held in a fixed position during advancement of the needle and should be positioned so that the prescribed needle pathway courses through the center of the target. Appropriate position of the needle along the expected path should always be confirmed **(Fig. 18)**. The needle shaft will appear as an echogenic line between the parallel dotted lines on the screen.

The needle guide attachment can be particularly useful for guiding percutaneous access to lesions which can be visualized from a single small acoustic window. For example, US visualization of lesions located near the dome of the liver is often limited due to overlying ribs and interposed lung. In such cases, the needle guide device can delineate a safe approach for the needle from the sole US viewing site **(Fig. 19)**.

With the freehand method, more options are available in the selection of the skin entry site and needle path, thereby offering greater flexibility to the radiologist. Although technically more demanding, this method, once mastered, offers several advantages. The operator can select the appropriate needle entry and transducer viewing sites to reduce the length of the needle path, avoid overlying structures, and optimize needle visibility. Also, subtle adjustments can be made more easily in real time to compensate for deviation of the needle or patient movement. However, when separate appropriate entry and transducer sites cannot be identified, the freehand method may be quite difficult.

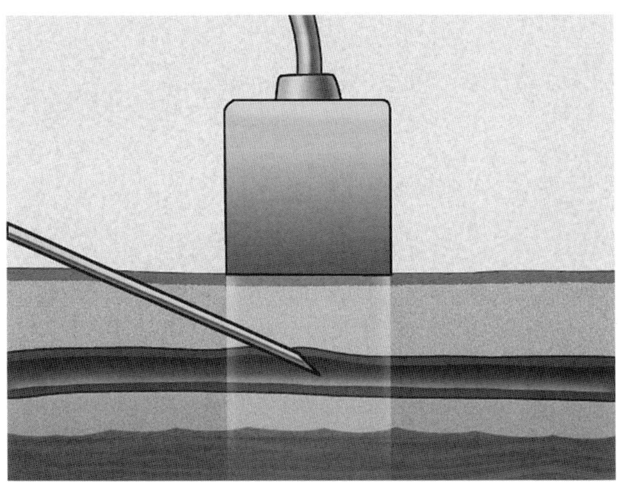

Figure 20. A linear array transducer is often preferred for US guidance of vascular access with the transducer oriented along the long axis of the vessel to be punctured.

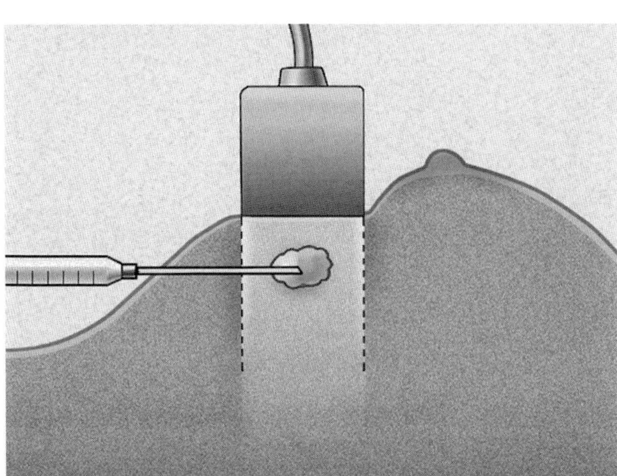

Figure 21. A linear array transducer is typically selected when performing US-guided breast procedures, with the transducer placed perpendicular to the skin surface, directly over the target lesion.

Transducers

The ideal transducer is one which will provide optimal visualization of the lesion and the needle. Consequently, the transducer used will vary with the target location and depth, and with the patient's body habitus. A 3.5 MHz sector array transducer is preferred for the majority of US-guided procedures in the abdomen and pelvis. It can be fitted with a needle guide attachment or used with the freehand technique. Commercially available sterile drapes or sleeves fit easily over the transducer. A 2.25 MHz transducer can be used when deep tissue penetration is necessary. Because needle visibility is a function of the transducer frequency, the highest frequency transducer that allows visualization of the target should be used.

When lesions in the superficial soft tissues are to be sampled, or superficial vascular structures cannulated, a high-resolution, 5–10 MHz linear array transducer is most often used **(Figs. 20, 21)**.[12] In these cases, the transducer is applied directly over the target or vessel and the needle is inserted obliquely so that it lies parallel to the transducer face (perpendicular to the US beam), appropriately deep to the skin surface **(Fig. 22)**.

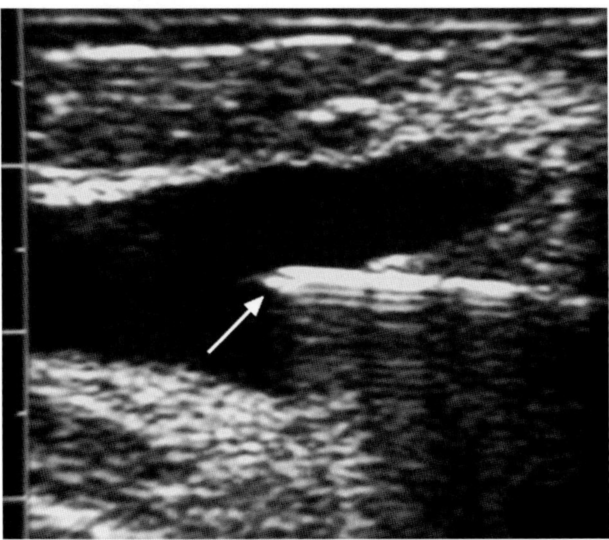

Figure 22. Fine needle aspiration of a breast cyst using US guidance. A linear array transducer is placed directly over the cyst. The echogenic needle (arrow) is seen entering the lesion.

Specially designed transducers are often well suited for other unique applications. Small footprint or "microcase" transducers are often used for procedures in pediatric patients, in the operating room, or when the target is located within small superficial parts. Transvaginal and transrectal transducers facilitate the performance of pelvic and prostate biopsies and aspirations.

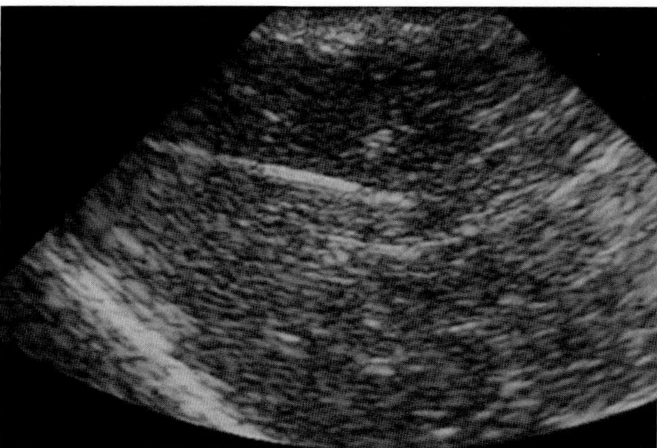

Figure 23. US image clearly depicting a standard 22-gauge Chiba needle.

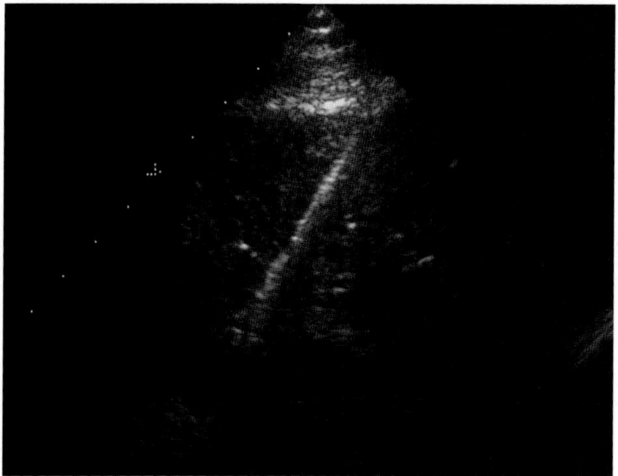

Figure 24. Excellent visualization of the needle course and tip during biopsy of a hypoechoic liver mass with a standard needle.

Needle Selection

The selection of needle size and type depends on the clinical indication, the target structure, and the indications for the procedure, such as aspiration, biopsy, or catheter placement. Manufacturers have developed scored needles, needles coated with reflective surfaces, helical and "screw-tip" stylets, and electronic needle tip enhancers, all of which may improve needle tip visibility. However, such needles are often more costly and are not necessary for successful performance of US-guided procedures **(Figs. 23, 24)**. The radiologist must work jointly with the pathologist in selecting the needle size and type best suited for each particular percutaneous fine needle aspiration or core biopsy.

Needle Entry And Transducer Viewing Sites

The optimal needle entry site is typically directly over the target so the needle pass is perpendicular and easily reproducible. US is used to determine the depth of the lesion from the needle entry site and to evaluate for any significant intervening structures. Color Doppler US is often useful to identify unsuspected vascular structures in the intended needle path.[13] The location for optimal transducer position from which to view the approach of the needle as it is advanced toward the target is then selected. The viewing site is determined on the basis of the location of the lesion and the needle entry site.

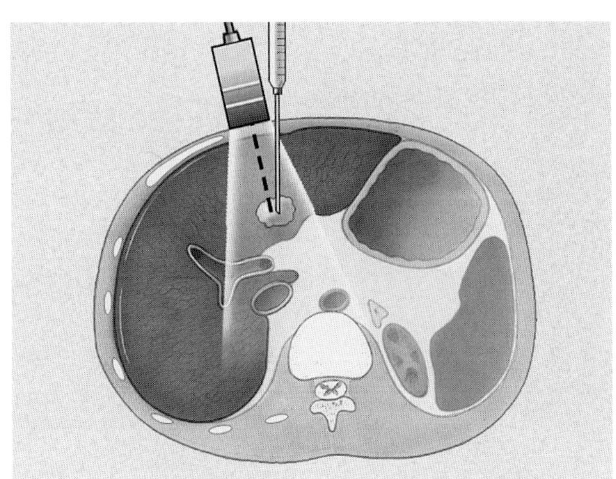

Figure 25. Diagram illustrates the effect of the transducer viewing site on needle visibility. The selected needle entry site is directly over the lesion, so the length of the needle pass is minimized and the needle path is more easily maintained. Initially, the transducer is placed too close to the needle entry site, making the needle less conspicuous by US.

Some important physical principles must be remembered whenever US is used for needle guidance. The greater the angle of incidence between the needle shaft and the insonant US beam, the brighter the specular reflection and the greater the visibility of the needle. In fact, the needle shaft is best seen when it is perpendicular to the insonant US beam. Therefore, the transducer viewing site should be an appropriate distance away from the needle entry site such that the angle between the US beam and the needle shaft approaches 90 degrees, thereby increasing needle visibility. For this reason, when a sector array transducer is used, the deeper the target is from the skin surface, the farther apart the needle entry site and the transducer viewing site should be (**Figs. 25, 26**).

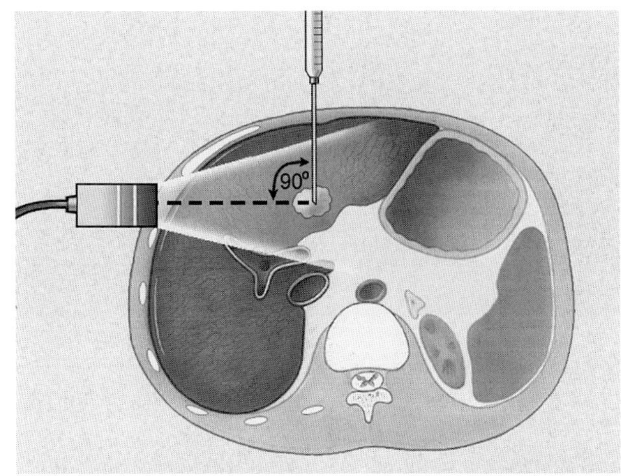

Figure 26. By moving the transducer viewing site farther from the needle entry site, the angle between the insonant sound beam and the needle shaft approaches 90 degrees, enhancing needle visibility.

The US image, including the depth, gain, and focal zone settings, should be adjusted so that visualization of the tissues through which the needle passes is optimized. The needle can be identified as a brightly echogenic structure, provided that it is positioned centrally within the plane of section defined by the sound beam emanating from the transducer. Misalignment of the ultrasound beam relative to the needle shaft is a common cause of inadequate needle visualization.

Improving Needle Visualization

After careful selection of the needle entry site and the transducer viewing site, the most important factor affecting visibility of the needle is the alignment of the needle relative to the US beam. If the needle is not readily visible, its alignment with the transducer should be checked and various maneuvers attempted to optimize visualization.

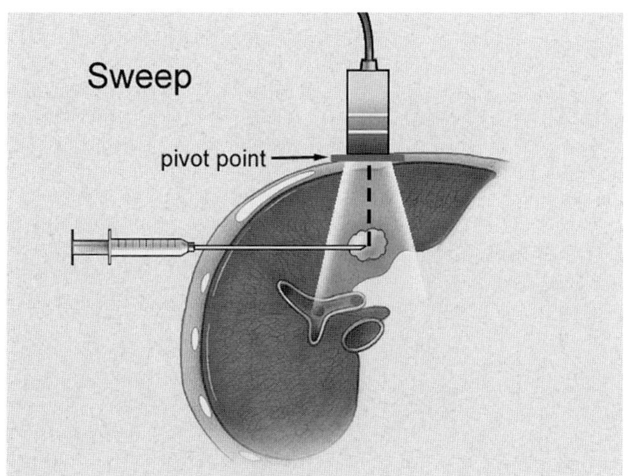

Figure 27. Diagram indicating the pivot point at which the transducer is moved to perform the sweep maneuver.

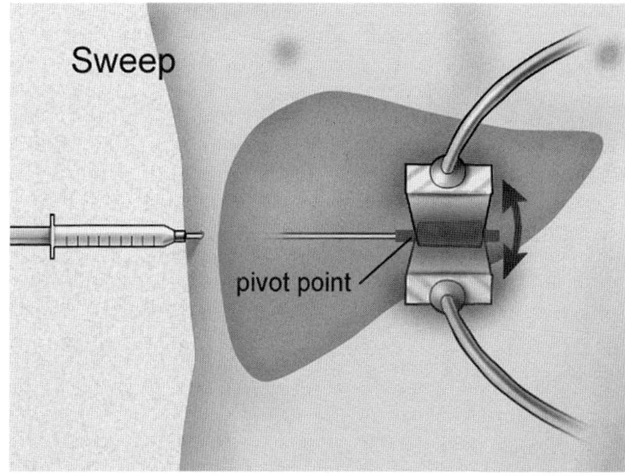

Figure 28. Overhead view illustrates the sweeping motion, scanning from above to below, used to locate the needle and evaluate its position relative to the target lesion.

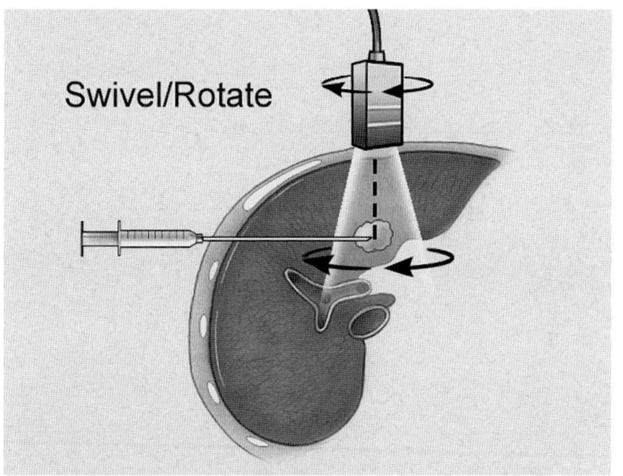

Figure 29. By swiveling along the long axis of the transducer, the needle shaft and tip can be better visualized.

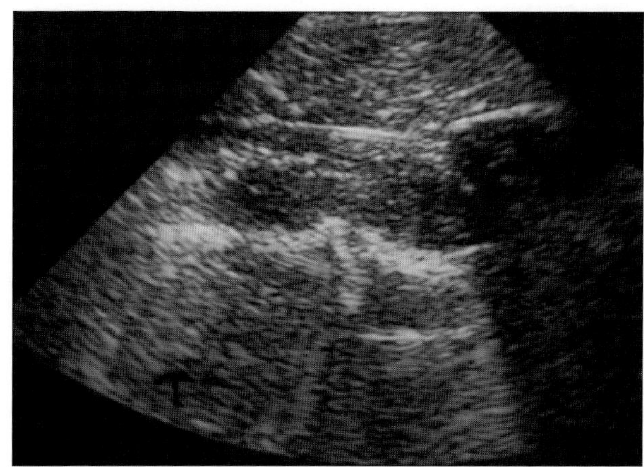

Figure 30. Poor alignment of the transducer with the needle—the echogenic needle shaft is shown but the needle tip is not well seen.

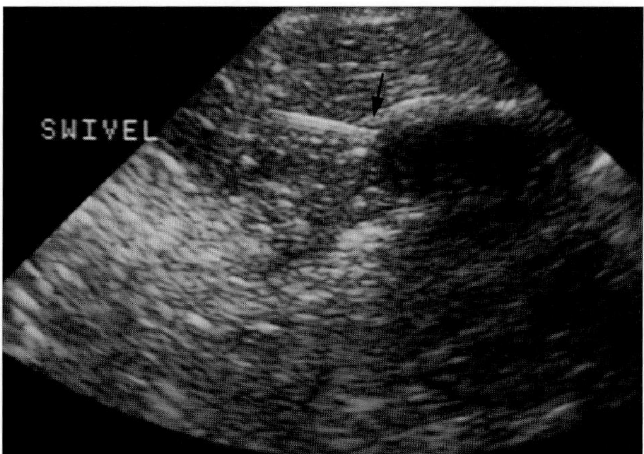

Figure 31. By swiveling the transducer, there is improved alignment with the needle—the tip is well seen (arrow) as it approaches the target lesion.

Three specific motions of the transducer should be used. A gradual *sweep* or scan from above to below the imaging plane is used to find the needle **(Figs. 27, 28)**. Once localized, *rotating* or swiveling along the long axis of the transducer improves longitudinal alignment of the sound beam with the needle shaft **(Figs. 29–31)**.

Rocking the transducer by pressing the edge of the transducer face into the skin surface alters the incident angle and provides maximal visualization of the needle shaft and tip **(Fig. 32)**.

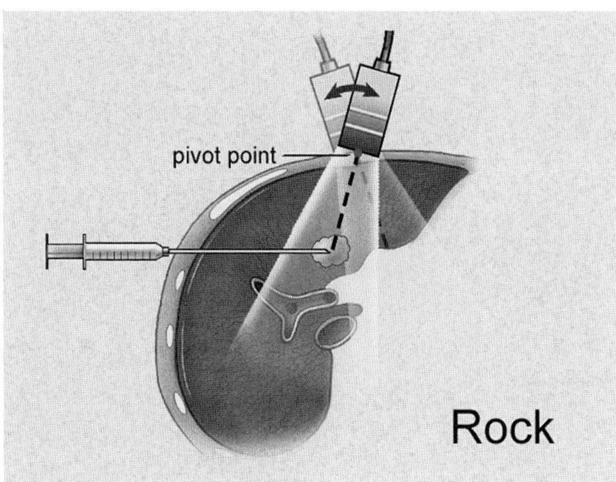

Figure 32. The rocking maneuver is used to optimize visibility of the needle tip.

Continuous real-time evaluation of the needle throughout insertion is the most accurate way to verify needle position. An "in-and-out" or jiggling motion of the needle increases reflectivity and is often useful in locating the echogenic needle tip. The use of color Doppler US may be helpful during such maneuvers, because the movement of the needle results in color motion artifact.[13]

Conclusion

US guidance for diagnostic and therapeutic interventional procedures is a useful, widely applied technique. It has been shown to be accurate, safe, and expeditious. Compared to CT guidance, US guidance of percutaneous procedures may be underused because many radiologists are not familiar with the techniques used to optimize needle visualization. Successful US guidance of interventional procedures is possible with an understanding of the sonographic maneuvers and with skilled operator experience.

References

1. Dodd GD III, Esola CC, Memel DS, et al. Sonography: the undiscovered jewel of interventional radiology. Radiographics 1996; 16:1271–1288.

2. Matalon TA, Silver B. US guidance of interventional procedures. Radiology 1990; 174:43–47.

3. McGahan JP, ed. Interventional ultrasound. Baltimore: Williams & Wilkins, 1990.

4. Fornage BD, Coan JD, David CL. Ultrasound-guided needle biopsy of the breast and other interventional procedures. Radiol Clin North Am 1992; 30:167–185.

5. Boland GW, Lee MJ, Leung J, Mueller PR. Percutaneous cholecystostomy in critically ill patients: early response and final outcome in 82 patients. AJR 1994; 163:339–342.

6. Alexander AA, Eschelman DJ, Nazarian LN, Bonn J. Transrectal sonographically guided drainage of deep pelvic abscesses. AJR 1994; 162:1227–1230.

7. Fleischer AC, Burnett LS, Jones HW III, Cullinan JA. Transrectal and transperineal sonography during guided intrauterine procedures. J Ultrasound Med 1995; 14:135–138.

8. Skolnick ML. The role of sonography in the placement and management of jugular and subclavian central venous catheters. AJR 1994; 163:291–295.

9. Paulson EK, Kliewer MA, Hertzberg BS, et al. Ultrasonographically guided manual compression of femoral artery injuries. J Ultrasound Med 1995; 14:653–659.

10. Shiels WE, Babcock DS, Wilson JL, Burch RA. Localization and guided removal of soft-tissue foreign bodies with sonography. AJR 1990; 155:1277–1281.

11. Silver B, Metzger TS, Matalon TA. A simple phantom for learning needle placement for sonographically guided biopsy. AJR 1990; 154:847–848.

12. Rizzatto G, Solbiati L, Croce F, Derchi LE. Aspiration biopsy of superficial lesions: ultrasonic guidance with a linear array probe. AJR 1987; 148:623–625.

13. Longo JM, Bilbao JI, Barettino MD, et al. Percutaneous vascular and nonvascular puncture under US guidance: role of color Doppler imaging. Radiographics 1994; 14:959–972.

Endnotes

Figures 12 and 24 courtesy of Kenyon Kopecky, M.D., Indiana University School of Medicine.

Figures 14 and 15 courtesy of Scott Trerotola, M.D., Indiana University School of Medicine.

Figures 7, 13, and 18 courtesy of Jeet Sandhu, M.D., University of North Carolina School of Medicine.

TUTORIAL 3
PERCUTANEOUS LIVER BIOPSY

Shailendra Chopra, M.D., M.R.C.P., F.R.C.R., Christine C. Esola, M.D., and Gerald D. Dodd III, M.D.

Introduction

The subjects addressed in this tutorial include:
1. Hepatic anatomy relevant to percutaneous biopsy
2. Indications, contraindications, and patient preparation
3. Instrumentation
4. Guidance methods and technique
5. Postprocedure care and complications.

Percutaneous liver biopsy is a relatively easy and reliable method of obtaining hepatic tissue for histologic or cytopathologic diagnosis. While it has been performed blindly in cases of diffuse liver disease for over a hundred years, in the last decade imaging guidance has made it possible to target small focal lesions.

Hepatic Anatomy

Position of Liver

The liver is situated in the right upper quadrant of the abdomen below the right dome of the diaphragm. The exact position of the liver is somewhat variable, depending on the size of the liver, the degree to which the lungs are inflated, and the build of the patient. The dome of the right lobe is surrounded by the base of the right lung, descending into the anterior, posterior, and lateral costophrenic recesses. The inferior margin of the right lobe follows the position of the 11th rib. The left lobe and a part of the right lobe extend below the costal margin. The gallbladder lies in the interlobar fissure between the anterior segment of the right lobe and the medial segment of the left lobe.

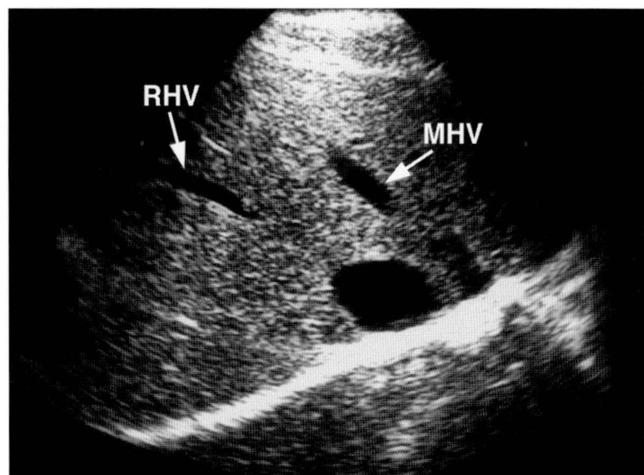

Figure 1. Right and middle hepatic veins (arrows).

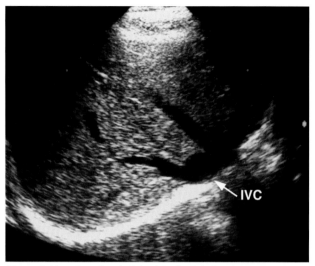

Figure 2. Hepatic veins draining into the inferior vena cava (arrow).

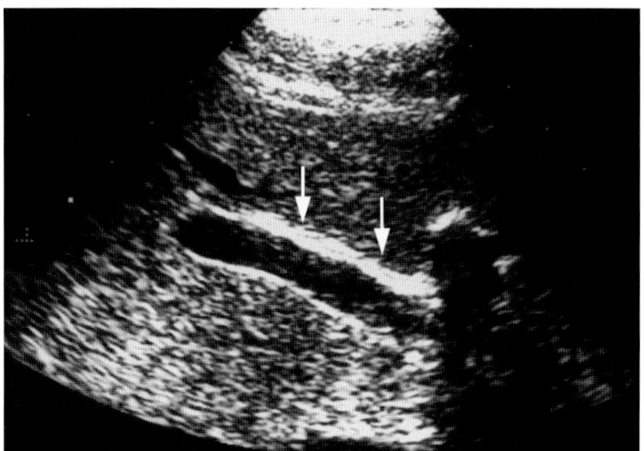
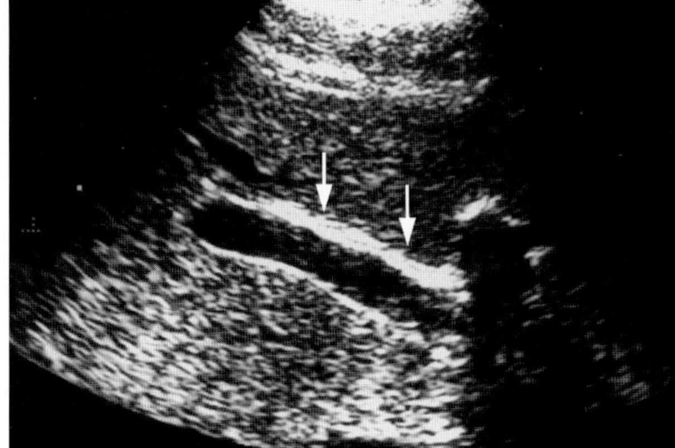

Figure 3. Portal vein at the porta hepatis (arrows).

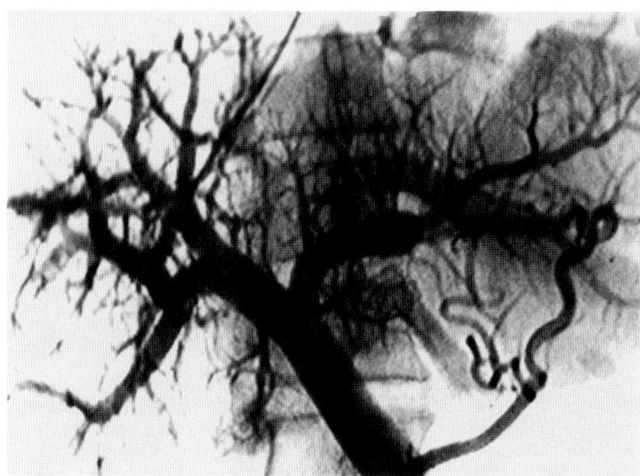

Figure 4. Direct portogram obtained during transjugular intrahepatic portosystemic shunt placement demonstrates the portal vein branching pattern.

Venous Anatomy

Apart from forming the basis for the Couinaud classification of hepatic segmental anatomy, the hepatic and portal venous systems in the liver are important to the interventionalist performing a liver biopsy. To reduce the risk of postprocedural hemorrhage, the large vessels within the liver must be avoided. The vessels within the liver provide convenient landmarks that are helpful in localizing, with ultrasound, small lesions revealed on computed tomography (CT) scanning. The right, middle, and left hepatic veins run in the interlobar and intersegmental fissures and drain into the inferior vena cava **(Figs. 1, 2)**. The portal vein enters the liver through the porta hepatis and quickly divides into the right and left branches, which run in an inclined horizontal plane **(Figs. 3, 4)**. All these vessels subdivide and rapidly become smaller in caliber as they approach the periphery of the liver **(Fig. 5)**.

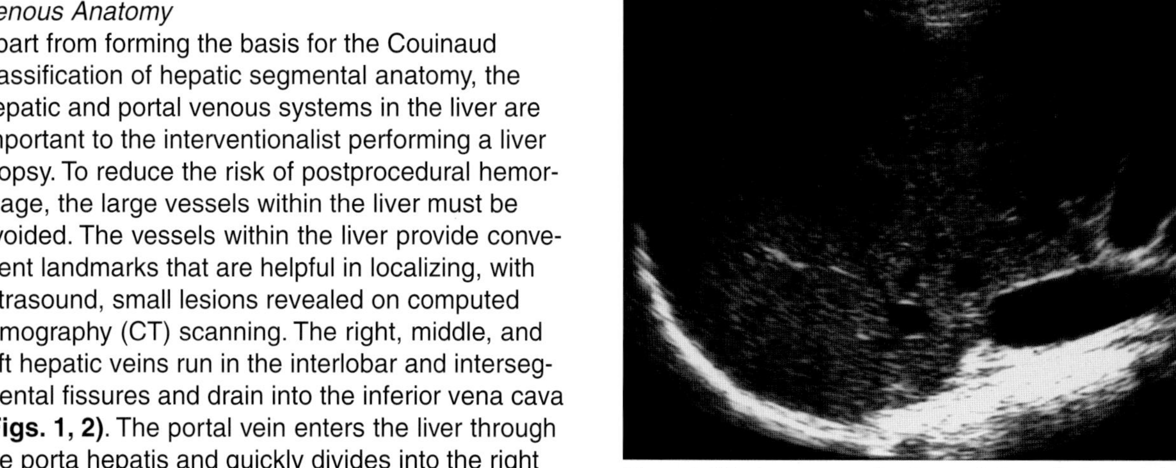

Figure 5. US shows a paucity of vessels towards the periphery of the liver.

Indications For Liver Biopsy

Diffuse Disease
- Chronic hepatitis
- Cirrhosis
- Metabolic liver disease
- To assess efficacy of treatment for any of the above
- Hepatic transplant rejection

Focal Disease
- Liver mass in patients with newly diagnosed malignancy
- New liver mass in patients with known malignancy
- Liver mass in patients with cirrhosis
- Unexplained liver mass

Figure 6.

Contraindications To Liver Biopsy

Absolute Contraindications
- None

Relative Contraindications
- Patient-Related:
  - Coagulopathy PT >15 sec, PTT >45 sec, platelets <50,000/mm^3
  - Uncooperative patient
- Lesion-Related:
  - Suspected hemangioma
  - Hypervascular lesion at the surface of the liver

Figure 7.

Patient Preparation For Liver Biopsy

At The Time Of Appointment
- Review indications
- Review previous images
- Review lab results
- Arrange for cytopathology if required

On The Day Of Procedure
- Nothing by mouth for 8 hours
- Procedure explained to the patient
- Informed consent obtained
- Baseline pulse, blood pressure, and temperature
- Review images again
- Decide between fine needle and core biopsy

Figure 8.

Indications

Indications for liver biopsy are shown in **Figure 6**. Random biopsy for diffuse liver disease is usually carried out without imaging guidance, although imaging guidance is suggested if attempts at blind biopsy have failed, the liver is small, or the patient is morbidly obese. Biopsy of focal liver lesions must be performed under imaging guidance to have any realistic chance of success.

Contraindications

There are no absolute contraindications to liver biopsy. The relative contraindications are shown in **Figure 7**. Coagulopathy increases the risk of significant intraperitoneal hemorrhage.[1,2] Patients with coagulopathies should receive transfusion of fresh frozen plasma and/or platelets as appropriate. Because of the short physiological half-life of these blood products, it is important to schedule the biopsy within 3–4 hours of the transfusion. In those patients with an uncorrectable coagulopathy, transjugular liver biopsy should be considered an alternative to transhepatic biopsy **(see SCVIR Syllabus Volume II, *Portal Hypertension: Options for Diagnosis and Treatment*)**. Sedation may be required in patients who are unable to cooperate. General anesthesia is rarely needed. Hemangiomas are notorious for bleeding after biopsy, but in our experience this is most likely to occur if a surface hemangioma is biopsied directly without a mantle of normal liver between the lesion and the puncture site in the liver capsule. In fact, it is advisable to have such a mantle in all lesions. Even when lesions are at the liver surface, it is possible to go through a mantle of normal liver parenchyma by adjusting the position of the transducer.

Patient Preparation

Before scheduling a patient for biopsy, the indications, possible contraindications, coagulation study results, and the previous imaging studies should be reviewed and any relative contraindications addressed **(Fig. 8)**. Unless the patient is admitted for some other reason, all imaging-guided liver biopsies in our institution are performed on an outpatient basis. The patient comes to the department the day of the biopsy after having fasted for 8 hours. After informed consent is obtained, the patient is connected to an electronic monitor and baseline pulse, blood pressure, and temperature readings are recorded. Hemodynamic status is monitored throughout the procedure.

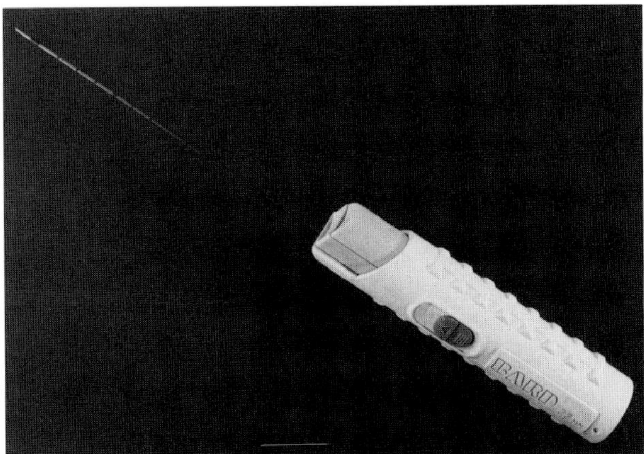

Figure 9. MaxCore disposable core biopsy gun (Bard, Covington, GA).

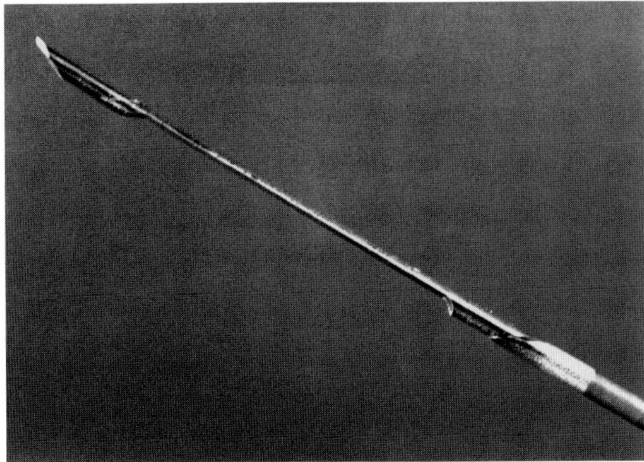

Figure 10. Tip of the core biopsy needle.

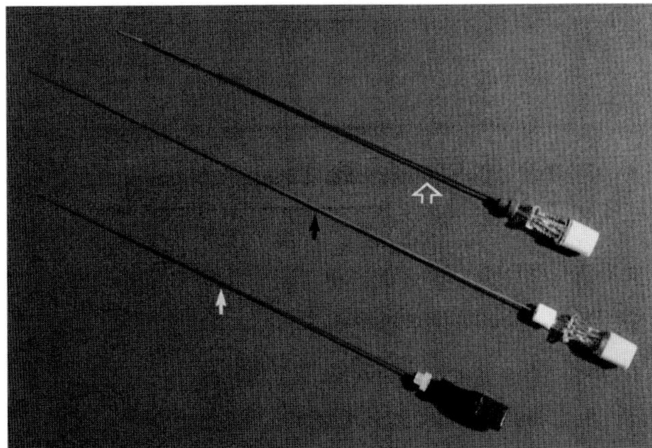

Figure 11. Chiba-type needle (Manan Medical Products, Northbrook, IL), white arrow; Crown biopsy needle (Medi-Tech, Watertown, MA), black arrow; and Greene biopsy needle (Cook, Bloomington, IN), open arrow.

Instrumentation

Any of the large number of soft-tissue biopsy needles can be used for percutaneous liver biopsy. Menghini-type suction needles are used extensively by hepatologists for blind liver biopsies. However, for imaging-guided biopsies, smaller caliber needles are preferred. Automated core biopsy systems with 15–18-gauge needles are used for random liver biopsy and biopsy of relatively larger lesions **(Figs. 9, 10)**.[3] These have the advantage of being quick and providing large tissue samples. Chiba-type needles with and without cutting edges and/or echogenic tips are used for fine-needle aspiration **(Figs. 11, 12)**. These needles vary from 18- to 22-gauge in caliber. They can be used for any type of lesion but are particularly useful for the biopsy of small lesions which are close to large vessels. However, the tissue samples are relatively small and more than one pass is often required to obtain adequate tissue.

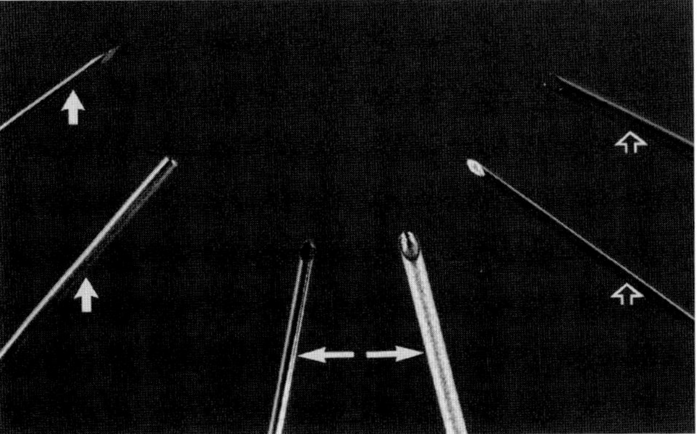

Figure 12. Tips of Chiba (short arrows), Greene (long arrows), and Crown (open arrows) needles and their stylets.

Advantages Of Ultrasound As a Guiding Modality
• Real-time capability • Multiplanar capability • Doppler capability • Portability • No ionizing radiation • Speed • Low cost

Figure 13.

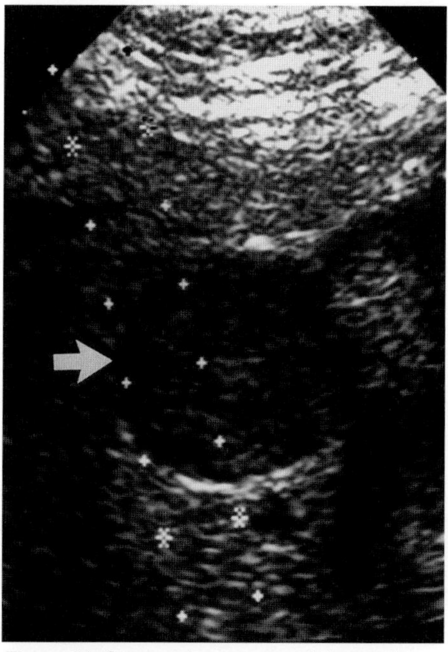

Figure 14. Gray-scale sonographic image in preparation for biopsy of a hypoechoic liver lesion (arrow) using a needle guide (dashed line).

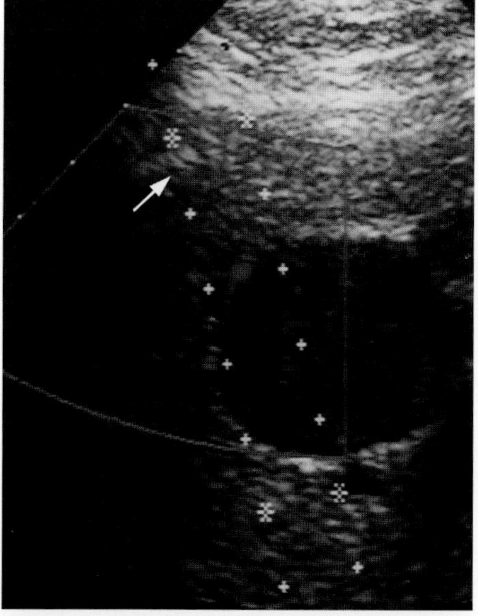

Figure 15. Color Doppler image shows flow (arrow) in the path which was not visible on the gray-scale image.

Guidance Methods and Technique

A number of imaging modalities have been used for liver biopsy. Ultrasound and CT are the most common. In rare instances fluoroscopy is used, but its use is actually limited to random liver biopsy because guided biopsy is not possible with fluoroscopy. Only a few reports of the use of magnetic resonance (MR) imaging to guide liver biopsy have appeared in the literature. Although developments in instrument design will make MR-guided biopsies generally more feasible in the future, the relative ease of ultrasound and CT guidance will probably limit its use to those lesions which are detectable only by MR imaging. This tutorial will address ultrasound- and CT-guided biopsies.

Ultrasound-Guided Liver Biopsy

Ultrasound is a simple, quick, and effective method of providing imaging guidance for liver biopsy.[4,5] In our institution almost all liver biopsies are performed under ultrasound guidance.

Advantages

Figure 13 lists the advantages of ultrasound as a guiding modality. The real-time capability of ultrasound makes the procedure quick and reliable because the needle tip and its movement can be accurately and confidently visualized throughout the procedure. The multiplanar capability of ultrasound gives flexibility of approach, making it possible to biopsy lesions which would otherwise be considered beyond reach. Color Doppler identifies major vessels in the biopsy path so they can be avoided **(Figs. 14, 15)**.

Limitations
Limitations of ultrasound are primarily related to operator variability and small acoustic windows which can make biopsy difficult. Ultrasound-guided biopsy requires experience. However, by standardizing the various aspects of the procedure and using needle guides for all liver biopsies, we have made the procedure less operator-dependent in our institution. Severe obesity leads to considerable degradation of the ultrasound image and may make a liver lesion biopsy impossible under ultrasound guidance.

Technique—Freehand or Needle Guide?
Ultrasound-guided liver biopsy can be performed with either freehand or needle guide techniques. Freehand technique provides a greater freedom of choice in needle placement and better needle visibility **(Fig. 16)**. The advantages of the needle guide technique are its accuracy, quicker needle localization, and the relative ease of learning the technique. The modern needle guides supplied by the various ultrasound manufacturers are fairly accurate **(Figs. 17–19)**. The procedure using a needle guide can be performed by one person but the presence of an assistant improves the success rate and speed of the procedure **(Figs. 20, 21)**. The operator holds the transducer and directs while the assistant, under direction from the operator, places the needle. Because the operator's task is the most critical, the more experienced radiologist usually takes that role while the assistant can be a resident or fellow in an academic setting or a technician or nurse in a private practice setting.

Technique—Preliminary Sonogram
A preliminary ultrasound examination is performed in all patients to localize the lesion and select an appropriate path. The highest frequency transducer that provides adequate visualization of the target lesion is used. This ranges from 2.5 MHz for deeply situated lesions in obese patients to 5 MHz for superficial lesions in very thin patients. In most patients 3.5 MHz is satisfactory. The ideal lesion for this procedure is an easily visualized lesion in the middle of a liver lobe. The majority of small lesions seen on CT scans can be visualized with ultrasound with a diligent search. It is essential to have the CT images at hand and refer to them frequently. The relationship of the lesion to the branching points of major vessels can be used to localize small lesions. In patients with a liver mass and portal vein thrombosis, it is preferable to biopsy the portal vein thrombus because it often gives the diagnosis and helps stage the malignancy **(Figs. 22, 23)**.[6]

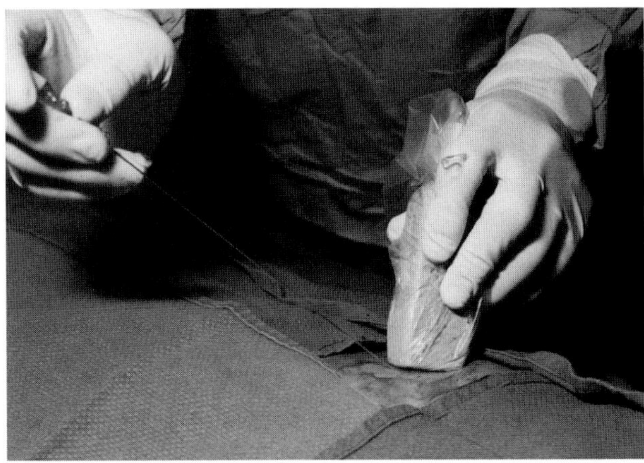

Figure 16. Freehand biopsy.

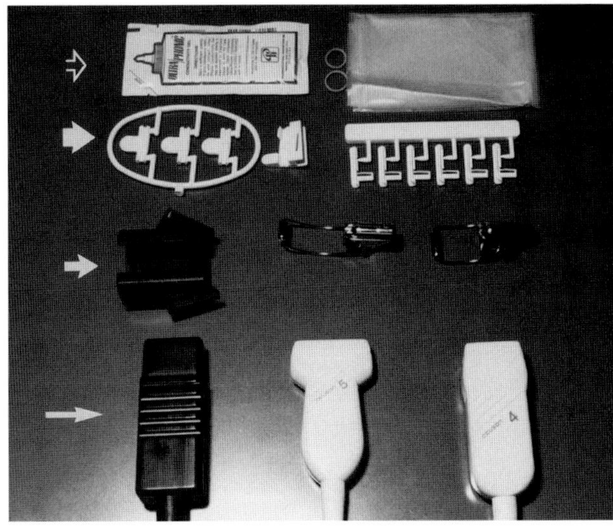

Figure 17. Various types of transducers (long arrow) with corresponding needle guides (short arrow), attachments (thick arrow), and transducer cover and gel (open arrow).

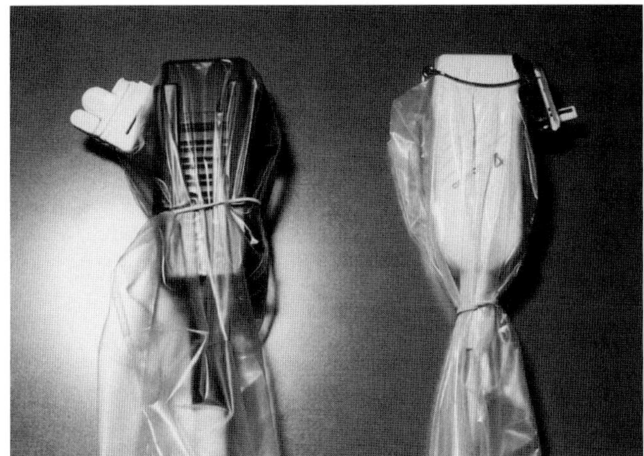

Figure 18. Needle guides mounted on transducers.

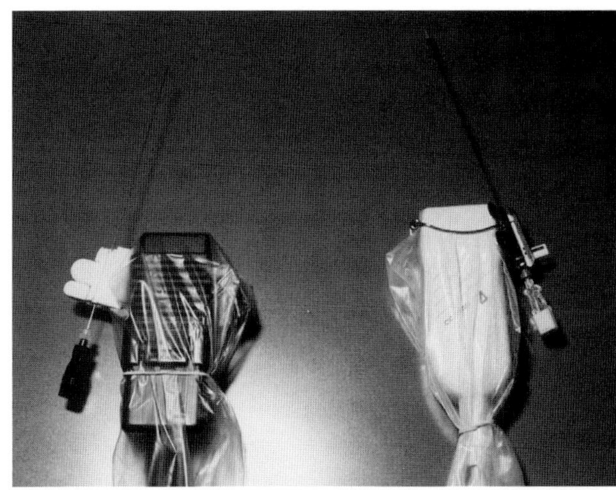

Figure 19. Transducer, needle guide, and needle assembly.

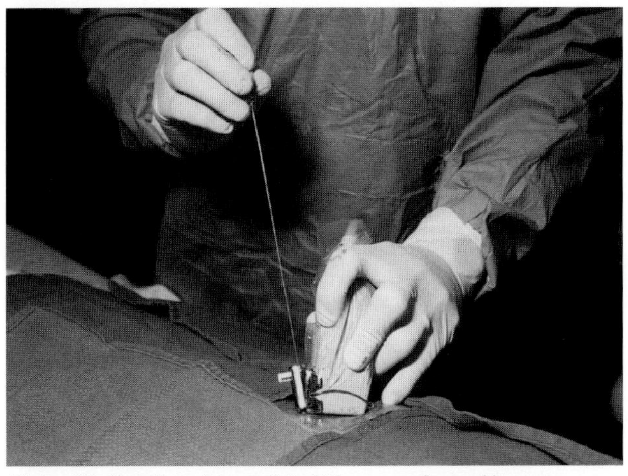

Figure 20. Needle guide assisted biopsy performed by one person.

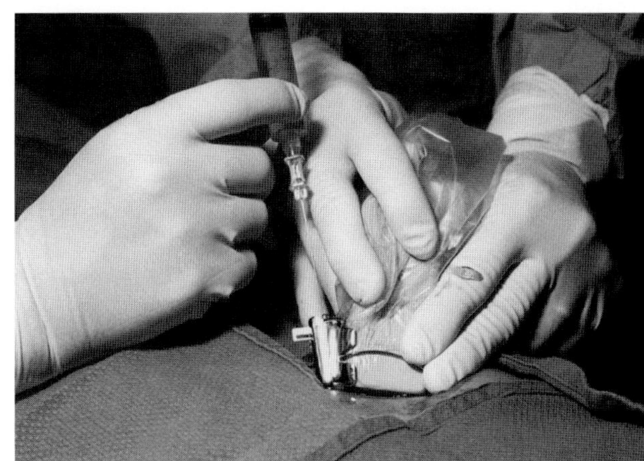

Figure 21. Needle guide assisted biopsy performed by two people.

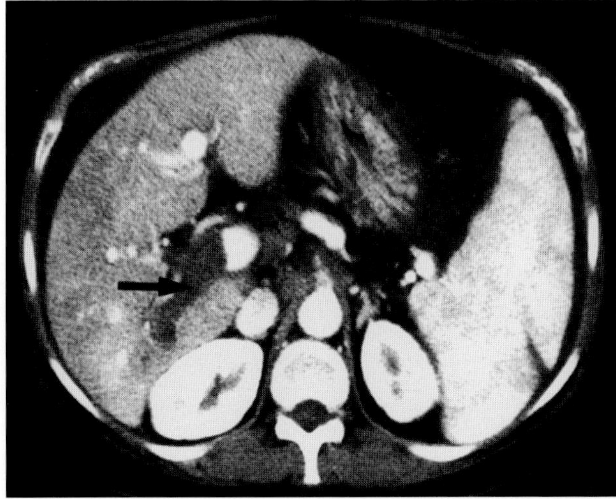

Figure 22. CT scan shows portal vein thrombus (arrow).

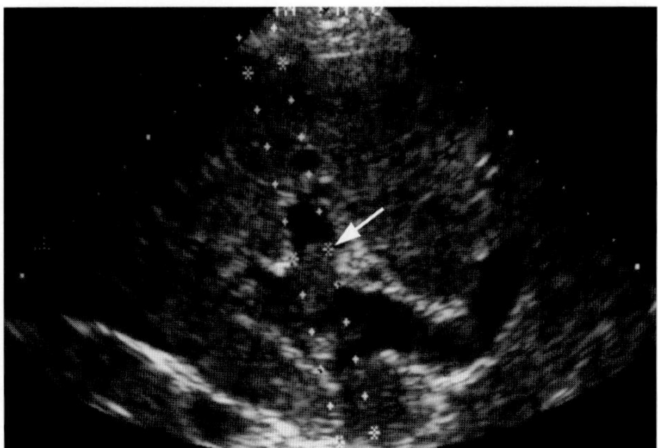

Figure 23. Same patient as in Figure 22. Ultrasound image shows the planned biopsy path into the right portal vein thrombus (arrow).

Ideal Biopsy Path
• Subcostal approach • Avoid pleural space • No large vessels in the way • 1–2-cm mantle of normal liver between the surface and the lesion

Figure 24.

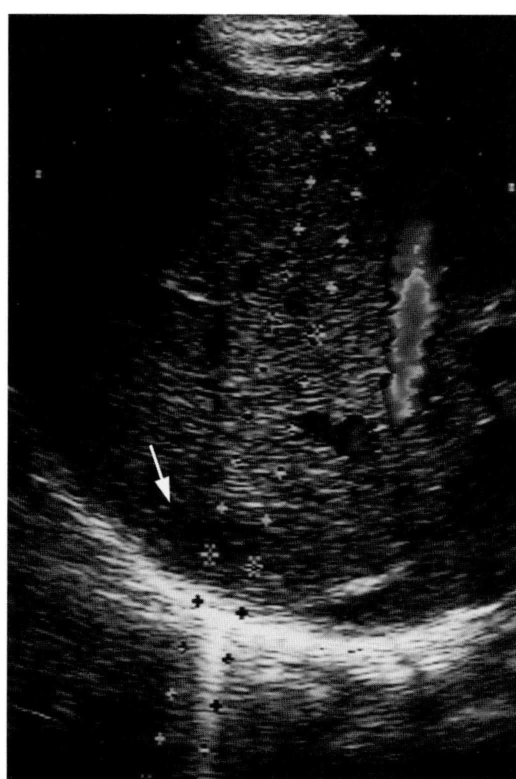

Figure 25. Color Doppler with no vessels seen in the path to the lesion (arrow).

Technique—Selection of the Biopsy Path

Figure 24 delineates the characteristics of an ideal biopsy path for a hepatic lesion. A subcostal approach completely avoids the pleural space and the intercostal vessels. Even lesions in the dome of the right lobe of the liver can usually be visualized subcostally by having the patient take a deep breath and angling the transducer superiorly. However, sometimes a lesion is not visualized subcostally. In such patients the lowest possible intercostal approach is used and it is imperative that the puncture site be in the lower part of the intercostal space, just superior to the upper border of the lower rib, to avoid injury to the intercostal neurovascular bundle. Color Doppler is always used to make sure that no significant vessels are in the biopsy path or within the area of the lesion to be biopsied **(Fig. 25)**. To decrease the risk of hemorrhage, an effort is made to select a path that interposes at least 2–3 cm of liver parenchyma between the puncture site on the liver surface and the lesion. Even with surface lesions this can usually be accomplished by modifying the direction of the ultrasound beam.

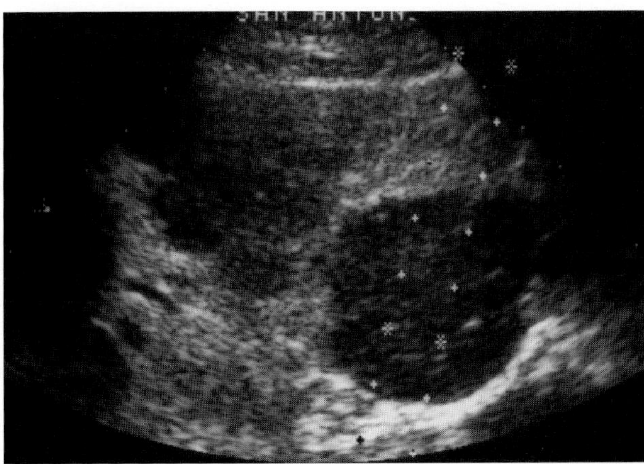

Figure 26. An optimized image.

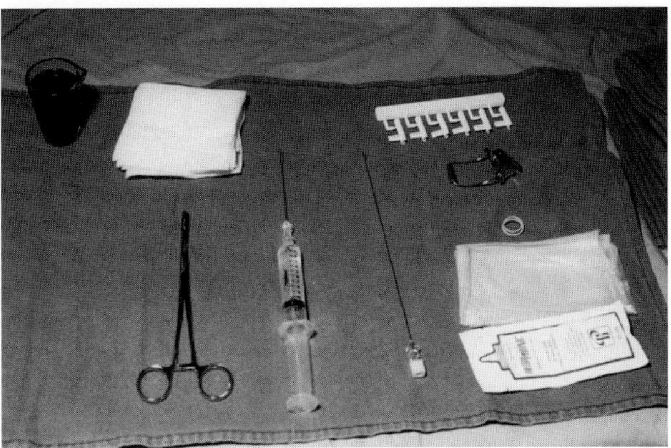

Figure 27. Tray setting for an ultrasound-guided biopsy procedure.

Technique—Optimizing the Image

Once the lesion or biopsy area has been selected, it is important to optimize the image to improve sonographic visualization of the lesion and the needle **(Fig. 26)**. As mentioned earlier, the transducer frequency should be appropriate to the depth of the lesion and the size of the patient. A depth should be selected so that the lesion and the biopsy path fill the image on the monitor and not much of the area deep to the lesion is seen. The focal zone is moved to the level of the superficial margin of the lesion.

Technique—Supplies and Site Preparation

Tray setting: The sterile supplies in an ultrasound biopsy set are shown in **Figure 27**.

Site preparation: The patient's skin around the selected site of entry is cleaned with povidone-iodine solution and draped with sterile towels. The transducer is covered with a sterile soft plastic probe cover and the needle guide is attached. In our institution, sterile gown, gloves, mask, and goggles to provide asepsis and reverse isolation are standard for operators performing any biopsy procedure.

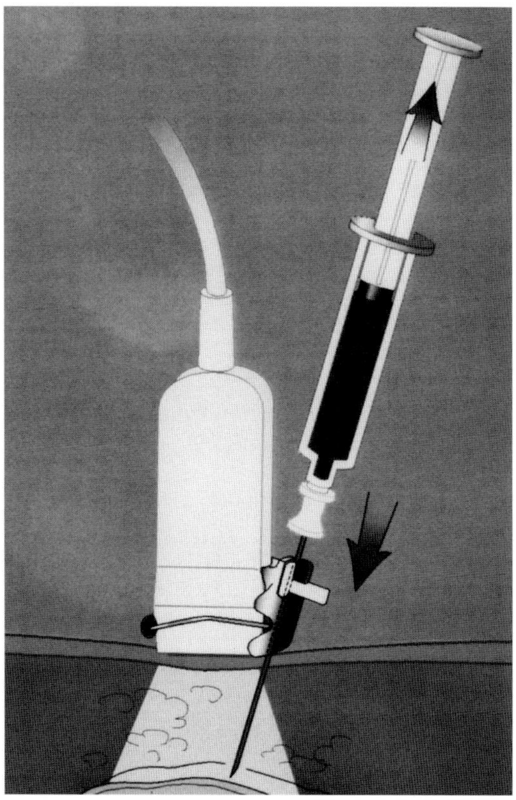

Figure 28. Local anesthesia—introduction of the needle.

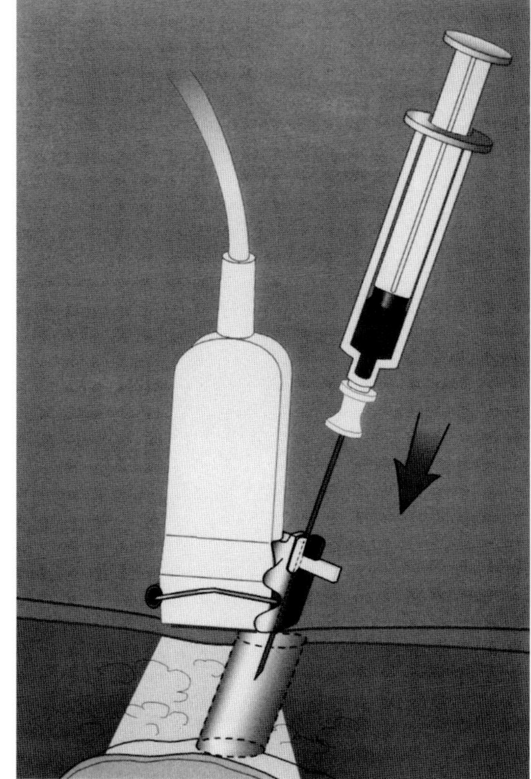

Figure 29. Local anesthesia—cylinder of anesthesia.

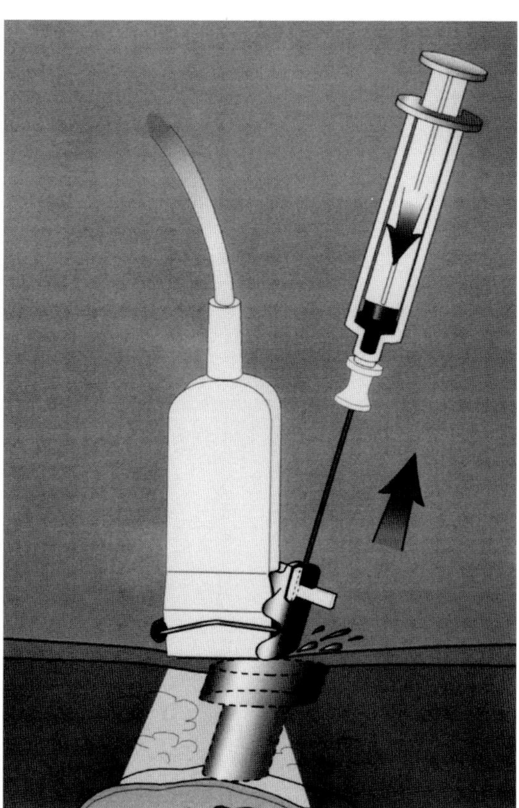

Figure 30. Local anesthesia—dermal and subcutaneous anesthesia.

Technique—Local Anesthesia

Sterile gel is spread on the selected area, then the transducer is placed on the skin and fine adjustments are made to obtain an accurate path to the lesion as shown by the electronic guide on the screen. While the transducer is held in place, a 22-gauge spinal needle mounted on a 10-mL syringe filled with 1% lidocaine is advanced through the needle guide into the subcutaneous tissue. The progress of the local anesthetic needle is monitored up to the liver capsule, which is not punctured **(Fig. 28)**. After ensuring that no blood can be aspirated, the needle is withdrawn while a bolus of lidocaine is injected in the biopsy track, producing a subcutaneous cylinder of local anesthesia **(Fig. 29)**. The needle is then reintroduced into the skin and a local anesthetic solution injected to produce dermal anesthesia **(Fig. 30)**.

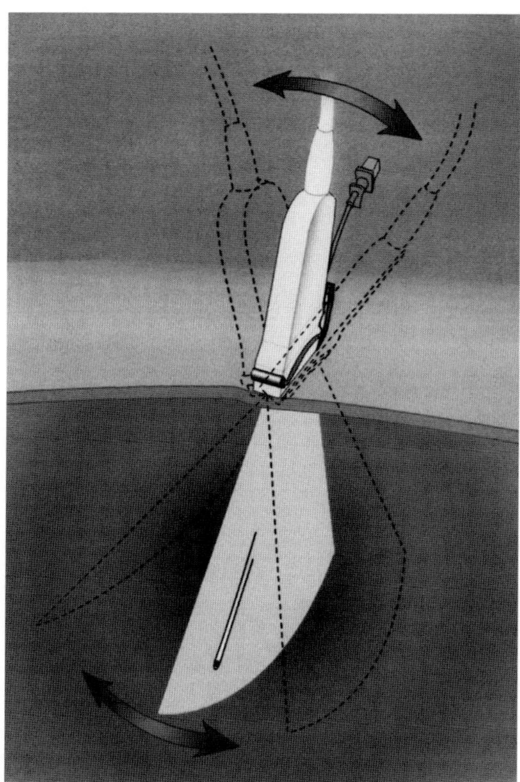

Figure 31. Rocking movements of the transducer to find the needle tip.

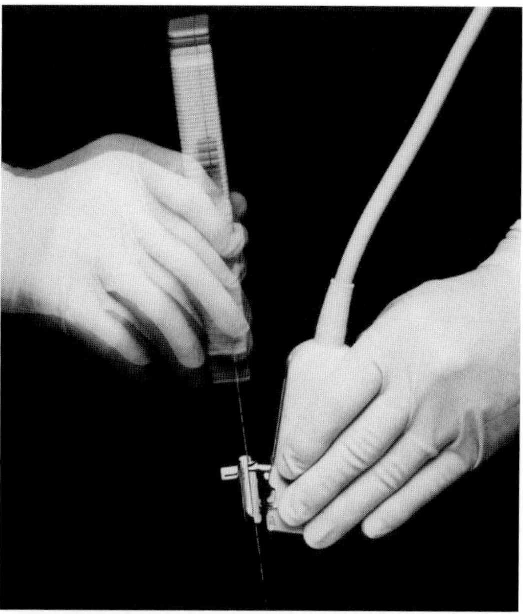

Figure 32. In-and-out movement of the needle to facilitate imaging of the needle tip.

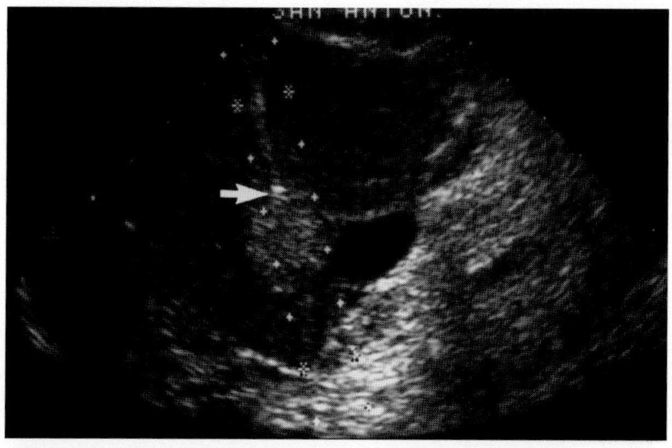

Figure 33. Needle placement at the periphery of the lesion (arrow).

Technique—Needle Placement

While the operator holds the transducer steadily in place, the assistant introduces the biopsy needle into the needle guide. After ascertaining that the skin is anesthetized, the skin is punctured with the needle. For this step it is important to hold the needle as close to the skin entry site as possible to prevent the needle from bending. The patient is asked to stop breathing, and the liver capsule is punctured and the needle introduced into the liver and advanced to the lesion under real-time guidance. If at any time the needle tip is lost from view, fine adjustments are made in the transducer orientation by rocking it until the needle tip comes back into view **(Fig. 31)**. Simultaneous, rapid, in-and-out movements of the needle help identify the tip more clearly **(Fig. 32)**. The needle is advanced until the tip is just outside the margin of the lesion **(Fig. 33)**.

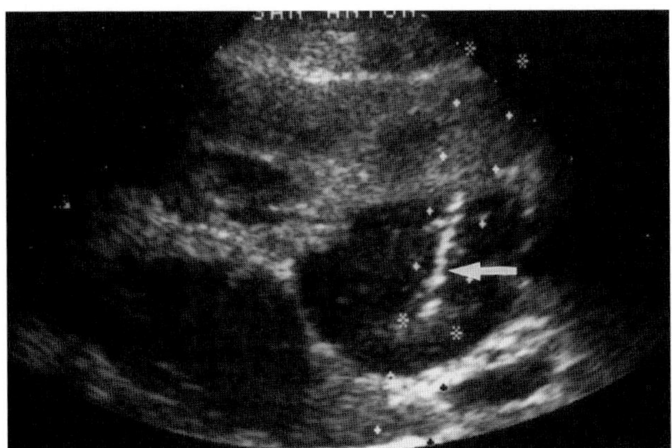

Figure 34. Core biopsy being performed (arrow).

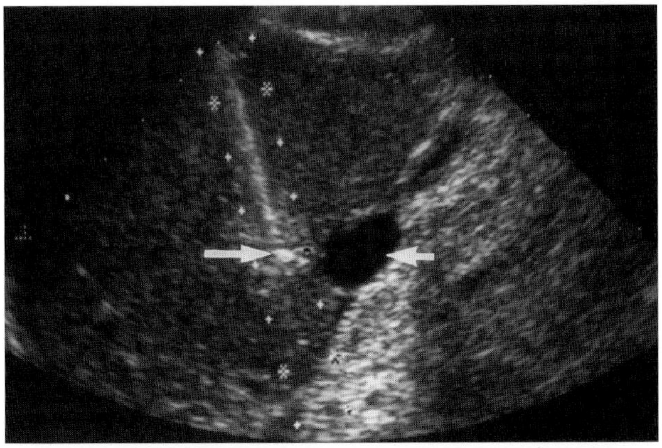

Figure 35. Fine needle biopsy of the lesion shown in Figure 34 with the needle (left arrow) advanced into the lesion. Continuous real-time monitoring of the needle position ensures its accurate position and prevents inadvertent entry into the inferior vena cava (right arrow).

Technique—Obtaining the Tissue

Once the needle tip is placed appropriately, the tissue sample is obtained. It is a matter of pressing a button with the core biopsy gun. The excursion of the biopsy tip of the needle varies between different types of guns but is a maximum of 2.5 cm. It is therefore imperative to make sure that there is no vessel or liver capsule within 2.5 cm distal to the needle tip to prevent vascular injury **(Fig. 34)**. If a fine aspiration needle is used, the needle is moved in and out and rotated at the same time. The real-time image of the moving needle tip is observed to make sure that it stays within the lesion **(Fig. 35)**.

Immediate Patient Care and Specimen Handling

As soon as the needle is removed, the biopsy track is examined with color Doppler to ensure that it is not actively bleeding **(Fig. 36)**. Cores obtained with a core biopsy needle are sent for pathological examination in formalin. If lymphoma is suspected, at least one core should be sent to the laboratory in normal saline for flow cytometry. If required, touch preparations may be obtained by the cytopathologist on site. Samples obtained with fine needle aspiration are given at once to the cytopathologist, who makes slides immediately and saves some of the material for cell block preparation.

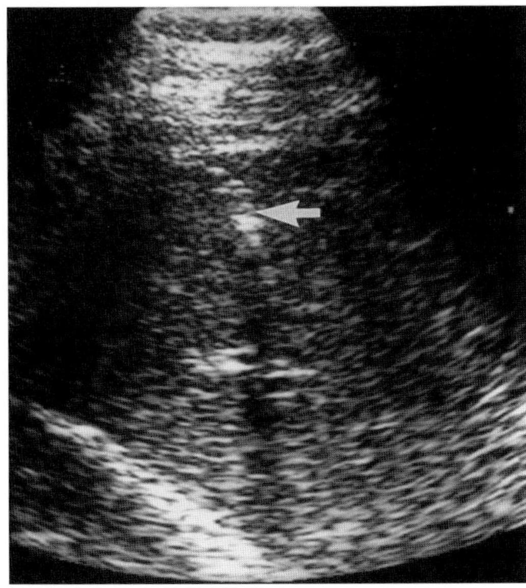

Figure 36. Needle track after biopsy (arrow).

Advantages Of CT As a Guiding Modality

- Lesion may be visualized only by CT
- Less operator-dependent

Figure 37.

Limitations Of CT As a Guiding Modality

- Biopsy is blind
- Lesions may not be visible without intravenous contrast material
- Only one plane of sectioning is available
- It may be impossible to avoid the pleural space to reach lesions high in the dome of the diaphragm
- It may be impossible to avoid small but significant vessels
- Respiratory motion may interfere with accurate localization of a small lesion
- Ionizing radiation

Figure 38.

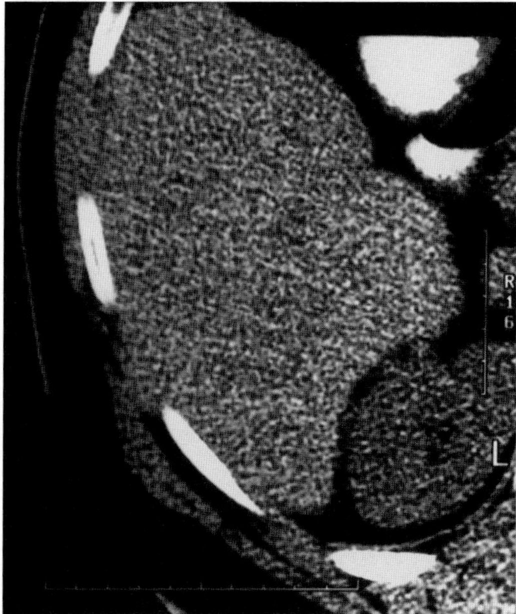

Figure 39. No lesion seen on a noncontrast CT scan.

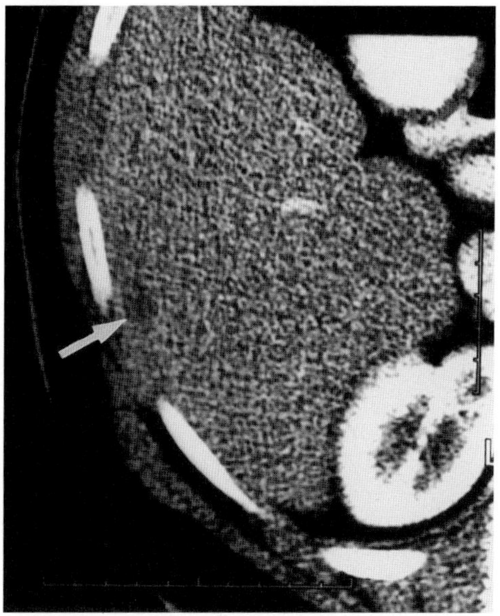

Figure 40. Lesion seen on a contrast-enhanced CT scan (arrow).

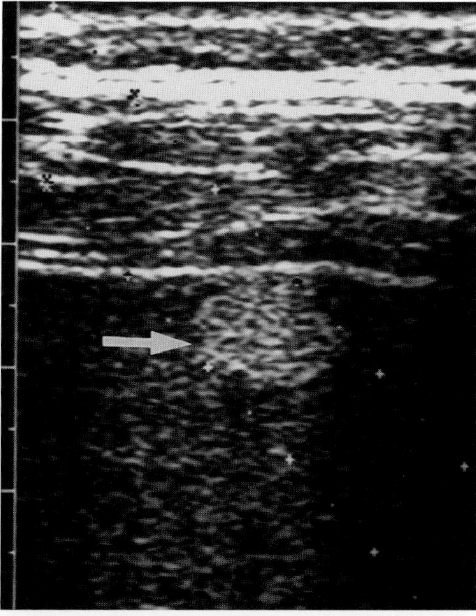

Figure 41. Lesion seen clearly on ultrasound for biopsy (arrow).

CT-Guided Liver Biopsy

Advantages and Limitations

CT is used to guide liver biopsies in a number of centers.[7,8] The advantages of CT-guided biopsy are shown in **Figure 37**. This method is particularly useful for lesions seen only by CT scanning. Also, it is less operator-dependent than ultrasound. However, CT has some limitations **(Fig. 38)**. It does not provide real-time guidance. Lesions that are not visible without injection of contrast material may not be suitable for CT-guided biopsy **(Figs. 39–41)**. The lack of multiplanar sectioning capability makes it difficult to target lesions high in the liver, although this problem can be partially offset by tilting the gantry. Respiratory motion makes accurate targeting of small lesions difficult. Ionizing radiation exposures may become considerable if multiple attempts are required to obtain adequate tissue. In our institution, we use ultrasound guidance for all liver biopsy procedures except those where the lesion is visible only by CT scanning.

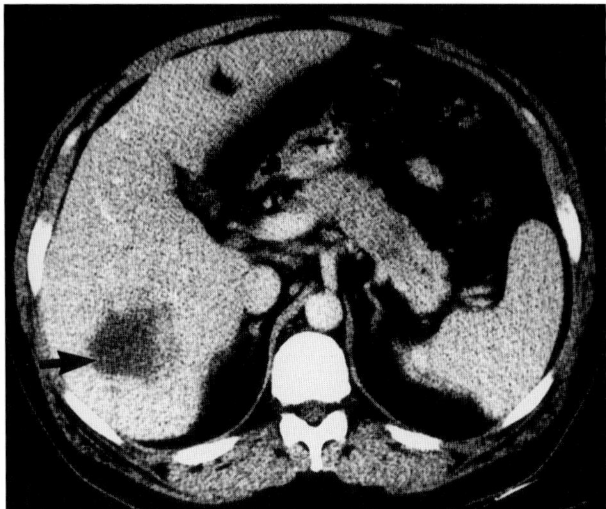

Figure 42. Lesion in the posterior segment of the right hepatic lobe (arrow).

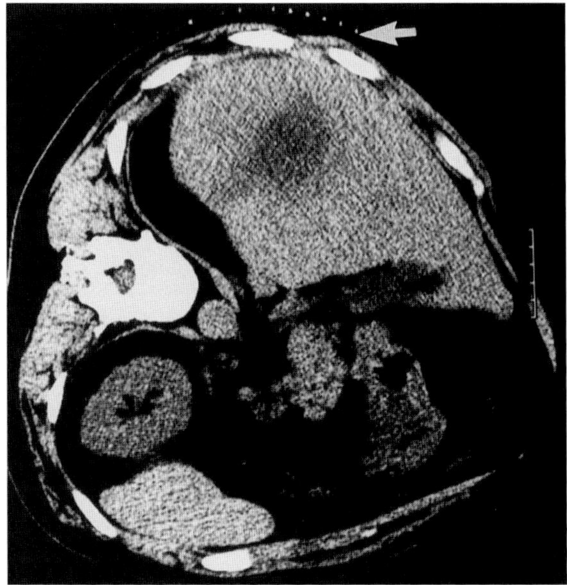

Figure 43. Decubitus positioning of the patient with a localizing grid (arrow).

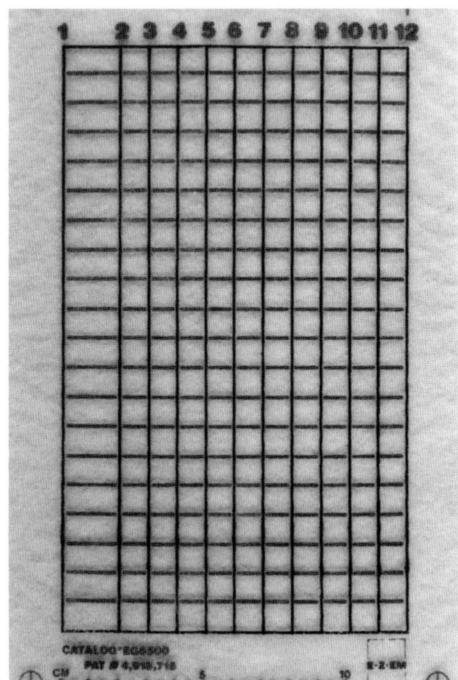

Figure 44. Commercially available localizing grid.

Localizing Cuts

The patient is placed in a position that makes the lesion easily approachable **(Figs. 42, 43)**. A radio-paque localizing grid is placed over the expected region of the lesion. These grids are commercially available **(Fig. 44)** but a rough version can be prepared with sheathed needles or expired vascular catheters stuck between two layers of sticky tape **(Fig. 45)**. Contiguous 5-mm-thick slices are then obtained through the area of the lesion. The line of the grid closest to the lesion with no lung or ribs in the path is selected. The level of the section is shown on the skin by the laser localizer on the CT gantry.

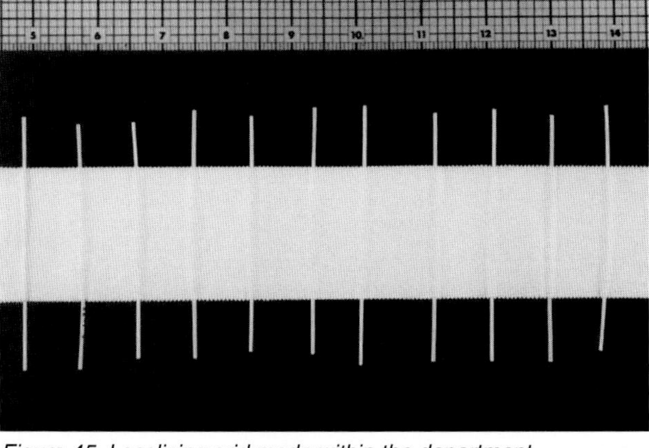

Figure 45. Localizing grid made within the department.

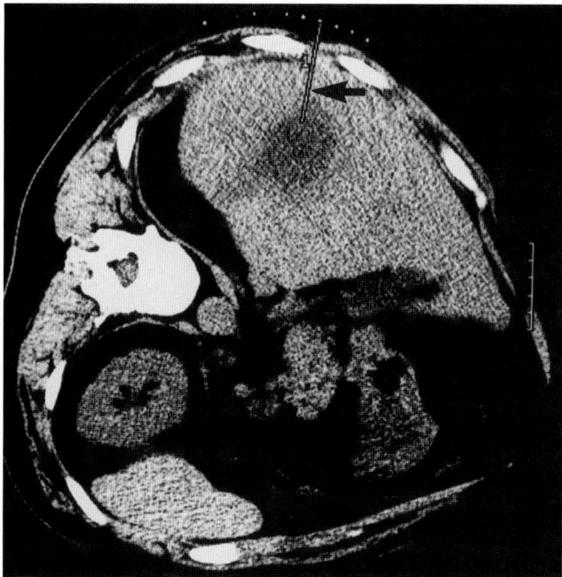

Figure 46. Line (arrow) drawn from the grid to the lesion.

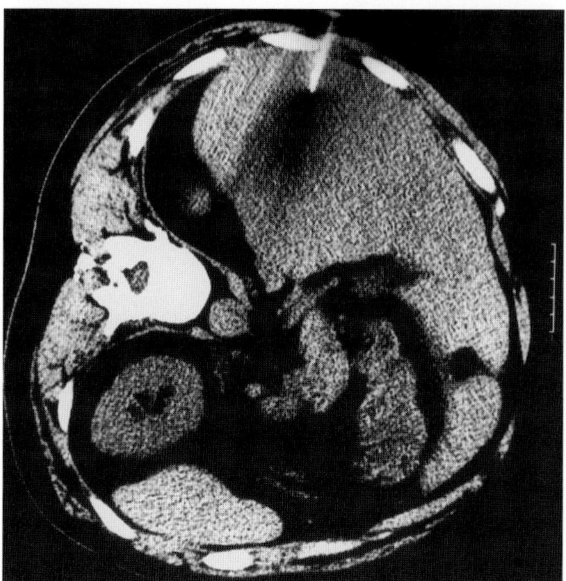

Figure 47. Needle tip in the desired location.

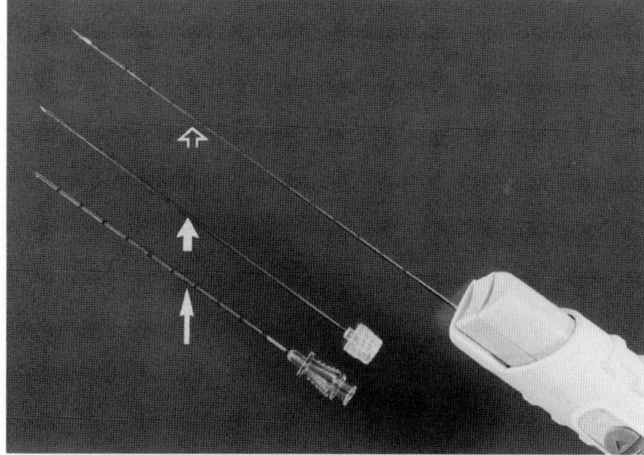

Figure 48. Outer needle (long arrow), stylet (short arrow), and core biopsy needle (open arrow) are parts of a coaxial automated biopsy system.

The point where the laser intersects the selected grid line is marked as the skin entry site. The depth of the lesion and the angle of the biopsy path are determined from the localizing images **(Fig. 46)**.

Fine Needle Aspiration

Biopsy site preparation is performed as described in the section on ultrasound-guided biopsy. Local anesthetic is injected into the skin and subcutaneous tissue. The distance between the skin entry site and the edge of the lesion is marked on the needle. If a fine needle is used, the biopsy needle is inserted into the skin at the selected angle and advanced the measured distance with the patient suspending respiration in the same phase as for the localizing scan. Contiguous 5-mm CT sections are then taken, centered around the lesion to confirm the position of the needle tip within the lesion **(Fig. 47)**. If the needle is not in the optimal position, it is withdrawn into the subcutaneous tissue and reinserted after the desired correction has been made. If an end-cutting needle is used, tissue is obtained by making in-and-out excursions with the needle as described for ultrasound-guided biopsy, making sure that the excursions are short enough to stay within the mass.

Core Biopsy

For core biopsies, automated systems are available where the core biopsy gun can be attached to the needle after the needle tip has been positioned in the lesion. Some automated systems have a coaxial outer needle that is first placed into the lesion **(Fig. 48)**. After the correct positioning of its tip within the lesion is confirmed, the biopsy needle is advanced into the outer coaxial needle and a biopsy taken. The tissue obtained is processed in the same way as for ultrasound-guided biopsy.

Postprocedure Care
Patients are observed for 4 hours and vital signs are recorded at regular intervals. Patients are allowed to eat and are given bathroom privileges under supervision. At the end of 4 hours, one of the radiologists sees the patient and, if the postprocedure period has been uneventful, discharges the patient home with the instructions to come to the emergency department in case of severe abdominal pain.

Complications
The complication rate for liver biopsy is low and has been reported as 0.1%–1% in various series. Most complications occur within the first 3 hours after the procedure. Complications are relatively more frequent in patients with severe liver disease, coagulopathy, or ascites, and especially after the biopsy of hypervascular liver masses and tumors at the surface of the liver. Mortality is extremely rare, having been reported in 9 out of 100,000 patients in a large series of blind liver biopsies.

Pain is the most common complication and is experienced when the biopsy needle traverses the liver capsule. It may persist at the biopsy site for a short while after the procedure and frequently radiates to the right shoulder. Postprocedure pain in the right shoulder may be due to the needle traversing a slip of the diaphragm. However, it is usually due to irritation of the diaphragm from minor oozing from the biopsy site. An ultrasound of the right upper quadrant in such patients usually shows no abnormality.

Persistent severe pain may suggest more serious complications. Hemoperitoneum is the most common and can largely be prevented by paying attention to details. Color Doppler should be used while planning the approach to avoid any major vessels in the biopsy path. Immediately after the biopsy, the track should be examined with color Doppler to detect any oozing from the puncture site on the liver surface **(Fig. 49)**. Oozing usually stops spontaneously, but it is wise to exert local pressure over the site with the transducer in an attempt to hasten the process. Biliary peritonitis is rare but occurs more commonly in the presence of biliary obstruction. Tumor seeding is extremely rare. Injury to the surrounding viscera should not occur with imaging-guided biopsy. With lesions high in the dome of the right lobe, it may not be possible to avoid traversing the pleural space under CT guidance. In such cases a subcostal approach under ultrasound guidance can be used as an alternative.

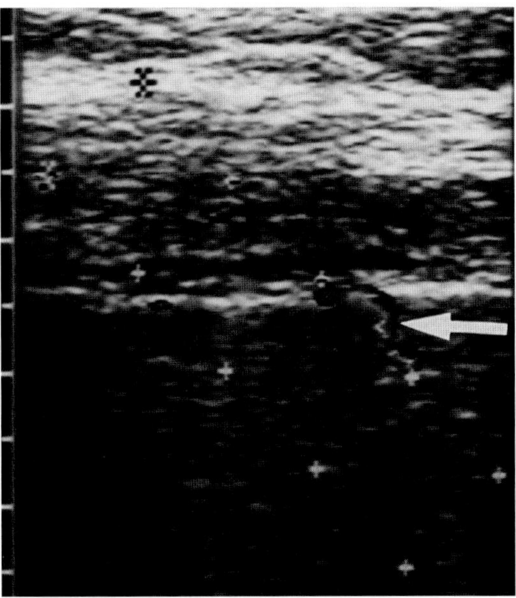

Figure 49. Color Doppler shows oozing from the biopsy site (arrow).

Although ascites has been considered a relative contraindication to percutaneous liver biopsy, a comparative analysis of complications in patients with and without ascites showed no significant difference in complication rate.[9] Ascites in and of itself should not be considered a contraindication to percutaneous liver biopsy, although it may make the biopsy technically more difficult. Patients with severe uncorrectable coagulopathies have a higher risk of complications. In these patients, several alternatives exist to the standard biopsy technique described in this tutorial. In cases where a nondirected liver biopsy is needed for histological evaluation of diffuse liver disease, a transjugular approach to the liver can minimize the complication rate from the underlying coagulopathy.[10]

The availability of transjugular cutting core biopsy needles has increased the success rate of transjugular liver biopsies and provides sufficient material for adequate pathologic analysis. When a focal lesion is present in the liver and imaging guidance is required, a percutaneous approach can still be used in patients with severe coagulopathy. Bleeding complications can be minimized by embolizing the biopsy track with Gelfoam (Upjohn, Kalamazoo, MI) and/or thrombin to decrease any bleeding from the biopsy site.[11,12] In addition, the use of color Doppler ultrasound during the biopsy enables the operator to avoid any vessels in the biopsy path.

Conclusion

Imaging-guided liver biopsy is a relatively safe technique which can be performed as an outpatient procedure. CT and ultrasound are both suitable modalities for providing imaging guidance. Each has its advantages and limitations. The choice of modality will depend on local experience and the specific needs of the patient. In our institution, ultrasound guidance is used in almost all imaging-guided liver biopsy procedures. In any case, attention to detail is important for accuracy and avoiding complications.

References

1. Silverman SG, Mueller PR, Pfister RC. Hemostatic evaluation before abdominal interventions: an overview and proposal. AJR 1990; 154:233–238.

2. Rapaport SI. Assessing hemostatic function before abdominal interventions. AJR 1990; 154:239–240.

3. Hopper KD, Abendroth CS, Sturtz KW, Matthews YL, Stevens LA, Shirk SJ. Automated biopsy devices: a blinded evaluation. Radiology 1993; 187:653–660.

4. Reading CC, Charboneau JW, James EM, Hurt MR. Sonographically guided percutaneous biopsy of small (3 cm or less) masses. AJR 1988; 151:189–192.

5. Dodd GD III, Esola CC, Memel DS, et al. Sonography: the undiscovered jewel of interventional radiology. Radiographics 1996; 16:1271–1288.

6. Dodd GD III, Carr BI. Percutaneous biopsy of portal vein thrombus: a new staging technique for hepatocellular carcinoma. AJR 1993; 161:229–233.

7. Martino CR, Haaga JR, Bryan PJ, LiPuma JP, El-Yousef SJ, Alfidi RJ. CT-guided liver biopsies: eight years experience. Work in progress. Radiology 1984; 152:755–757.

8. Welch TJ, Sheedy PF, Johnson CD, Johnson CM, Stephens DH. CT-guided biopsy: prospective analysis of 1,000 procedures. Radiology 1989; 171:493–496.

9. Little AF, Ferris JV, Dodd GD III, Baron RL. Image-guided percutaneous hepatic biopsy: effect of ascites on the complication rate. Radiology 1996; 199:79–83.

10. Jackson JE, Adam A, Allison DJ. Transjugular and plugged liver biopsies. Baillieres Clin Gastroenterol 1992; 6:245–258.

11. Smith TP, McDermott VG, Ayoub DM, Suhocki PV, Stackhouse DJ. Percutaneous transhepatic liver biopsy with tract embolization. Radiology 1996; 198:769–774.

12. Zins M, Vilgrain V, Gayno S, et al. US-guided percutaneous liver biopsy with plugging of the needle track: a prospective study in 72 high-risk patients. Radiology 1992; 184:841–843.

Endnote

Figures 24, 25, 34–38 from Dodd GD III, Esola CC, Memel DS, et al. Sonography: the undiscovered jewel of interventional radiology. Radiographics 1996; 16:1271–1288. Used with permission.

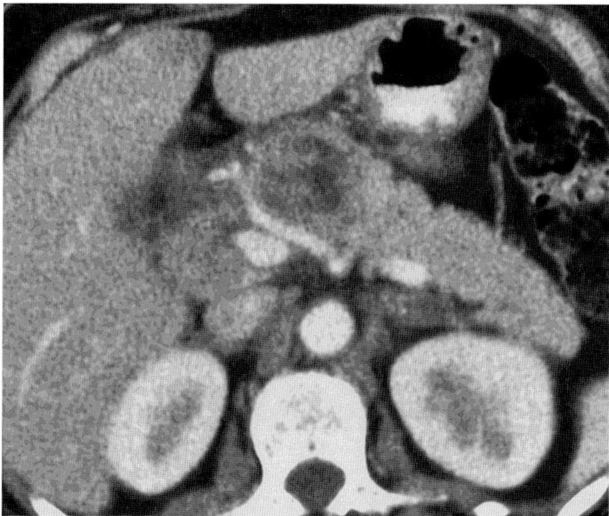

Figure 1. Mass in the head of the pancreas.

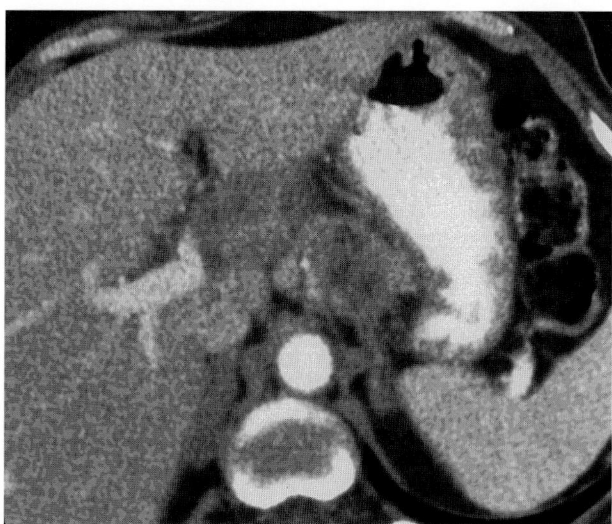

Figure 2. Adenopathy in the porta hepatis indicates metastatic disease precluding a curative surgical resection. Biopsy is warranted in this case to confirm the diagnosis of pancreatic adenocarcinoma.

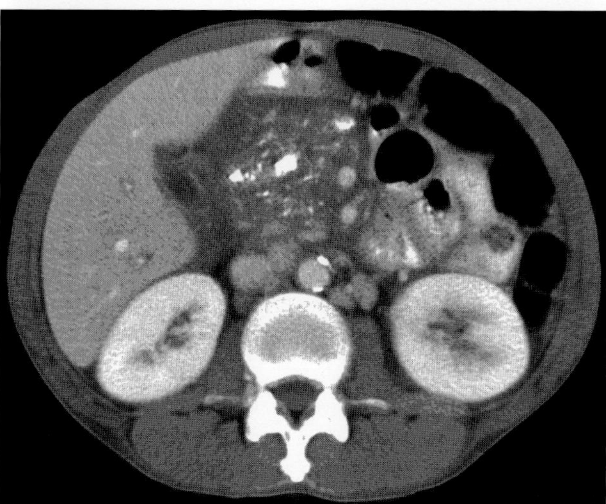

Figure 3. Computed tomography scan demonstrates changes of chronic pancreatitis which could be confused with a pancreatic mass.

TUTORIAL 4
PANCREATIC BIOPSY

Joseph L. Higgins, Ph.D., M.D.

Introduction

The subjects addressed in this tutorial include:

1. Indications for percutaneous pancreatic biopsy
2. Imaging guidance
3. Patient preparation
4. Biopsy technique
5. Specimen evaluation
6. Complications.

Percutaneous biopsy of the pancreas is performed primarily to obtain tissue to confirm the diagnosis of pancreatic adenocarcinoma, especially in patients with suspected unresectable disease **(Figs. 1, 2)**.[1] Biopsy of pancreatic masses can also be performed to characterize other types of pancreatic lesions, such as pseudocyst, abscess, cystadenocarcinoma, or to differentiate chronic pancreatitis from neoplasm **(Fig. 3)**.[2] Pancreatic biopsy to assess pancreatic transplant grafts for rejection is an increasingly common procedure.[3] Multiple factors have played a role in the increasing use of imaging-guided biopsy, including improved lesion detectability, advances in needle biopsy systems, and improvements in and wider availability of cytologic evaluation of the biopsy specimen. Over the years, the accuracy of fine-needle percutaneous biopsy in the setting of suspected malignancy has increased to 80%–95%[4,5] with few serious complications.

Interestingly, new technical developments with spring-loaded cutting needles have rejuvenated interest in the use of larger needles which can provide material for histopathologic rather than cytologic examination. Larger specimen size should also decrease the number of biopsies that yield insufficient or inadequate specimens.

Localization

Accurate localization of the target lesion is the crux of a successful imaging-guided biopsy. The imaging modality chosen for pancreatic biopsy, as for all percutaneous biopsies, depends on which modality best demonstrates the lesion. Equal facility with ultrasound (US) and computed tomography (CT) biopsy techniques allows the radiologist to provide rapid and cost-effective service. CT localization for percutaneous pancreatic biopsy may be preferred because it offers the versatility of either an anterior or posterior approach, and CT scanning often demonstrates lesions that are not clearly defined by US **(Fig. 4)**.[5–9] CT better defines the relationship of the pancreatic mass to surrounding structures, but it is limited by its inability to continuously monitor needle position and inability to provide complex angles due to limited gantry tilt.

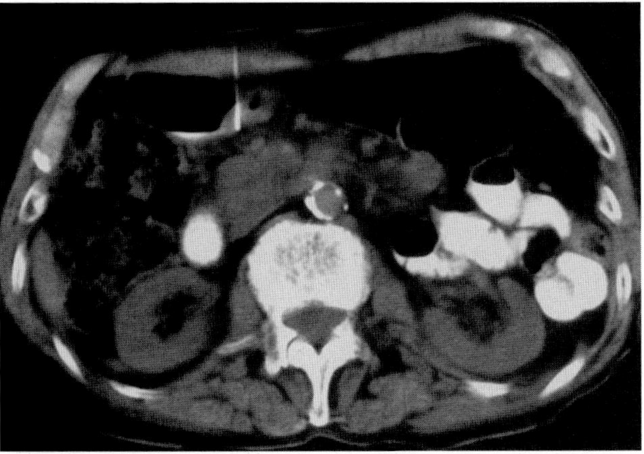

Figure 4. Biopsy performed under CT guidance because US could not adequately delineate the mass secondary to surrounding bowel gas.

Although US provides greater flexibility in guidance, the utility of US is sometimes compromised by the presence of overlying intestinal gas and acoustic shadowing from the anterior ribs. Visualization of lesions in the tail of the pancreas with US may be particularly difficult with anterior scanning, and a posterior approach may not resolve this limitation because of the small acoustic window afforded by intercostal or transsplenic scanning of the pancreas.

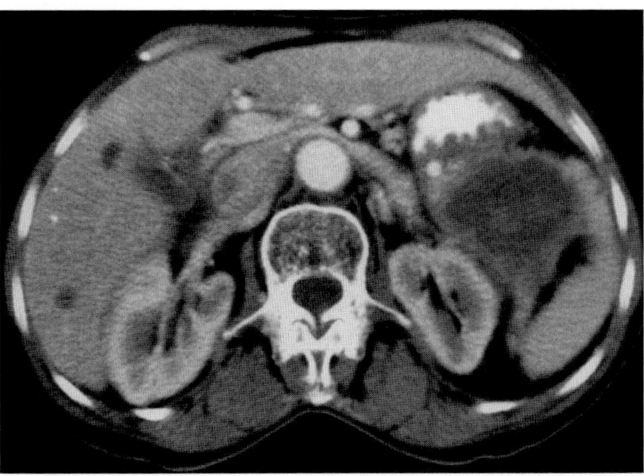

Figure 5. Pancreatic tail mass and metastatic lesions in the liver. The mass is surrounded by the liver, spleen, kidney, and stomach, making a biopsy in this transaxial plane difficult.

A recent series of over 250 percutaneous pancreatic biopsies reported more than 90% sensitivity and accuracy for combined results of CT- and US-guided procedures.[5] The individual sensitivity and accuracy for CT were both approximately 85%, while for US they were both approximately 95%. This series also indicated better accuracy with larger needles (16–19 gauge) than with fine needles (20–22 gauge)—92% versus 85%. This is the largest reported study to date and the combined results are a significant improvement over results reported earlier.[10,11] The combined accuracy for CT- and US-guided percutaneous pancreatic biopsy is higher than that reported for fluoroscopic localization following endoscopic retrograde cholangiopancreatography[12] or transhepatic cholangiography.[6,8,13] Given the flexibility of US, the ability to perform the biopsy faster with US, and the greater sensitivity and accuracy of US compared to CT guidance, the biopsy should initially be attempted under US guidance if the lesion is well seen **(Figs. 5, 6)**, and CT reserved for lesions poorly delineated by US.

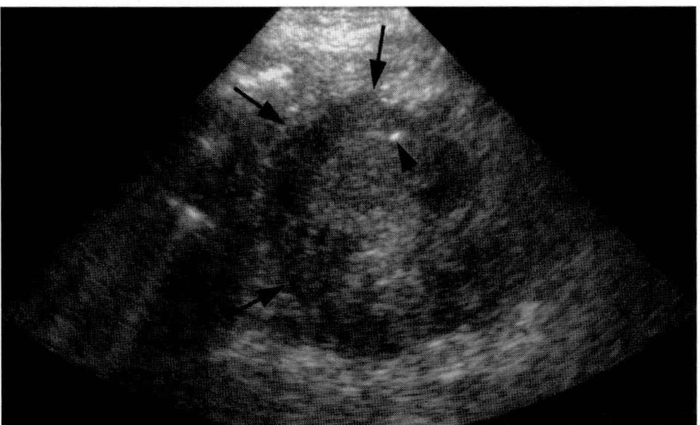

Figure 6. Longitudinal US clearly defines the mass (arrows). The angled subcostal approach available with US guidance avoids any surrounding structures. The echogenic dot (arrowhead) in the mass is the tip of the biopsy needle.

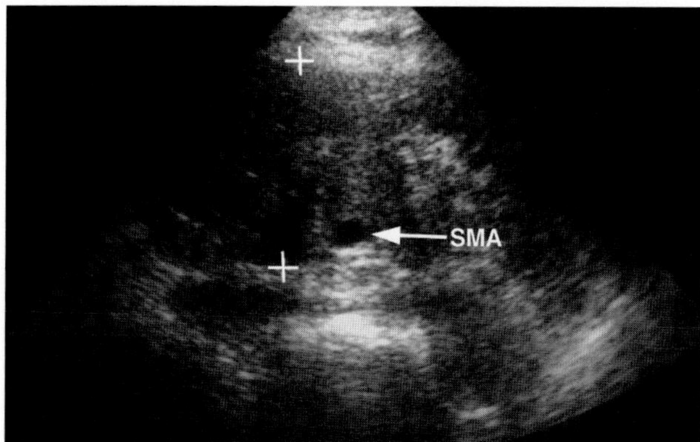

Figure 7. Transverse US demonstrates a mass in the head of the pancreas (between cursors). SMA=superior mesenteric artery.

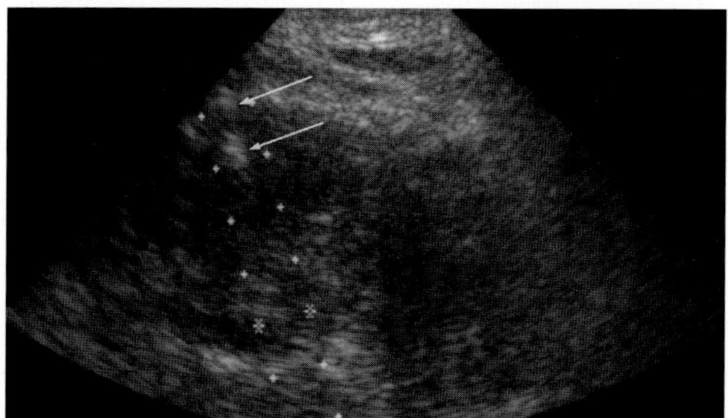

Figure 8. Biopsy of the mass with a needle guide shows the expected path of the needle (between the cursor lines) and the needle (arrows) between the lines.

US Guidance

The principles of US-guided needle biopsy have been reviewed in **Tutorials 1–3** on liver biopsy and US guidance for interventional procedures, and those same principles apply to pancreatic biopsies. Biopsies can be performed with either the freehand or needle-guided technique. The value of the needle guide is that it shows where the needle should be, and the relationship of the needle trajectory to adjacent structures can be determined **(Figs. 7, 8)**. Needle localization is improved with use of small in-and-out movements of the needle[14,15] or use of needles with echogenic tips.[16] Color Doppler may assist in determining needle position.[17]

CT Guidance

CT localization is often used for percutaneous biopsy of the pancreas.[18–21] CT often provides visualization of lesions that are not clearly defined by US. In rare instances, it is not possible to verify the exact position of the needle tip with CT guidance; specifically, this occurs in those situations where the combination of lesion position, patient size, needle length, and gantry aperture diameter do not allow the patient to be repositioned within the CT scanner for repeat studies.

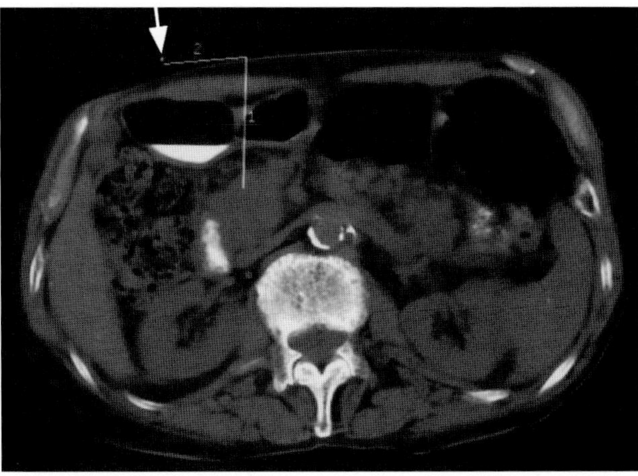

Figure 9. Appropriate measurements are obtained from the skin marker (arrow) as a guide.

For localization with CT, the patient is placed in the position that should optimize target lesion localization. A transaxial plane for biopsy is selected from diagnostic images and a grid or marker is placed on the patient's skin at that level **(Fig. 9)**.[22] A repeat scan with the marker in place allows for precise definition of the puncture site, the depth of the target lesion, and the degree of angulation of the needle track in that transaxial plane. A scan can be obtained with the small lidocaine needle in place to confirm appropriate positioning and angulation **(Fig. 10)**. Once the needle is inserted with aseptic technique, the tip position is verified by repeat scanning at the same transaxial plane **(Fig. 11)**.

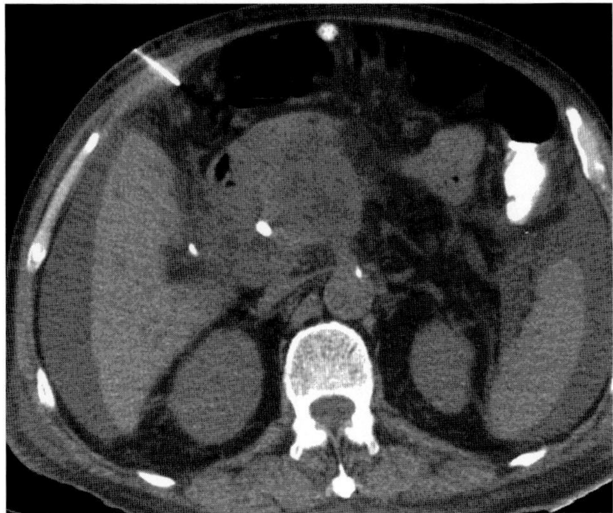

Figure 10. Repeat scan with the lidocaine needle in place in another patient confirms the expected trajectory and location.

Angulation of the needle course in a cephalad or caudad direction is sometimes necessary to avoid puncturing intervening structures. This is not a problem with real-time US guidance. Tilting the scanner gantry during localization with CT may be required to ensure that the needle path is free of intervening structures.[23] When gantry tilt is used, the target is localized directly and the needle is inserted in the same plane as the plane of gantry tilt.

Fluoroscopic Guidance

Occasionally, biliary drainage will have been performed on the patient before a histologic diagnosis was obtained. Fluoroscopic guidance in conjunction with a cholangiogram can be used to guide the pancreatic biopsy **(Figs. 12–14)**. The cholangiogram is obtained to identify the level of obstruction, and correlation with CT scans is done to locate the biopsy site directly over the mass. The needle is advanced parallel to the fluoroscopic beam until angled fluoroscopy determines that the tip of the needle is at the target site, which will usually be the biliary drain. Obviously, this technique is better suited for larger masses. Although the chances of traversing adjacent structures are greater with this approach, the consequences of inadvertent puncture of the bowel are minimal with the small-gauge needles used for aspiration biopsies.

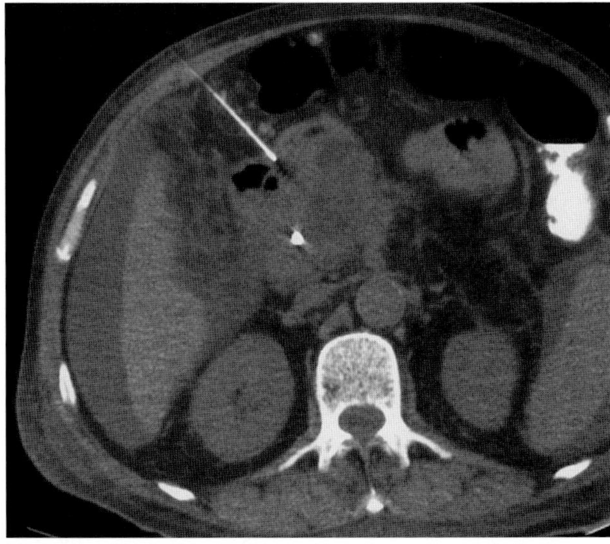

Figure 11. Biopsy needle inserted into the mass parallel to the lidocaine needle to the predetermined depth.

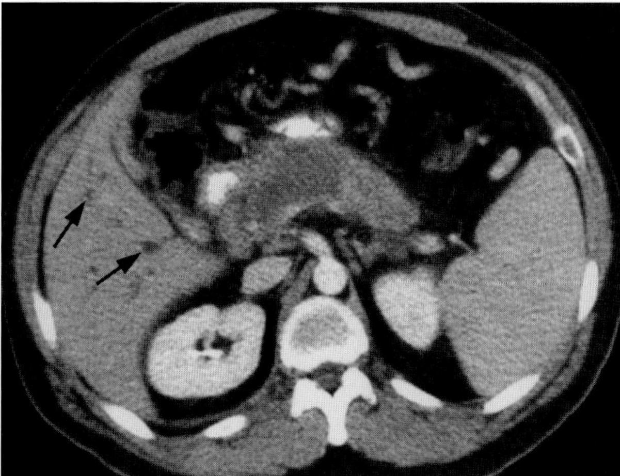

Figure 12. CT scan in a patient with jaundice shows a pancreatic mass in the head and neck of the gland with associated biliary obstruction (arrows).

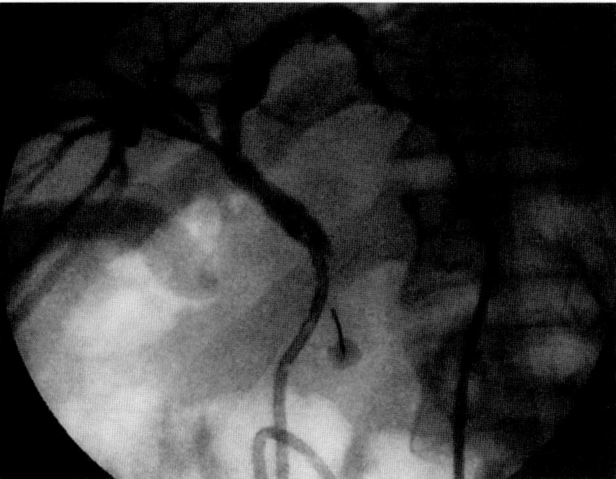

Figure 13. Cholangiogram after biliary drainage depicts the site of obstruction which correlates with the location of the mass seen on the CT scan. A skin site is chosen directly over the mass and the needle is advanced parallel to the image intensifier.

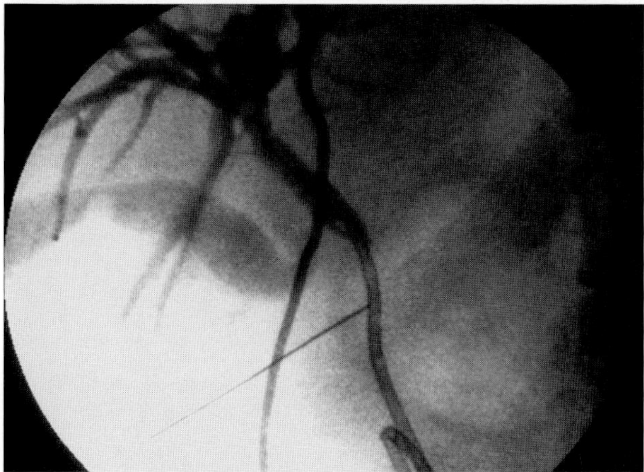

Figure 14. Angled fluoroscopy confirms the appropriate depth of the biopsy needle. Samples demonstrated pancreatic adenocarcinoma.

Patient Preparation

Because accurate localization of the target lesion and precise positioning of the biopsy needle is required for successful biopsy, patient cooperation is of paramount importance for this procedure. If cooperation cannot be assured in apprehensive or pediatric patients, heavy sedation may be required. If the patient still cannot cooperate, the procedure may have to be aborted. Both inpatients and outpatients can undergo percutaneous biopsy procedures. Careful monitoring of patients in both categories is required for 2 to 4 hours following biopsy, after which outpatients can be discharged with instructions to return for any changes in status. Acquisition of a screening history for possible coagulation disorders and recent use of aspirin or other medications that decrease platelet function should precede all pancreatic biopsies.[24] Laboratory evaluation should include a complete blood cell count with platelet quantification and prothrombin and partial thromboplastin times. An attempt to correct abnormal bleeding parameters should be made before the biopsy procedure.

Patient preparation prior to percutaneous biopsy is usually minimal. Fasting is advisable in patients as it helps decrease the amount of bowel gas. Informed consent should be obtained in all patients before any sedative medications are administered. Before the aspiration or biopsy, prophylactic antibiotics should be given to any patients with suspected infected lesions.

Biopsy Technique

Following lesion localization and selection of a puncture site for percutaneous biopsy, the skin is marked and cleaned with an antiseptic preparation. The puncture site is draped, and local anesthesia is given. A small skin dermatotomy facilitates needle placement. The need for patient cooperation is most important during needle placement, which should be done during suspended respiration. With US guidance, the needle tip position can be monitored continuously during placement. As continuous visualization is not possible with CT guidance, the needle should be advanced to the predetermined depth in a single smooth movement. Shallow respiration is then resumed during repeat scanning to define the needle tip position. Ideal positioning of the needle tip for percutaneous biopsy will depend in part on the radiographic appearance of the lesion. Biopsy should be performed from the periphery of a more solid, potentially neoplastic lesion and from the center of a more cystic or inflammatory lesion.

Two basic types of biopsy needles are available: aspiration and cutting needles. The specifics of the biopsy technique are determined in large part by the type of needle that is selected for use. In general, fine needles (22–20 gauge) should be used when there is a risk of entering a vital structure, such as a major blood vessel or bowel loop. Although attempts should be made to avoid any intervening normal structures, the deep location of the pancreatic mass may make this impossible **(Fig. 15)**. Many of the surrounding intervening structures such as the liver, stomach, small bowel, and large bowel can be traversed safely by a fine needle during percutaneous biopsy **(Figs. 16–17)**. If possible, the spleen should be avoided because of the risk of splenic laceration and hemorrhage. In certain cases where the pancreatic mass is difficult to visualize or biopsy, biopsy of alternative locations may yield the same information **(Figs. 18–20)**.

Needle sets are commercially available that facilitate the performance of coaxial and modified coaxial biopsy techniques. The Greene biopsy set (Cook, Bloomington, IN) contains a larger spinal needle for lesion localization and a fine-caliber Greene needle for biopsy.[25] Biopsy sets are also available for a modified coaxial technique. The vanSonnenberg biopsy set (Cook) contains a fine needle with a detachable hub, a larger needle for stabilization of the target lesion, and a fine Chiba needle for aspiration biopsy. The latter type of system allows initial localization of the target lesion with a fine needle.[26]

Lightweight, disposable spring-loaded biopsy guns have been developed by several manufacturers. We prefer to use an 18-gauge biopsy gun when lesion size, location, and needle path allow its use. The nondetachable needle version can easily be used with US guidance. For CT-guided procedures, a detachable needle version is advantageous because it allows a coaxial approach for needle placement. Without the protruding handle and handle weight, rescanning for needle tip localization is easier because there is no interference from the gantry and inadvertent needle movement is minimized. It is preferable to use core biopsy sets only when there is a clear path to the lesion.

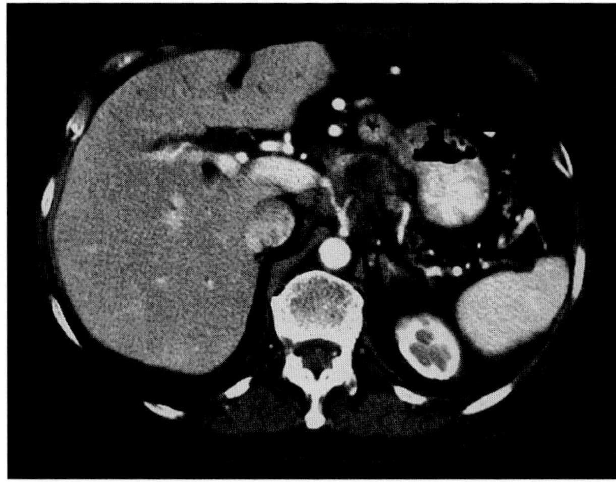

Figure 15. Deep location of a pancreatic mass which has extended around the celiac axis. Biopsy from an anterior approach may be limited by the stomach and duodenum, while a posterior approach may be difficult because of the vertebral column.

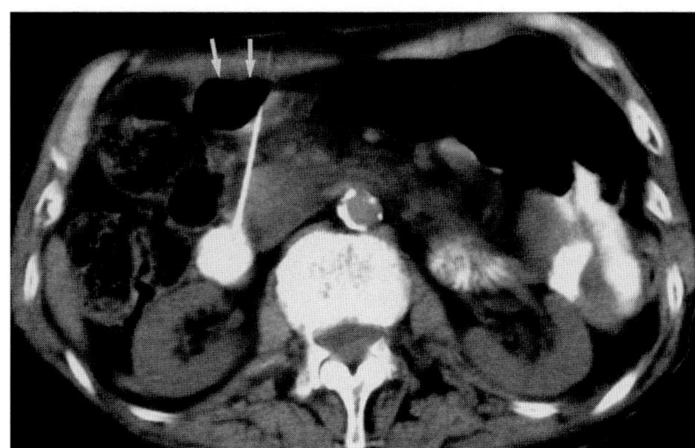

Figure 16. During positioning of the needle for biopsy of the pancreatic head mass, the biopsy needle transgressed the first portion of the duodenum (arrows) and the tip was inadvertently advanced into the second portion of the duodenum. The patient had no complications from the biopsy.

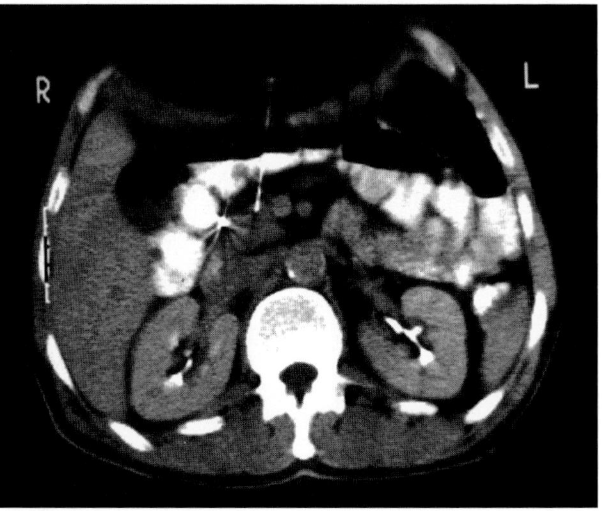

Figure 17. The needle passes through the transverse colon during biopsy of the pancreatic head.

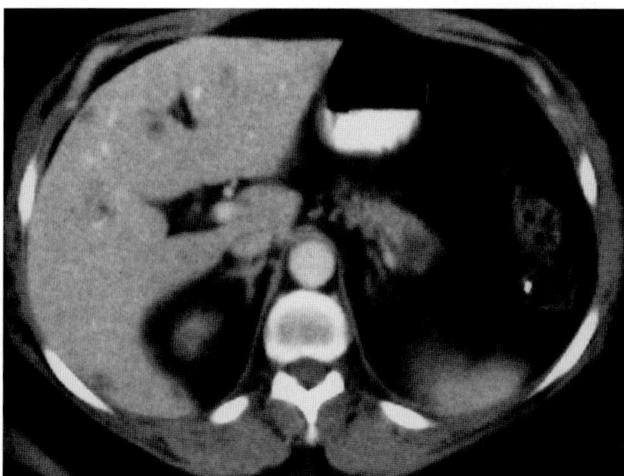

Figure 18. Obese patient (10 cm from the skin surface to the abdominal wall musculature) with a small pancreatic tail mass and liver metastases.

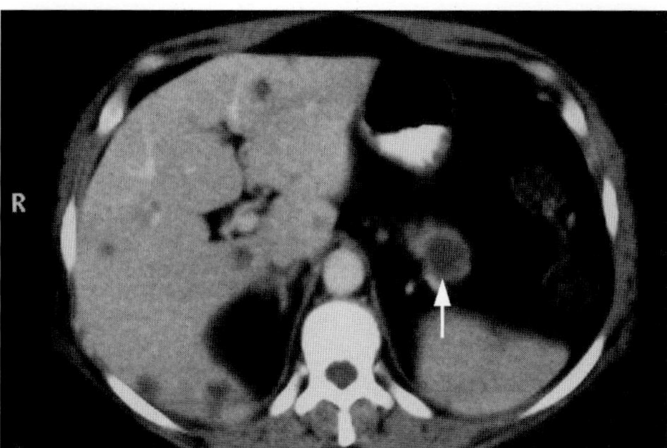

Figure 19. Sequential inferior image better displays the 2-cm pancreatic tail mass (arrow).

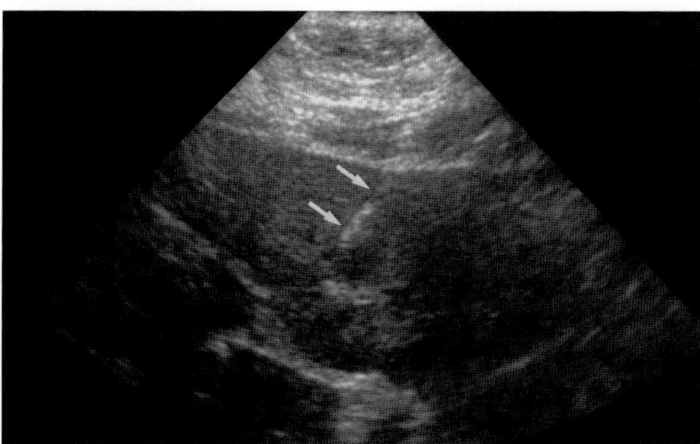

Figure 20. US unable to locate the pancreatic mass. A lesion in the left lobe of the liver was biopsied on this transverse US of the liver with the biopsy needle (arrows) advancing into the lesion.

Precise positioning of the needle tip within the target lesion can be optimized by paying attention to detail during the procedure. The creation of a small skin nick at the puncture site with a scalpel blade decreases resistance and deviation of the needle path during passage through the skin and subcutaneous tissues. Stabilizing the needle at the puncture site in the skin with one hand while advancing it with the other hand facilitates needle placement, especially when a fine needle is used. If the needle is to be advanced without continuous visualization, as with CT localization, having an observer monitor the needle angulation is often helpful. In such a situation, the observer is positioned so as to clearly visualize the needle and its relationship to the patient's skin surface and to the table top.

The technique and principles of aspiration biopsies with Chiba-type needles and core biopsies with a cutting needle have been reviewed in the tutorial on biopsy overview **(see Tutorial 1)** and those same principles apply to pancreatic biopsies.[27–29]

Evaluation of the Specimen

The final step of percutaneous biopsy is processing the specimen. This must be done carefully to maximize the success of the procedure. The presence of a cytologist during the procedure ensures adequate treatment of the specimen. However, a cytologist is not always available, and familiarity with a variety of methods for handling the biopsy material is beneficial.

The aspirated material is expelled from the syringe onto the frosted glass slides and is spread out with the edge of a second glass slide, taking care to distribute the cellular material. The slides are then quickly fixed in 95% ethanol for Papanicolaou staining. This method of rapid fixation preserves nuclear detail.[30,31] Ethanol fixation can be continued for 24 hours to allow for transport of the material.[32] Alternatively, air-drying of the slides can be done, followed by Wright-Giemsa or May-Grunwald-Giemsa staining to preserve the tissue pattern and permit staining of the tissue stroma.

Residual material within the needle and syringe should be expelled with use of sterile nonbacteriostatic saline or a solution of 50% Ringer's and 50% ethanol. This material can then be processed as a cell block.

When cutting or large needles are used, core biopsy fragments of tissue are obtained for histologic examination. These tissue fragments should be fixed immediately in formalin.

Chemical analyses and bacteriologic studies are of value when fluid is aspirated. Fluid carcinoembryonic antigen (CA), viscosity, and cytology will reliably differentiate mucinous tumors from pseudocysts and serous cystadenomas.[33] Malignant cystic neoplasms may be distinguished from benign cystic lesions using CA 15-3, CA 72-4, and cytology.[34,35]

Complications

Significant complications of pancreatic biopsy include pancreatitis, peritonitis or sepsis, and needle track or cutaneous seeding.[36–38] Out of six reported deaths as a result of percutaneous biopsy of the pancreas, five resulted from pancreatitis and one from sepsis.[39,40] A recent series of 269 pancreatic biopsies performed under CT and US guidance reported no deaths and an overall major complication rate of approximately 1%, which included pancreatitis and pancreatic duct laceration.[4] Mesenteric hematomas have also been reported.[41,42] It has been suggested that the risk of pancreatitis increases with biopsy of lesions 3 cm or smaller.[40] However, this is anecdotal and there are no reported series to support this observation. In general, lesions in this size range are more likely to be resectable and biopsy is not usually considered.

Although many different types of complications have been reported with percutaneous biopsy of the pancreas, these complications occur infrequently. Serious complications associated with percutaneous biopsy procedures are rare. The mortality rate associated with the procedure, particularly with the use of fine needles, is also low. Careful attention to patient selection, preprocedural laboratory evaluation, and lesion localization and needle placement should minimize these complications.

Conclusion

Imaging-guided biopsy of the pancreas is a common procedure because of its high rate of diagnostic accuracy and its low rate of complications. Percutaneous biopsy is often performed to confirm the diagnosis of unresectable ductal adenocarcinoma. Accurate lesion localization with US or CT is the cornerstone of a successful procedure. Successful performance of these procedures requires close cooperation between the patient, radiologist, pathologist, and referring clinician.

References

1. Cameron JL. The current management of carcinoma of the head of the pancreas. Annu Rev Med 1995; 46:361–370.

2. DelMashio A, Vanzulli A, Sironi S, et al. Pancreatic cancer versus chronic pancreatitis: diagnosis with CA 19-9 assessment, US, CT, and CT-guided fine-needle biopsy. Radiology 1991; 178:95–99.

3. Gaber AO, Gaber LW, Shokouh-Amiri MH, Hathaway D. Percutaneous biopsy of pancreas transplants. Transplantation 1992; 54:548–550.

4. Burbank F, Kaye K, Belville J, Ekuan J, Blumenfeld M. Image-guided automated core biopsies of the breast, chest, abdomen, and pelvis. Radiology 1994; 191:165–171.

5. Brandt KR, Charboneau JW, Stephens DH, Welch TJ, Goellner JR. CT- and US-guided biopsy of the pancreas. Radiology 1993; 187:99–104.

6. Hall-Craggs MA, Lees WR. Fine-needle aspiration biopsy: pancreatic and biliary tumors. AJR 1986; 147:399–403.

7. Cope C, Marinelli DL, Weinstein JK. Transcatheter biopsy of lesions obstructing the bile ducts. Radiology 1988; 169:555–556.

8. Teplick SK, Haskin PH, Kline TS, Sammon JK, Laffey PA. Percutaneous pancreaticobiliary biopsies in 173 patients using primarily ultrasound fluoroscopic guidance. Cardiovasc Intervent Radiol 1988; 11:26–28.

9. Hancke S, Holm HH, Koch F. Ultrasonically guided percutaneous fine-needle biopsy of the pancreas. Surg Gynecol Obstet 1975; 140:361–364.

10. Saini S, Ferrucci JT Jr. Percutaneous biopsy of pancreatic and peripancreatic masses. Semin Intervent Radiol 1985; 2:254–263.

11. Taavitsainen M, Koivuniemi A, Bondestam S, Kivisaari L, Tierala E. Ultrasonically guided fine-needle aspiration biopsy in focal pancreatic lesions. Acta Radiol 1987; 28:541–543.

12. Freeny PC, Kidd R, Ball TJ. ERCP-guided percutaneous fine-needle pancreatic biopsy. West J Med 1980; 132:283–287.

13. Freeny PC, Lawson TL. Adenocarcinoma of the pancreas. In: Freeny PC, Lawson TL, eds. Radiology of the pancreas. New York: Springer-Verlag, 1982; 397–496.

14. Bisceglia M, Matalon TA, Silver B. The pump maneuver: an atraumatic adjunct to enhance US needle tip localization. Radiology 1990; 176:867–868.

15. Matalon TA, Silver B. US guidance of interventional procedures. Radiology 1990; 174:43–47.

16. McGahan JP. Laboratory assessment of ultrasonic needle and catheter visualization. J Ultrasound Med 1986; 5:373–377.

17. Longo JM, Bilbao JI, Barettino MD, et al. Percutaneous vascular and nonvascular puncture under US guidance: role of color Doppler imaging. Radiographics 1994; 14:959–972.

18. Charboneau JW, Reading CC, Welch TJ. CT and sonographically guided needle biopsy: current techniques and new innovations. AJR 1990; 154:1–10.

19. Gazelle GS, Haaga JR. Guided percutaneous biopsy of intraabdominal lesions. AJR 1989; 153:929–935.

20. Welch TJ, Sheedy PF II, Johnson CD, Johnson CM, Stephens DH. CT-guided biopsy: prospective analysis of 1,000 procedures. Radiology 1989; 171:493–496.

21. Haaga JR, Alfidi RJ. Precise biopsy localization by computed tomography. Radiology 1976; 118:603–607.

22. Wittenberg J, Mueller PR, Ferrucci JT Jr. Percutaneous core biopsy of abdominal tumors using 22-gauge needles: further observations. AJR 1982; 139:75–80.

23. Yueh N, Halvorsen RA, Letourneau JG, Crass JR. Gantry tilt technique for CT-guided biopsy and drainage. J Comput Assist Tomogr 1989; 13(1):182–184.

24. Silverman SG, Mueller PR, Pfister RC. Hemostatic evaluation before abdominal interventions: an overview and proposal. AJR 1990; 154:233–238.

25. Greene RF. Transthoracic needle aspiration. In: Athanasoulis CA, Pfister RC, Greene RE, Roberson GH, eds. Interventional radiology. Philadelphia: W.B. Saunders Company, 1982; 587–634.

26. vanSonnenberg E, Lin AS, Casola G, Nakamoto SK, Wing VW, Cubberly DA. Removable hub needle system for coaxial biopsy of small and difficult lesions. Radiology 1984; 152:226.

27. Fagelman D, Chess Q. Non-aspiration fine-needle cytology of the liver: a new technique for obtaining diagnostic samples. AJR 1990; 155:1217–1219.

28. Hopper KD, Abendroth CS, Sturtz KW, Matthews YL, Shirk SJ. Fine-needle aspiration biopsy for cytopathologic analysis: utility of syringe handles, automated guns, and the nonsuction method. Radiology 1992; 185:819–824.

29. Kinney TB, Lee MJ, Filomena CA, et al. Fine-needle biopsy: prospective comparison of aspiration versus nonaspiration techniques in the abdomen. Radiology 1993; 186:549–552.

30. Jacobsen GK. Aspiration biopsy cytology. In: Holm HH, Kristensen JK, eds. Ultrasonically guided puncture technique. Philadelphia: W.B. Saunders Company, 1980.

31. Soost HJ. Requirements in gaining and treating biopsy material. In: Anacker H, Gullotta U, Rupp N, eds. Percutaneous biopsy and therapeutic vascular occlusion. New York: Thieme-Stratton, 1980.

32. Kline TS. Handbook of fine-needle aspiration biopsy cytology. St. Louis: C.V. Mosby Company, 1981; 1–7.

33. Lewandrowski KB, Southern JF, Pins MR, Compton CC, Warshaw AL. Cyst fluid analysis in the differential diagnosis of pancreatic cysts: a comparison of pseudocysts, serous cystadenomas, mucinous cystic neoplasms, and mucinous cystadenocarcinoma. Ann Surg 1993; 217:41–47.

34. Rubin D, Warshaw AL, Southern JF, Pins M, Compton CC, Lewandrowski KB. Expression of CA 15.3 protein in the cyst contents distinguishes benign from malignant pancreatic mucinous cystic neoplasms. Surgery 1994; 115:52–55.

35. Alles AJ, Warshaw AL, Southern JF, Compton CC, Lewandrowski KB. Expression of CA 72-4 (TAG-72) in the fluid contents of pancreatic cysts: a new marker to distinguish malignant pancreatic cystic tumors from benign neoplasms and pseudocysts. Ann Surg 1994; 219:131–134.

36. Ferrucci JT Jr, Wittenberg J, Mueller PR, et al. Diagnosis of abdominal malignancy by radiologic fine-needle aspiration biopsy. AJR 1980; 134:323–330.

37. Rashleigh-Belcher HJ, Russell RC, Lees WR. Cutaneous seeding of pancreatic carcinoma by fine-needle aspiration biopsy. Br J Radiol 1986; 59:182–183.

38. Smith FP, MacDonald JS, Schein PS, Ornitz RD. Cutaneous seeding of pancreatic cancer by skinny needle aspiration biopsy. Arch Intern Med 140:855.

39. Smith EH. Complications of percutaneous abdominal fine-needle biopsy. Radiology 1991; 178:253–258.

40. Levin DP, Bret PM. Percutaneous fine-needle aspiration biopsy of the pancreas resulting in death. Gastrointest Radiol 1991; 16:67–69.

41. Yankaskas BC, Staab EV, Craven MB, Blatt PM, Sokhandan M, Carney C. Delayed complications from fine-needle biopsies of solid masses of the abdomen. Invest Radiol 1986; 21:325–328.

42. McLoughlin MJ, Ho CS, Langer B, McHattie J, Tao LC. Fine-needle aspiration biopsies of malignant lesions in and around the pancreas. Cancer 1978; 41:2413–2419.

Endnotes

Figures 15 and 17 courtesy of Kenyon Kopecky, M.D., Indiana University School of Medicine.

Figures 4–9, 12–14, 16, and 18–20 courtesy of Jeet Sandhu, M.D., University of North Carolina School of Medicine.

TUTORIAL 5
ADRENAL BIOPSY

C. Humberto Carrasco, M.D., William R. Richili, M.D., David D. Lawrence, M.D., and Kimberly A. Waugh, M.D.

Introduction

The subjects addressed in this tutorial include:

1. Incidence and characterization of adrenal masses
2. Indications for adrenal needle biopsy
3. Technique of adrenal biopsy
4. Results of adrenal biopsy
5. Complications of adrenal biopsy.

The routine use of ultrasound (US), magnetic resonance (MR) imaging, and computed tomography (CT) scanning to evaluate various disorders has led to increased detection of adrenal masses. Adrenal lesions were demonstrated in 3.38% of a large series of CT studies performed for various indications. These lesions were incidental discoveries unrelated to the indications for which the studies were performed in 0.42% of the cases.[1] However, adrenal masses are discovered most often in oncology patients. Adrenal masses as small as 0.5 cm are routinely demonstrated, and improvement in image resolution is likely to increase the rate of their detection.

In a selected review of the literature, CT evidence of adrenal metastases was reported in 3.0% to 6.4% of patients with non-small cell carcinoma of the lung.[2] CT scanning has also demonstrated ipsilateral adrenal metastases in 2% to 6% of patients with renal carcinoma.[3,4] However, it should be stressed that most adrenal lesions are benign, even in patients with an underlying malignancy.

CT and MR imaging are used to discriminate benign from malignant adrenal masses. Lesion size and stability,[1,5,6,7] CT attenuation values,[8,9,10] and various MR techniques, pulse sequences, magnet field strengths, and methods of quantitative and qualitative assessment[11–16] are criteria that have been used to categorize adrenal masses.

Size has been used to assess adrenal neoplasms because most lesions larger than 3 cm are malignant. However, size at discovery is not an accurate indicator of biologic behavior and cannot be used solely to exclude metastatic disease.[17] In one series of oncology patients, metastatic disease was found in 13% of the smaller (<3 cm) masses.[18] Lesion stability is another unreliable indicator of whether or not a tumor is benign; primary malignancies and metastatic lesions may remain stable for long periods of time.[10] CT and MR characterization of adrenal neoplasms is based on the premise that benign adrenal cortical cells, in contrast to malignant ones, have a relatively high lipid content.[19] However, fat may be present within a carcinoma.[20]

Many retrospective studies using different criteria to assess the CT attenuation values of adrenal lesions have been inconclusive in characterizing adrenal lesions.[8,9,10,21] A prospective study evaluating the relative signal strengths of MR T1- and T2-weighted images in lung cancer patients with adrenal masses concluded that the technique was not accurate enough to replace biopsy.[22] However, chemical shift MR imaging may be more reliable in distinguishing benign from malignant adrenal lesions.[11,14,15,16]

Indications For Adrenal Needle Biopsy

Obtaining accurate tissue diagnosis is vital for accurate evaluation of adrenal masses. Needle biopsy, a routine procedure since the 1970s, is the most practical technique for tissue acquisition.

The principal indication for adrenal needle biopsy is to determine the nature of an adrenal mass in patients with potentially curable extra-adrenal malignancy. Biopsy can also document the presence of nonsurgical disease before toxic antineoplastic therapy is initiated. Bronchogenic carcinoma, renal carcinoma, and melanoma are the most common primary tumors metastasizing to the adrenal gland. Occasionally, needle biopsy is needed for tissue diagnosis of a suspected unresectable adrenal carcinoma. Sometimes the adrenal gland is the only gross site of involvement by lymphoma. Rarely, it is the site of infectious processes such as histoplasmosis or tuberculosis.

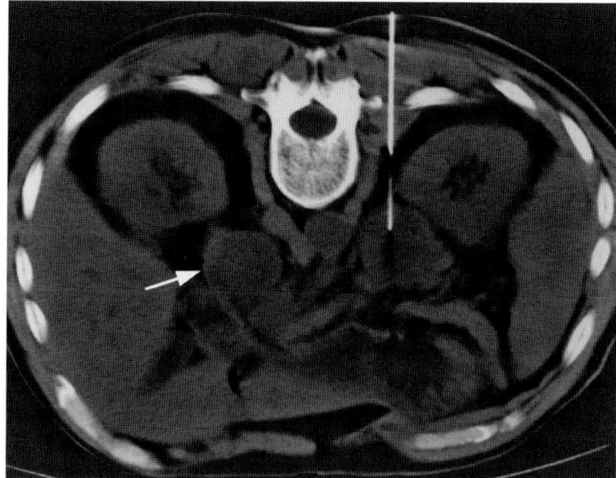

Figure 1. Carcinoma metastatic to the adrenal gland. The large lesion facilitates a direct translumbar approach. A coaxial needle technique is used. Note the contralateral adrenal mass (arrow).

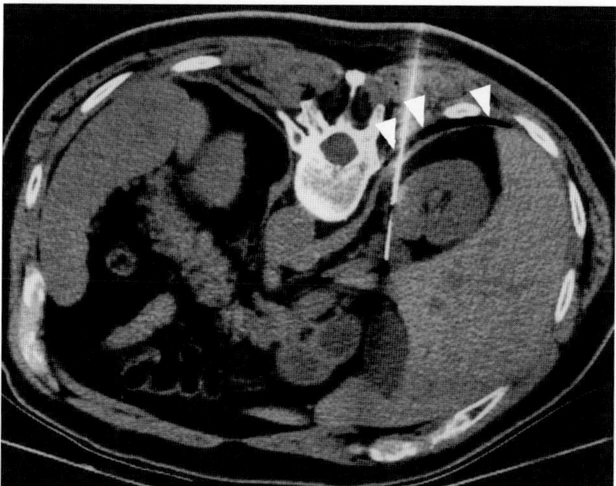

Figure 2. Adrenal cortical nodule. The needle path is through the posterior costophrenic angle of the right lung (arrowheads), diaphragm, and kidney.

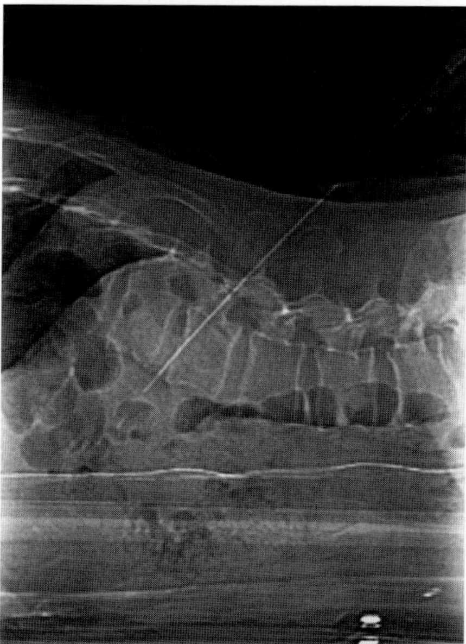

Figure 3. Digital scout film shows an angled needle approach. The needle entry site is at the level of the nadir of the lumbar curvature. The needle tip is in the adrenal lesion. A coaxial needle technique is used.

Patients with functioning primary adrenal neoplasms usually undergo biochemical characterization of the tumor and resection; however, tissue diagnosis may still be required in cases of unresectable disease. In patients with incidentally discovered adrenal lesions, tissue diagnosis is indicated for the larger (>3 cm) masses given the higher incidence of malignancy among these lesions. Otherwise, various algorithms involving endocrinologic, radiologic, and nuclear scintigraphic modalities have been proposed for work-up of incidental adrenal lesions.[23,24,25]

Preprocedural Considerations

The procedure is performed in an outpatient setting. Routine coagulation studies are not required for needle biopsy. Anticoagulation should be reversed and any known coagulopathies should be corrected.

Patients are advised to keep to a liquid diet for 6 hours before the procedure. After informed consent is obtained, an intravenous line is started for the administration of sedatives, analgesics, and any other required medications. Patients must be sedated before the procedure is begun, and routine monitoring, including blood pressure measurements, pulse oximetry, and cardiac monitoring, is maintained throughout the procedure. Previous imaging studies should be reviewed. Pheochromocytoma is a rare entity, but if it is suspected, a thorough biochemical work-up should be done to avoid performing a needle biopsy that could result in a severe hypertensive crisis.

Technique

US guidance is used mainly for needle biopsy of larger lesions, but CT remains the preferred guidance modality, particularly for small lesions.[26,27]

The retroperitoneal location of the adrenal glands, where they are surrounded by the liver, spleen, pancreas, kidneys, lungs, inferior vena cava, and abdominal aorta makes access by needle biopsy relatively difficult. The simplest, most direct, translumbar approach is possible when the adrenal mass is relatively large **(Fig. 1)**. However, this approach is often hindered by the interposition of the lungs, the transgression of which may result in a pneumothorax **(Fig. 2)**.

The needle biopsy technique favored at our institution is the angled translumbar approach under CT guidance without angulation of the CT gantry.[28] The patient lies on the CT scanner in the prone position with the affected side toward the operator **(Fig. 3)**. The contralateral decubitus position is used if the patient is unable to lie prone.

A 20- to 30-cm segment of radiopaque angiographic catheter overlying the paraspinal muscles just lateral to the transverse processes is taped to the patient's back so that it extends from the lower rib cage to the upper lumbar area on the side of the lesion. Scans of the upper abdomen (10-mm-thick every 10 mm) which include the adrenal mass and the posterior insertions of the diaphragm are obtained. Breathing instructions are not required because respiratory motion of retroperitoneal structures is negligible. A point directly overlying the adrenal lesion is marked on the skin to serve as the needle entry site, if the lung base is not interposed. Transgression of the diaphragm should be avoided because it is difficult to achieve adequate local anesthesia of this muscle and transgression of the pleural space may induce a pneumothorax.

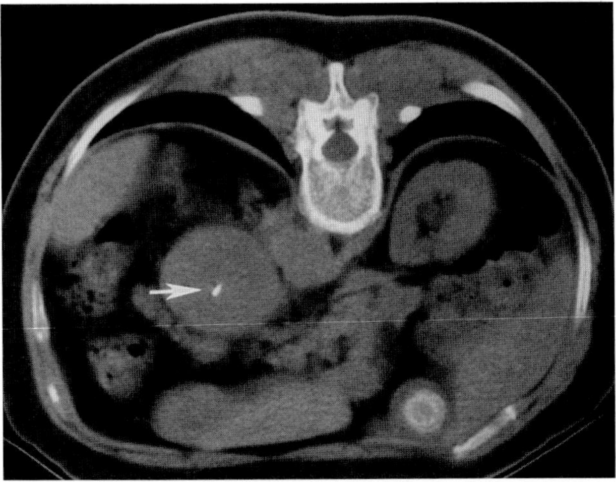

Figure 4. Metastatic endometrial carcinoma. The CT scan was obtained near the needle tip within the lesion (arrow). Steep needle angulation avoids the lung.

When there is interposition of the lung bases, a second skin point is marked caudal to the 12th rib (and the insertion of the diaphragm) in a vertical plane between the psoas muscle and the kidney. This point will be the needle entry site for the angled approach. Generally, the needle entry site for an angled approach should be as caudal as possible and preferably just cephalad to the nadir of the lumbar curvature **(Figs. 3, 4)**. The planned needle path is through the retroperitoneal fat between the psoas muscle and the kidney. When this approach is not feasible, a path through the psoas muscle is chosen. Obviously, a transrenal path is best avoided.

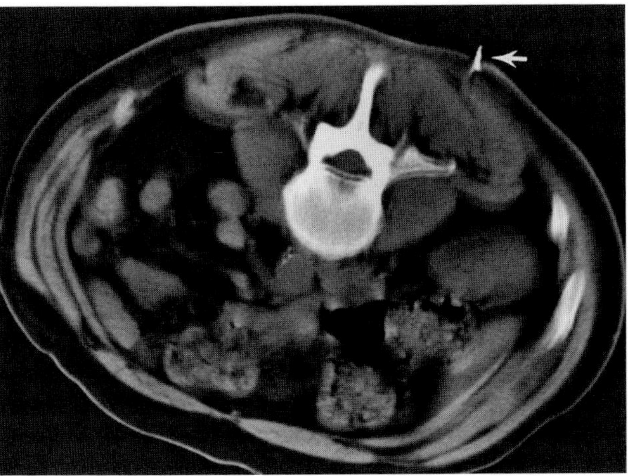

Figure 5. Metastatic bronchogenic carcinoma. An angled needle approach is being used. Caudal needle entry site (arrow) near the lower pole of the right kidney. CT scans in the following figures follow the needle path from entry to target.

The needle path angle and length from the skin to the target can be obtained by applying the Pythagorean theorem,[28] but precise calculations are hampered by the lumbar curvature. Path angle and length are more easily estimated by measuring the lesion's depth from a point directly over the lesion then measuring the distance from this point to the needle entry site.

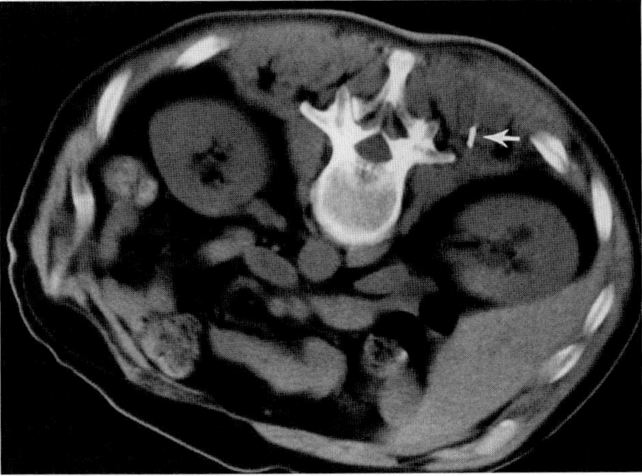

Figure 6. Same patient as in Figure 5. The needle (arrow) went through the lumbar musculature.

To perform the needle biopsy, a coaxial needle technique is used, with an 18-gauge thin-walled guide needle and a 22-gauge beveled biopsy needle. Depending on the length of the needle path, the needle lengths are 10 or 15 cm for the guide needle and 20 or 25 cm for the biopsy needle, which should be at least 10 cm longer than the guide needle. An automated 20-gauge core biopsy system 20 or 25 cm in length is available for when tissue cores are required.

Following antiseptic cleansing of the skin entry site, local anesthesia with 1% Xylocaine without epinephrine is administered. The 18-gauge needle is inserted percutaneously to a depth of 1 or 2 cm at the estimated angle and pointing in the direction of the skin mark overlying the adrenal lesion.

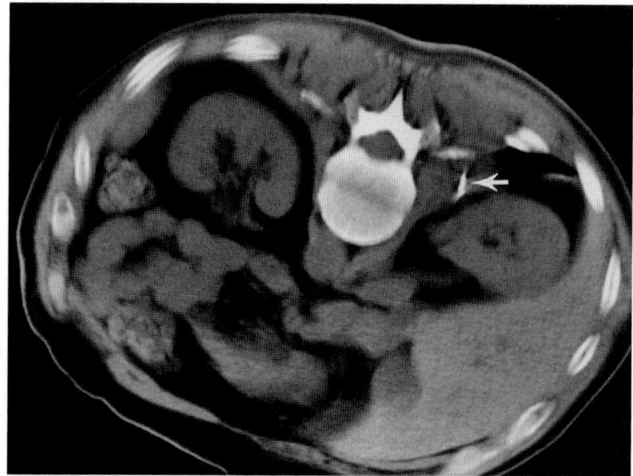

Figure 7. Same patient as in Figure 5. The needle (arrow) is in a plane anterior to the diaphragmatic insertion.

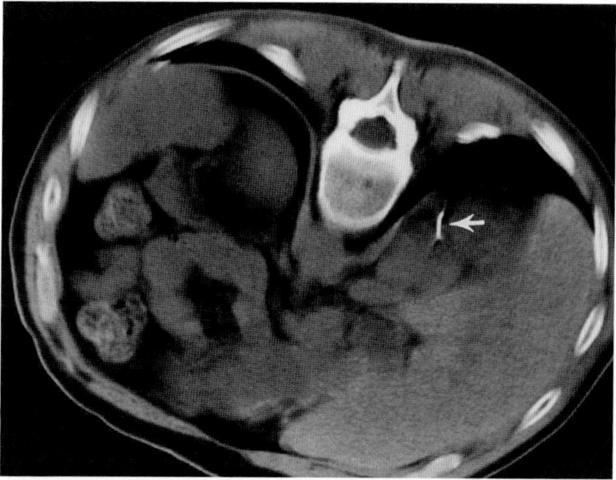

Figure 8. Same patient as in Figure 5. The needle (arrow) is medial to the upper pole of the right kidney and enters the adrenal mass.

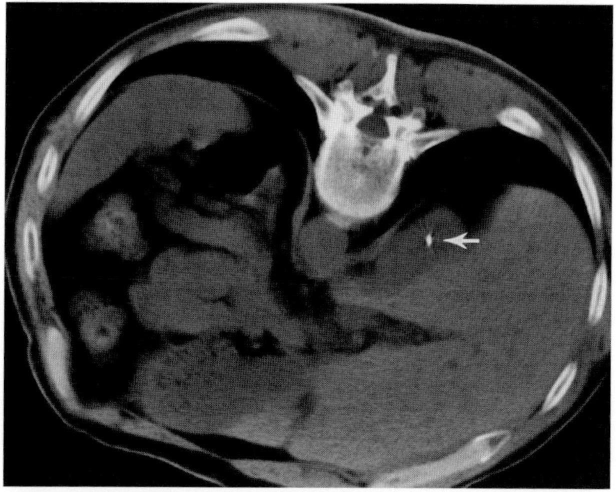

Figure 9. Same patient as in Figure 5. A scan near the needle tip (arrow) shows it to be located within the adrenal mass. The base of the right lung has not been transgressed.

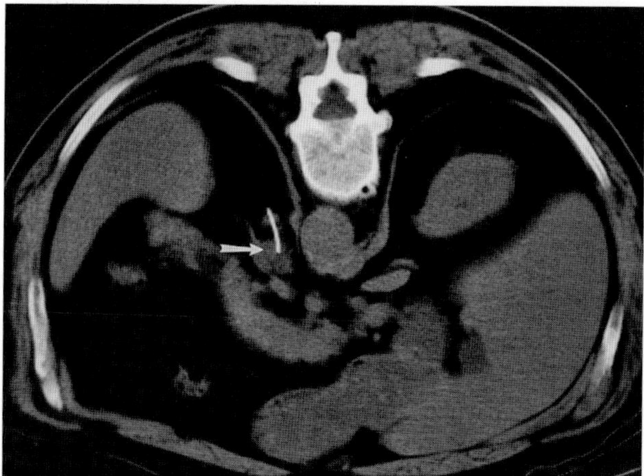

Figure 10. Adrenal cortical nodule. A slight misalignment of the guide needle was corrected by bending the tip of the biopsy needle (arrow).

While additional local anesthetic is injected, the 22-gauge needle is advanced with a coaxial technique approximately 5 cm toward the target. Bending the tip of the 22-gauge needle beforehand with a hemostat permits directional control of the needle.[29] Sequential CT scans are obtained to assess and correct the needle path; however, ill effects usually do not occur if the needle adopts an unfavorable path. Once the needle tip is within or at the edge of the target **(Figs. 5–9)**, the 18-gauge guiding needle is advanced over the 22-gauge needle until its tip is just caudal to the lesion. A needle path that is slightly off target can be corrected by the curve of the needle tip **(Fig. 10)**.

Verifying the angled 22-gauge needle tip position within small lesions may require thin (3 or 5 mm) scans to exclude deceptive needle placement caused by volume averaging.

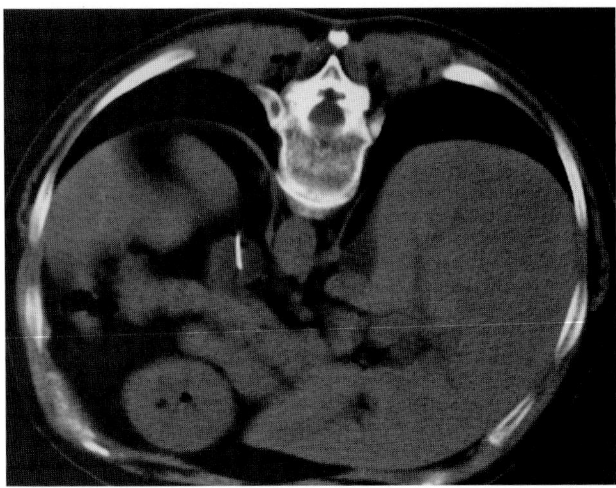

Figure 11. Adrenal cortical nodule. The tip of the (bent) biopsy needle is within the adrenal mass.

Once the needle tip is within the target **(Fig. 11)** or just in front of it **(Fig. 12)**, it is connected to a 10- or 20-mL syringe. Lesional tissue is aspirated as the needle is moved gently through short in-and-out excursions while maintaining its tip within the lesion. The biopsy needle is then withdrawn and the guide needle left in place. The aspirated material is processed promptly to prevent clotting and air drying artifacts. Additional specimens are easily obtained by reinserting the biopsy needle through the guide needle and repeating the aspiration. It may or may not be necessary to verify the needle tip position again, depending on the size of the mass and the proximity of the guide needle tip to the lesion.

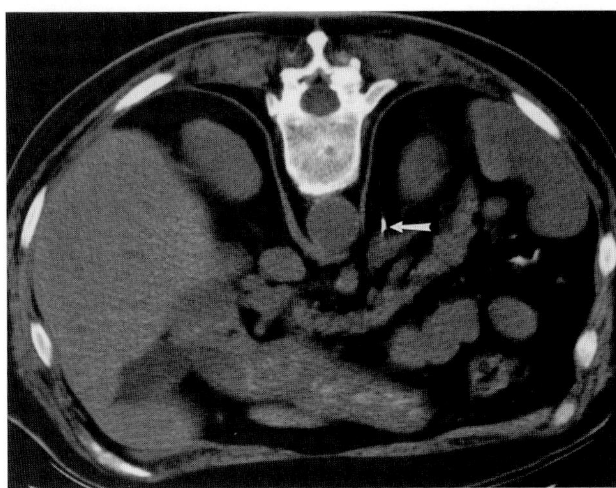

Figure 12. Adrenal cortical nodule. The tip of the biopsy needle is just posterior and caudal to the adrenal lesion (arrow). A biopsy was performed without repeating the scan after advancing the needle.

Tissue for histologic analysis and electron microscopy can be obtained with the 20-gauge, automated, slotted needle, which is coaxially inserted through the guide needle **(Fig. 13)**. The tip of the slotted needle's inner stylet may be bent slightly (keeping the slot on the convex side) to modify its final location and improve tissue acquisition. Both needles are withdrawn once sufficient tissue for diagnosis has been obtained.

Results

Reported accuracy rates for needle biopsy of adrenal lesions are generally around 90%,[30,31] a figure that is influenced by selection bias and cytologic diagnostic criteria. Needle aspirates of adrenal masses are best classified as metastatic lesions, primary adrenal lesions, and nondiagnostic aspirates.[3] Metastatic disease can be diagnosed with a very high level of confidence. The specificity of adrenal needle biopsy for metastatic disease is near 100% because metastatic processes have distinct cytologic features.[30,31] Nondiagnostic aspirates are devoid of recognizable diagnostic material. In such cases, the biopsy should be repeated, if possible.

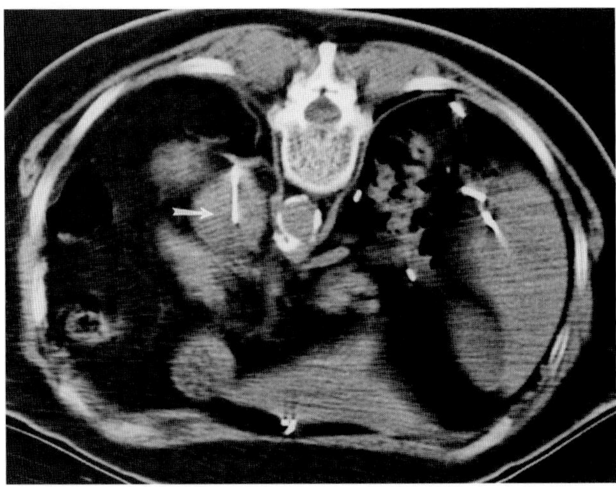

Figure 13. Metastatic renal carcinoma. Immediate cytological analysis of the aspirate was nondiagnostic. A diagnostic tissue core for histology was obtained with a 20-gauge automated slotted needle (arrow).

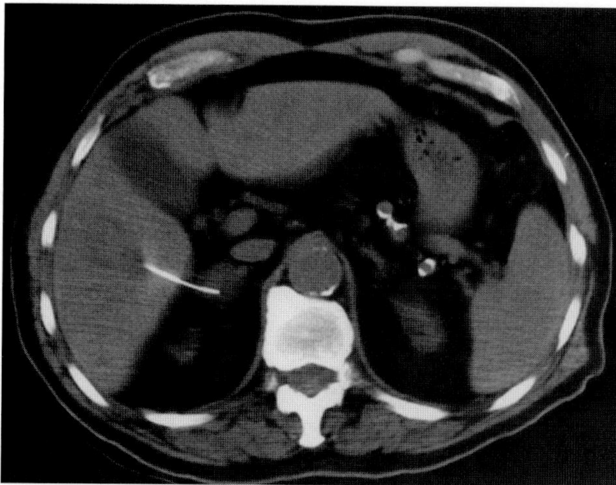

Figure 14. Adrenal cyst biopsy from a lateral transhepatic approach. Misalignment of the guide needle was corrected by bending the tip of the 22-gauge biopsy needle.

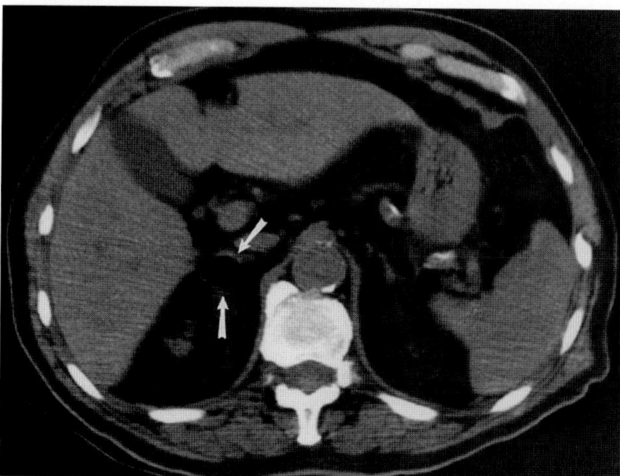

Figure 15. Following aspiration of serous cyst fluid, a small amount of air was injected to document the diagnosis (arrows).

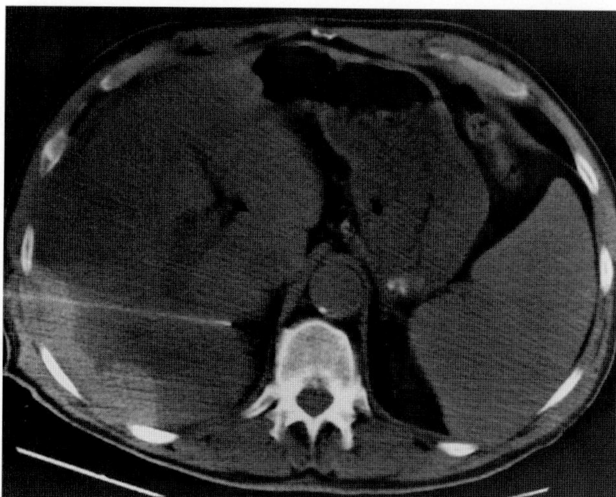

Figure 16. Adrenal cortical nodule. Lateral transhepatic approach with a single 22-gauge needle. The adrenal biopsy was complicated by a hepatic subcapsular hematoma.

Of 116 CT-guided needle biopsies of adrenal lesions performed during the last three and a half years, six (5%) were considered nondiagnostic, three included aspiration of residual masses in treated lymphoma patients, necrotic tissue from what was likely an adrenal infarction, and necrotic tissue with only a few atypical cells (probably necrotic metastasis). There were 46 (40%) aspirates that yielded benign adrenal cortical cells; however, metastatic disease was diagnosed on subsequent needle biopsy in one of these patients. Metastatic disease from various primary neoplasms and lymphoma was diagnosed in 57 (49%) of the biopsies. In addition, there was one myelolipoma, two adrenal carcinomas, one benign spindle cell lesion, one pheochromocytoma, and two cysts. Needle biopsy of the patient with unsuspected pheochromocytoma resulted in vascular instability which was managed successfully. Diagnostic CT air cystography **(Figs. 14, 15)** was performed in the cysts following aspiration of serous fluid.

The presence of benign adrenal cortical tissue in a needle biopsy sample, although highly predictive of benignity, does not completely exclude the presence of metastatic disease.[32] Aspirates of benign cortical cells may occasionally be obtained in cases of metastatic lesions and should be interpreted with caution. In addition, differentiation of benign from malignant adrenal cortical neoplasms may be difficult due to the lack of clearly distinguishing cytologic and histologic features.[33,34,35]

Complications

A total complication rate of 8.4% with a 3.6% rate of major complications was reported for needle biopsy of adrenal lesions. This complication rate was comparable to an overall complication rate of 5.3% noted from a review of the literature.[36] Most of the complications are secondary to needle transgression of adjacent organs. These complications include hepatic **(Fig. 16)** and renal hemorrhage, pneumothorax, and pancreatitis.[31,36,37] Isolated instances of needle track seeding of tumor and secondary abscess have been reported.[36,38,39]

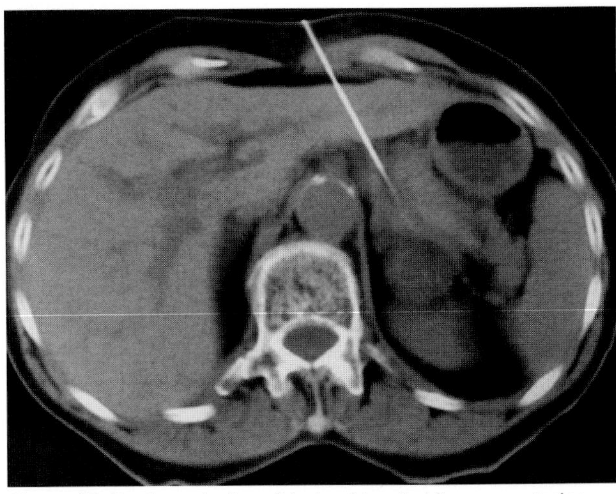

Figure 17. Benign spindle cell lesion biopsied from an anterior transhepatic and transpancreatic coaxial approach.

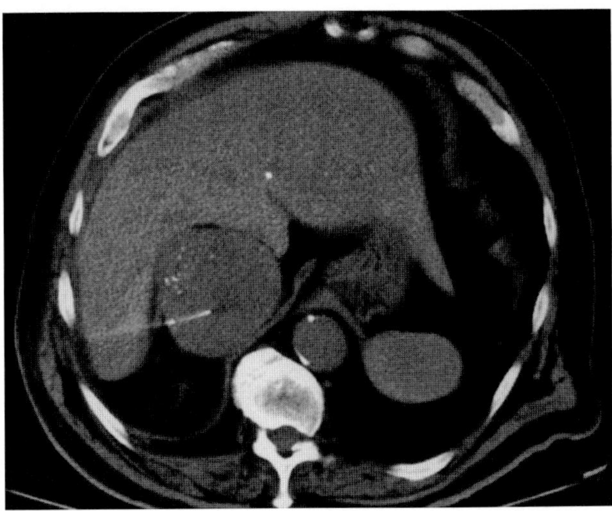

Figure 18. Adrenal cortical neoplasm. The large size of the mass simplifies needle biopsy through a lateral transhepatic approach.

Conclusion

Because of the risk of pneumothorax from the direct posterior approach, other approaches and techniques have been evaluated to ensure safe adrenal needle biopsies. Unfortunately, some of these techniques carry a high risk of more severe complications such as pancreatitis, especially when the anterior, transhepatic approach to the left adrenal gland is used **(Fig. 17)**.[37]

The anterior and lateral transabdominal approaches usually result in a more complicated procedure compared with the posterior translumbar approach. Transgression of peritoneal surfaces and the diaphragm is more painful than needle passage through the lumbar and paraspinal musculature and posterior retroperitoneal fat. Pain causes sudden respiratory motion which contributes to needle deflection. This problem is most pronounced with the lateral transhepatic (and transdiaphragmatic) approach to small right-sided adrenal lesions, which often requires multiple passes for proper needle placement.[40] Transhepatic biopsy of large masses is relatively simple **(Fig. 18)**, but the risk of increased pain and hepatic hemorrhage remains.

The ipsilateral decubitus position displaces the lung bases cephalad and permits a direct translumbar approach without lung puncture.[41] However, patient positioning and approach may be cumbersome. Angulation of the CT gantry permits visualization of the needle path,[33,34] but if needle angles greater than the maximum CT gantry angulation are used, the CT gantry should be maintained in its vertical, neutral position. In certain cases, intentional widening of the paraspinal tissues can be performed by injecting saline through a small-gauge needle to optimize and increase the biopsy path as well as avoid traversing the lung.

The angled approach to the adrenal gland minimizes the risk of complications because it avoids transgression of adjacent organs. In addition, it is much less painful for the patient than the transperitoneal approach.

References

1. Herrera MF, Grant CS, van Heerden JA, Sheedy PF, Ilstrup DM. Incidentally discovered adrenal tumors: an institutional perspective. Surgery 1991; 110:1014–1021.

2. Hillers TK, Sauve MD, Guyatt GH. Analysis of published studies on the detection of extrathoracic metastases in patients presumed to have operable non-small cell lung cancer. Thorax 1994; 49:14–19.

3. Kletscher BA, Qian J, Bostwick DG, Blute ML, Zincke H. Prospective analysis of the incidence of ipsilateral adrenal metastasis in localized renal cell carcinoma. J Urol 1996; 155:1844–1846.

4. Gill IS, McClennan BL, Kerbl K, Carbone JM, Wick M, Clayman RV. Adrenal involvement from renal cell carcinoma: predictive value of computerized tomography. J Urol 1994; 152:1082–1085.

5. Hussain S, Belldegrun A, Seltzer SE, Richie JP, Gittes RF, Abrams HL. Differentiation of malignant from benign adrenal masses: predictive indices on computed tomography. AJR 1985; 144:61–65.

6. Bernardino ME. Management of the asymptomatic patient with a unilateral adrenal mass. Radiology 1988; 166:121–123.

7. Wood DE, Delbridge L, Reeve TS. Surgery for adrenal tumours: is surgery for the small incidental tumour appropriate? Aust N Z J Surg 1987; 57:739–742.

8. Lee MJ, Hahn PF, Papanicolaou N, et al. Benign and malignant adrenal masses: CT distinction with attenuation coefficients, size, and observer analysis. Radiology 1991; 179:415–418.

9. Korobkin M, Brodeur FJ, Yutzy GG, et al. Differentiation of adrenal adenomas from nonadenomas using CT attenuation values. AJR 1996; 166:531–536.

10. Singer AA, Obuchowski NA, Einstein DM, Paushter DM. Metastasis or adenoma? Computed tomographic evaluation of the adrenal mass. Cleve Clin J Med 1994; 61:200–205.

11. Korobkin M, Dunnick NR. Characterization of adrenal masses (Comment). AJR 1995; 164:643–644.

12. Mitchell DG, Crovello M, Matteucci T, Petersen RO, Miettinen MM. Benign adrenocortical masses: diagnosis with chemical shift MR imaging. Radiology 1992; 185:345–351.

13. Reinig JW, Stutley JE, Leonhardt CM, Spicer KM, Margolis M, Caldwell CB. Differentiation of adrenal masses with MR imaging: comparison of techniques. Radiology 1994; 192:41–46.

14. Bilbey JH, McLoughlin RF, Kurkjian PS, et al. MR imaging of adrenal masses: value of chemical-shift imaging for distinguishing adenomas from other tumors. AJR 1995; 164:637–642.

15. Mayo-Smith WW, Lee MJ, McNicholas MM, Hahn PF, Boland GW, Saini S. Characterization of adrenal masses (<5 cm) by use of chemical shift MR imaging: observer performance versus quantitative measures. AJR 1995; 165:91–95.

16. McNicholas MM, Lee MJ, Mayo-Smith WW, Hahn PF, Boland GW, Mueller PR. An imaging algorithm for the differential diagnosis of adrenal adenomas and metastases. AJR 1995; 165:1453–1459.

17. Hussain S, Belldegrun A, Seltzer SE, Richie JP, Abrams HL. CT diagnosis of adrenal abnormalities in patients with primary nonadrenal malignancies. Eur J Radiol 1986; 6:127–131.

18. Candel AG, Gattuso P, Reyes CV, Prinz RA, Castelli MJ. Fine needle aspiration biopsy of adrenal masses in patients with extraadrenal malignancy. Surgery 1993; 114:1132–1136.

19. Korobkin M, Giordano TJ, Brodeur FJ, et al. Adrenal adenomas: relationship between histologic lipid and CT and MR findings. Radiology 1996; 200:743–747.

20. Ferrozzi F, Bova D. CT and MR demonstration of fat within an adrenal cortical carcinoma. Abdom Imaging 1995; 20:272–274.

21. Korobkin M, Brodeur FJ, Francis IR, Quint LE, Dunnick NR, Goodsitt M. Delayed enhanced CT for differentiation of benign from malignant adrenal masses. Radiology 1996; 200:737–742.

22. Burt M, Heelan RT, Coit D, et al. Prospective evaluation of unilateral adrenal masses in patients with operable non-small cell lung cancer. Impact of magnetic resonance imaging. J Thorac Cardiovasc Surg 1994; 107:584–588.

23. Kloos RT, Gross MD, Francis IR, Korobkin M, Shapiro B. Incidentally discovered adrenal masses. Endocr Rev 1995; 16:460–484.

24. Staren ED, Prinz RA. Selection of patients with adrenal incidentalomas for operation. Surg Clin North Am 1995; 75:499–509.

25. Gajraj H, Young AE. Adrenal incidentaloma. Br J Surg 1993; 80:422–426.

26. Montali G, Solbiati L, Bossi MC, De Pra L, Di Donna A, Ravetto C. Sonographically guided fine needle aspiration of adrenal masses. AJR 1984; 143:1081–1084.

27. Kojima M, Saitoh M, Itoh H, Ukimura O, Ohe H, Watanabe H. Percutaneous biopsy for adrenal tumors using ultrasonically guided puncture. Tohoku J Exp Med 1994; 172:333–343.

28. vanSonnenberg E, Wittenberg J, Ferrucci JT Jr, Mueller PR, Simeone JF. Triangulation method for percutaneous needle guidance: the angled approach to upper abdominal masses. AJR 1981; 137:757–761.

29. Carrasco CH, Wallace S, Charnsangavej C. Aspiration biopsy: use of a curved needle. Radiology 1985; 155:254.

30. Saboorian MH, Katz RL, Charnsangavej C. Fine needle aspiration cytology of primary and metastatic lesions of the adrenal gland. Acta Cytol 1995; 39:843–851.

31. Welch TJ, Sheedy II PF, Stephens DH, Johnson CM, Swensen SJ. Percutaneous adrenal biopsy: review of a 10-year experience. Radiology 1994; 193:341–344.

32. Silverman SG, Mueller PR, Pinkney LP, Koenker RM, Seltzer SE. Predictive value of image-guided adrenal biopsy: analysis of results of 101 biopsies. Radiology 1993; 187:715–718.

33. Candel AG, Gattuso P, Reyes CV, Prinz RA, Castelli MJ. Fine-needle aspiration biopsy of adrenal masses in patients with extraadrenal malignancy. Surgery 1993; 114:1132–1137.

34. Wadih GE, Nance KV, Silverman JF. Fine-needle aspiration cytology of the adrenal gland: fifty biopsies in 48 patients. Arch Pathol Lab Med 1992; 116:841–847.

35. Medeiros LJ, Weiss LM. New developments in the pathologic diagnosis of adrenal cortical neoplasms: a review. Am J Clin Pathol 1992; 97:73–83.

36. Mody MK, Kazerooni EA, Korobkin M. Percutaneous CT-guided biopsy of adrenal masses: immediate and delayed complications. J Comput Assist Tomogr 1995; 19:434–439.

37. Kane NM, Korobkin M, Francis IR, Quint LE, Cascade PN. Percutaneous biopsy of left adrenal masses: prevalence of pancreatitis after anterior approach. AJR 1991; 157:777–780.

38. Voravud N, Shin DM, Dekmezian RH, Dimery I , Lee JS, Hong WK. Implantation metastasis of carcinoma after percutaneous fine-needle aspiration biopsy. Chest 1992; 102:313–315.

39. Masmiquel L, Hernandez-Pascual C, Simo R, Mesa J. Adrenal abscess as a complication of adrenal fine-needle biopsy. Am J Med 1993; 95:244–245.

40. Price RB, Bernardino ME, Berkman WA, Sones PJ Jr, Torres WE. Biopsy of the right adrenal gland by the transhepatic approach. Radiology 1983; 148:566.

41. Heiberg E, Wolverson MK. Ipsilateral decubitus position for percutaneous CT-guided adrenal biopsy. J Comput Assist Tomogr 1985; 9:217–218.

TUTORIAL 6
EVALUATION AND MANAGEMENT OF ABDOMINAL ABSCESSES

Rajiv Sawhney, M.D.

Introduction

The subjects addressed in this tutorial include:

1. Indications for percutaneous abscess drainage
2. Technique for performing percutaneous abscess drainage
3. Postprocedure catheter management
4. Potential complications of percutaneous abscess drainage
5. Outcome of percutaneous abscess drainage.

Percutaneous management is widely accepted as the first-line treatment in patients with abdominal abscesses. In the past, infected fluid collections were only treated surgically. Because of advances in imaging technology and percutaneous techniques over the past decade, these collections are now routinely drained by interventional radiologists, with open surgical drainage reserved only for the most complex cases. The percutaneous approach brings about complete resolution of the abscess in most cases; in other cases it allows for simpler, safer definitive surgical procedures once the acute process has been addressed. Abnormal fluid collections in the peritoneal cavity, liver, spleen, pancreas, kidneys, and other areas within the retroperitoneal space can be successfully approached percutaneously.

Patient Selection

Clinically, patients with abscesses may present with fever, elevated white blood cell count, pain, fullness, or abnormalities related to mass effect from the collection. Patients can be placed on antibiotics empirically, and a search for the cause of the patient's symptoms is usually undertaken with computed tomography (CT) or ultrasound (US) imaging. Most patients with abdominal abscesses should be considered for percutaneous management as long as the collection can be safely accessed percutaneously.[1] Simple, unilocular, superficial collections are ideal for percutaneous drainage. However, successful drainage can also be achieved with deeper collections and certain multilocular abscesses if a safe route exists. Interloop abscesses, phlegmonous collections, and collections with extensive loculations are generally difficult to treat successfully with percutaneous techniques.[2,3] In patients with fungal abscesses, infected hematomas, and large enteric fistulas, percutaneous drainage may temporize the clinical situation and improve the patient's surgical status. If the patient is overtly septic, the diagnosis must be made quickly and drainage performed emergently.

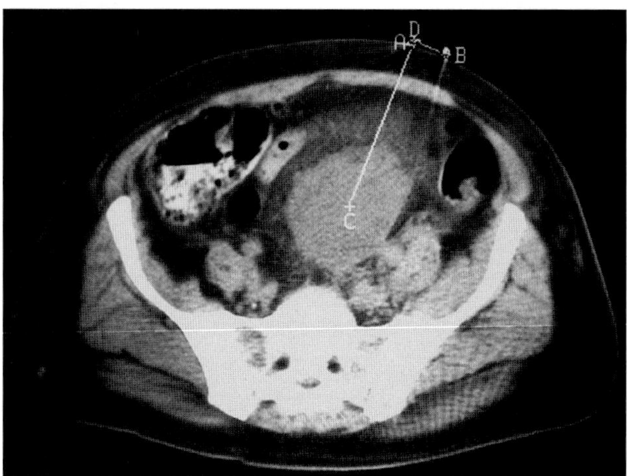

Figure 1. Percutaneous access route, angle of approach, and depth assessed using CT.

Patient Preparation

Ideally, prior to the procedure, the patient should be kept fasting or on a clear liquid diet and have intravenous access. Coagulation studies should be performed and significant coagulopathy corrected. Broad spectrum antibiotic coverage helps protect against acute sepsis during the procedure. Appropriate cardiopulmonary monitoring and conscious sedation are recommended.

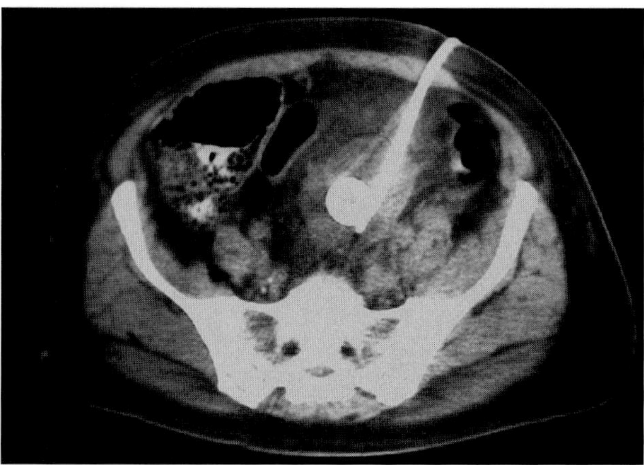
Figure 2. Same patient as in Figure 1. Drainage catheter placed using trocar technique.

Procedure Planning

Debate continues regarding the best imaging modality to guide abscess drainage. Almost all patients will have had a diagnostic CT scan. If the fluid collection is easily visualized by ultrasound and a safe route is shown on the diagnostic CT scan, an US-guided puncture with fluoroscopic monitoring should be used. CT guidance should be reserved for complicated cases. New magnetic resonance (MR) imaging units with interventional capabilities will allow for the addition of MR multiplanar imaging as another means to approach these collections.

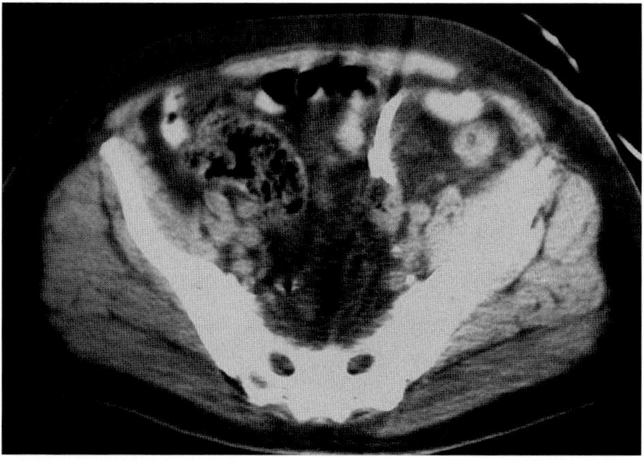
Figure 3. Same patient as in Figure 1. Immediate post-drainage image shows no residual cavity.

When planning the percutaneous access route, the shortest and most direct route into the collection is generally chosen. Obviously, the chosen route must not involve transgressing intervening vital structures such as bowel, uninvolved solid organs, pleura, or vessels. Appropriate depths and angles for catheter insertion are measured **(Figs. 1–3)**. US has the advantage of allowing real-time visualization of the needle as it is being placed.

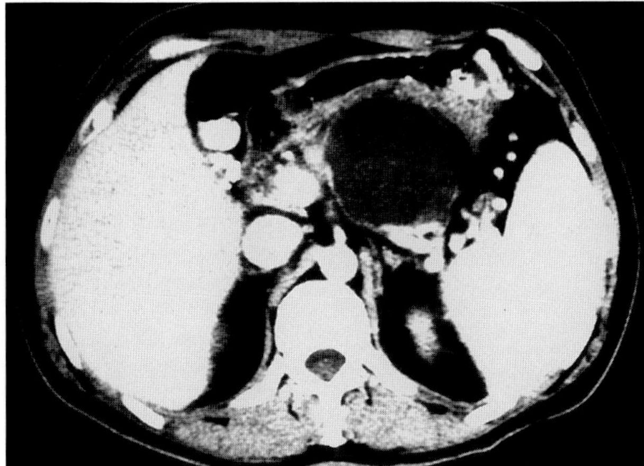

Figure 4. CT scan shows an infected pancreatic pseudocyst.

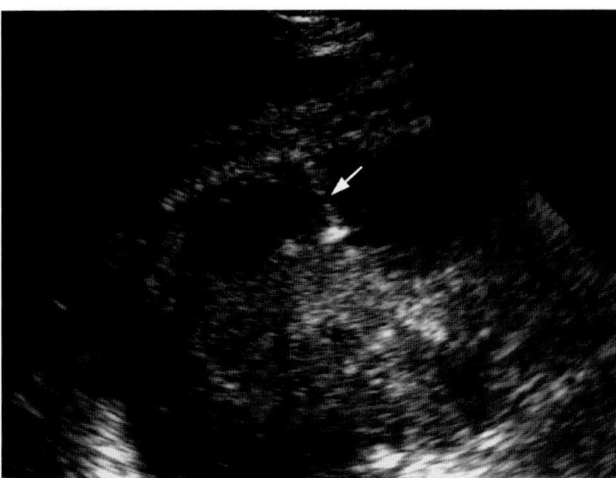

Figure 5. Percutaneous transgastric US-guided drainage was performed. Sonogram shows the needle (arrow) entering the collection, which is filled with internal echoes.

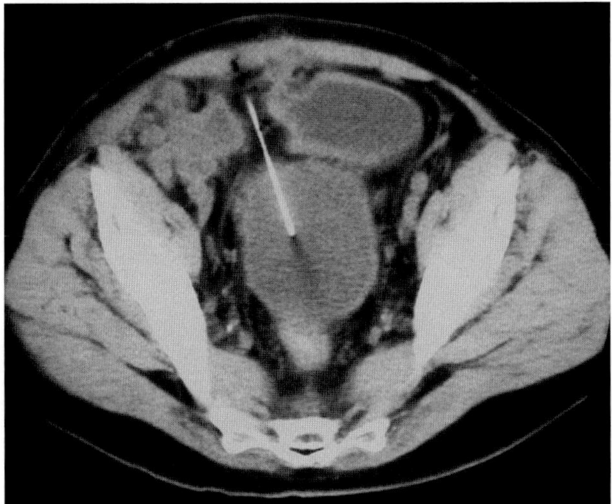

Figure 6. CT-guided abscess drainage with the needle advanced into the abscess, avoiding the bowel and bladder.

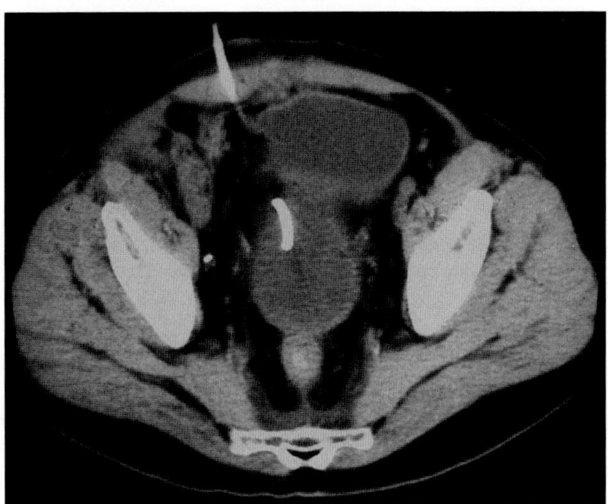

Figure 7. Same patient as in Figure 6. Placement of a drainage catheter.

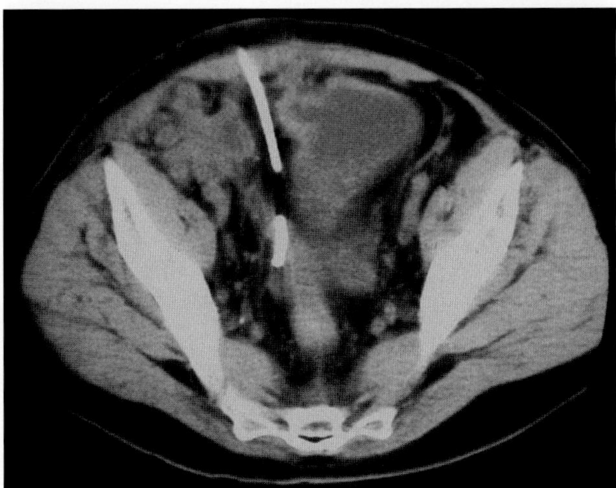

Figure 8. Same patient as in Figure 6. Immediate post-drainage image demonstrates evacuation of the abscess cavity.

Technical Details

Catheters are usually placed under CT or US guidance **(Figs. 4–8)**, or by catheterizing a preexisting cutaneous track. Because ultrasound guidance permits direct real-time access into the collection, it is especially useful for more superficial collections. CT guidance is preferred for deep collections because CT more precisely delineates adjacent bowel loops, organs, and vascular structures. Operator preference also influences the imaging guidance of choice. Once a wire has been advanced into the collection, further dilation and catheter placement can be performed under fluoroscopy. If a percutaneous fistula exists, contrast material can be injected and a wire and catheter can be advanced from the skin through the track and positioned within the cavity under fluoroscopy.

Following sterile preparation and draping of the skin entry site, local anesthesia is administered and one of the two following basic techniques is used to access the collection:

1. Seldinger technique. A needle is placed percutaneously into the collection, a wire is advanced through the needle, the track is dilated, and the drainage catheter is advanced over the wire into the collection **(Figs. 9–15)**.
2. Tandem trocar technique. A localizing needle is placed percutaneously into the collection, and the drainage catheter with a sharp inner stylet is then advanced adjacent and parallel to the needle into the collection.

In a technically difficult abscess drainage, access to the collection can be achieved with CT guidance and a wire coiled in the cavity. The patient is then transferred to a fluoroscopic room for completion of the procedure under fluoroscopic guidance. This method may be most appropriate for small collections or very heavy patients where the risk of wire dislodgement during track dilation or catheter placement is significant.

Once a wire has been placed into the collection, one must decide which catheter to place for drainage. Numerous types of drainage catheters are available: locking Cope loop or straight catheters, with or without parallel sump channels, and in sizes ranging from 6 to 30 F. In most cases, an 8–10-F Cope loop catheter will provide adequate drainage. Catheters can always be exchanged for the next larger size as needed. Sump catheters are advantageous when suction is used to aid drainage because their design minimizes the chance of the catheter side-holes becoming blocked by tissue. The larger catheters are generally used for drainage of thick, viscous fluid collections. Occasionally, multiple catheters are needed for especially thick fluid collections or multiloculated collections in which septa cannot be broken up with wire or catheter manipulation. Once the catheter is placed into the collection, an initial fluid sample is collected for appropriate laboratory studies. A sample should always be sent for culture and sensitivity (C&S) with immediate Gram stain. Obviously, C&S is vitally important to identify the bacterial pathogen appropriately and to ensure proper antibiotic selection. If an anaerobic infection is suspected, all of the air should be expressed from the syringe or sample container before it is sent to the lab. Once a sample has been obtained, complete evacuation of the fluid is then recommended. If any question exists as to whether the collection is infected and needs to be drained, diagnostic aspiration can be performed and the fluid sent for bacteriologic analysis first. If the fluid is infected, drainage can then be performed.

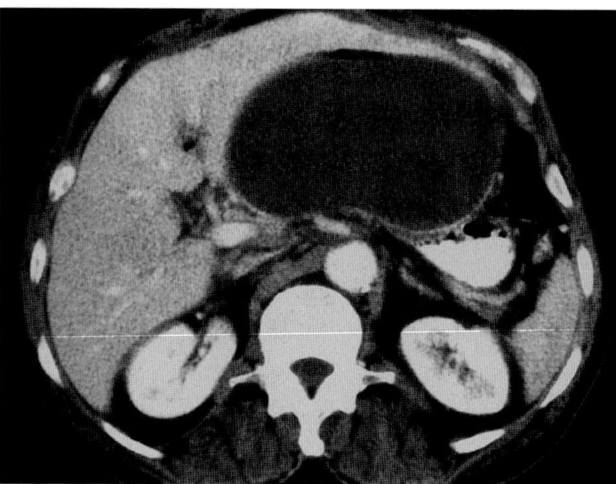

Figure 9. Large abscess thought to be secondary to a perforated duodenal ulcer.

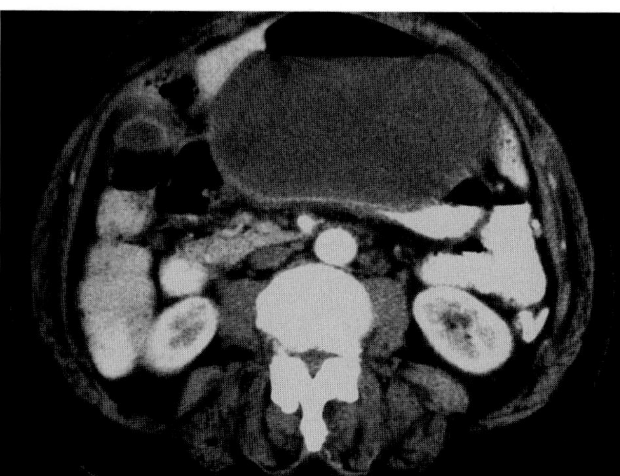

Figure 10. Same patient as in Figure 9. Inferior image shows the large collection.

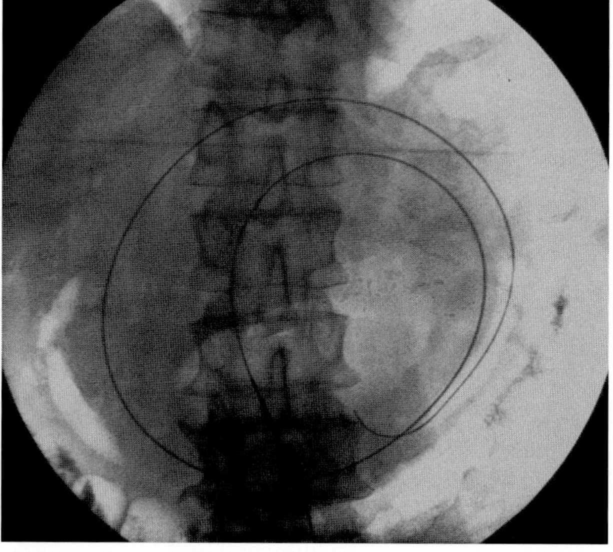

Figure 11. Same patient as in Figure 9. Fluoroscopic image following US-guided puncture and wire advancement into the collection.

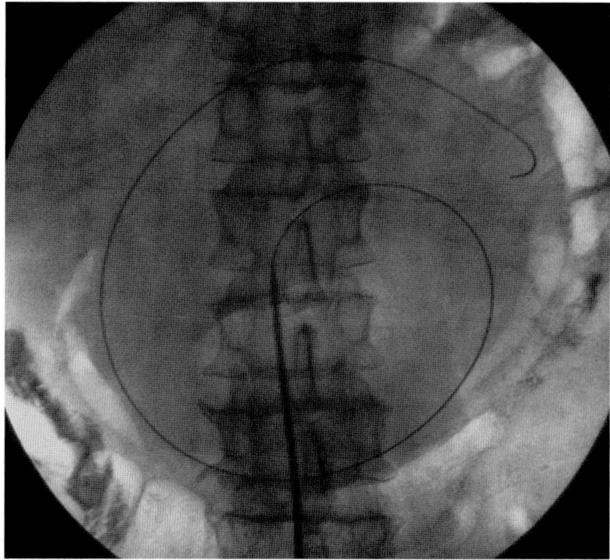

Figure 12. Same patient as in Figure 9. Dilation performed over the wire under fluoroscopy.

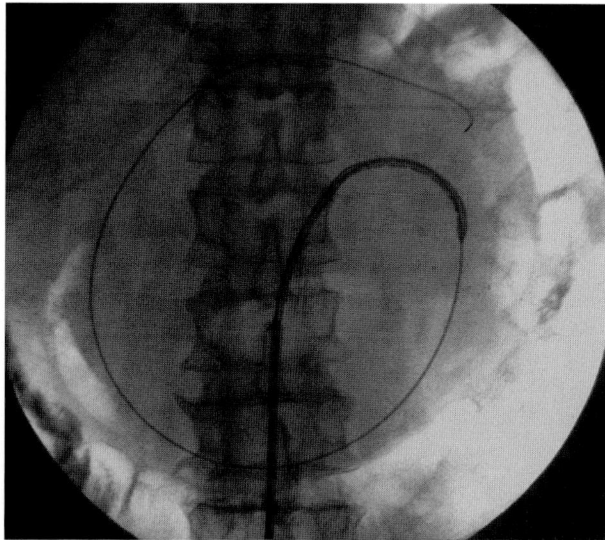

Figure 13. Same patient as in Figure 9. Advancement of the drainage catheter over the wire.

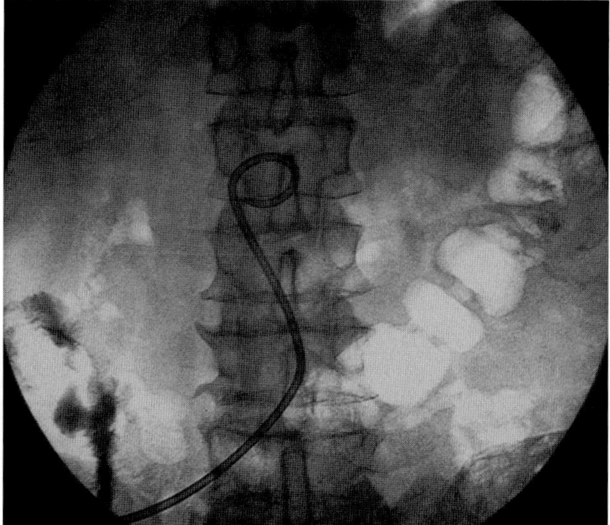

Figure 14. Same patient as in Figure 9. Drainage catheter in place; turbid fluid was aspirated.

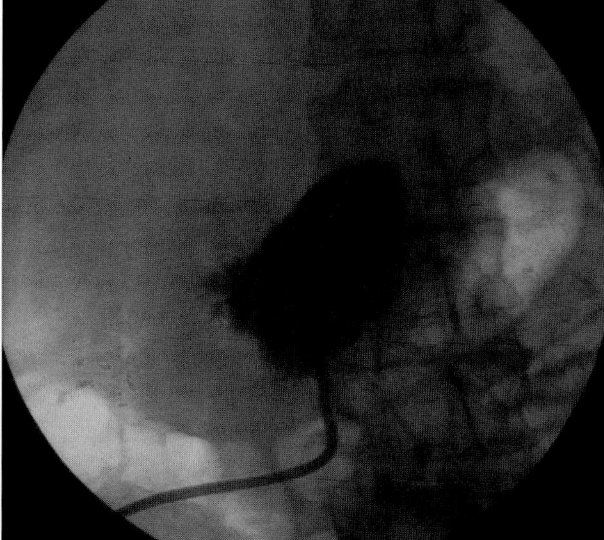

Figure 15. Same patient as in Figure 9. Catheter sinogram performed 3 days after initial catheter placement. The cavity is smaller and no fistulous communication is seen.

Some interventionalists advocate initial gentle irrigation of the cavity with saline to help remove most of the purulent material.[4] Others do not irrigate, thereby avoiding possible overdistention and septicemia.[5] A small volume of contrast material can be injected to aid in optimal positioning of the catheter within the dependent portion of the cavity.[6] The catheter is then secured to the skin with suture material and tape, or with any one of a variety of retention devices, and left in place for continued drainage.

Ongoing Catheter Management

The interventional radiology service is responsible for the important ongoing care and management of drainage catheters. Such care includes bedside saline flushes to maintain tube patency, monitoring of daily tube output, and tube checks and changes in the interventional suite. The catheters can be left to gravity drainage or J-P bulb suction. If there is communication with the bowel or biliary tree, suction should definitely be applied. If the patient's clinical status does not improve within 2 or 3 days, a repeat CT scan should be obtained to ensure that no undrained collections remain. When sepsis has improved, patients routinely return for a catheter sinogram 2 to 3 days after initial catheter placement to check tube position and to evaluate for possible fistulous communications between the cavity and bowel, biliary system, or pancreatic duct **(Fig. 15)**.

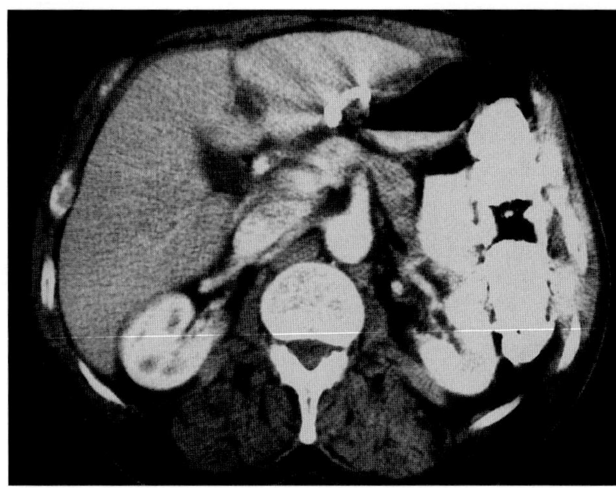

Figure 16. Same patient as in Figure 9. CT image obtained 1 week after initial drainage of the abscess shows no significant residual fluid collection.

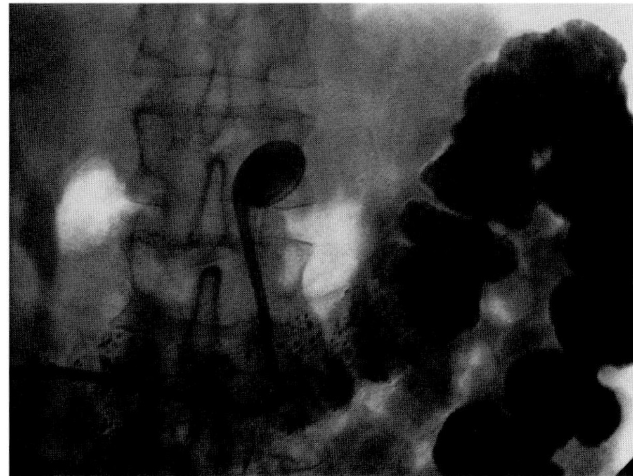

Figure 17. Same patient as in Figure 9. Tube check following the CT scan shows no residual cavity. The patient was clinically well and the catheter was removed.

Drainage catheters are removed when certain criteria of successful, complete drainage have been met **(Figs. 16, 17)**. These include:

1. Patient clinically well—afebrile, normalized white blood cell count;
2. No undrained fluid on CT or US evaluation;
3. Tube output <10 mL/day;
4. No residual cavity or fistula seen on tube check.

If catheter output suddenly decreases or stops, a tube check should be performed to confirm tube patency and location. The tube may become dislodged from the cavity, become occluded by debris, or kink. Tube replacement or repositioning should be performed as needed.

If the patient does not improve or worsens clinically, repeat CT imaging should be performed to determine the degree of drainage and assess for the presence of other undrained collections. Additional tubes may be required for complex collections. Surgery may be necessary if sepsis continues and adequate drainage cannot be achieved because of thick, necrotic material or evidence of multiple interloop abscesses.

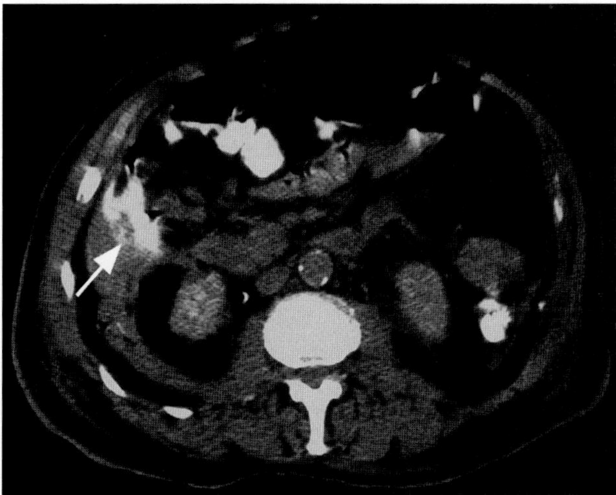

Figure 18. CT scan of a patient after right colon surgery. There is evidence of an anastomotic leak with an abscess cavity, which is beginning to fill with bowel contrast (arrow).

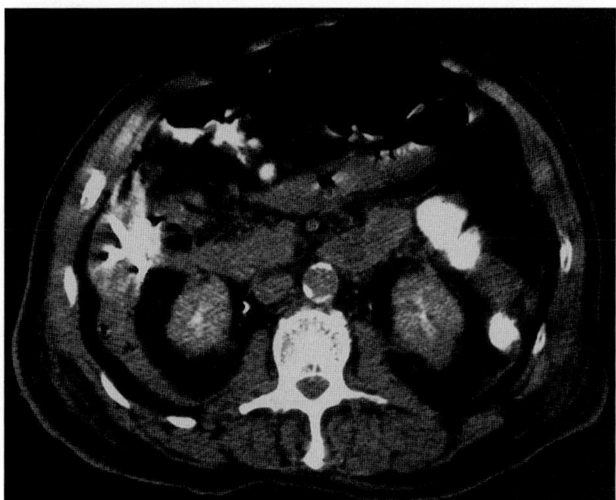

Figure 19. Same patient as in Figure 18. Drainage catheter placed percutaneously using the tandem trocar technique.

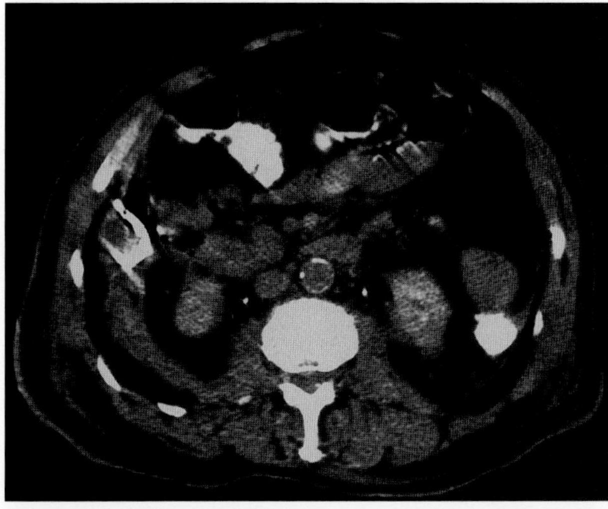

Figure 20. Same patient as in Figure 18. Catheter in place for prolonged continuous drainage.

Enteric fistulas, which are abnormal communications between the gastrointestinal tract and the abscess cavity and/or the skin, require somewhat different percutaneous management **(Figs. 18–20)**. Most fistulas develop after abdominal surgeries and are often due to anastomotic breakdown with leaks resulting in abscess formation. Fistulas can also result from malignancy or inflammatory conditions such as Crohn's disease.

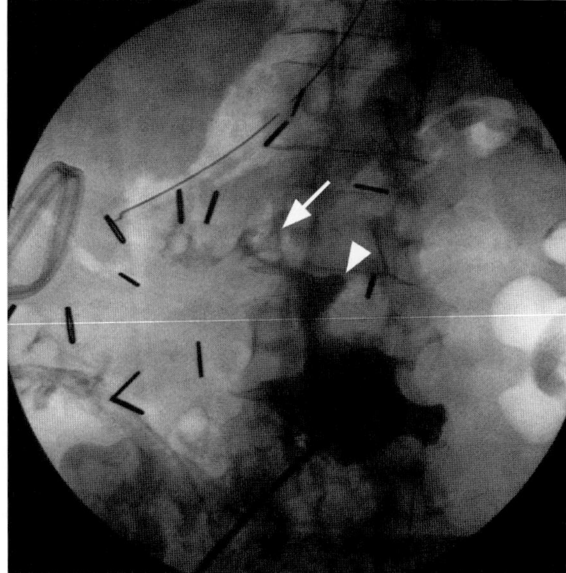

Figure 21. Patient after small bowel surgery with continued drainage from the surgical wound. Percutaneous sinogram demonstrates an abscess cavity, a smaller cavity (arrowhead), and faint opacification of the small bowel (arrow), confirming a bowel leak.

The search for a fistulous track should be prompted by persistent high output from the drainage catheter. Fistulas can be located by injecting contrast material through the tube 2–3 days after the initial drainage procedure, when the patient's sepsis has improved. If a fistula is suspected clinically and no communication is seen on the sinogram, gentle probing with angiographic catheters and/or wires may help identify the fistulous track.[6] The goal is to externalize the fistula to the skin in a controlled manner by placing the drainage catheter immediately adjacent to the site of bowel leak, thereby allowing the fistula to involute over time **(Figs. 21, 22)**. Output from the catheter is characteristically of higher volume and of longer duration for fistula treatment than for routine abscess drainage. Appropriate control of bowel effluent and parenteral nutrition along with catheter drainage aid in the closure of the fistula.[7,8]

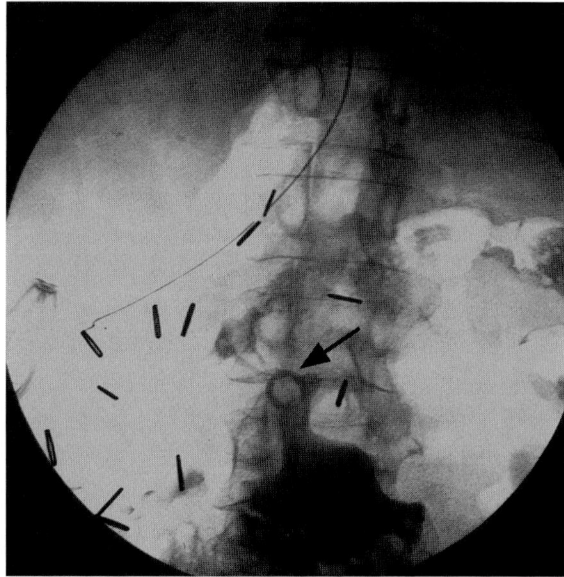

Figure 22. A wire and catheter were manipulated through the track into the smaller cavity and placed adjacent to the site of the bowel leak (arrow) to optimize fibrosis of the fistula. The catheter was slowly backed out of the track over time.

Complications

Major and minor complications are seen in approximately 10% or fewer of cases.[3,9] Most complications are due to sepsis occurring during percutaneous drainage and can be minimized by using broad spectrum antibiotic coverage prior to the procedure, avoiding overdistention of the cavity, and adhering to sterile technique during tube flushes, checks, and changes. Complications can also occur related directly to catheter placement and include vessel injury, bowel injury, solid organ injury, and transgression of the pleura with contamination of the pleural space.[2,4] These complications can be avoided with careful preprocedural planning of the puncture site, angle, and depth.

Results

Success rates for percutaneous management should include cases where percutaneous drainage resulted in complete cure as well as those cases in which percutaneous management of abscesses allowed clinical stabilization via treatment of the acute process so that a simpler, definitive surgical procedure could be performed electively. Reported success rates of percutaneous drainage of abdominal abscesses have been 70%–100%.[1–4,9,10,11] Successful percutaneous treatment of enteric fistulas has been reported in 57%–84% of cases.[6,7,12]

References

1. Jaques P, Mauro M, Safrit H, Yankaskas B, Piggott B. CT features of intraabdominal abscesses: prediction of successful percutaneous drainage. AJR 1986; 146:1041–1045.

2. Clark RA, Towbin R. Abscess drainage with CT and ultrasound guidance. Radiol Clin North Am 1983; 21(3):445–459.

3. vanSonnenberg E, Mueller PR, Ferrucci JT. Percutaneous drainage of 250 abdominal abscesses and fluid collections. Part I: Results, failures, and complications. Radiology 1984; 151:337–341.

4. vanSonnenberg E, Ferrucci JT, Mueller PR, Wittenberg J, Simeone JF. Percutaneous drainage of abscesses and fluid collections: technique, results, and applications. Radiology 1982; 142:1–10.

5. Kerlan RK, Pogany AC, Jeffrey RB, Goldberg HI, Ring EJ. Interventional radiology rounds: radiologic management of abdominal abscesses. AJR 1985; 144:145–149.

6. Kerlan RK, Jeffrey RB, Pogany AC, Ring EJ. Abdominal abscess with low-output fistula: successful percutaneous drainage. Radiology 1985; 155:73–75.

7. LaBerge JM, Kerlan RK, Gordon RL, Ring EJ. Nonoperative treatment of enteric fistulas: results in 53 patients. J Vasc Interv Radiol 1992; 3:353–357.

8. McLean GK, Mackie JA, Freiman DB, Ring EJ. Enterocutaneous fistulae: interventional radiologic management. AJR 1982; 138:615–619.

9. Lambiase RE, Deyoe L, Cronan JJ, Dorfman GS. Percutaneous drainage of 335 consecutive abscesses: results of primary drainage with 1-year follow-up. Radiology 1992; 184:167–179.

10. Jeffrey RB, Federle MP, Tolentino CS. Periappendiceal inflammatory masses: CT-directed management and clinical outcome in 70 patients. Radiology 1988; 167:13–16.

11. Sacks D, Banner MP, Meranze SG, Burke DR, Robinson M, McLean GK. Renal and related retroperitoneal abscesses: percutaneous drainage. Radiology 1988; 167:447–451.

12. Lambiase RE, Cronan JJ, Dorfman GS, Paolella LP, Haas RA. Postoperative abscesses with enteric communication: percutaneous treatment. Radiology 1989; 171:497–500.

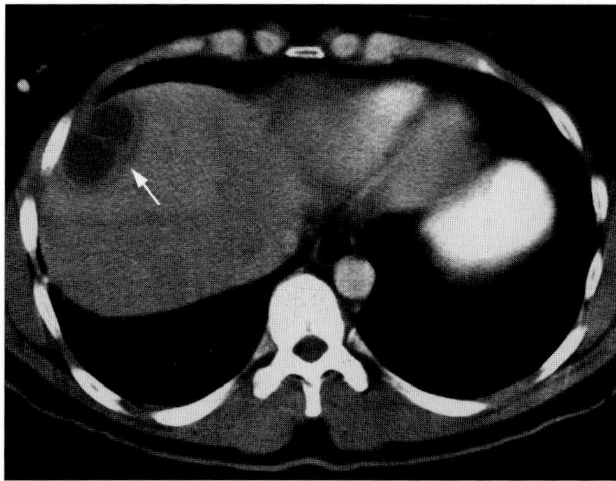

Figure 1. CT scan shows a pyogenic hepatic abscess (arrow).

TUTORIAL 7
HEPATIC ABSCESS: PERCUTANEOUS DRAINAGE

Steven Souza, M.D.

Introduction

The subjects addressed in this tutorial include:

1. Manifestations and treatment of pyogenic hepatic abscesses
2. Manifestations and treatment of amebic abscesses
3. Manifestations and treatment of hydatid cysts.

Pyogenic Abscess

Hepatic abscess remains a serious condition with high mortality despite advances in diagnosis and treatment. Worldwide, *Entamoeba histolytica* is the most common cause of hepatic abscess, whereas in developed countries, pyogenic hepatic abscess is more common **(Fig. 1)**.[1] Fungal abscess of the liver is uncommon. It typically occurs in immunocompromised patients and presents with characteristic microabscesses.

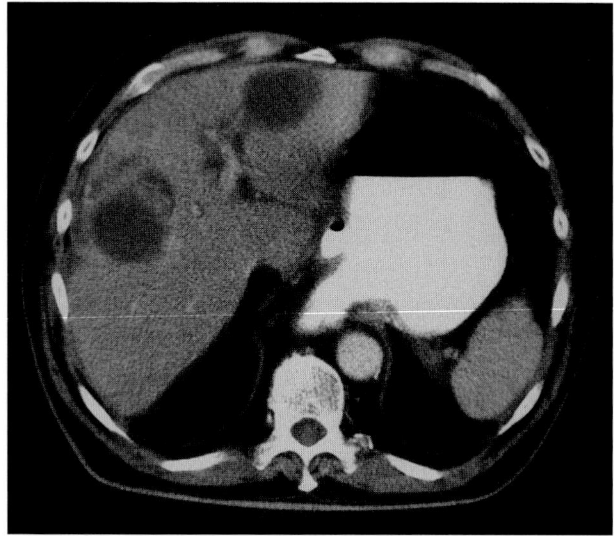

Figure 2. CT scan identifies abscesses in both the right and left lobes of the liver. Both were drained percutaneously.

Etiology

In developed countries, most hepatic abscesses result from ascending cholangitis complicating biliary obstruction **(Figs. 2, 3)** or are cryptogenic in origin. Historically, intestinal causes of pyogenic hepatic abscess were the most common etiology. These included portal vein seeding from appendicitis, diverticular disease, inflammatory bowel disease, splanchnic pyophlebitis, and colonic carcinoma. With improved antibiotics and diagnosis, these causes have decreased in frequency. Other etiologies of pyogenic abscess include arterial seeding secondary to systemic bacteremia, hepatic injury from penetrating trauma, postoperative abscess formation, or contiguous spread from adjacent infection.

Secondary pyogenic hepatic abscess occurs due to infection of pre-existing hepatic abnormalities including tumors **(Fig. 4)**, hematoma **(Fig. 5)**, congenital cysts, and amebic or parasitic cysts.

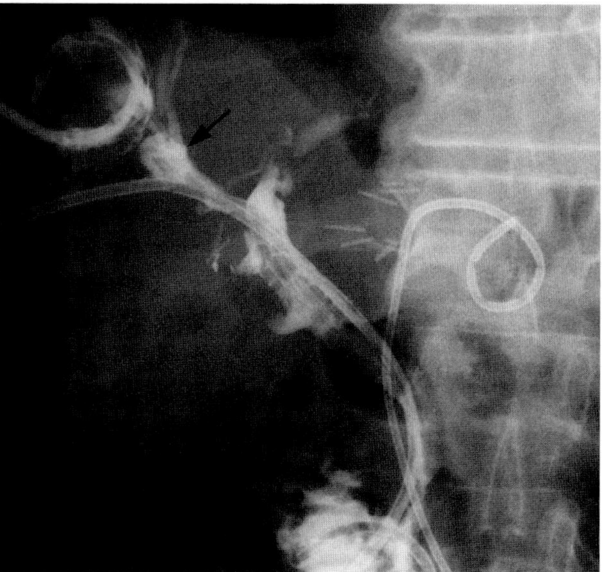

Figure 3. Same patient as in Figure 2. After drainage of the abscess, a sinogram obtained through the right catheter (arrowhead) demonstrates communication with the right hepatic duct (arrow). A biliary drainage catheter was placed because of ampullary stenosis and common bile duct stones.

Clinical Manifestations[1–3]

Clinical manifestations of pyogenic hepatic abscess include an elevated white blood cell count in 75%–90% of cases, fever in 70%–80%, chills, malaise, weight loss, right upper quadrant pain, and tender hepatomegaly. Jaundice may occur in patients with associated biliary obstruction. Because clinical findings and imaging studies are nonspecific, diagnostic aspiration with Gram staining is recommended prior to drainage to confirm that the hepatic lesion is an abscess. Patients with a pancreatobiliary source of the abscess usually demonstrate a predominance of gram-negative rods, most commonly *Escherichia coli*. Mixed flora or anaerobic isolates suggest a colonic source. Cytology is helpful when infected tumor is a diagnostic consideration.

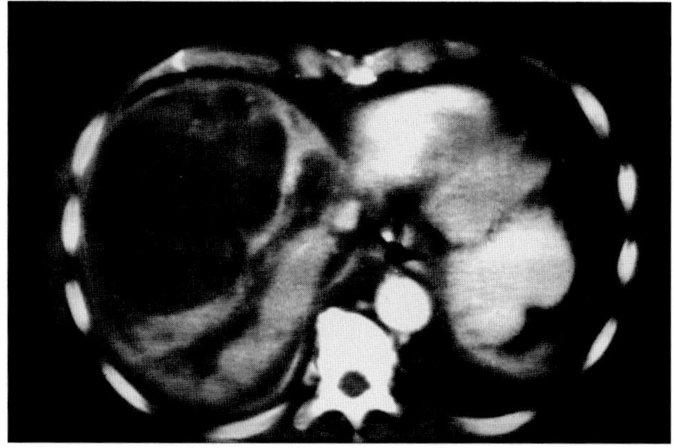

Figure 4. CT scan shows an infected hepatic metastasis.

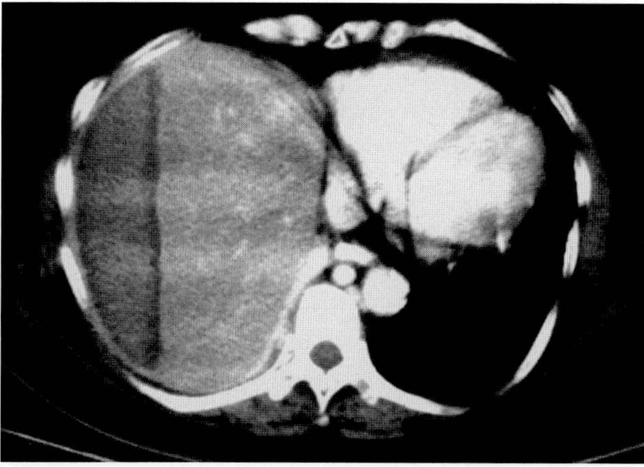

Figure 5. CT scan shows an infected right subcapsular hematoma.

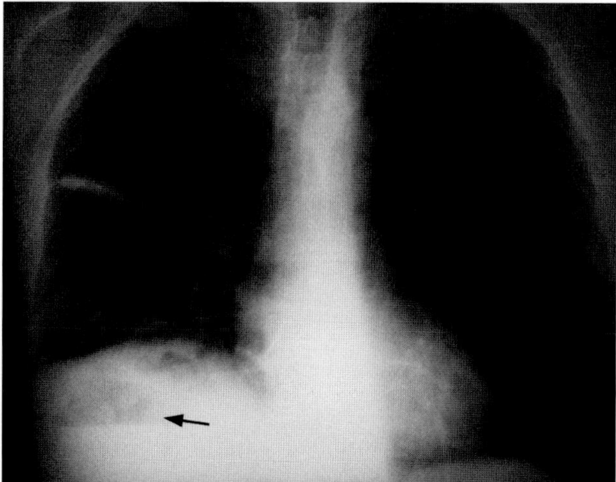

Figure 6. Chest radiograph shows an elevated right hemidiaphragm, right lower lobe atelectasis, and air in a hepatic abscess (arrow).

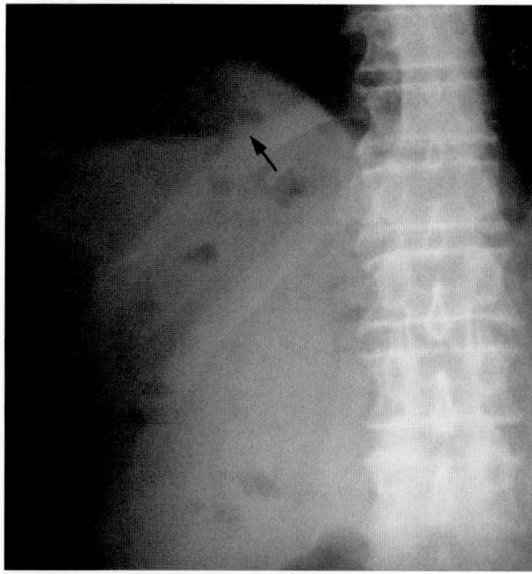

Figure 7. Abdominal radiograph shows air over the liver shadow which may represent abscesses or air in the biliary tree (arrow).

Radiographic Findings

Plain films often show elevation of the right hemidiaphragm, with or without right lower lobe atelectasis and a pleural effusion **(Fig. 6)**. A mass or loculated collection of air within the liver **(Fig. 7)** is sometimes seen.

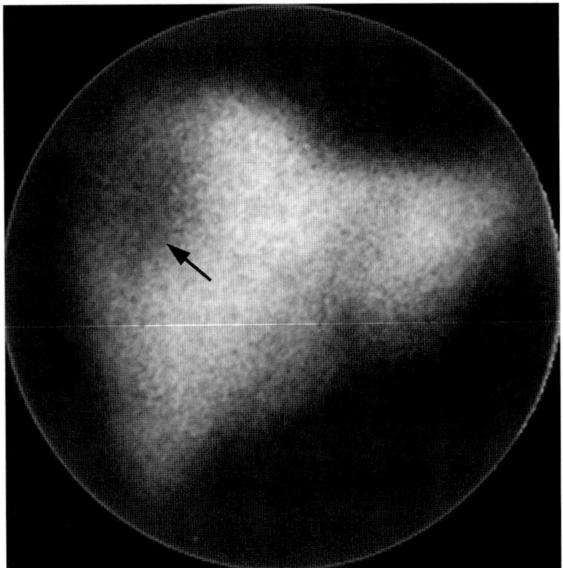

Figure 8. Technetium-99m labeled sulfur colloid scan shows a focal photopenic area along the superior aspect of the right lobe (arrow).

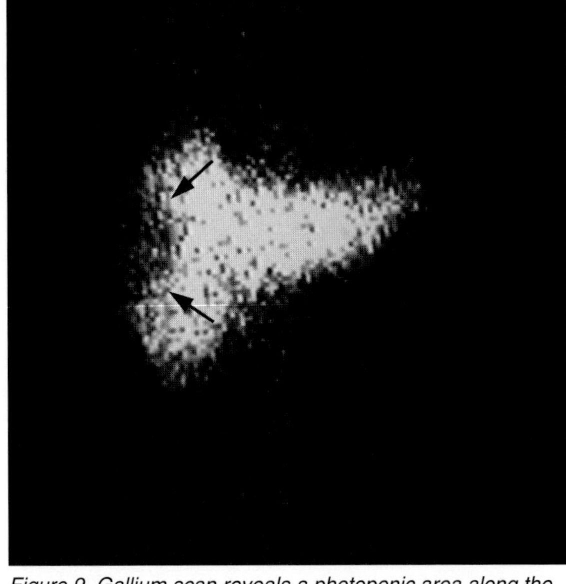

Figure 9. Gallium scan reveals a photopenic area along the lateral aspect of the right lobe of the liver (arrows) in this patient with an amebic abscess.

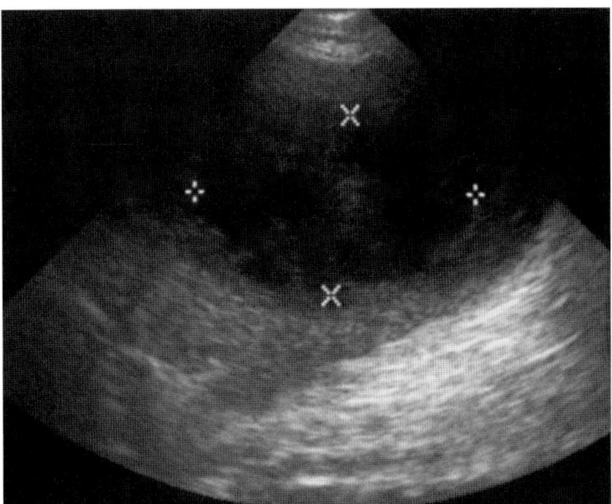

Figure 10. Longitudinal ultrasound demonstrates a hypoechoic area with echogenic material in the cavity and associated septations compatible with a complex pyogenic abscess.

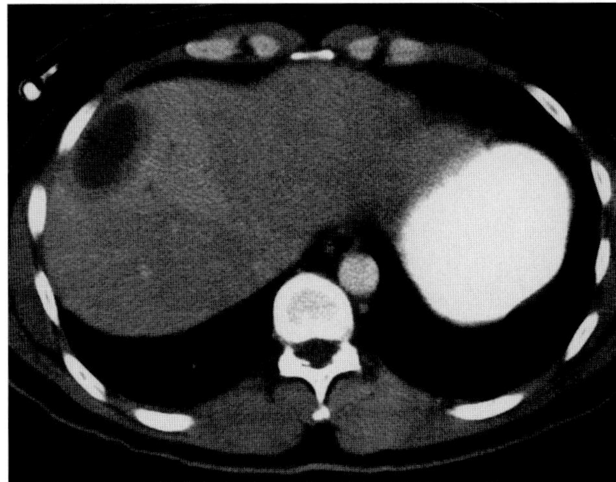

Figure 11. CT scan delineates a low-density cavity in the dome of the liver with a surrounding area of low attenuation. The abscess has a uniform appearance.

The role of nuclear medicine in the diagnosis of hepatic abscess has diminished since the advent of computed tomography (CT) scanning and ultrasound (US) evaluation. Hepatic abscesses typically appear as one or more focal defects on sulfur-colloid scans **(Fig. 8)**. A focal "hot spot" is seen on gallium scans; however, this finding is nonspecific because tumors also concentrate gallium. Amebic abscesses do not accumulate gallium **(Fig. 9)**. Indium-labeled white blood cells are concentrated in hepatic abscesses.

US generally shows a poorly marginated hypoechoic cavity with internal echoes **(Fig. 10)**. If gas is present, the lesion may appear very echogenic.

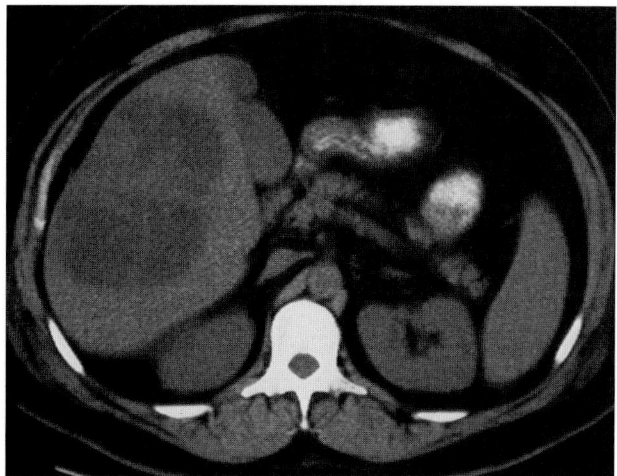

Figure 12. CT scan shows a complex pyogenic hepatic abscess with increased density and thick septation.

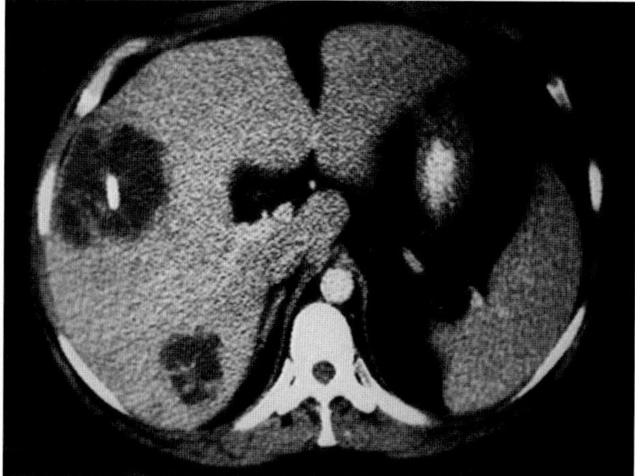

Figure 13. CT scan shows multiple low-density areas in the liver indicative of multiple abscesses.

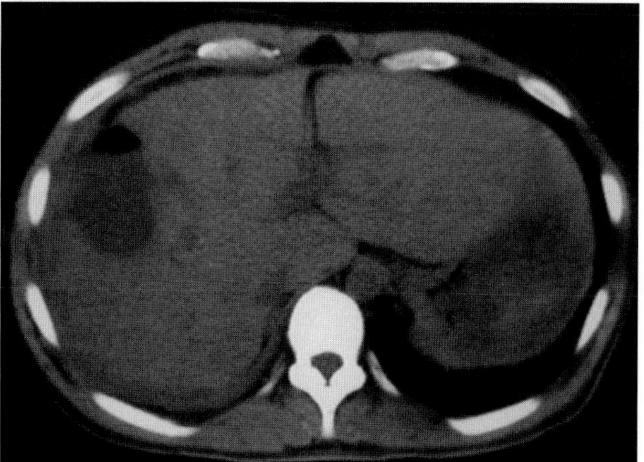

Figure 14. CT scan shows air in simple pyogenic abscesses.

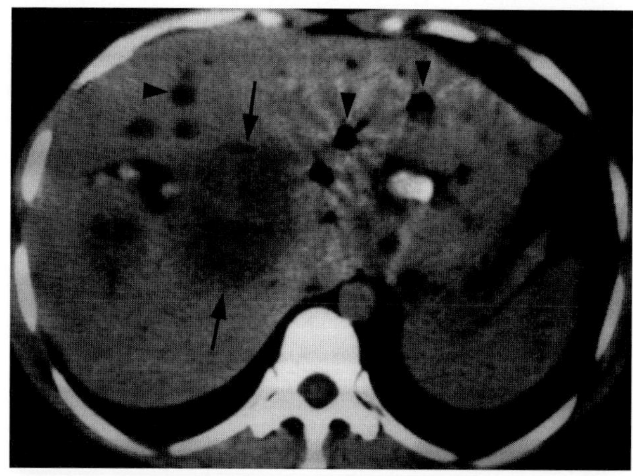

Figure 15. Transverse CT scan of the liver reveals air in a complex pyogenic abscess (arrows) and biliary system (arrowheads).

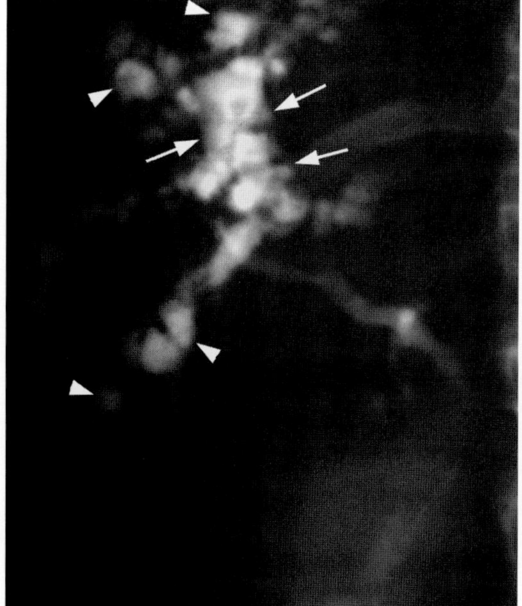

Figure 16. Cholangiogram of a complex pyogenic abscess (arrows) in a patient with acquired immunodeficiency syndrome demonstrates communication with the biliary system, which has numerous outpouches (arrowheads) possibly representing suppurative cholangitis.

CT findings vary from a low attenuating cavity **(Fig. 11)** to a complex heterogeneous mass **(Fig. 12)**. Abscesses are often multiple **(Fig. 13)**. Gas is seen in 20% of cases **(Figs. 14, 15)** and reflects infection with a gas-forming organism or fistulous communication to the bowel or biliary tree. Rim enhancement is rare but a hypodense rim surrounding the lesion is fairly suggestive of pyogenic or amebic abscesses. Pyogenic abscesses in immunocompromised patients may have a bizarre appearance **(Fig. 16)**.

The differential diagnosis of pyogenic hepatic abscess includes necrotic neoplasm, hematoma, complicated cysts, amebic abscess, and hydatid cyst.[4]

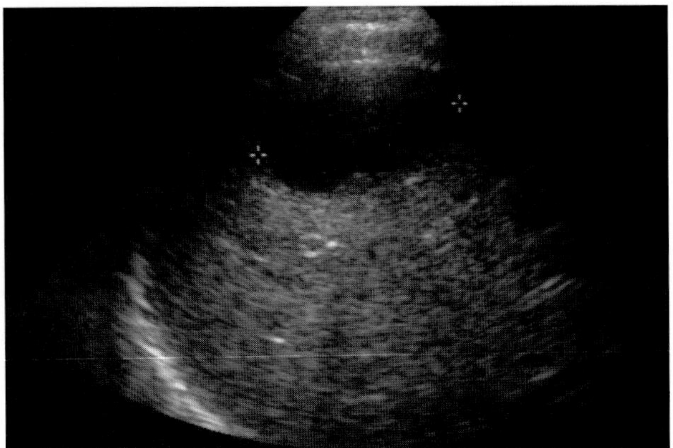

Figure 17. Transverse sonogram shows a 5-cm pyogenic abscess.

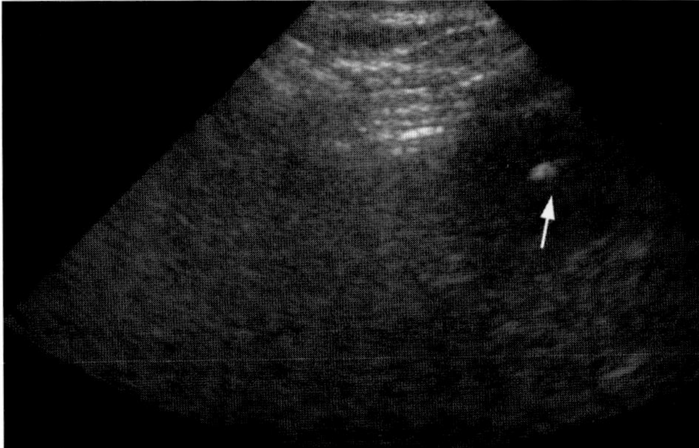

Figure 18. Same patient as in Figure 17. Tip of aspiration needle in the collection (arrow).

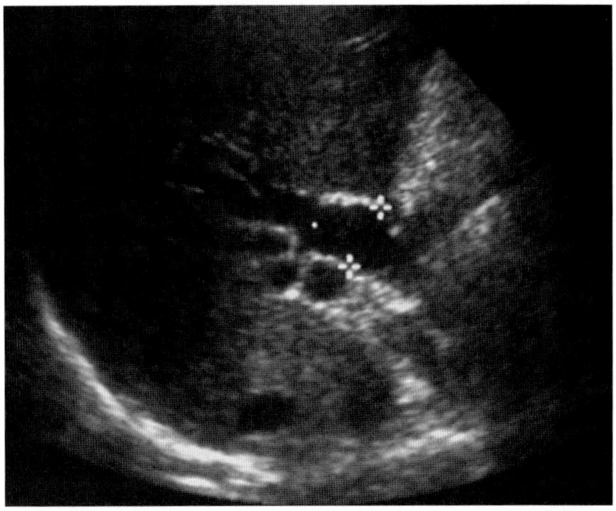

Treatment

Treatment consists of antibiotic therapy and drainage.[5,6] Abscesses smaller than 3 cm in diameter will usually resolve with antibiotic therapy alone. If a diagnostic aspiration is performed in such small lesions and purulent material is obtained, the collection should be aspirated fully and antibiotics continued. In the past, external drainage via a percutaneous catheter was the means of treating these pyogenic abscesses. However, needle aspiration alone is adequate in selected cases where a unilocular abscess smaller than 5 cm is present; success rates of over 90%–95% have been reported, which compare favorably with catheter drainage **(Figs. 17, 18)**.[7,8] Percutaneous placement of a drainage catheter should be considered in abscesses larger than 5 cm and in complex abscesses.[9] Air-containing abscesses should be drained rather than aspirated because a fistula from the abscess may be present which may need to be controlled.

When the abscess is secondary to biliary obstruction, the biliary system must be decompressed **(Figs. 19, 20)**. Fungal microabscesses usually do not require drainage. Pyogenic microabscesses, as in **Figure 20**, are usually not amenable to individual drainage because of their size and multiplicity; however, treatment of the biliary obstruction will result in resolution of the abscesses.

Figure 19. Longitudinal US of the porta hepatis demonstrates that the common bile duct (between calipers) is dilated to 11 mm in diameter.

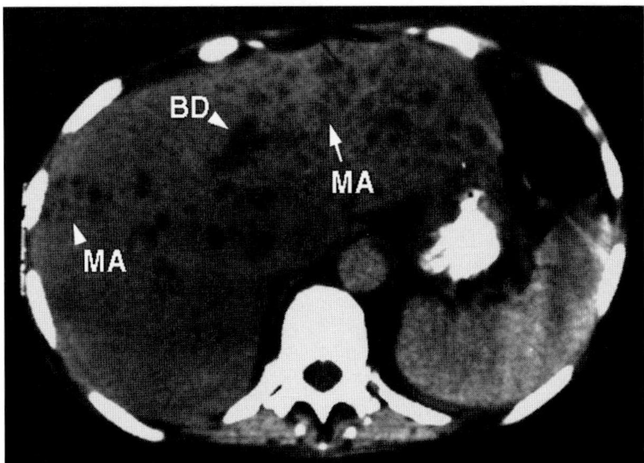

Figure 20. Microabscesses from biliary obstruction. MA=microabscess; BD=bile duct dilatation.

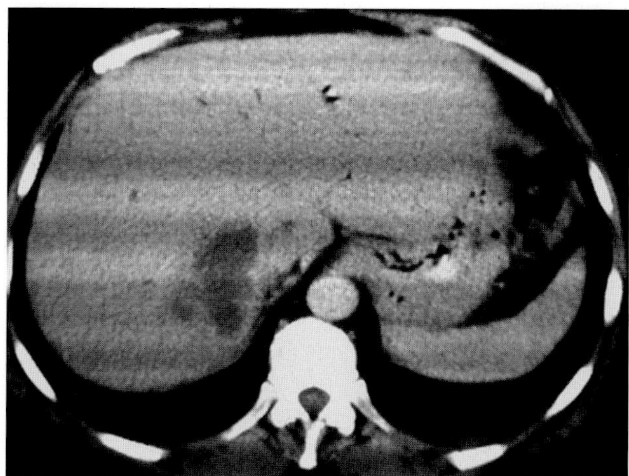

Figure 21. CT scan shows a low-density collection suggestive of a pyogenic abscess in the dome of the liver.

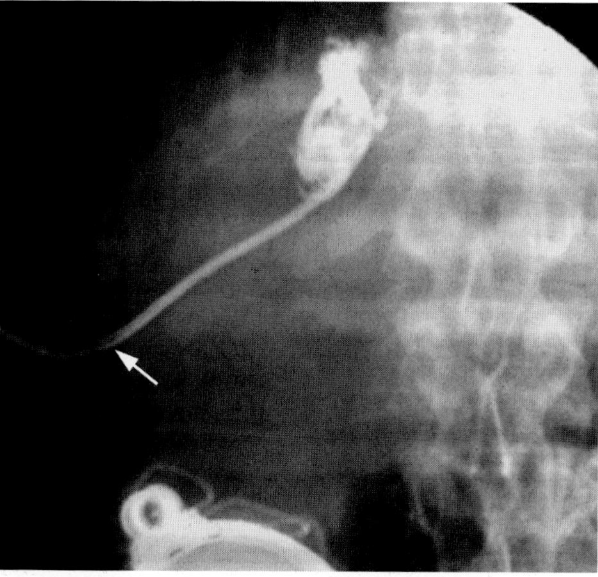

Figure 22. Same patient as in Figure 21. Catheter sinogram after drainage of the abscess shows the oblique course from the skin puncture site (arrow) to the collection in the dome of the liver.

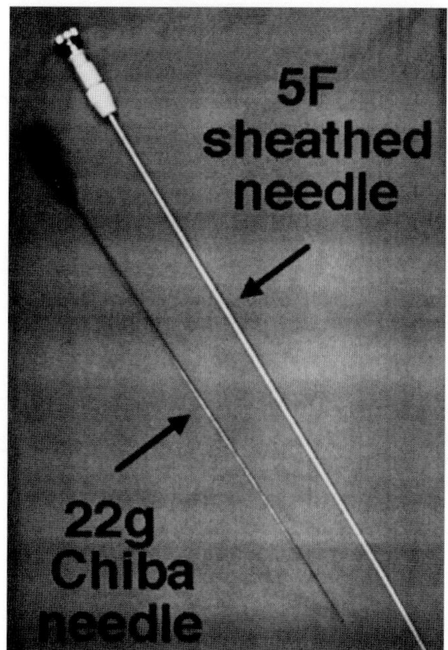

Figure 23. 5-F sheath needle and 22-gauge Chiba needle.

Either US or CT imaging can be used to guide abscess drainage. US is quicker, nonionizing, provides real-time guidance, and is more flexible, permitting an oblique approach to lesions in the dome of the liver **(Figs. 21, 22)**. CT scanning better defines the entire abdominal and pelvic anatomy, is not limited by bowel gas artifact from the often coexisting ileus, and frequently reveals the underlying cause of the abscess.

Technique[9,10]

Diagnostic puncture is often performed with a 22-gauge needle. Placement of a larger needle or a 5-F catheter may be required to aspirate viscous fluid **(Fig. 23)**. The pleura, bowel, and adjacent viscera are avoided, and when possible, a segment of normal liver parenchyma is traversed to decrease the risk of peritoneal spillage. Gram stain is performed on the aspirated material to confirm pyogenic abscess prior to drainage. Drainage can be accomplished with simple aspiration or placement of one or more drainage catheters.

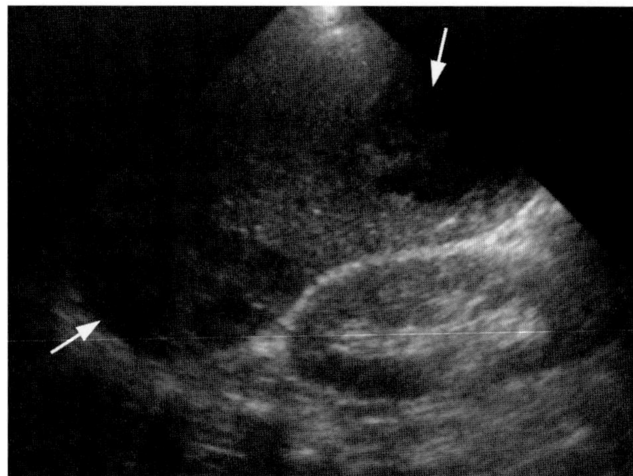

Figure 24. Two separate complex pyogenic abscesses demonstrated by US (arrows).

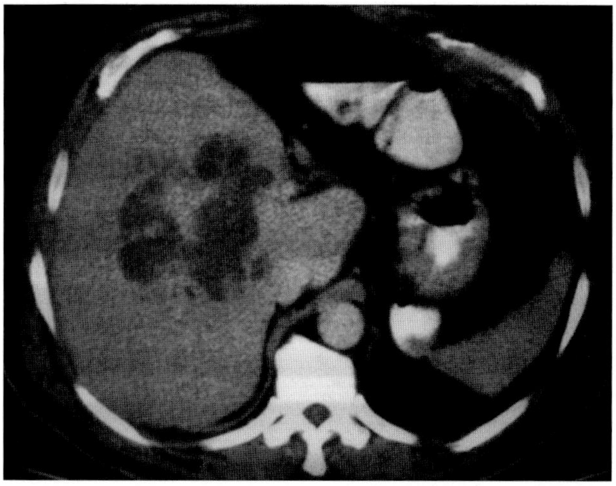

Figure 25. Complex pyogenic abscess with septations and loculations noted on the CT scan in another patient.

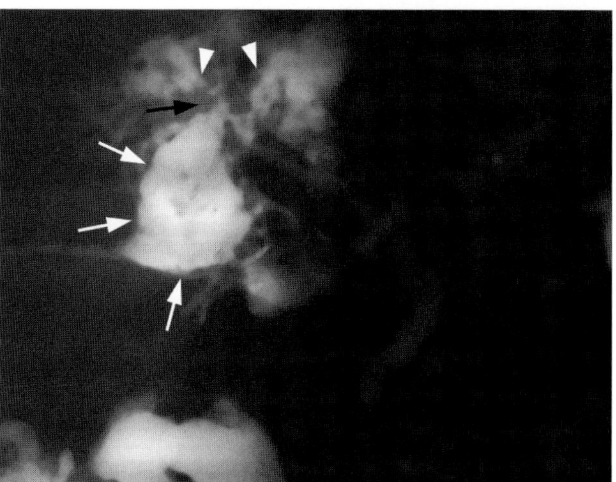

Figure 26. Sinogram obtained after catheter drainage of a liver abscess in another patient reveals a small residual cavity (white arrows), but there is a fistula (black arrow) to the biliary tree (arrowheads).

Aspiration without prolonged catheter placement is appropriate if the lesion is unilocular and well defined, smaller than 5 cm in diameter, and does not communicate with the biliary system or bowel. When a catheter is placed, the collection is completely aspirated and the cavity irrigated with a volume of normal saline or an antiseptic solution that is approximately two thirds the volume of the original cavity. Irrigation is repeated until the return fluid is clear, then a sinogram is obtained to assess for any communication to the biliary system or bowel. If no fistula is present, the catheter is removed. Follow-up US or CT imaging is performed in a few days to confirm resolution. Several reports have now shown that needle aspiration of liver abscesses, with associated antibiotic therapy without catheter placement, is sufficient to treat the abscess.[7,8]

Placement of an indwelling drainage catheter is indicated when the abscess is multiloculated, ill defined, larger than 5 cm in diameter, or if a fistula is demonstrated **(Figs. 24–26)**. An indwelling catheter can be placed either by the Seldinger or trocar technique. The trocar technique may be appropriate in large collections with a straightforward access route. It is typically easier and faster than the Seldinger technique, and is usually performed under CT guidance.

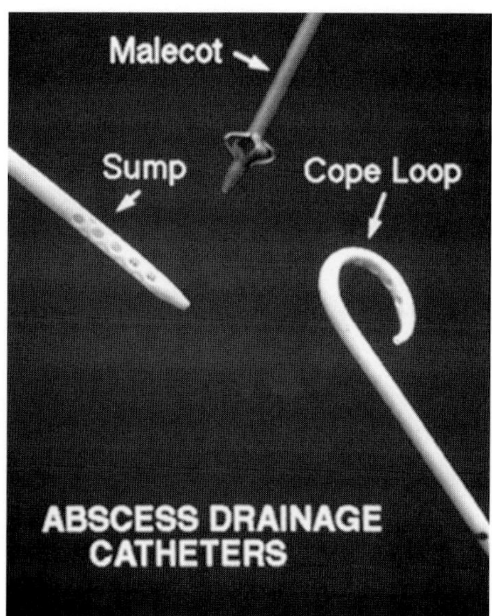

Figure 27. Drainage catheters.

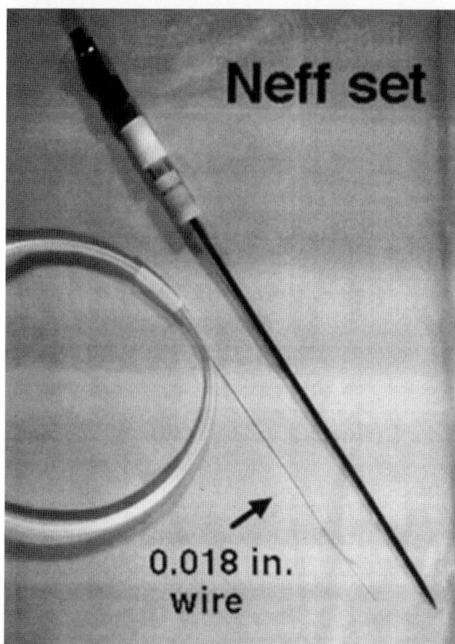

Figure 28. Neff set (Cook, Bloomington, IN).

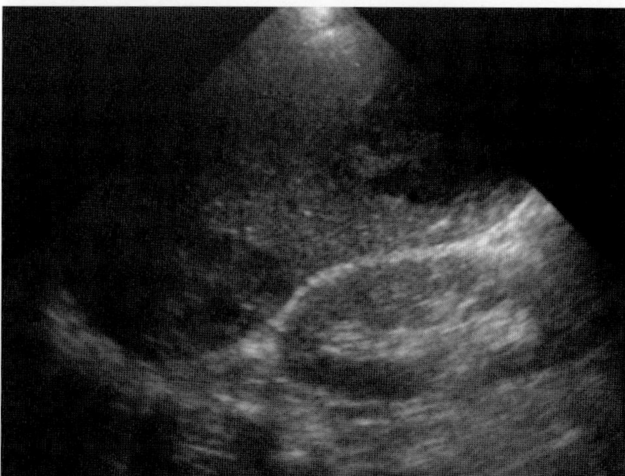
Figure 29. Two separate abscesses are present on this longitudinal US of the right lobe of the liver.

The Seldinger technique involves initial puncture with a 5-F needle sheath or 22-gauge needle in conjunction with an upsizing system, followed by placement of an 0.035-inch wire into the cavity. Typically, a floppy-tipped guide wire is coiled in the cavity, the catheter is advanced, and then a stiffer wire can be introduced. Over this, the track is dilated with Teflon dilators. Numerous drainage catheters are available and the choice of catheter depends on the location and viscosity of the fluid to be drained. For less viscous collections, 8–12-F Cope nephrostomy tubes are frequently placed, while 12–16-F sumps are used for more viscous collections **(Fig. 27)**.

When the abscess is deep or difficult to reach, initial puncture with a 22-gauge needle may be preferred. Once position is confirmed, a conversion system such as a Neff set or Cope set is used to gain access with a 5-F catheter **(Fig. 28)**. Although complex abscesses may occasionally require multiple catheters to resolve completely, the numerous cavities within a multiloculated complex abscess communicate with each other in most cases and a single catheter in the largest, most dependent cavity will drain the entire collection. In cases of multiple abscesses, drainage of each abscess is required **(Fig. 29)**. The entire procedure can be accomplished under US or CT guidance, or the patient can be transferred to a fluoroscopy room for catheter placement once the needle and guide wire are positioned in the collection.

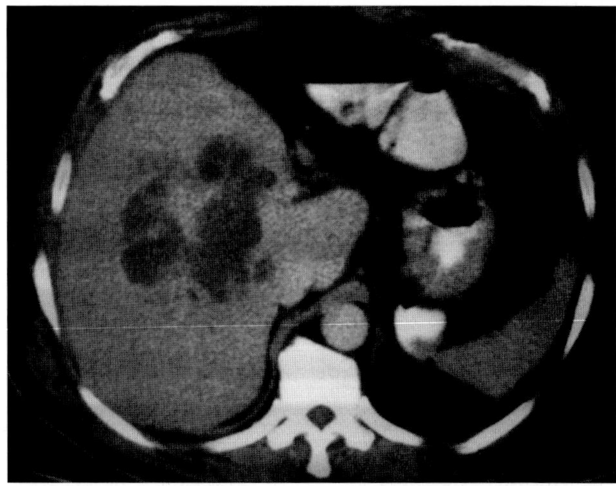

Figure 30. Multiseptated abscess in the right lobe of the liver seen previously in Figure 25.

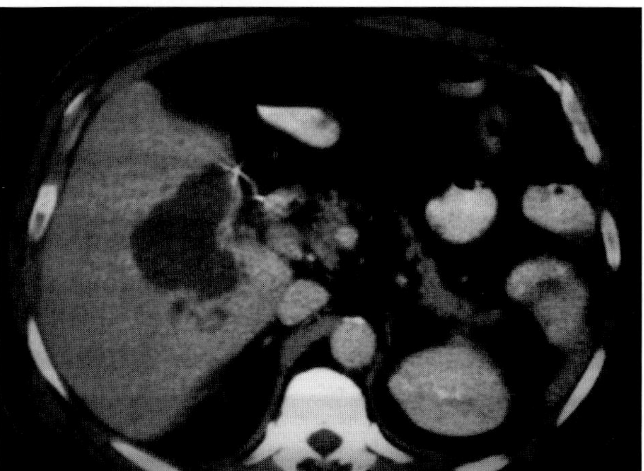

Figure 31. Same patient as in Figure 30. On a caudal image, the lower portion of the abscess appears less septated than the superior portion.

Once the catheter is in place, the collection is aspirated completely and irrigated with normal saline until clear. Care should be taken not to overdistend the cavity, to reduce the risk of inducing septicemia. Low intermittent suction is used for Cope catheters while continuous suction is applied to sumps. Septations within complex cavities generally break down with guide wire manipulations or during irrigation. When the largest loculation is drained, adjacent ones often decompress into that cavity and generally respond to drainage with a single catheter **(Figs. 30–32)**.

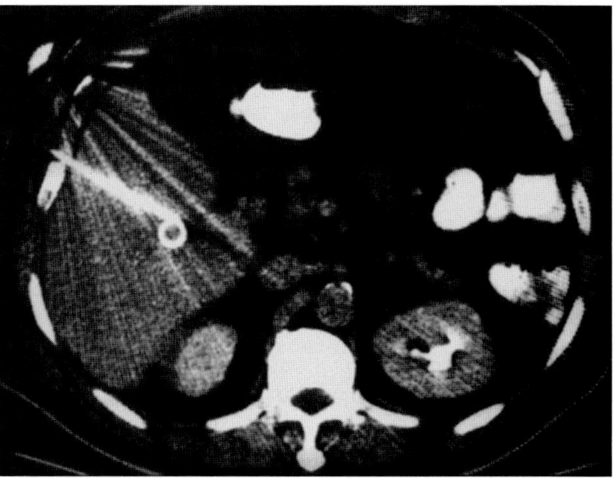

Figure 32. After a simple drainage catheter was placed in the lower dependent portion of the abscess, a follow-up CT scan demonstrates complete evacuation and resolution of the previously identified complex pyogenic abscess.

Percutaneous drainage of pyogenic hepatic abscesses with or without biliary communication have similar rates of cure, although the duration of drainage is longer with biliary fistulas. Abscesses with extrahepatic biliary communication—essentially infected bilomas—all require drainage as well as biliary decompression **(Figs. 33–37)**.

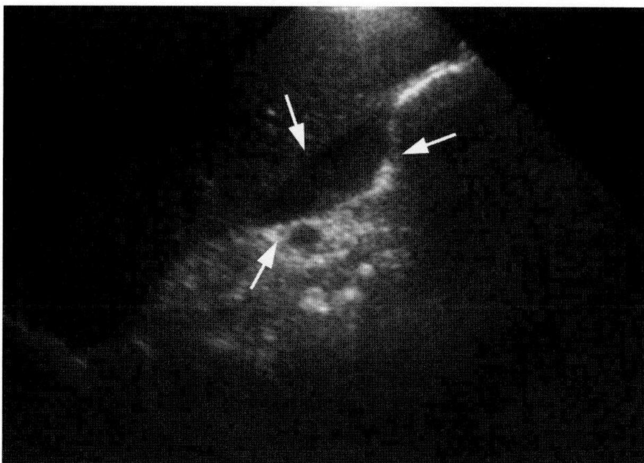

Figure 33. Sonographic evaluation of a patient after laparoscopic cholecystectomy identifies a subhepatic fluid collection (arrows) on this longitudinal US of the right lobe of the liver.

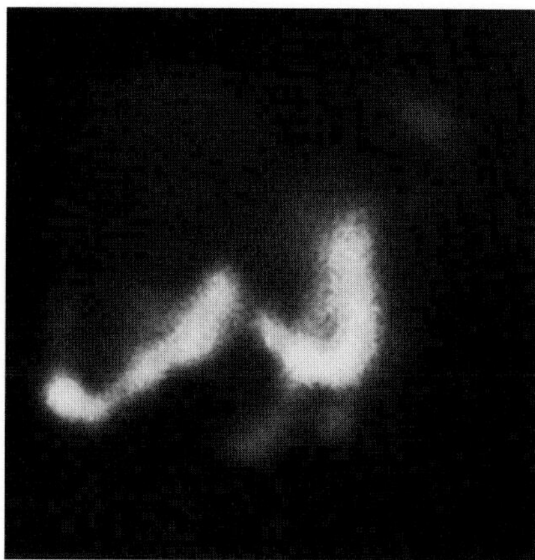

Figure 34. Same patient as in Figure 33. Dimethyl acetanilide iminodiacetic acid (HIDA) scan confirms extravasation of the tracer into the subhepatic space indicating bile leak.

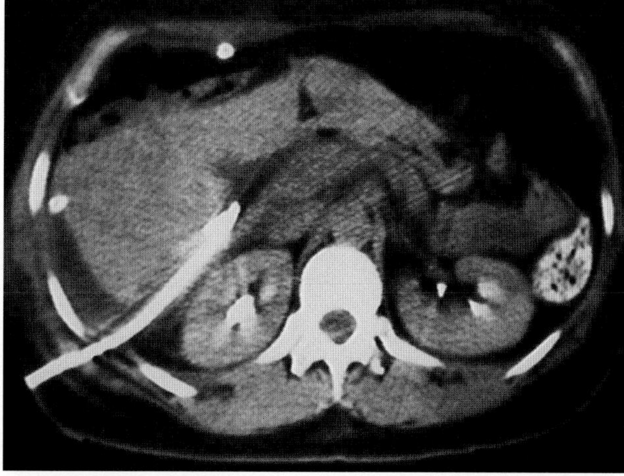

Figure 35. Same patient as in Figure 33. Follow-up CT scan indicates complete drainage of the biloma. With persistent output from the drainage catheter, biliary diversion, either percutaneously or endoscopically, will be required to allow the fistula to close and heal.

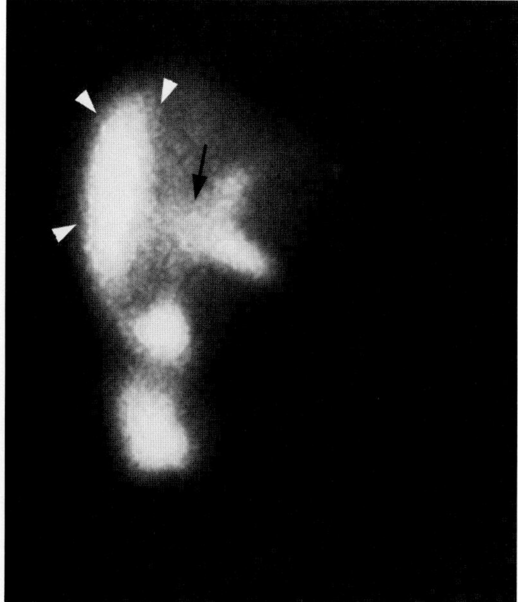

Figure 36. In another patient with hepatic trauma, the HIDA scan demonstrates leakage of bile from the right hepatic duct (arrow) into the subphrenic space (arrowheads).

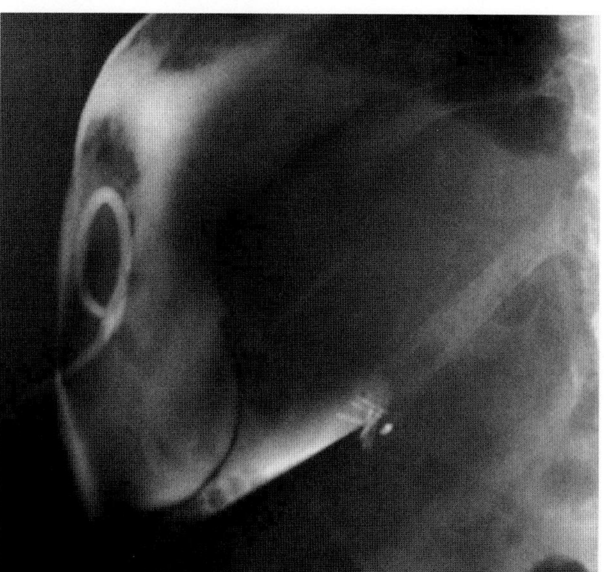

Figure 37. Same patient as in Figure 36. Sinogram after catheter drainage of the subphrenic bilious collection.

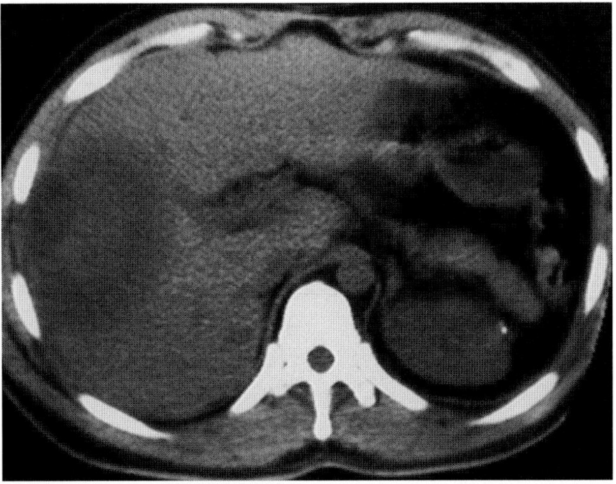

Figure 38. CT scan of a patient with right upper quadrant pain and fevers reveals a heterogeneous area in the right lobe of the liver without well-defined margins and lacking the low, near water, density characteristic of a true abscess.

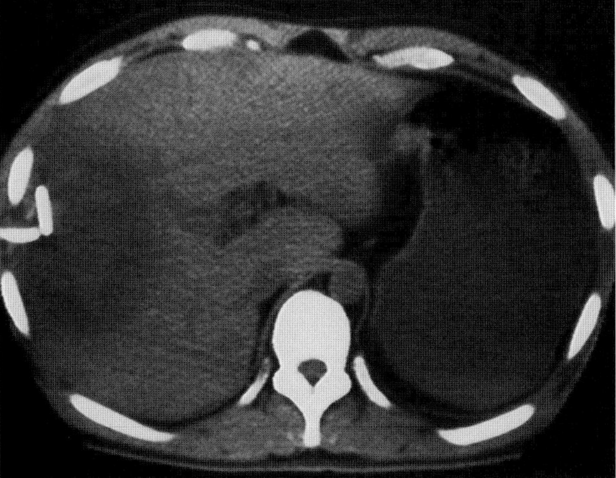

Figure 39. Same patient as in Figure 38. Drainage catheter placed in the abnormal area of the liver.

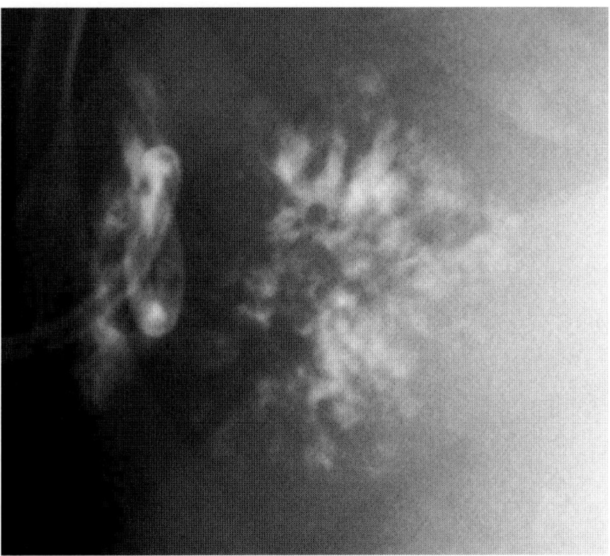

Figure 40. Same patient as in Figure 38. Catheter sinogram demonstrates no definite cavity and extension of contrast material into multiple small channels interdigitating with hepatic parenchyma consistent with a phlegmon.

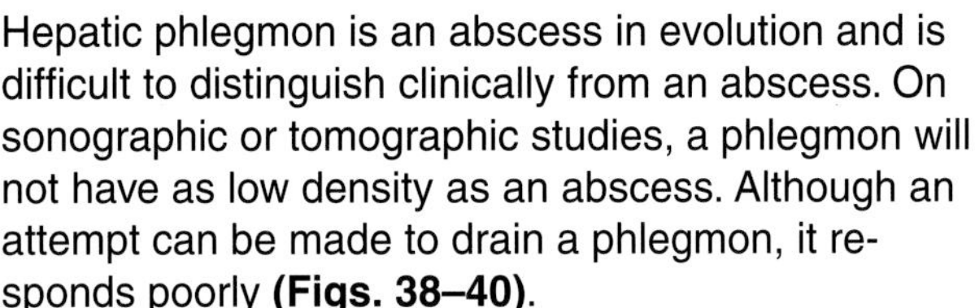

Hepatic phlegmon is an abscess in evolution and is difficult to distinguish clinically from an abscess. On sonographic or tomographic studies, a phlegmon will not have as low density as an abscess. Although an attempt can be made to drain a phlegmon, it responds poorly **(Figs. 38–40)**.

Follow-up

The patient's temperature and white blood cell count are followed, and output from the drainage tube is monitored. Analgesics may be required. A repeat US or CT study is obtained after 3–4 days to confirm adequate drainage. The drainage catheter may need to be repositioned in a more dependent portion of the abscess, or a second catheter may be required to obtain adequate drainage **(Fig. 41)**. A sinogram is obtained to assess for a fistula prior to drain removal.

When the cavity has collapsed, the drainage is insignificant, and the white blood cell count and temperature have been normal for 48 hours, the drains are removed. Percutaneous drainage requires an average of 7–10 days, longer if a fistula is associated with the abscess.

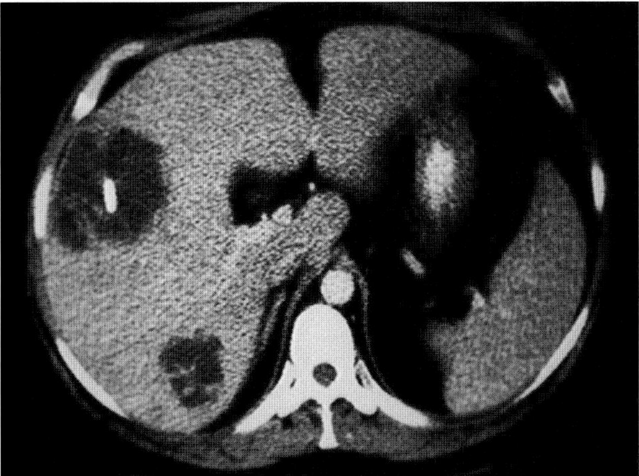

Figure 41. Follow-up CT scan after drainage of an abscess in the anterior segment of the right lobe indicates lack of resolution of the abscess cavity as well as enlargement of the second abscess in the posterior segment of the right lobe which required another catheter.

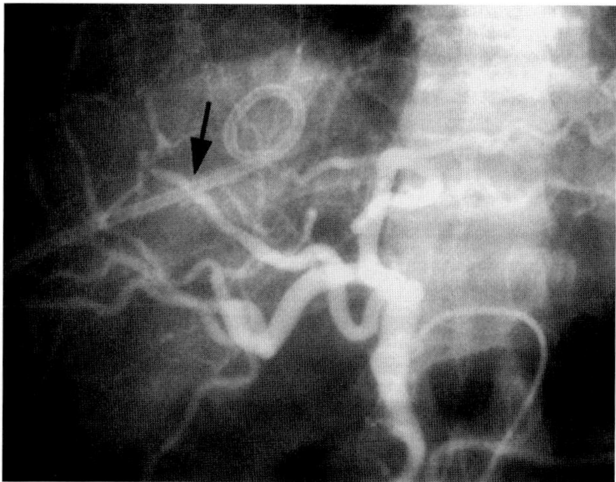

Figure 42. Hepatic arteriogram obtained in a patient with significant bleeding from the drainage catheter. Although active extravasation is not identified, the drain is in close proximity to an arterial branch (arrow).

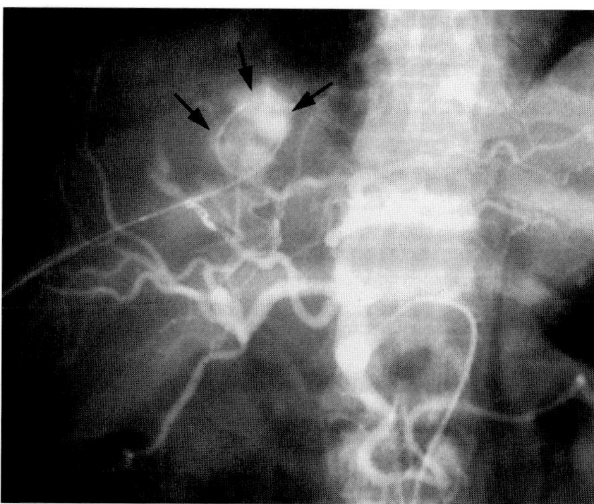

Figure 43. Same patient as in Figure 42. Repeat arteriogram obtained after the drainage catheter was removed over a wire now demonstrates extravasation of contrast material into the abscess cavity (arrows). Successful embolization was performed to control the active extravasation.

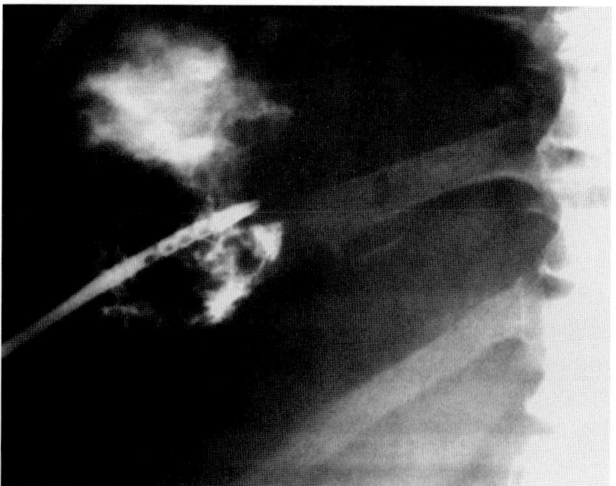

Figure 44. Sinogram after drainage of an infected metastatic lesion for palliation.

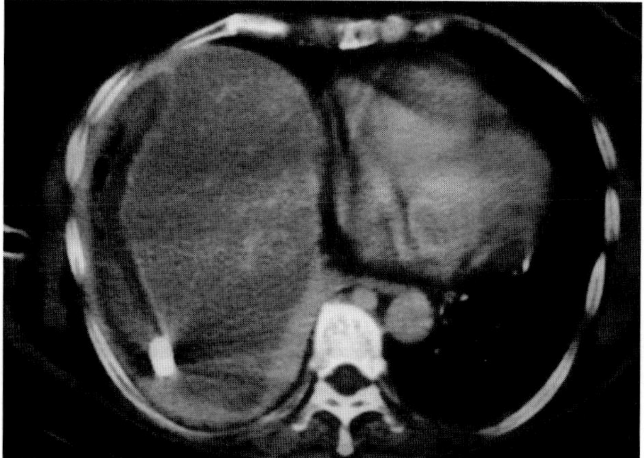

Figure 45. CT scan after drainage of an infected hematoma demonstrates poor resolution of the lesion due to the thick, viscous, dense nature of the hematoma.

Complications

Bacteremia with transient chills and fever is the most common complication, occurring in 10% of cases. Sepsis, hemorrhage, pneumothorax, and bowel injury rarely occur. However, because of the risk of septicemia, all patients suspected of having an abscess should receive antibiotics prior to any aspiration or drainage. Delayed complications are empyema, peritonitis, and arterial fistula **(Figs. 42, 43)**. The incidence of complications is reduced if simple needle aspiration without tube placement is performed.

Failure of percutaneous abscess drainage is secondary to inadequate drainage, persistent fistula, infected tumor **(Fig. 44)**, or hematoma **(Fig. 45)**.

Summary

The goal of drainage should be defined—cure, temporization, or palliation. Temporization is improvement in the patient's condition prior to adjunctive surgery to correct the underlying cause. Palliation is symptomatic relief in patients with limited life expectancy. Curative drainage is achieved in 80%–85% of cases, with partial success (temporization or palliation) in another 5%–10%. Secondary hepatic abscesses are likely to respond more poorly to percutaneous drainage because of the nature of the primary disease.

The advantages of the percutaneous approach are that general anesthesia and extensive surgical exploration can be avoided, guidance provides a safe access route, and multiple collections can be drained. Many of the contraindications to surgery in very ill patients do not preclude percutaneous drainage. The procedure is tolerated well, the success rate is high, and morbidity and mortality rates are low. If percutaneous treatment fails, surgery is not precluded. However, the role of surgical colleagues in the management of these complex problems should not be minimized. The underlying cause of the abscess—colon carcinoma, diverticulitis, appendicitis, cholecystitis, etc—often requires surgical correction.

Echinococcal Cysts

Etiology

Echinococcus granulosis is the most common form of hydatid disease in humans. The primary hosts are dogs and other carnivores. The adult tapeworm lives in the host's intestines, the eggs being expelled in the feces. The intermediate hosts, sheep and humans, are contaminated when the parasitic eggs are ingested. The embryo leaves the intestine of the intermediate host and reaches the liver through the portal vein. The lung is the second most common site of infection. Endemic areas include the Mediterranean, the Middle East, Australia, New Zealand, South America, and parts of North America (California, Arizona, Utah, and the Mississippi Valley).

Echinococcus multilocularis is less common and produces a tumor-like infiltration of the liver parenchyma. This form is seen in Central Europe, Russia, the Middle East, Japan, and Alaska. The primary host is the fox, with wild rodents serving as the intermediate host. Multiple tiny cysts produce an infiltrating process that produces a heterogeneous mass on US or CT evaluation which is often misdiagnosed as a tumor.

Diagnosis and Radiographic Findings

Diagnosis depends on serologic tests, which are 65%–85% sensitive, and imaging studies. US and CT appearances have been classified into five types.[11] Types II, III, and V show an undulating membrane, multiseptated cysts, and a calcified cyst, respectively. Although these are the more specific radiographic appearances, these findings are rarely seen. The most common appearance is that of a simple cyst, perhaps with minimal debris, or a complex mass, respectively, for types I and IV. These two nonspecific radiographic patterns are more common, and the patient is often diagnosed with simple cysts, hepatic abscess, or tumor in nonendemic areas.

Clinical Manifestations[12]

Most patients are asymptomatic, but some may present with pain, usually in the right upper quadrant, a mass, fever, or cholangitis. Because both clinical symptoms and imaging studies are usually nonspecific, a high degree of suspicion is necessary to make the diagnosis. Hydatid disease should be considered in patients who have recently been in endemic areas, or who have a history of hydatid disease. Serologic studies should be obtained, but these do not necessarily exclude the diagnosis because of the high false-negative rate.

Treatment

Conventional therapy is surgical resection.[12] The role of aspiration and percutaneous drainage and sclerosis is controversial but with further experience will likely become the indicated therapy for type I cysts.[13–15] Some physicians recommend percutaneous treatment as an alternative to surgery. Others reserve it for difficult diagnostic cases, cases where recurrent disease after surgery is suspected, and for nonsurgical candidates. Most hydatid cyst aspirations will actually be performed for other apparent indications because the diagnosis is not suspected outside of endemic areas, and the symptoms and radiographic findings are nonspecific. Medical therapy is somewhat controversial, and can be used in nonsurgical candidates or for recurrent disease.

Aspiration is performed under CT or US guidance. To minimize the risk of peritoneal spillage, care should be taken to traverse a segment of liver parenchyma rather than make a direct transperitoneal puncture, The aspirated cyst fluid is centrifuged and the sediment stained. Drainage can be performed by placing a small catheter, usually 5–8 F, in the cavity, which is then aspirated until dry. A cystogram is obtained to evaluate for biliary communication or peritoneal leakage. The cyst is then sclerosed with alcohol, hydrogen peroxide, or hypertonic saline.

Complications

The major risk of hydatid cyst puncture is the potential for anaphylaxis or peritoneal dissemination. Many cases have been reported of echinococcal cyst drainage without significant complication when a transhepatic route is used and care is taken to avoid dissemination.[14,15] Pretreatment with steroids is helpful to decrease the risk of anaphylaxis when hydatid disease is suspected. Serologic titers should be measured in any patient suspected of having echinococcal disease, and if aspiration or drainage is being considered the patient should be placed on an antiparasitic agent such as mebendazole or albendazole prior to the procedure.

Amebic Abscess

Etiology

Amebiasis is caused by the protozoan *Entamoeba histolytica*. It primarily involves the colon, but hepatic abscess is the most common extraintestinal manifestation. Most individuals infected with *Entamoeba histolytica* are asymptomatic carriers. Invasion of the colonic epithelium results in gastrointestinal symptoms that range from mild diarrhea to severe dysentery, and occurs in approximately 10% of infected individuals. The parasites travel to the liver via the portal system, where hepatic abscesses slowly develop in 3%–9% of patients.

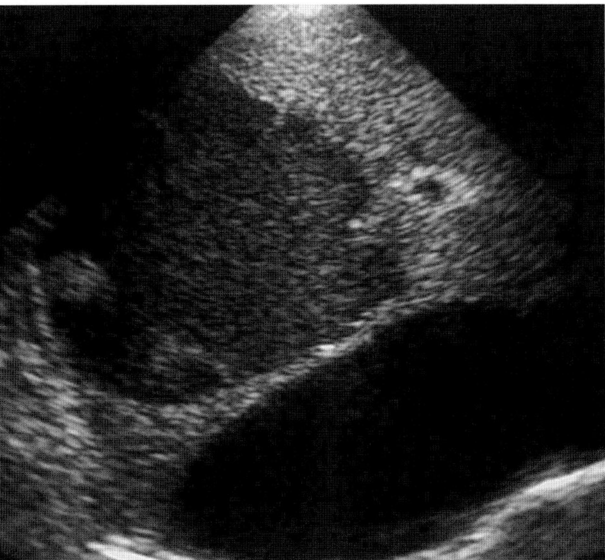

Figure 46. Right lobe amebic abscess in a subdiaphragmatic position.

Clinical Manifestations

Nearly all patients with amebic hepatic abscess manifest pain, generally in the right upper quadrant. Fever is seen in 75% of cases, with cough, shoulder pain, and weight loss being less common. A left lobe abscess results in epigastric or chest pain. Amebic pericarditis occurs in 3% of patients, is associated with left lobe abscess, and carries a 30% mortality rate.

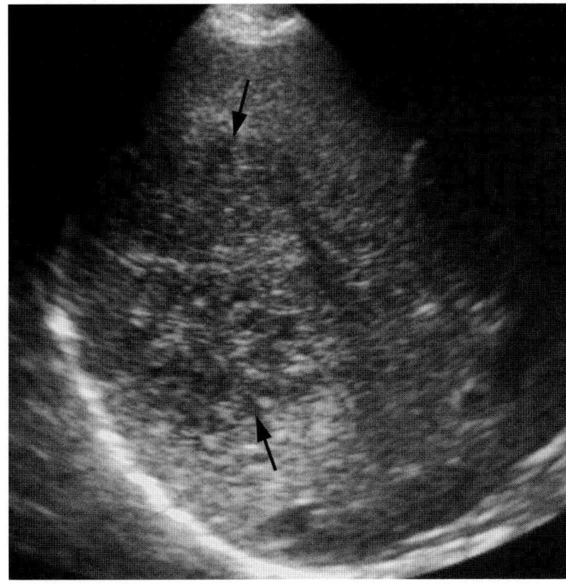

Figure 47. Early amebic abscess (arrows) on US shows heterogeneous echotexture to the right lobe of the liver without a well-defined collection.

Radiographic Findings

Chest radiographs commonly show elevation of the right hemidiaphragm, often with atelectasis at the right base and an effusion. US and CT images typically demonstrate a solitary, well-defined abscess in the posterior aspect of the right lobe, adjacent to the liver capsule **(Fig. 46)**. Amebic abscesses often display diffuse, homogeneous low-level echoes in the collection. Early amebic abscesses demonstrate heterogeneous changes in the echotexture of the hepatic parenchyma **(Fig. 47)**. Left lobe abscesses are less common. Direct extension into the pleural cavity occurs in 10%–20% of amebic abscesses.

Diagnosis

The diagnosis should be suspected in patients who have recently been in endemic areas—the tropics and subtropics, most notably Mexico. Serologic tests are positive in 90% of cases. When imaging and serologic tests are nondiagnostic, aspiration is helpful to exclude tumor or pyogenic abscess. Amebae live in the capsule of the abscess and biopsy of the wall is required to demonstrate active amebae **(Fig. 48)**. Rarely will amebae be seen in the aspirate.

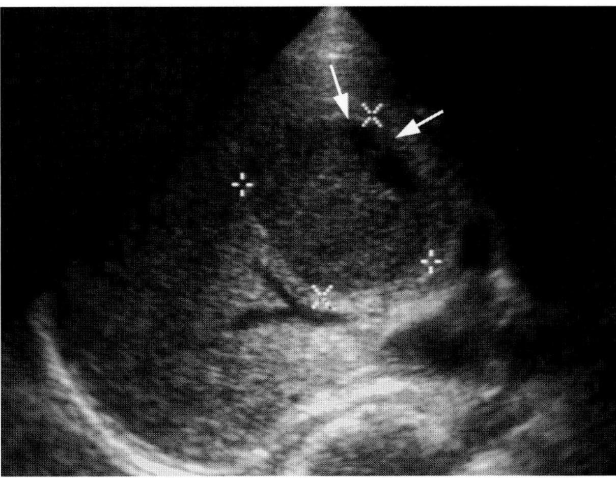

Figure 48. The capsule (arrows) around an amebic abscess is where the biopsy or aspiration should be directed.

Treatment

Amebic abscess responds well to medical therapy with metronidazole. Iodoquinol can also be given in conjunction with metronidazole. The role of aspiration and percutaneous drainage remains controversial.[16–20] Diagnostic aspiration may be used to differentiate amebic from pyogenic abscess when clinical, laboratory, and imaging findings are nondiagnostic. The aspirate in approximately half of amebic abscesses is suggestive of pyogenic abscess rather than having the classic "anchovy paste" appearance. Laboratory studies of the aspirate are essential.

Summary

Follow-up imaging studies often show that the abscesses are slow to resolve and can even worsen in appearance despite clinical improvement. This is not an indication for drainage. Almost all amebic abscesses will resolve with appropriate antibiotic therapy. Rupture of an amebic hepatic abscess into the peritoneal cavity or thorax occurs in approximately 2% of patients, and still generally responds well to medical therapy. Percutaneous drainage does play a role in the treatment of complicated amebic abscesses. Drainage is reserved for those patients who do not respond to amebicidal therapy, where superinfection occurs, when a fistula to bowel or the biliary system develops, and when pericardial rupture is threatened.

References

1. Seeto RK, Rockey DC. Pyogenic liver abscess: changes in etiology, management, and outcome. Medicine 1996; 75:99–113.

2. Hashimoto L, Hermann R, Grundfest-Broniatowski S. Pyogenic hepatic abscess: results of current management. Am Surg 1995; 61:407–411.

3. Farges O, Leese T, Bismuth H. Pyogenic liver abscess: an improvement in prognosis. Br J Surg 1988; 75:862–865.

4. Barreda R, Ros PR. Diagnostic imaging of liver abscesses. Crit Rev Diagn Imaging 1992; 33:29–58.

5. Lambiase RE, Deyoe L, Cronan JJ, Dorfman GS. Percutaneous drainage of 335 consecutive abscesses: results of primary drainage with 1-year follow-up. Radiology 1992; 184:167–179.

6. vanSonnenberg E, D'Agostino HB, Casola G, Halasz NA, Sanchez RB, Goodacre BW. Percutaneous abscess drainage: current concepts. Radiology 1991; 181:617–626.

7. Baek SY, Lee MG, Cho KS, Lee SC, Sung KB, Auh YH. Therapeutic percutaneous aspiration of hepatic abscesses: effectiveness in 25 patients. AJR 1993; 160:799–802.

8. Giorgio A, Tarantino L, Mariniello N, et al. Pyogenic liver abscesses: 13 years of experience in percutaneous needle aspiration with US guidance. Radiology 1995; 195:122–124.

9. Johnson RD, Mueller PR, Ferrucci JT, et al. Percutaneous drainage of pyogenic liver abscesses. AJR 1985; 144:463–467.

10. Wong KP. Percutaneous drainage of pyogenic liver abscesses. World J Surg 1990; 14:492–497.

11. el-Tahir MI, Omojola MF, Malatani T, al-Saigh AH, Ogunbiyi OA. Hydatid disease of the liver: evaluation of ultrasound and computed tomography. Br J Radiol 1992; 65:390–392.

12. Safioleas M, Misiakos E, Manti C, Katsikas D, Skalkeas G. Diagnostic evaluation and surgical management of hydatid disease of the liver. World J Surg 1994; 18:859–865.

13. Bastid C, Azar C, Doyer M, Sahel J. Percutaneous treatment of hydatid cysts under sonographic guidance. Dig Dis Sci 1994; 39:1576–1580.

14. Bret PM, Fond A, Bretagnolle M, et al. Percutaneous aspiration and drainage of hydatid cysts in the liver. Radiology 1988; 168:617–620.

15. Giorgio A, Tarantino L, Francica G, et al. Unilocular hydatid liver cysts: treatment with US-guided double percutaneous aspiration and alcohol injection. Radiology 1992; 184:705–710.

16. Ralls PW, Barnes PF, Johnson MB, De Cock KM, Radin DR, Halls J. Medical treatment of hepatic amebic abscess: rare need for percutaneous drainage. Radiology 1987; 165:805–807.

17. Van Allan RJ, Katz MD, Johnson MB, Laine LA, Liu Y, Ralls PW. Uncomplicated amebic liver abscess: prospective evaluation of percutaneous therapeutic aspiration. Radiology 1992; 183:827–830.

18. vanSonnenberg E, Mueller PR, Schiffman HR, et al. Intrahepatic amebic abscesses: indications for and results of percutaneous catheter drainage. Radiology 1985; 156:631–635.

19. Ken JG, vanSonnenberg E, Casola G, Christensen R, Polansky M. Perforated amebic liver abscesses: successful percutaneous treatment. Radiology 1989; 170:195–197.

20. Singh JP, Kashyap A. A comparative evaluation of percutaneous catheter drainage for resistant amebic liver abscesses. Am J Surg 1989; 158:58–62.

TUTORIAL 8
DRAINAGE OF DEEP PELVIC ABSCESSES INCLUDING TRANSGLUTEAL, TRANSRECTAL, AND TRANSVAGINAL APPROACHES

Jeet Sandhu, M.D.

Introduction

The subjects addressed in this tutorial include:

1. Etiology of deep pelvic abscesses
2. Approaches to drainage of deep pelvic abscesses
3. Results of deep pelvic abscess drainage.

The technique of percutaneous abscess drainage has been established as a safe, effective, minimally invasive means of treating infectious collections in almost all parts of the body.[1,2] The critical issue determining the feasibility of percutaneous abscess drainage is safe access to the collection. To perform safe percutaneous drainage, a clear path from the skin to the collection must exist with no intervening structures that could be traversed or damaged by the drainage catheter.

This same issue complicates drainage of pelvic abscesses because a simple anterior or anterolateral route cannot be used in most cases because of intervening structures such as the bladder, uterus, neurovascular structures, and small bowel or colon. Because of these intervening structures, alternative access routes must be considered for effective percutaneous drainage of pelvic abscesses.

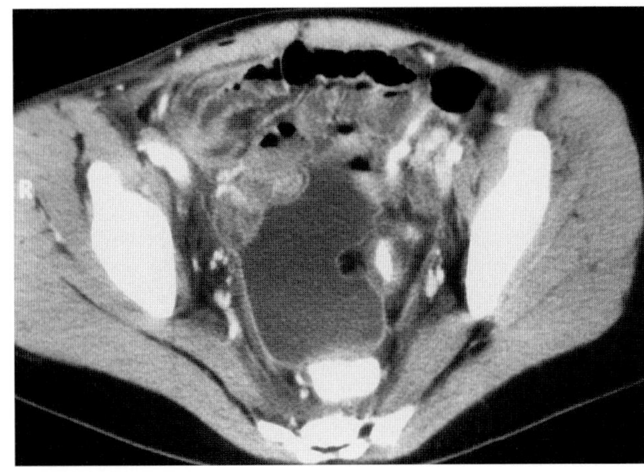

Figure 1. Deep pelvic abscess.

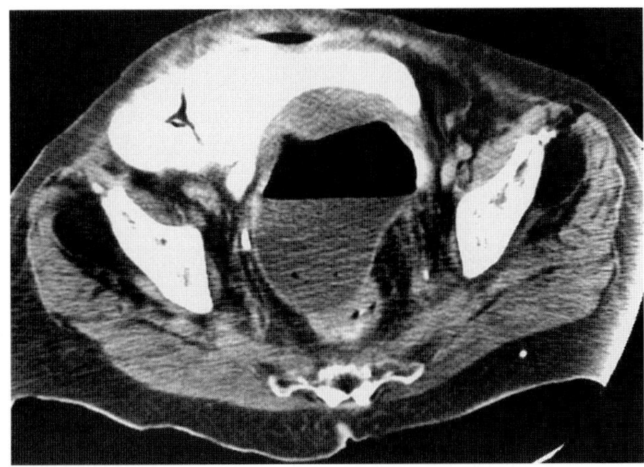

Figure 2. Abscess in the pouch of Douglas with air in the collection. This patient had a large fistula to the colon from diverticulitis.

Etiology

Because of the dependent location of the pelvis, especially the pouch of Douglas, it is not surprising that pelvic abscesses occur frequently, as any intraperitoneal free fluid tends to collect in the pelvis. One study of 335 abscesses throughout the body found that almost 25% of the abscesses were located in the pelvis.[2]

Pelvic abscesses most frequently occur postoperatively, after bowel resections for malignant or benign disease, after gynecologic or urologic procedures such as cystectomy or hysterectomy, and after appendectomy. In the series described by Lambiase, 71% of the pelvic abscesses occurred after surgery.[2] Spontaneous causes of pelvic abscesses include diverticulitis, appendicitis, and inflammatory bowel disease, especially Crohn's disease.[3] Pelvic hematomas from pelvic trauma or surgery can become infected and lead to pelvic abscesses. Iatrogenic injury to the bowel from colonoscopy or polypectomy may also cause pelvic abscesses.

Clinical Signs and Symptoms

As with abscesses elsewhere in the body, patients typically present with fever, leukocytosis, and pain. Symptoms specific to a pelvic abscess may include intractable diarrhea, tenesmus, and pain on voiding.

The radiographic appearance of pelvic abscesses is similar to that of abscesses elsewhere in the body. Most abscesses appear as a unilocular fluid collection with an enhancing rim **(Fig. 1)**. Infiltration and stranding of the adjacent soft tissues and fat planes are commonly seen. Air may be present in the fluid collection and usually suggests the possibility of a fistulous communication to the bowel and less often represents gas-forming organisms **(Fig. 2)**.

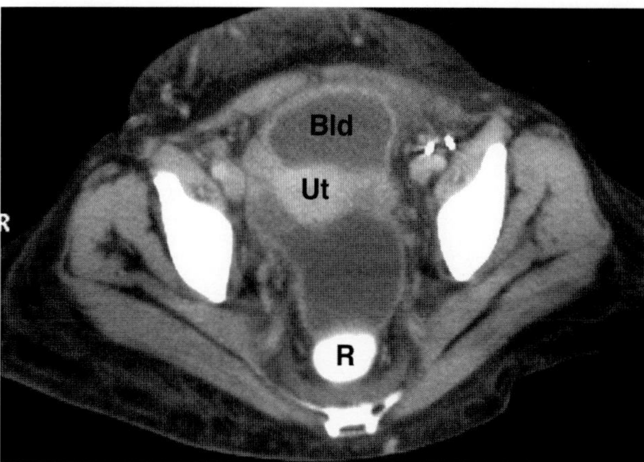

Figure 3. Postoperative fluid collection in the pouch of Douglas with an enhancing rim suggestive of an abscess. R=rectum; Bld=bladder; Ut=uterus.

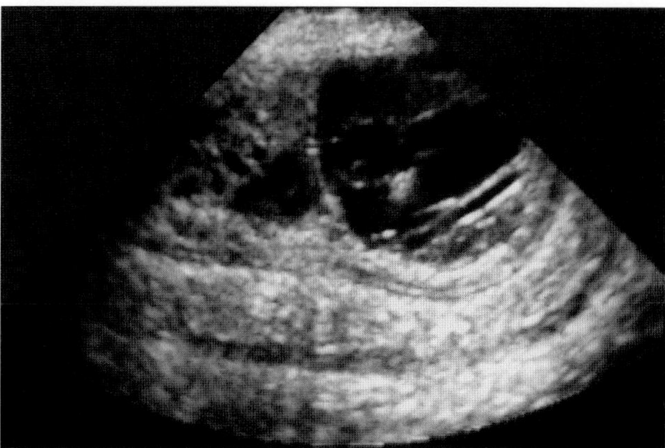

Figure 4. Same patient as in Figure 3. Endovaginal scan demonstrates multiple thick septations with a multiloculated appearance.

Although the abscess may appear unilocular on computed tomography (CT) evaluation **(Fig. 3)**, ultrasound examination of the same collection frequently demonstrates a more complex appearance with multiple septations and loculations **(Fig. 4)**. This multiloculated appearance should not be a deterrent to percutaneous drainage because most of these cavities will communicate with each other and placement of a drainage catheter in the largest cavity usually leads to adequate resolution of the entire abscess.

Preprocedural Evaluation

As with other interventional procedures, informed consent should be obtained from the patient or appropriate guardian or family member. Any coagulopathy should be corrected as much as possible. Ideally, the prothrombin time should be less than 16 seconds, and fresh frozen plasma or vitamin K should be used as needed to normalize it. In addition, the platelet count should be greater than 50,000. Before a suspected infected collection is drained, the patient should receive intravenous antibiotics to minimize the risk of systemic bacteremia. All previous imaging studies should be reviewed to determine the optimal access route and to avoid transgressing any vital intervening structures.

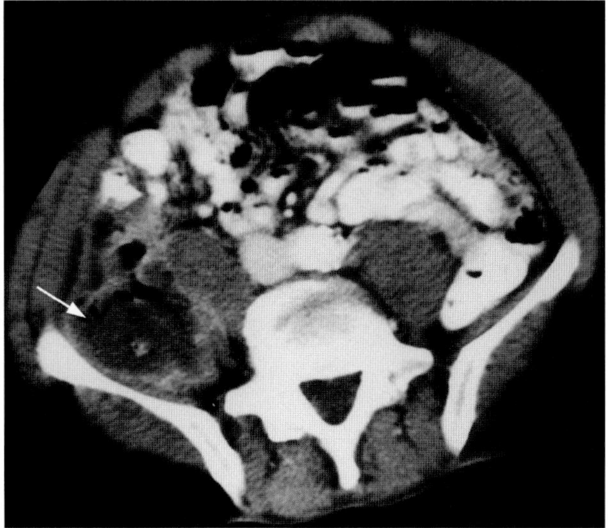

Figure 5. Right iliacus abscess from appendicitis. An angled approach (arrow) immediately above the iliac wing allows an anterior approach and avoids any intervening structures.

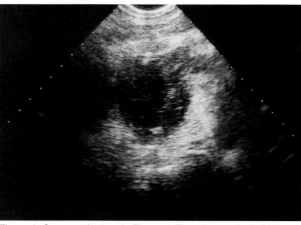

Figure 6. Same patient as in Figure 5. The abscess is well visualized with sonography, which can be used for needle guidance into the collection.

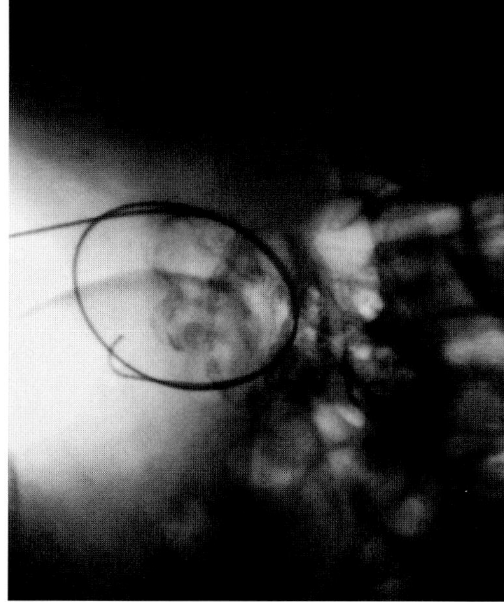

Figure 7. Same patient as in Figure 5. Wire coiled in the collection.

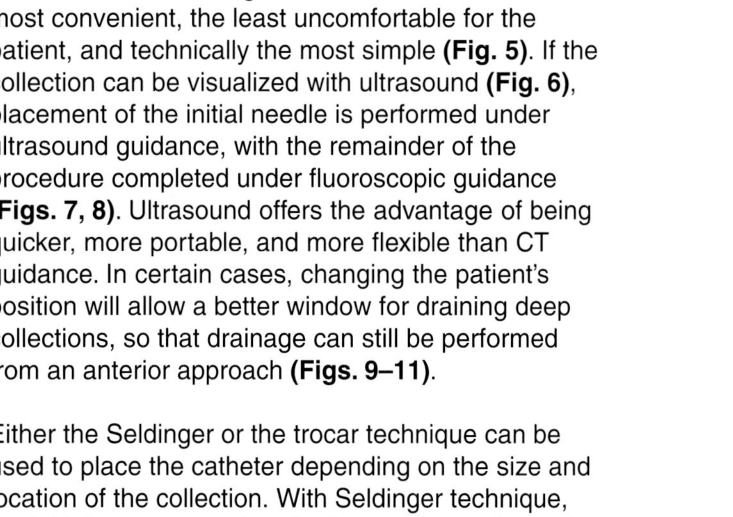

An access route into the pelvic abscess through the anterior or anterolateral abdominal wall is the preferred route for draining the abscess because it is the most convenient, the least uncomfortable for the patient, and technically the most simple **(Fig. 5)**. If the collection can be visualized with ultrasound **(Fig. 6)**, placement of the initial needle is performed under ultrasound guidance, with the remainder of the procedure completed under fluoroscopic guidance **(Figs. 7, 8)**. Ultrasound offers the advantage of being quicker, more portable, and more flexible than CT guidance. In certain cases, changing the patient's position will allow a better window for draining deep collections, so that drainage can still be performed from an anterior approach **(Figs. 9–11)**.

Either the Seldinger or the trocar technique can be used to place the catheter depending on the size and location of the collection. With Seldinger technique, the initial puncture and aspiration can be performed with small 21- or 22-gauge needles followed by conversion to standard 0.035-inch or 0.038-inch wires with use of a Cope, Neff, or Accustick set. If the collection is particularly viscous or no fluid can be aspirated through the small needle after its location within the collection has been confirmed, initial access can be obtained with an 18-gauge needle and direct placement of an 0.038-inch or 0.035-inch wire.

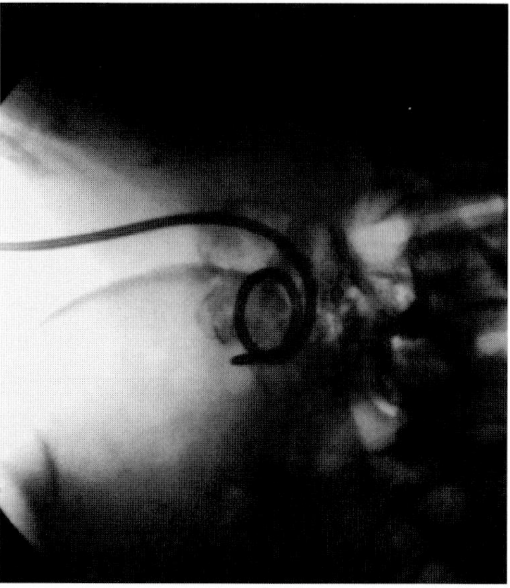

Figure 8. Same patient as in Figure 5. Placement of an 8-F locking Cope loop drainage catheter which successfully resolved the abscess. No fistula was present on the sinogram.

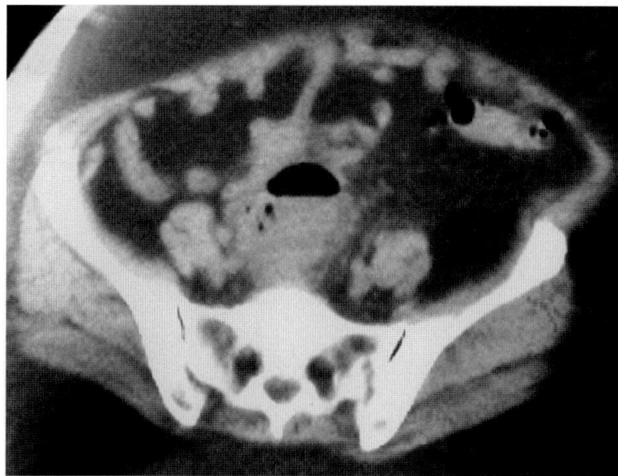

Figure 9. Deep diverticular abscess with limited pathway to the collection.

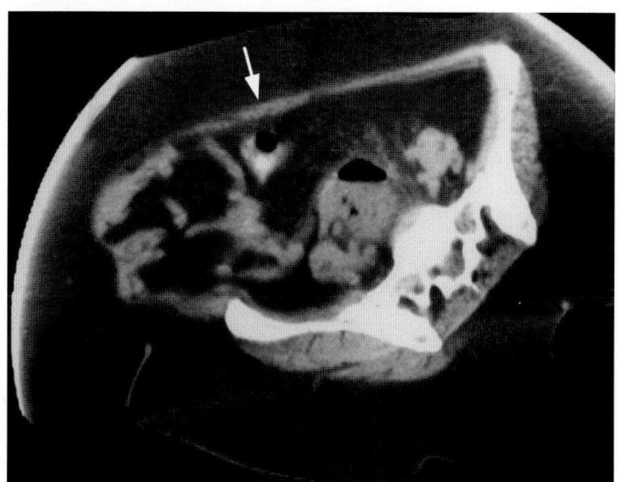

Figure 10. Placing the patient in the right posterior oblique position shifts away many of the intervening structures, especially the colon (arrow), and provides a good window for drainage of the collection.

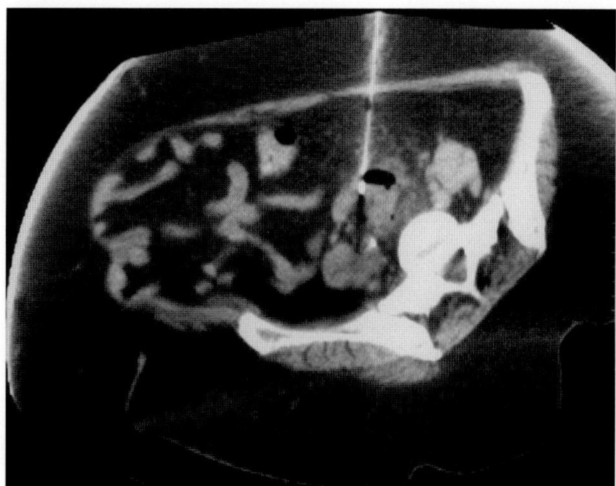

Figure 11. Successful drainage of the collection.

Catheter Management

Regardless of the access route, several general principles govern catheter management. Once the catheter has been inserted into the abscess cavity, all of the material is aspirated. For most collections, an 8-F catheter will suffice, but larger catheters can be placed if needed. A locking catheter may be helpful to prevent inadvertent removal or expulsion of the catheter. This is especially important for endocavitary drainages because there are minimal means of securing the catheter externally. The abscess cavity is irrigated with aliquots of sterile saline, approximately half of the initial volume of the cavity, until the return is clear. To minimize the risk of inducing systemic bacteremia, a small amount of contrast material is injected to confirm appropriate catheter placement, but a complete initial sinogram is not obtained at that time.

The catheter should be flushed with 5–10 mL of sterile saline at least twice a day to maintain catheter patency. The daily output of the catheter is recorded. If the patient has not become afebrile and clinically stable within 48 to 72 hours, a repeat CT scan should be obtained to evaluate for any undrained or residual collections. Once the catheter output has decreased to less than 10 mL per day, catheter removal can be considered. Before the catheter is removed, a contrast sinogram should be obtained to exclude any fistulous communication as well as to assess the size of the cavity. If no fistula is seen and the cavity size conforms to the catheter loop size, the catheter may be removed. Fistulas are rarely identified on the initial sinogram, which is why a complete sinogram is not obtained at the time of initial catheter drainage.

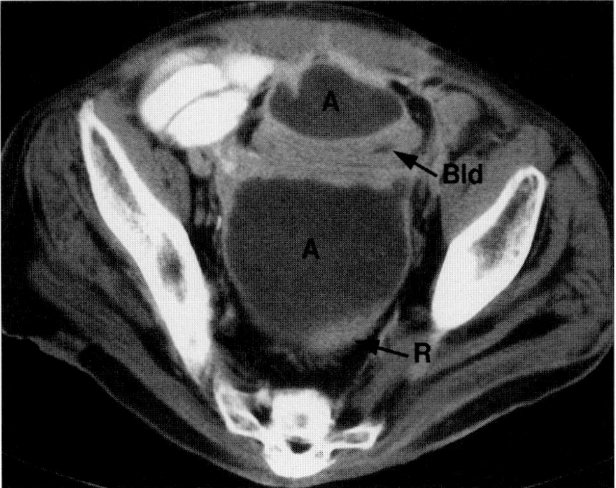

Figure 12. Patient with two separate abscesses (A). The one anterior to the bladder (Bld) can be drained from an anterior approach. An anterior approach is not possible for the posterior collection due to numerous overlying and intervening structures. R=rectum.

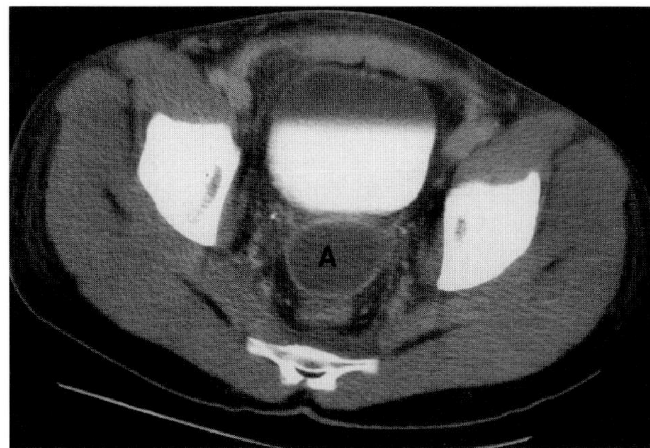

Figure 13. Appendiceal abscess (A).

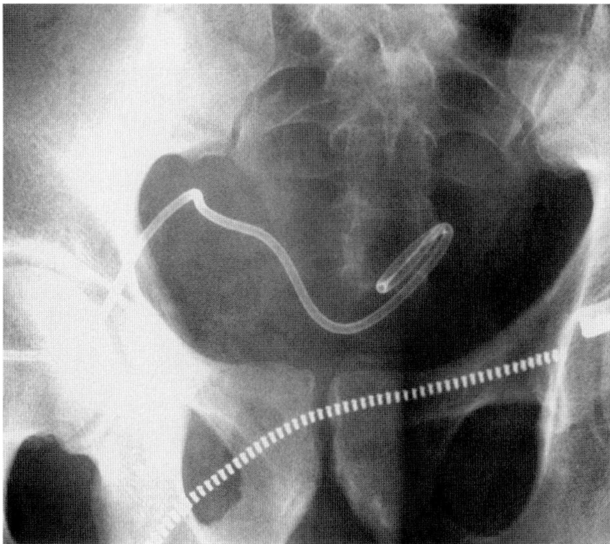

Figure 14. Same patient as in Figure 13. Placement of a drainage catheter into the collection from a transgluteal approach. Note the desired position immediately adjacent to the sacrum.

Transgluteal Drainage

As noted previously, no safe anterior access route exists for some pelvic abscesses **(Fig. 12)**. In such cases, the transgluteal or transsciatic approach can be used to access deep pelvic abscesses via the greater sciatic foramen.[4] Because of the complex anatomy of the greater sciatic foramen and the need for precise needle deployment, at least the initial needle and wire placement must be performed under CT guidance. Although the procedure can be completed under CT guidance, it is better to complete the catheter insertion, dilation, and guide wire exchange under fluoroscopic guidance to prevent buckling of the wire and catheters in the tissues of the buttock **(Figs. 13, 14)**.

The piriformis muscle **(Fig. 15)** courses through the sciatic foramen and is an important landmark in preventing injury to other structures in the sciatic foramen. The superior and inferior gluteal arteries and veins and the internal pudendal artery are located in the cephalad aspect of the greater sciatic foramen. The greater sciatic foramen also contains the sciatic nerve, which runs immediately posterior to the ischial spine.

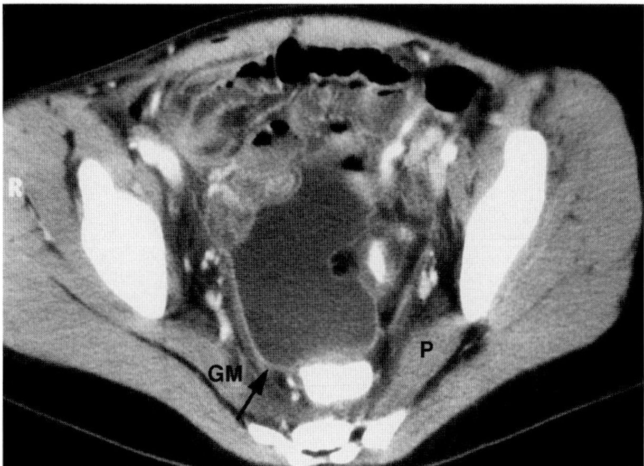

Figure 15. Piriformis (P) and gluteus medius (GM) muscles. A transgluteal drainage could be performed at this level from the right side (arrow) but could not be performed on the left due to the piriformis.

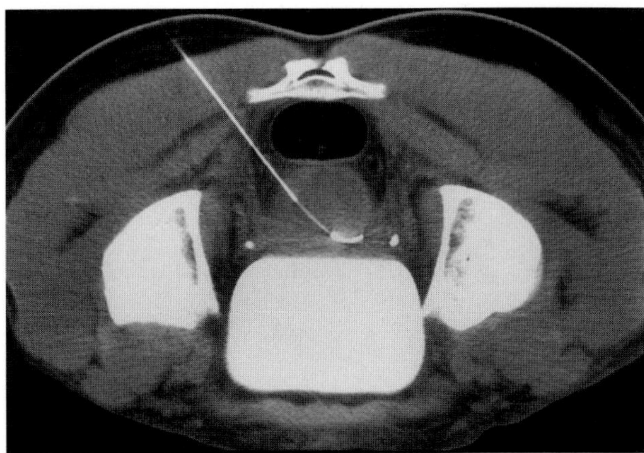

Figure 16. Transgluteal drainage of an appendiceal abscess.

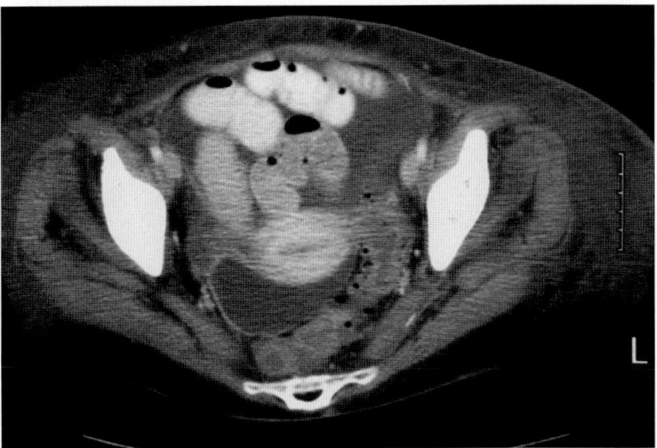

Figure 17. Abscess at the level of the piriformis.

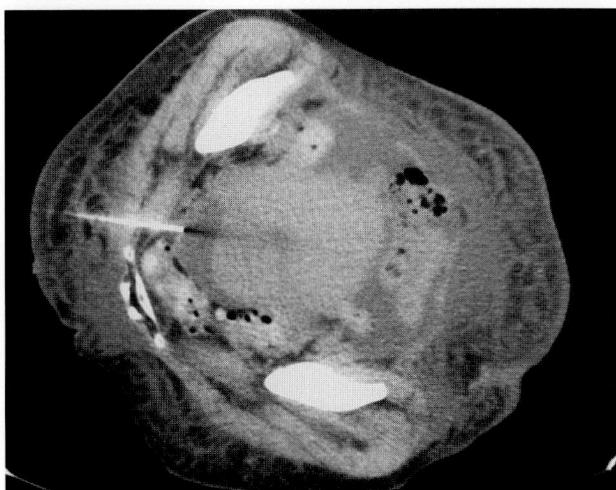

Figure 18. Transgluteal drainage through the inferior edge of the piriformis without complication.

Because most of the neurovascular structures are located superior and lateral to the piriformis muscle, every attempt should be made to stay inferior to the piriformis muscle and as adjacent to the sacrum as possible when performing a transgluteal drainage **(Fig. 16)**. If this pathway is followed, the neurovascular structures can be avoided. Occasionally the needle transgresses the piriformis muscle when it enters the collection **(Figs. 17, 18)**. This approach may be necessitated by the cephalad location of the abscess and usually does not cause any serious problems. However, catheters immediately adjacent to or through the piriformis muscle have a higher incidence of persistent pain.

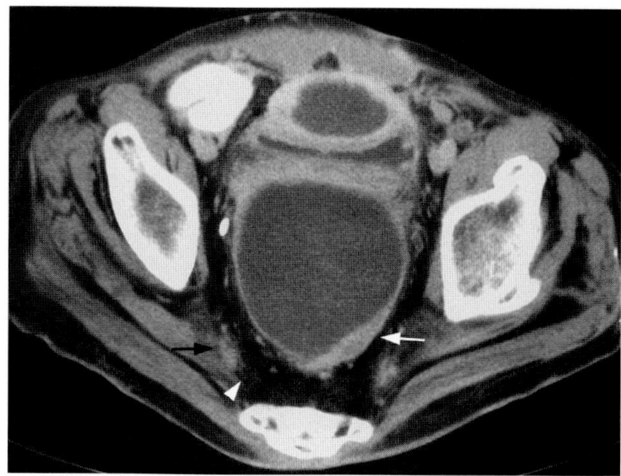

Figure 19. The transgluteal approach on the left is limited by the intervening rectum (white arrow). The inferior gluteal vessels (black arrow) are perilously close to the path for transgluteal drainage (arrowhead) on the right.

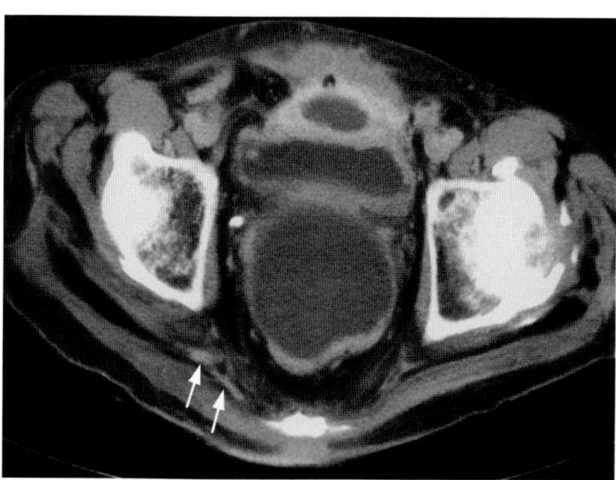

Figure 20. Same patient as in Figure 19. A more inferior image shows the inferior gluteal vessels again (arrows).

In the series described by Butch et al, transgluteal drainage was technically successful in 100% of cases and resulted in cure of the abscess in 80% of cases.[4] Despite the technical and therapeutic success of transgluteal drainage of pelvic abscesses, significant problems are associated with this approach. Numerous vascular structures run through the sciatic foramen and the possibility always exists that one of the vessels may be injured during the transgluteal drainage procedure **(Figs. 19, 20)**. This consideration is not theoretical; actual injury to branches of the internal iliac artery has occurred secondary to transgluteal drainage.[5]

In addition to complications from the procedure itself, transgluteal drainage is relatively painful for patients. Butch et al found that 20% of patients had persistent pain after catheter insertion.[4] This was likely related to irritation of the sacral plexus or sciatic nerve by the catheter. After removal of the catheter the symptoms resolved without any untoward sequelae. During transgluteal drainage, catheter insertion itself induces significant pain and a considerable amount of intravenous sedation is required. Because the catheter exits in the immediate lower lateral aspect of the gluteal muscles, it may be uncomfortable and inconvenient for the patient to sit or lie down with the catheter in place. The fascial planes and muscular contractions of the gluteal muscles may cause the catheter to become kinked and dysfunctional, resulting in suboptimal drainage. Because of these drawbacks to the transgluteal approach, a group of authors concluded that "...it [transgluteal drainage] is now considered a method of last resort."[6]

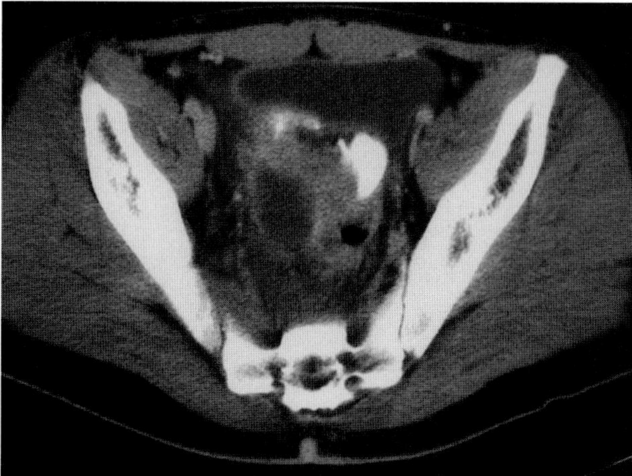

Figure 21. 4-cm pelvic abscess. An anterior approach is not possible, and the location high in the pelvis precludes a transgluteal approach.

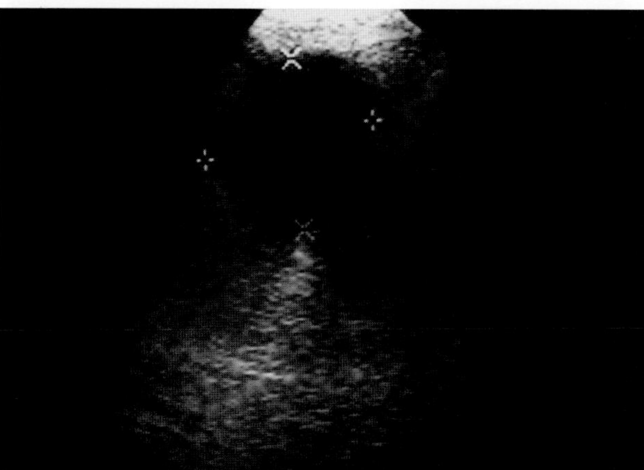

Figure 22. Same patient as in Figure 21. The collection could be visualized transrectally by ultrasound, and transrectal drainage was performed.

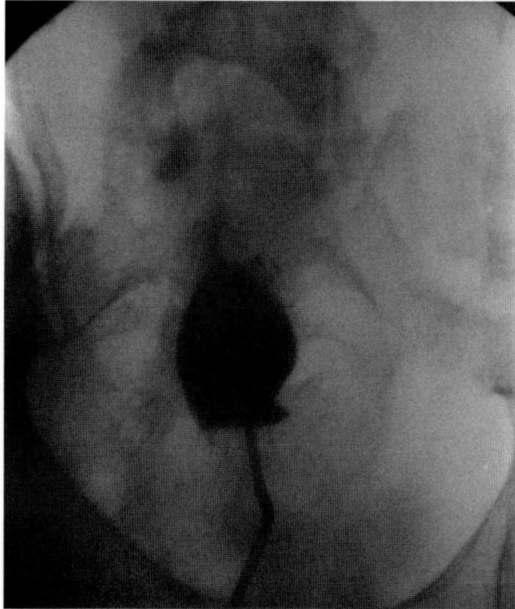

Figure 23. Same patient as in Figure 21. Contrast sinogram confirms the appropriate location of the catheter after transrectal drainage of the collection. The initial injection shows no fistula but the patient was found to have an appendiceal fistula on his follow-up sinogram.

Endoluminal Drainage

Endoluminal drainage via a transvaginal or transrectal approach is the preferred technique for draining deep pelvic abscesses.[7,8] Even if it is thought that transgluteal drainage should or could be performed, certain collections are totally inaccessible even from a transgluteal route because of their location. This leaves an endoluminal approach as the only alternative for nonsurgical drainage of such abscesses **(Figs. 21–23)**. Consequently, the ability to perform endocavitary drainages is an important skill, and the remainder of this tutorial will be devoted to the techniques of transrectal and transvaginal drainage.

Surgical transrectal and transvaginal drainage of pelvic abscess are well-established techniques.[9,10] Despite the utility of surgical drainage, there are significant limitations to this approach. Surgical drainage requires that the abscess can be palpated through the vaginal or rectal wall. Surgical drainage is more invasive than simple percutaneous catheter placement because it requires an incision large enough to permit the introduction of a finger into the cavity. Many of the early surgical procedures were beset by failure due to closure of the track or expulsion of the drains, and daily digital or instrumental dilation of the track was recommended until the cavity was completely evacuated.[10] Catheter-based drainage has obviated the need for daily dilation and surmounted many of the other problems associated with surgical transrectal drainage.

Mauro and Jaques were the first radiologists to perform a catheter-based transrectal drainage.[11] The initial radiologic procedures relied on fluoroscopic guidance with visualization of the abscess bulging into the rectum. The addition of endoluminal ultrasound has circumvented the need to visualize the abscess bulging into the rectum or vagina.

Nosher first described the use of ultrasound guidance to perform a transrectal drainage.[12] With the use of transabdominal ultrasound through a distended bladder, he was able to guide a catheter into the abscess collection from a transrectal approach. Since the early description of the technique, transrectal drainage of pelvic abscesses has been described using fluoroscopic,[13] CT,[14] and endorectal ultrasound guidance.[15,16] Transvaginal drainage of deep pelvic abscesses via endovaginal ultrasound guidance has also become a well-established technique.[17–21]

Transrectal and Transvaginal Drainage

Numerous factors will determine the route of drainage—transrectal versus transvaginal—and the mode of guidance—fluoroscopy versus endoluminal ultrasound versus transabdominal ultrasound.

In certain patients, especially small children, the endovaginal probe is too large to be placed either endovaginally or endorectally due to the patient's small size **(Fig. 24)**. In these patients, transrectal drainage can still be performed but transabdominal ultrasound guidance in conjunction with transrectal digitally assisted needle advancement is used.[12,22] With this approach, a finger is placed into the rectum to localize the abscess. With the use of transabdominal ultrasound, the needle is advanced alongside the finger into the collection and a drainage catheter is placed with standard techniques from a transrectal approach. Because the small size of these patients makes visualization of the rectal finger and the needle relatively easy, transabdominal ultrasound almost always identifies and delineates the collection.

Obviously, either transvaginal or transrectal drainage can be performed in females while only a transrectal approach can be used in males. In female patients, if the abscess collection is anterior to the vagina, a transrectal approach would not be warranted because the vagina or cervix may have to be traversed to reach the collection. In these cases, the transvaginal approach should be used. Conversely, presacral abscesses should always be accessed from a transrectal approach; an endovaginal approach would necessitate crossing the rectum, which should be avoided. If a collection can be approached either transvaginally or transrectally, the route of access will depend on operator and patient preference. The approach that provides the shortest distance and safest path to the collection should be chosen. However, transvaginal drainage should be avoided in premenarchal and virginal females because of the psychosocial issues involved. Since transrectal drainages are a bit easier to perform from a technical standpoint, it may be reasonable, all other factors being equal, to drain the collection from a transrectal approach.

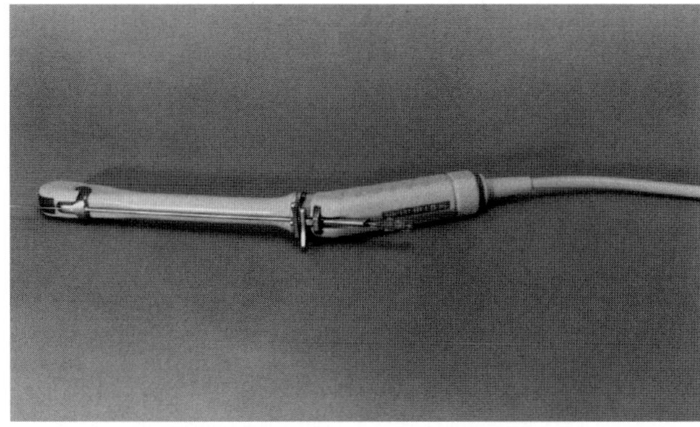

Figure 24. Endovaginal probe with needle guide.

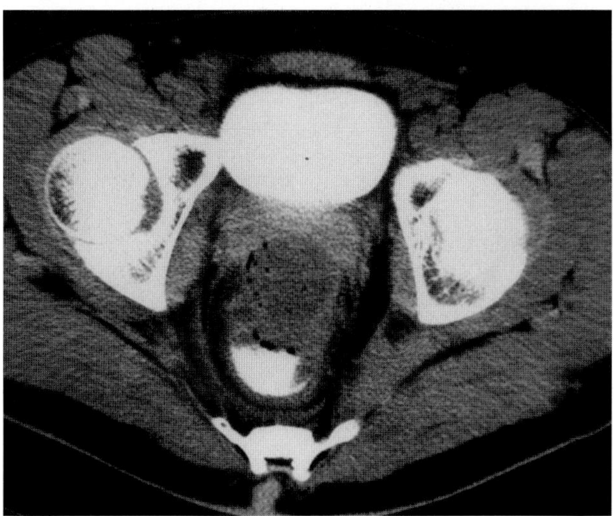

Figure 25. Inferior extent of a large pelvic abscess at the level of the seminal vesicles and fovea capitalis of the femoral head.

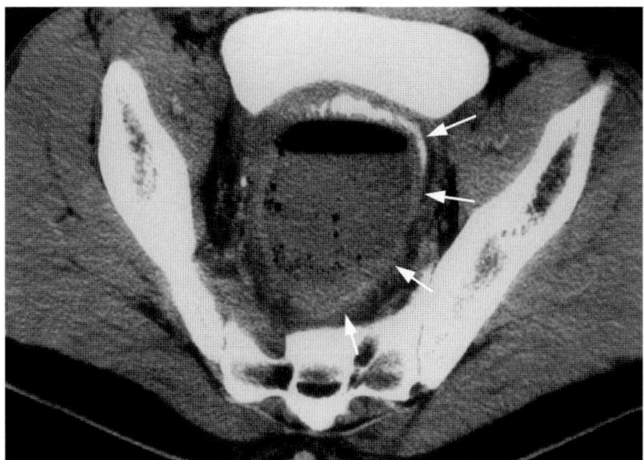

Figure 26. Same patient as in Figure 25. More superior extent of the pelvic abscess. Given the large size and intimate relationship of the abscess to the rectum, a fluoroscopically guided transrectal drainage can easily be performed. Using the mid femoral head as a landmark from the CT scan, the abscess can be entered safely. The rectum and sigmoid colon (arrows) are draped around the abscess.

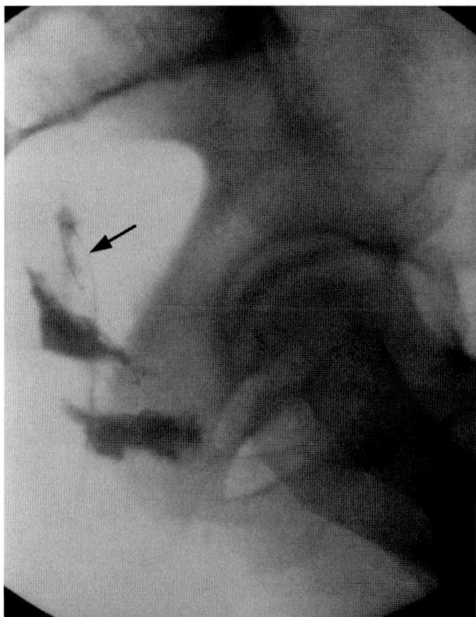

Figure 27. Same patient as in Figure 25. Lateral fluoroscopic view during fluoroscopically guided transrectal drainage of the collection. Contrast material injected through the transrectal hemostatic sheath outlines the rectum. A 21-gauge needle is inserted over a mandril wire (arrow) to the appropriate puncture level (top of femoral head) and directed anteriorly through the rectal wall into the collection.

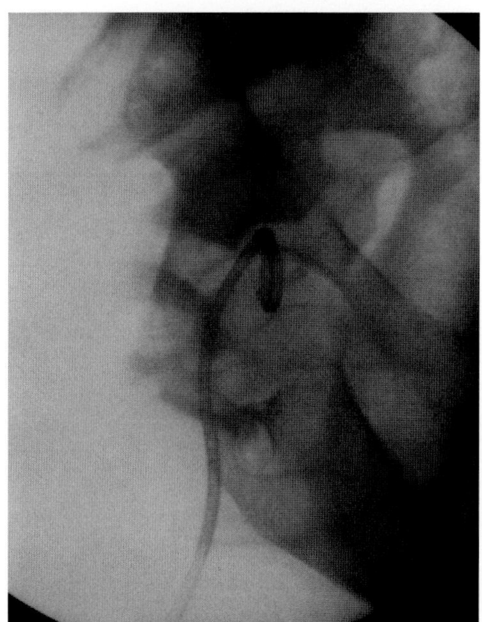

Figure 29. Same patient as in Figure 25. 8-F locking pigtail catheter advanced over the wire in the abscess.

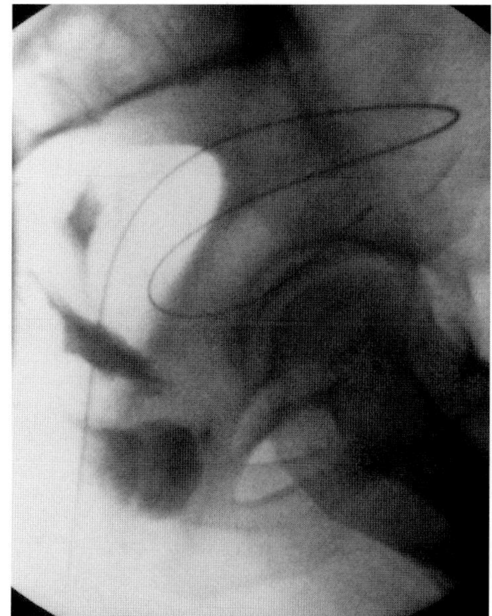

Figure 28. Same patient as in Figure 25. Wire coiled in the abscess collection after the needle was advanced.

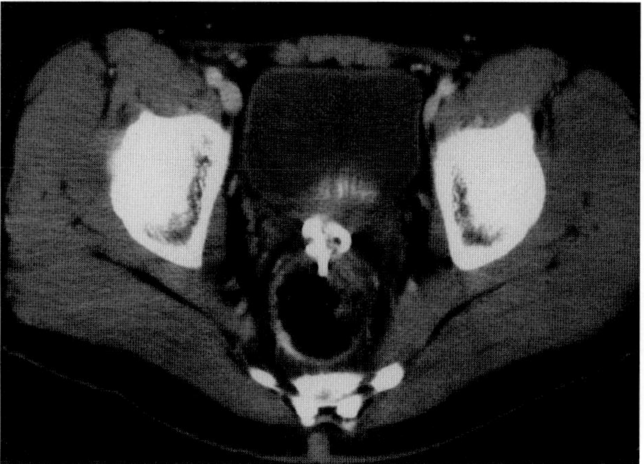

Figure 30. Same patient as in Figure 25. Follow-up CT scan after drainage of the abscess depicts resolution of the abscess, with the transrectal catheter in place.

Fluoroscopic Guidance

Certain collections are large enough **(Figs. 25, 26)** that the entire drainage procedure can be performed under fluoroscopic guidance without the use of endoluminal or transabdominal ultrasound. The appropriate puncture level can be determined from landmarks on the CT study. When a fluoroscopic-guided puncture is performed, a hemostatic sheath is inserted into the rectum to protect the anal verge and rectal mucosa. A small amount of contrast material is injected through the hemostatic sheath to delineate the rectum, and a needle (18–22 gauge) is inserted through the sheath over a wire and directed appropriately based on the CT findings **(Fig. 27)**. With a short thrust, the needle is inserted into the collection and the wire advanced through the needle after the return of pus is confirmed **(Fig. 28)**.

Depending on the viscosity of the fluid, an 8–12-F locking pigtail catheter can then be placed over the guide wire into the collection **(Fig. 29)**. Clinical and radiographic follow-up is performed to document resolution of the abscess **(Fig. 30)**.

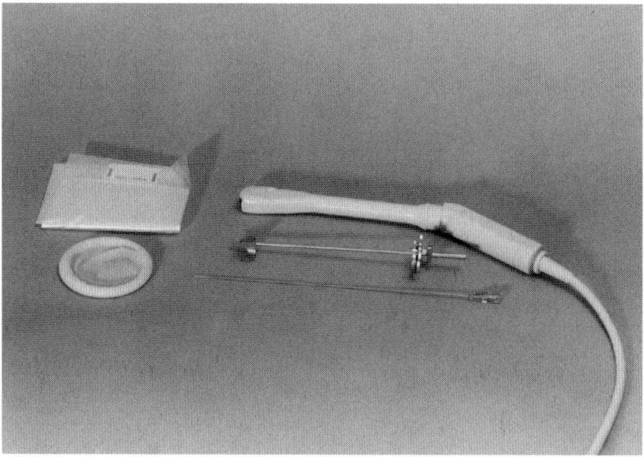

Figure 31. Components for endoluminal drainage. Clockwise starting from the lower left: condom for probe; sleeve to cover the transducer; endocavitary probe; needle guide; 20-gauge 20-cm-long puncture needle.

Transrectal Drainage

In cases where smaller collections are present and fluoroscopic guidance alone is insufficient, endorectal ultrasound guidance can be used for placement of the needle into the collection. No special patient preparation is needed for transrectal drainage. Cleansing enemas are not needed because most patients are postoperative and probably are not eating. Even in patients who are not postoperative, the underlying clinical problem causing the abscess produces symptoms such that the patient is not eating very much, either. As a result, the amount of feces in the rectum is usually minimal.

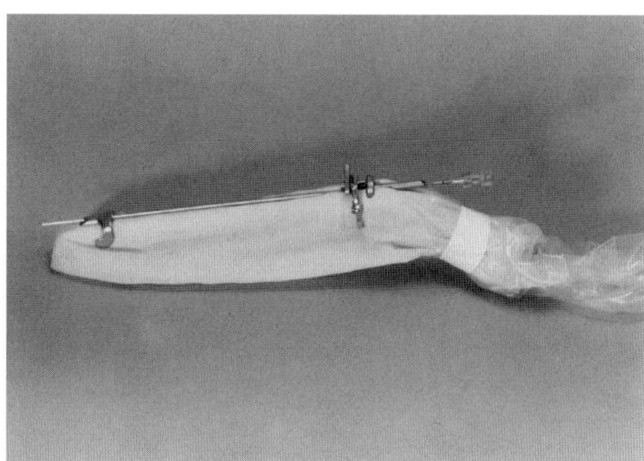

Figure 32. Components assembled for needle puncture.

The patient is placed in a left lateral decubitus position. The perianal area is cleaned with Betadine and a drape is placed over the anal orifice. Gel is placed in the condom and the probe is covered with the condom and secured **(Fig. 31)**. The probe is then inserted into the rectum to evaluate the relationship of the abscess to the rectum and to determine whether a clear and safe path exists for placement of the needle. If it is determined that the abscess is accessible, the probe is removed and the needle guide is attached **(Fig. 32)**. Because of the needle guide needed for transrectal and transvaginal drainages, 20–30-cm-long needles 18–20 gauge in diameter are required. The 18–20-gauge needle is then inserted through the needle guide. On the monitor, the dashed line will indicate the expected course of the needle **(Fig. 33)**. The needle or trocar sheath is then advanced through the needle guide until the tip of the needle is in the collection **(Fig. 34)**. It is important to avoid the prostate when advancing the needle. The stylet is removed and fluid or pus is aspirated. This initial aspirate should be saved for microbiologic analysis. With the probe still in place, a guide wire is advanced through the needle and coiled in the collection. Because the probe is still in place, the wire can be seen to enter the collection **(Fig. 35)**.

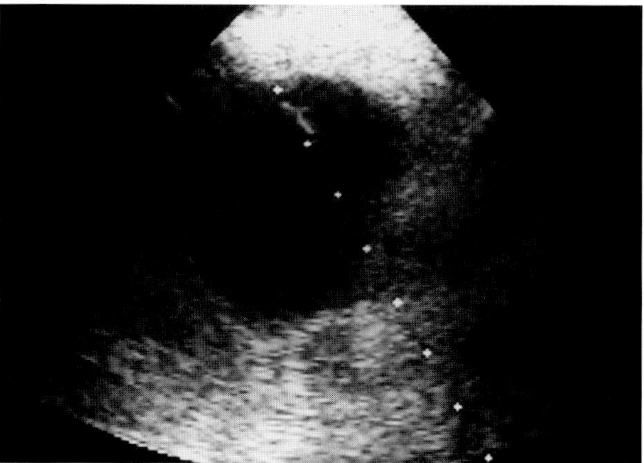

Figure 33. Needle advancing along the expected puncture course for drainage of a pelvic abscess.

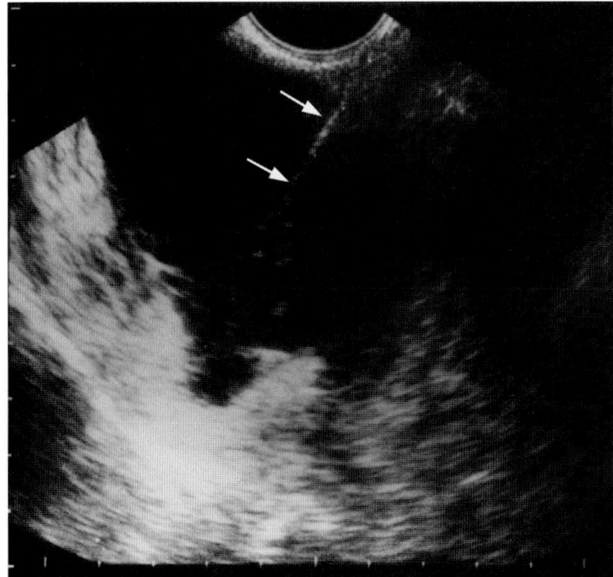

Figure 34. Needle (arrows) in a collection through which a wire has been advanced.

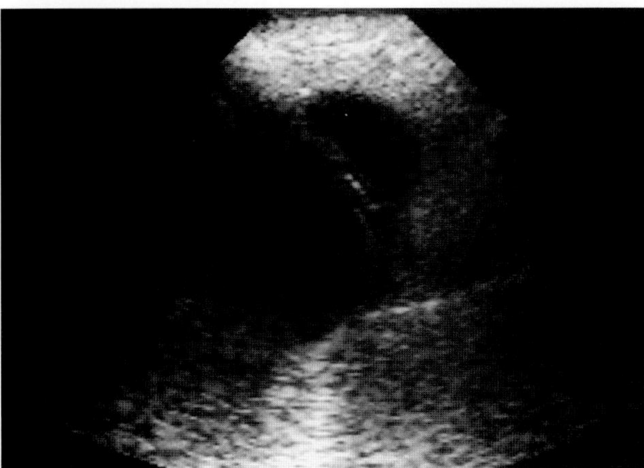

Figure 35. Wire coiled in the cavity.

The appropriate location of the wire in the collection can also be observed fluoroscopically, and ideally the procedure is performed on a fluoroscopy table with the ultrasound machine there. Having both ultrasound and fluoroscopy available eliminates the need to transport the patient and risk inadvertent wire dislodgement. The needle is removed over the wire. The endocavitary probe is then removed over the wire while the wire is kept in position within the abscess cavity. The remainder of the procedure can then be completed in standard fashion with the use of fascial dilators to enlarge the transrectal puncture site to the appropriate size. A locking pigtail catheter is then placed within the cavity, which is evacuated and irrigated in normal fashion, after which the catheter is placed to bulb suction. Catheter management is as previously described.

Some controversy exists concerning the need for catheter drainage versus simple needle aspiration of the abscess.[6,21] Kuligowska et al aspirate and lavage the collection from a transrectal approach without placing a catheter. Abscess aspiration and lavage is performed in conjunction with a course of intravenous and oral antibiotics. In their paper, 28 of 33 collections resolved without any additional treatment. Although simple aspiration and lavage works well, it should probably be reserved for smaller unilocular collections with no evidence of internal septations. Complex abscess collections should have catheter drainage to ensure complete evacuation of all components of the cavity.

Feld et al used the patient's clinical history and the character of the aspirate to decide whether to perform an aspiration or place a catheter. If the aspirated material was purulent or the clinical history was strongly suspicious for infection, a catheter was placed. If the aspirated material was not grossly purulent and the clinical suspicion for infection was moderate to low, only an aspiration was performed. In half of the patients in whom aspiration was performed and the material was not thought to be infected, the culture results were actually positive. Therefore, the character of the aspirated fluid is not a reliable indicator for determining whether or not to place a catheter. Because placement of a catheter is only minimally more involved than needle aspiration alone, catheter placement can be performed pending the culture results.

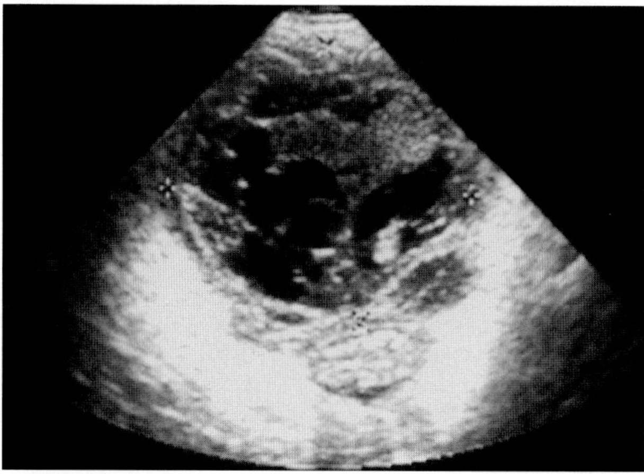

Figure 36. Endovaginal sonogram of a complex infected hematoma.

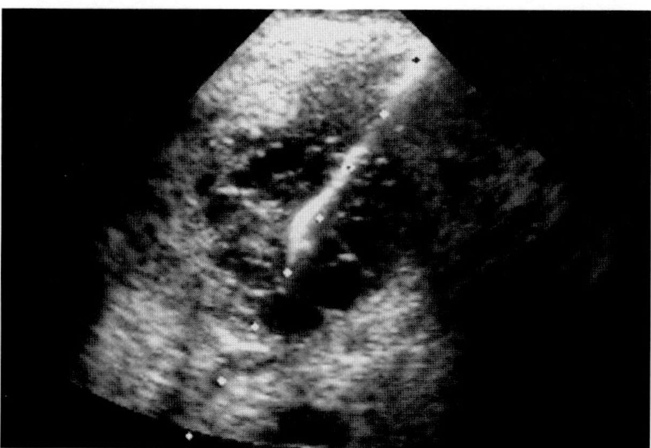

Figure 37. Transvaginal insertion of a needle into the collection. Some pus and old blood were obtained.

The other rationale for catheter placement is that any enteric fistula will be controlled and possibly even treated with the catheter in place. In one series, fistulas were present in 36% of the abdominal abscesses that were drained.[23] Although the number of fistulas associated with pelvic abscesses is not known, if a fistula is present, the abscess will likely recur with simple aspiration alone. Catheter placement with follow-up sinography will identify any fistula, and external drainage of the fistula may allow healing and preclude the necessity of surgical intervention.

Transvaginal Drainage

Many of the same principles apply to transvaginal drainage as to transrectal drainage. The probe and needle guide are prepared in the same fashion. The patient is placed supine with the legs placed to the side in a flexed position. The introitus is cleansed with Betadine and a drape is placed over the vaginal orifice. The probe is inserted and the needle advanced through the needle guide until it is within the collection **(Figs. 36, 37)**. The cervix should always be avoided when planning the needle trajectory. The guide wire is then coiled in the collection and the probe and needle are removed **(Fig. 38)**. Unlike the rectum with its relatively thin, compliant walls, the vaginal walls are much more elastic and thus resistant to dilation and even initial needle entry. Also, because of the distance between the rectal or vaginal orifice and the puncture site, there is a significant gap in which buckling of the wire and catheter may occur. A relatively stiff wire such as the Amplatz Super Stiff wire (Medi-Tech, Boston Scientific Corporation, Watertown, MA) should be used.

A straightened Colapinto needle can be used to provide enough rigidity to the guide wire to allow sufficient dilation of the vaginal wall for placement of a catheter.[24] An alternative is to use a trimmed van Andel 8-F catheter mounted on the inner metal stiffener of the locking pigtail catheter as the fascial dilator **(Fig. 39)**. Because of the noncompliant elastic nature of the vaginal tissues, fluoroscopic guidance is mandatory to prevent inadvertent loss of access due to buckling or kinking of the guide wire.

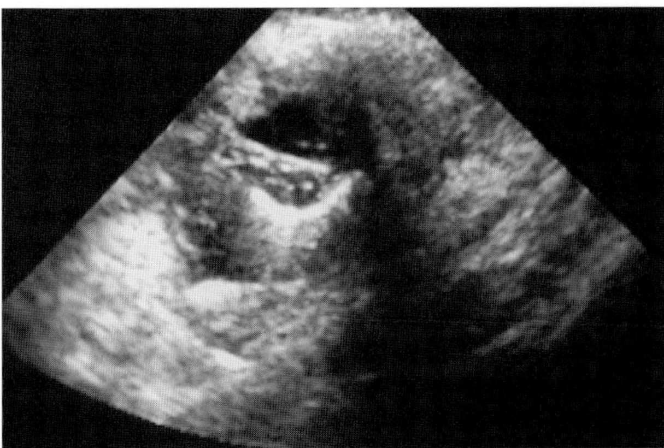

Figure 38. Wire coiled in the collection. Prolonged drainage of the collection eventually resulted in resolution of the hematoma.

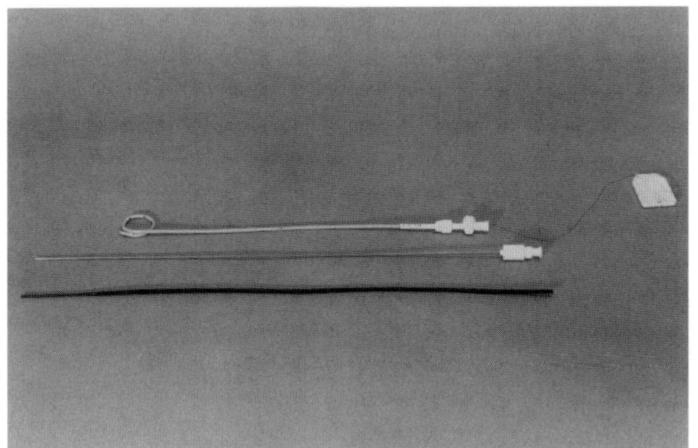

Figure 39. 8-F van Andel catheter (bottom) can be mounted on the stiffener of the drainage catheter and used as a dilator. The metal cannula provides support and stability.

Results

As noted previously, almost any pelvic abscess is accessible from a transvaginal or transrectal approach. Complications attributable to the transvaginal or transrectal approach are minimal and the catheter placement is well tolerated by patients. There has been one report of a vaginal fistula after endovaginal drainage.[21] The success rates for endocavitary drainage vary from 80%–100%.[15,16,19,21] The abscess will be treated in most cases but the patient may still require surgery for other reasons such as appendectomy, bowel resection, or treatment of a persistent fistula. In patients who eventually require surgical treatment, initial abscess drainage can facilitate and simplify the surgical approach and often converts a multistage procedure into a single-stage operation. Abscess drainage will also improve the patient's condition for surgery.

Causes of drainage failure include drainage of tumors, hematomas, or complex abscesses with significant undrained components. Most enteric fistulas can be controlled and even treated but those from Crohn's disease may require surgical bowel resection to resolve the underlying cause of the abscess. Postoperative abscesses, diverticulitis, and appendiceal abscesses are almost always treated with catheter drainage alone. So far, there have been no reports of superinfection of noninfected collections from a transvaginal or transrectal drainage. As noted by Finne, the natural pressure gradients during defecation tend to force fluid and abscess contents from the collection into the rectum instead of vice versa.[9]

Transrectal and transvaginal drainage of deep pelvic abscesses expands the interventional arsenal and provides a safe, relatively noninvasive, and well-accepted alternative to surgical drainage of the abscess.

References

1. vanSonnenberg E, D'Agostino HB, Casola G, Halasz NA, Sanchez RB, Goodacre BW. Percutaneous abscess drainage: current concepts. Radiology 1991; 181:617–626.

2. Lambiase RE, Deyoe L, Cronan JJ, Dorfman GS. Percutaneous drainage of 335 consecutive abscesses: results of primary drainage with 1-year follow-up. Radiology 1992; 184:167–179.

3. Schechter S, Eisenstat TE, Oliver GC, Rubin RJ, Salvati EP. Computerized tomographic scan-guided drainage of intraabdominal abscesses. Preoperative and postoperative modalities in colon and rectal surgery. Dis Colon Rectum 1994; 37:984–988.

4. Butch RJ, Mueller PR, Ferrucci JT, et al. Drainage of pelvic abscesses through the greater sciatic foramen. Radiology 1986; 158:487–491.

5. Malden ES, Picus D. Hemorrhagic complication of transgluteal pelvic abscess drainage: successful percutaneous treatment. J Vasc Interv Radiol 1992; 3:323–328.

6. Kuligowska E, Keller E, Ferrucci JT. Treatment of pelvic abscesses: value of one-step sonographically guided transrectal needle aspiration and lavage. AJR 1995; 164:201–206.

7. Jaques PF, Mauro M. Drainage of pelvic abscesses through the greater sciatic foramen. Radiology 1986; 160:278–279.

8. Fabiszewski NL, Sumkin JH, Johns CM. Contemporary radiologic percutaneous abscess drainage in the pelvis. Clin Obstet Gynecol 1993; 36:445–456.

9. Finne III CO. Transrectal drainage of pelvic abscesses. Dis Colon Rectum 1980; 23:293–297.

10. Walker AP, Condon RE. Peritonitis and intraabdominal abscesses. In: Schwartz SI, Shires GT, Spencer FC, eds. Principles of surgery. 5th edition. New York: McGraw-Hill, 1989: 1460–1489.

11. Mauro MA, Jaques PF, Mandell VS, Mandel SR. Pelvic abscess drainage by the transrectal catheter approach in men. AJR 1985; 144:477–479.

12. Nosher JL, Needell GS, Amorosa JK, Krasna IH. Transrectal pelvic abscess drainage with sonographic guidance. AJR 1986; 146:1047–1048.

13. Carmody E, Thurston W, Yeung E, Ho CS. Transrectal drainage of deep pelvic collections under fluoroscopic guidance. Can Assoc Radiol J 1993; 44:429–433.

14. Gazelle GS, Haaga JR, Stellato TA, Gauderer MW, Plecha DT. Pelvic abscesses: CT-guided transrectal drainage. Radiology 1991; 181:49–51.

15. Bennett JD, Kozak RI, Taylor BM, Jory TA. Deep pelvic abscesses: transrectal drainage with radiologic guidance. Radiology 1992; 185:825–828.

16. Alexander AA, Eschelman DJ, Nazarian LN, Bonn J. Transrectal sonographically guided drainage of deep pelvic abscesses. AJR 1994; 162:1227–1230.

17. Nosher JL, Winchman HK, Needell GS. Transvaginal pelvic abscess drainage with US guidance. Radiology 1987; 165:872–873.

18. Abbitt PL, Goldwag S, Urbanski S. Endovaginal sonography for guidance in draining pelvic fluid collections. AJR 1990; 154:849–850.

19. vanSonnenberg E, D'Agostino HB, Casola G, Goodacre BW, Sanchez RB, Taylor B. US-guided transvaginal drainage of pelvic abscesses and fluid collections. Radiology 1991; 181:53–56.

20. VanDerKolk HL. Small, deep pelvic abscesses: definition and drainage guided with an endovaginal probe. Radiology 1991; 181:283–284.

21. Feld R, Eschelman DJ, Sagerman JE, Segal S, Hovsepian DM, Sullivan KL. Treatment of pelvic abscesses and other fluid collections: efficacy of transvaginal sonographically guided aspiration and drainage. AJR 1994; 163:1141–1145.

22. Pereira JK, Chait PG, Miller SF. Deep pelvic abscesses in children: transrectal drainage under radiologic guidance. Radiology 1996; 198:393–396.

23. Kerlan RK, Jeffrey RB Jr, Pogany AC, Ring EJ. Abdominal abscess with low-output fistula: successful percutaneous drainage. Radiology 1985; 155:73–75.

24. Eschelman DJ, Sullivan KL. Use of a Colapinto needle in US-guided transvaginal drainage of pelvic abscesses. Radiology 1993; 186:893–894.

Endnote

Figures 17 and 18 courtesy of Mark Wilson, M.D., University of Michigan School of Medicine.

TUTORIAL 9
MANAGING COMPLICATIONS OF ACUTE PANCREATITIS

Albert A. Nemcek, Jr., M.D., and
Robert L. Vogelzang, M.D.

Introduction

The subjects addressed in this tutorial include:
1. Etiologies and pathogenesis of acute pancreatitis
2. Clinical and laboratory manifestations of acute pancreatitis
3. Imaging of the pancreas
4. Complications of acute pancreatitis
5. Indications for percutaneous interventional therapy
6. Technique for aspiration and drainage of pancreatic fluid collections.

Acute pancreatitis is a common disease that can have a markedly variable clinical course. Mild cases typically require only conservative medical therapy for uneventful recovery without detectable sequelae, whereas severe acute pancreatitis is among the most challenging of human afflictions. With its propensity to lead to a plethora of local and systemic complications, it taxes the abilities and resources of multiple medical disciplines and exacts a considerable toll in morbidity and mortality. The optimal therapeutic approach to severe acute pancreatitis remains controversial and uncertain. In this regard the role of interventional radiology is no exception: while much data supports a place for interventional techniques in the management of complicated acute pancreatitis, agreement as to their utility in individual situations is far from uniform.

This situation has been compounded by literature which has been confusing and inconsistent in applying clinical and morphological definitions and in which there is a relative dearth of prospective comparative studies. Meaningful study and application of therapy for acute pancreatitis and communication between medical specialties requires a comparison of "apples with apples." Recognition of this fact has led to attempts to define more clearly the terminology used to classify acute pancreatitis. It is therefore important to begin this tutorial with a prelude on what is currently a widely accepted classification system, and to describe the clinical, pathological, and radiological correlates of that system.[1,2] This groundwork serves as preparation for a discussion of the use of interventional radiology in the treatment of complications of acute pancreatitis.

Etiologies and Pathogenesis

Acute pancreatitis is defined as the abrupt onset of an inflammatory process of pancreatic tissue. The majority of cases can be linked to precipitating factors.[3] Broad categories of such factors include mechanisms that obstruct the pancreatic duct orifice and/or overdistend the pancreatic duct, exposure to alcohol and other toxins or drugs, traumatic causes (including blunt abdominal trauma and iatrogenic trauma such as abdominal surgery or endoscopic retrograde cholangiopancreatography [ERCP]), metabolic abnormalities, inherited causes, infections, vascular etiologies, and miscellaneous conditions. Considerable variation in etiology exists, related to geographical and other factors, but gallstones and alcoholism are the two most important causes in most series.

Contrasted with this wide array of well-established etiologic factors is a limited understanding of how these factors actually trigger acute pancreatitis.[4] The initial changes are believed to occur within the acinar cells of the pancreas, and to involve inappropriate intraglandular activation of a variety of pancreatic enzymes. In some cases, inflammation remains confined to the gland, while in others (again for poorly understood reasons) local spread of digestive enzymes affects peripancreatic tissues, and in still others release of toxins into the peritoneal space and/or the bloodstream leads to systemic complications and multiorgan failure.

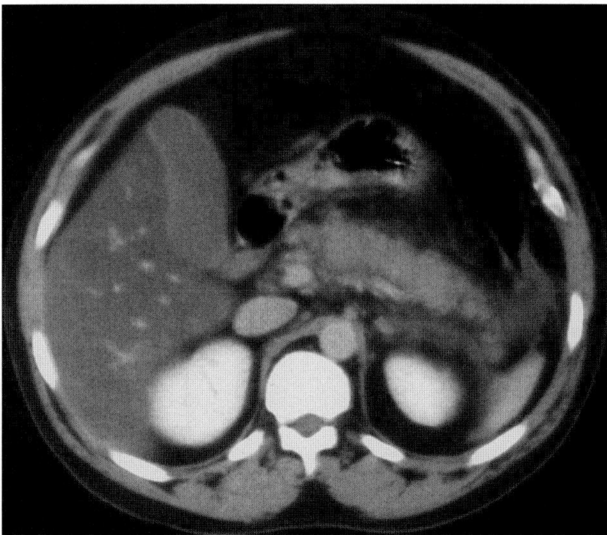

Figure 1. CT scan shows mild pancreatitis in a 34-year-old man. The pancreas is enlarged and soft-tissue stranding is seen in the peripancreatic fat of the anterior pararenal space. Note also the relative low density of the liver resulting from ethanol exposure.

Presentation and Laboratory Features

Acute pancreatitis usually manifests as the abrupt onset of abdominal pain. Physical findings can vary from mild abdominal tenderness to rebound tenderness and guarding. Signs and symptoms which commonly accompany pancreatitis include nausea and vomiting, fever, and tachycardia. Laboratory findings include elevation of serum or urinary amylase—thought to be sensitive, although nonspecific, especially in the early stages of the disease—and lipase—which has somewhat greater sensitivity and specificity than amylase and is more useful after the acute stage because it remains elevated for a longer period of time. Leukocytosis is common. Other biochemical tests for pancreatitis such as serum C-reactive protein have been proposed as measures of the severity of pancreatitis, but these have not yet found widespread use.

Whether based on clinical or pathologic criteria, the severity of pancreatitis represents a continuum. Nevertheless, it is useful to classify acute pancreatitis into two main categories of severity, *mild* and *severe*.

Most cases of acute pancreatitis are mild. They are associated with little or no systemic organ dysfunction and demonstrate prompt (within 48 to 72 hours) resolution of symptoms, physical signs, and laboratory abnormalities following conservative therapy. Pathologically, mild pancreatitis is characterized by interstitial edema and white blood cell infiltration. Necrosis of pancreatic tissue is unusual and, if present, generally confined to small foci. Pancreatic and peripancreatic fat necrosis may be present but is usually not marked. Imaging findings may be normal or they may show minimal changes confined to the pancreas or immediately adjacent fat **(Fig. 1)**.

Severe acute pancreatitis is associated with more pronounced symptomatology, physical findings, and laboratory abnormalities. It is accompanied by organ failure and/or a variety of local complications as discussed below. Pathologically, some degree of pancreatic necrosis is typical, although interstitial pancreatitis without significant necrosis may occasionally progress to severe acute pancreatitis as well. Most often, the manifestations of severe pancreatitis develop soon after the onset of the disease; a delayed progression from mild acute pancreatitis is unusual.

CT Severity Index				
Grade	**Definition**	**Points**	**% Necrosis**	**Points**
A	Normal	0	none	0
B	Focal or diffuse enlargement of gland	1	<30%	2
C	Pancreatic gland abnormalities associated with peripancreatic inflammation	4	30%–50%	2
plus				
D	Fluid collection in one location	3	>50%	6
E	Two or more fluid collections and/or gas within or adjacent to pancreas	4		

Figure 2.

The interventional radiologist should be aware that a variety of systems have been developed to grade the severity of acute pancreatitis.[5–11] Such systems can be used to provide prognostic information, to compare results of therapy, and to guide management. The Ranson criteria, for example, are based on eleven early objective clinical and laboratory features. As the number of Ranson criteria present rises, so does the risk of mortality or of complications requiring prolonged intensive care; the presence of more than three Ranson criteria indicates severe acute pancreatitis. A grading system based on computed tomography (CT) findings, the "CT severity index," has also been proposed. It assigns scores on a 0–10 scale based on a combination of grade and estimated percent necrosis **(Fig. 2)**.[12]

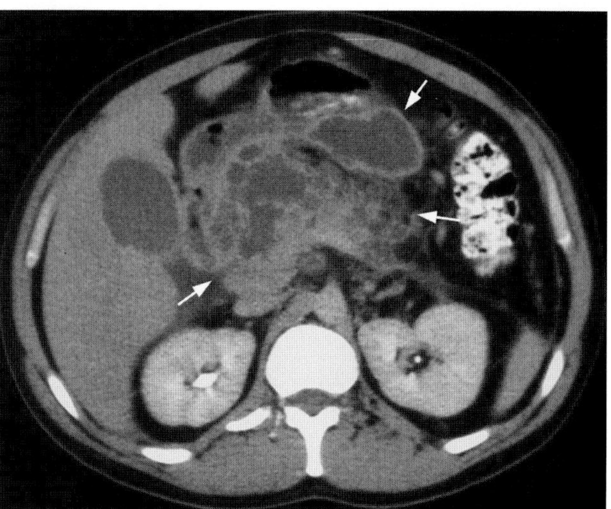

Figure 3. CT scan shows a complex multilocular fluid collection (arrows) posterior to the stomach.

Imaging

Several imaging methods can be useful in evaluating acute pancreatitis. Currently, dynamic contrast-enhanced CT scanning is widely considered the modality of choice for imaging of acute pancreatitis and its complications. It is ideally performed at peak arterial enhancement of the pancreas following large volume bolus or bolus and rapid infusion of contrast material, using thin (5 mm) cuts or thinly collimated spiral CT reconstructions. **Figure 3** is a CT scan of a 31-year-old man with severe acute pancreatitis.

CT scanning readily detects abnormalities in all but the mildest forms of pancreatitis (in which the need for imaging is limited anyway), can detect most complications, and provides convincing and repeatable delineation of the entire pancreas, of surrounding tissues, and of the extent, location, and size of peripancreatic fluid collections.

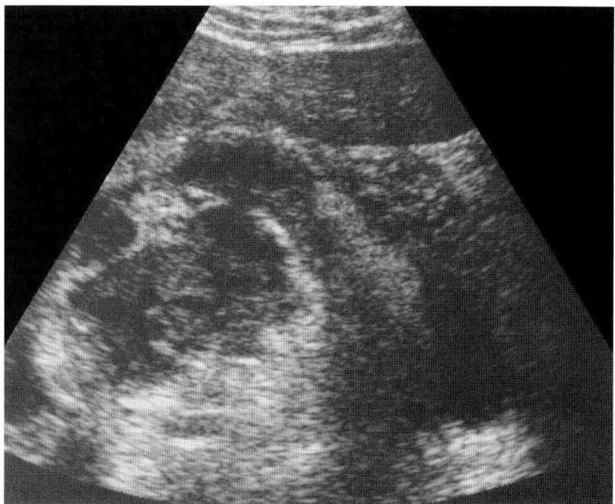

Figure 4. Same patient as in Figure 3. Although the sonogram is of good quality, the delineation of the fluid collections and their relationship to adjacent structures is better appreciated on the CT scan.

Other imaging tests can be useful in specific situations. Ultrasonography is portable and inexpensive and shows gallstones and other biliary abnormalities readily. However, it is operator-dependent and frequently provides only limited visualization of the pancreas and peripancreatic fluid collections **(Fig. 4)**.

Indications for Imaging in Acute Pancreatitis
(a) confirmation of an uncertain clinical diagnosis (or establishment of an alternate diagnosis) (b) assessment for causes of pancreatitis (eg, gallstones) (c) evidence of severe pancreatitis (d) mild pancreatitis failing to respond rapidly (48–72 hrs) to conservative therapy (e) clinical signs or symptoms of a complication of pancreatitis, whether or not initial imaging studies have been obtained and regardless of initial findings (f) follow-up of patients who show clinical improvement but in whom initial imaging studies showed more severe grades of acute pancreatitis (grade D–E pancreatitis or CT Severity Index scores of 3–10); Balthazar et al recommend follow-up at 7–10 days or prior to discharge of such patients to confirm resolution of findings, because some complications can become manifest on imaging prior to development of clinical signs (g) as a guide to interventional therapy

Figure 5.

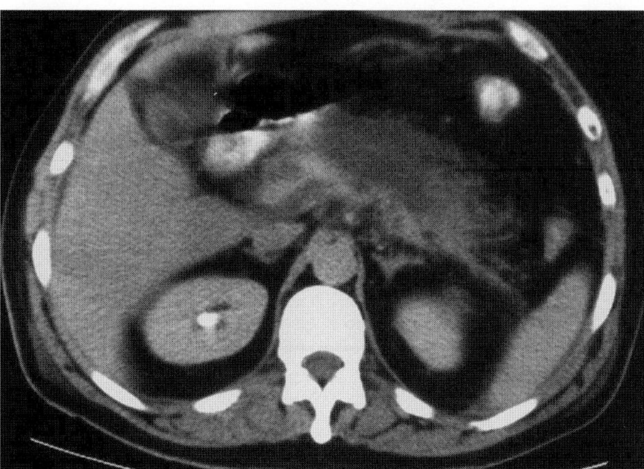

Figure 6. CT scan shows an acute peripancreatic fluid collection.

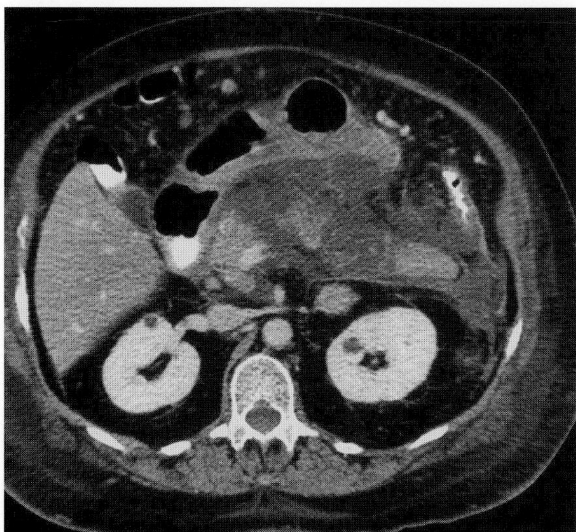

Figure 7. Another example of an acute fluid collection adjacent to the pancreas from pancreatitis. Note the lack of a wall which distinguishes this from a pseudocyst.

ERCP is being used more routinely in acute pancreatitis. It provides detailed evaluation of the status of the pancreatic and biliary ducts, and can be used therapeutically in appropriate circumstances.[13,14] Arteriography can evaluate and treat vascular complications of pancreatitis. Finally, early results of magnetic resonance (MR) imaging have been encouraging.[15] MR imaging may assume a larger role in the future, particularly if experimental data suggesting that iodinated contrast material may exacerbate severe pancreatitis prove to have clinical relevance.[16]

Because mild pancreatitis typically resolves with conservative therapy, imaging is not required in all cases of pancreatitis. While imaging will generally include CT scanning, the exact method should be tailored to the specific clinical setting. Indications for imaging are listed in **Figure 5.**[2]

Complications of Acute Pancreatitis

Acute Fluid Collections

About 40% of patients develop peripancreatic fluid collections early in the course of acute severe pancreatitis. These typically occur adjacent to the pancreas, within the anterior pararenal space of the retroperitoneum, or, less commonly, within the pancreatic substance. Being rich in pancreatic enzymes, the collections can dissect into distant locations such as the posterior pararenal space or mediastinum, or into adjacent organs such as the spleen, the liver, or the bowel wall.

On CT scanning and when otherwise uncomplicated, these collections have ill-defined borders and low attenuation **(Figs. 6, 7)**. Acute peripancreatic fluid collections may be mixed with variable degrees of hemorrhage, fat necrosis, and tissue edema and inflammation to give a heterogeneous appearance to peripancreatic tissues. These areas of heterogeneity have been referred to in the past as phlegmons. However, it is now recommended that the term phlegmon be abandoned because of its past history of ambiguous usage. More than half of acute fluid collections can be expected to resolve spontaneously. Those which persist may form pseudocysts or pancreatic abscesses.

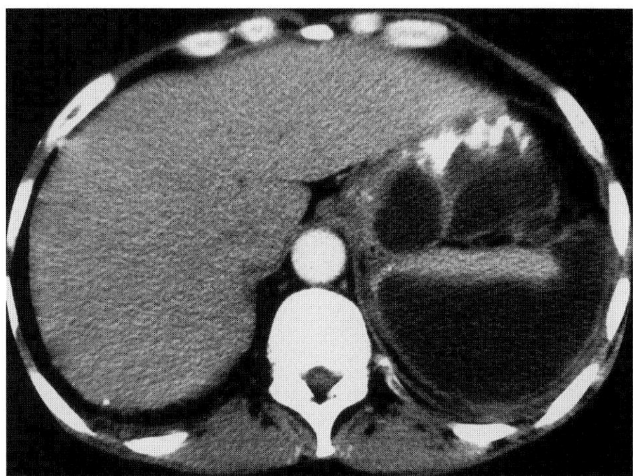

Figure 8. CT scan shows well-defined fluid collections with thin walls, the largest of which involves the spleen.

Pancreatic Pseudocyst

A pseudocyst is a collection of pancreatic enzymes encapsulated by a nonepithelialized wall of fibrous or granulation tissue. An acute pseudocyst is one of the possible outcomes of unresolved acute pancreatic fluid collections. A pseudocyst can be distinguished from a fluid collection by the presence of a wall and by a time course (required for the wall to develop) of at least 4 weeks duration. Pseudocysts can also result from pancreatic trauma or chronic pancreatitis, in the latter instance forming a chronic pseudocyst. A pseudocyst will generally appear on imaging studies as a well-defined, round or ovoid fluid collection with a wall of variable thickness **(Figs. 8–11)**.

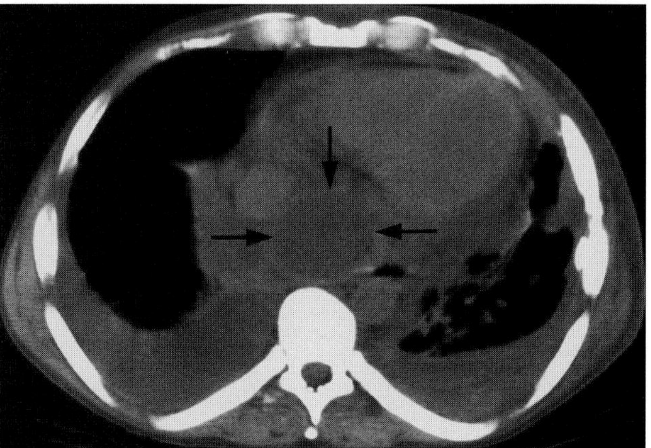

Figure 9. CT scan from a 27-year-old man with alcoholic pancreatitis shows a pseudocyst in an unusual location, the middle mediastinum (arrows).

Pseudocysts are most often sterile, but they may have bacteria present as contaminants. If frank pus is present, the collection is more properly called a pancreatic abscess; for this reason, it has been suggested that the term "infected pseudocyst" be abandoned. About half of all acute pseudocysts resolve without drainage.

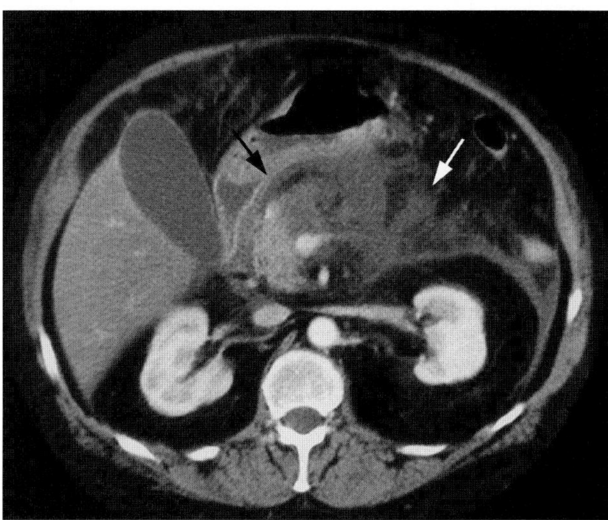

Figure 10. CT scan shows an acute peripancreatic fluid collection (arrows).

Pancreatic Abscess

A pancreatic abscess is a collection of pus within the abdomen which arises as a consequence of acute pancreatitis or pancreatic trauma. Abscesses generally arise near the pancreas. By definition little or no necrosis is associated with abscesses, and they are thought most likely to result from the progression of limited necrosis to liquefaction and secondary infection. It is important for both therapeutic and prognostic purposes to distinguish pancreatic abscess from infected pancreatic necrosis (discussed below). Pancreatic abscesses tend to occur late after the onset of severe acute pancreatitis, frequently after the same 4-week time span which distinguishes pseudocysts.

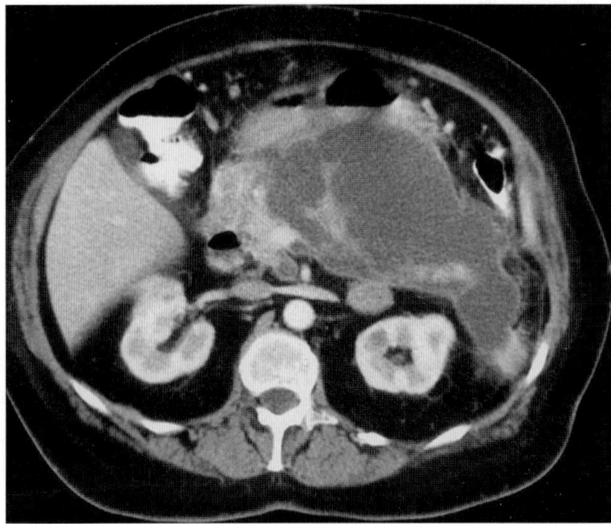

Figure 11. Same patient as in Figure 10. Evolution of an acute peripancreatic fluid collection into a pancreatic pseudocyst as seen on a scan obtained 4 weeks later.

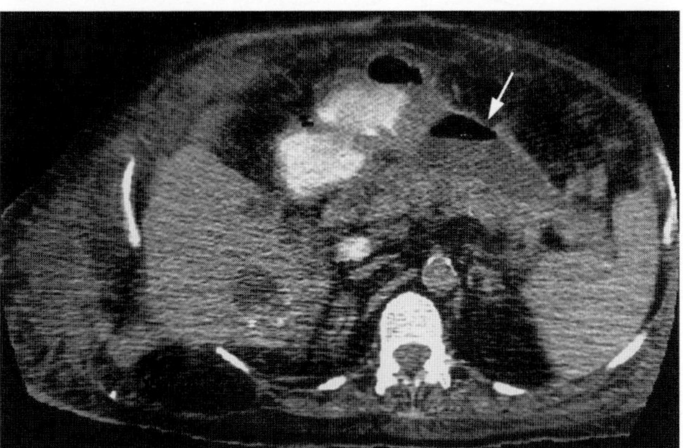

Figure 12. CT scan shows a collection of fluid and gas (arrow) anterior to the pancreas in a 65-year-old woman who developed acute pancreatitis following renal transplantation and immunosuppression; on needle aspiration, the contents of this collection were grossly purulent.

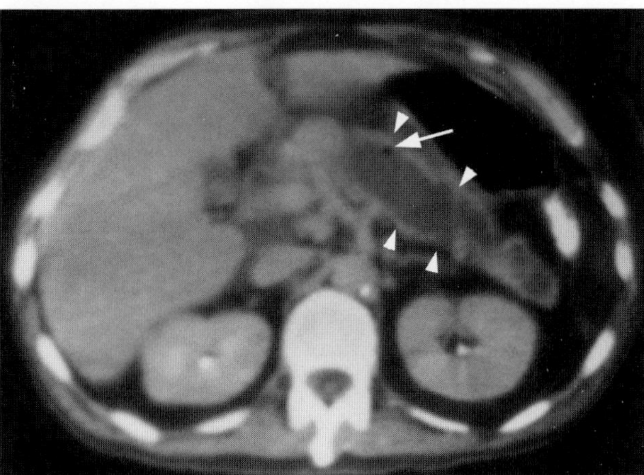

Figure 13. CT scan shows pancreatic necrosis. Note the low attenuation of the entire body and tail of the pancreas (arrowheads); a small locule of gas is also present within the low density (arrow). Review Figure 10, which reveals evidence of pancreatic necrosis, with the pancreatic parenchyma in the pancreatic neck failing to enhance to the same degree as the pancreatic head.

On CT scans, pancreatic abscesses appear as focal collections of low attenuation. While they tend to have a thick wall and may contain gas bubbles as a sign of infection, these findings need not be present, nor are they specific: pseudocysts may have a thick wall, and may have gas bubbles as a result of communication with the gastrointestinal tract **(Fig. 12)**.

When abscesses arise following surgical therapy for pancreatitis, the term "postoperative abscess," rather than "pancreatic abscess," is favored.

Pancreatic Necrosis

Pancreatic necrosis is defined as the presence of diffuse or focal areas of nonviable pancreatic tissue. The greater the clinical severity of pancreatitis, the more likely the presence of pancreatic necrosis. Contrast-enhanced CT scanning is currently the test of choice for demonstration of the presence and extent of pancreatic necrosis. Normally, the pancreatic parenchyma increases its density from a baseline of about 30–50 Hounsfield units (HU) to about 100–150 HU following bolus contrast enhancement. As a rule of thumb, the pancreas enhances to a density similar to that of the spleen **(Fig. 13)**.

Reliable diagnosis of pancreatic necrosis requires the presence of focal or diffuse well-marginated regions of nonenhanced pancreatic parenchyma on CT scanning, larger than 3 cm in diameter or involving more than 30% of the gland.[12] While smaller regions of necrosis can occur, the sensitivity and specificity of CT scanning in detecting such limited necrosis drops. It is also recognized that pancreatic necrosis may be associated with a variable degree of peripancreatic fat necrosis, which in unusual instances may form loculated collections of thick material.

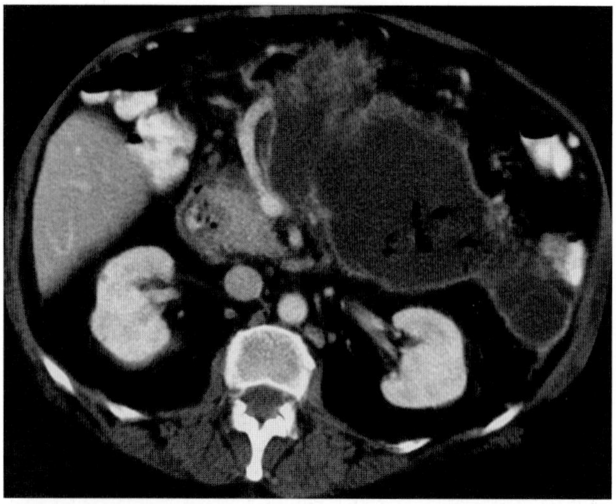

Figure 14. Same patient as in Figure 10, 2 weeks after the later image. CT scan shows a collection of gas and fluid in the anterior pararenal space.

Infected Necrosis

Infected necrosis occurs when nonviable pancreatic and/or peripancreatic tissue becomes secondarily infected. On imaging, the condition may be indicated by the findings of pancreatic necrosis in combination with pancreatic or peripancreatic gas. In the absence of gas, no specific imaging features are found. Nevertheless, the distinction is critical: infected necrosis significantly increases the mortality rate of pancreatitis and, in most if not all cases, demands surgical intervention. Percutaneous needle aspiration and culture of suspicious areas allows this distinction to be made and, as a result, has become an important procedure in the management of severe pancreatitis.

In this case **(Fig. 14)**, the combination of imaging findings which included evidence of necrosis, and the clinical findings of fever, rigors, and a white blood cell count of 19,600/mm^3 suggested the presence of infected necrosis. Aspiration of the fluid yielded brownish, thick fluid that was culture positive for *Klebsiella pneumoniae*; although the patient did show some initial clinical benefit from catheter drainage of the collection, she eventually required surgical debridement.

Other Complications

In addition to the variable combinations of fluid, necrotic tissue, and infection which can result from severe acute pancreatitis, interventional radiologists should be cognizant of other potential complications they may be called upon to evaluate or treat.

The mass effect of pancreatitis-associated inflammation and fluid collections may cause complications, including venous occlusion and secondary development of varices or splenic infarction, and biliary or gastrointestinal tract obstruction. While these complications will not be discussed in this tutorial, the interventional radiologist may play a role (for example, biliary drainage) in certain occurrences of such complications.

The release of pancreatic enzymes into pancreatic and peripancreatic tissue may cause damage to the walls of adjacent blood vessels, especially the splenic and gastroduodenal arteries and their branches. This damage can result in frank bleeding, a development which can be recognized on CT scanning by the presence of high-attenuation material within or around the pancreas. Pseudoaneurysms may also occur; if large, these can be recognized on CT scanning as rounded, enhancing collections larger than adjacent blood vessels. Arteriography reliably demonstrates pseudoaneurysms or active bleeding, and in turn can be used for selective embolotherapy.[17–20]

Therapy For Acute Pancreatitis

This tutorial is not the forum for a detailed discussion of the many therapies which have been used in the setting of acute pancreatitis. The local and systemic manifestations of pancreatitis typically require timely and consistent cooperation among a variety of medical specialties. The many therapies proposed and used attest, in part, to the great variety of adverse consequences which can be associated with acute pancreatitis, as well as to the lack of any clearly and uniformly successful treatment algorithm.

It is also important to remember that many current therapeutic approaches to pancreatitis focus not on treatment of the primary cascade of events by which pancreatitis evolves, but on minimizing the effects or complications of the primary disorder.[4] This approach has been referred to and should be thought of as "damage control" rather than "damage prevention,"[21] and certainly is an apt description of the role of interventional techniques even at their most successful.

Indications for Percutaneous Interventional Therapy

Depending on their particular skills and training, interventional radiologists may become involved in treating acute pancreatitis in a variety of ways. For instance, they may provide venous access for fluid and electrolyte management, administration of medications, and provision of parenteral nutrition; they may treat associated or predisposing biliary pathology via biliary interventions; or they may manage vascular complications of pancreatitis through diagnostic arteriography and endovascular intervention. The remainder of this tutorial will concentrate on intervention for the treatment of fluid collections associated with acute pancreatitis. The primary decisions concerning these fluid collections revolve around if and when to aspirate and/or drain them.

Indications For Needle Aspiration
The main purpose of percutaneous needle aspiration of fluid collections is to confirm or refute clinically suspected infection.[22,23] Noninfected and otherwise asymptomatic fluid collections should typically be observed, because many such collections resolve spontaneously. Conversely, pancreatitis associated with infection mandates aggressive therapy, including percutaneous and/or surgical drainage and possible surgical debridement.

Because clinical and laboratory signs of infection such as elevated white blood cell count and fever can accompany sterile pancreatitis, these signs cannot be relied upon solely to guide timing of diagnostic aspiration. On the other hand, early detection of infection and timely intervention, prior to development of a frankly septic picture, offers the best chance for optimal management. Consequently, it is important to maintain a high level of suspicion for infection and a low threshold for performing needle aspiration, as long as the latter can be done relatively safely. Initial aspiration is also useful for confirming that there is drainable fluid within the collection, because CT scanning alone is not always reliable for that purpose. Aspiration is generally performed with 18–22-gauge needles. Specimens should be sent for Gram stain, and for aerobic and anaerobic bacterial, mycobacterial, and fungal cultures.[2] Most positive aspirates will yield coliform bacteria.[24]

Indications For Drainage
Several considerations enter into the decision to attempt drainage of fluid collections associated with acute pancreatitis.[2,25–27] Because most acute fluid collections and as many as half of all pseudocysts (particularly when smaller than 5–6 cm in diameter) resolve spontaneously, the mere presence of a technically drainable collection is not an indication for drainage.[2,28]

At the other end of the spectrum, infected necrosis may be associated with some drainable fluid, but such collections may also contain large fragments of necrotic pancreas and fat which cannot be drained even by very large tubes. **Figures 15–17** were obtained following drainage of the acute pancreatic collection shown in **Figure 6**, and illustrate this point. Surgical debridement offers the only possibility of cure in such collections, although debate persists and investigations continue as to whether percutaneous drainage may be a beneficial temporizing measure in some cases where palliation could improve the patient's overall clinical condition.

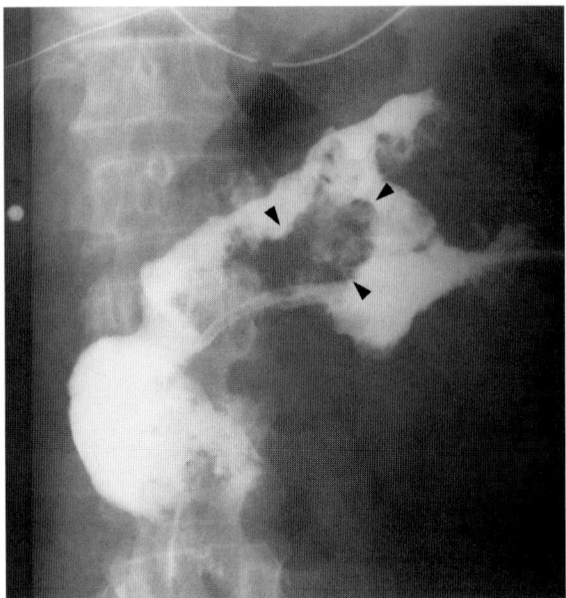

Figure 15. Sinogram shows a large irregular filling defect (arrowheads) and debris within the drainage cavity.

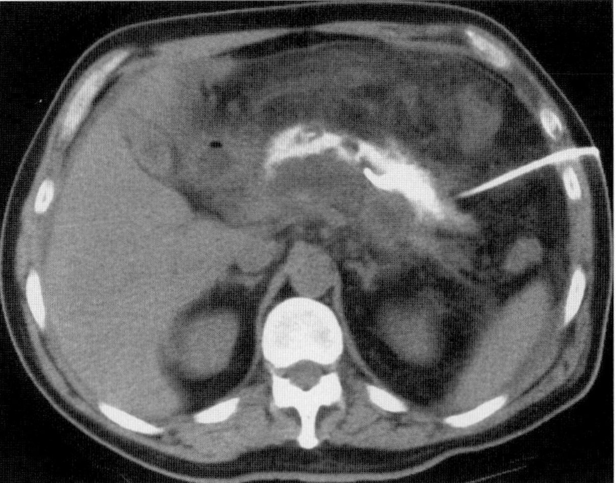

Figure 16. CT scan following injection of contrast material into the collection shows little debris.

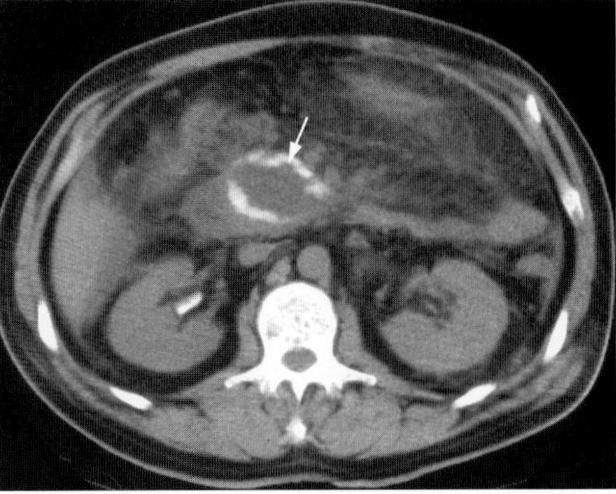

Figure 17. Same patient as in Figure 16. On a more caudal cut a large solid fragment (arrow) is outlined by contrast material.

Between these two extremes are collections which can be considered candidates for percutaneous drainage, in which a reasonable chance of a beneficial outcome exists. Included in this group are infected collections not associated with significant pancreatic necrosis (ie, pancreatic abscesses) or acute fluid collections or pseudocysts associated with adverse clinical sequelae: pain, gastrointestinal tract obstruction, or biliary obstruction. Some authors also consider enlarging pseudocysts or pseudocysts involving contiguous organs as potential indications, as these are associated with increasing complications over time.[2,27]

One other category of patients in whom drainage may be indicated is patients who develop postoperative peripancreatic abscesses. Because necrotic tissue has already been debrided, percutaneous drainage should achieve better success rates than preoperative attempts to drain devitalized tissue and solid and semi-solid debris.[25,29]

Even in cases with seemingly good indications for drainage, it is important to understand and to communicate to the patient and referring physician(s) several important points. First, even if successful, drainage may be prolonged (weeks to months) and require aggressive and frequent tube management and repeated imaging. Second, associated problems—such as pancreatic ductal stenosis or obstruction—frequently require additional therapy. Finally, development of complications of drainage or lack of clinical response may mandate different approaches to therapy at any time (including placement of additional tubes).

Contraindications

General contraindications to percutaneous drainage of pancreatic fluid collections include severe and uncorrectable coagulopathy and lack of a safe access route to the collection. Drainage is also contraindicated in collections associated with evidence of recent or active bleeding or with an arterial pseudoaneurysm.

As mentioned earlier, pancreatic collections associated with excessive solid debris and significant necrosis respond poorly to drainage. Such patients should be treated surgically.[2,25,29–31] The degree to which some patients in this category—specifically those who are critically ill, clinically unstable, and very poor surgical risks—may improve their clinical status and their surgical risk with percutaneous drainage is debatable.[25,29] Drainage in such patients should be performed with an anticipation of high failure rates and with the understanding that lack of response may mandate more aggressive therapy despite risks. Multiple and/or multilocular collections also respond poorly to drainage, although the placement of additional catheters can sometimes address this problem.

Preprocedural Care

Before aspiration or drainage of pancreatic fluid collections is attempted, radiographic studies and the clinical indications for the procedure should be reviewed carefully. Preprocedural laboratory studies should include coagulation studies as well as baseline laboratory data such as white blood cell count and differential, which will be used in assessing the patient's response to therapy. If the indication for drainage is suspicion of an infected fluid collection and the fluid aspirated is not grossly purulent, drainage may be deferred pending results of Gram stain and culture of aspirated fluid. Intravenous access should be established for administration of medications during the procedure. Antibiotics should be started as appropriate, guided by fluid or blood cultures.

Technical Aspects of Drainage

While CT scanning is generally favored over ultrasound for delineation of fluid collections, access to such collections can be achieved with use of either method. If the collection to be aspirated and/or drained and a safe path of access are readily visualized by ultrasound, this method of guidance has clear advantages, including real-time observation of the needle during its passage and portability (making it easy to combine with subsequent fluoroscopic manipulations or allowing bedside procedures in patients too ill to be moved safely). Conversely, if the collection and/or the path to it are poorly visualized by ultrasound, CT guidance is preferable. CT guidance also has potential advantages with multilocular or complex collections, in that it can more readily identify collections undrained by an initial tube.

Given the retroperitoneal location of the pancreas, the propensity for pancreatic fluid collections to dissect to sometimes remote anatomic locations, and the frequently complex and multilocular nature of pancreatic fluid collections, choosing a path or paths for access can be quite challenging. The optimal path involves several considerations, including technical ease, safety, patient comfort, the size of the collection, and the ability of the catheter location to facilitate drainage and future catheter manipulations during what is often a prolonged course.[2,26,32] In general, the shortest path to the collection that crosses the fewest and least critical structures or anatomic spaces is best. Large blood vessels must be avoided because of the risk of bleeding complications. The colon should also be avoided because of its high bacterial content and consequent risk of infectious complications.

Wittich et al have provided a good review of anatomic considerations applicable to drainage in pancreatitis.[32] Because peripancreatic fluid often dissects along the left anterior pararenal space and may displace the colon anteriorly, a common drainage route is a left posterolateral approach via the retroperitoneum. Transperitoneal approaches are also acceptable, as they have not yielded prohibitive rates of peritoneal contamination. With use of a transperitoneal route, it makes sense to approach the collection where it is close to or in contact with the parietal peritoneum. Frequently, such approaches cross the transverse mesocolon, or gastrocolic or gastrosplenic ligaments. Solid organs should be avoided if possible; however, collections high in the lesser sac may require a route through the left lobe of the liver. Successful transsplenic drainage has also been reported in exceptional circumstances.

Many pancreatic and lesser sac fluid collections lie immediately behind the stomach. Here, a transgastric route may be used. Indeed, reports in the literature support this route. Conversion to completely internal drainage is also advocated, based on the surgical model of long-term drainage of pseudocysts via cystogastrostomy. Potential advantages include minimizing the inconvenience of prolonged external drainage and decreasing the risks of developing a pancreaticocutaneous fistula or secondary infection of a previously noninfected collection.[33] While the evidence supporting these purported advantages is debatable,[2,27] and while this route may be associated with technical difficulties such as tube dislodgement and problematic guide wire and catheter manipulation, the transgastric route is a viable option, particularly if no other routes are available.

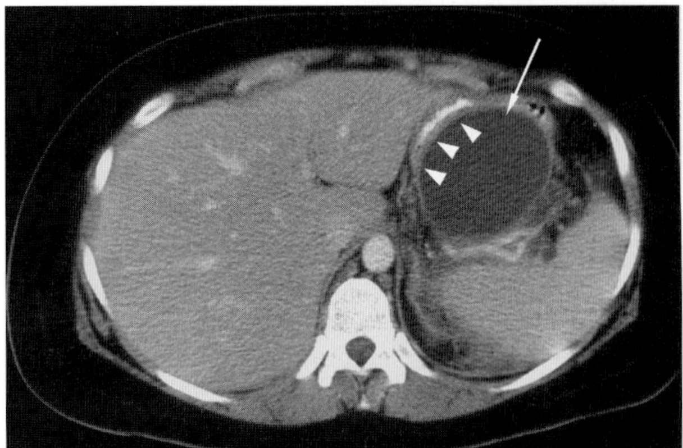

Figure 18. CT shows a pancreatic pseudocyst, with compression of the stomach by the pseudocyst (arrowheads). A possible transgastric drainage route is apparent (arrow).

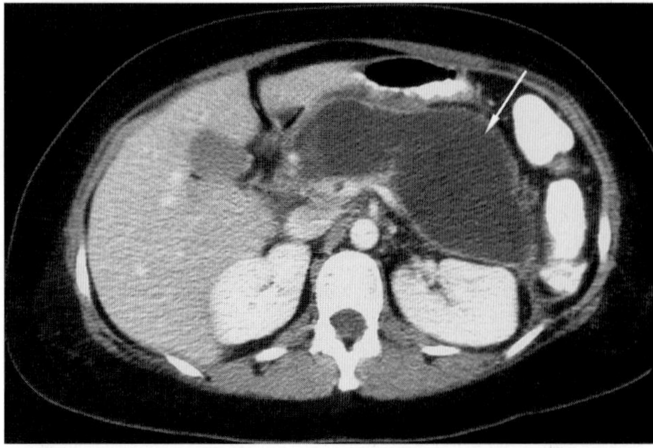

Figure 19. Same patient as in Figure 18. A more inferior CT scan shows a pancreatic pseudocyst. A possible anterior transperitoneal drainage route is apparent (arrow).

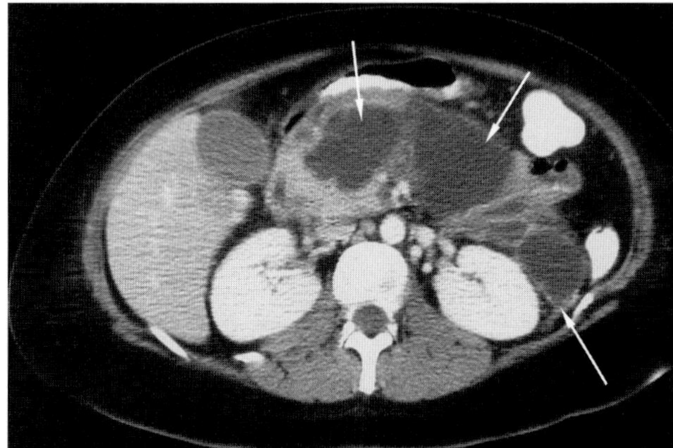

Figure 20. Same patient as in Figure 18. A more caudal image shows pancreatic pseudocysts. Several possible drainage routes are apparent (arrows).

Figures 18–20 are CT scans, from cephalad to caudad, of a pancreatic pseudocyst in a 30-year-old woman with gallstone pancreatitis. Although she had no clinical signs of infection, she had severe abdominal discomfort and nausea believed to be related to compression of the stomach by the pseudocyst, and was referred for drainage to relieve these symptoms. Several potential drainage routes are suggested by the scans, including transgastric, anterior transperitoneal, and posterior routes.

In this case, the route chosen took advantage of the left posterior-inferior retroperitoneal extension of the collection and anterior displacement of the colon. Under sonographic guidance, an 18-gauge Seldinger needle was passed into the collection, then a wire and catheter passed under fluoroscopic guidance were coiled behind the compressed stomach and a drain was placed **(Figs. 21, 22)**. **Figures 23–25** are CT scans of the same patient, running caudad to cephalad, which show the course of the drainage catheter shortly after drainage; the patient's symptoms improved significantly following drainage. **Figures 26** and **27** show other examples of drainage routes.

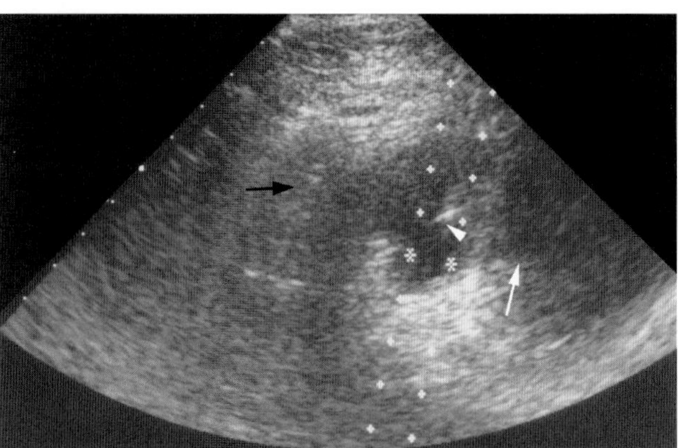

Figure 21. Same patient as in Figure 18. Sonogram shows needle placement into the pseudocyst. Black arrow=colon; white arrow=left kidney; arrowhead=needle tip.

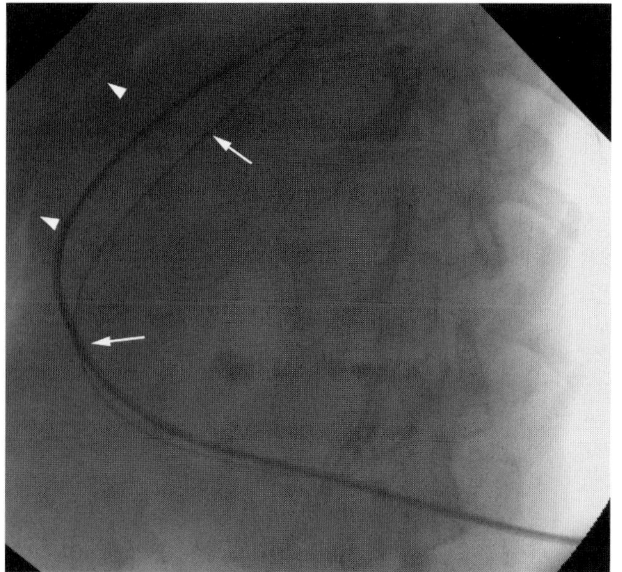

Figure 22. Same patient as in Figure 18. Wire and catheter (arrows) coiled in the pseudocyst, behind the compressed stomach (arrowheads).

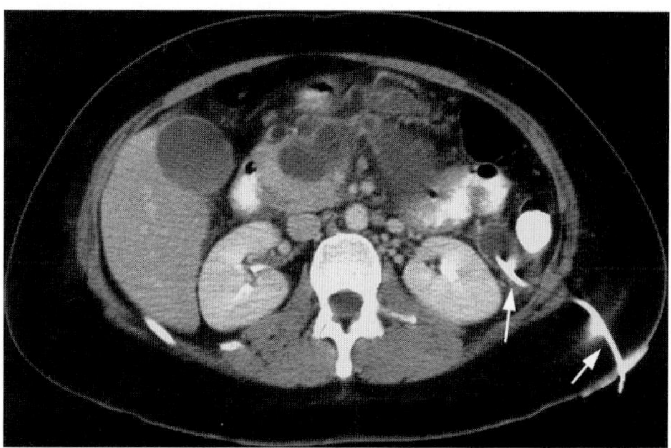

Figure 23. Same patient as in Figure 18. CT scan after pseudocyst drainage shows the course of the drainage catheter (arrows).

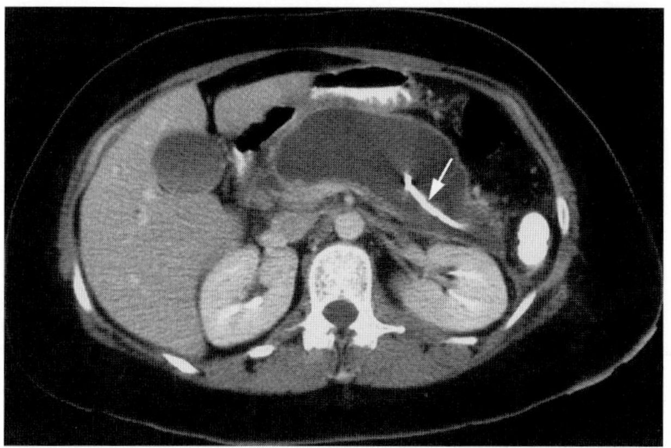

Figure 24. Same patient as in Figure 18. A more superior cut from a CT scan after pseudocyst drainage shows the course of the drainage catheter (arrow).

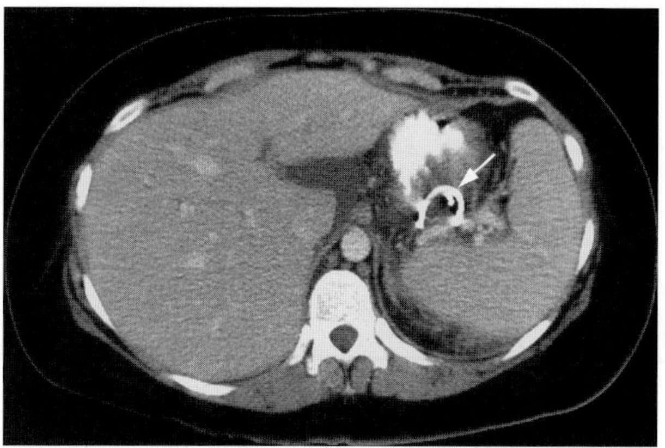

Figure 25. Same patient as in Figure 18. A more superior cut from a CT scan after pseudocyst drainage shows the course of the drainage catheter (arrow).

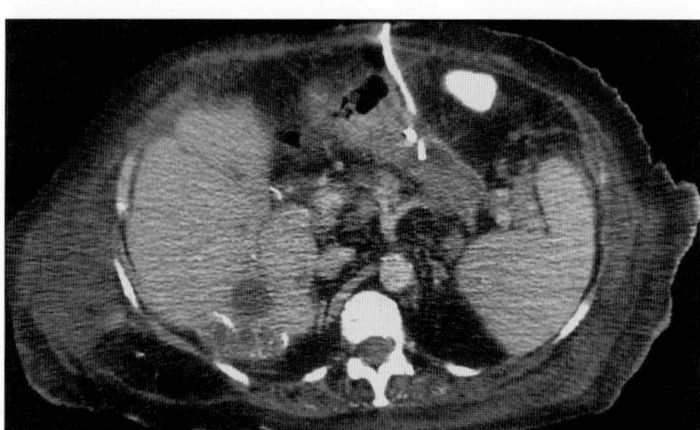

Figure 26. Same patient as in Figure 12. CT scan shows an anterior route through the gastrocolic ligament.

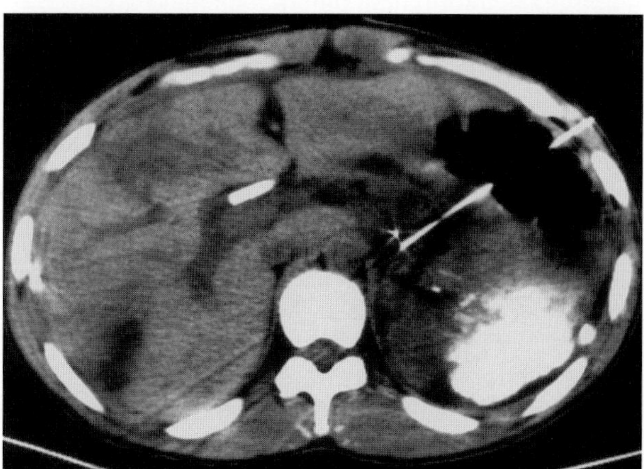

Figure 27. CT scan shows a transgastric route in a patient who developed a peripancreatic lesser sac collection following abdominal trauma.

We prefer to use the Seldinger technique for drainage of pancreatic fluid collections, because we believe it provides some margin for error in initial needle passage into the collection; however, other investigators routinely use the trocar technique, particularly when collections are large and easily accessible.[2,26,27] When the route to the collection appears technically difficult, we typically start with a 20-gauge needle. Once the needle is positioned adequately, an 0.018-inch wire is placed within the collection, followed by a transitional dilator to permit positioning of larger diameter wires, progressive track dilation, and drainage catheter placement. If the route to the collection is more straightforward, we often avoid the intermediate step of a transitional dilator by using an 18-gauge Seldinger needle **(Figs. 28, 29)**.

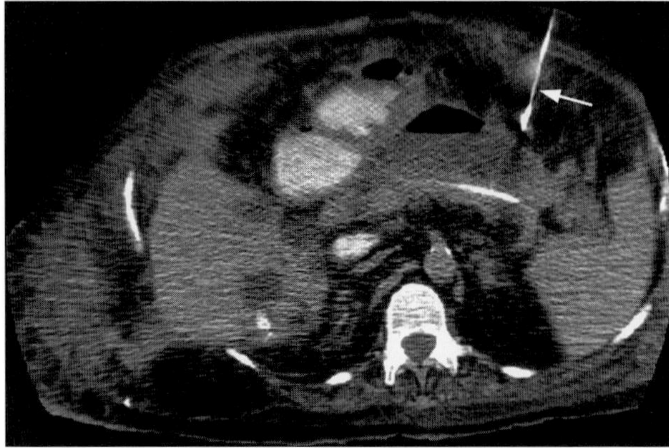

Figure 28. Same patient as in Figure 12. A 20-gauge needle (arrow) has been advanced most of the way toward the pancreatic abscess.

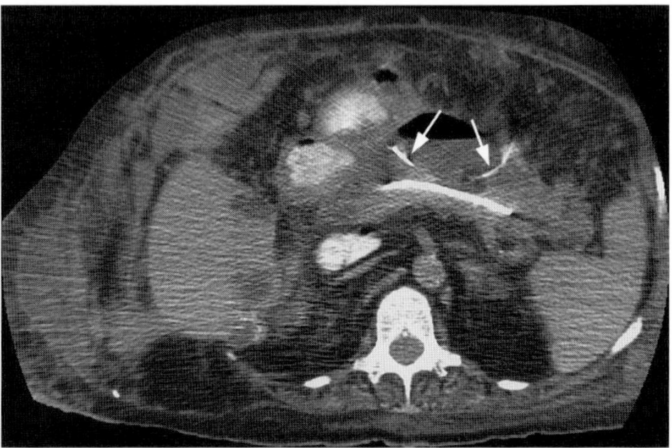

Figure 29. After the needle has been advanced slightly compared to Figure 28, an 0.018-inch wire (arrows) is coiled within the collection prior to track dilation and drainage.

The size of the initial catheter is chosen based on the character of the fluid aspirated from the collection.[26,27] If the fluid is relatively thin, an 8–12-F drainage catheter often suffices. For thicker collections, progressively larger catheters are placed, either immediately or after a period of track maturation. For very thick collections with abundant debris, upsizing to 24–30-F catheters can be done without hesitation. The catheter should be manipulated into the largest portion of the collection, if possible. Once the catheter is in position, it can be secured to an adhesive disk placed on the patient's skin, after which a dressing is applied and the catheter is allowed to drain to gravity. We do not routinely attach the catheter to a suction device, although this is an option others use.[26]

Pitfalls

Several potential pitfalls illustrate the need for the interventional radiologist to synthesize clinical and radiographic information before aspirating and/or draining collections assumed to result from pancreatitis.[26]

As mentioned earlier, pancreatitis can be associated with vascular complications that require different therapies.[17–20] Interventional radiologists should maintain a high level of vigilance for signs of vascular complications, because drainage of actively bleeding lesions can be catastrophic.[34]

It is also important to be aware that not all peripancreatic fluid collections are the result of pancreatitis. For example, cystic pancreatic neoplasms can mimic pancreatic pseudocysts, as can enteric duplications or mesenteric cysts **(Fig. 30)**. Further, even if pancreatitis is present, other important imaging features should not be missed **(Fig. 31)**.

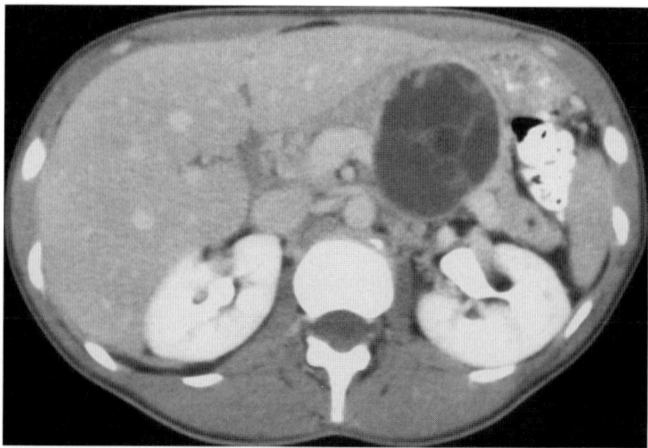

Figure 30. CT scan of a cystic-appearing peripancreatic collection in a 36-year-old woman who was referred for "pseudocyst drainage." Because the patient lacked any clear antecedent clinical history of pancreatitis, the lesion was biopsied and discovered to be a mucinous cystadenocarcinoma of the pancreas.

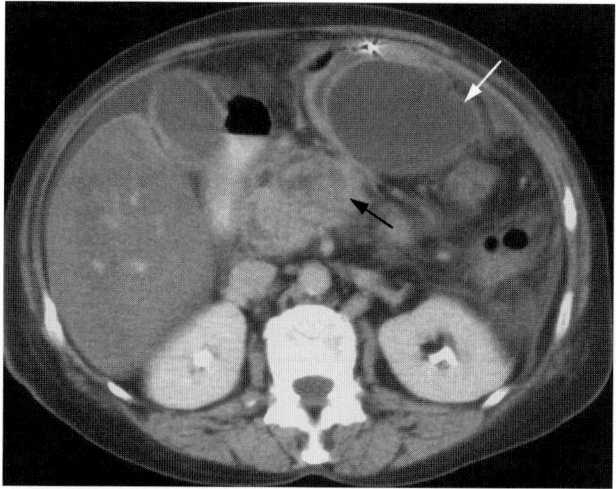

Figure 31. CT scan of a pancreatic pseudocyst (white arrow) in an elderly woman; review of the scan also shows the pancreatic head adenocarcinoma (black arrow) which led to the pancreatitis.

Postprocedure Tube Management

At the time of initial drainage, especially when the fluid collection is infected, we generally perform only gentle manipulations and small injections of contrast material to avoid precipitating sepsis. However, as opposed to other abdominal drainages, which may require only conservative postprocedural care and follow-up, optimal management of pancreatic drainage requires a very active and aggressive approach.[26,27]

Because of the thick, viscous nature of many pancreatic fluid collections, we typically strive to maintain patency of drains and to optimize drainage by flushing and irrigating the collection copiously and frequently once drainage has been established. Vigorous flushing is performed as often as once a day and consists of instilling and aspirating saline until clear. Volumes used for this irrigation should be gauged according to the cavity size so as not to overdistend the collection and cause contamination of previously uninvolved tissues and spaces. The amount injected into the tube should be aspirated back; if this is difficult, a fluoroscopic tube check is needed, along with possible repositioning of the catheter to optimize drainage. In addition, we routinely order that the catheter be flushed every nursing shift with 5–10 mL of sterile saline to maintain patency. The amount of catheter output should be monitored, and the patient's clinical status should be followed closely.

Fluoroscopic catheter checks with injection of contrast material are also performed on a regular basis. If the catheter is draining well and the patient is doing well or is at least stable clinically, catheter checks can be done once a week or, later on, less frequently. Indications for more frequent catheter checks include a change in the volume or character of the drainage (particularly if abrupt) or clinical deterioration. Because many pancreatic fluid collections are large and irregularly shaped, the optimal position for catheter drainage often changes over time, necessitating catheter change and/or repositioning. Similarly, if drainage increases in viscosity or if the catheter occludes frequently, a larger bore catheter may be needed.

As mentioned earlier, periodic CT scanning is also important for managing pancreatic drainage to evaluate cavity size, catheter position, and the development of new pancreatic fluid collections. Obviously, the potential benefit of CT scanning needs to be weighed against its relatively higher cost.

Complications and Sequelae of Drainage

Reported complications of percutaneous drainage of fluid collections associated with pancreatitis have varied, and comparison between different series is difficult because definitions are not applied uniformly.[2,26,27] In a review by Freeny, an overall complication rate of 15% was reported, with a major complication rate of 9%, no mortality related directly to drainage, and an overall mortality, mostly related to multisystem organ failure, of 4%.[27]

These complication rates compare favorably to surgical rates. In D'Agostino's review, for example, morbidity and mortality rates associated with percutaneous drainage of pseudocysts were 16% and 1%, respectively, compared to 28% and 5% for surgical drainage.[26] For drainage of pancreatic abscesses or collections associated with necrosis, morbidity and mortality rates were 29% and 11%, respectively, for percutaneous drainage compared to 60% and 27% for surgical drainage.

Specific complications include infection of a previously sterile collection; this has been reported to occur in 8% of pseudocysts, a frequency quite similar to that reported for spontaneous infection of untreated pseudocysts.[2] Treatment consists of instituting appropriate antibiotics and maintaining drainage. Contamination of previously uninvolved spaces such as the left pleural space (with high left upper quadrant collections) and the peritoneal space can also occur. Pleural space transgression can also result in pneumothorax. In the acute setting, sepsis can be precipitated as a result of release of infected material into the systemic circulation. The risk of sepsis can be minimized by avoiding vigorous or prolonged catheter manipulations and irrigation immediately after drainage. Drainage of infected material or pancreatic enzymes along the catheter track to the skin can result in cellulitis.

Hemorrhagic complications can develop following drainage of nonhemorrhagic collections as a result of progression of the pancreatitis; however, they can also occur due to traversal of vascular structures or as a result of draining actively hemorrhagic collections. Both of these complications should be minimized with the use of optimal pre-drainage imaging.

Catheter problems such as dislodgement, cracking, or kinking may prolong drainage; these can be minimized through careful catheter management and patient education. Prophylactic catheter changes may also be helpful when drainage is prolonged, not only to prevent the previously mentioned problems but to decrease the occurrence of catheter lumen and side-hole encrustation and occlusion.

Inadvertent traversal of the gastrointestinal tract can be avoided by carefully selecting and checking the route used to drain the collection. Such complications can often be managed conservatively with continued catheter drainage and bowel rest.

During the course of catheter drainage, fistulas to the gastrointestinal tract or the pancreatic duct may develop. Most of the former close spontaneously with continued drainage. Closure of pancreatic duct fistulas depends on several factors, the most important of which is the status of the duct between the site of leakage and the duodenum.[27] If the duct is obstructed, significantly strictured, or transected, the fistula will remain open until the problem is corrected. If the duct is otherwise relatively normal, successful closure may occur with continued drainage. Residual infection, continued active pancreatitis, and steroid therapy also contribute to continued patency. Management of such fistulas includes optimization of drainage (by placing the catheter near the site of leakage), pancreatic "rest" by means of total parenteral nutrition or a low fat diet, and administration of octreotide, a somatostatin analog that works by decreasing pancreatic exocrine secretion. The presence of a fistula to the pancreatic duct typically prolongs drainage, often to several weeks or months duration.[35]

Preparation For Catheter Removal

As drainage progresses and the cavity decreases in size, it may be reasonable to decrease the catheter size (particularly if a very large catheter has been in place). Indications for catheter removal include diminution of drainage to minimal amounts (usually less than 10–20 mL per day), collapse of the cavity to a size corresponding to that of the drainage catheter, and lack of communication with adjacent structures such as the gastrointestinal tract or pancreatic duct. We do not routinely cap catheters for a trial period, although this is an option if there is any question as to the advisability of removing the catheter. Gradual catheter removal may also be helpful, to allow the catheter track to close in a progressive fashion.

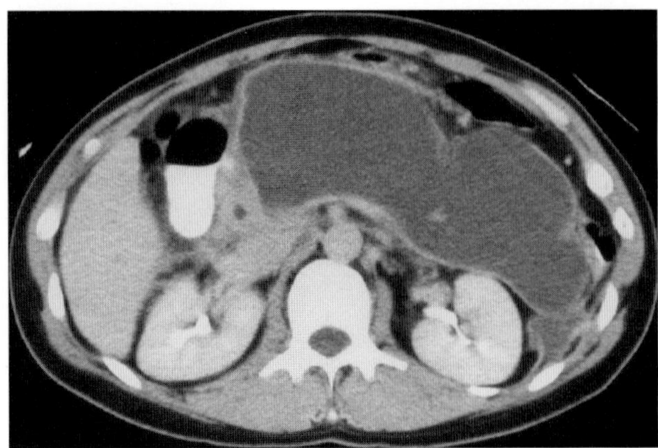

Figure 32. CT scan shows a pancreatic pseudocyst that resulted from iatrogenic trauma.

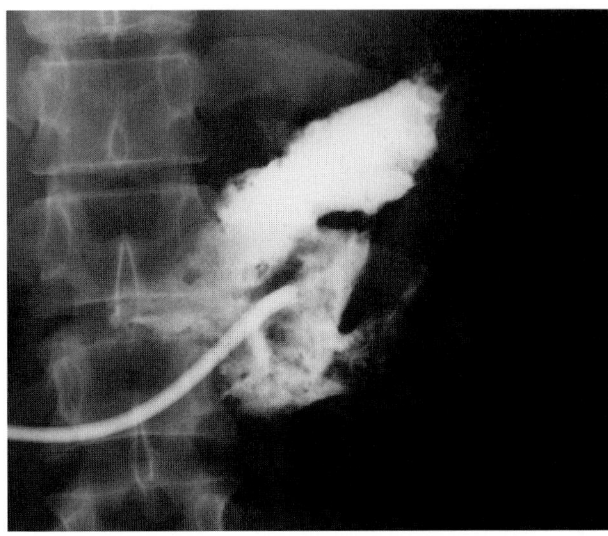

Figure 33. Same patient as in Figure 32. Catheter sinogram after drainage of the pseudocyst reveals the pseudocyst cavity.

Figures 32–39, obtained during the course of drainage of a pancreatic pseudocyst in a 34-year-old man who developed pancreatitis following ERCP, illustrate many of the principles discussed above. **Figure 32** shows a very large, symptomatic pancreatic pseudocyst. A relatively small (10 F) tube was placed within the collection from an anterior approach, and a tube check 1 month later showed a moderate sized, irregular cavity with some debris **(Fig. 33)**. Although a CT scan obtained 5 weeks later showed no other fluid collections and a well-positioned tube **(Fig. 34)**, the cavity had failed to shrink. The tube was therefore upsized first to a 14-F and then, 6 days later, to a 24-F catheter **(Fig. 35)**. Frequent irrigation was performed during this time, yielding particulate debris.

Four days later the cavity had diminished in size and was free of further debris, but a communication with the pancreatic duct had become apparent **(Fig. 36)**. The 24-F tube was downsized to a 10-F tube which could be positioned better in the smaller cavity **(Fig. 37)**. One month later, a repeat tube check showed virtually no residual cavity, but the communication with the pancreatic duct persisted **(Figs. 38, 39)**. Despite a good clinical response to the pseudocyst drainage, this patient eventually required distal pancreatectomy because of the pancreatic duct abnormality. Long-term stent placement of the pancreatic duct, via either the drainage track or ERCP, is another potential therapeutic option in such cases, although long-term data on the effectiveness of this approach are lacking.

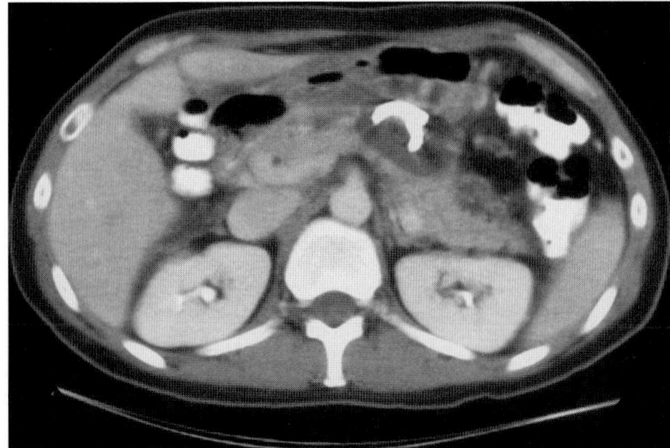

Figure 34. Same patient as in Figure 32. CT scan obtained after pseudocyst drainage.

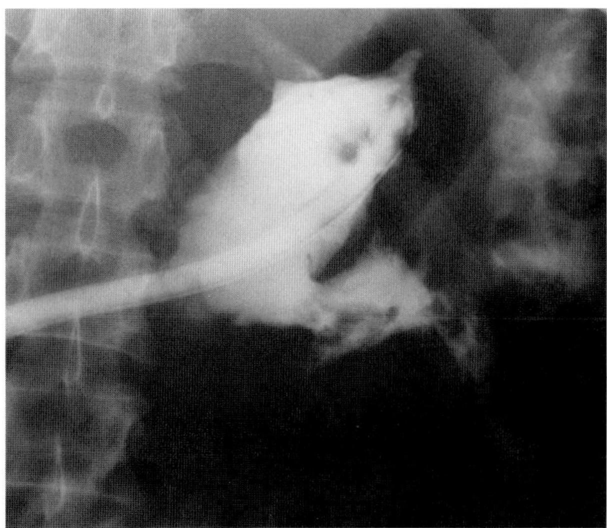

Figure 35. Same patient as in Figure 32. Catheter sinogram, large-bore tube.

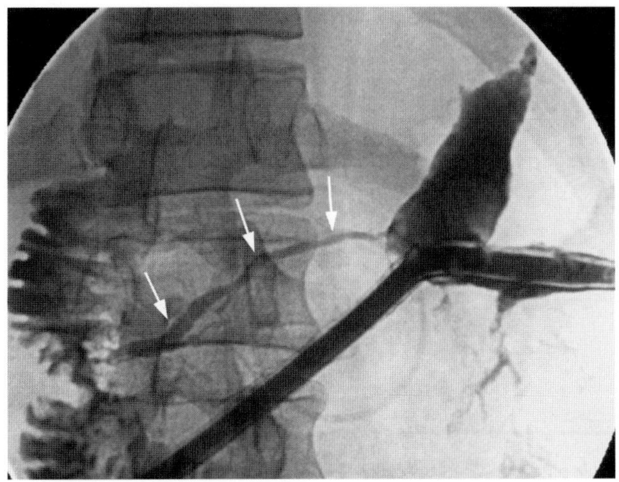

Figure 36. Same patient as in Figure 32. Catheter sinogram with pancreatic duct fistula. A communication with the pancreatic duct has become apparent (arrows).

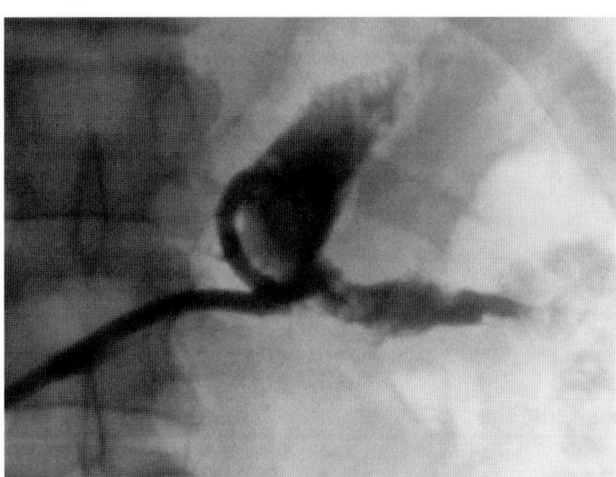

Figure 37. Same patient as in Figure 32. Catheter sinogram.

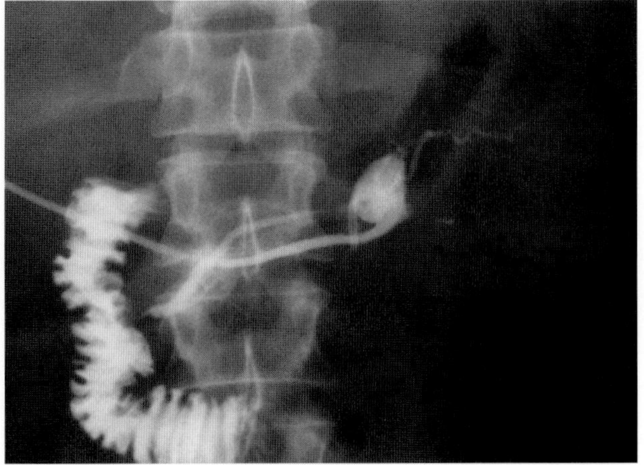

Figure 38. Same patient as in Figure 32. Catheter sinogram shows almost no residual cavity. The pancreatic duct still fills, however.

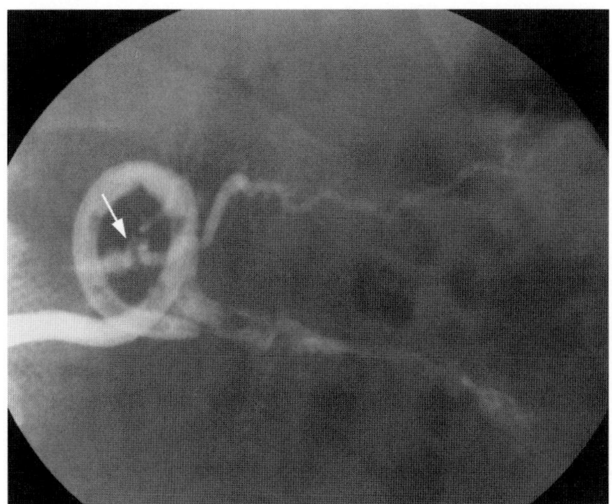

Figure 39. Same patient as in Figure 32. Catheter sinogram. On a close-up view, the pancreatic duct shows some irregularity (arrow).

Results of Interventional Radiology in Pancreatitis

In assessing the utility of catheter drainage of fluid collections associated with pancreatitis, the problems alluded to in the introduction to this tutorial become apparent: lack of adequate comparative clinical trials of therapeutic options for pancreatitis, inconsistent and ambiguous classification of treated patients, and differing definitions of success. Nevertheless, experience with these techniques continues to accumulate and some general statements regarding their effectiveness can be made.

Overall success rates for pancreatic drainage in reviews of multiple series fall in the range of 70%–80%, with recurrence rates of 15%–20%, although the range of individual studies shows considerable variation.[2,25–27,29] In general, the success rates are lower and recurrence rates higher than for surgical series, but percutaneous drainage also has lower rates of morbidity and mortality.

As would be expected, success rates for percutaneous drainage of noninfected fluid collections and pseudocysts are relatively high, with rates of about 90%, while abscesses and infected necrosis give progressively lower rates of success and higher rates of recurrences.[25,26,29] In D'Agostino's review of the literature, for example, patients with pancreatic abscess or infected necrosis had successful percutaneous drainage in just less than 50% of cases (compared to a 72% surgical rate) and recurrence or reoperation rate of 39% (close to the surgical rate of 38%).[26] Comparison to endoscopic series is thus far limited, in part because of lower numbers of patients treated by endoscopic means and in part because a smaller proportion of fluid collections are amenable to endoscopic drainage.

Summary

Imaging-guided drainage of fluid collections associated with acute pancreatitis offers several attractive features: it is minimally invasive, relatively safe (particularly in gravely ill patients at high risk for surgery), and tolerated well by most patients. It rarely precludes other therapies, and, with proper patient selection, seems to be efficacious. However, drainage of fluid collections associated with pancreatitis has not achieved the same success rates as for drainage of other abdominal fluid collections. While a great deal remains to be learned about its proper role, particularly with regard to its use as an effective "temporizing" measure in patients who will still require surgical therapy, interventional radiologists seem likely in the foreseeable future to continue to participate in the management of this difficult and often frustrating clinical problem.

Despite the best efforts of skilled practitioners from multiple disciplines, pancreatitis will continue to be a challenging and often frustrating clinical problem. Keys to success include effective communication and cooperation among many disciplines—internal medicine, critical care, surgery, gastroenterology, diagnostic and interventional radiology, nursing, nutritional support, pulmonary care, and anesthesiology. Thoughtful review of the literature, proper classification of the complications of pancreatitis, and continued improvement of technical skills and knowledge of the clinical and radiological features of this complex disorder will help the interventional radiologist play an important role in its management.

References

1. Bradley III EL. A clinically based classification system for acute pancreatitis. Arch Surg 1993; 128:586–590.

2. Balthazar EJ, Freeny PC, vanSonnenberg E. Imaging and intervention in acute pancreatitis. Radiology 1994; 193:297–306.

3. Steinberg W, Tenner S. Acute pancreatitis. N Engl J Med 1994; 330:1198–1210.

4. Berk JE. The management of acute pancreatitis: a critical assessment as Dr. Bockus would have wished. Am J Gastroenterol 1995; 90:696–703.

5. Blamey SL, Imrie CW, O'Neill J, Gilmour WH, Carter DC. Prognostic factors in acute pancreatitis. Gut 1984; 25:1340–1346.

6. Knaus WA, Draper EA, Wagner DP, Zimmerman JE. APACHE II: a severity of disease classification system. Crit Care Med 1985; 13:818–829.

7. Larvin M, McMahon MJ. APACHE II score for assessment and monitoring of acute pancreatitis. Lancet 1989; 2:201–205.

8. Ranson JH. Etiological and prognostic factors in human acute pancreatitis: a review. Am J Gastroenterol 1982; 77:633–638.

9. Ranson JH. The current management of acute pancreatitis. Adv Surg 1995; 28:93–112.

10. Wilson C, Heath DI, Imrie CW. Prediction of outcome in acute pancreatitis: a comparative study of APACHE II, clinical assessment, and multiple factor scoring systems. Br J Surg 1990; 77:1260–1264.

11. Calleja GA, Barkin JS. Acute pancreatitis. Med Clin North Am 1993; 77:1037–1056.

12. Balthazar EJ, Robinson DL, Megibow AJ, Ranson JH. Acute pancreatitis: value of CT in establishing prognosis. Radiology 1990; 174:331–336.

13. Neoptolemos JP, London NJ, Carr-Locke DL. Assessment of main pancreatic duct integrity by endoscopic retrograde pancreatography in patients with acute pancreatitis. Br J Surg 1993; 80:94–99.

14. Huibregtse K, Smits ME. Endoscopic management of diseases of the pancreas. Am J Gastroenterol 1994; 89(8 Suppl):S66–S77.

15. Saifuddin A, Ward J, Ridgway J, Chalmers AG. Comparison of MR and CT scanning in severe acute pancreatitis: initial experiences. Clin Radiol 1993; 48:111–116.

16. Foitzik T, Bassi DG, Schmidt J, et al. Intravenous contrast medium accentuates the severity of acute necrotizing pancreatitis in the rat. Gastroenterol 1994; 106:207–214.

17. Boudghéne F, L'Herminé C, Bigot J. Arterial complications of pancreatitis: diagnostic and therapeutic aspects in 104 cases. J Vasc Interv Radiol 1993; 4:551–558.

18. Mauro MA, Schiebler ML, Parker LA, Jaques PF. The spleen and its vasculature in pancreatitis: CT findings. Am Surgeon 1993; 59:155–159.

19. Vujic I. Vascular complications of pancreatitis. Radiol Clin North Am 1989; 27:81–91.

20. Mauro MA, Jaques P. Transcatheter management of pseudoaneurysms complicating pancreatitis. J Vasc Interv Radiol 1991; 2:527–532.

21. Warshaw AL. Damage prevention versus damage control in acute pancreatitis. Gastroenterology 1993; 104:1216–1219.

22. Gerzof SG, Banks PA, Robbins AH, et al. Early diagnosis of pancreatic infection by computed tomography-guided aspiration. Gastroenterology 1987; 93:1315–1320.

23. Hiatt J, Fink AS, King W, Pitt HA. Percutaneous aspiration of peripancreatic fluid collections: a safe method to detect infection. Surgery 1987; 101:523–530.

24. Howard TJ, Wiebke EA, Mogavero G, et al. Classification and treatment of local septic complications in acute pancreatitis. Am J Surg 1995; 170:44–50.

25. Lee MJ, Rattner DW, Legemate DA, et al. Acute complicated pancreatitis: redefining the role of interventional radiology. Radiology 1992; 183:171–174.

26. D'Agostino HB, Fotoohi M, Aspron MM, Oglevie S, Kinney T, Rose S. Percutaneous drainage of pancreatic fluid collections. Semin Intervent Radiol 1996; 13:101–136.

27. Freeny PC. Percutaneous management of pancreatic fluid collections. Baillieres Clin Gastroenterol 1992; 6:259–272.

28. Vitas GJ, Sarr MG. Selected management of pancreatic pseudocysts: operative versus expectant management. Surgery 1992; 111:123–130.

29. Lambiase RE. Percutaneous abscess and fluid drainage: a critical review. Cardiovasc Intervent Radiol 1991; 14:143–157.

30. Feig BW, Pomerantz RA, Vogelzang R, Rege RV, Nahrwold DL, Joehl RJ. Treatment of peripancreatic fluid collections in patients with complicated acute pancreatitis. Surg Gynecol Obstet 1992; 175:429–436.

31. Rattner DW, Legermate DA, Lee MJ, Mueller PR, Warshaw AL. Early surgical debridement of symptomatic pancreatic necrosis is beneficial irrespective of infection. Am J Surg 1992; 163:105–109.

32. Wittich GR, Goodacre BW, Walter RM, Karnel F. Anatomic access to pancreatic fluid collections. Semin Intervent Radiol 1995; 12:191–198.

33. Grosso M, Gandini G, Cassinis MC, Regge D, Righi D, Rossi P. Percutaneous treatment (including pseudocystogastrostomy) of 74 pancreatic pseudocysts. Radiology 1989; 173:493–497.

34. Lee MJ, Saini S, Geller SC, Warshaw AL, Mueller PR. Pancreatitis with pseudoaneurysm formation: a pitfall for the interventional radiologist. AJR 1991; 156:97–98.

35. Freeny PC, Lewis GP, Traverso LW, Ryan JA. Infected pancreatic fluid collections: percutaneous catheter drainage. Radiology 1988; 167:435–441.

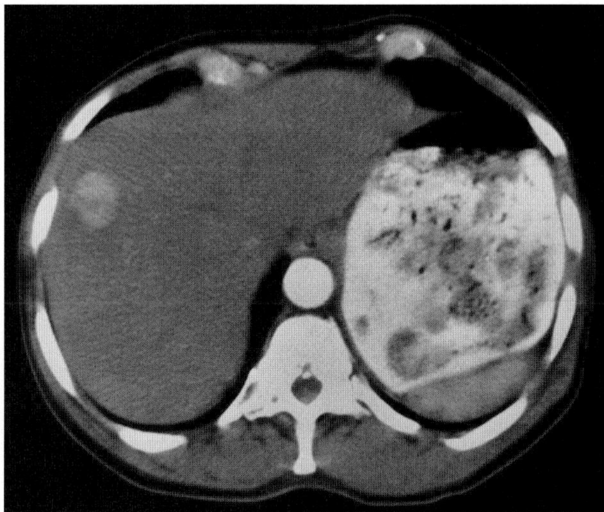

Figure 1. Small HCC detected by dual-phase contrast-enhanced computed tomography (CT) scanning, hepatic arterial phase.

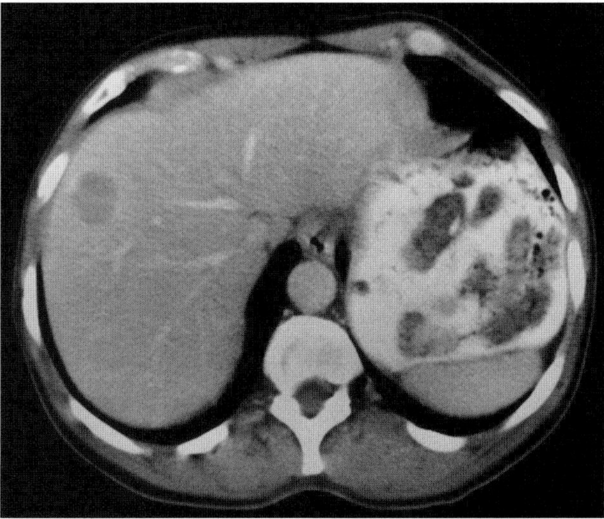

Figure 2. Same patient as in Figure 1. Small HCC detected by dual-phase contrast-enhanced CT scanning now seen in the portal venous phase.

TUTORIAL 10
PERCUTANEOUS ETHANOL ABLATION THERAPY OF HEPATOCELLULAR CARCINOMA

Richard D. Redvanly, M.D., and Ricardo Lencioni, M.D.

Introduction

The subjects addressed in this tutorial include:

1. Rationale for nonsurgical management of hepatocellular carcinoma (HCC)
2. Mechanism of action
3. Patient selection, indications, and contraindications
4. Technique
5. Evaluation of treatment efficacy
6. Results
7. Complications.

Rationale for Nonsurgical Management of HCC

HCC is one of the most common neoplasms worldwide and occurs in association with cirrhosis in over 80% of patients. Many patients with cirrhosis undergo screening procedures that permit the early detection of HCC. Presently, measurement of serum alpha-fetoprotein (AFP) levels and hepatic sonography are the most common screening techniques used to detect early HCC. As a result of widespread screening programs, the detection of HCC while it is still small and unifocal has increased significantly **(Figs. 1, 2)**. Unfortunately, only 30% of patients with HCC are suitable candidates for hepatic resection.[1]

Surgery in many patients with HCC is precluded because of severe hepatic dysfunction secondary to underlying cirrhosis. These patients have little functional reserve and would be at high risk for postoperative hepatic failure. Also, because of the associated cirrhosis, these patients are at high risk for the development of future tumors. That is, the initial lesion may be the prelude to other lesions. The metachronous nature of HCC in patients with cirrhosis must be considered when treatment options are weighed, and continued surveillance is necessary even after successful therapy. Because of the significant underlying hepatic disease, treatment methods that result in minimal damage to uninvolved hepatic parenchyma are best for the majority of patients with HCC.

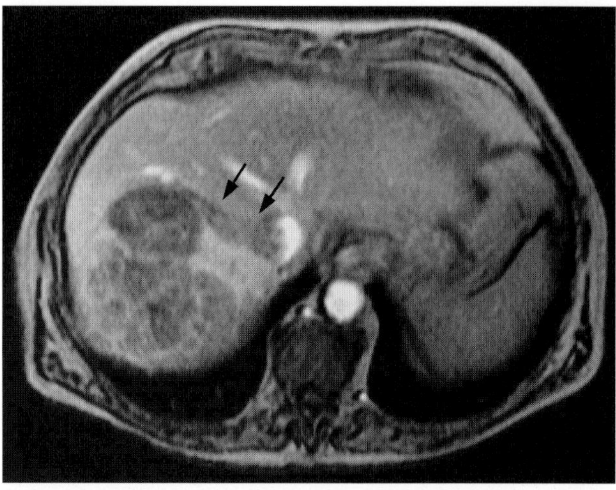

Figure 3. T1-weighted magnetic resonance (MR) image of HCC with hepatic vein and inferior vena cava invasion (arrows).

Percutaneous ethanol ablation therapy (PEAT) has proven to be a safe, effective, inexpensive treatment option for patients with cirrhosis and HCC.[2] Furthermore, it is minimally invasive and results in minimal damage to healthy hepatic parenchyma. Thus, PEAT can be performed on patients with Childs A–C cirrhosis and can be repeated for recurrent disease as well as new lesions.[2]

Mechanism of Action

Absolute ethanol destroys tumor tissue mainly because of the dehydrating and denaturing effects it has on protein.[3] In addition, ethanol has a thrombotic effect on tissue. As to the tumor, ethanol exerts tumoricidal and thrombotic effects locally. Homogeneous diffusion of ethanol throughout the tumor is necessary for complete tumor necrosis. Thus, tumor size, the presence or absence of internal septations, the volume of ethanol injected, and accurate needle placement into various portions of the tumor are important factors that determine whether the tumor will be successfully ablated.

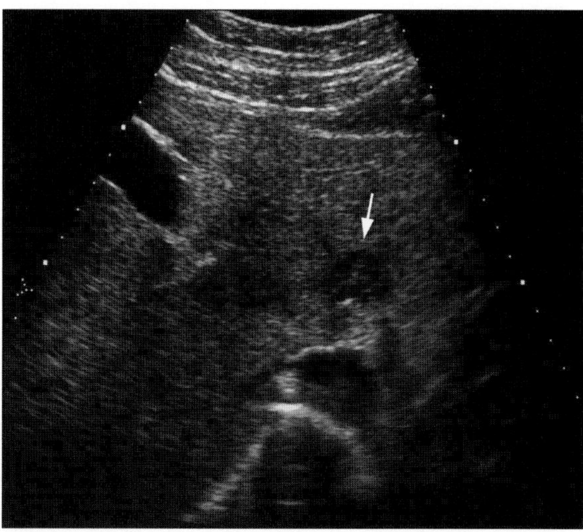

Figure 4. Same patient as in Figure 3. Ultrasound (US) examination of a small (1 cm in diameter) unifocal HCC that is optimal for PEAT (arrow).

Patient Selection

Patients with HCC are considered for PEAT if the tumor is not resectable. This can be because of severe hepatic dysfunction associated with cirrhosis, concomitant medical illnesses increasing the surgical risk, or patient refusal of surgery. PEAT can also be used as palliative therapy. Patients with multifocal or diffuse HCC, extrahepatic metastases, or vascular invasion are excluded from PEAT **(Fig. 3)**, and other therapies such as hepatic chemoembolization should be considered.

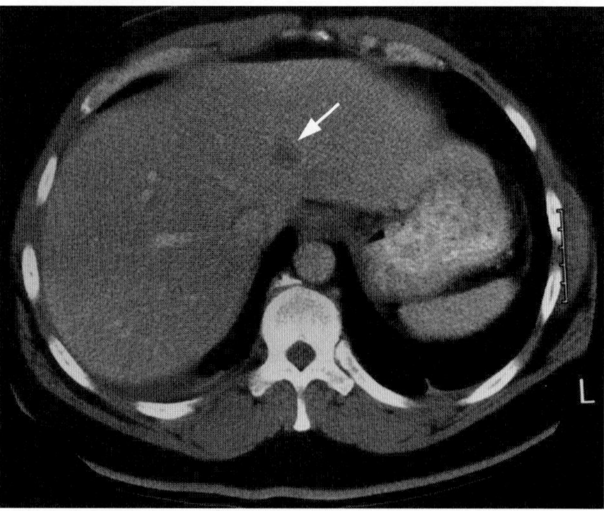

Figure 5. Same patient as in Figure 3. CT scan confirms the presence of a 1-cm HCC (arrow).

The highest possibility of cure is when treating a solitary HCC smaller than 3 cm in diameter **(Figs. 4, 5)**. Treatment of larger lesions has been undertaken but is less successful. This is most likely related to the internal characteristics of larger tumors which affect the distribution of injected ethanol so that small peripheral neoplastic nodules or portions of the tumor isolated by septa receive inadequate amounts of the ethanol for adequate treatment. Multiple synchronous lesions can be treated but most investigators perform PEAT on patients with three or fewer lesions.

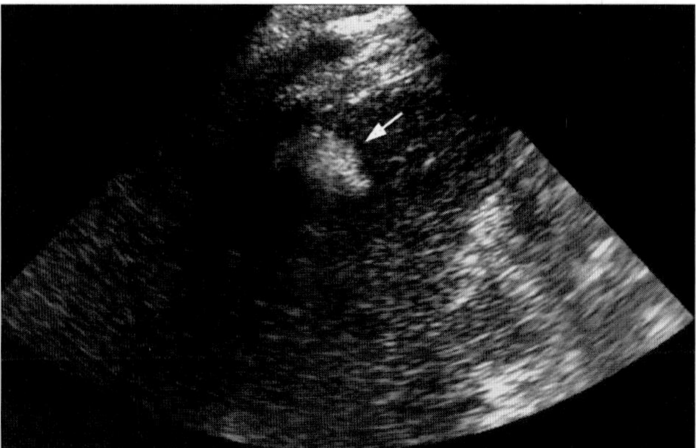

Figure 6. US following PEAT shows that the tumor has become hyperechoic and is obscured by ethanol (arrow).

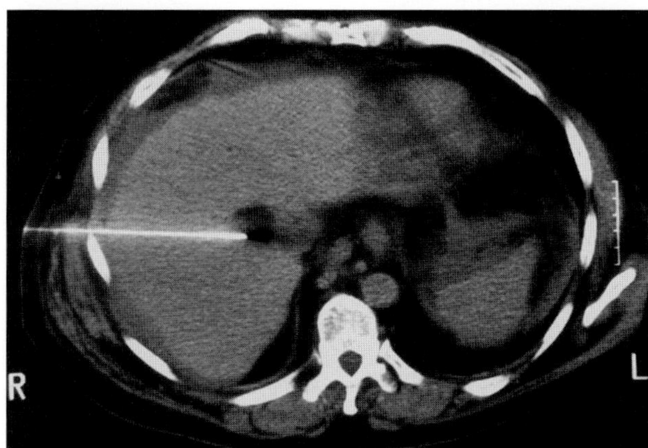

Figure 7. CT scan of needle placement and ethanol injection during PEAT.

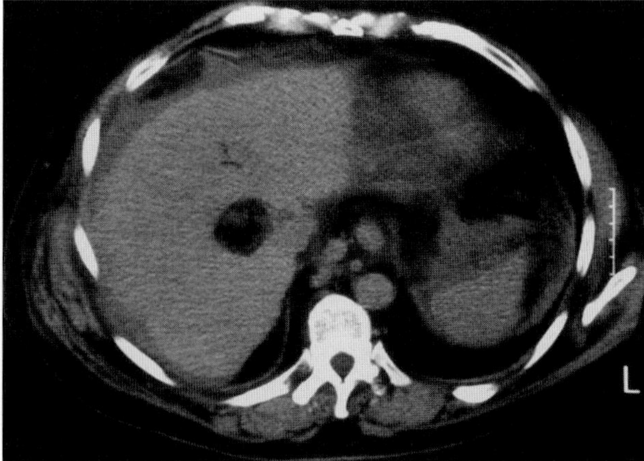

Figure 8. Same patient as in Figure 7. CT scan of an adequately ablated tumor shows a hypodense area equal in size to the tumor before PEAT.

Patients with a marked bleeding diathesis and/or thrombocytopenia (platelet count $<50,000/mm^3$) are not suitable candidates unless this condition can be corrected with transfusions of fresh frozen plasma or platelets.

Technique

PEAT can be performed with either ultrasound (US) or computed tomography (CT) guidance. US guidance has the advantage of real-time monitoring which allows precise placement of the needle into specific portions of the tumor. US also permits direct visualization of the diffusion of ethanol, and the procedure can usually be performed more quickly. However, lesions become markedly hyperechoic and heterogeneous on US following ethanol injection, which often obscures the margins of the lesion as well as the lesion itself **(Fig. 6)**, making it difficult to identify untreated portions of the tumor during PEAT.

Although US can be used to guide PEAT, CT guidance has several distinct advantages. During PEAT, the tumor is easier to identify after injection of ethanol. CT guidance also permits direct visualization of areas of tumor necrosis and identification of potentially untreated areas within the tumor **(Figs. 7, 8)**.[4] Although the choice of imaging guidance is largely dependent on the preference and skill of the radiologist, the ability of CT imaging to identify treated and untreated portions of the tumor is a significant advantage over US that may result in more effective tumor ablation.

Once the tumor is localized, the size is determined and the tumor volume calculated. The total volume of ethanol needed is calculated according to the equation: $V = 4/3\ \pi\ (r + 0.5\ cm)^3$ where V is the total volume of injected ethanol and r is the radius of the tumor. The addition of 0.5 cm provides a safety margin based on the principle that a small amount of surrounding tissue at the periphery of the lesion as well as the lesion itself must be destroyed to ensure complete tumor necrosis.

To inject ethanol, 18–22-gauge spinal needles or customized needles with multiple side-holes are used. A method of multiple needle insertion is used to inject ethanol into various sites within the tumor. The needle is placed into a specific portion of the lesion, approximately 1 mL of ethanol is injected, the needle is rotated about 60 degrees, and the process is repeated. Then the needle is withdrawn 5 mm and the entire process is repeated. This process of injection, rotation, and incremental needle retraction can be repeated after the needle has been passed into another portion of the tumor **(Fig. 9)**. At the end of the retraction, the needle is left in place for at least 60 seconds in order to decrease the chance of ethanol reflux into the peritoneal cavity.

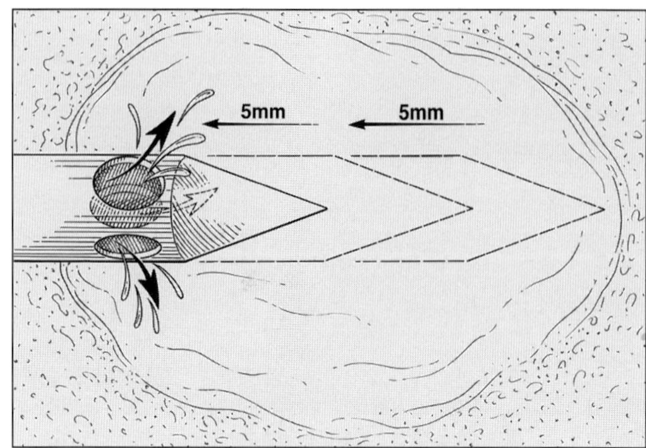

Figure 9. Schematic illustration of PEAT technique.

The total number of treatment sessions required depends on the size of the tumor and the amount of ethanol injected during each session. Ideally, the total calculated dose should be administered over as short a time as possible so that any remaining viable tumor can be quickly ablated. For small lesions (≤3 cm), ethanol injected in doses of 2–12 mL has proven successful, is well tolerated, and can be performed in a few treatment sessions. However, successful ablation of larger lesions is more difficult and requires numerous treatment sessions when small doses of ethanol are used. To ablate larger tumors (>3 cm) in a similar period of time, larger volumes of ethanol must be injected during each session. Ethanol can be safely injected in volumes as large as 40 mL per treatment session.[5] By administering larger volumes of ethanol, larger tumors can be treated in fewer sessions. Furthermore, because the total dose is administered over a short time period, the possibility of leaving residual viable tumor is diminished.

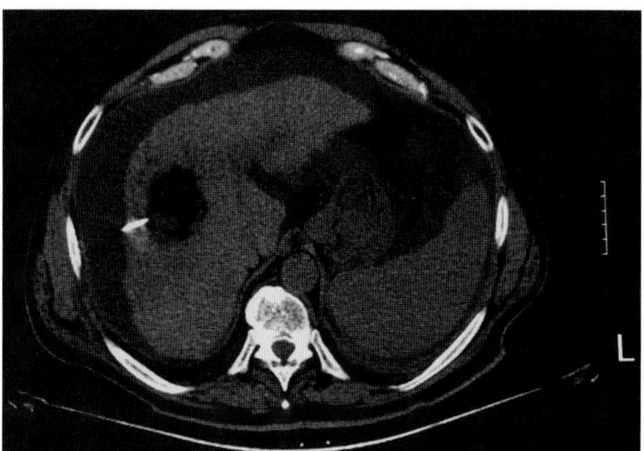

Figure 10. CT appearance during PEAT demonstrates the hypoattenuating treated tumor.

Evaluation of Efficacy

Immediately following PEAT, repeat CT scans of the lesion(s) are obtained. With CT scanning, a large hypodense area representing tumor necrosis is seen within the treated lesion immediately after ethanol injection **(Fig. 10)**. If a necrotic area equal in size to the original lesion is observed, the treatment is complete. Foci of inadequately treated tumor are readily identified as persistent areas of nodularity on immediate postablation CT scans and require additional treatment **(Figs. 11, 12)**.[6] If PEAT is performed with use of US guidance, color and/or power Doppler evaluation of tumor vascularity immediately following tumor ablation can help evaluate the efficacy of PEAT **(Figs. 13, 14)**.

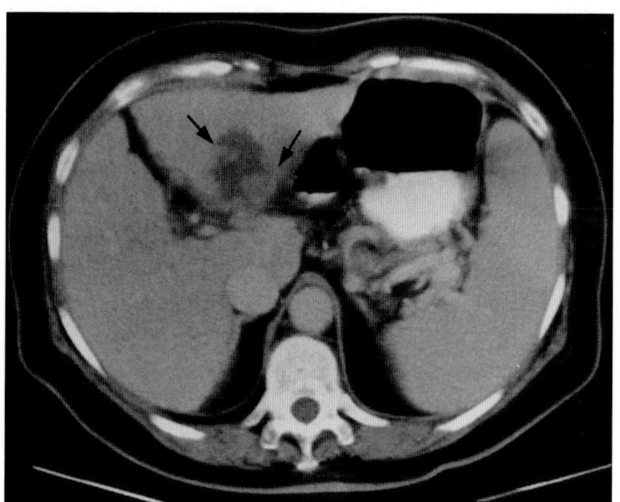

Figure 11. CT scan shows persistent areas of soft-tissue nodularity immediately following PEAT that represent untreated viable tumor (arrows).

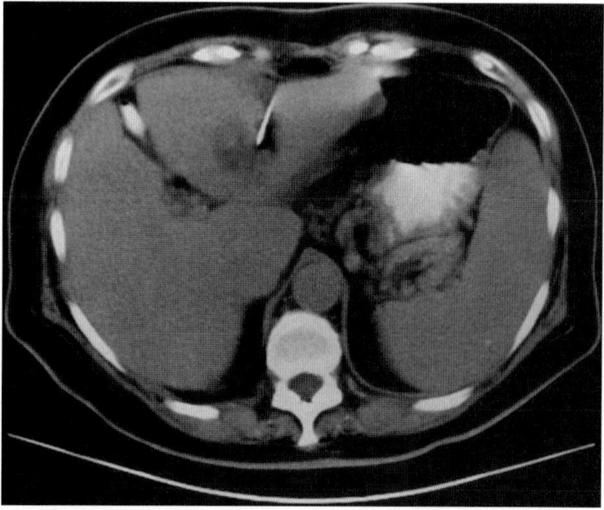

Figure 12. Same patient as in Figure 11. Nodular tissue in the periphery of the lesion was targeted for further ablation.

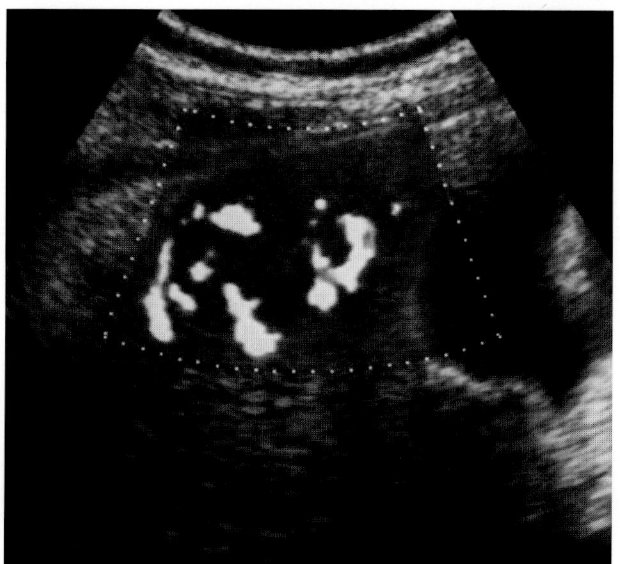

Figure 13. Power Doppler before treatment shows tumor vascularity.

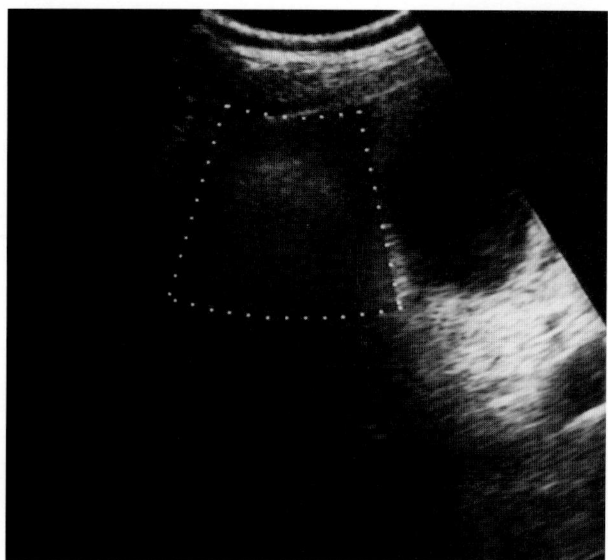

Figure 14. Same patient as in Figure 13. Following PEAT, no vascularity is detected within the HCC with power Doppler US.

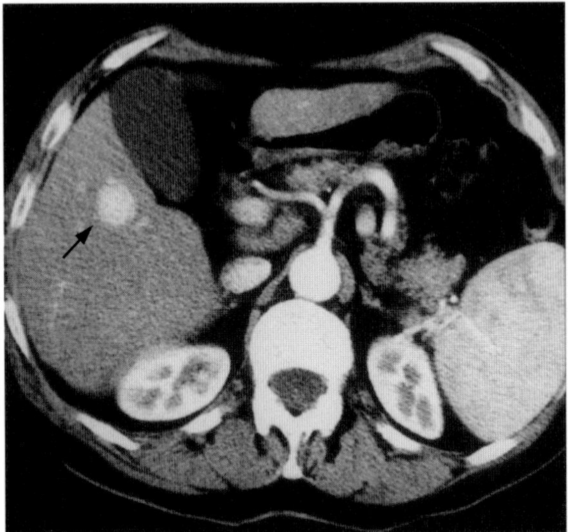

Figure 15. Contrast-enhanced CT scan demonstrates enhancing HCC (arrow).

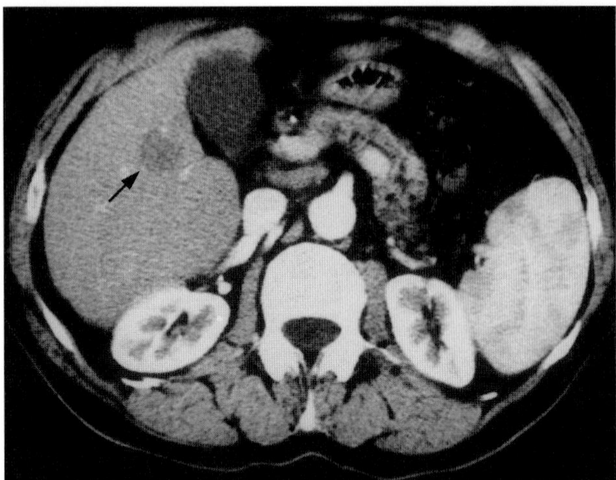

Figure 16. Same patient as in Figure 15. Following PEAT, a contrast-enhanced CT scan demonstrates lack of enhancement which correlates with complete tumor necrosis (arrow).

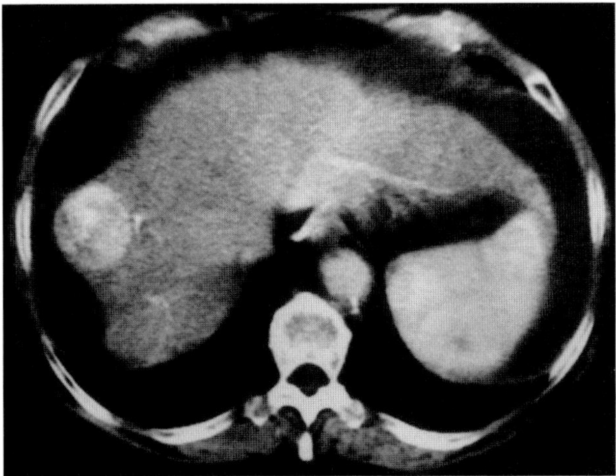

Figure 17. Contrast-enhanced CT scan demonstrates enhancing HCC.

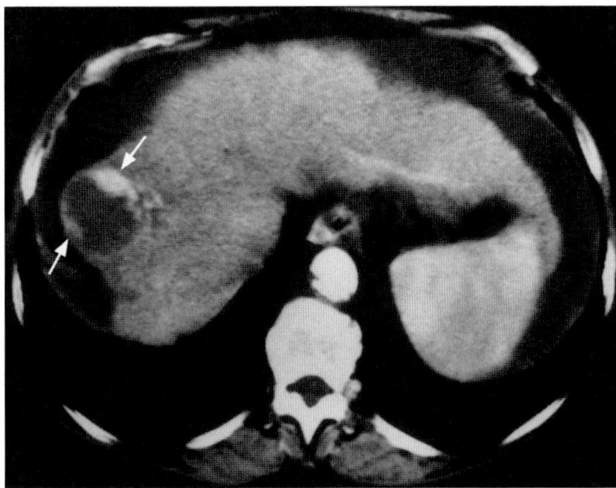

Figure 18. Same patient as in Figure 17. Contrast-enhanced CT scan shows foci of enhancement representing persistent viable tumor which should be targeted for repeat PEAT (arrows).

Following PEAT, a combination of imaging techniques, measurement of serum AFP, and percutaneous biopsy determines if the tumor is completely necrotic and detects any recurrence. Contrast-enhanced CT scanning is used most often to detect foci of viable tumor. Completely necrotic tumors lack enhancement on contrast-enhanced CT scans **(Figs. 15, 16)**, whereas areas of residual or recurrent tumor typically demonstrate foci of enhancement. These areas, if present, should be specifically targeted for percutaneous biopsy and repeat PEAT **(Figs. 17, 18)**.

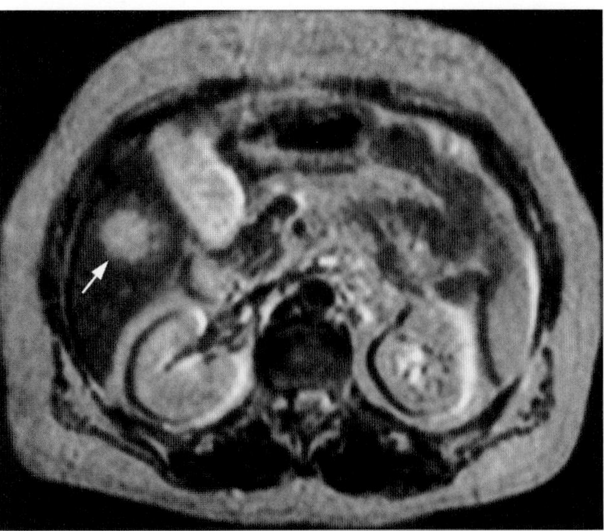

Figure 19. T2-weighted MR image of HCC before treatment has high signal intensity (arrow).

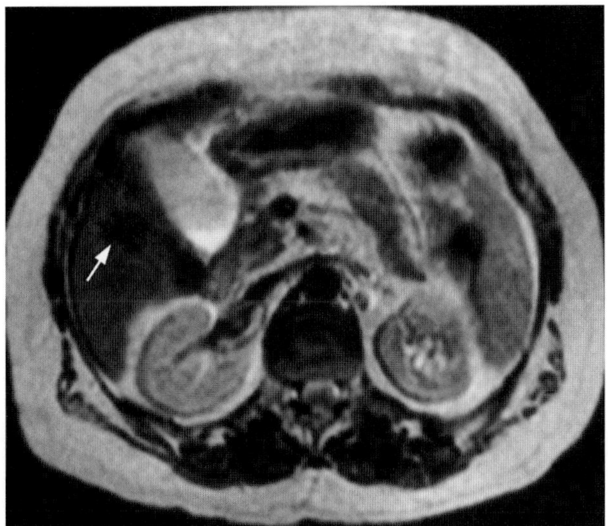

Figure 20. Same patient as in Figure 19. Following PEAT, T2-weighted MR image shows that the tumor has very low signal intensity (arrow).

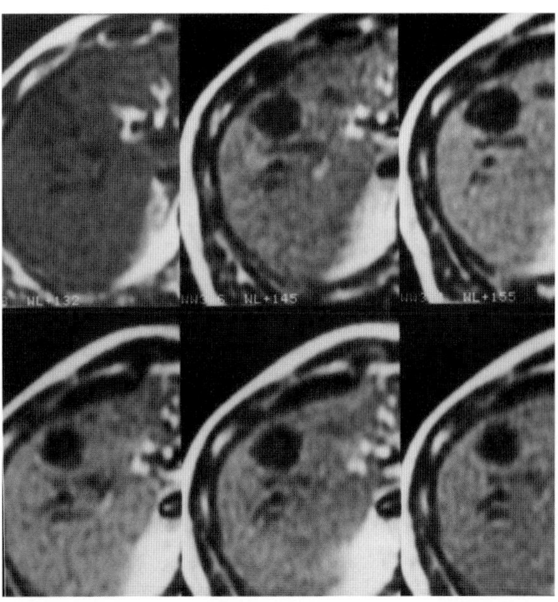

Figure 21. Following PEAT, no enhancement is detected on a dynamic gadolinium-enhanced T1-weighted MR image, representing complete tumor ablation.

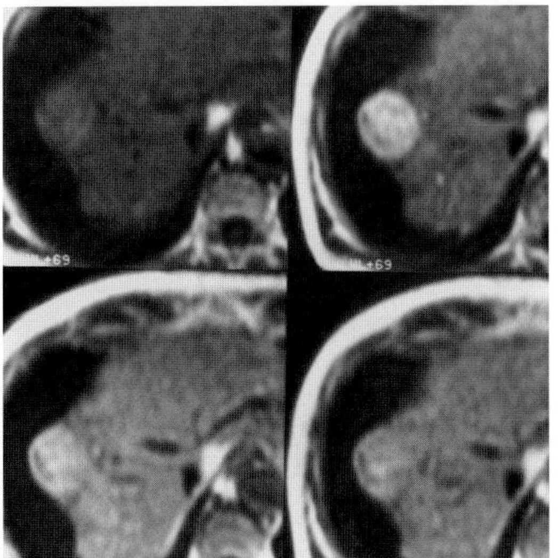

Figure 22. Dynamic gadolinium-enhanced T1-weighted image demonstrates homogeneously enhancing HCC.

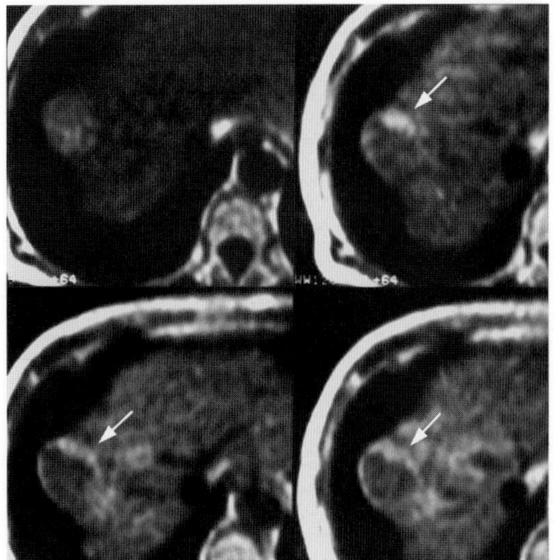

Figure 23. Same patient as in Figure 22. Following PEAT, a rim of enhancement is detected within the HCC on this dynamic gadolinium-enhanced T1-weighted MR image. This represents persistent viable tumor (arrows).

Alternatively, magnetic resonance (MR) imaging can be performed to detect foci of viable tumor, which demonstrate high signal intensity on T2-weighted sequences prior to ablation. Following PEAT, completely necrotic lesions are of low signal intensity on T2-weighted images, whereas lesions with viable tumor continue to demonstrate foci of increased signal intensity **(Figs. 19, 20)**.[7] On dynamic gadolinium-enhanced T1-weighted images, completely necrotic tumors lack enhancement while areas of viable tumor demonstrate foci of enhancement **(Figs. 21–23)**.[8]

Serum AFP should be measured routinely. Serum AFP levels decrease after successful tumor ablation; increases suggest recurrent disease. However, evaluation of serum AFP is useful only if it is elevated prior to therapy.

Long-term Survival Rate Based on Lesion Size					
Lesion Size (cm)	*Survival Rate (%)*				
	1-year	2-year	3-year	4-year	5-year
<3	97	92	68	57	40
3–5	94	77	57	45	37
>5	85	73	53	30	30
multiple	94	82	47	36	28

Figure 24.

Long-Term Survival Rate Based on Lesion Size, Number, and Childs Class[2]					
Lesion Size (cm)	*Survival Rate (%)*				
	1-year	2-year	3-year	4-year	5-year
A, ≤5	98	91	79	70	47
A, single <3	99	96	86	69	48
A, single 3–5	97	86	70	51	44
A, multiple	94	83	68	46	36
B, ≤5	93	78	63	37	29
B, multiple	93	78	59	17	0
C, ≤5	64	12	0	0	0

Figure 25.

A simple follow-up protocol includes contrast-enhanced CT scanning, measurement of serum AFP levels, and biopsy 1 month after completion of treatment. If the biopsy is negative for viable tumor, serum AFP levels and contrast-enhanced CT scans are obtained at 3 months. If the lesion demonstrates enhancement or the serum AFP levels rise, then biopsy and additional ablation are performed. If these studies do not indicate recurrent tumor, contrast-enhanced CT scanning, measurement of serum AFP levels, and biopsy are performed at 6 months, 1 year, and at yearly intervals thereafter. If viable tumor is identified at any time, PEAT can be repeated.

Long-Term Results

Long-term survival rates in patients with HCC treated with PEAT are related to the number of lesions, tumor size, and degree of underlying cirrhosis. In general, the best result is obtained in the patient with a solitary small tumor (≤3 cm in diameter) and minimal hepatocellular dysfunction (ie, Childs A cirrhosis). As expected, outcomes are poor in patients with large tumors (≥5 cm) and/or vascular invasion, and in those with multiple tumors (>3). Patients with Childs C cirrhosis tend to do poorly regardless of the size or number of lesions, since the prognosis in these patients is primarily related to the complications of portal hypertension. In patients with large solitary tumors, segmental chemoembolization followed by interval PEAT may be more effective than ethanol ablation alone.

The 5-year survival rates according to lesion size and number, and Childs classification are shown in **Figures 24** and **25.** Survival rates following PEAT compare favorably to those of surgical resection, which are: 1-year=81%; 2-year=73%; 3-year=44%; and 4-year=44%.[9]

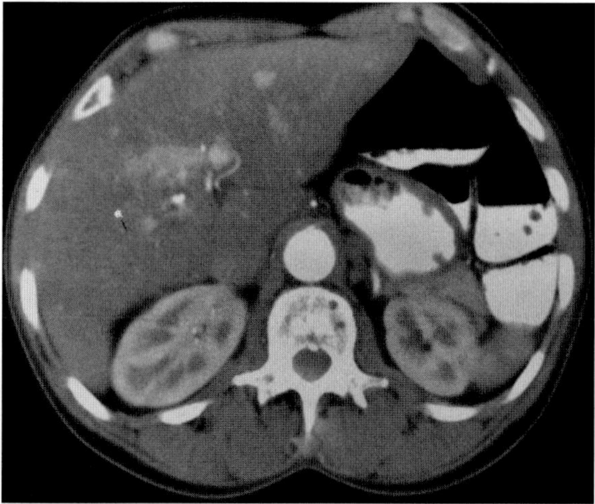

Figure 26. CT follow-up of a patient with HCC treated with PEAT. Hepatic arterial phase images show multiple enhancing lesions representing recurrent HCC in different segments of the liver.

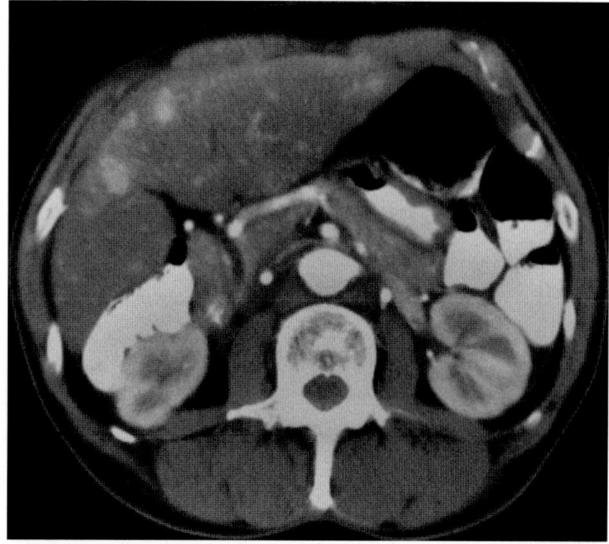

Figure 27. Same patient as in Figure 26.

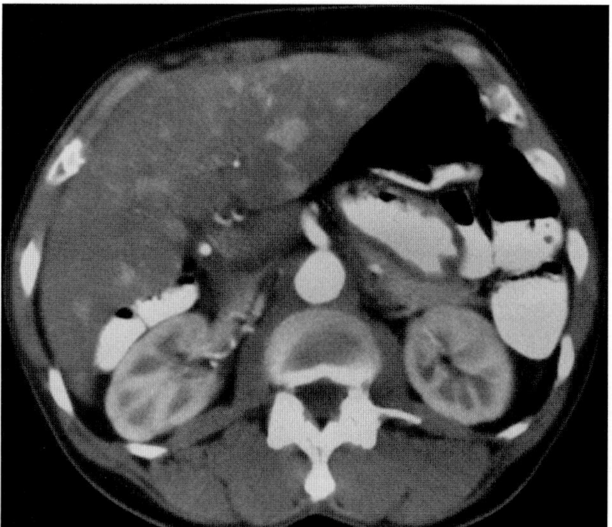

Figure 28. Same patient as in Figure 26.

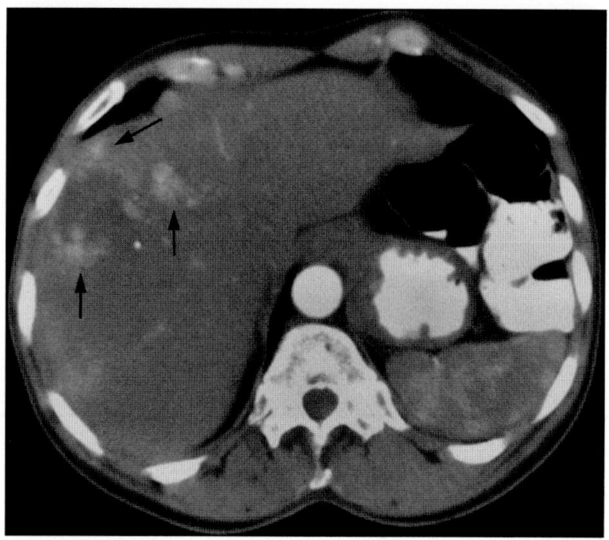

Figure 29. CT scan demonstrates locally recurrent tumor (arrows) following PEAT. Note the hypodense area which was the site of the previous tumor.

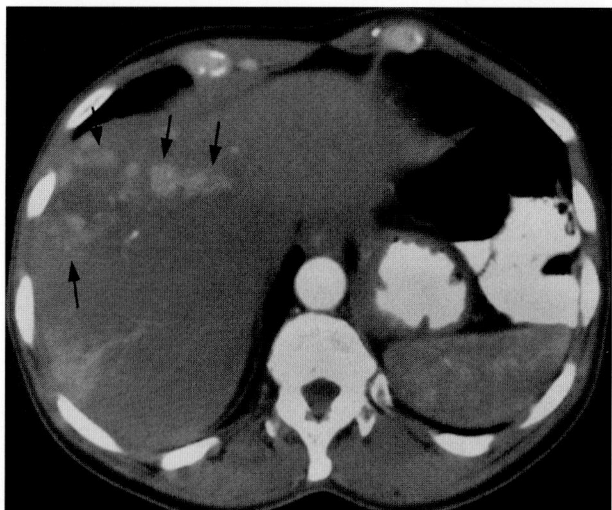

Figure 30. Same patient as in Figure 29. CT scan demonstrates locally recurrent tumor and enhancing tumor thrombus (arrows).

Tumor recurrence is common following PEAT. Recurrence rates are higher in patients with multiple lesions and more advanced cirrhosis. The 5-year tumor recurrence rate is approximately 83%.[2] Most recurrent lesions are distinct new tumors in portions of the untreated liver **(Figs. 26–28)**. Local tumor recurrence is approximately 17% at 5 years **(Figs. 29, 30)**.[2] In both circumstances, the recurrent tumor can be retreated successfully. The high recurrence rate underscores the importance of continued follow-up with periodic imaging studies and serum AFP measurements.

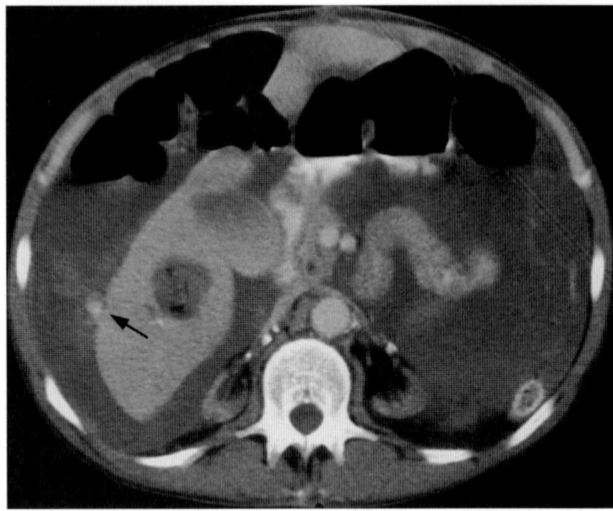

Figure 31. Intraperitoneal hemorrhage following PEAT. Arrow shows bleeding site.

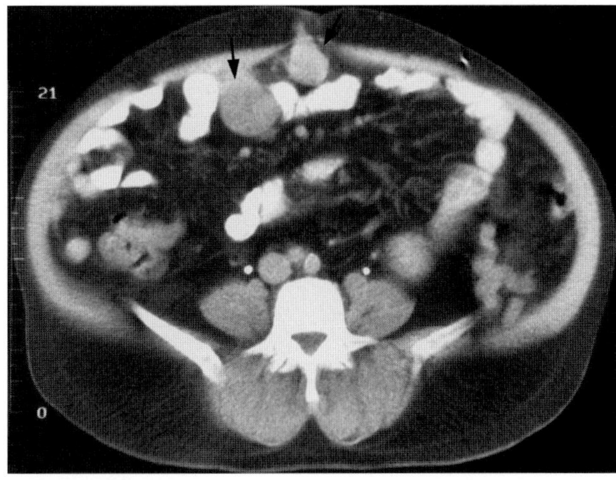

Figure 32. Intraperitoneal metastases along the path of the needle track (arrows).

Safety and Complications

Minor complications are common. They are more frequent when treating larger tumors and are primarily related to the use of larger volumes of ethanol and greater tumor necrosis.[4] Pain and fever should be expected and can be managed conservatively. Peritoneal reflux of ethanol along the needle track may cause pain and is related to the size of the needle, tumor location, and the rate of injection.[10] To minimize peritoneal reflux, ethanol should be injected slowly and the needle left in place for several minutes. Mild, transient elevations in serum liver transaminases frequently occur but are less than those observed with arterial chemoembolization or hepatic resection. Ethanol intoxication, which is usually mild and transient, may occur. Small right-sided pleural effusions and pneumothorax occasionally occur.

Major complications are unusual. Massive liver necrosis and death probably related to reflux of ethanol into portal vein branches is extremely rare.[11] Other rare complications include intraperitoneal hemorrhage, peritoneal tumor seeding, and jaundice due to bile duct injury **(Figs. 31, 32)**.[12,13] Theoretically, intraperitoneal bleeding and tumor seeding should be rare because ethanol that refluxes back along the needle track exerts a thrombotic and tumoricidal effect.

PEAT in Other Tumors

Although PEAT can be used to treat other hepatic neoplasms, notably metastases, the results have not been as good as with HCC.[14] This is likely due to the consistency of adenocarcinoma metastases, which are much harder than HCC. Because of the hard consistency, the ethanol does not diffuse throughout the tumor but rather spreads along the periportal spaces, resulting in more complications. If amenable to surgery, colorectal metastases should be treated with hepatic resection; otherwise, hepatic chemoembolization should be considered.

Conclusion

PEAT is a viable option for the treatment of HCC and should be strongly considered in those patients who have a small solitary lesion and are not candidates for surgical resection.

References

1. Shiina S, Niwa Y, Omata M. Percutaneous ethanol injection therapy for liver neoplasms. Semin Intervent Radiol 1993; 10:57–68.

2. Livraghi T, Giorgio A, Marin G, et al. Hepatocellular carcinoma and cirrhosis in 746 patients: long-term results of percutaneous ethanol injection. Radiology 1995; 197:101–108.

3. Livraghi T, Solbiati L. Percutaneous ethanol injection in liver cancer: method and results. Semin Intervent Radiol 1993; 10:69–77.

4. Redvanly RD, Chezmar JL. Percutaneous ethanol ablation therapy of malignant hepatic tumors using CT guidance. Semin Intervent Radiol 1993; 10:82–87.

5. Redvanly RD, Chezmar JL, Strauss RM, Galloway JR, Boyer TD, Bernardino ME. Malignant hepatic tumors: safety of high-dose percutaneous ethanol ablation therapy. Radiology 1993; 188:283–285.

6. Joseph FB, Baumgarten DA, Bernardino ME. Hepatocellular carcinoma: CT appearance after percutaneous ethanol ablation therapy (work in progress). Radiology 1993; 186:553–556.

7. Sironi S, Livraghi T, Angeli E, et al. Small hepatocellular carcinoma: MR follow-up of treatment with percutaneous ethanol injection. Radiology 1993; 187:119–123.

8. Bartolozzi C, Lencioni R, Caramella D, Mazzeo S, Ciancia EM. Treatment of hepatocellular carcinoma with percutaneous ethanol injection: evaluation with contrast-enhanced MR imaging. AJR 1994; 162:827–831.

9. Castells A, Bruix J, Bru C, et al. Treatment of small hepatocellular carcinoma in cirrhotic patients: a cohort study comparing surgical resection and percutaneous ethanol injection. Hepatology 1993; 18:1121–1126.

10. Vehmas T. Reflux of ethanol during experimental liver ethanol injections. Invest Radiol 1992; 27:918–921.

11. Taavitsainen M, Vehmas T, Kauppila R. Fatal liver necrosis following percutaneous ethanol injection for hepatocellular carcinoma. Abdom Imaging 1993; 18:357–359.

12. Cedrone A, Rapaccini GL, Pompili M, Grattagliano A, Aliotta A, Trombino C. Neoplastic seeding complicating percutaneous ethanol injection for treatment of hepatocellular carcinoma. Radiology 1992; 183:787–788.

13. Koda M, Okamoto K, Miyoshi Y, Kawasaki H. Hepatic vascular and bile duct injury after ethanol injection therapy for hepatocellular carcinoma. Gastrointest Radiol 1992; 17:167–169.

14. Livraghi T, Vettori C, Lazzaroni S. Liver metastases: results of percutaneous ethanol injection in 14 patients. Radiology 1991; 179:709–712.

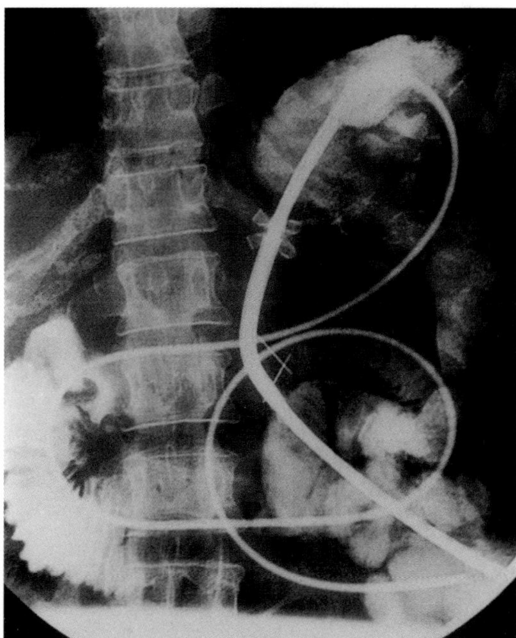

Figure 1. Gastrojejunostomy.

TUTORIAL 11 RADIOGRAPHICALLY GUIDED PERCUTANEOUS GASTROSTOMY AND GASTROJEJUNOSTOMY

Curtis A. Lewis, M.D.

Introduction

The subjects addressed in this tutorial include:

1. Indications for and contraindications to enteral feeding tube placement
2. Review of techniques of inserting gastrostomy and gastrojejunostomy tubes
3. Complications associated with inserting gastrostomy and gastrojejunostomy tubes
4. Expected outcomes.

The placement of gastrostomies and gastrojejunostomies by radiologists is becoming a more common practice **(Fig. 1)**.[1–5] The use of imaging to assist in the placement of these tubes results in fewer complications and higher success rates when compared to surgically placed enteral tubes.[1,3-10,11,12,13]

Indications

The placement of enteral tubes is indicated for decompression of gastroenteric contents (10% of cases), or more commonly, to provide nutritional support in patients unable to maintain their nutritional status orally (90% of cases).[1–4,9,11,13–15] The other means of nutritional support in the latter patient population is parenteral feeding, which is significantly more costly and is associated with more long-term complications than enteral feeding.[1,13] In patients who do not suffer from malabsorption secondary to short gut, malabsorption syndromes, or bowel obstruction, enteral feedings provide a more physiologic means of delivering nutrients than parenteral feedings.[16]

Contraindications

Contraindications to the placement of a gastrostomy or gastrojejunostomy tube are either absolute or relative **(Fig. 2)**.[1,2,4,9,14,17] Because placement of these tubes is rarely done emergently, many of the relative contraindications can be corrected, allowing the procedure to be performed. If the tube is being placed for decompression of gastric contents (obstruction) and the jejunostomy limb of the gastrojejunostomy tube is long enough to be placed beyond a proximal obstructing lesion, then gastric obstruction should not be considered a contraindication. Conditions such as total gastrectomy and severe abdominal skin burns obviously preclude gastrostomy or gastrojejunostomy tube placement. However, imaging-guided direct jejunostomy or percutaneous duodenostomy may be performed in these patients[15,18] **(See Tutorial 12)**.

Contraindications to Gastrostomy or Gastrojejunostomy

Relative

1. Correctable coagulopathy
2. Overlying viscera
3. Ascites
4. Prior gastric surgery
5. Peritoneal dialysis
6. Ventriculoperitoneal shunt
7. Gastric outlet obstruction
8. Dermatologic abnormality

Absolute

1. Uncorrected coagulopathy
2. Portal hypertension with gastric varices
3. Extensive abdominal burns
4. Gastric carcinomatosis
5. Total gastrectomy

Figure 2.

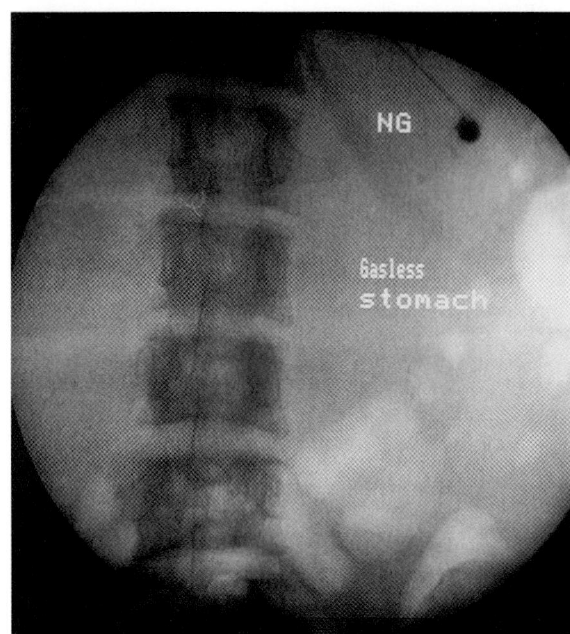

Figure 3. Nasogastric tube in a decompressed stomach.

Procedure

Preprocedural Considerations

Before an enteral tube is placed, it is important that the patient be evaluated to ensure that the tube requested is appropriate and indicated. A brief history and physical examination should be performed to identify any contraindications (relative or absolute) that might delay or preclude tube placement. Contraindications that can be rectified should be identified and corrected (ie, coagulopathy). The procedure and its immediate and long-term complications should be explained to the patient or care-giver when informed consent is obtained. This is particularly important because many of these patients are debilitated or suffer from neurologic deficits that prevent them from understanding the potential complications and care requirements associated with these devices.

Patients are kept fasting for 12 to 24 hours prior to the procedure.[1,24] Laboratory tests are evaluated with special attention to prothrombin time, partial thromboplastin time, and the platelet count. A nasogastric (NG) tube is placed first **(Fig. 3)**.[1,2,4,12,13,15] However, if such placement is difficult, the tube can be inserted at the time of the procedure. In patients with esophageal obstructions, the use of fluoroscopy and, possibly, selective angiographic catheters and hydrophilic wires may be required to traverse the obstruction and place a tube into the stomach. This can usually be done with a minimum of time and difficulty. Some radiologists will have contrast material placed into the gastrointestinal tract the evening before the procedure so the colon will be more easily visualized.[12,19] It is also important that patients arrive in the interventional radiology suite with adequate intravenous (IV) access.

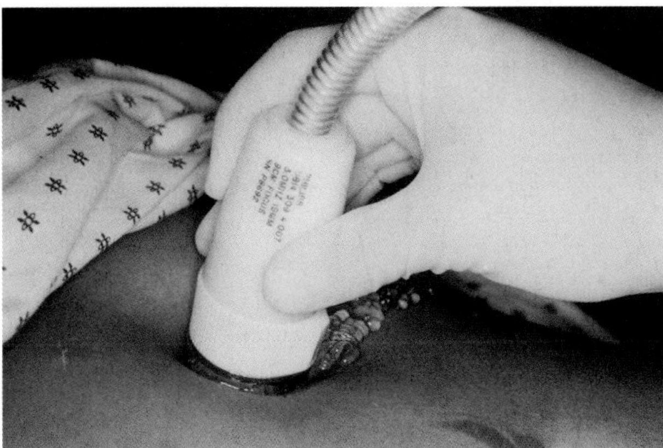

Figure 4. Limited ultrasound examination performed to localize the liver edge.

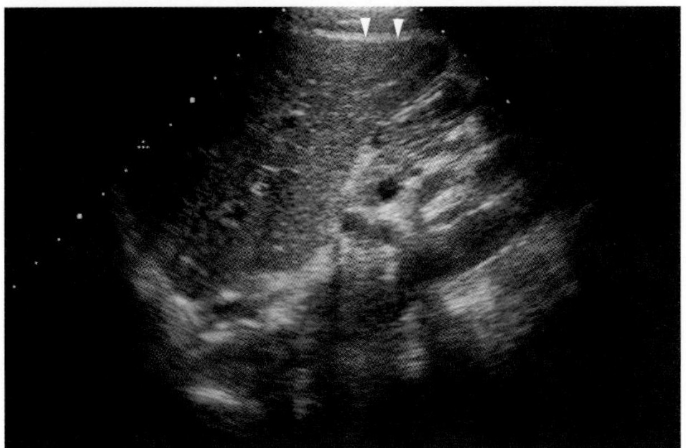

Figure 5. Sonogram demonstrates the left lobe of the liver (arrowheads).

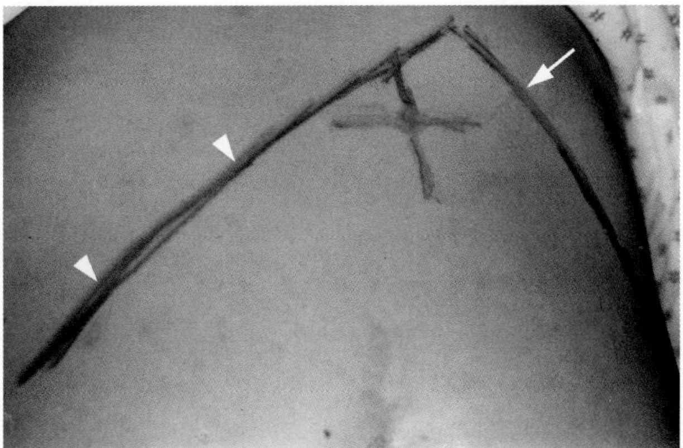

Figure 6. Abdomen marked with the liver edge (arrowheads) and left costal margin (arrow).

Procedural Considerations

Previous imaging studies should be evaluated to identify anatomical variations or variations due to surgery that could alter or prevent adequate approach to the stomach.[2–5,9,12,14,15,19,20] A limited ultrasound examination performed immediately prior to the procedure can help localize and mark the liver edge and identify any hepatosplenomegaly **(Figs. 4–6)**. Although traversing the liver with a tube may be inconsequential, it is preferable not to do so, if possible. In addition to the liver edge, the left costal margin is localized and marked **(Fig. 6)**. Before beginning it is also advisable to examine the abdomen with fluoroscopy, checking for the presence of marked gaseous distention of either the small bowel or colon that could delay the procedure or necessitate placement of a rectal tube for decompression. The patient is then prepared with use of a surgical antiseptic over most of the anterior abdomen and lower chest wall. Although no studies documenting the effectiveness of preprocedural antibiotics prior to a gastrostomy have been done and considerable controversy exists over their use in this situation, prophylactic antibiotic coverage can be administered before the procedure, usually cefazolin. The patient is maintained on IV fluids during the procedure and sedated with IV midazolam and fentanyl. The procedure can be performed with local anesthesia only (2% lidocaine) at the site of tube insertion if the patient is unstable or does not desire IV sedation.

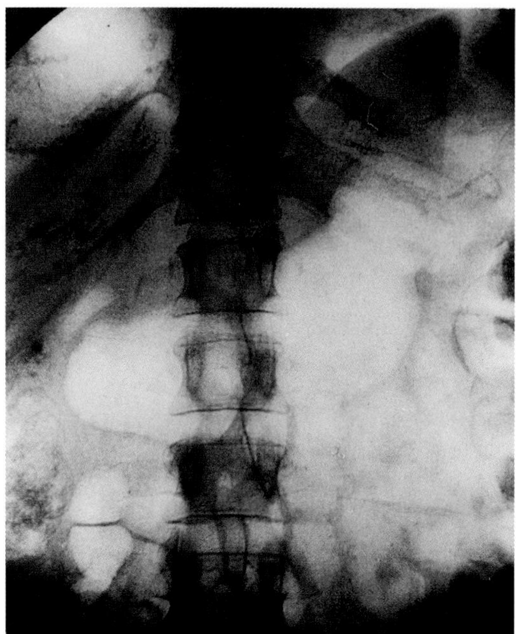

Figure 7. Stomach insufflated with air.

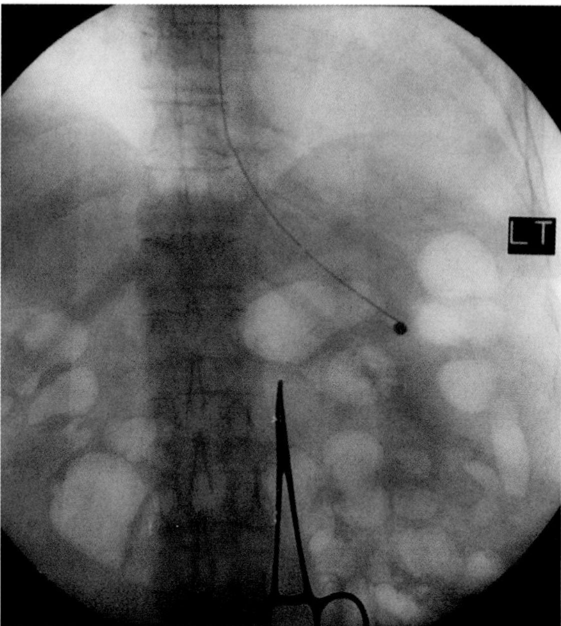

Figure 8. Decompressed stomach prior to insufflation with air. Note the position of the hemostat.

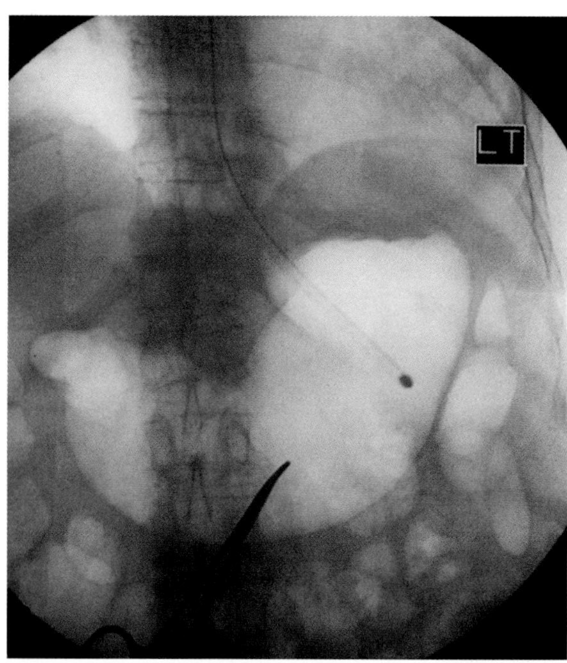

Figure 9. Stomach insufflated with air. The hemostat tip has not moved from its position in Figure 8 and marks an appropriate puncture site.

After the abdomen has been prepared and draped, the indwelling NG catheter is connected to a 60-mL syringe and room air insufflated into the stomach under direct fluoroscopic observation, facilitating excellent visualization of the stomach **(Fig. 7)**. As the stomach becomes distended it displaces other air-filled structures such as the colon and small bowel. Expansion of the stomach will not only alter its size but also its relative position **(Figs. 8, 9)**. Frequently this change in position will allow the procedure to be performed in a patient who was initially thought to have poor access (ie, intrathoracic stomach). Should insufflated air escape into the small bowel, glucagon can be administered to reduce peristalsis and prevent gastric decompression.[1,4,12,14,19] However, administration of glucagon will make it more difficult to pass a jejunostomy tube through the pylorus and will decrease peristaltic assistance in advancing the tube through the duodenum into the jejunum.

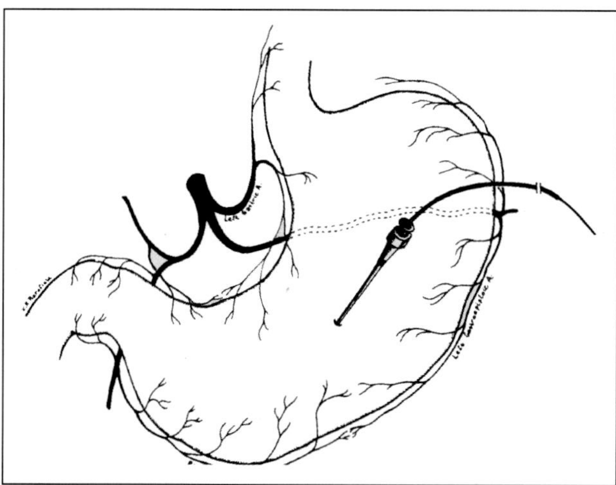

Figure 10. Illustration demonstrates the location and angulation of the puncture.

After the stomach has been distended adequately, a site for the gastrostomy or gastrojejunostomy is selected with the aid of hemostats and fluoroscopy. The location for puncture should be between the mid body of the stomach and the junction of the body and antrum. The puncture should enter the stomach equidistant from the greater and lesser curvatures. A puncture in this location will enter anteriorly and distant from the right and left gastroepiploic arteries and the left gastric artery, which course along the greater and lesser curvatures, respectively **(Fig. 10)**.[4,5] In addition, this site should lie at least 2 cm below the rib margin and not over the liver edge. Placement of the tube close to the rib margin could lead to increased discomfort for the patient.

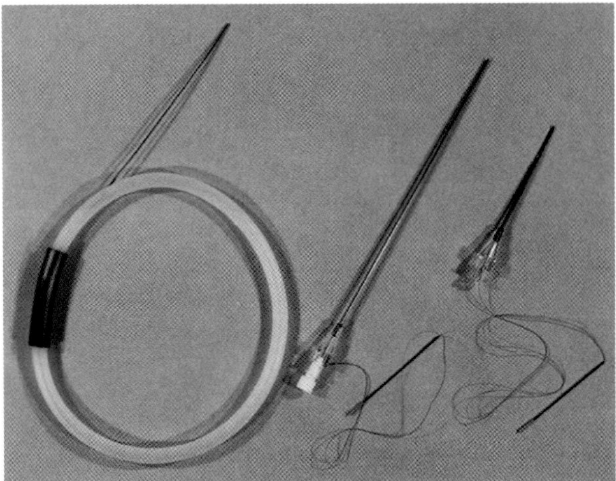

Figure 11. Cook Cope gastrointestinal suture anchor set.

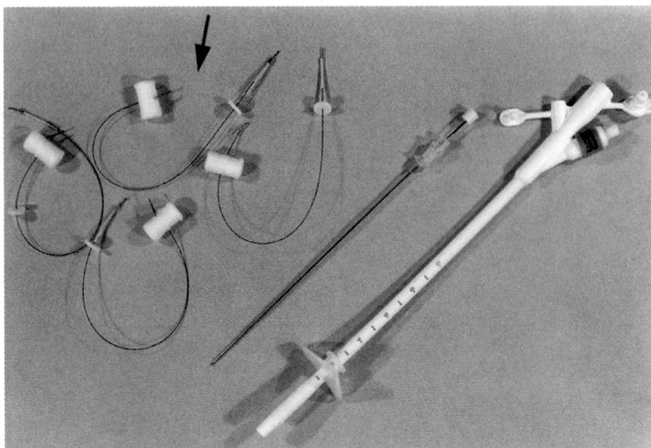

Figure 12. Brown/Mueller T-Fasteners (arrow) included with the Flexiflo gastrostomy tube (Ross Laboratories, Columbus, OH).

When the appropriate puncture site has been selected, the region is anesthetized with lidocaine. A Cope gastrointestinal suture anchor set (Cook, Bloomington, IN) **(Fig. 11)** or its equivalent (Brown/ Mueller T-Fastener [Medi-Tech, Boston Scientific Corporation, Watertown, MA]) **(Fig. 12)** can then be used to attach the stomach firmly to the anterior abdominal wall. Although gastropexy is not an absolute requirement, it will facilitate the procedure by allowing the advancement of dilators, sheaths, and tubes without the risk of displacing the stomach.[1,2,4,11,15,19] Although the absolute need for gastropexy remains contested and enteral tube placement can be performed without gastropexy, the use of gastropexy may reduce leakage of gastric contents into the peritoneum and decrease complications associated with early tube dislodgement.[1–4,11] Gastropexy is performed with a 17- or 18-gauge needle pre-loaded with an anchor which is attached to a suture. The needle is advanced through the skin and can be seen to indent the anterior stomach wall **(Fig. 13)**. When the needle can be seen entering the stomach, its position can be verified by the aspiration of air followed by injection of contrast material to demonstrate the gastric rugae **(Fig. 14)**. Advancement of a wire through the shaft of the needle deposits the anchor into the stomach **(Figs. 15, 16)**. With firm retraction on the thread the stomach is pulled up to the anterior abdominal wall and sutured into place **(Figs. 17, 18)**.

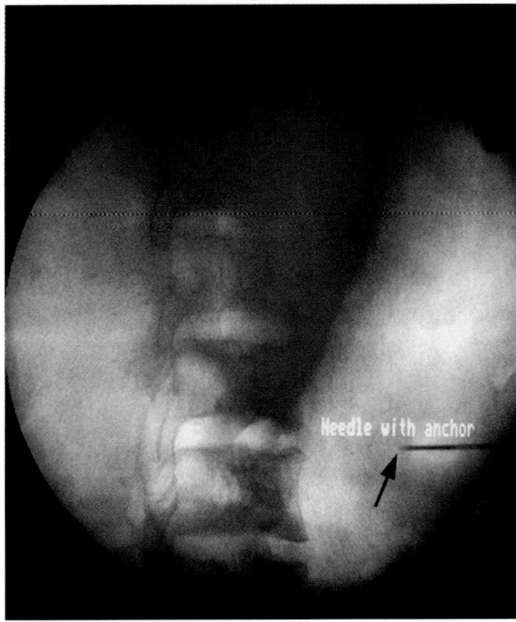

Figure 13. Needle in the stomach with tenting of the stomach wall (arrow).

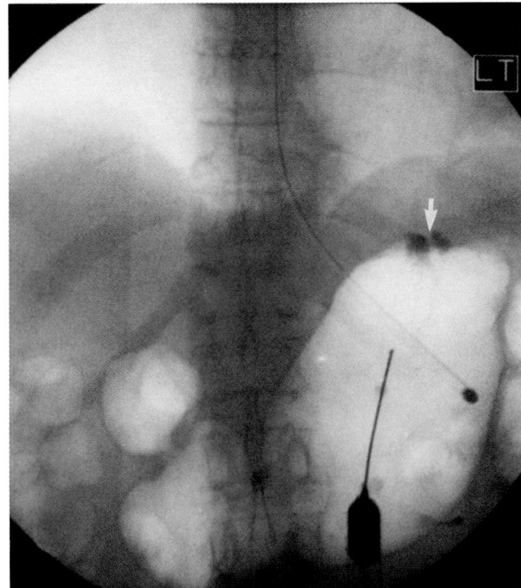

Figure 14. Syringe injecting contrast material to verify that the needle is in the stomach. Contrast material is seen in the fundus (arrow).

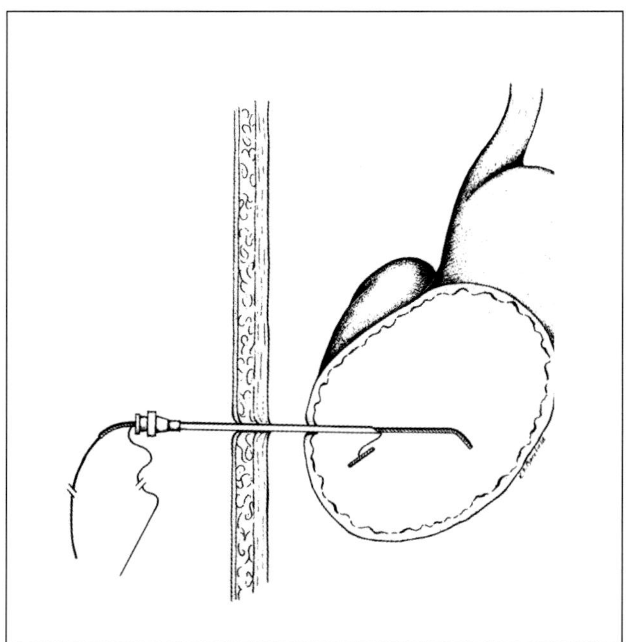

Figure 15. Illustration of a wire depositing the anchor into the stomach.

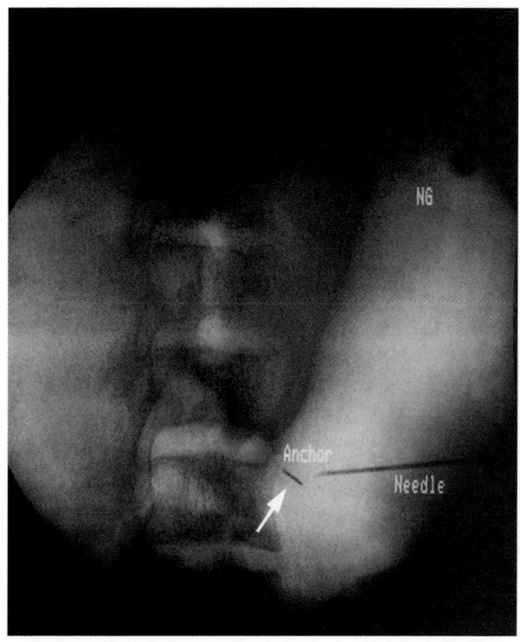

Figure 16. Anchor dangling from the tip of the needle (arrow).

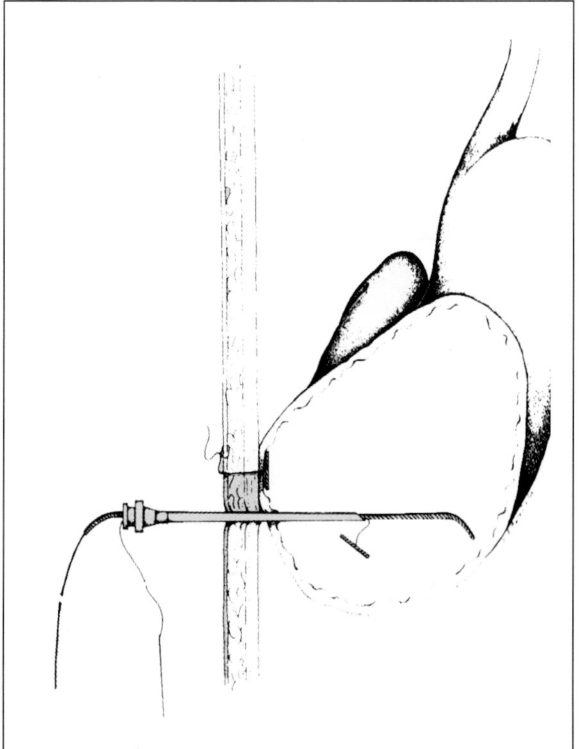

Figure 17. Illustration demonstrates retraction of the stomach to the anterior abdominal wall by the first anchor. A second anchor is being placed.

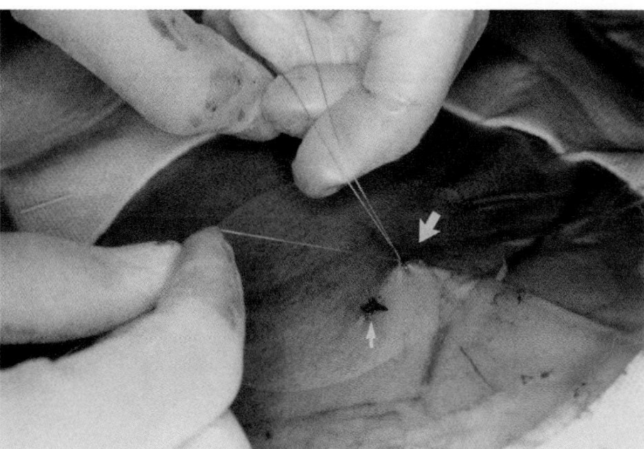

Figure 18. Suturing a second anchor to the skin on the abdominal wall (large arrow). Small arrow=first anchor suture.

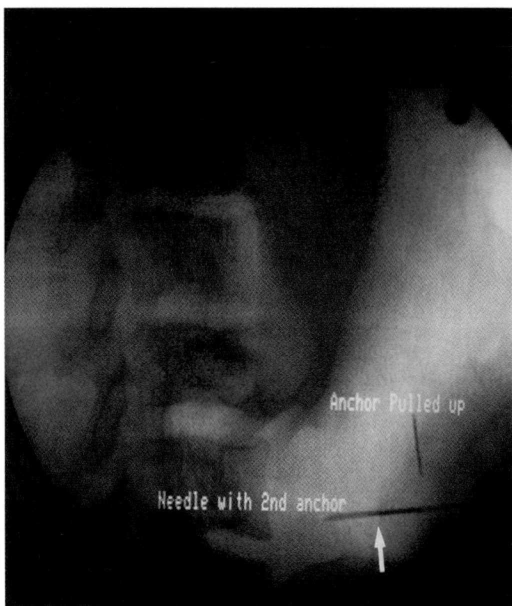

Figure 19. Second needle pass with the second anchor being placed (arrow).

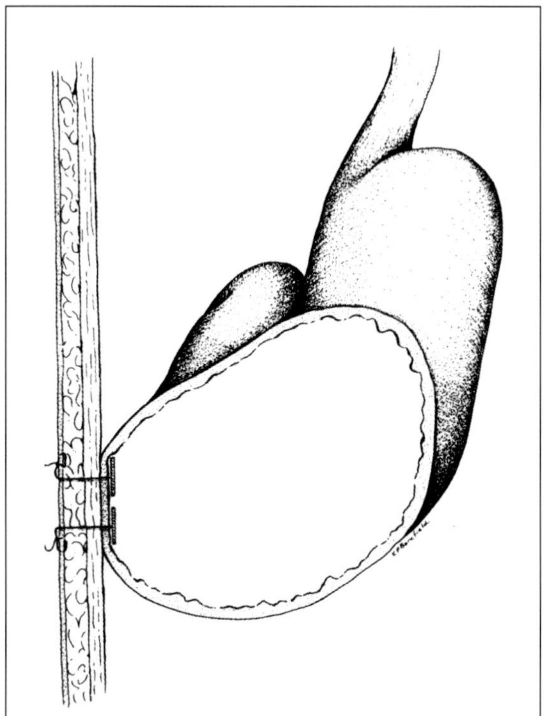
Figure 20. Illustration shows apposition of the stomach to the abdominal wall following placement of a second anchor.

Two to three anchors are generally placed to assure that the stomach is adequately secured, although a simple gastrostomy can be performed with only one anchor. For a gastrojejunostomy, at least two anchors should be used because of the larger tube sizes **(Figs. 19–21)**.

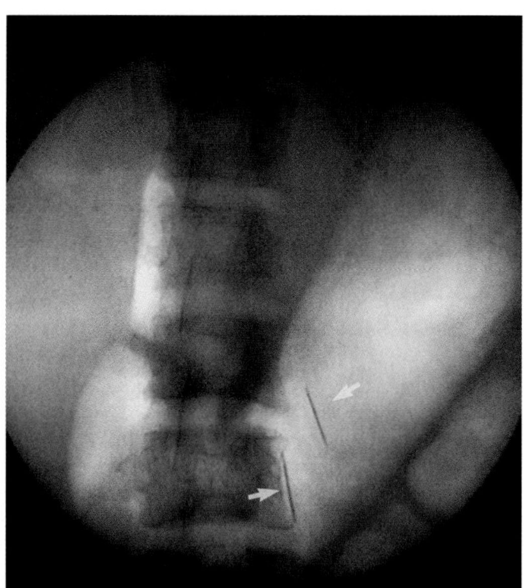
Figure 21. Both anchors in place (arrows).

Once the gastropexy has been completed, a location between the anchors is selected as the site for final tube placement. Angulation of the needle for this final puncture is important because it will affect the outcome of the procedure. A near perpendicular approach **(Fig. 22)** is optimal for placement of gastrostomies and will facilitate conversion of a gastrostomy to a jejunostomy or gastrojejunostomy. Slight angulation (with the needle tip pointing toward the antrum) will aid in placement of gastrojejunostomies and jejunostomy tubes **(Fig. 23)**. In patients who will have a tube placed with a fundal loop component, slight angulation toward the fundus may be helpful if the fundal loop is formed at the beginning of the procedure **(Fig. 24)**. However, ease of placement, time required, and overall success rates are improved if the initial approach is angled toward the antrum and the fundal loop formed at the end of the procedure.

For gastrostomies, a wire is advanced into the stomach and the track is dilated with use of a balloon or multiple dilators.[1,2] The gastrostomy tube **(Fig. 25)** is then prepared and advanced over the wire into the stomach.

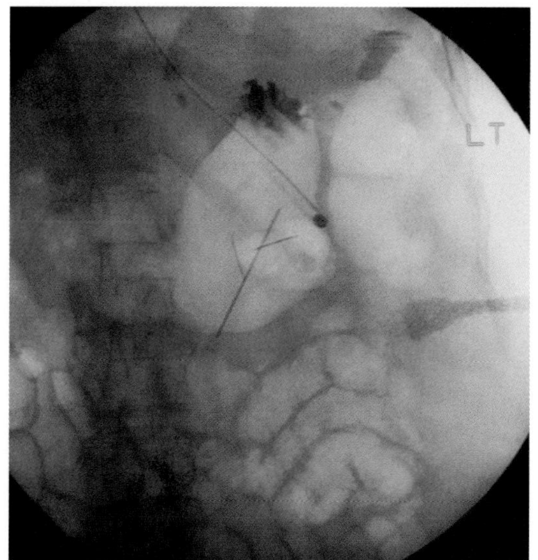

Figure 22. Near perpendicular approach of the final needle, between the two previously placed anchors.

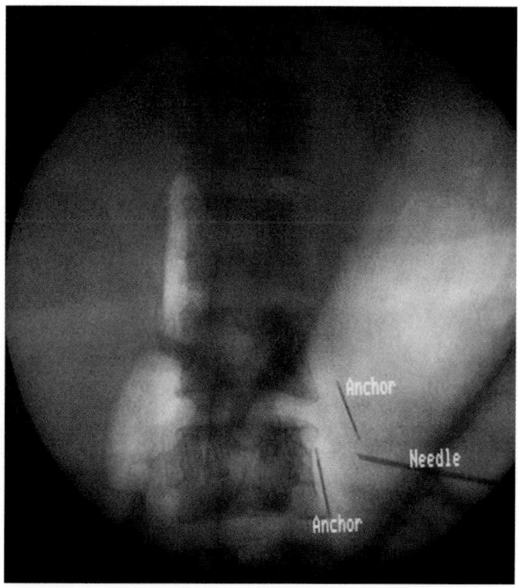

Figure 23. The tip of the needle directed toward the antrum of the stomach assists in jejunostomy and gastrojejunostomy tube placements.

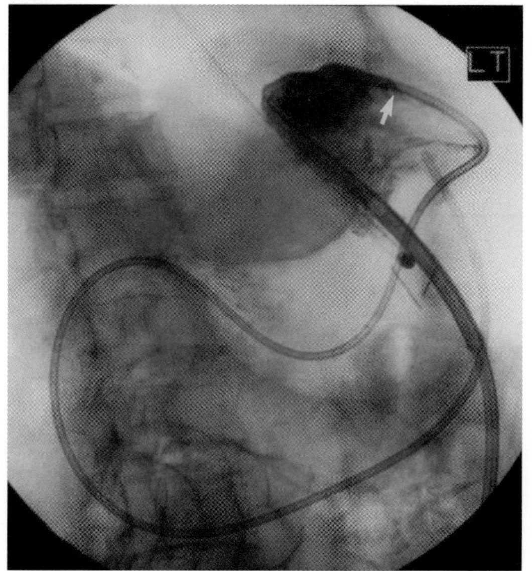

Figure 24. Gastrojejunostomy with fundal loop (arrow).

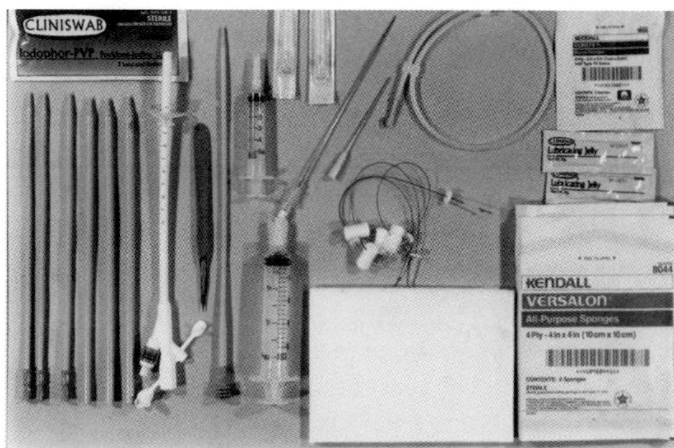

Figure 25. Flexiflo gastrostomy tube set with dilators, gastropexy anchors, and other useful sundries.

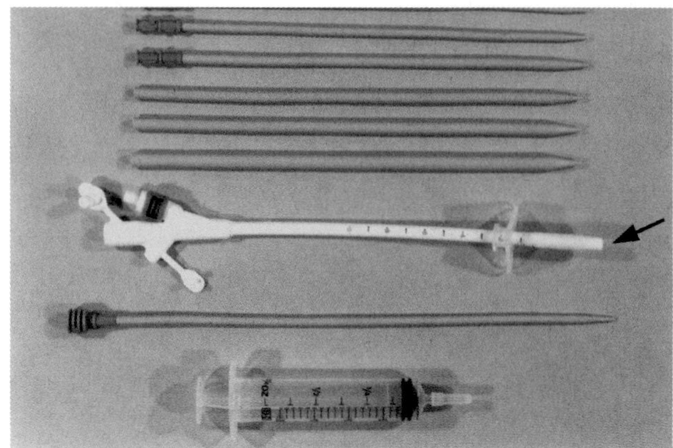

Figure 26. Close-up of the gastrostomy tube, dilators, and obturator for placing the tube (arrow).

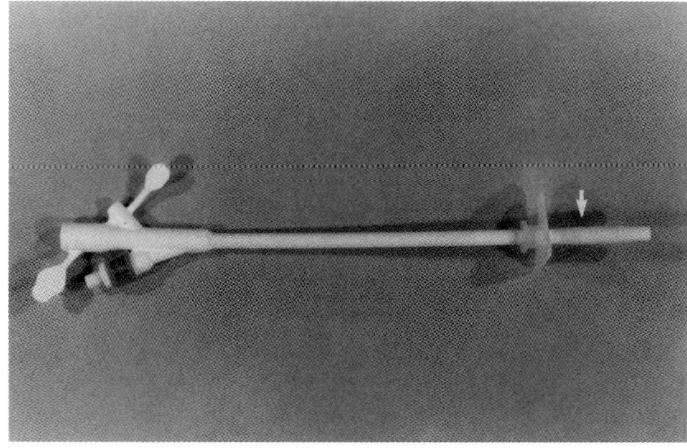

Figure 27. Flexiflo gastrostomy tube with deflated balloon (arrow).

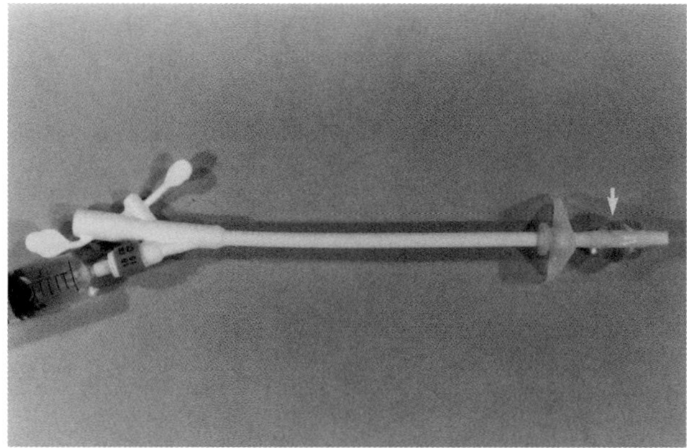

Figure 28. Flexiflo gastrostomy tube with partially inflated balloon (arrow).

A retention device consisting of a Silastic mushroom, a Malecot anchor, or a balloon is then formed to prevent accidental dislodgement of the tube **(Figs. 26–30)**. Injection of contrast material through the tube will verify the appropriate position. A single anteroposterior (AP) film at this point can be used to document the tube placement and position.

Gastrojejunostomies and jejunostomies are slightly more difficult and time-consuming to insert than gastrostomies.[1,15] These tubes should be placed in patients who are at risk of aspiration or who have an obstructing lesion in the duodenum or proximal jejunum.[1,3,12,13,15,16] Successful placement of a jejunal tube beyond an obstruction would permit feeding. Negotiating the pylorus, duodenum, and proximal jejunum can be arduous. Placement of a jejunal tube begins with the initial puncture because a puncture directed toward the antrum can greatly facilitate the advancement of the wire through the pylorus and into the duodenum. As mentioned earlier, the use of glucagon will make advancement of a wire through the pylorus and duodenum more difficult because the peristalsis and relaxation of the pylorus that aid passage of a wire into the proximal jejunum are impeded by glucagon. The use of a selective catheter such as a Kumpe catheter (Cook) or a 6-F dilator with an angled tip **(Fig. 31)** can greatly facilitate advancement of a wire through the pylorus, which is generally directed slightly superiorly and posteriorly **(Fig. 32)**. Injection of both air and contrast material can assist in identifying the entrance into the pyloric channel and will often stimulate peristalsis and relaxation of the pylorus **(Fig. 33)**.

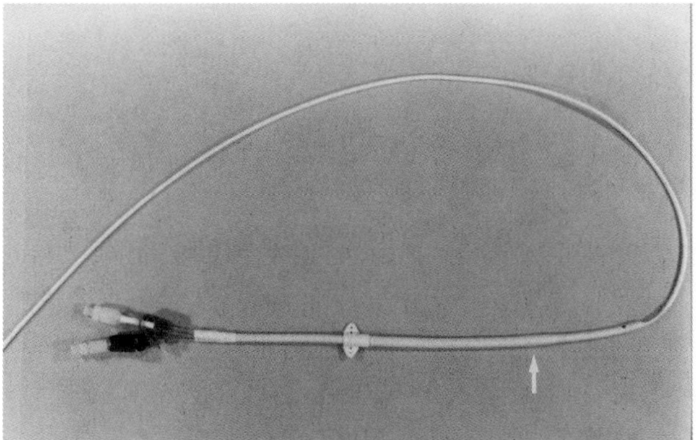

Figure 29. Carey-Alzate-Coons gastrojejunostomy tube with an unformed Malecot anchor (arrow).

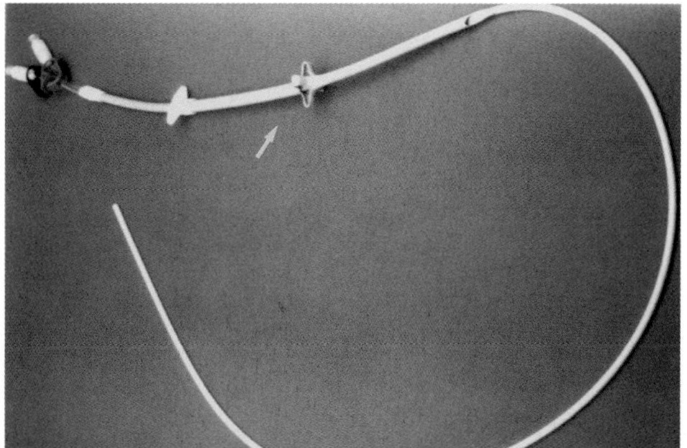

Figure 30. Carey-Alzate-Coons gastrojejunostomy tube with a formed Malecot anchor (arrow).

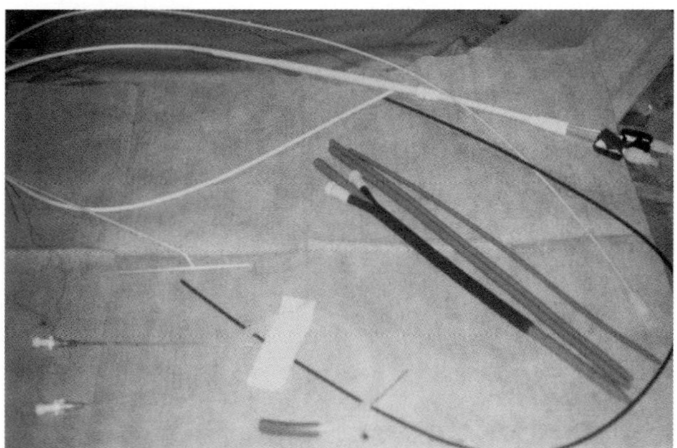

Figure 31. Carey-Alzate-Coons gastrojejunostomy set complete with tube, selective catheters, wires, fascial dilators, and peel-away sheath.

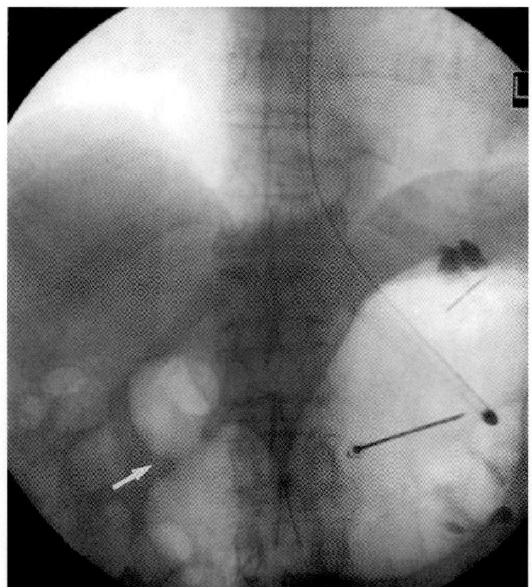

Figure 32. Gas-filled stomach demonstrates that the pyloric channel is directed superiorly (arrow).

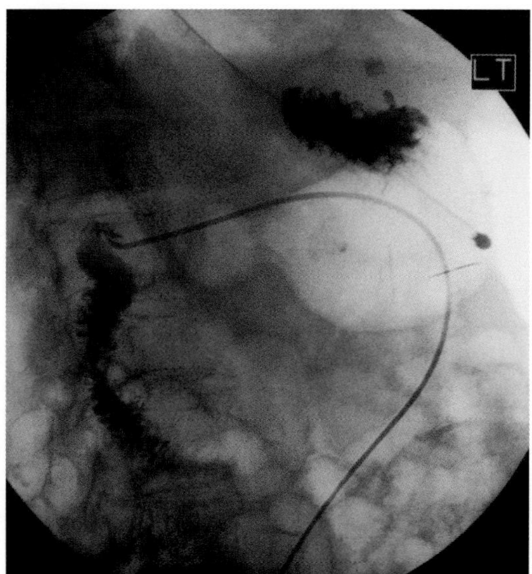

Figure 33. Injection of contrast material and air help identify and negotiate the pylorus and duodenal bulb.

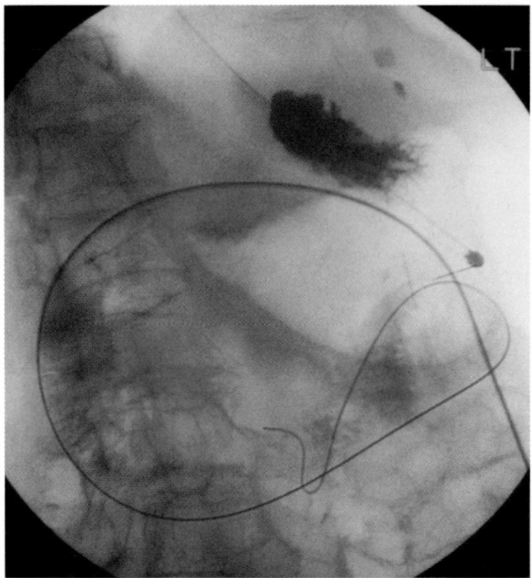

Figure 34. Wire and catheter advanced to the ligament of Treitz.

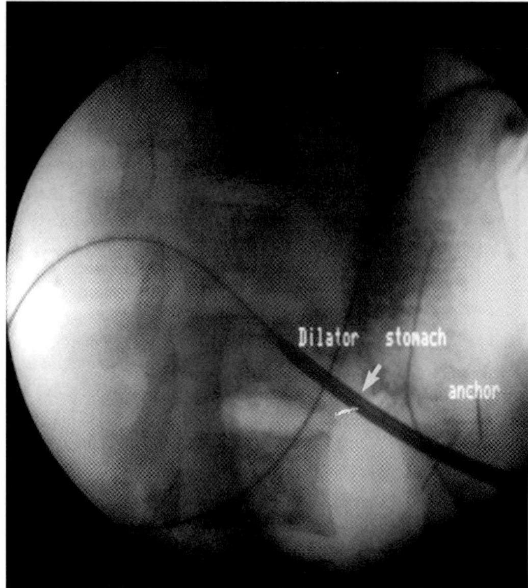

Figure 35. Fascial dilator (arrow) being advanced over a wire to dilate the subcutaneous track and stomach wall.

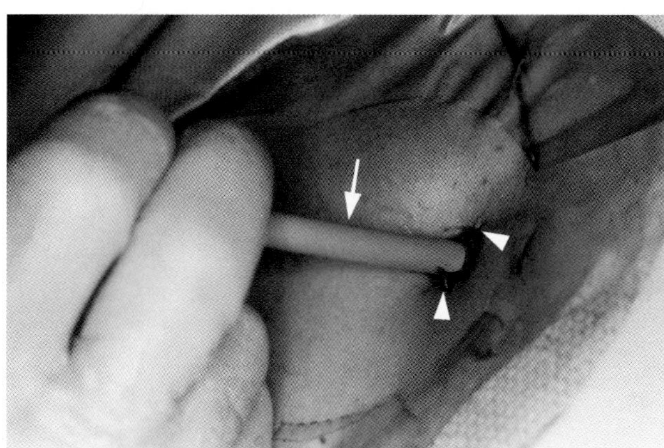

Figure 36. Fascial dilator (arrow) being advanced through the skin. Arrowheads show the retention anchor sutures.

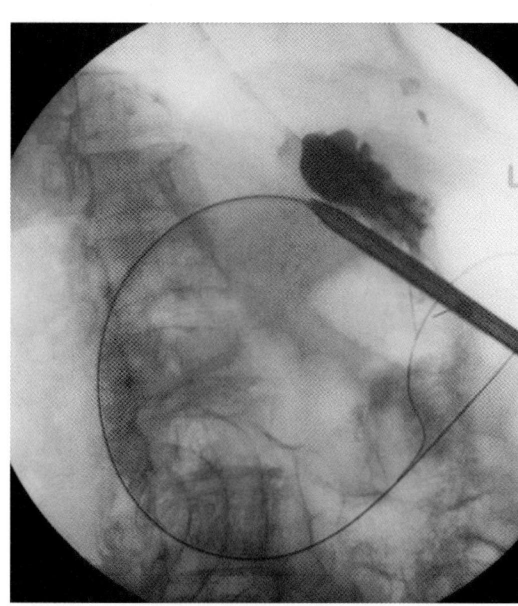

Figure 37. Peel-away sheath being advanced over the dilator and wire into the stomach.

Once the wire has been advanced into the duodenum, a 100-cm-long selective catheter and exchange wire are used to negotiate the remainder of the duodenum and proximal jejunum. Again, the injection of air and contrast material can help identify the course of the bowel and promote peristalsis, facilitating advancement of the wire into the jejunum beyond the ligament of Treitz **(Fig. 34)**. When sufficient wire has been passed into the jejunum, the selective catheter is removed, and the subcutaneous track and stomach wall are dilated in a similar manner as described for placement of gastrostomy tubes **(Figs. 35, 36)**.

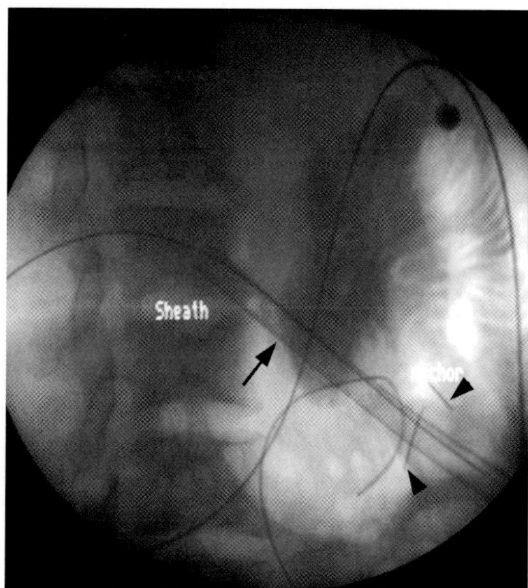

Figure 38. Peel-away sheath (arrow) and retention anchors (arrowheads) in place.

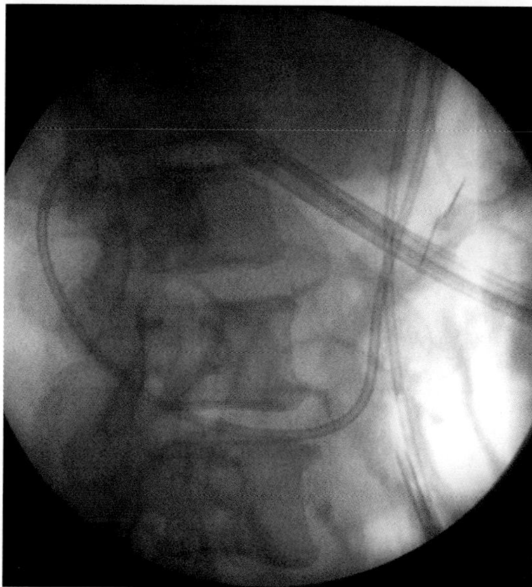

Figure 40. Catheter in place after the wire has been withdrawn and the distal tip is in the jejunum.

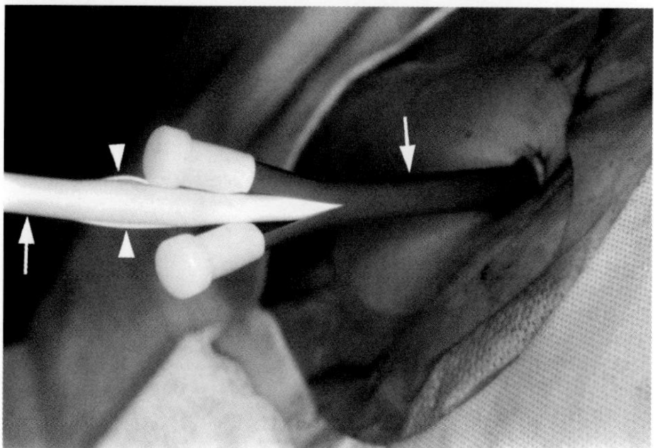

Figure 42. Peel-away sheath (right arrow) with a gastrojejunostomy tube (left arrow) being advanced over the wire. Note the slits (arrowheads) of the Malecot anchor.

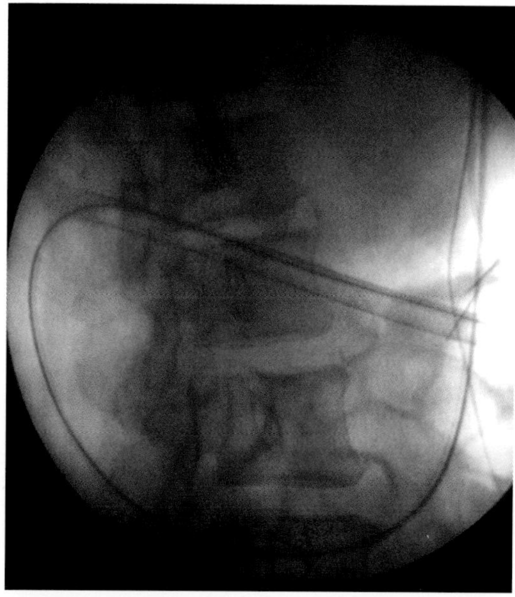

Figure 39. Catheter advanced over the wire through the sheath into the jejunum beyond the ligament of Treitz.

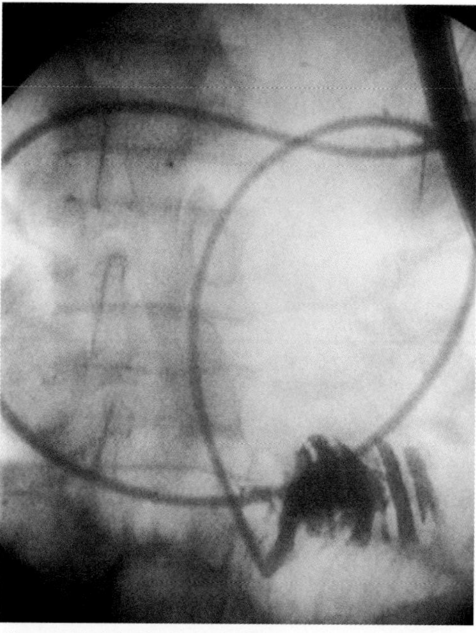

Figure 41. Injection of contrast material confirms the position of the distal tip in the jejunum beyond the ligament of Treitz.

The final dilation is performed with a peel-away sheath that may vary in size from 14 to 24 F depending on the particular jejunostomy or gastrojejunostomy tube being used **(Figs. 37, 38)**. Once the sheath has been advanced into the stomach, the tube is advanced slowly over the wire until its tip rests in the jejunum beyond the ligament of Treitz **(Figs. 39–42)**.

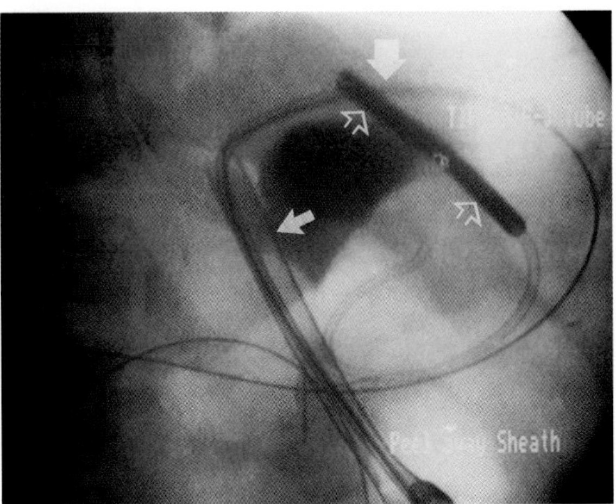

Figure 43. Peel-away sheath (arrow) redirected to the fundus of the stomach (wide arrow) to assist in the formation of a fundal loop. A nasogastric feeding tube is in place (open arrows).

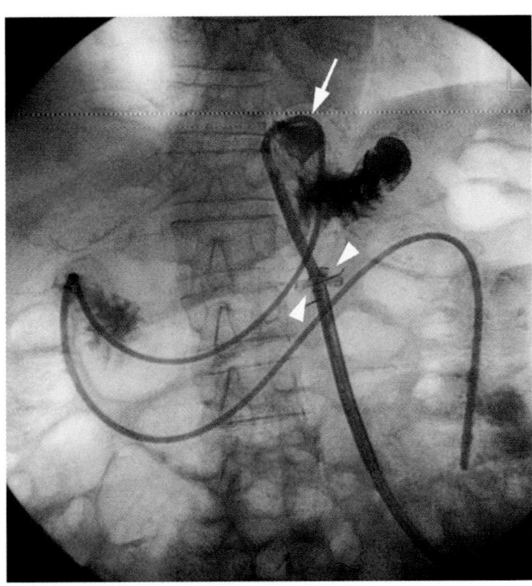

Figure 44. Fundal loop (arrow) and formed Malecot anchor (arrowheads).

If the tube requires the formation of a fundal loop, the indwelling sheath is withdrawn slightly and redirected toward the fundus of the stomach **(Fig. 43)**. The tube is then advanced into the fundus while it is being turned clockwise. This action results in the formation of a fundal loop **(Fig. 44)**. The peel-away sheath is then removed and the tube retention device deployed as described for the placement of gastrostomy tubes **(Fig. 45)**.

The tube can be temporarily sutured to the skin or attached to a retention disk to prevent accidental dislodgement before a well-developed subcutaneous track has formed **(Figs. 46, 47)**. Vaseline gauze can also be wrapped around the tube to seal the entrance site in the skin. The ports of the tube are then injected with contrast material to verify their final positioning. Again, a single AP film can be obtained to verify placement and positioning **(Fig. 48)**. The tube should be flushed vigorously with saline and the entry site dressed. The procedure is then terminated.

These same principles can be employed to place enteral feeding tubes in children[4,12] as well as to place gastric buttons and skin-level devices for enteral feeding.[21,22]

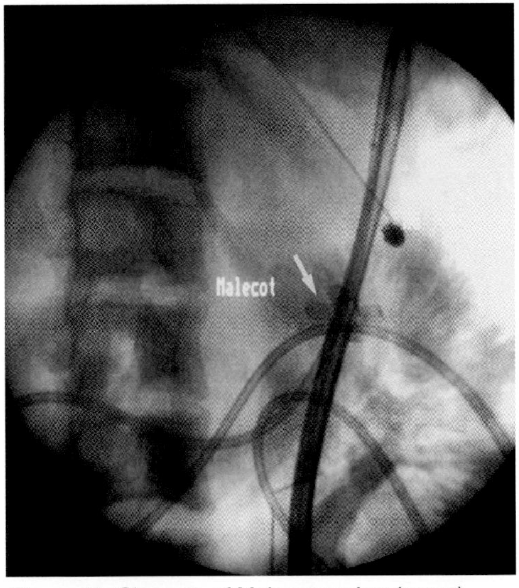

Figure 45. Close-up of Malecot anchor (arrow).

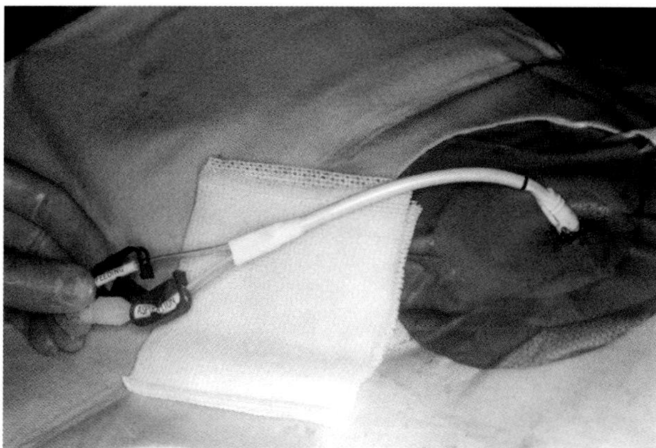

Figure 46. Gastrojejunostomy catheter in position demonstrates two ports: gastric (aspiration) port and jejunal (feeding) port.

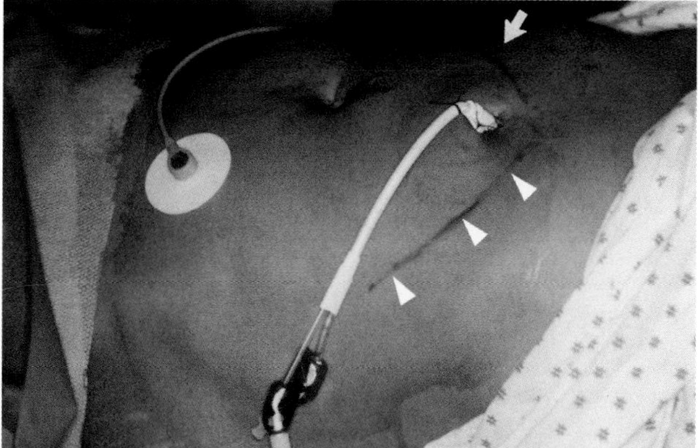

Figure 47. Location of the final exit from the anterior abdominal wall. Arrow=liver margin; arrowheads=left costal margin.

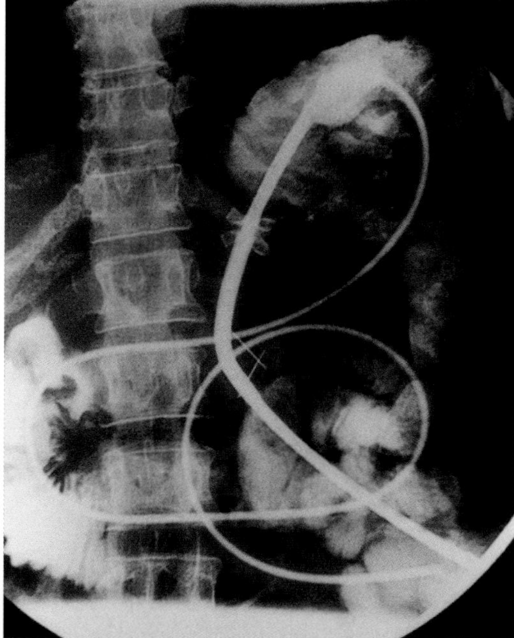

Figure 48. AP abdominal film with contrast verifies the final positions of the gastric and jejunal ports.

Postprocedural Considerations

Postprocedure orders should not allow use of the gastric port for 12–24 hours following placement. The jejunal port should also not be used during this time unless the tip is beyond the ligament of Treitz and only limited use is required. It is also necessary to specify what can and cannot be administered through the ports. Crushed medications should not be given through jejunostomy ports; because of their length and smaller caliber these tubes can easily become occluded. Crushed medications can be given through gastric ports if they are crushed finely and the tube is liberally flushed with saline or water beforehand and afterwards. Orders are written to monitor vital signs and observe the patient for signs of peritonitis. An abdominal film can be obtained the following day to assess the amount of free air and check for the presence of ileus. The gastropexy sutures are usually cut within 14 days, after a well-developed track has formed. If the tube becomes dislodged after this time, it is usually easy to slide a new tube through the track.

Complications

Because most of these procedures are performed in patients who are either very elderly or significantly debilitated, appropriate personnel and equipment for monitoring must be available during and immediately after the procedure. Complications of imaging-guided enteral tube placement are relatively few and can be divided into procedural and postprocedural complications and further divided into major and minor categories.[11,14,23] Overall, the morbidity and mortality rates for imaging-guided techniques are approximately 10%–20% and less than 2%, respectively, which compare favorably with surgical rates of approximately 13%–23% and 2%–6%.[5,6,10,11,12,14] Procedural complications are usually problems associated with gaining access to the stomach. These include inadvertent puncture of structures lying in the left upper quadrant of the abdomen, such as the liver, spleen, small bowel, and colon, or puncture of a vessel such as the left gastric artery, the right or left gastroepiploic arteries, or the superior epigastric artery. Less commonly, the splenic, hepatic, or superior mesenteric arteries, or the aorta, is punctured. Puncture of the accompanying venous structures is also possible.[1,3–5,15] All of these complications can be avoided with the use of appropriate preprocedural imaging as well as the use of imaging guidance during the procedure. However, if any of these complications do occur, they are generally self-limited and of little consequence if they are identified early (prior to dilations) and if the patient's preprocedural coagulation factors are normal or have been corrected.

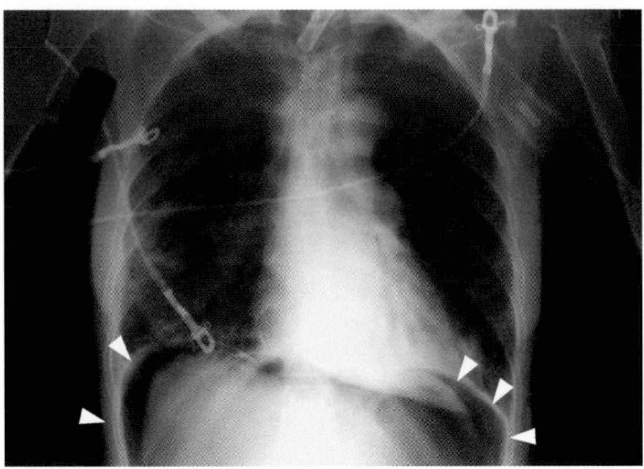

Figure 49. Pneumoperitoneum (arrowheads).

Other complications that can occur at the time of tube placement include aspiration, hypotension, vasovagal reactions, dyspnea, and over-sedation resulting in decreased oxygenation, arrhythmias, and myocardial infarction.[1,3–5] Again, many of these complications can be avoided or treated successfully if they are recognized early and the appropriate personnel are available.

An occurrence which can be problematic is pneumoperitoneum **(Fig. 49)**. A small pneumoperitoneum is not uncommon; however, a large pneumoperitoneum can either be benign or signify a significant underlying complication **(Fig. 50)**.[2,4,9,24] Another procedure-related complication is malpositioning of the tube. The tube may be inadvertently placed into the peritoneal cavity, posterior to the stomach, or it may be partially placed into the stomach with part of the tube either anterior or posterior to the stomach cavity. With the use of imaging to confirm the position of needles and catheters at several points during the procedure, these complications are nearly nonexistent. One of the more significant complications is the development of peritonitis, which most commonly occurs after spillage of gastric contents into the peritoneal cavity during the procedure or by a partially or completely malpositioned enteric tube.[1,3–5,13,16]

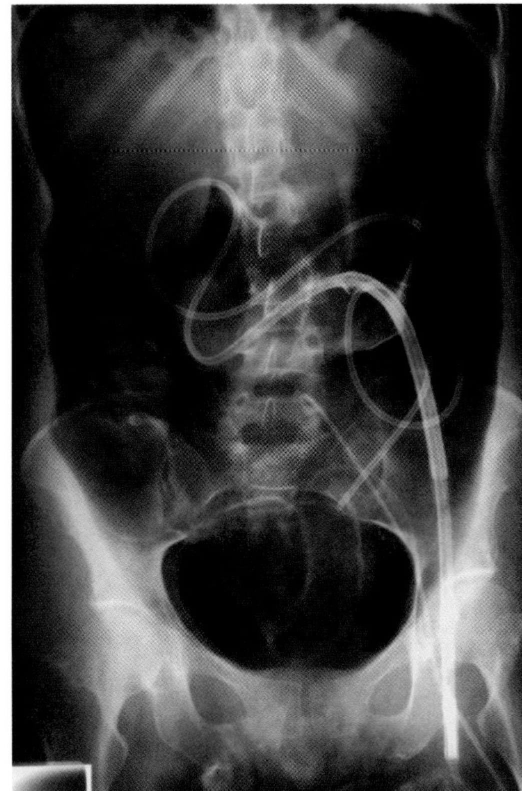

Figure 50. Large tension pneumoperitoneum.

Postprocedure complications include wound and stomal infections, which can easily be treated with local cleansing and frequent dressing changes. More advanced wound infections may require local debridement of tissue and antibiotics, or rarely, surgical intervention.[1–4,13] The most frequent postprocedure complications involve malfunctioning of the tube secondary to clogging by inspissated feedings and/or improperly crushed medications.[2,4,9] This problem can usually be resolved by vigorous flushing of the tube with a 5-mL syringe. If this is unsuccessful, then injection of carbonated liquids into the tube can often reestablish patency. The passage of a wire through the lumen may also reestablish patency. If all these procedures fail, then replacement of the tube over a wire in a dual-lumen tube or through a well-developed track can be accomplished without difficulty.

Probably the second most common delayed complication is accidental dislodgement of the tube.[2,4,12] This problem is best avoided by securing the tube adequately at the time of placement. This is accomplished through successful deployment of the retention device and by securing the tube with a retention disk or suturing the tube directly to the skin. In extremely combative patients, restraints may be necessary to prevent this complication. Appropriate anchoring of the tube will also decrease the incidence of tube migration. It is necessary to pay careful attention to details before, during, and after the procedure to reduce the risk and sequelae of complications. Patients should be followed routinely after placement until the anchor sutures are cut. This is usually done after about 2 weeks, thus permitting adequate development of a subcutaneous track. This postprocedure follow-up is an integral component of the procedure. It permits early identification and treatment of complications. Most complications will be apparent within the first week, and if treatment is instituted early they are easily corrected.

Results

Since the early description of imaging-guided gastrostomies,[1–3,5,13] successful placement of enteric tubes by radiologists has now been established.[1–5,25,26] High success rates (greater than 95%) and low complication rates have been documented.[1,2] In addition, the overall cost-effectiveness and timeliness of the procedure in the hands of a qualified radiologist favors imaging-guided placement of these tubes.[9,19]

References

1. Ho CS, Yeung EY. Percutaneous gastrostomy and transgastric jejunostomy. AJR 1992; 158:251–257.

2. O'Keeffe F, Carrasco CH, Charnsangavej C, Richli WR, Wallace S, Freedman RS. Percutaneous drainage and feeding gastrostomies in 100 patients. Radiology 1989; 172:341–343.

3. Halkier BK, Ho CS, Yee AC. Percutaneous feeding gastrostomy with the Seldinger technique: review of 252 patients. Radiology 1989; 171:359–362.

4. Yeung EY, Ho CS. Percutaneous radiologic gastrostomy. Baillieres Clin Gastroenterol 1992; 6:297–317.

5. Ho CS, Yee AC, McPherson R. Complications of surgical and percutaneous nonendoscopic gastrostomy: review of 233 patients. Gastroenterology 1988; 95:1206–1210.

6. Darcy MD. Comparison of radiological, endoscopic and surgical enteral access procedures. Semin Intervent Radiol 1996; 13:289–297.

7. Shellito PC, Malt RA. Tube gastrostomy: techniques and complications. Ann Surg 1985; 201:180–185.

8. Wasiljew BK, Ujiki GT, Beal JM. Feeding gastrostomy: complications and mortality. Am J Surg 1982; 143:194–195.

9. Foutch PG, vanSonnenberg E, Casola G, D'Agostino H. Nonsurgical gastrostomy: x-ray or endoscopy. Am J Gastroenterol 1990; 85:1560–1563.

10. Rogers DA, Bowden TA. Gastrostomy: operative or nonoperative? Surg Clin North Am 1992; 72:515–524.

11. Saini S, Mueller PR, Gaa J, et al. Percutaneous gastrostomy with gastropexy: experience in 125 patients. AJR 1990; 154:1003–1006.

12. Towbin RB, Ball WS, Bisset III GS. Percutaneous gastrostomy and percutaneous gastrojejunostomy in children: antegrade approach. Radiology 1988; 168:473–476.

13. Alzate GD, Coons HG, Elliott J, Carey PH. Percutaneous gastrostomy for jejunal feeding: a new technique. AJR 1986; 147:822–825.

14. vanSonnenberg E, Wittich GR, Cabrera OA, et al. Percutaneous gastrostomy and gastroenterostomy: 2. Clinical experience. AJR 1986; 146:581–586.

15. Coleman CC, Coons HG, Cope C, et al. Percutaneous enterostomy with the Cope suture anchor. Radiology 1990; 174:889–891.

16. Olson DL, Krubsack AJ, Stewart ET. Percutaneous enteral alimentation: gastrostomy versus gastrojejunostomy. Radiology 1993; 187:105–108.

17. Hicks ME, Darcy MD. Percutaneous fluoroscopic gastrostomy: general considerations. Semin Intervent Radiol 1996; 13:281–287.

18. Sheeran SR, Hallisey MJ. Direct approaches to the small bowel: direct percutaneous jejunostomy and percutaneous translumbar duodenostomy. Semin Intervent Radiol 1996; 13:339–344.

19. Brown AS, Mueller PR, Ferrucci JT. Controlled percutaneous gastrostomy: nylon T-fastener for fixation of the anterior gastric wall. Radiology 1986; 158:543–545.

20. Malden ES, Hicks ME. Gastrostomy in the postoperative stomach. Semin Intervent Radiol 1996; 13:309–316.

21. Vesely TM, Hovsepian DM. Skin-level gastrostomy devices. Semin Intervent Radiol 1996; 13:329–337.

22. Shike M, Wallach C, Gerdes H, Hermann-Zaidins M. Skin-level gastrostomies and jejunostomies for long–term enteral feeding. J Parenteral Enteral Nutr 1989; 13:648–650.

23. Kanterman RY, Darcy MD. Complications of the fluoroscopically guided percutaneous gastrostomy. Semin Intervent Radiol 1996; 13:317–327.

24. Kealey WD, McCallion WA, Boston VE. Tension pneumoperitoneum: a potentially life-threatening complication of percutaneous endoscopic gastrojejunostomy. J Pediatr Gastroenterol Nutr 1996; 22:334–335.

25. Darcy MD. Radiological percutaneous transgastric jejunostomy. Semin Intervent Radiol 1996; 13:299–307.

26. vanSonnenberg E, Wittich GR, Brown LK, et al. Percutaneous gastrostomy and gastroenterostomy: 1. Techniques derived from laboratory evaluation. AJR 1986; 146:577–580.

TUTORIAL 12
DIRECT PERCUTANEOUS JEJUNOSTOMY

Allen A. Currier, Jr., M.D., and Michael J. Hallisey, M.D.

Introduction

The subjects addressed in this tutorial include:

1. Indications and contraindications for direct percutaneous jejunostomy (DPJ)
2. Technique for establishing DPJ
3. Outcome of DPJ.

Many surgical and percutaneous techniques have evolved for the establishment of enteral and parenteral feeding in patients unable to maintain adequate oral intake. Surgical jejunostomy has morbidity and mortality rates reported to be as high as 50% and 10%, respectively.[1] The advent of laparoscopic jejunostomy minimizes the morbidity and mortality but is still quite invasive compared with DPJ.[2] DPJ is an alternative in these patients, who are generally poor surgical candidates.

Indications and Contraindications

Chronic aspiration is a serious and potentially life-threatening condition. Aspiration is the most common reason for DPJ placement. Previous gastric surgery or resection is also a common indication. Abnormal stomach position that makes percutaneously placed endoscopic gastrostomy difficult, duodenal or gastric outlet obstruction, and recurrent inadvertent gastrojejunal tube dislodgement are less common indications. An absolute contraindication is a coagulopathy or overlapping colonic loops. Ascites is a relative contraindication as the major concern is contamination of fluid by leakage of bowel contents.

Patient Preparation

Twelve hours before the procedure, the patient is given an oral dose of 50 mL of dilute water-soluble contrast material (eg, Gastrografin) to opacify the colon. On arrival at the interventional radiology suite, the patient is given 1 gram of cefazolin sodium intravenously for antimicrobial prophylaxis. Two additional doses are given at 12-hour intervals if the patient remains hospitalized.

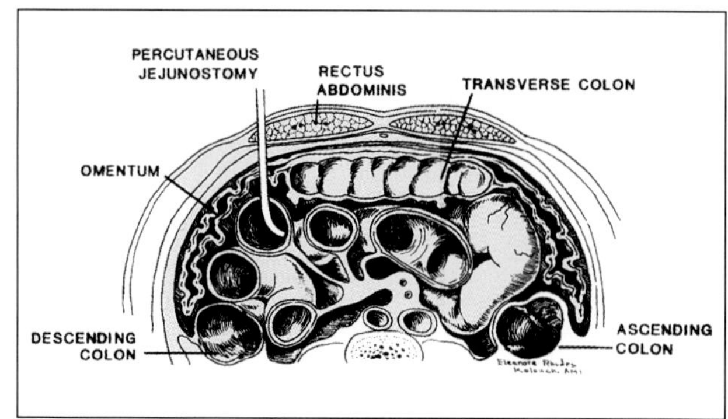

Figure 1. Axial anatomy and desired catheter position.

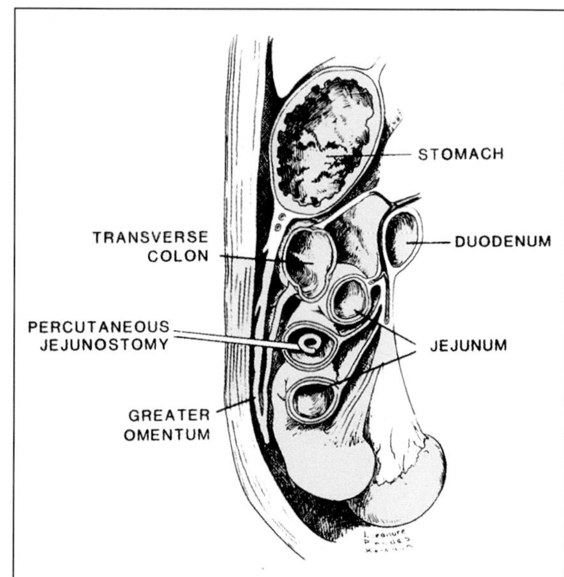

Figure 2. Sagittal view of the jejunal loop puncture at the antimesenteric side.

Technique[3]

The left upper abdomen is prepared with the standard sterile technique. A nasogastric tube is placed into the duodenum (if possible), and air is insufflated into the proximal jejunum. When the proximal loop is identified, the skin site is anesthetized with lidocaine. The site should be to the left of midline but within the rectus abdominis muscle to avoid the superior epigastric artery and vein. **Figures 1** and **2** show the jejunal anatomy and position of the DPJ tube. A dose of 1 mg glucagon is then given intravenously. A 17-gauge needle is used to puncture the loop; the needle should be kept perpendicular to the skin to optimize entry into the antimesenteric side of the jejunum. When air is withdrawn from the needle, the position is confirmed with air or contrast material injection.

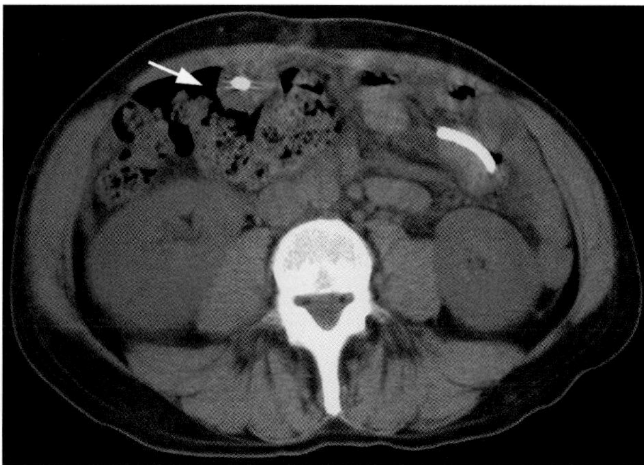

Figure 3. Jejunal loop anchored to the anterior abdominal wall (arrow).

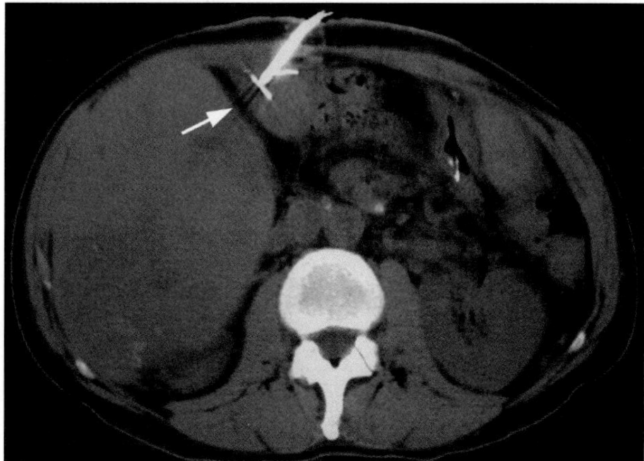

Figure 4. Jejunal loop anchored to the anterior abdominal wall (arrow).

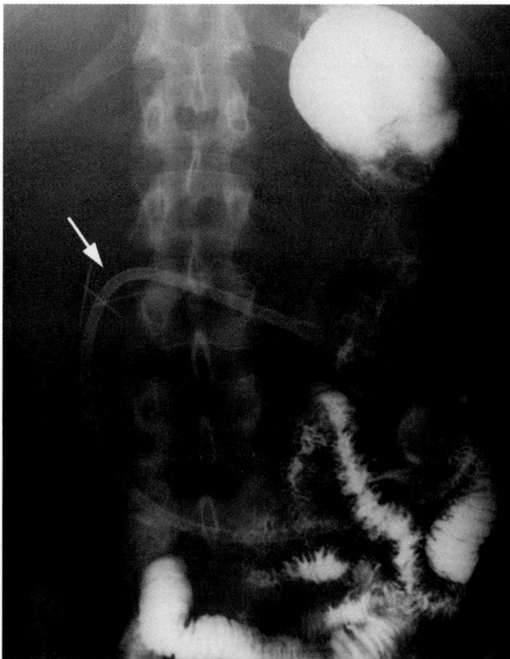

Figure 5. DPJ tube in the jejunum. Arrow indicates the entrance site with suture anchors.

An 0.035-inch stiff hydrophilic guide wire is placed through the needle into the distal jejunum, and the needle is removed. An angled hydrophilic 5-F catheter is introduced over the wire, and the wire is removed. Next, a stiff guide wire is placed through the catheter, and the catheter is removed. Two to four gastrointestinal suture anchors are then placed near the entry site and used to pull the jejunal loop up to the anterior abdominal wall **(Figs. 3, 4)**. Fascial dilators are used to dilate the track to between 8 and 14 F, depending on the size of the feeding tube required.

Finally, a locking pigtail loop catheter is placed over the wire and its position confirmed with contrast material injection **(Fig. 5)**. The catheter is sutured to the skin, and the site is covered with sterile dressings. Small, dilute feedings can begin within 24 hours.

Results

The reported success rates are 60%–100%,[3–5] but the total number of patients who have undergone this procedure is small. Occasionally, the patient's anatomy makes the jejunum inaccessible for the percutaneous puncture. One major complication was related to premature release of the gastrointestinal anchors, which permitted the feeding solution to fill the peritoneal cavity.

Conclusion

Direct percutaneous jejunostomy provides an alternative approach to enteral feedings in patients who are not candidates for standard PEG placement or an open surgical procedure.

References

1. Adams MB, Seabrook GR, Quebbeman EA, Condon RE. Jejunostomy: a rarely indicated procedure. Arch Surg 1986; 121:236–238.

2. Reed DN. Percutaneous peritoneoscopic jejunostomy. Surg Gynecol Obstet 1992; 174:527–529.

3. Hallisey MJ, Pollard JC. Direct percutaneous jejunostomy. J Vasc Interv Radiol 1994; 5:625–632.

4. Gray RR, Ho CS, Yee A, Montanera W, Jones DP. Direct percutaneous jejunostomy. AJR 1987; 149:931–932.

5. Coleman CC, Coons HG, Cope C, et al. Percutaneous enterostomy with the Cope suture anchor. Radiology 1990; 174:889–891.

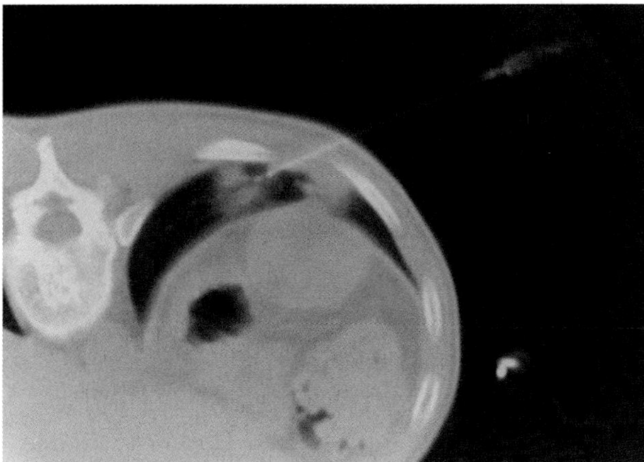

Figure 1. CT guidance used to biopsy a lesion not visible on fluoroscopy.

TUTORIAL 13 TRANSTHORACIC NEEDLE BIOPSY

Dewey J. Conces, Jr., M.D.

Introduction

The subjects addressed in this tutorial include:

1. Indications and contraindications for transthoracic needle aspiration biopsy (TNAB)
2. Procedure planning
3. Technique of fluoroscopically guided TNAB
4. Technique of computed tomography-guided TNAB
5. Complications.

TNAB is a reliable technique which can be used to diagnose both benign and malignant disease of the thorax.[1,2] Lesions in the lung, mediastinum, hilum, pleura, and chest wall can be biopsied. Even lesions as small as 5 mm can be biopsied successfully.[3] The majority of TNAB procedures can be performed on an outpatient basis, which makes the procedure very cost-effective.[4,5]

An absolute contraindication to TNAB is a totally uncooperative patient. Relative contraindications include severe bullous emphysematous disease, pulmonary arterial hypertension, and severe uncorrectable coagulation disorders. TNAB is usually performed under either fluoroscopic or computed tomographic guidance, although ultrasound may be the method of choice in some cases. This tutorial only discusses fluoroscopic and computed tomography (CT) biopsy techniques.

Pre-Biopsy Planning

In planning a TNAB, the radiographic studies of the lesion should be reviewed to determine which imaging modality—fluoroscopy or CT—is best suited for guiding the biopsy. We prefer to use fluoroscopy to guide the biopsy of lung nodules because it is quicker and less expensive. For lung lesions that cannot be seen on fluoroscopy, CT guidance is used **(Fig. 1)**. Lesions involving the mediastinum, hilum, and chest wall are typically biopsied under CT guidance. The ability of CT to clearly define the various structures in these regions makes it ideally suited to guide biopsies of lesions located in these areas.

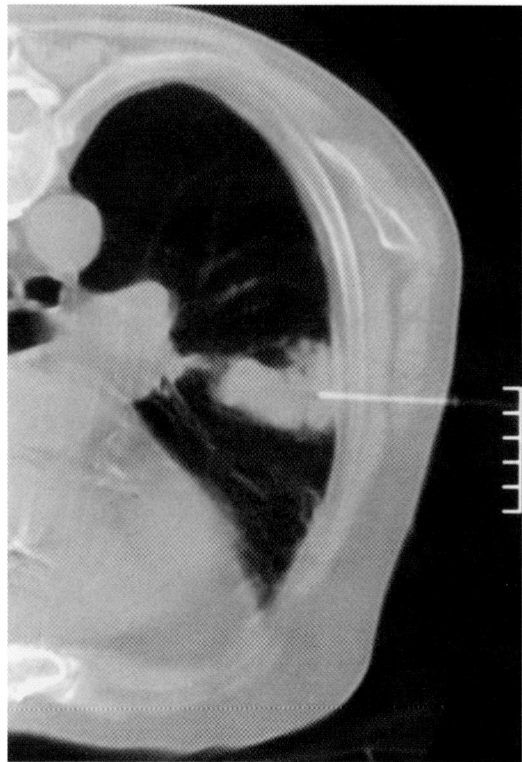

Figure 2. Lateral approach used so that aerated lung is not traversed by the biopsy needle.

Lung lesions that are visible on a chest radiograph can usually be biopsied with the use of fluoroscopy. At times a lesion may only be visible on the posteroanterior (PA) projection. In these cases, with use of information obtained from a CT scan—the depth from the skin surface and relationship to the trachea and spine—fluoroscopic biopsy can be performed. Some lesions that are visible on a chest radiograph, particularly small nodules or nodules with indistinct borders, may not be visible on fluoroscopy. If there is a question as to whether a lesion will be visible on fluoroscopy, the patient can undergo fluoroscopy prior to the biopsy to assess the visibility of the lesion.

The biopsy approach selected is usually the route that has the shortest distance from the skin to the lesion. An anterior or posterior approach is usually taken, although in some cases a lateral approach may be best **(Fig. 2)**. Another factor to consider is the number of pleural surfaces that will be traversed by the needle. These should be kept to a minimum to decrease the risk of post-biopsy pneumothorax. Occasionally, however, the ideal needle trajectory may traverse multiple pleural surfaces.

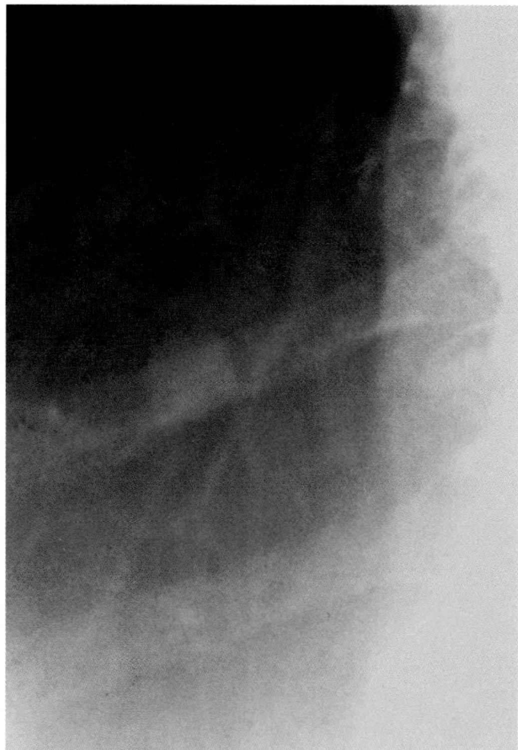

Figure 3. The rib overlies the nodule during quiet respiration.

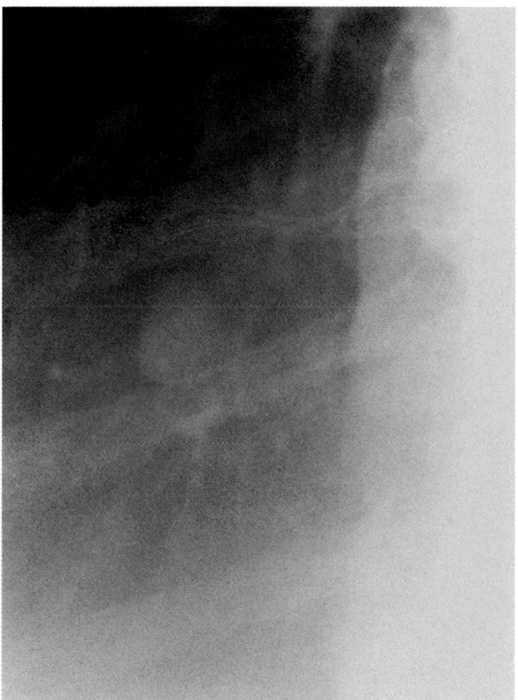

Figure 4. Tilting the fluoroscopic table cephalad projects the lesion off of the rib.

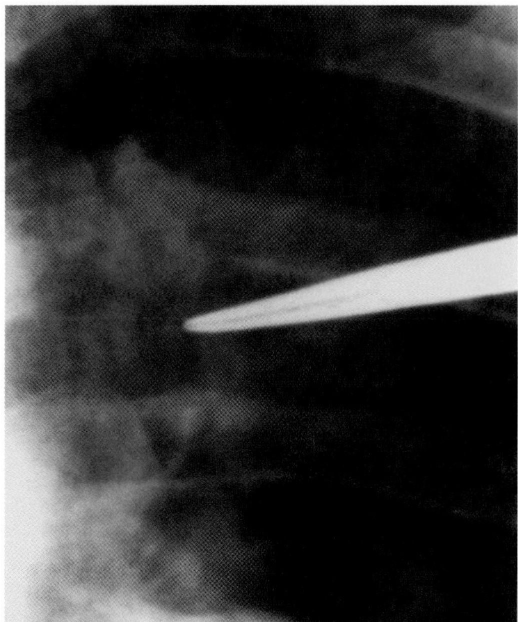

Figure 5. Entrance site marked with a hemostat.

Fluoroscopic Biopsy

After the approach for the biopsy has been determined, the patient is placed on the fluoroscopy table in the appropriate position. With use of either C-arm or biplane fluoroscopy, the lesion is localized. The relationship of the lesion to the overlying ribs and its movement during respiration are assessed. Fluoro-scopy is initially performed with the tube perpendicular to the chest wall, and a route between the overlying ribs is identified. If the lesion is located behind a rib, the tube is angled to project the lesion off of the rib **(Figs. 3, 4)**. With use of a hemostat as a pointer, the skin entrance site is localized and marked on the skin with a permanent marker **(Fig. 5)**.

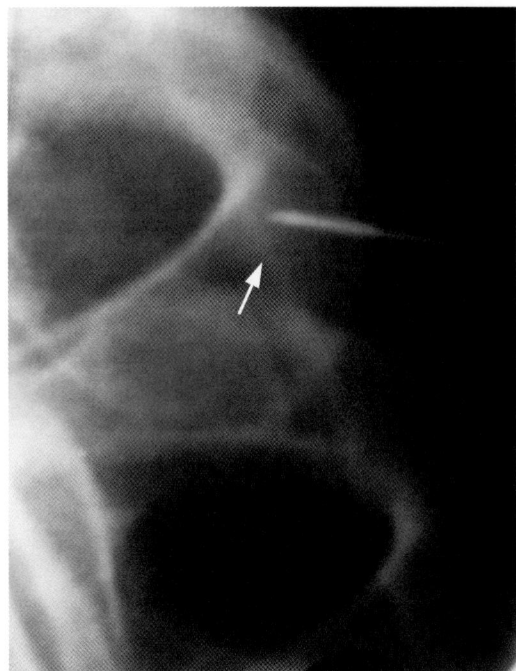

Figure 6. The tip of the anesthetic needle is advanced to a location immediately adjacent to the parietal pleura (arrow).

After the entrance site is prepared with an antiseptic, the skin and subcutaneous tissues are infiltrated with local anesthetic. The initial anesthetic is administered to a level short of the parietal pleura; this depth is determined from measurements obtained from CT images or chest radiographs. The fluoroscopy tube is positioned so that it projects perpendicular to the needle and tangential to the parietal pleura. The anesthetic needle is then advanced to a position just beneath the parietal pleura **(Fig. 6)**, where additional anesthetic is injected to anesthetize the parietal pleura. The fluoroscopic unit can then be aligned along the axis of the anesthetic needle to confirm the adequacy of the biopsy approach **(Fig. 7)**.

Many different types of biopsy needles are available and the choice of needle is based on personal preference. We have had excellent success using a coaxial needle system consisting of a 19-gauge guide needle and a 22-gauge Greene biopsy needle. Initially, the guide needle is inserted through the skin and advanced deep enough to stabilize the needle. The alignment of the needle in relation to the lesion is checked with fluoroscopy **(Fig. 8)**. If misalignment is present, the needle is adjusted and the alignment rechecked. When proper alignment is achieved, the needle is advanced a short distance and the alignment rechecked. This process is repeated until the needle is in the intercostal muscle. A clue that the guide needle is in the intercostal muscle is that the needle will move in the opposite direction of the lung during respiration. Angled fluoroscopy can also be used to check the depth of the needle. Once the intercostal muscle is reached, tangential fluoroscopy is used to guide the advancement of the needle to a subpleural location.

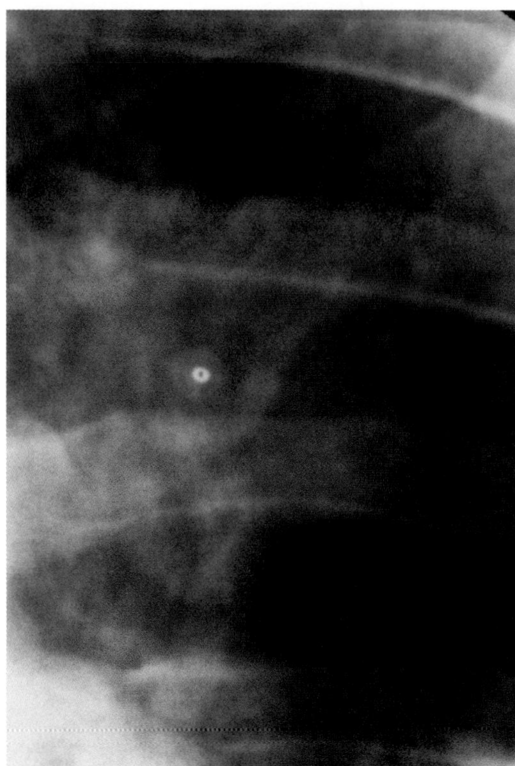

Figure 7. Anesthetic needle viewed along its axis confirms the intended biopsy approach.

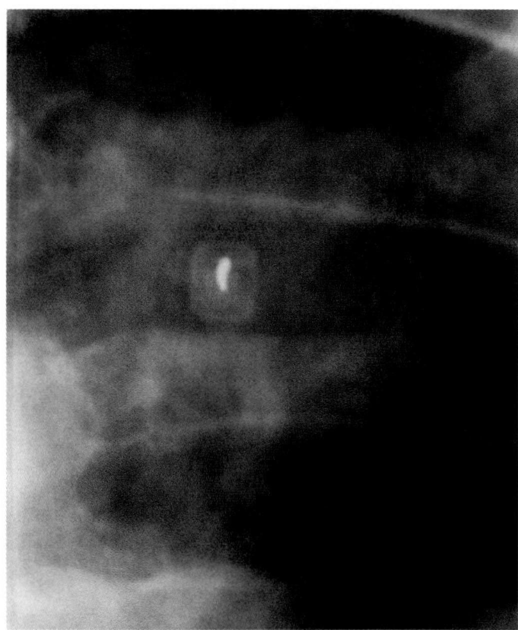

Figure 8. Fluoroscopy used to guide the guide needle.

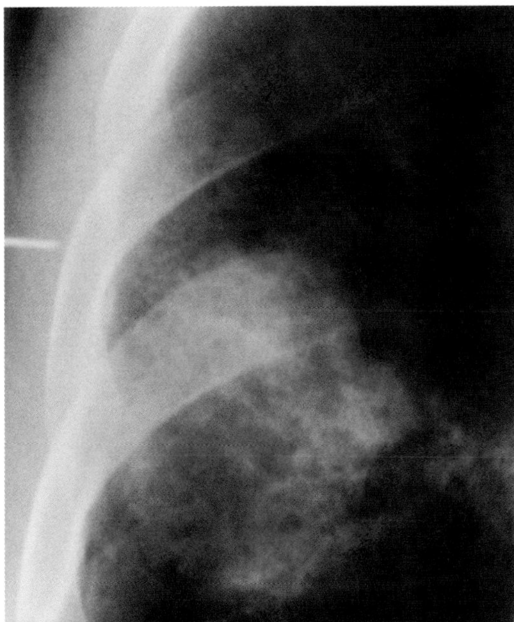

Figure 9. The mass is located inferior to the guide needle during inspiration.

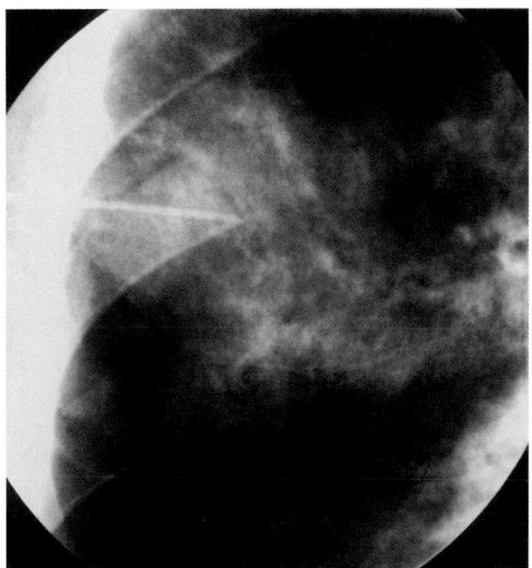

Figure 10. During expiration, the position of the mass allows the guide needle to be placed in the center of the mass.

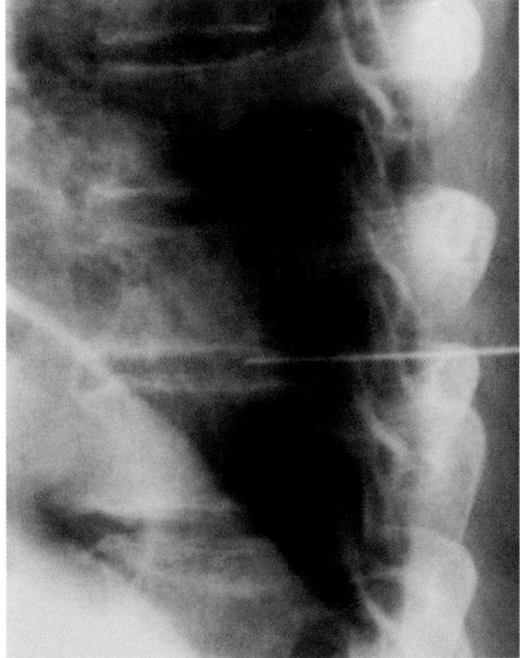

Figure 11. Tip of the biopsy needle positioned at the posterior aspect of the mass.

Several practice breath-holding sessions are then performed to align the needle and the lesion in the proper phase of respiration **(Figs. 9, 10)**. During suspended respiration, the guide needle is advanced a short distance into the lung. After the patient is allowed several shallow respirations, the needle is further advanced during suspended respiration while oblique or lateral fluoroscopy is used to guide the depth of advancement until the lesion is reached. Anteroposterior fluoroscopy is performed to control the course of the needle, with adjustments in the needle position made as necessary.

The tip of the guide needle is positioned either within the lesion or immediately adjacent to the leading edge of the lesion **(Fig. 11)**. A biopsy of the margins of the lesion often has a greater yield than biopsy of the center because necrosis may be present in the central portions of the lesion.

Sampling of the lesion is performed next. The biopsy needle is attached to a 10-mL syringe which has had all of the air expressed from it. During suspended respiration, the stylet of the guide needle is removed and the biopsy needle is immediately inserted into the guide needle. The biopsy needle is then advanced to the end of the guide needle, and resistance is usually felt when contact is made with the lesion. However, with some cancers and areas of infection, no resistance to the needle can be discerned.

The position of the needle tip can be confirmed with oblique or lateral fluoroscopy. Suction is then applied by the syringe and the needle is advanced into the lesion with multiple short, rapid, reciprocating movements. The sampling is observed with fluoroscopy to ensure that the needle does not extend beyond the far side of the lesion. Suction is released before the needle is withdrawn from the guide needle to prevent the sample from being aspirated in the syringe. The stylet is reinserted into the guide needle, which is left in place. The patient is instructed to remain still and breathe shallowly. The syringe is detached from the biopsy needle and filled with air. It is then reattached and the sample expressed onto a sterile slide.

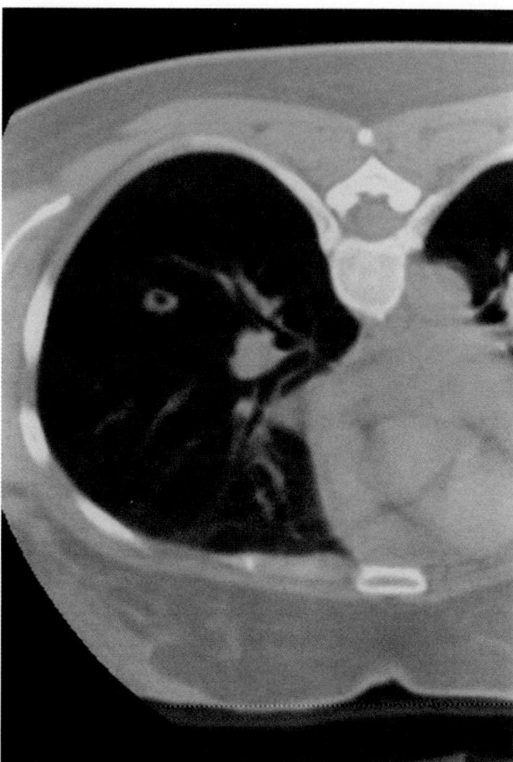

Figure 12. CT scout images locate the lesion and identify possible biopsy approaches.

We typically take three initial samples. They are prepared with a rapid stain and reviewed by the cytologist who is in attendance during the procedure. If the sample is deemed adequate by the cytologist, no further sampling is required. If the samples are inadequate or the cytologist requests additional material for special stains or microbiologic processing, the biopsy is repeated. The cycle of sampling and reviewing specimens is continued until an adequate sample is obtained. Once the cytologist indicates that the sample is adequate, the guide needle is removed while the patient suspends respiration.

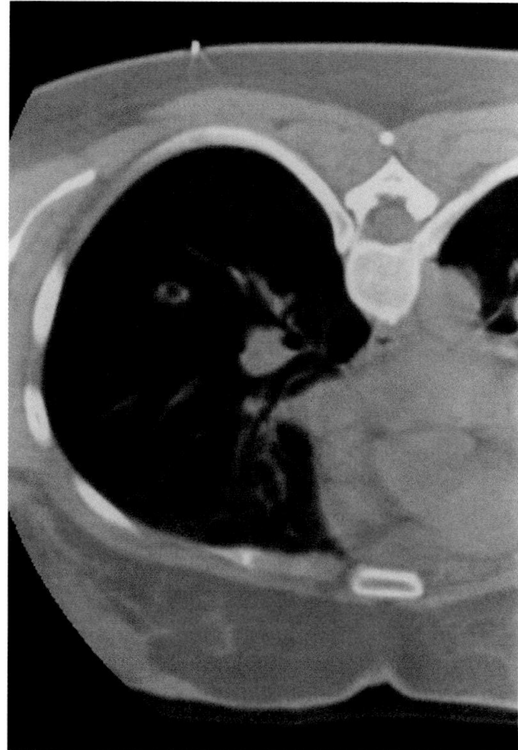

Figure 13. Skin entrance site marked with a metallic marker.

After needle removal, the patient is monitored for a period of time to exclude the development of a pneumothorax, the most common complication following TNAB.[6] The lungs are examined fluoroscopically before the patient is removed from the fluoroscopy table to evaluate for a rapidly occurring pneumothorax. If no pneumothorax is detected, the patient is transferred to a gurney with the biopsied side in a dependent position. An immediate PA chest radiograph is obtained. If no pneumothorax is identified, the patient remains at rest on the gurney with the dependent side down for 1 hour.[7] Another chest radiograph is obtained in an hour and if no pneumothorax is detected, the patient is allowed to ambulate. A final 4-hour post-biopsy film is obtained, and if no pneumothorax is identified at that time, the patient is discharged.[6]

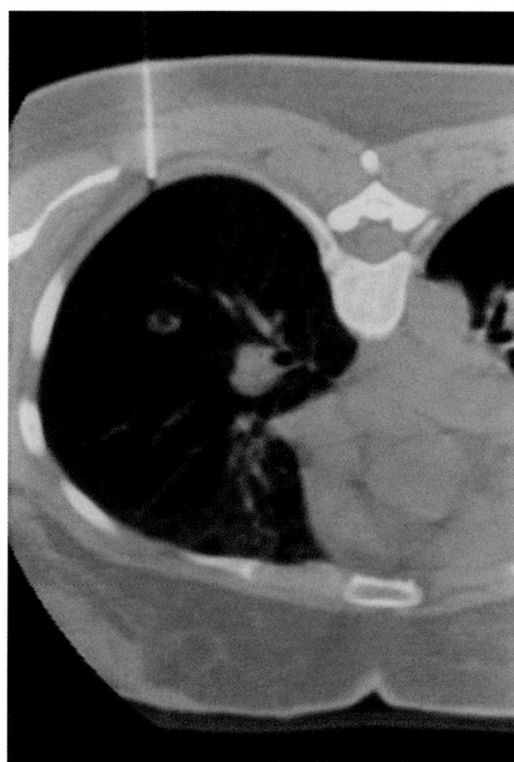

Figure 14. Guide needle advanced to a subpleural location.

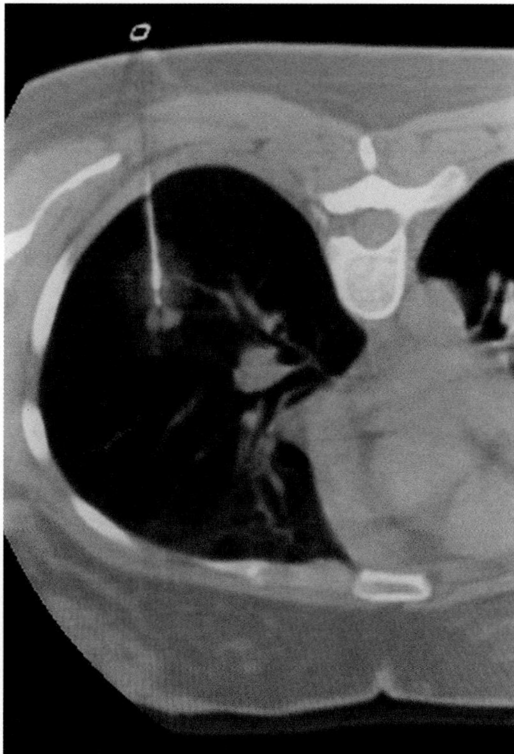

Figure 15. Guide needle positioned immediately adjacent to the lesion. A small contusion is present around the distal aspect of the guide needle.

Management of any pneumothorax that develops will depend on several factors including the size and growth rate of the pneumothorax, the clinical symptoms, and the presence of underlying pulmonary disease. The patient's travel distance and the proximity of medical facilities to the patient's home will also influence treatment of the pneumothorax. Management ranges from additional observation to the insertion of a small-caliber chest tube.[8,9]

CT-Guided Biopsy

The patient is positioned on the CT table according to the planned biopsy approach. Several contiguous CT scans are then taken through the lesion. If it is necessary to identify adjacent vascular structures, intravenous contrast material can be administered. The preliminary slices are reviewed to identify a level at which no overlying bony structures are impeding access to the lesion **(Fig. 12)**.

Once the entrance site has been chosen, the distance from the midline is measured and a lead shot placed on the site. A scan is obtained to confirm the location of the entrance site **(Fig. 13)**. The site is then prepared antiseptically and local anesthetic administered.

The guide needle is inserted into the chest wall and, with serial CT scans for guidance, the needle is aligned and advanced until its tip is in a subpleural location **(Fig. 14)**. Additional anesthetic can be administered through the guide needle if pain is felt as the needle is advanced. During suspended respiration, the guide needle is advanced through the pleura and into the lung, then advanced incrementally as its position is confirmed with repeat scans.

When the tip of the guide needle abuts the lesion, samples are obtained **(Fig. 15)**. When the sample is deemed adequate by the cytologist, the needle is removed. If lung parenchyma was traversed by the guide needle, serial chest radiographs are obtained following the same protocol used for fluoroscopic biopsies. If aerated lung was never entered, a single post-biopsy chest radiograph is adequate.

During CT-guided biopsies, identification of the needle tip may be problematic. The CT level and width should be changed as needed to best demonstrate the biopsy needle and the lesion to be sampled.[10] The tip of the needle often produces a shadowing artifact.[11] Needle tip location can also be suggested by adjacent CT slices that do not show the needle tip.

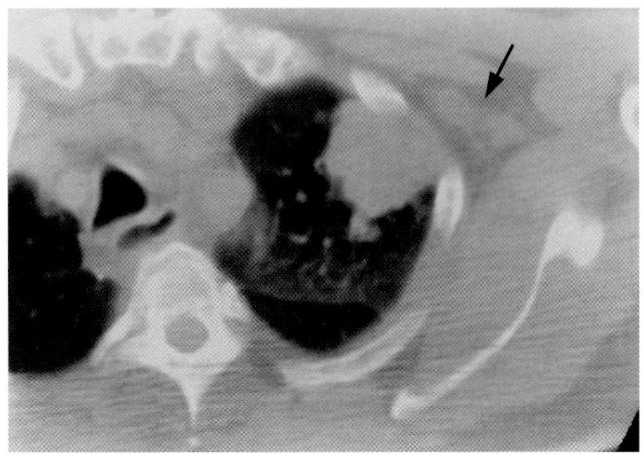

Figure 16. When the patient's arms are down, the axillary vein and artery (arrow) are located in the intended biopsy route.

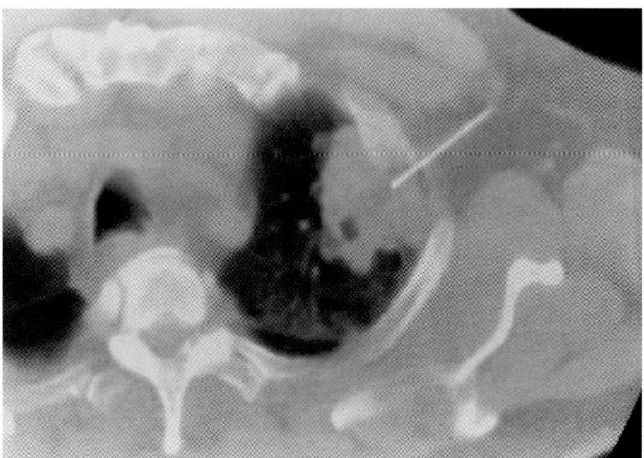

Figure 17. When the patient's arms are raised, the axillary vessels move superiorly, allowing biopsy of the left upper lobe mass.

If overlying skeletal structures interfere with the biopsy, tilting the CT gantry may provide an approach to the lesion.[12] Tilting the CT gantry is analogous to the tilt used in fluoroscopic biopsies to expose the lesion from behind the overlying ribs. This tilt technique is somewhat more cumbersome with CT because it is not possible to image along the needle in real time as can be done with fluoroscopy. Positioning the patient's arm either up or down can also alter the anatomy, allowing a biopsy to be performed **(Figs. 16, 17)**.

When mediastinal structures are biopsied, an effort should be made to avoid transgressing the visceral pleura. Anterior mediastinal masses can be biopsied from a parasternal approach, which avoids the lung. However, when this approach is taken, the internal mammary vessels must be identified and avoided **(Fig. 18)**.

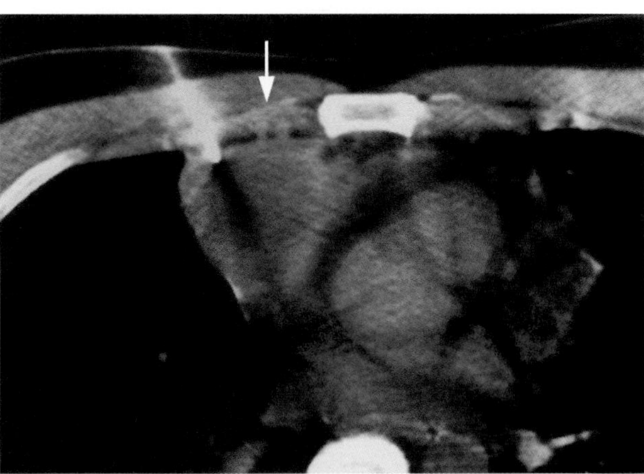

Figure 18. Guide needle inserted lateral to the internal mammary vessels (arrow).

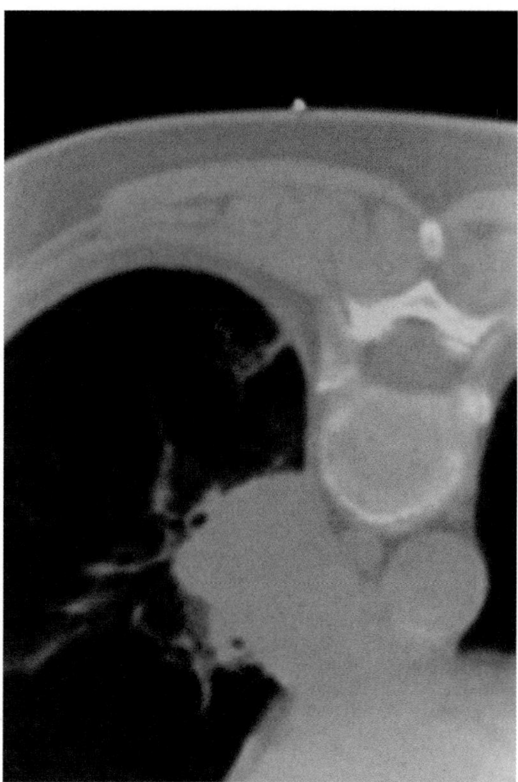

Figure 19. Scout image taken prior to biopsy of a paraesophageal mass. Minimal soft tissue is present in the paraspinal lesion.

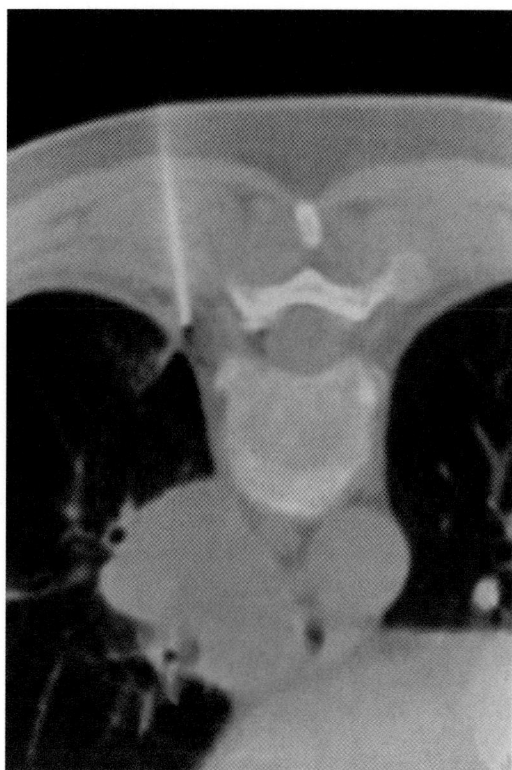

Figure 20. Guide needle placed in a subpleural location and a mixture of anesthetic and saline solution injected.

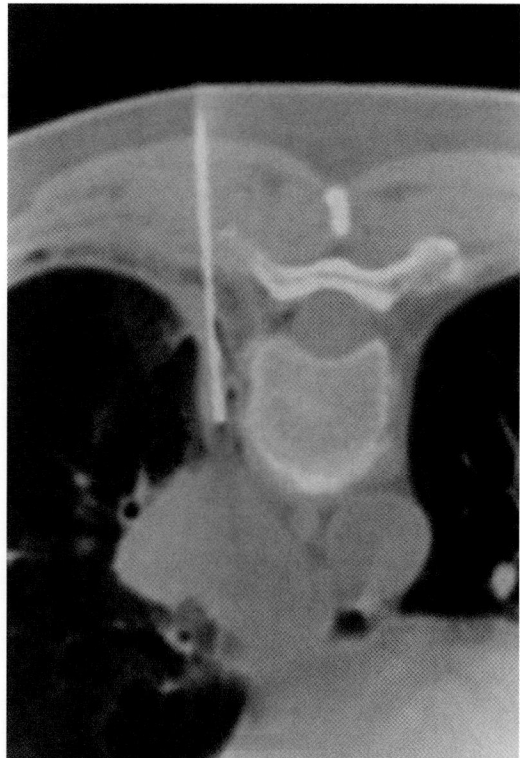

Figure 21. Widened paraspinal space permits biopsy of a mediastinal mass without traversing the lung.

The injection of a saline and anesthetic solution into the paraspinal soft tissues will elevate the pleura off the spine and provide a route through which posterior mediastinal masses can be biopsied without traversing the pleura **(Figs. 19–21)**.[13] Other techniques to avoid penetrating the visceral pleura include a pleural space approach through a pleural effusion, induced controlled pneumothorax, lateral decubitus positioning, and direct semicoronal scanning to guide suprasternal biopsies.[14]

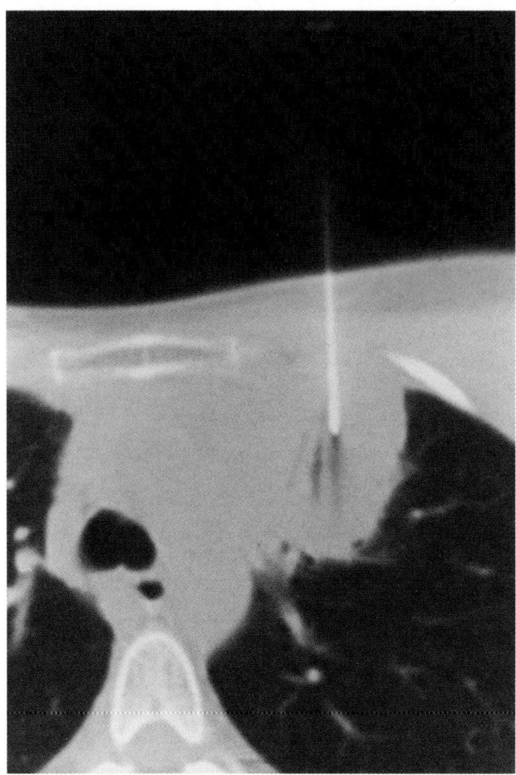

Figure 22. Air-filled tracks produced during biopsy of a firm mass. Angling the biopsy needle increased the amount of tissue obtained.

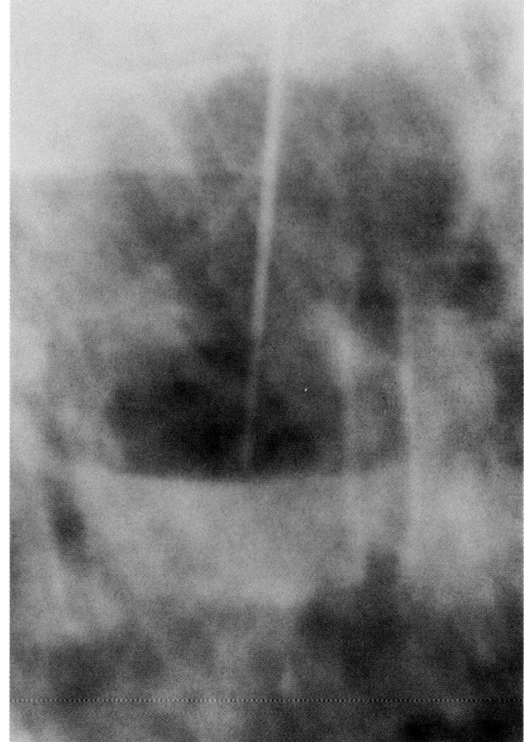

Figure 23. Biopsy needle advanced into the fluid within a lung abscess.

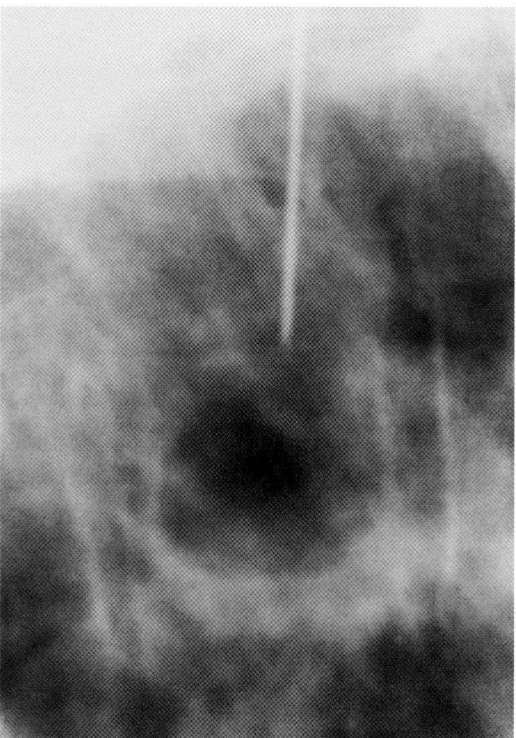

Figure 24. Abscess cavity following aspiration of fluid. Biopsy of the wall of the abscess can now be performed without the fear of diluting abscess fluid specimens with blood.

Lesion Sampling

In some firm lesions, serial samples show decreasing cellularity caused by a track which forms along the path of the needle. This problem can be eliminated by angling the guide needle in different directions when sampling **(Fig. 22)**. When lung abscesses are aspirated, the central fluid should be removed before the abscess wall is sampled **(Figs. 23, 24)**.This will limit the amount of blood present in the sample, which makes it difficult to identify organisms. When sampling parenchymal opacities that are possibly infectious in origin, we never inject saline into the lesion as recommended by some authors.[15,16] It is our belief that saline injection dilutes the number of organisms in a given sample volume and reduces the chance of identifying any organisms.[17]

Complications

As noted earlier, the most common complication of TNAB is pneumothorax, which occurs in 10%–60% of cases with about 8% of these cases requiring tube evacuation. The management and evaluation of pneumothoraces will be discussed in **Tutorial 14**. Another frequent sequela of biopsy is hemoptysis, which occurs in about 5% of cases. Post-biopsy hemoptysis is almost always self-limited and is more frightening to the patient than it is significant. The possibility of a pneumothorax or hemoptysis should always be discussed with the patient prior to the procedure. Other complications such as infection, neoplastic seeding of the track, or air embolism are quite rare. The overall mortality for lung biopsy varies depending on the series but is in the range of 0.01% to 0.05%.[20]

Conclusion

TNAB is a cost-effective, safe, accurate, and minimally invasive means of evaluating parenchymal abnormalities and nodules. The success of TNAB ultimately depends on the skill of the cytologist interpreting the samples. A team approach to TNAB in which the cytologist is in attendance at the biopsy has been shown to improve the diagnostic yield of the procedure.[1,18] The use of a coaxial needle biopsy technique optimizes this interaction because additional material can be readily obtained to ensure that the sample is adequate. The ability to obtain samples for special stains as well as electron microscopy and microbiologic studies increases the diagnostic accuracy of TNAB.[1,19]

References

1. Conces DJ, Schwenk GR, Doering PR, Glant MD. Thoracic needle biopsy: improved results utilizing a team approach. Chest 1987; 91:813–816.

2. Khouri NF, Stitik FP, Erozan YS, et al. Transthoracic needle aspiration biopsy of benign and malignant lung lesions. AJR 1985; 144:281–288.

3. Westcott JL, Rao N, Colley DP. Transthoracic needle biopsy of small pulmonary nodules. Radiology 1997; 202:97–103.

4. Stevens GM, Jackman RJ. Outpatient needle biopsy of the lung: its safety and utility. Radiology 1984; 151:301–304.

5. Poe RH, Kallay MC. Transthoracic needle biopsy of lung in nonhospitalized patients. Chest 1987; 92:676–678.

6. Perlmutt LM, Braun SD, Newman GE, Oke EJ, Dunnick NR. Timing of chest film follow-up after transthoracic needle aspiration. AJR 1986; 146:1049–1050.

7. Moore EH, Shepard JA, McLoud TC, Templeton PA, Kosiuk JP. Positional precautions in needle aspiration lung biopsy. Radiology 1990; 175:733–735.

8. Conces DJ, Tarver RD, Gray WC, Pearcy EA. Treatment of pneumothoraces utilizing small caliber chest tubes. Chest 1988; 94:55–57.

9. Perlmutt LM, Braun SD, Newman GE, et al. Transthoracic needle aspiration: use of a small chest tube to treat pneumothorax. AJR 1987; 148:849–851.

10. Yankelevitz DF, Henschke CI, Davis SD. Appropriate window and level settings in CT-guided biopsies. J Thorac Imaging 1994; 9:108–111.

11. Yankelevitz DF, Henschke CI. Needle-tip localization for CT-guided biopsies. J Thorac Imaging 1993; 8:241–243.

12. Stern EJ, Webb WR, Gamsu G. CT gantry tilt: utility in transthoracic fine-needle aspiration biopsy. Work in progress. Radiology 1993; 187:873–874.

13. Lenglinger FX, Zisch RJ. Technique to avoid iatrogenic pneumothorax during biopsy of mediastinal lesions. Radiology 1994; 193:878–879.

14. Bressler EL, Kirkham JA. Mediastinal masses: alternative approaches to CT-guided needle biopsy. Radiology 1994; 191:391–396.

15. Zavala DC, Schoell JE. Ultrathin needle aspiration of the lung in infectious and malignant disease. Am Rev Resp Dis 1981; 123:125–131.

16. Castellino RA, Blank N. Etiologic diagnosis of focal pulmonary infection in immunocompromised patients by fluoroscopically guided percutaneous needle aspiration. Radiology 1979; 132:563–567.

17. Conces DJ, Clark SA, Tarver RD, Schwenk GR. Transthoracic aspiration needle biopsy: value in the diagnosis of pulmonary infections. AJR 1989; 152:31–34.

18. Austin JH, Cohen MB. Value of having a cytopathologist present during percutaneous fine-needle aspiration biopsy of lung: report of 55 cancer patients and meta-analysis of the literature. AJR 1993; 160:175–177.

19. Davidson DD, Conces DJ, Goheen MP, Clark SA. Comparative ultrastructure of needle aspiration biopsy and surgical resection specimens of lung tumors. Ultrastructural Path 1992; 16:505–519.

20. Weisbrod GL. Transthoracic needle biopsy. World J Surg 1993; 17: 705–711.

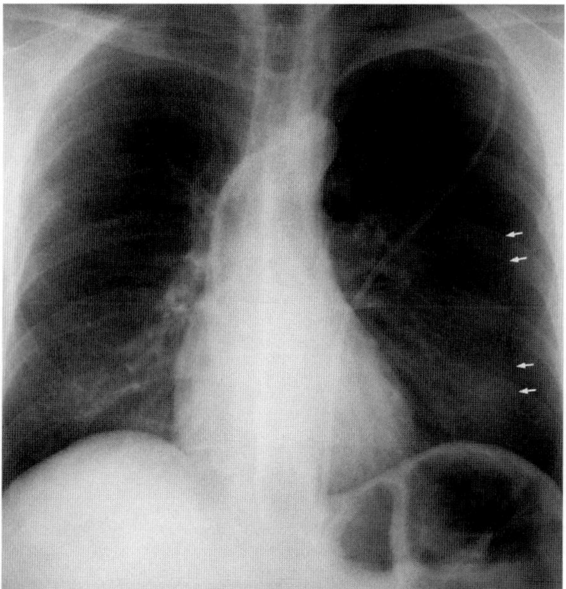
Figure 1. Left pneumothorax (arrows) following placement of a dual-lumen catheter into the superior vena cava from a left subclavian venous approach.

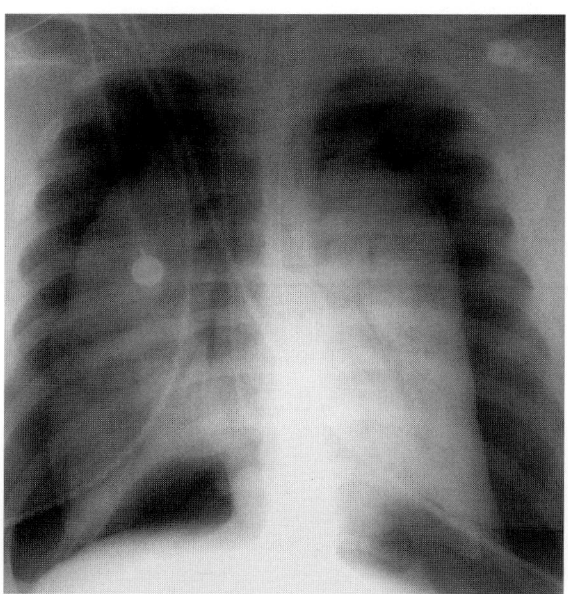
Figure 2. Bilateral pneumothoraces in a patient with severe acute respiratory distress syndrome.

TUTORIAL 14
EVALUATION AND TREATMENT OF PNEUMOTHORAX

L. Alden Parker, M.D., and
David L. Levin, Ph.D., M.D.

Introduction

The subjects addressed in this tutorial include:
1. Etiology of pneumothoraces
2. Management of pneumothoraces
3. Outcome of chest tube placement.

Etiology

Pneumothorax can occur from a variety of causes. Primary spontaneous pneumothorax results from the rupture of a subpleural bleb in patients without other underlying lung disease. There is a strong male predominance, with most individuals being between 20 and 40 years of age. It is more frequent in smokers. Secondary spontaneous pneumothorax can be seen in patients with a variety of underlying diseases, including chronic obstructive pulmonary disease, asthma, granulomatous disease, and pulmonary fibrosis.

Pneumothorax can also have iatrogenic or traumatic causes. It can be seen following transthoracic needle or transbronchial biopsy, or with central line placement **(Fig. 1)**. Pneumothorax is also seen as a complication of positive pressure ventilation **(Fig. 2)**. Blunt trauma usually leads to pneumothorax by a sudden increase in intra-alveolar pressure causing dissection of air from a ruptured alveolus through the pulmonary interstitium into the pleural space. Direct laceration of the lung parenchyma from an adjacent rib fracture is a less common mechanism.[1,2]

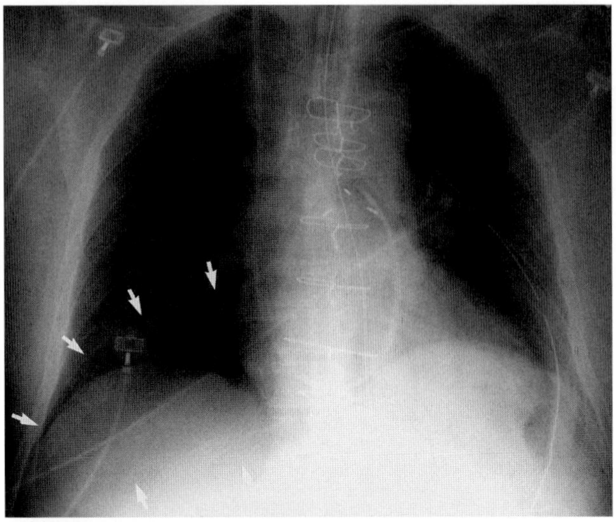

Figure 3. Hyperlucency at the right base (arrows) with the patient recumbent suggests pneumothorax.

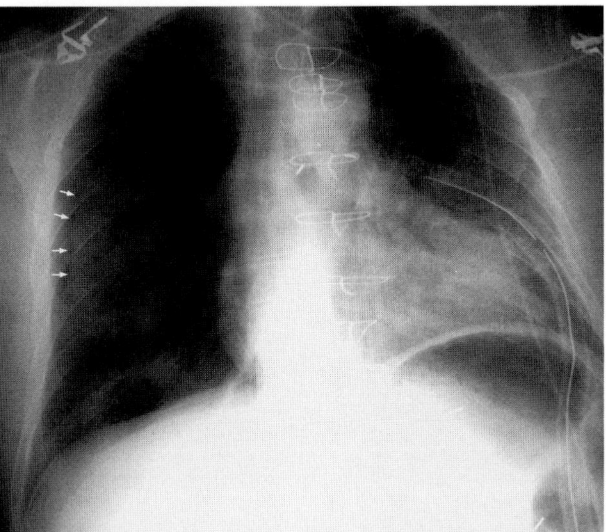

Figure 4. Pleural edge (arrows) easily seen with the patient semi-erect.

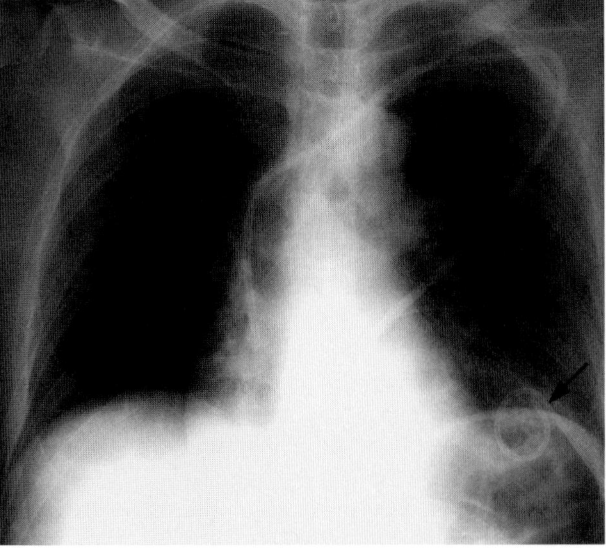

Figure 5. Same patient as in Figure 1. Re-expansion of the left lung following placement of a pigtail catheter (arrow). The catheter was inserted low on the anterior axillary line to avoid the subcutaneous track of a recently placed subclavian venous catheter and to position it in the "high point" with the patient recumbent.

Diagnosis

Clinical symptoms include dyspnea and pleuritic chest pain. Symptoms are usually more prominent with larger pneumothoraces or in patients with underlying lung disease. Dyspnea may resolve without intervention. Although physical findings may suggest pneumothorax, the diagnosis is made radiographically. In otherwise healthy patients, this is done with an erect posteroanterior (PA) inspiratory chest radiograph.[3,4] In the debilitated patient, the examination at the bedside should be done with the patient in the decubitus position with the affected side up, using a horizontal x-ray beam.[3] In this situation a semi-erect anteroposterior chest film will underestimate the magnitude of the pneumothorax **(Figs. 3, 4)**.

Management

The indications for intervention include increasing size of a pneumothorax on serial chest radiographs and/or substantial dyspnea. Most physicians will have an absolute size criterion which warrants the placement of a chest tube. Although this varies, most will intervene when a pneumothorax approaches 25% to 35% of the volume of the hemithorax.[5,6] In general, a small pneumothorax that is stable in size on an upright PA chest radiograph 2 hours (or more) after transthoracic needle biopsy will not require treatment. On the other hand, if it is definitely increasing in size, intervention is appropriate even if the patient is asymptomatic. A tension pneumothorax always requires decompression.

Several approaches can be used for chest tube placement.[5] Most commonly, catheters are placed in the second or third anterior intercostal space at the midclavicular line. In women, an anterior or mid-axillary line approach may be desirable to avoid traversing breast tissue.[5] A low anterior approach may also be desirable in the recumbent patient as this will be the "high point" of the chest **(Fig. 5)**.

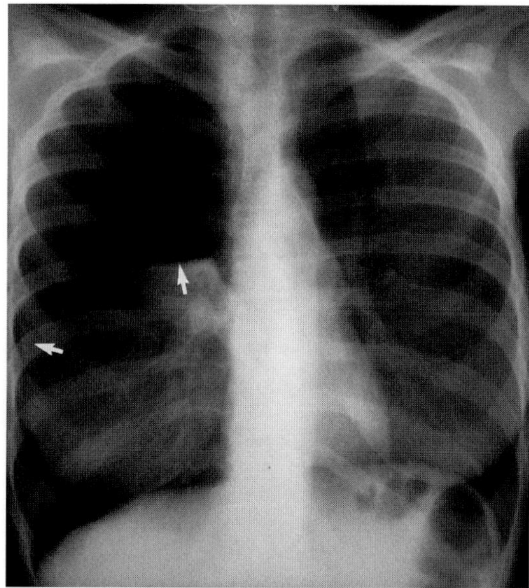

Figure 6. Large right pneumothorax (arrows) in a young patient with acquired immunodeficiency syndrome.

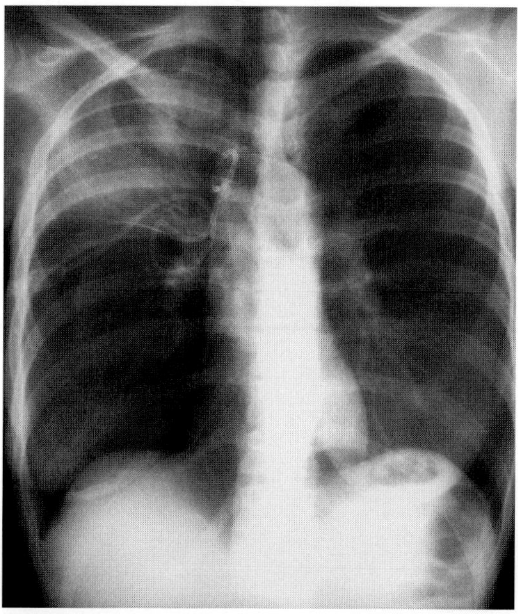

Figure 7. Patchy air-space filling in the right upper lobe represents re-expansion pulmonary edema.

Technique

The chest tube and trocar or entry needle are advanced over the superior margin of the rib and angled so that the tip travels toward the apex of the lung. Entrance into the pleural space is confirmed by aspiration of air. The chest tube is then advanced into the pleural space if a trocar system is used. Alternatively, a modified Seldinger technique can be used with a floppy-tipped wire and standard self-retaining pigtail catheter. At this point, 3 mL of lidocaine can be instilled through the chest tube to reduce the pain from irritation of the pleural surface. After the chest tube is secured, the pneumothorax should be aspirated manually, and the catheter attached to a Pleurevac (Deknatel, Inc., Fall River, MA) for drainage on wall suction. In general, fluoroscopy is sufficient for placement of catheters and drainage of pleural air collections. Occasionally, CT guidance may be necessary for drainage of loculated pneumothoraces. A single unit device which attaches to the chest wall and contains a catheter and check valve is also commercially available.[7] In an emergency, a patient can be stabilized with an Amplatz arterial sheath (Medi-Tech, Boston Scientific Corporation, Watertown, MA) or a 16-gauge Angiocath (Becton Dickinson, Sandy, UT) inserted into the second interspace and connected to a three-way stopcock for manual aspiration during transport to the interventional suite. Rarely, re-expansion pulmonary edema can occur following rapid re-expansion of a large pneumothorax **(Figs. 6, 7)**.

Outcome

Small chest tubes have a high success rate. In one study, 28 of 30 pneumothoraces following transthoracic needle biopsy were successfully treated with a small-bore chest tube alone.[6] The mean duration of drainage was 2 days. After the pneumothorax has resolved completely, the chest tube can be placed on the waterseal. If no air leak is evident and the lung remains expanded, the chest tube can be removed. In general, a bronchopleural fistula will seal more rapidly if pleural apposition can be achieved by re-establishing negative intrapleural pressure. Selected patients can also be managed as outpatients with the chest tube connected to a Heimlich valve.[5] However, this device has the disadvantage of being connected backwards easily and a tension pneumothorax can result.

References

1. Dowdeswell IRG. Pleural disease. In: Stein JH, ed. Internal medicine. 3rd edition. Boston: Little, Brown and Company, 1990; 737–744.

2. Fraser RG, Pare PD. Synopsis of diseases of the chest. 2nd edition. Philadelphia: W.B. Saunders Company, 1994; 878–881.

3. Beres RA, Goodman LR. Pneumothorax: detection with upright versus decubitus radiography. Radiology 1993; 186:19–22.

4. Hall FM. Radiographic diagnosis of pneumothorax. Radiology 1993; 188:583.

5. Klein JS, Schultz S, Heffner JE. Interventional radiology of the chest: image-guided percutaneous drainage of pleural effusion, lung abscess, and pneumothorax. AJR 1995; 164:581–588.

6. Casola G, vanSonnenberg E, Keightley A, Ho M, Withers C, Lee AS. Pneumothorax: radiologic treatment with small catheters. Radiology 1988; 166:89–91.

7. Molina PL, Solomon SL, Glazer HS, Sagel SS, Anderson DJ. A one-piece unit for treatment of pneumothorax complicating needle biopsy: evaluation in 10 patients. AJR 1990; 155:31–33.

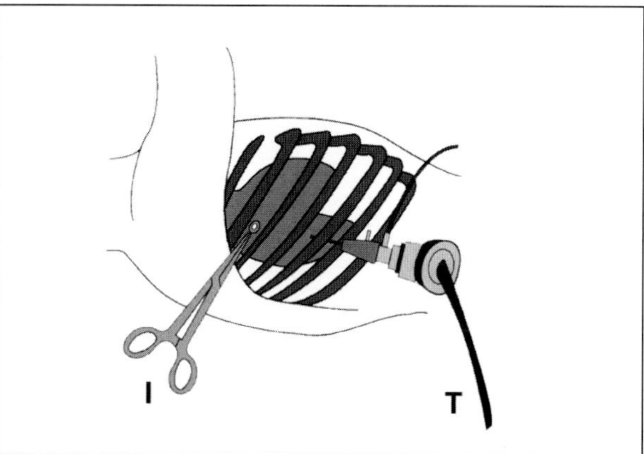

Figure 1. Schematic of the thoracoscopic procedure in which a thoracoscope (T) and endoscopic instruments (I) are inserted into the pleural space through small incisions.

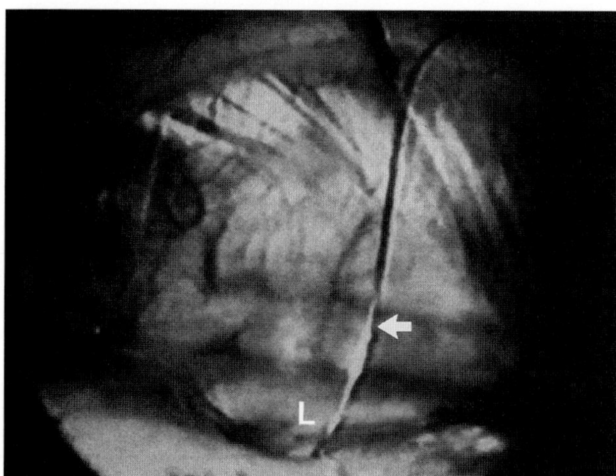

Figure 2. Intraoperative photograph of the pleural space at thoracoscopy. A hookwire (arrow) placed preoperatively under computed tomography guidance crosses the pleural space and extends into the lung (L), marking an occult pulmonary nodule.

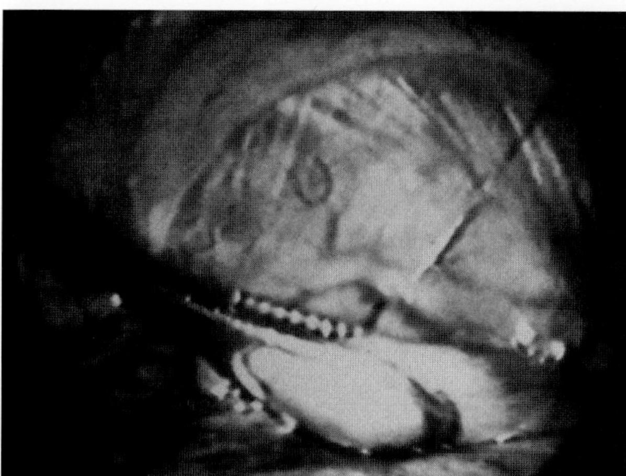

Figure 3. The localizing wire within a pulmonary nodule is engaged by surgical forceps.

TUTORIAL 15 PREOPERATIVE LOCALIZATION OF PULMONARY NODULES FOR THORACOSCOPIC RESECTION

Ana M. Salazar, M.D., and Rosita M. Shah, M.D.

Introduction

The subjects addressed in this tutorial include:
1. Indications for video-assisted thoracoscopic surgery
2. Management of pulmonary nodules
3. Preoperative planning and localization
4. Technique
5. Complications.

Video-assisted thoracoscopic surgery (VATS) is used widely in the management of intrathoracic pathology, having replaced standard open thoracotomy in many instances with a significant reduction in surgical morbidity. Pleural, mediastinal, and parenchymal processes, including small pulmonary nodules, can be diagnosed and treated with endoscopic surgical techniques. Resection of small pulmonary nodules is facilitated by preoperative localization under radiographic guidance.

Indications for VATS

The surgical techniques used in VATS permit visualization of the intrathoracic cavity, including the pleural space and the surfaces of the lung and mediastinum **(Figs. 1–3)**. Procedures facilitated by VATS include drainage of empyema and hemothorax, staging of neoplastic involvement in the pleural space, treatment of pleurodesis, biopsy and therapeutic resection of superficial mediastinal masses and pulmonary nodules, and biopsy of parenchymal lung disease.[1,2]

Indications for Nodule Resection by VATS

Nodule resection by VATS is an alternative to open lung biopsy for the diagnosis of pulmonary nodules when conventional diagnosis by fine needle aspiration (FNA) fails, or small lesion size limits the yield from FNA. The diagnostic accuracy of FNA for lesions smaller than 1 cm in diameter is approximately 74%.[3] VATS is also useful for performing wedge resection of previously diagnosed isolated nodular pulmonary metastases in certain cancers, and can be used for parenchymal sparing resection of primary bronchogenic carcinoma in patients with limited pulmonary reserve.

Management of Metastases and Bronchogenic Carcinoma

Resection of isolated or limited pulmonary metastases is accepted management in certain malignancies, including osseous or soft-tissue sarcomas, adenocarcinomas of renal or thyroid origin, seminoma, and malignant melanoma. Moderate improvement in 5-year survival, approaching 40%–50%, is reported in patients with osteosarcomas and genitourinary malignancies.[4] Limited resection of bronchogenic carcinoma may be the only surgical option for attempted cure in patients with synchronous or metachronous lesions and limited pulmonary reserve.

Preoperative Planning in VATS

When one of the previously discussed indications is present, preoperative planning is essential. For successful thoracoscopic resection, the surgeon must be able to visualize or palpate the lesion. This may be difficult where access is limited, where deep nodules cannot be seen or palpated, and where changes in the relationship of a parenchymal nodule to superficial landmarks have occurred due to complete lung collapse. Nodules adjacent to or on the pleural surface, and subpleural nodules in the anterior and lateral lung are usually easily amenable to unassisted resection by VATS techniques. Resection of small, nonpalpable peripheral lesions is facilitated by preoperative wire localization.[5]

Indications for Preoperative Localization Procedures

Preoperative localization is indicated and may facilitate resection of pulmonary nodules when one of the following conditions is present: 1) peripheral nodule <1 cm in diameter; 2) peripheral nodule >1 cm deep to the pleura (but not deeper than 3–4 cm); 3) nodule in a posterobasal location; 4) multiple lesions; or 5) coexisting lung disease or pulmonary fibrosis.[5] **Figure 4** demonstrates a nodule localized in the right lower lobe, which is a particularly difficult area to access thoracoscopically.

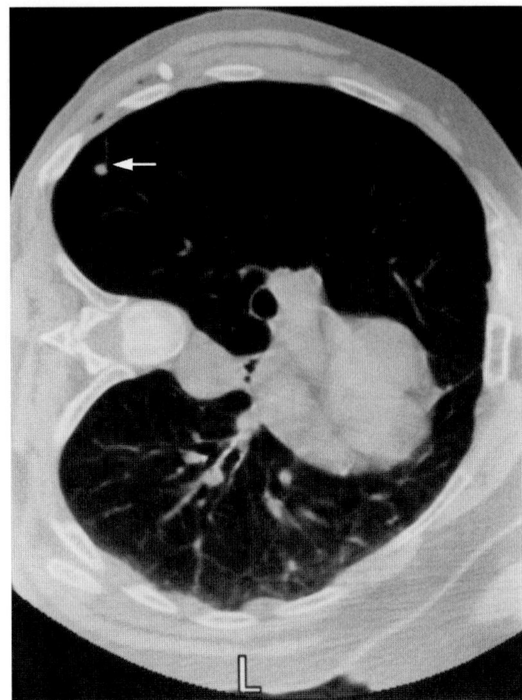

Figure 4. Small nodule in a difficult location for VATS (arrow).

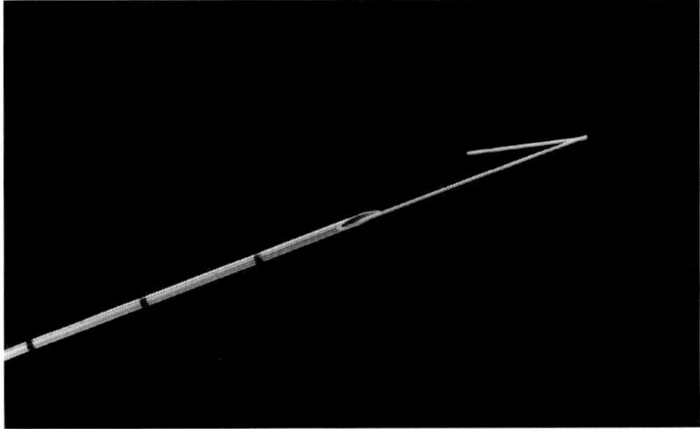

Figure 5. Open Kopans hookwire (Cook, Bloomington, IN).

Hookwires Used in Preoperative Localization
• Mack 1992 Sadowsky (Ranfac) • Plunkett 1992 Hawkins III (Medi-Tech, Boston Scientific Corporation, Watertown, MA) • Templeton 1992 Homer (Mitek Surgical Products, Glenfalls, NY) • Shah 1993 Kopans (Cook) • Sheppard 1994 Kopans (Cook) • Gossot 1994 Nycomed (Paris, France)

Figure 6.

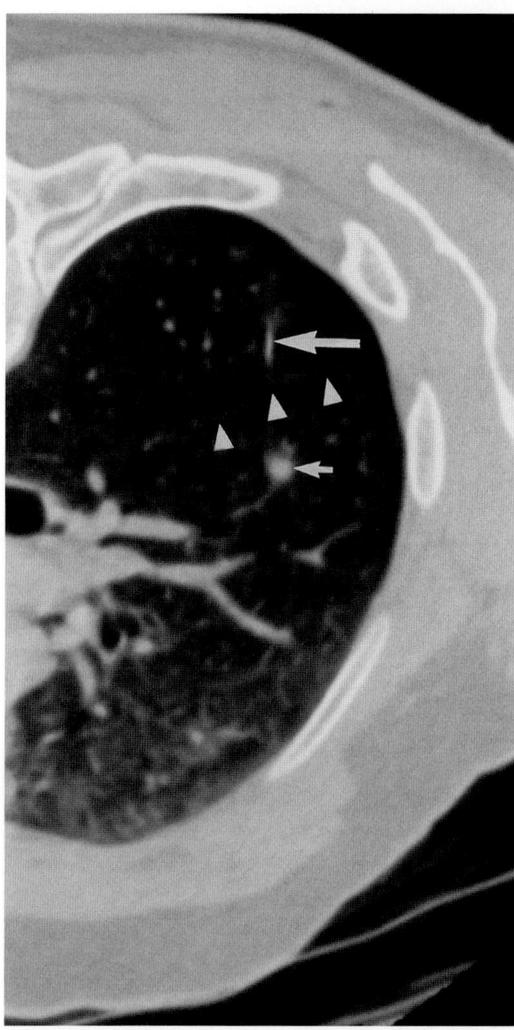

Figure 7. Transfissural needle route (long arrow) required to localize a pulmonary nodule (short arrow) located subpleurally relative to the fissure (arrowheads).

Preoperative Localization Methods

The first radiographically guided procedures were reported in 1992 by Mack et al, using methylene blue dye for pleural staining and a hookwire breast localizing system (Sadowsky, Ranfac Corporation, Avon, MA).[6] Several authors have since described their experiences and methods for preoperative localization using various localizing wires with or without pleural staining. As with the localization of breast masses, spring hookwires are used routinely because of their greater flexibility and fixation **(Figs. 5, 6)**. A recent effort to improve the wire flexibility necessary for pulmonary needle localization has been to replace the shaft of the localizing wire with a nylon suture.[7]

Preoperative Localization with Methylene Blue Dye

Methylene blue dye may be used in combination with hookwire placement to provide surgical guidance in the event of wire dislodgement. Lenglinger and Wicky have used methylene blue dye without hookwire placement and had similar success rates to wire localization.[8,9] A potential problem with this technique is the potential for dye diffusion in the event of a long delay between the localization and the time of surgery. Several authors have reported significant pleural pain associated with the instillation of methylene blue dye.[5]

Procedure

The procedure for nodule localization with VATS is similar whether a localizing wire or methylene blue dye is used and is independent of the choice of localizing wire. Pulmonary nodule localization is an extension of the techniques used in lung FNA and breast localization procedures.

Guidance with CT is preferred over fluoroscopy because it better demonstrates the anatomy and fissural planes. The shortest transthoracic distance between the chest wall and nodule is chosen for the introducer path to minimize the amount of resected parenchyma. This may even require a transfissural route **(Fig. 7)**.

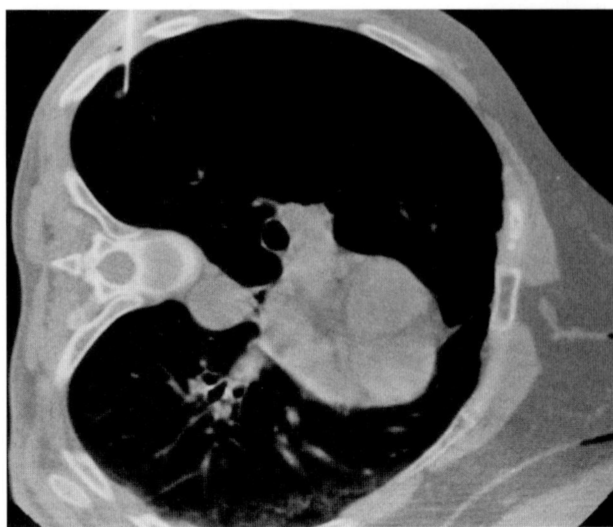

Figure 8. Patient placed in the left lateral decubitus position to permit perpendicular entry of the introducer.

The patient is positioned to permit perpendicular entry of the introducer at the skin surface **(Fig. 8)**.

The introducer needle and an occluding stylet are advanced in a fashion similar to that for CT-guided lung biopsy. Satisfactory needle position is achieved when the needle tip is within a 1-cm radius of the nodule or when the needle has advanced through the nodule with the tip approximately 1 cm beyond the nodule. The obturating stylet is then exchanged for the localizing wire, and the needle introducer is removed while the position of the localizing wire is maintained **(Fig. 9)**.[5] The wire is left unanchored to prevent inadvertent dislodgement during patient transport and surgical positioning.

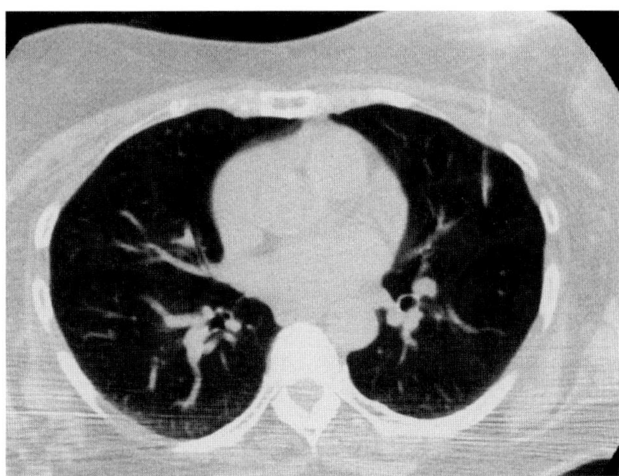

Figure 9. Wire correctly positioned through an 8-mm left upper lobe nodule.

Communication with the surgeon is essential to describe the wire course and location of the wire tip. The patient should be transported to the operating room for the VATS immediately after the localization procedure to minimize the risk of wire dislodgement; however, inadvertent delays of 4 to 6 hours have been followed by successful thoracoscopic resection.

Complications

Preoperative wire dislodgement occurs in 6%–20% of cases. The presence of a hemorrhagic pleural stain at surgery may facilitate resection in these cases, but a time delay between wire placement and surgery should be avoided. Pneumothorax occurs with 30%–100% frequency but is usually asymptomatic. The occurrence of pneumothorax does not preclude surgery. If necessary, symptomatic pneumothorax can be treated with a small-caliber chest tube or a Heimlich valve apparatus. Subsequent re-expansion of the lung allows the procedure to proceed. Other complications include pleural pain, which occurs in 5%–10% of cases, and parenchymal hemorrhage, in 5%–35% of cases, which is usually asymptomatic **(Fig. 10)**. VATS is unsuccessful in 12% of cases, usually because of posterobasal location or nodules that are too deep.

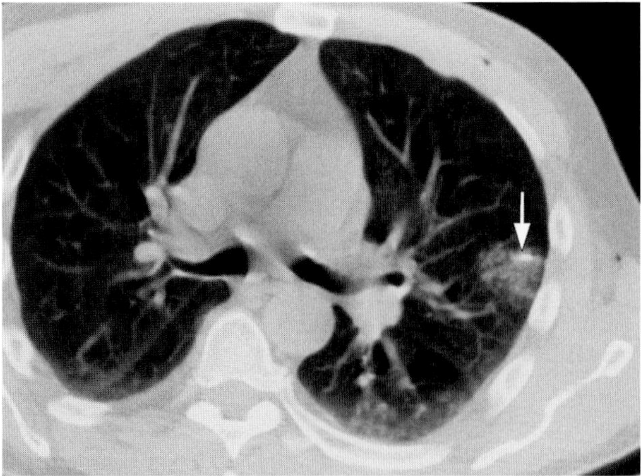

Figure 10. Small amount of parenchymal hemorrhage at the time of introducer (arrow) placement.

Conclusion

An aggressive approach to the diagnosis and management of pulmonary nodules is permitted by VATS. Resection of these nodules can be facilitated by preoperative localization and should be considered when dealing with small, deep nodules. The techniques of preoperative localization are analogous to those of CT-guided FNA biopsies with an important exception: a transfissural route is not prohibitive. Any spring hookwire can be used, alone or in combination with methylene blue dye. It is important that the external wire be left unanchored to prevent dislodgement. The rates of pneumothorax and hemorrhage do not exceed those of FNA.

References

1. Landreneau RJ, Hazelrigg SR, Ferson PF, et al. Thoracoscopic resection of 85 pulmonary lesions. Ann Thorac Surg 1992; 54:415–420.

2. Menzies R, Charbonneau M. Thoracoscopy for the diagnosis of pleural disease. Ann Intern Med 1991; 114:271–276.

3. vanSonnenberg E, Casola G, Ho M, et al. Difficult thoracic lesions: CT-guided biopsy experience in 150 cases. Radiology 1988; 167:457–461.

4. Mountain CF, McMurtrey MJ, Hermes KE. Surgery for pulmonary metastasis: a 20-year experience. Ann Thorac Surg 1984; 38:323–330.

5. Shah RM, Spirn PW, Salazar AM. Localization of peripheral pulmonary nodules for thoracoscopic excision: value of CT-guided wire placement. AJR 1993; 161:279–283.

6. Mack MJ, Gordon MJ, Postma TW, et al. Percutaneous localization of pulmonary nodules for thoracoscopic lung resection. Ann Thorac Surg 1992; 53:1123–1124.

7. Kanazawa S, Ando A, Yasui K, Tanaka A, Hiraki Y. Localization of pulmonary nodules for thoracoscopic excision: use of newly developed hookwire system. Cardiovasc Intervent Radiol 1995; 18:122–124.

8. Lenglinger FX, Schwarz CD, Artman W. Localization of pulmonary nodules before thoracoscopic surgery: value of percutaneous staining with methylene blue. AJR 1994; 163:297–300.

9. Wicky S, Mayor B, Cuttat JF, Schnyder P. CT-guided localizations of pulmonary nodules with methylene blue injections for thoracoscopic resections. Chest 1994; 106:1326–1328.

Endnotes

Figures 1–3 from Shah et al. Sem US CT MRI 1995; 16:5. Used with permission.

Figure 5 courtesy of Cook, Bloomington, IN.

TUTORIAL 16
PERCUTANEOUS DRAINAGE OF INTRATHORACIC FLUID COLLECTIONS

Jeffrey S. Klein, M.D., and
Scott Schultz, M.D.

Introduction

The subjects addressed in this tutorial include:

1. Indications for percutaneous drainage of intrathoracic fluid collections
2. Etiologies and types of intrathoracic fluid collections
3. General drainage techniques
4. Drainage of empyema
5. Drainage of malignant effusion
6. Drainage of hepatic hydrothorax
7. Drainage of lung abscess
8. Drainage of pericardial effusion.

The percutaneous drainage of intrathoracic fluid collections is an extension of similar techniques used to drain abdominal fluid collections and abscesses. The use of imaging guidance and smaller catheters has provided an efficacious alternative to the traditional surgical approaches, especially with empyemas. In many cases, percutaneous therapy can totally obviate the need for surgical intervention. In those cases where surgery is still required, initial percutaneous drainage may simplify and expedite the surgical approach.

The most common indication for drainage of intrathoracic fluid collections is treatment of an empyema or parapneumonic pleural effusion. Historically, an empyema has been described as a grossly purulent fluid collection in the pleural space. Currently, most individuals would extend that definition to include loculated pleural fluid that shows a positive Gram stain or grows pathogenic material on culture. If the aspirated fluid falls into any of these categories, percutaneous drainage should be pursued. Empyemas commonly develop as an extension of pneumonia. They may also occur secondary to recent surgery, or may be produced by super-infection of a prior hemo- or hydrothorax.

Although empyemas may develop in conjunction with pneumonia, a parapneumonic effusion is much more likely to develop. Up to 40% of patients with a community-acquired pneumonia may develop a parapneumonic effusion.[1] Although the vast majority of these parapneumonic effusions will resolve with only antibiotic therapy, a small percentage of them may progress to a chronic organized pleural fluid collection despite antibiotic therapy. These exudative parapneumonic effusions are characterized by a low pH (<7.20), elevated lactate dehydrogenase (>1000 IU/L), or low glucose (<40 mg/dL). Effusions demonstrating any of these characteristics should be considered for percutaneous drainage as they are unlikely to resolve with antibiotic therapy alone and may lead to chronic pleural abnormalities.

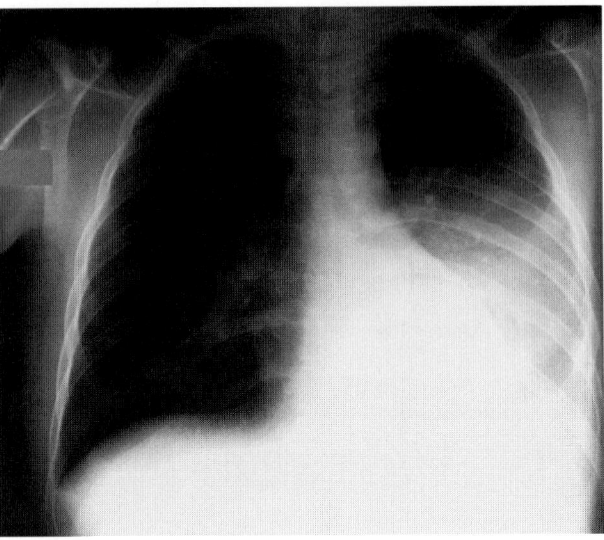

Figure 1. Posteroauterior (PA) chest radiograph shows opacity in the left lower lung field.

General Drainage Techniques

Seldinger or trocar technique can be utilized to insert a catheter into the fluid collection. Fluoroscopy or ultrasound (US) can be used for large collections. US is especially useful when portability is an issue. Computed tomography (CT) scanning can be utilized in those cases where an access route may be difficult or multiple catheters may be required. CT very readily distinguishes the pleural fluid from underlying pulmonary consolidation and can identify multiple loculated components which may not be appreciated as well with fluoroscopy or US.

The catheter size selected for insertion will vary depending on the character of the aspirated fluid. For relatively free-flowing, more serous fluid, 8–10-F catheters are adequate, while very thick, viscous fluid may require larger catheters up to 30 F in size. If possible, the catheter should be placed in the dependent portion of the cavity to optimize drainage. Once catheter drainage is minimal (less than 10 mL per day), and repeat imaging has confirmed resolution of the pleural fluid collection, the catheter can be removed. The presence of persistent pleural fluid may indicate undrained components or particularly thick, viscous material not amenable to drainage. In these situations, repeat imaging with manipulation of the pre-existing catheter or placement of additional catheters should be considered. The intracavitary administration of urokinase may facilitate breakdown of adhesions and septations and enhance the percutaneous drainage **(see Teaching File 31)**.

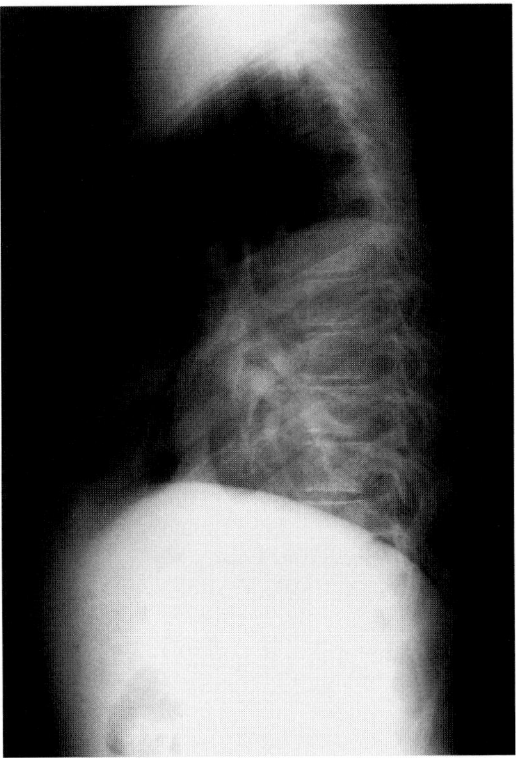

Figure 2. Same patient as in Figure 1. Lateral radiograph of the peripheral opacity has an appearance that could suggest either an empyema or a lung abscess.

CT-Guided Empyema Drainage

Imaging-guided percutaneous drainage is an accepted technique in the nonsurgical management of infected pleural fluid collections. The procedure is well tolerated and safe with a high success rate in patients with a relatively short duration of symptoms and exudative or early fibrinopurulent parapneumonic effusions.[2]

An example of a parapneumonic empyema amenable to percutaneous drainage is shown in **Figures 1–4**. A 30-year-old patient with a large left-sided pleural collection **(Figs. 1, 2)** has a lenticular fluid collection with enhancing pleural layers on contrast-enhanced CT scanning **(Fig. 3)**. A scan obtained after trocar placement of a 12-F drainage catheter **(Fig. 4)** shows complete evacuation of the collection.

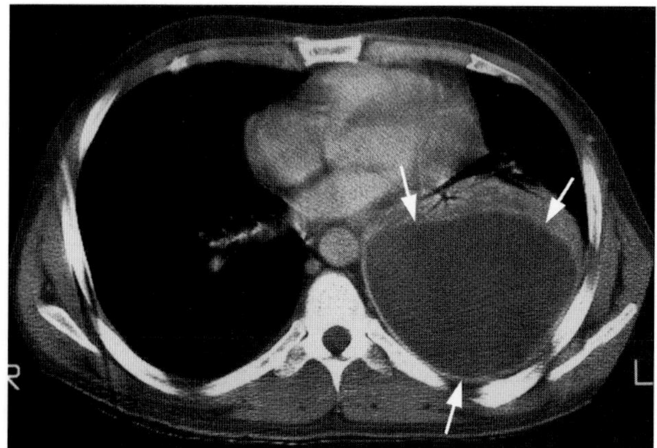

Figure 3. Same patient as in Figure 1. CT scan shows the split pleura sign (arrows) confirming a pleural fluid collection which is highly suggestive of an empyema.

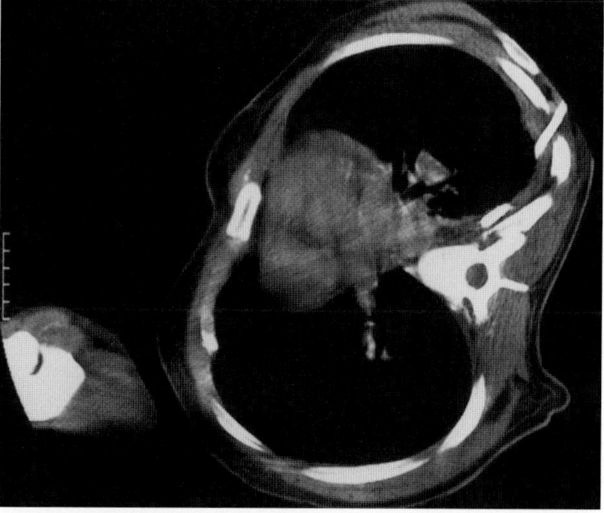

Figure 4. Same patient as in Figure 1. After catheter drainage, CT scan shows evacuation of the collection.

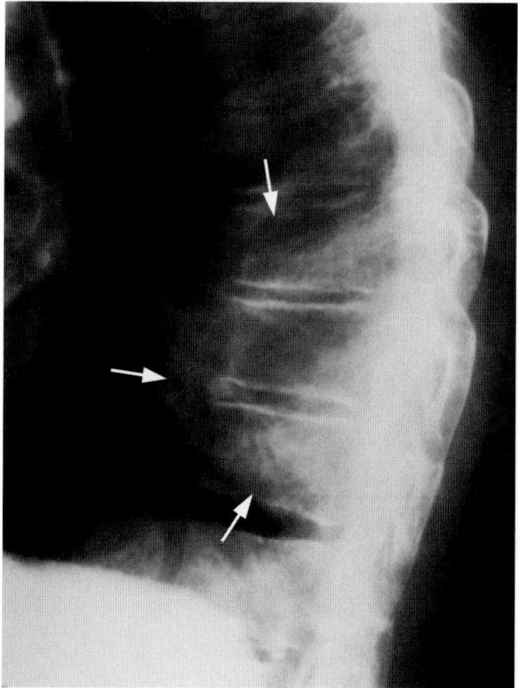

Figure 5. Lateral spot film shows a lenticular collection (arrows).

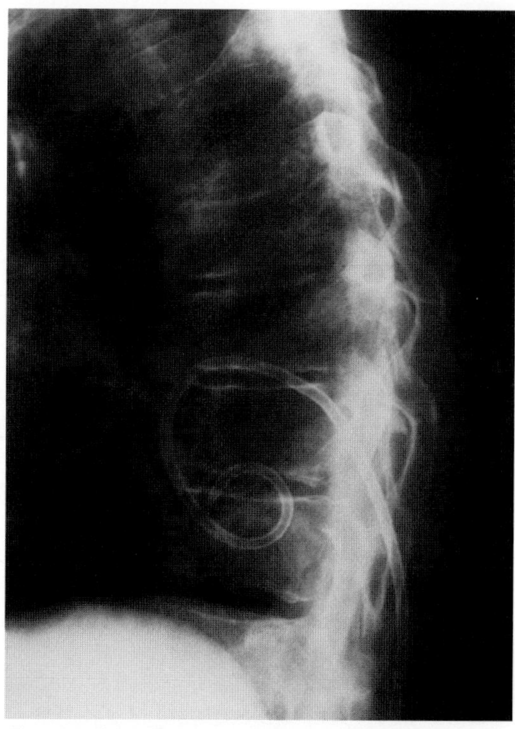

Figure 6. Same patient as in Figure 5. Spot film after placement of a drainage catheter into the collection.

Fluoroscopically Guided Empyema Drainage
Pleural fluid collections that have a large area of contact with the chest wall are easily drained under real-time fluoroscopic guidance. A lateral spot film **(Fig. 5)** obtained immediately prior to catheter placement shows a lenticular-shaped posterior collection with smooth margins and obtuse angles where it contacts the chest wall. After trocar placement of the pigtail drainage catheter and aspiration of 60 mL of pus, a repeat film **(Fig. 6)** shows the catheter tip in the inferior portion of the collapsed empyema cavity.

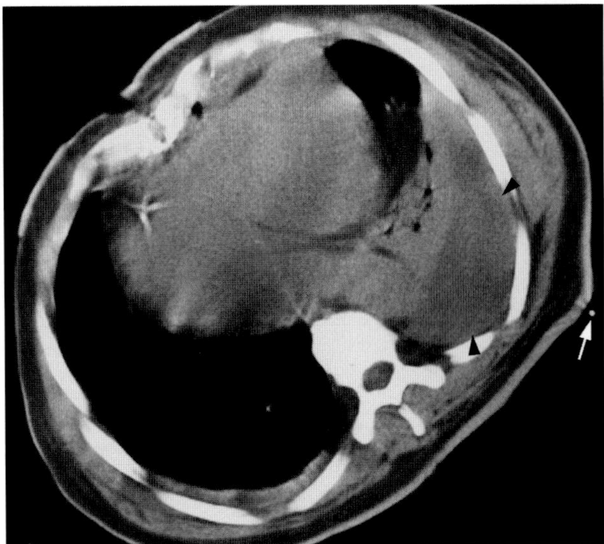

Figure 7. CT scan shows a left pleural fluid collection (arrowheads); a skin marker (arrow) has been placed to direct the puncture.

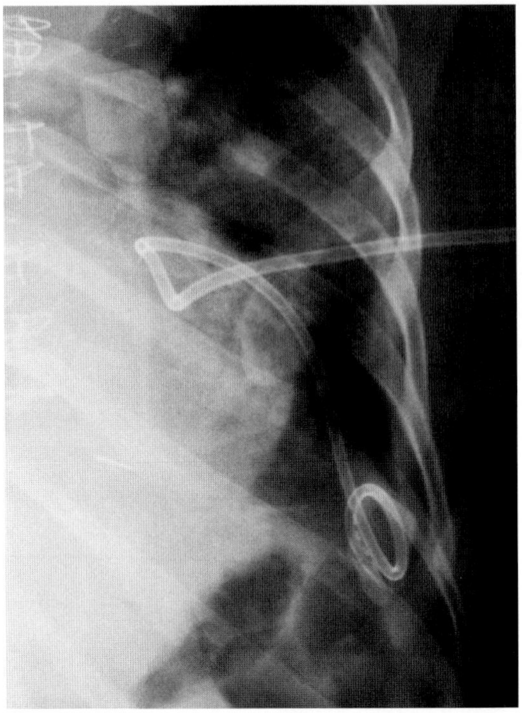

Figure 8. Same patient as in Figure 7. Spot radiograph after catheter placement demonstrates how fluoroscopy was able to direct catheter positioning into the dependent portion of the collection.

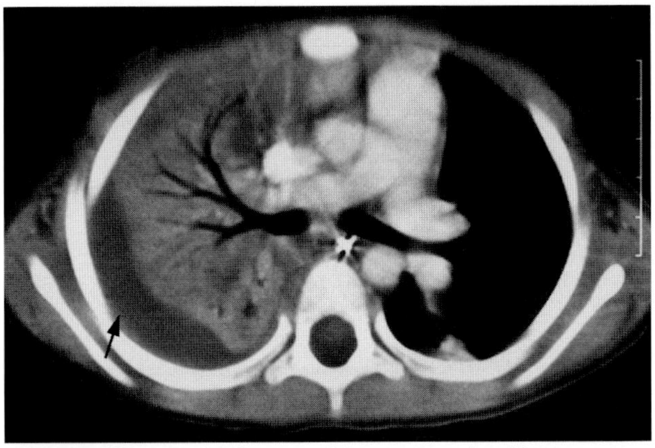

Figure 9. CT scan of right upper lobe pneumonia with an adjacent parapneumonic collection (arrow).

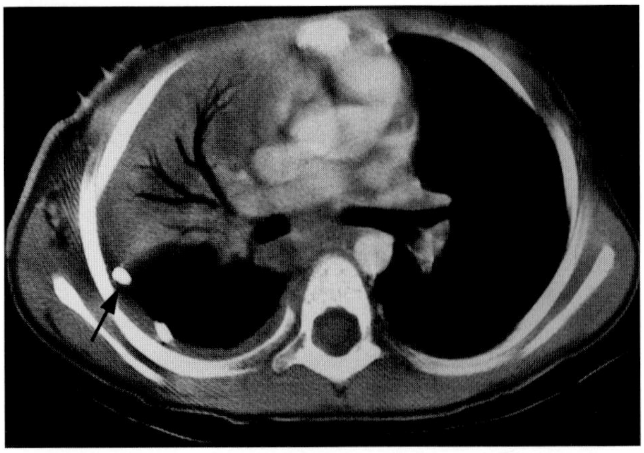

Figure 10. CT scan after drainage and urokinase administration over a 3-day period. Arrow shows the catheter location in the nearly resolved pleural collection with persistent pulmonary consolidation.

Combined CT-Fluoroscopic Drainage of Empyema

CT and fluoroscopy can play complementary roles in the drainage of infected pleural fluid collections. This combination is utilized when it is necessary to visualize the course of guide wires and catheters in real time, especially when a catheter is placed using a Seldinger technique. In a mechanically ventilated patient with a post-sternotomy Aspergillus empyema, a CT scan **(Fig. 7)** shows a left pleural effusion with the desired puncture site denoted by a skin marker. A spot film after fluoroscopic placement of a pigtail drainage catheter **(Fig. 8)** shows the catheter tip in a dependent position.

Empyema Drainage Using Intrapleural Urokinase

Percutaneous drainage of a parapneumonic effusion that has progressed to a fibrinopurulent or organized stage requires large drainage catheters and intrapleural fibrinolytic therapy in hopes of avoiding open surgical drainage.[3,4] In a child with a right upper lobe pneumococcal pneumonia, a CT scan **(Fig. 9)** following an unsuccessful diagnostic thoracentesis shows a parapneumonic effusion with a slightly convex contour towards the lung suggesting early loculation. Repeat CT scanning after pleural catheter placement and three daily instillations of 50,000 U urokinase **(Fig. 10)** shows near complete resolution of the effusion.

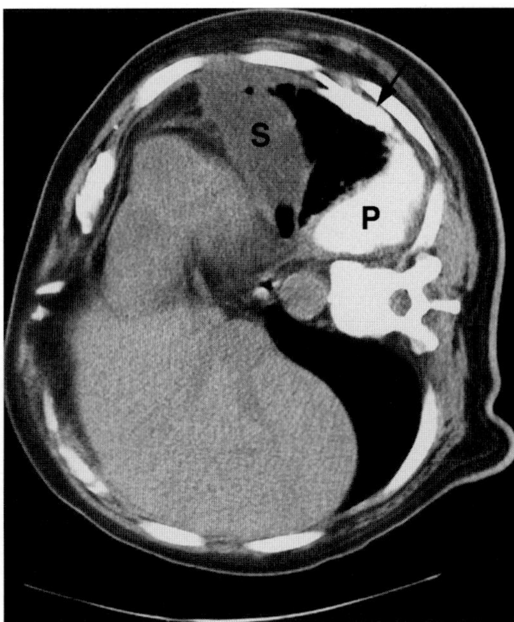

Figure 11. Injection of contrast material via the indwelling drainage tube (arrow) into a posterior locule (P) identifies an undrained second subpulmonic locule (S) that does not communicate with the first locule.

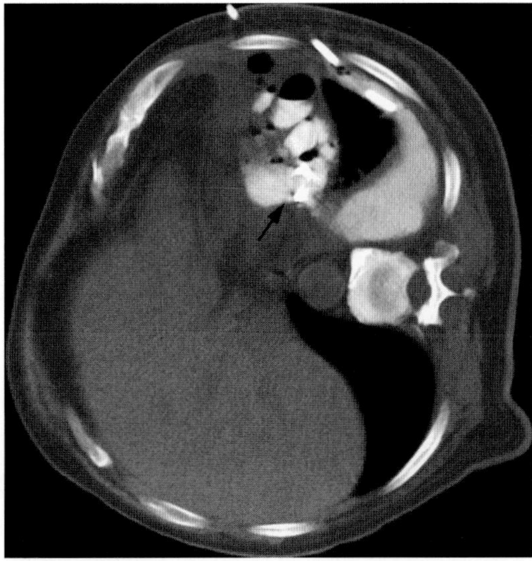

Figure 12. A second drainage catheter placed under CT guidance shows a multiseptated collection (arrow).

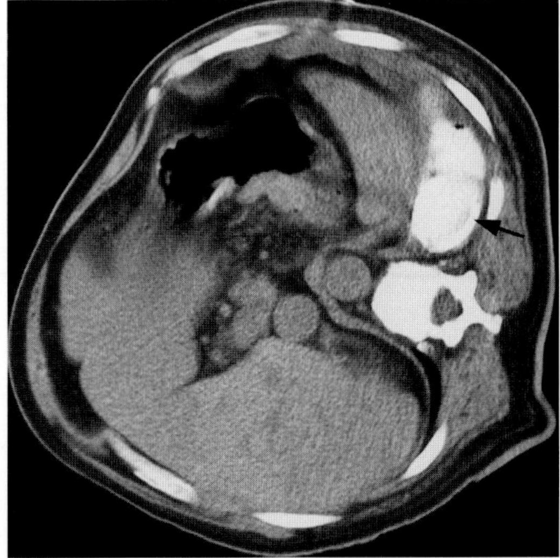

Figure 13. Replacement of the initial catheter over a wire into a more dependent part of the first collection (arrow).

Catheter Manipulation and Additional Catheter Placement For Failed Drainage

Techniques used to manage patients with failed catheter drainage of empyema include catheter exchange and manipulation, fibrinolytic therapy, and placement of additional catheters into undrained locules. In a patient with persistent fever following pleural drainage, a CT scan obtained in the right decubitus position following intrapleural contrast material injection via the indwelling catheter demonstrates inadequate drainage of the empyema with a single catheter **(Fig. 11)**. A second drainage catheter was then placed into the undrained locule with contrast material injection **(Fig. 12)**. Finally, the first catheter was exchanged over a guide wire for a new catheter **(Fig. 13)** placed dependently into the posterior collection. In any patient with persistent clinical symptoms and unresolved pleural fluid, repeat imaging with catheter manipulation or additional catheter placement should be performed to maximize drainage. Daily assessment of the catheter drainage and patient response should be done to ensure adequate response and to determine the need for additional interventions.

Failure to drain an infected pleural effusion adequately may result from 1) catheter occlusion, kinking, or malposition; 2) a thick or multiloculated collection not amenable to small-bore catheter drainage; or 3) the development of a fibrous pleural peel that precludes adequate lung re-expansion and obliteration of the pleural space. Following attempted fluoroscopic drainage of a parapneumonic empyema, no fluid returned from the drainage catheter despite apparent adequate positioning of the catheter **(Fig. 14)**. A CT scan **(Fig. 15)** showed the catheter tip in an extrathoracic position within the subscapular tissues. Only after all of these possibilities have been considered should the drainage be deemed a failure. If the fluid does not resolve despite adequate tube size, position, and patency, other options should be considered, including surgical intervention. Retrospective studies evaluating the success of percutaneous drainage procedures indicate that they are successful in 72%–88% of cases.[2,5,6] These rates are comparable to large-bore surgical thoracostomy tube drainage.

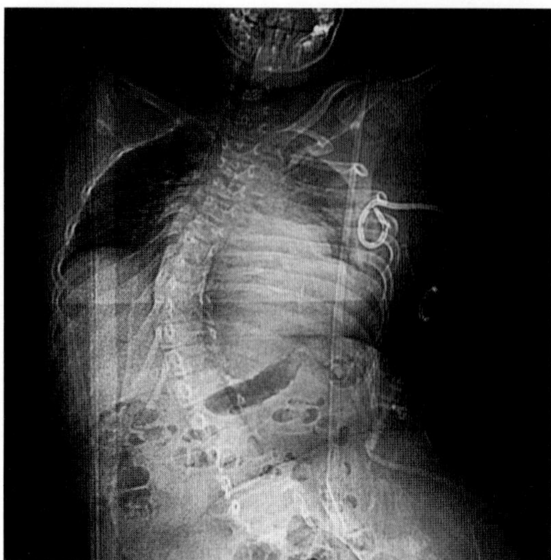

Figure 14. Scout view shows the catheter projecting over the left effusion.

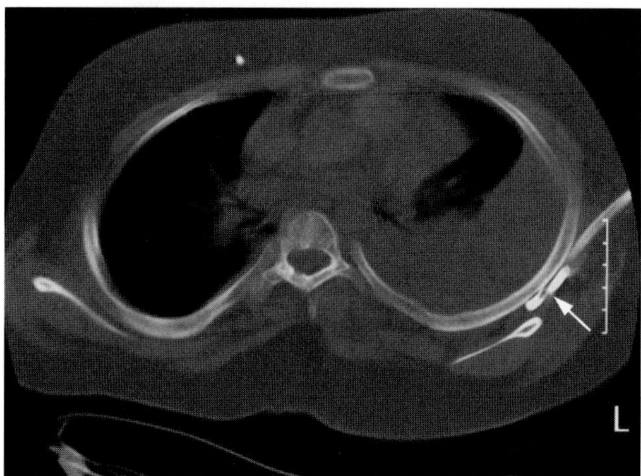

Figure 15. Same patient as in Figure 14. CT scan at the level of the pigtail catheter tip shows extrathoracic catheter location (arrow).

US-Guided Drainage of Malignant Pleural Effusion

In the patient with a malignant effusion, US-guided catheter drainage is a safe, well tolerated, and effective alternative to large-bore thoracostomy or open drainage.[7] Most malignant pleural effusions are due to pleural metastases from lung or breast carcinoma, or to lymphomatous involvement of the pleural space in patients with lymphoma. Patients with malignant pleural effusions can be quite symptomatic with shortness of breath and difficult respirations due to the compressive effects of the usually large pleural fluid collection on the adjacent pulmonary parenchyma. In addition, the pleural fluid may restrict diaphragmatic movements contributing to the shortness of breath and dyspnea. In these patients, evacuation of the pleural fluid may result in significant symptomatic relief. Because there is a very high recurrence rate with simple tube drainage, pleurodesis should be considered in those patients with a predicted life span greater than 1–2 months to prevent reaccumulation of the fluid which may require repeat drainage.

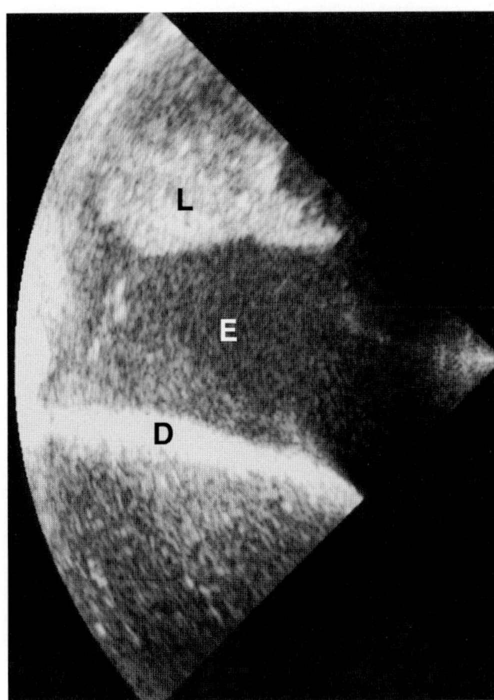

Figure 16. US shows a malignant pleural effusion (E), collapsed lung (L), and diaphragm (D). (The image has been rotated to mimic the sitting position).

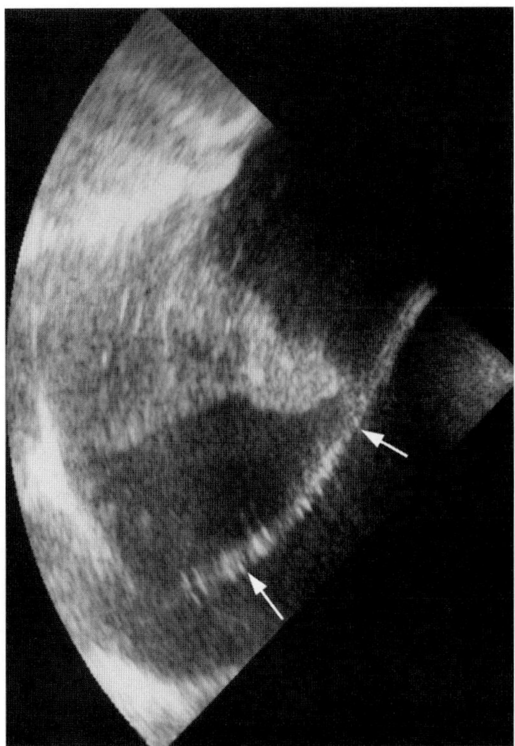

Figure 17. US image of dependent catheter placement (arrows).

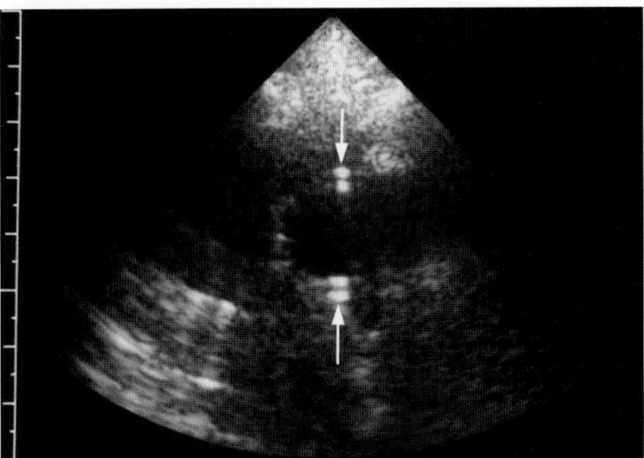

Figure 18. US-guided catheter placement in another patient with malignant effusion. Note the appearance of the pigtail catheter tip after catheter placement (arrows).

Because most of these pleural fluid collections are free-flowing, US guidance with the patient sitting upright allows for easy placement of the catheter into the dependent portion of the pleural space **(Fig. 16)**. With use of a freehand technique, the pigtail drainage catheter **(Fig. 17)** is placed into the pleural space under real-time visualization and advanced into a dependent position. In another patient undergoing US-guided drainage of a malignant effusion, the pigtail catheter tip **(Fig. 18)** is seen on US as a pair of opposing parallel echogenic lines which represent the walls of the hollow rounded catheter tip. The initial quantity of fluid removed should be limited to 1.5 L to avoid the possibility of pulmonary edema due to re-expansion.

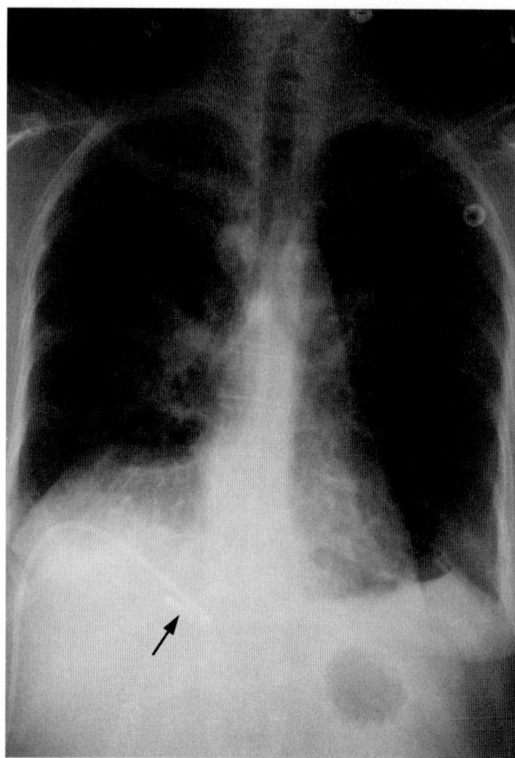

Figure 19. Radiograph after catheter placement shows the catheter (arrow) in the medial costophrenic sulcus in this patient with subpulmonic effusion and lymphangitic carcinomatosis.

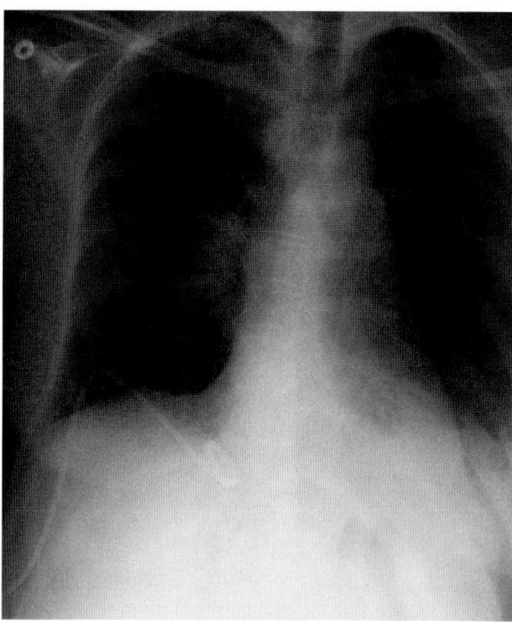

Figure 20. Film obtained after drainage shows resolution of the subpulmonic effusion.

Drainage and Sclerosis of Subpulmonic Malignant Effusion

In patients with recurrent malignant effusion and a life expectancy exceeding 1–2 months, transcatheter pleural sclerosis using doxycycline, bleomycin, or talc slurry is an effective palliative therapy to prevent fluid reaccumulation.[8] Effective sclerosis requires the coaptation of the visceral and parietal pleural layers. After the initial catheter placement, fluid output and chest radiographic findings should be monitored daily to confirm re-expansion of the lung and resolution of the pleural fluid. Once the output is less than 100 mL /day, sclerosis can be considered. This usually occurs within 5 days of catheter placement.[9] In a patient with a right subpulmonic malignant effusion and lymphangitic carcinomatosis from ovarian carcinoma **(Fig. 19)**, a pigtail drainage catheter is seen in a dependent position. After catheter output has decreased to <100 mL/day and the subpulmonic effusion has resolved radiographically **(Fig. 20)**, the pleural space is sclerosed with doxycycline. The exact sclerosant chosen will vary depending on availability and operator preference but talc appears to be the agent of choice.[10]

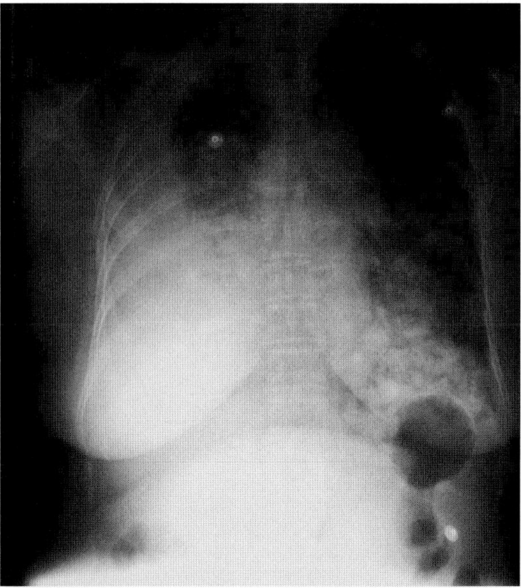

Figure 21. Chest film shows lung metastases and a large right effusion resulting in dyspnea. Catheter drainage was requested to palliate the patient's symptoms.

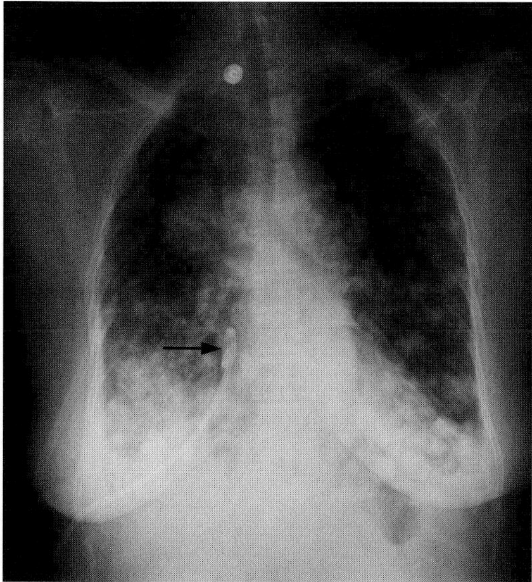

Figure 22. Follow-up PA chest film shows a right pleural catheter (arrow) with diminished effusion, but the catheter tip projects anterior and superior to the remaining effusion.

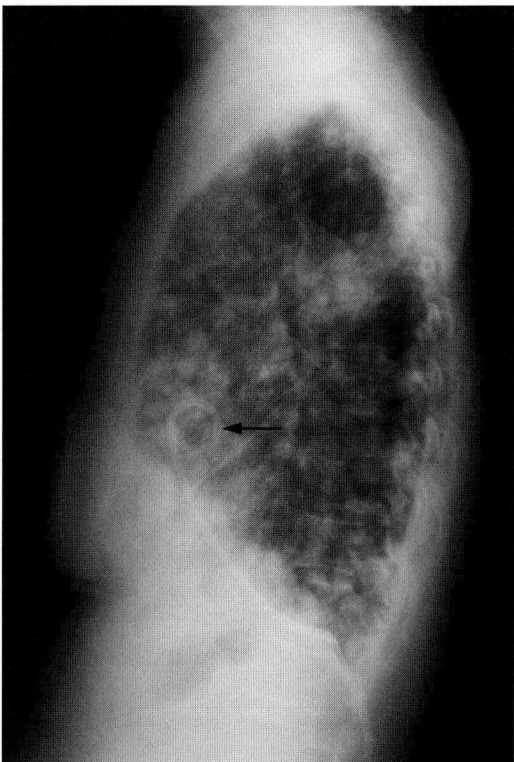

Figure 23. Lateral chest film confirms the location of the drainage catheter (arrow) above the remaining fluid. The catheter in this position will not evacuate the residual fluid and pleurodesis will be suboptimal.

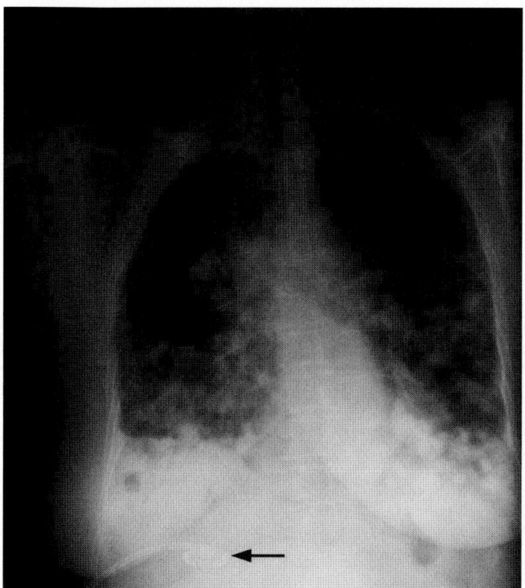

Figure 24. Catheter (arrow) repositioned into a more dependent portion of the effusion with improved drainage.

Repositioning of Pleural Catheter to Enhance Malignant Effusion Drainage

US-guided malignant effusion drainage and sclerosis is approximately 70%–92% effective in the management of malignant effusions. Successful therapy requires a patent catheter which is positioned dependently in the pleural space to evacuate the pleural space completely. Residual fluid may dilute the sclerosant and result in inadequate pleurodesis. Occasionally, a catheter placed into a large effusion **(Fig. 21)** requires repositioning as fluid is drained and the drainage catheter tip is suboptimally positioned anteriorly or in the oblique fissure **(Figs. 22, 23)**. After repositioning the catheter fluoroscopically with use of a tip-deflecting guide wire **(Fig. 24)**, the catheter is positioned dependently to enhance further drainage.

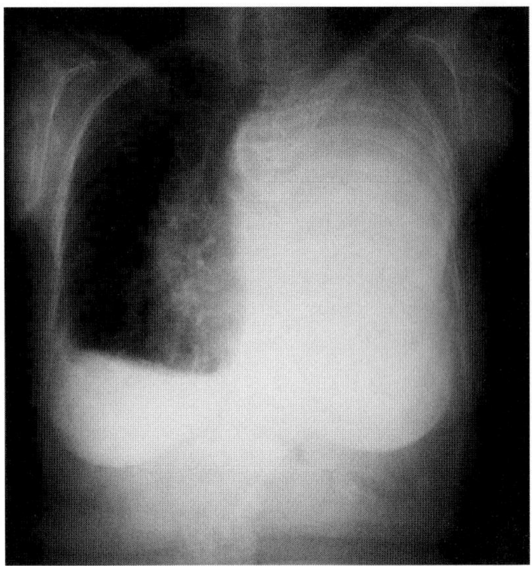

Figure 25. Chest radiograph of an opacified left hemithorax due to malignant effusion.

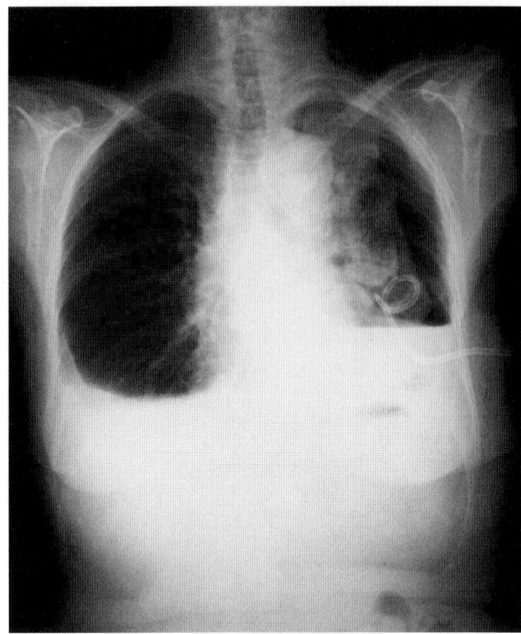

Figure 26. Film after catheter placement shows persistent hydropneumothorax and lung collapse despite –30-cm H_2O suction.

Failed Malignant Effusion Drainage Due to Pleural Peel

Unsuccessful malignant pleural effusion drainage can result from 1) tube or catheter malfunction or misplacement; 2) inability to evacuate complex (ie, multiloculated) malignant effusion; or 3) inability of the underlying lung to re-expand due to endobronchial obstruction, lymphangitic carcinomatosis, or a thick pleural peel.[11] In a patient with bronchogenic carcinoma and a large malignant left effusion from pleural tumor infiltration **(Fig. 25)**, catheter drainage results in a large left hydropneumothorax **(Fig. 26)** from incomplete lung re-expansion due to a thick visceral pleural peel. The hydropneumothorax persisted despite prolonged drainage with –30-cm H_2O suction applied to the drainage catheter. Because of the inability to fully re-expand the lung, sclerosis cannot be performed. Pneumothoraces may be seen in about one third of patients undergoing tube drainage for malignant effusions and is usually due to the inability of the noncompliant lung to re-expand.[12] With prolonged tube drainage and suction, 80% of cases will eventually re-expand and sclerosis can be carried out. In the remaining 20%, the lung never re-expands; these patients are not candidates for sclerosis. Despite the large pneumothoraces, the drainage catheter can be safely removed without inducing an enlarging or tension pneumothorax. Since the fluid will re-accumulate, it may be reasonable to leave a tube in place and allow periodic drainage if the fluid recurs very rapidly. Despite these shortcomings, small-bore tube drainage and subsequent pleurodesis should be considered in patients with malignant pleural effusions.

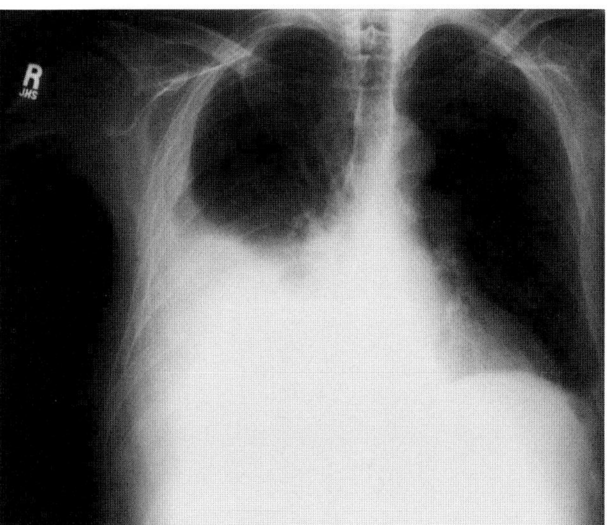

Figure 27. Chest film of a large right effusion due to hepatic hydrothorax.

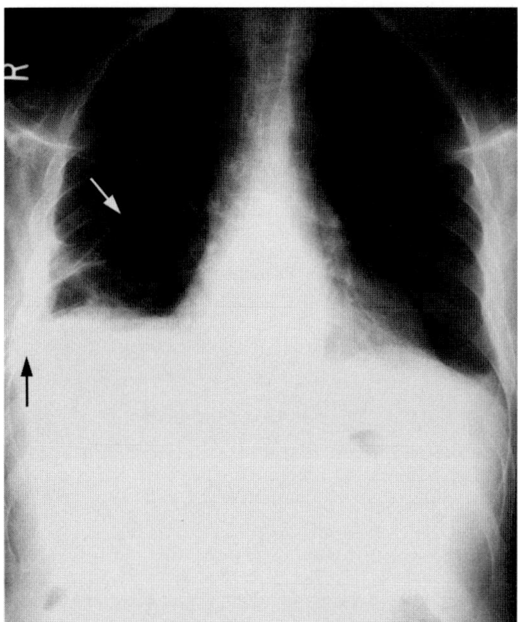

Figure 28. Same patient as in Figure 27. After placement of two large-bore drainage tubes in the right pleural space (arrows), decreased effusion is seen.

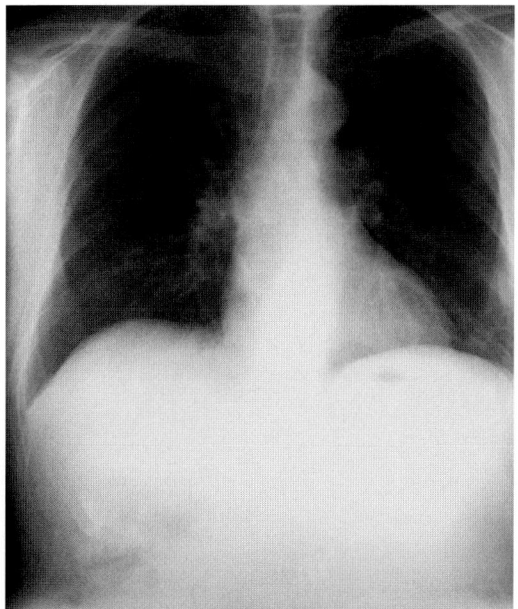
Figure 29. Same patient as in Figure 27. Chest film 4 months after sclerosis shows resolution of the right effusion.

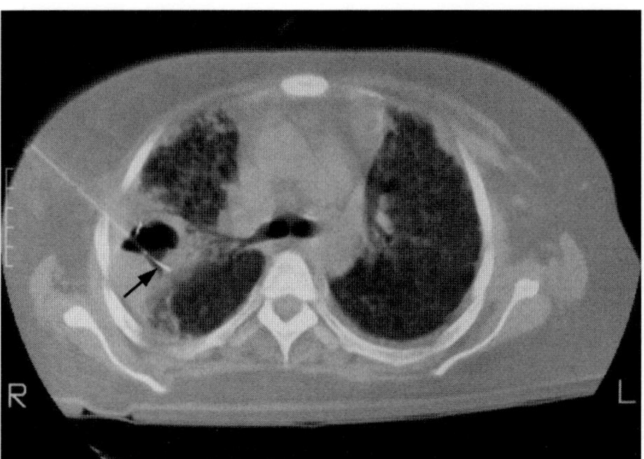

Figure 30. CT scan shows the needle and wire (arrow) in the lung absess.

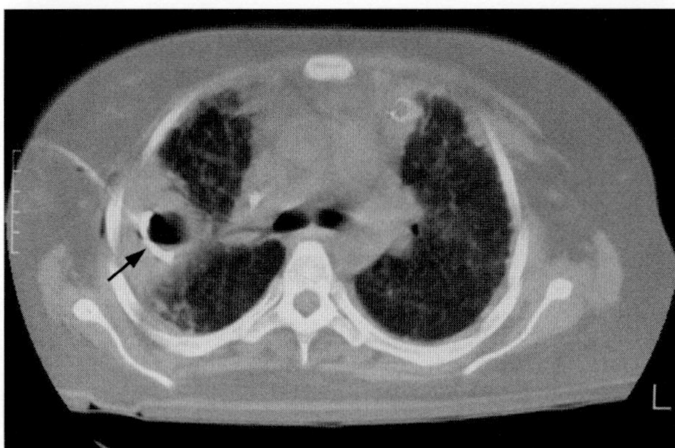

Figure 31. CT scan with the catheter in a dependent part of the abscess (arrow).

Percutaneous Drainage and Sclerosis of Hepatic Hydrothorax

Transdiaphragmatic extension of peritoneal or hepatic fluid complicating liver failure can produce an intractable right pleural effusion **(Fig. 27)**. Percutaneous drainage and sclerosis using small-diameter catheters or larger bore thoracostomy-type tubes (Thal-Quik, Cook, Inc.) **(Fig. 28)** can be used for evacuation of fluid and subsequent sclerotherapy to prevent fluid reaccumulation **(Fig. 29)**. Alternative treatment options include diuresis and protein repletion, peritoneojugular (LeVeen) shunt, and thoracoscopic or open surgical closure of peritoneal/right pleural fenestrations.[13] Transjugular intrahepatic portosystemic shunts (TIPS) have been shown to be effective in treating ascites and hepatic hydrothorax and should be considered initially, especially in those patients in whom sclerosis has already failed.[14,15]

CT-Guided Lung Abscess Drainage

For lung abscesses that fail to resolve with postural drainage and intravenous antibiotic therapy, percutaneous drainage using cross-sectional imaging guidance results in rapid clinical improvement with surgery avoided in up to 85% of patients.[16] Conservative measures will allow cure of the abscess in 80%–90% of cases[17] but when patients show no clinical or radiographic improvement or develop complications such as hemoptysis or bronchopleural fistula, drainage of the lung abscess should be considered. If an approach that avoids aerated lung is available, imaging-guided drainage offers numerous advantages when compared to surgical drainage or resection. With use of a Seldinger technique under CT guidance **(Fig. 30)**, a skinny needle is placed into the abscess an 0.018-inch guide wire is placed into the cavity. After dilation of the track, the catheter is placed **(Fig. 31)** with the pigtail drainage tip positioned dependently to promote drainage.

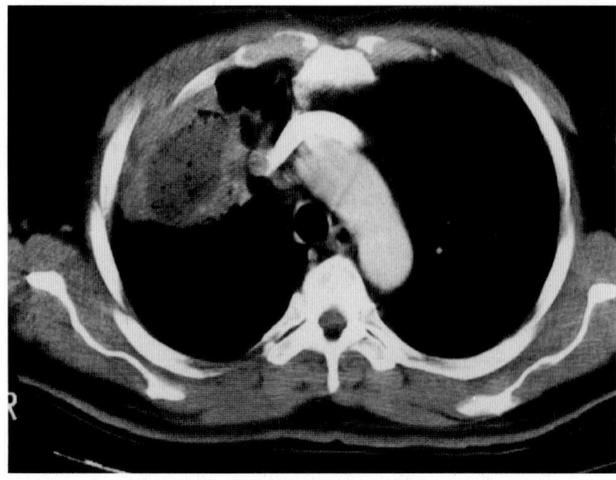

Figure 32. Intraparenchymal pulmonary abscess with a broad base of contact with the pleural surface and no intervening aerated lung between the puncture site and the abscess.

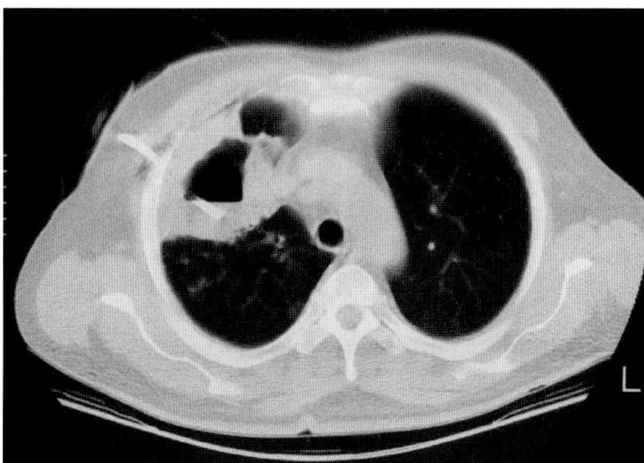

Figure 33. Same patient as in Figure 32. CT scan shows the catheter traversing the abscess/pleura interface.

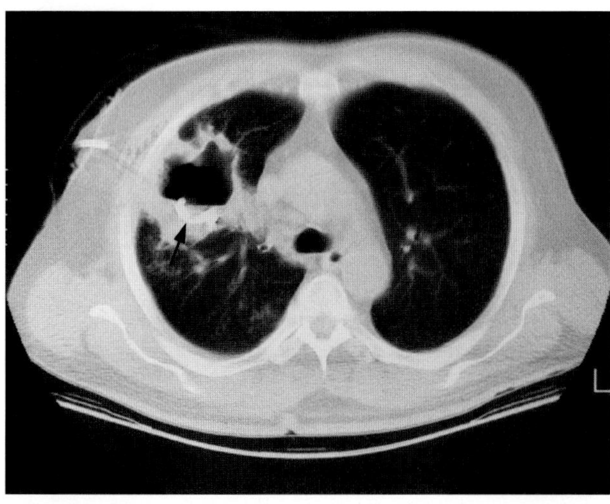

Figure 34. CT scan shows the catheter tip in the dependent part of the abscess cavity (arrow).

Trocar Drainage of Lung Abscess

CT-guided drainage of lung abscess using a trocar technique is best performed when a peripheral abscess **(Fig. 32)** contacts the chest wall, allowing for safe transpleural catheter placement.[18] Traversing intervening normal lung with the drainage catheter is associated with an increased incidence of complications including bleeding and bronchopleural fistula formation. After positioning of the patient to provide access to the collection while simultaneously avoiding dependent positioning of the normal lung, the chest wall and pleura are punctured with the inner trocar stylet and the catheter is advanced into the abscess **(Fig. 33)**. Once the stylet is removed and purulent fluid aspirated, the catheter is advanced and the pigtail tip placed dependently **(Fig. 34)**.

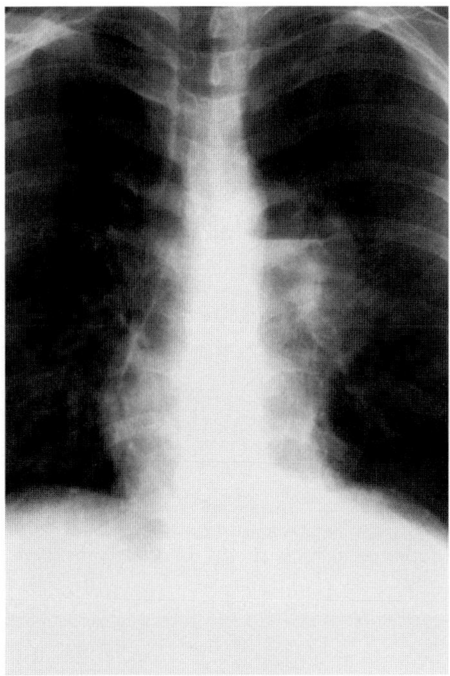

Figure 35. Frontal radiograph of a left paramediastinal lung abscess.

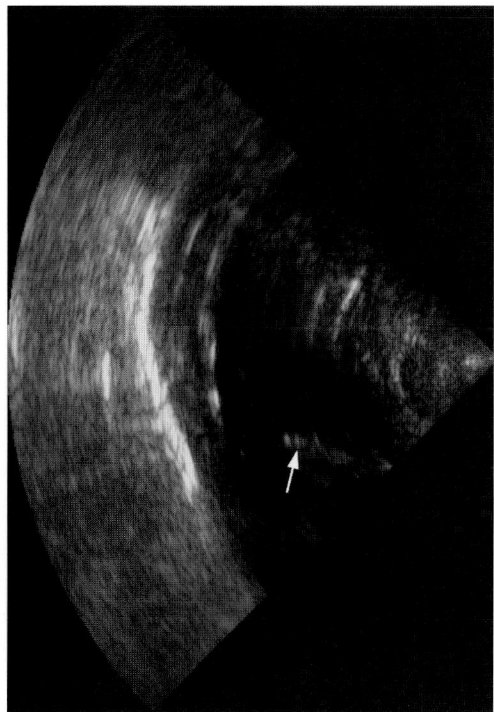

Figure 36. Same patient as in Figure 35. US shows the catheter in the abscess cavity (arrow).

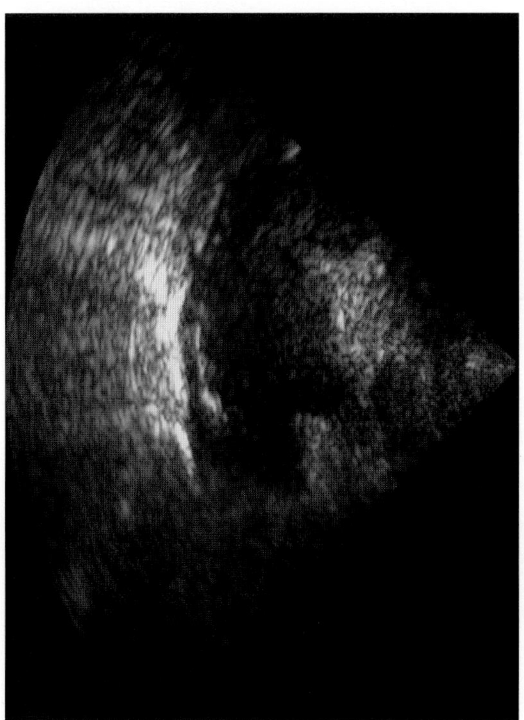

Figure 37. Same patient as in Figure 35. Follow-up US shows a decrease in the size of the abscess cavity.

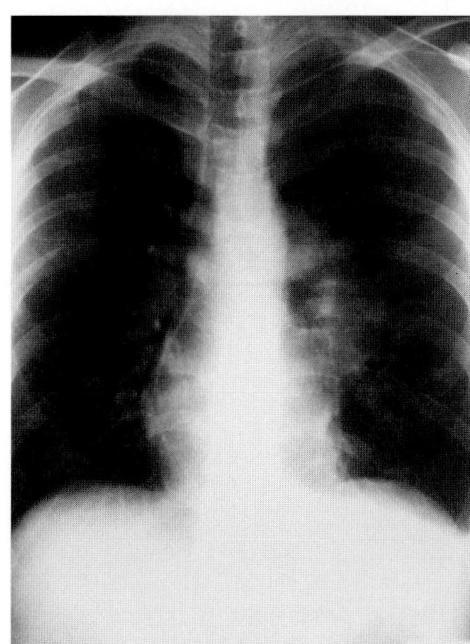

Figure 38. Same patient as in Figure 35. Frontal radiograph following abscess drainage demonstrates resolution of the paramediastinal lung abscess.

US-Guided Lung Abscess Aspiration and Drainage

Parenchymal collections with a large region of contact with the chest wall can be accessed using US guidance.[19] In a patient with a left paramediastinal lung abscess **(Fig. 35)**, real-time US-guided catheter placement **(Fig. 36)** is performed using a freehand technique. Purulent fluid is then aspirated, resulting in a decrease in the size of the abscess cavity as seen on US **(Fig. 37)** and postprocedure chest radiograph **(Fig. 38)**.

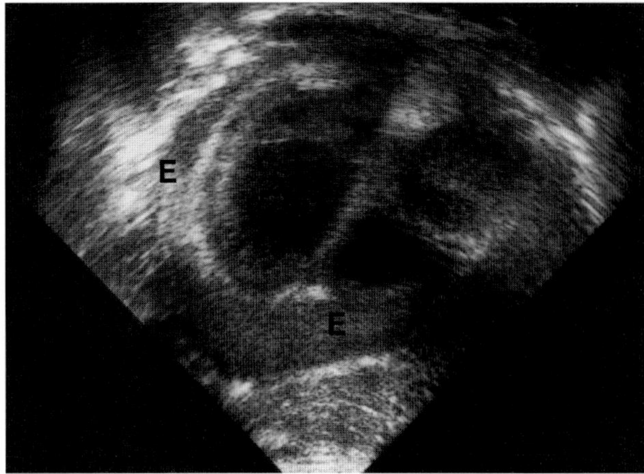

Figure 39. Transthoracic US of a large echogenic pericardial effusion (E).

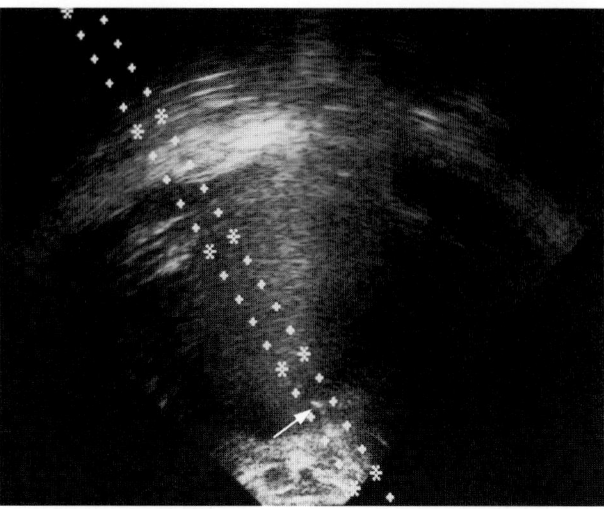

Figure 40. US during guided needle placement shows the sheathed needle (arrow) entering an echogenic collection inferior to the heart.

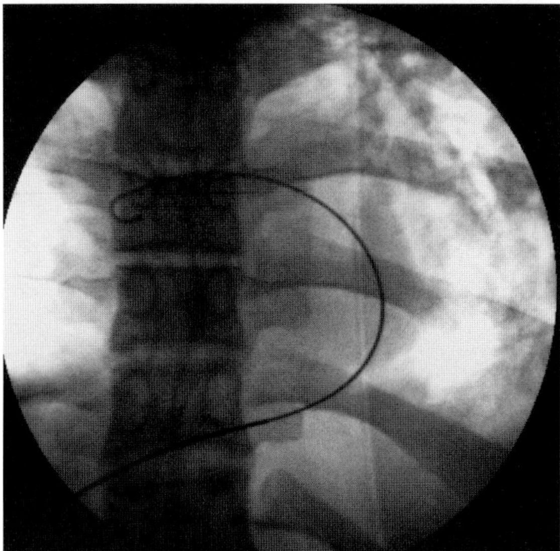

Figure 41. Fluoroscopic image of the wire placed through the sheath and coiled in the pericardial space.

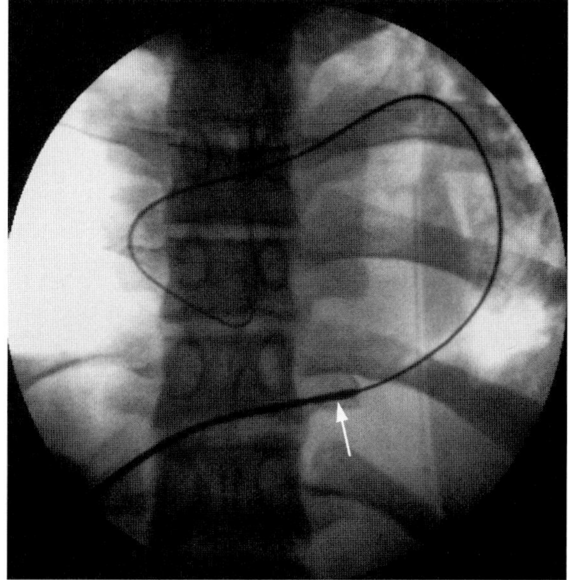

Figure 42. Fluoroscopic image of a dilator (arrow) advanced over the wire.

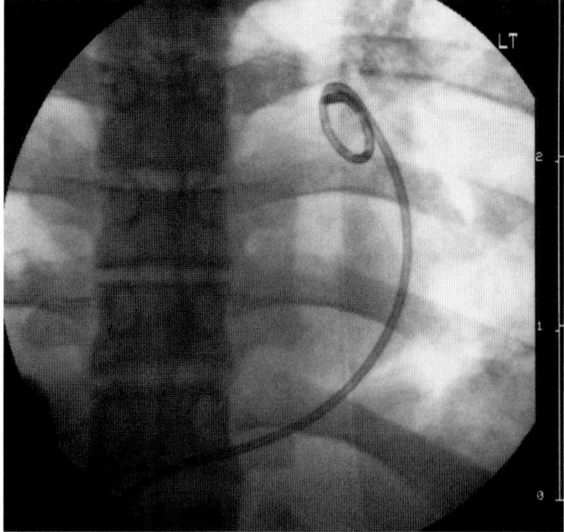

Figure 43. Final catheter position. 50 mL of purulent material was withdrawn.

Pericardial Effusion Drainage

Pericardial fluid drainage may be performed for pericardial tamponade or infectious pericarditis. A combined approach using US for puncture and fluoroscopy during track dilation and catheter placement can be safely utilized.[20] In a patient with an echogenic pericardial effusion due to pneumococcal pericarditis **(Fig. 39)**, a sheathed needle **(Fig. 40)** is placed inferior to the heart into the collection. Once the inner trocar is removed and fluid aspirated, a floppy guide wire **(Fig. 41)** is placed through the sheath into the pericardial space. The sheath is then removed and the track is dilated **(Fig. 42)** to accept the drainage catheter, which is advanced over the wire and left coiled in the pericardial space **(Fig. 43)**.

References

1. Light RW. Parapneumonic effusions and empyema. Clin Chest Med 1985; 6:55–62.

2. Silverman SG, Mueller PR, Saini S, et al. Thoracic empyema: management with image-guided catheter drainage. Radiology 1988; 169:5–9.

3. Moulton JS, Moore PT, Mencini RA. Treatment of loculated pleural effusions with transcatheter intracavitary urokinase. AJR 1989; 153:941–945.

4. Robinson LA, Moulton AL, Fleming WH, Alonso A, Galbraith TA. Intrapleural fibrinolytic treatment of multiloculated thoracic empyemas. Ann Thorac Surg 1994; 57:803–814.

5. O'Moore PV, Mueller PR, Simeone JF, et al. Sonographic guidance in diagnostic and therapeutic interventions in the pleural space. AJR 1987; 149:1–5.

6. Merriam MA, Cronan JJ, Dorfman GS, Lambiase RE, Haas RA. Radiographically guided percutaneous catheter drainage of pleural fluid collections. AJR 1988; 151:1113–1116.

7. Morrison MC, Mueller PR, Lee MJ, et al. Sclerotherapy of malignant pleural effusions through sonographically placed small-bore catheters. AJR 1992; 158:41–43.

8. Patz EF Jr, McAdams HP, Goodman PC, Blackwell S, Crawford J. Ambulatory sclerotherapy for malignant pleural effusions. Radiology 1996; 199:133–135.

9. Parker LA, Charnock GC, Delany DJ. Small bore catheter drainage and sclerotherapy for malignant pleural effusions. Cancer 1989; 64:1218–1221.

10. Hartman DL, Gaither JM, Kesler KA, Mylet DM, Brown JW, Mathur PN. Comparison of insufflated talc under thoracoscopic guidance with standard tetracycline and bleomycin pleurodesis for control of malignant pleural effusions. J Thorac Cardiovasc Surg 1993; 105:743–748.

11. Hausheer FH, Yarbro JW. Diagnosis and treatment of malignant pleural effusion. Semin Oncol 1985; 12:54–75.

12. Chang YC, Patz EF Jr, Goodman PC. Pneumothorax after small-bore catheter placement for malignant pleural effusions. AJR 1996; 166:1049–1051.

13. Mouroux J, Perrin C, Venissac N, Blaive B, Richelme H. Management of pleural effusion of cirrhotic origin. Chest 1996; 109:1093–1096.

14. Andrade RJ, Martin-Palanca A, Fraile JM, et al. Transjugular intrahepatic portosystemic shunt for the management of hepatic hydrothorax in the absence of ascites. J Clin Gastroenterol 1996; 22:305–307.

15. Kerlan RK Jr, LaBerge JM, Gordon RL, Ring EJ. Transjugular intrahepatic portosystemic shunts: current status. AJR 1995; 164:1059–1066.

16. vanSonnenberg E, D'Agostino HB, Casola G, Halasz NA, Sanchez RB, Goodacre BW. Percutaneous abscess drainage: current concepts. Radiology 1991; 181:617–626.

17. Yellin A, Yellin EO, Lieberman Y. Percutaneous tube drainage: the treatment of choice for refractory lung abscess. Ann Thorac Surg 1985; 39:266–270.

18. vanSonnenberg E, D'Agostino HB, Casola G, Wittich GR, Varney RR, Harker C. Lung abscess: CT-guided drainage. Radiology 1991; 178:347–351.

19. Yang PC, Luh KT, Lee YC, et al. Lung abscesses: US examination and US-guided transthoracic aspiration. Radiology 1991; 180:171–175.

20. Mostbeck GH, Korn M, Wittich GR, et al. The percutaneous ultrasonic-guided fluoroscopy-controlled drainage of pericardial fluids. Rofo Fortschr Geb Rontgenstr Neuen Bildgeb Verfahr 1991; 155:53–57.

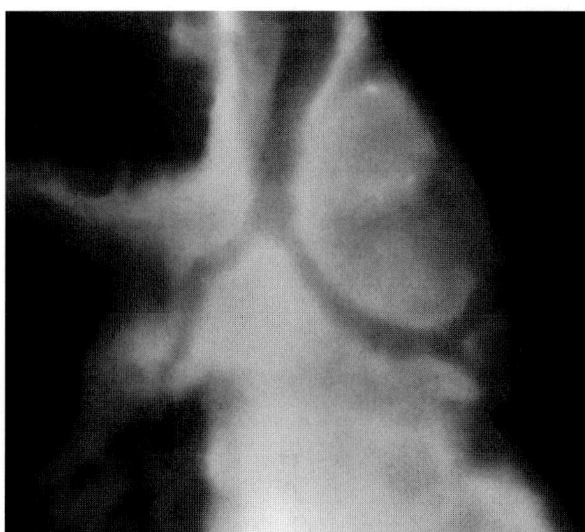

Figure 1. Tomogram demonstrates compression of the right upper lobe bronchus by bronchogenic carcinoma.

TUTORIAL 17
TRACHEAL AND ESOPHAGEAL STENT PLACEMENT

Robert D. Bloch, Ph.D., M.D.,
Bryan Peterson, M.D., and
Richard R. Saxon, M.D.

Introduction

The subjects addressed in this tutorial include:
1. Clinical presentation of patients with stenosis of the tracheobronchial tree
2. Stents
3. Technique of stent placement
4. Treatment of benign strictures
5. Results of stent placement for benign strictures
6. Treatment of malignant tracheobronchial strictures
7. Results of stent placement for malignant tracheobronchial obstructions
8. Malignant esophageal disease
9. Assessment of patients with esophageal obstruction or esophagorespiratory fistula
10. Therapeutic options for malignant esophageal disease
11. Materials
12. Patient selection
13. Techniques
14. Results
15. Clinical follow-up
16. Complications.

This tutorial discusses metallic stent placement as a treatment for obstructive disease of the tracheobronchial tree and esophagus. In many cases, stent placement is intended to palliate malignant and often terminal conditions. Noncovered or "bare" stents are used for benign stenosis and malignant compression of the trachea. When significant endoluminal tumor is present, covered stents may be used in the airway. Esophageal stent placement is generally performed for malignant disease, and both noncovered and covered stents are used.

Clinical Presentation and Assessment of Patients

Obstruction of the large airways by benign or malignant processes is associated with high morbidity and the risk of early death by gradual asphyxia. Patients commonly present with dyspnea, stridor, and recurrent infections. Benign tracheobronchial strictures are most often related to previous surgery (tracheostomy, anastomosis) or trauma. Other benign causes of obstruction include sarcoidosis, tuberculosis, vascular rings, and tracheobronchomalacia. Malignant obstructions may be extrinsic (compression, encasement) or intrinsic (endoluminal) in nature. While bronchoscopy, computed tomography (CT) scanning,[1] or conventional tomography can be useful in evaluating these lesions, most are initially diagnosed by chest radiography **(Fig. 1)**.

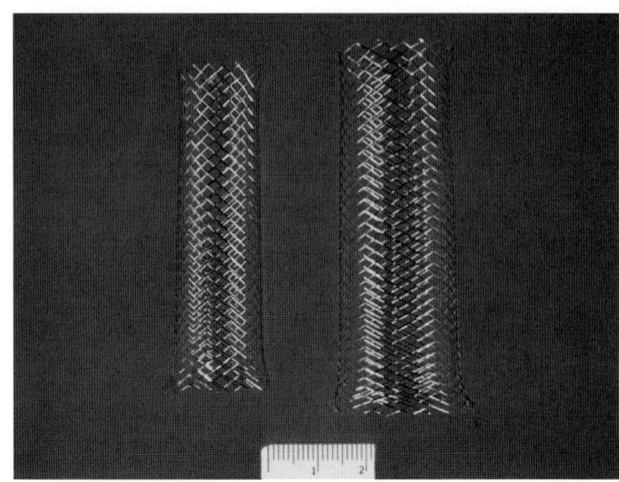

Figure 2. Wallstent for tracheal stent placement.

Materials

Stents may be placed through a rigid bronchoscope or an endotracheal tube. In the United States, the Gianturco-Rösch Z-stent (GRZ stent) (Cook, Bloomington, IN) and the Wallstent (Schneider, Minneapolis, MN) are currently the only devices approved by the Food and Drug Administration for tracheobronchial stent placement.[2–8] Other stents such as the Palmaz balloon expandable stent (Johnson & Johnson Interventional Systems, Warren, NJ), the self-expanding Strecker stent (Boston Scientific Corporation, Denmark), and Memotherm Nitinol stents (Angiomed, Karlsruhe, Germany) have been used in tracheobronchial strictures, particularly in Europe.[9]

Wallstent

The Wallstent device is composed of 20 surgical steel monofilaments 100 microns in diameter woven into a cylindrical tube **(Fig. 2)**. Stents range in size from 5 mm to 24 mm in diameter, and from 2 to 9 cm in length. Because the device is stretched longitudinally by the delivery system, it shrinks in length on deployment. The Wallstent delivery sheath is 7–9 F, depending on the stent diameter. The low radiopacity and shortening of the stent at deployment can make precise placement difficult. However, the Wallstent is very flexible, so it can conform to the curves of the airway. It has a tight lattice or weave, which may be an advantage in the treatment of malignant lesions, but it also has the potential to cause obstruction when it is placed over branching orifices of the airways.

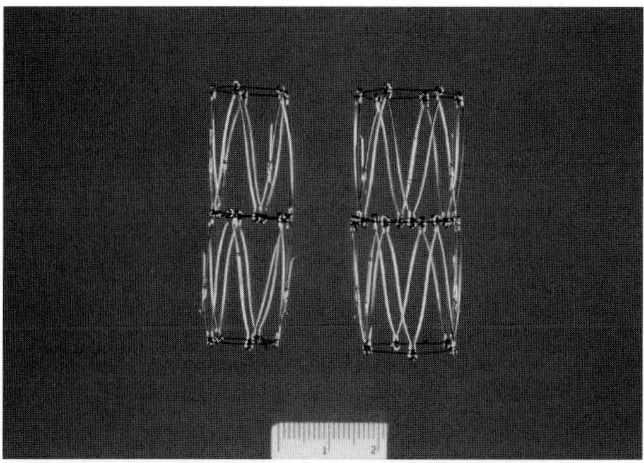

Figure 3. Gianturco-Rösch Z-stent, double-body type.

Gianturco-Rösch Z-Stent

The GRZ stent is constructed of 0.018-inch stainless steel wire in a double zigzag configuration. It is constrained to a given diameter by surgical nylon suture **(Fig. 3)**. Tracheobronchial Z-stents are available in a two-bodied stent configuration in diameters of 15–30 mm and lengths of 5 cm. Delivery sheaths range in size from 14 to 16 F. The GRZ stent is more rigid than the Wallstent, providing greater annular support; however, the stent can tolerate only slight curves. The GRZ stent is highly radiopaque, and does not change perceptively in length during deployment, allowing for precise placement.

Technique

Tracheobronchial stent placement is performed in the angiography suite with the patient under general anesthesia or deep sedation. Stents are most easily placed through an endotracheal tube with the patient in suspended respiration, or through a rigid bronchoscope or tracheostomy site. The airway is generally well visualized fluoroscopically and the stent can be delivered directly under fluoroscopic guidance without the use of endoscopy or skin markers. If the stenosis is difficult to see, the tracheobronchial tree may be opacified with Lipiodol (Laboratoire Guerbet, Aulnay-sous-Bois, France).[10]

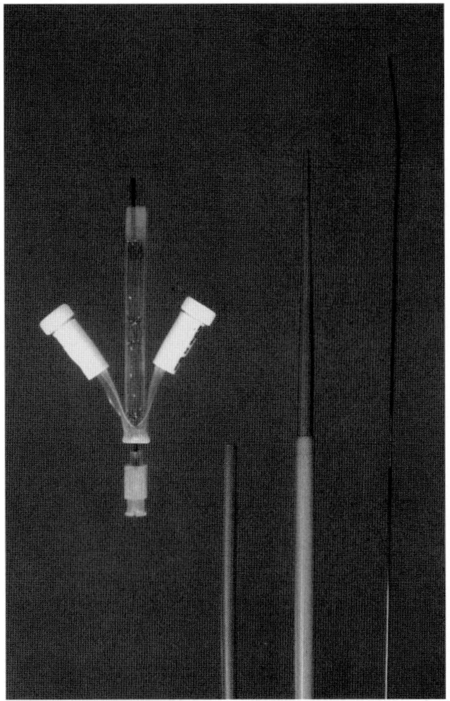

Figure 4. Equipment used to deploy tracheobronchial GRZ stents. From left to right: double-body GRZ stent collapsed inside the peel-away introducer; blunt end pusher; 14-F sheath and introducer; 0.038-inch Amplatz Super Stiff wire.

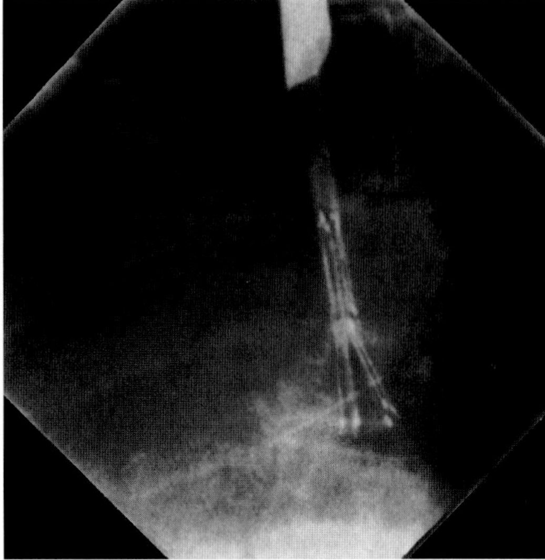

Figure 5. Endoscopic placement of a tracheal GRZ stent. The sheath is positioned across the lesion through a rigid endoscope. The stent is advanced through the sheath, and sheath and stent are positioned across the lesion and deployed with an unsheathing motion. A partially deployed stent is shown.

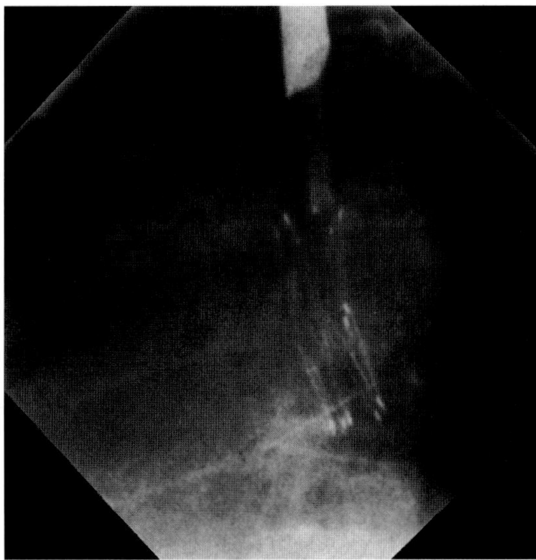

Figure 6. Final image after deployment of the tracheal GRZ stent demonstrates the deployed stent and the sheath inside the bronchoscope, above the stent.

Stent Delivery

The GRZ stent and the Wallstent are self-expanding and are deployed with an unsheathing motion. Equipment for deploying the GRZ stent is shown in **Figure 4**. The GRZ stent quickly expands to its full diameter **(Figs. 5, 6)**, and balloon dilation is required only for unusually tight or resistive lesions. Even tough, fibrotic lesions not amenable to balloon dilation will respond to the gradual outward force of the self-expanding stent **(Fig. 7)**. The Wallstent usually requires balloon dilation to reach its full outer diameter in the tracheobronchial tree. All stents initiate a mild foreign body sensation after placement which gradually resolves after several days. Patients should receive broad spectrum antibiotics before stent placement and should continue them for several days afterward.

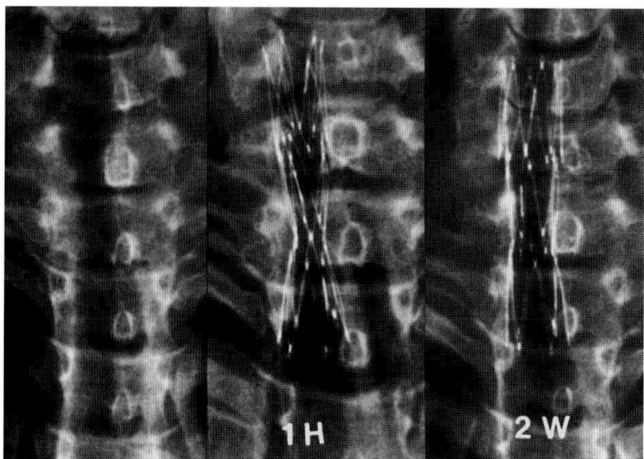

Figure 7. A fibrotic post-tracheostomy stricture is seen on the left. An hour after GRZ stent placement the lesion is incompletely expanded (middle image). The image on the right shows complete expansion of the lesion 2 weeks after stent placement due to the gradual outward force of the self-expanding stent.

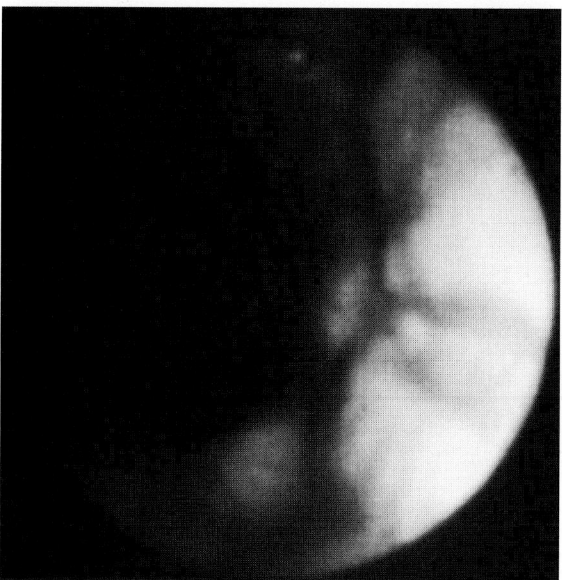

Figure 8. Bronchoscopy at 2 months after placement of a tracheal GRZ stent demonstrates only minimal inflammatory response to the stent.

Stent Sizing

Choosing the proper stent size prior to placement is critical. Helical CT scanning accurately depicts the airway and critical airway stenoses. However, conventional tomography of the mediastinum, or even a highly penetrated posteroanterior chest radiograph is generally all that is required. The stent selected should be 15%–20% wider than the adjacent normal tracheal lumen. It is important to realize that both the Wallstent and the GRZ stent are held in place by their outward force on the tracheal wall. Undersizing of the stent leads to weak outward pressure exerted by the stent, ineffective dilational force, and ultimately stent migration. Oversizing can lead to spontaneous fractures of the stent struts (GRZ). Oversizing may also result in tracheal wall perforation with perforation into adjacent tissues, hemorrhage, and in some cases, death.[11,12]

Silicone Versus Metal Stents

Rigid silicone stents have been in use for more than 25 years[13] and when placed appropriately are quite effective. However, the large outer diameter of these stents makes placement difficult, and traumatic placement may lead to uncontrollable bleeding, especially in the presence of endoluminal tumor. They are also prone to migrate when placed in short, conical stenoses.[14] The main disadvantage of the rigid silicone stents is their small internal to external diameter ratio; the large outer diameter makes placement difficult, and the small inner diameter may lead to early occlusion by mucus secretions. The smaller delivery catheters and less traumatic deployment of expandable metallic stents are distinct advantages over silicone stents.

Treatment of Benign Strictures

When possible, surgery is the primary therapy for benign strictures. If not amenable to surgery, recurrent benign strictures may be treated with repeated dilation procedures or silicone stent placement. Tracheostomy can be performed as a last resort for refractory benign strictures. While long-term patency remains unproven at this time, metallic stent placement is an attractive alternative therapy in benign airway disease.

Considerations in Tracheal Stent Placement

When placement of a tracheal stent is planned, long-term patency of the stent, biocompatibility, stent migration, patient pain, blockage of mucociliary transport, and crossing of bronchial orifices are issues to be considered. The GRZ stent has a low metal mass to surface area ratio which minimizes tissue interactions **(Fig. 8)**. The Wallstent also exhibits excellent biocompatibility, with a cellular covering seen at 3 weeks, and stable incorporation into the tracheal wall by 6 months.[5,10]

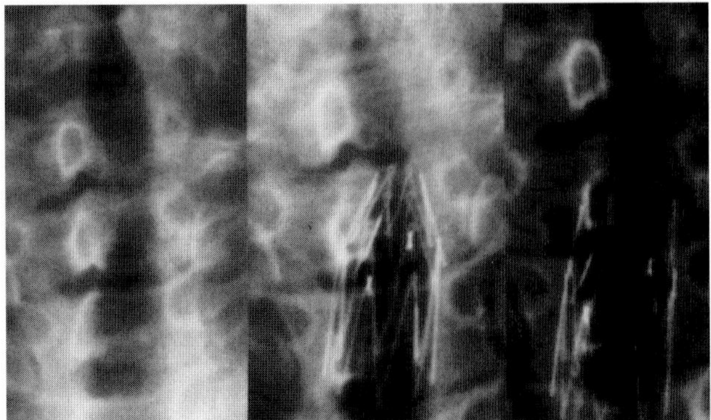

Figure 9. Positioning and deployment of a GRZ stent for a benign stricture in the subglottic trachea. Positioning at least 2 cm below the vocal cords is necessary for patient comfort and to maintain vocal cord function. In this case, caudad positioning slightly below the lesion resulted in improper centering and later in distal migration of the stent.

High Tracheal Lesions

High tracheal lesions usually occur postoperatively (eg, tracheostomy), and can be especially difficult to stent because of the close proximity of the vocal cords. Extension of the stent too far cephalad will alter the patient's speech and function of the larynx. For safe placement, the stent must be placed below the inferior margin of the cricoid cartilage, a distance approximately 2 cm below the level of the vocal cords **(Fig. 9)**.

Lung Transplant Stenoses

Tracheobronchial stenosis secondary to lung transplantation is being encountered more frequently as lung transplantation becomes more common. These post-transplant strictures are an indication for stent placement. Lung transplantation is done without anatomic restoration of the bronchial arterial blood supply. Ischemia of the donor tracheobronchial tree often occurs in the early post-transplant period and can lead to lethal dehiscence of the bronchial anastomosis or result in anastomotic bronchial stenosis. When severe, the bronchial stenosis leads to poor lung function, diminished mucociliary clearance, infection, and possible occlusion with subsequent atelectasis.

Dilation and silicone stent therapy have been integral parts of treatment for these anastomotic strictures. However, these therapies are not without serious potential drawbacks and offer little in the way of definitive treatment. Metallic stent therapy, primarily with Wallstents but also with other types of stents **(Fig. 10)**, has been used in transplant stenoses with good results.[15–17] However, the anastomotic region does have a greater tendency to develop a granulomatous or inflammatory reaction, which can lead to restenosis. These early recurrences can be managed with repeated balloon dilation, which permits the inflammatory stenosis to mature and stabilize.[5,15]

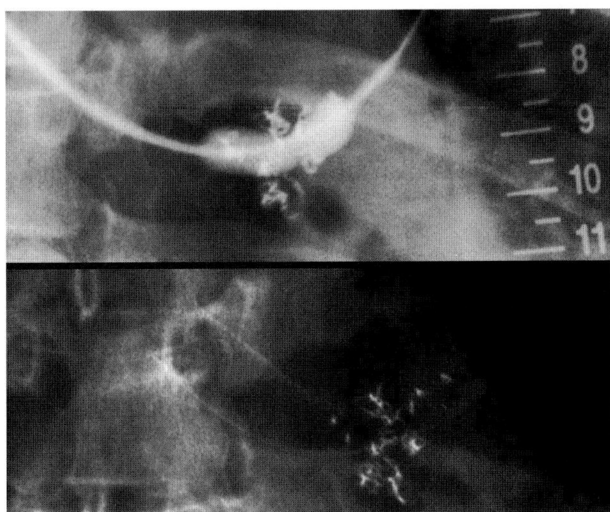

Figure 10. Placement of a 10-mm Wallstent at a left upper lobe bronchial anastomotic stricture.

Results of Stent Placement for Benign Disease

Rousseau has reported the largest experience in tracheobronchial stent placement for benign disease. In 50 patients, 34 Wallstents and 35 Gianturco stents were placed into the tracheobronchial tree. With a mean follow-up of 10.4 months (range 3–27 months), improvement in respiratory status was documented in 44 patients (89%).[5] In three of the six patients who did not show improvement, stent placement failure could be attributed to inadequate coverage of the lesion. After additional stent placement, these three patients responded well. In the three remaining failures, restenosis had developed in the stent; this was effectively treated with balloon dilation. After tracheal stent placement, significant granulation tissue, especially in the presence of inflammatory lesions, can develop. Carre has suggested that these granulation-induced stenoses be treated conservatively with repeated dilation or silicone stent placement until the granulomatous reaction subsides.[16]

Treatment of Malignant Strictures

Obstruction of the large airway from malignant processes presents a more common clinical problem. Localized large airway obstruction due to neoplasm may account for early death in nearly 40% of such patients.[18] Various methods have been used to treat these obstructions, including surgery, laser therapy, external radiation, and/or chemotherapy. Despite these therapies, tumor recurrence is likely and further options for palliation are limited. When these standard treatments have been exhausted, rigid silicone stents may be implanted to maintain airway patency.

Considerations for Stent Placement in Malignant Tracheobronchial Obstructions

Malignant airway obstruction by extrinsic compression or encasement may be treated with noncovered or “bare” metal stents. In these circumstances, the airway mucosa is generally preserved and the stent acts as a scaffold to maintain airway patency. Early stent failure has been observed in the presence of endoluminal tumor, with tumor protrusion through the stent struts and airway obstruction. These early failures led to the development of stents with both nonporous and semipermeable coverings.[3,6,19–21] In the short term, these covered stents have remained patent and blockade of the mucociliary transport mechanism has not been a clinical problem. Because orifices of branching airways should not be occluded by the covered stent, covered stents can only be used in the trachea and major bronchi. Stent placement at the carina with nonporous covered stents requires that the contralateral main bronchi remain unobstructed by the stent.

"Hinged" Covered Stents

Covered GRZ stents can be constructed with a "hinge" between two stent bodies, and then delivered so that the "hinge" is located along the lateral aspect of the airway at the junction of the trachea and main bronchus. This allows an opening in the covered stent to form, directed toward the contralateral main bronchus. Stent placement in the contralateral bronchus is done separately by placing a second stent through the opening of the first stent. The second stent must be placed in close apposition to the first stent to form the best seal and prevent tumor ingrowth **(Figs. 11–13)**.

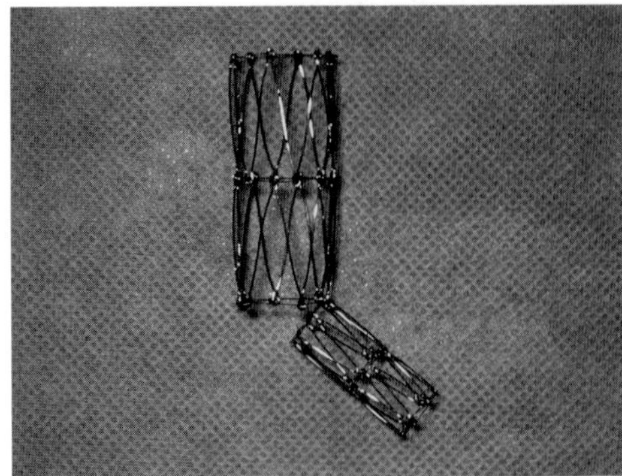

Figure 11. Noncovered hinged carinal Z-stent constructed from a large double-body Z-stent and a second, smaller double-body Z-stent attached on one side only. This can traverse the carina without obstruction of the contralateral bronchus, which can be treated separately.

Results

Early series using the original Gianturco Z-stents have demonstrated promising results, with efficacy and short-term patency rates similar to those for rigid silicone stents.[22–24] Moreover, complications are reduced compared to rigid silicone stents.

Patients with malignant disease obstructing the major airways have a short life expectancy. Tracheobronchial stent placement palliates airway obstruction and decreases patient suffering. The patients generally die from other manifestations of their malignancy. When treating any malignant stricture, it is important that the stent extend far enough above and below the lesion to account for progression of the disease. Recurrent obstruction from tumor growing beyond the stent margins may be treated by extension with additional stents, with care taken not to occlude the origins of crossing bronchi.

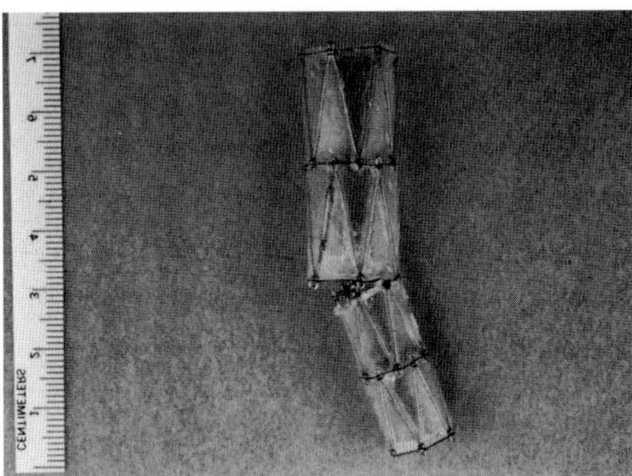

Figure 12. Covered hinged carinal Z-stent.

Conclusion—Tracheobronchial Stent Placement

Metallic self-expanding stents are a promising treatment for respiratory distress from both benign and malignant tracheobronchial obstructions confined to the mid and distal trachea and proximal mainstem bronchi.

During the short life expectancy of patients with malignancy, stents have worked well, with acceptable complication rates concerning migration, bleeding, and recurrent occlusion. Stents offer a relatively quick, atraumatic, and effective means to palliate a difficult clinical problem. Long-term biocompatibility of the metal stents has not been established in the tracheobronchial tree, and their use should be reserved for cases in which other treatment modalities have been exhausted. Further clinical trials with larger patient series will be required to determine if stents can be recommended as a first line of therapy.

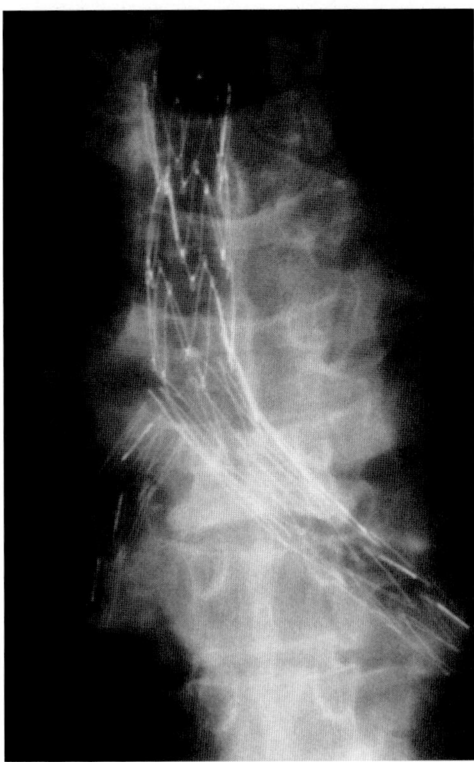

Figure 13. Stent treatment of a carinal mass. A hinged Z-stent is in the right mainstem bronchus with an additional Z-stent placed in the left mainstem bronchus through the hinged stent. This successfully palliated the patient's dyspnea.

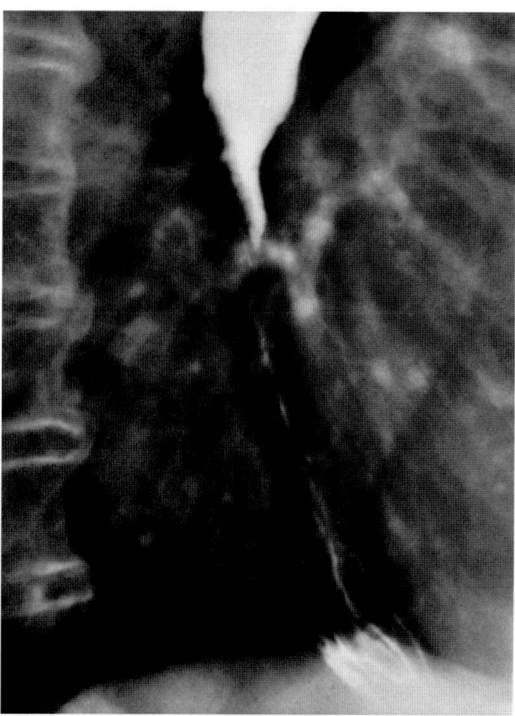

Figure 14. Primary squamous cell carcinoma causing a long, severe stricture of the mid and distal esophagus.

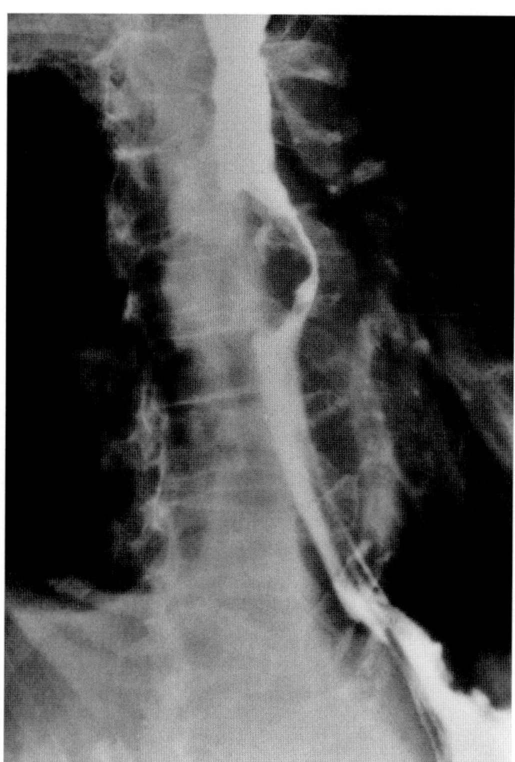

Figure 15. Extrinsic mass compressing the mid esophagus from lung cancer invading the mediastinum.

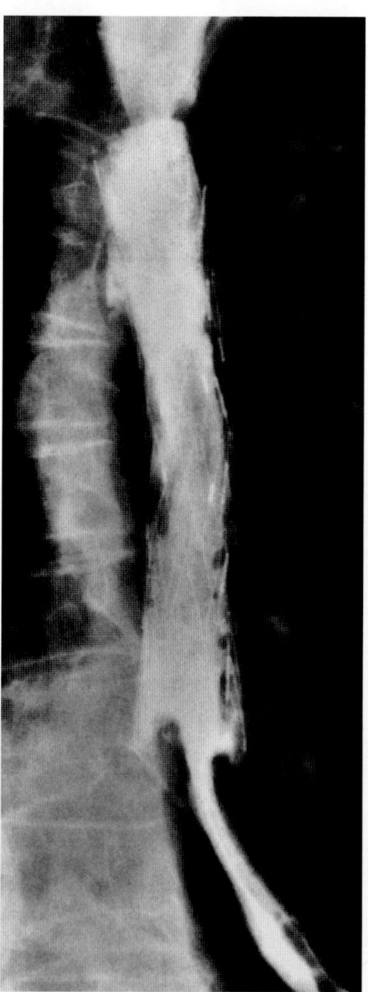

Figure 16. Same patient as in Figure 15. Barium swallow after esophageal stent placement shows resolution of the stricture.

Malignant Esophageal Disease

In the United States, 100,000 new cases of esophageal cancer are diagnosed each year. Squamous cell carcinoma accounts for the majority of cases of primary esophageal malignancy and occurs most often in the proximal and middle esophagus **(Fig. 14)**. However, adenocarcinoma involving the gastroesophageal junction is the most common form of neoplastic esophageal obstruction in our patient population. The esophagus may also be involved by direct extension of lung cancer **(Figs. 15, 16)** or by mediastinal metastases, leading to the development of esophageal obstruction or esophagorespiratory fistula (ERF).

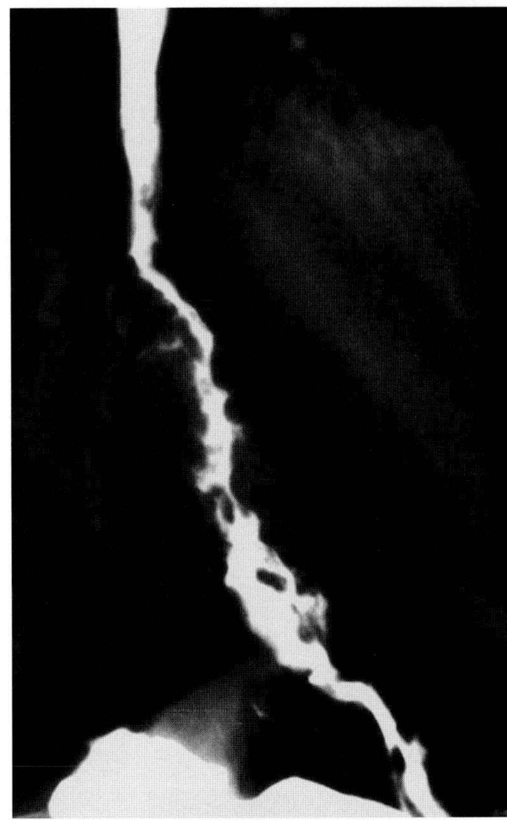

Figure 17. Primary adenocarcinoma of the distal esophagus. The patient had grade 3 dysphagia with difficulty swallowing solids and liquids.

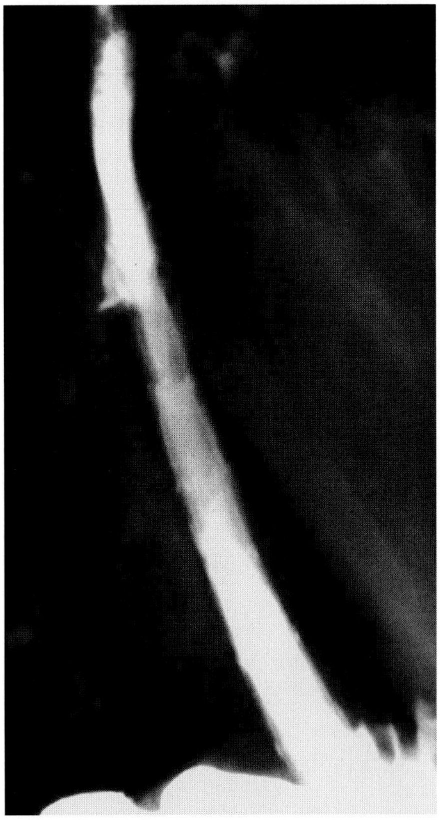

Assessment of Patients

The most common presentation of esophageal malignancy is progressive dysphagia. In primary and secondary esophageal carcinoma, tumor involvement is often extensive at the time of presentation and curative medical or surgical intervention is seldom possible.[25,26] The 1-year and 5-year survival rates for patients with primary esophageal cancer are 18% and 5%, respectively. Before embarking on a course of risky therapy, it must be ascertained that the patient's symptoms warrant aggressive intervention. Dysphagia is graded as: 0=no dysphagia; 1=dysphagia to normal solids; 2=dysphagia to soft solids; 3=dysphagia to solids and liquids; 4=inability to swallow saliva. Generally, patients with grade 3 or 4 dysphagia require aggressive intervention **(Figs. 17, 18)**.

Figure 18. Same patient as in Figure 17. After stent placement for the esophageal tumor, the patient's dysphagia resolved and he was able to tolerate a normal diet.

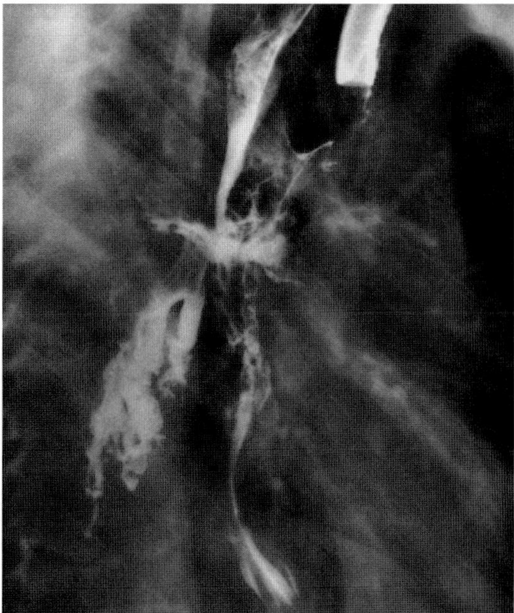

Figure 19. Esophageal carcinoma resulting in an esophagorespiratory fistula. Barium swallow demonstrates opacification of the bronchial tree.

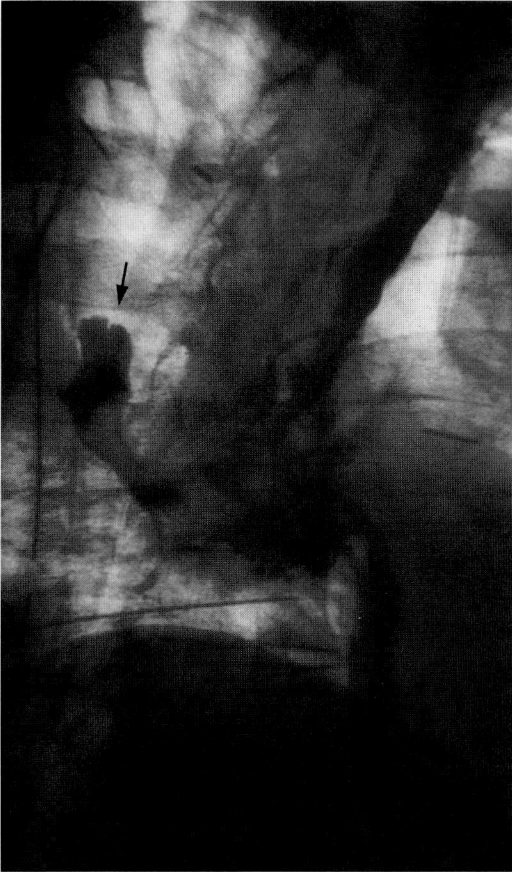

Figure 20. Recurrent adenocarcinoma of the distal esophagus with development of perforation and esophagopulmonary fistula. Note the contrast material extending toward the chest tube on the Gastrografin swallow (arrow).

Esophagorespiratory Fistula

One of the most severe and life-threatening complications of esophageal malignancy is the development of ERF or esophagopleural fistula (EPF). About 5%–10% of patients, particularly those with squamous cell carcinoma or lung cancer invading the mediastinum, will develop ERF **(Fig. 19)**. Patients with ERF usually suffer from a combination of aspiration, malnutrition, and sepsis.[27] The life expectancy after development of an ERF is usually less than 6 weeks. Patients with EPF develop recurrent empyema and sepsis **(Fig. 20)**.

Therapeutic Options

In patients with dysphagia whose disease is not amenable to surgery, the goal of therapy is to relieve the esophageal obstruction. A variety of treatments can be used. The traditional approach involves sequential dilation with bougies.[28–30] Chemotherapy and radiation administered together or separately have had limited success, often with no relief of dysphagia for weeks to months.[25–27,31,32] Palliative bypass surgery is rarely performed because of its high morbidity and mortality. Endoscopic therapy permits debulking of tumors with use of sclerosants, cryotherapy, photocoagulation, and lasers. A drawback to all of these therapies is the need for multiple costly treatment sessions.[33–37]

Rigid Prostheses

One alternative to repeated palliative endoscopic interventions which promises more lasting results is to relieve obstruction by placing esophageal endoprostheses. Rigid plastic endoprostheses have been used for years to treat malignant esophageal obstruction (MEO) and ERF. However, they have many drawbacks. Their rigidity, large outer diameter, and small inner diameter have caused numerous problems.[25–27,31–37] Insertion of these devices is often traumatic and esophageal perforation is common (5%–13% of cases). They are also prone to migrate and cause pressure necrosis and bleeding. Because of their 10–12-mm inner diameter, they can become obstructed by food, so patients are required to eat a soft diet. The overall complication rate associated with the use of these devices is 25%–40%.

Self-Expanding Stents

The recent development of large-diameter, self-expanding metallic stents has altered the management of unresectable esophageal carcinoma significantly. These stents can be placed easily on an outpatient basis and provide excellent symptomatic relief in more than 90% of patients, with much lower complication rates than for rigid endoprostheses.

In the last several years, a variety of covered and noncovered metallic esophageal stents have been developed **(Fig. 21)**. Most of our experience in the treatment of MEO and ERF has been with the Cook Esophageal Z-stent (Cook), which consists of five to seven interconnected 2-cm-long Z-stent bodies covered with a polyethylene membrane **(Fig. 22)**. This stent has an inner diameter of 18 mm with the stent bodies on either end flared to 25 mm, and it comes in lengths of 10–14 cm. Metal barbs are attached to the middle of the stent to prevent migration. The stent does not shorten and has excellent expansile force.

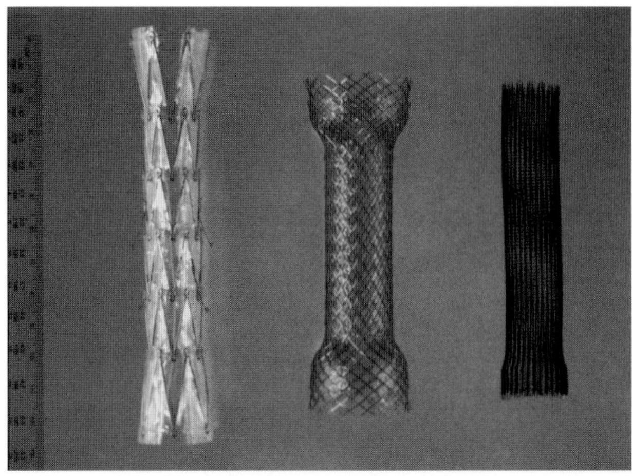

Figure 21. Three of the available metallic endoprostheses. From left to right: 1) Cook Esophageal Z-stent; 2) Schneider esophageal Wallstent; 3) Microvasive Ultraflex stent. Note that the Z-stent and Wallstent are covered while the Microvasive stent shown is the noncovered variety.

A similar stent is available from Wilson-Cook Medical, Inc. It differs from the Cook stent in that it lacks barbs and has a smaller flare. It also comes with a significantly different delivery system designed for endoscopic stent placement.

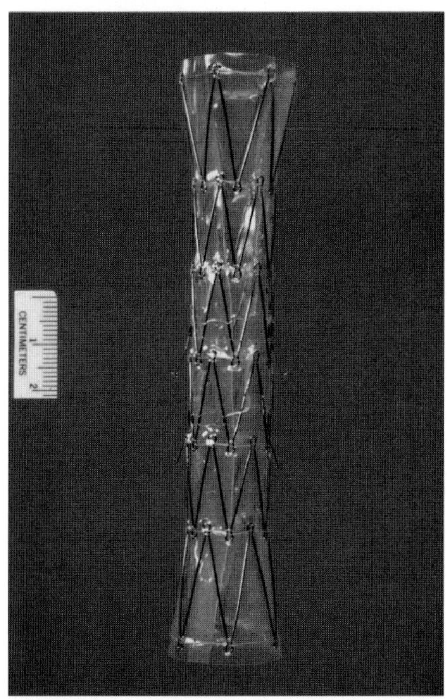

Figure 22. Cook Esophageal Z-stent.

The Wallstent Esophageal Prosthesis (Schneider) is a covered stent consisting of a proprietary polymer membrane sandwiched between two large-diameter Wallstents **(Fig. 21)**. This stent has a diameter of 18 mm along its shaft and 28 mm at either end. It comes in deployed lengths of 8, 10, and 13 cm. The stent shortens by 25%–30% when deployed. It has strong radial force and is simple to place. It is also possible to use noncovered versions of the Wallstent Endoprosthesis for palliation of esophageal obstruction. These are now available in sizes up to 24 mm in diameter and in a variety of lengths.

Two stents are available from Microvasive (Boston Scientific Corporation, Natick, MA). The Ultraflex stent is a noncovered device consisting of a single strand of Nitinol wire knitted to form a self-expanding stent **(Fig. 21)**. It has a diameter of 18 mm with a 21-mm proximal flare placement. This stent is more flexible but has less expansile force than other stents **(Figs. 23, 24)**. Balloon dilation of this stent is often required before and after stent placement. The stent is available in lengths of 10 and 15 mm. It also shortens considerably when deployed. The Ultraflex covered stent is similar except that it has a polymer covering along its shaft to prevent tumor ingrowth, and to potentially seal an ERF, which cannot be done with the noncovered variety.

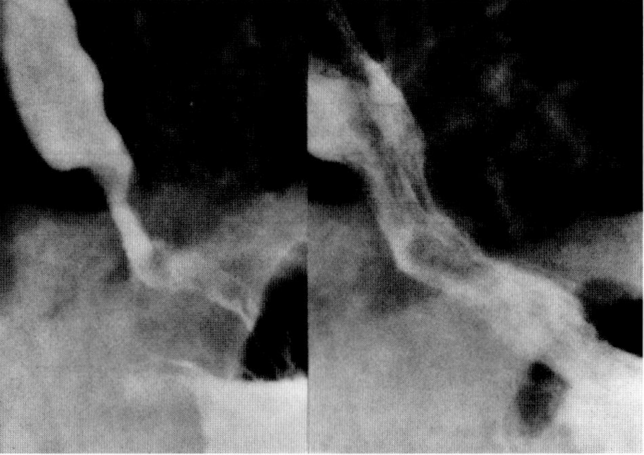

Figure 23. Distal adenocarcinoma of the esophagus with distal esophageal stricture (left). After placement of an Ultraflex stent (right), the obstruction is relieved as demonstrated on the barium swallow.

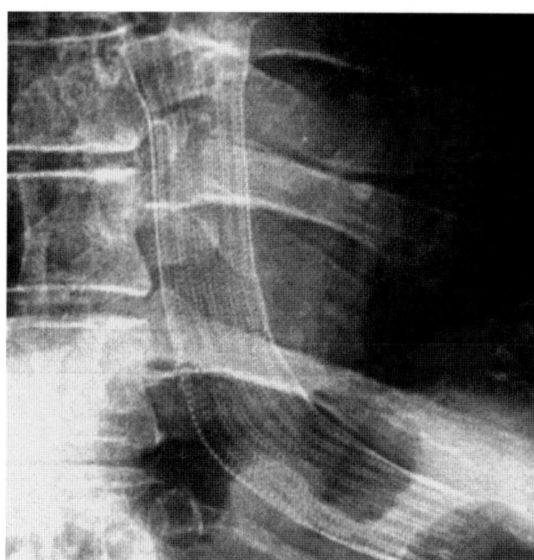

Figure 24. Same patient as in Figure 23. Magnified image after Ultraflex stent placement. Note the flexibility of the Ultraflex stent around the curved course of the distal esophagus and esophagogastric junction.

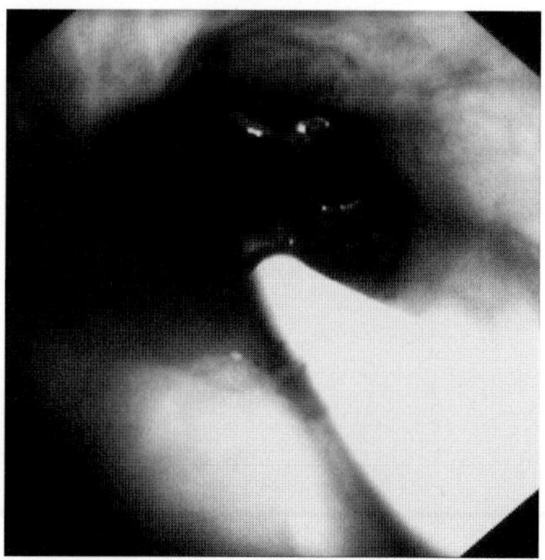

Figure 25. Endoscopic approach to placement of an Ultraflex endoprosthesis. Gastroenterologists typically traverse strictures and place stents using endoscopic guidance.

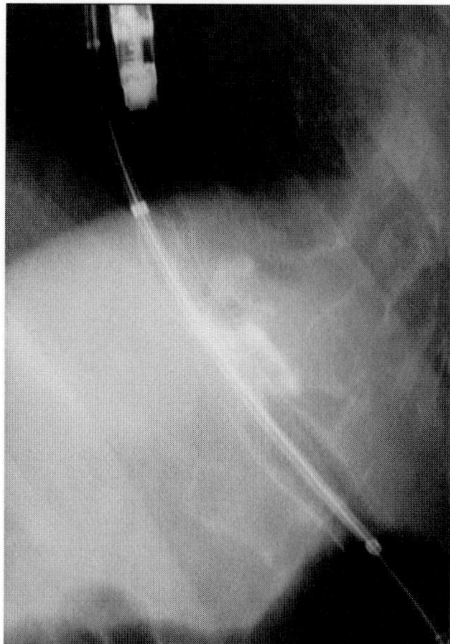

Figure 26. Correct placement of the stent is verified by fluoroscopy.

The EsophaCoil esophageal stent (InStent, Eden Prairie, MN) is another noncovered stent. It consists of a single piece of flattened Nitinol wire coiled to form a tube. It is available in diameters of 16 and 18 mm and lengths of 10 and 15 cm. It is a noncovered stent design with a very tight coil that is thought might prevent tumor ingrowth.

Patient Selection

Most patients with symptoms of moderate to severe (≥grade 2) MEO will benefit from stent placement. Stents are effective in relieving obstruction caused by both primary esophageal tumors and invasion or compression of the esophagus by adjacent tumors. Few problems are encountered in treating lesions throughout the esophagus. However, lesions in the proximal esophagus must be approached with care because the patient may experience a foreign body sensation which can be so severe as to require stent removal. Lesions requiring stent placement within 3 cm of the cricopharyngeal muscle should be avoided. Flexible stents should be used in the upper esophagus because they may be less likely to cause laryngeal compression and airway compromise.

Technique

The majority of our patients have been treated on an outpatient basis. Gastroenterologists often place stents themselves using endoscopic guidance and fluoroscopy **(Figs. 25, 26)**. However, all of the available stents are probably more easily placed with use of fluoroscopy. At our institution, patients usually have a barium swallow prior to stent placement to assess the length and location of the stricture or ERF. Endoscopy can be performed immediately prior to stent placement. It is most useful for identifying the proximal and distal tumor margins in patients with ERF by submucosal injections of iodinated contrast material. This obviates the need for intraluminal contrast material and the associated risk of aspiration.

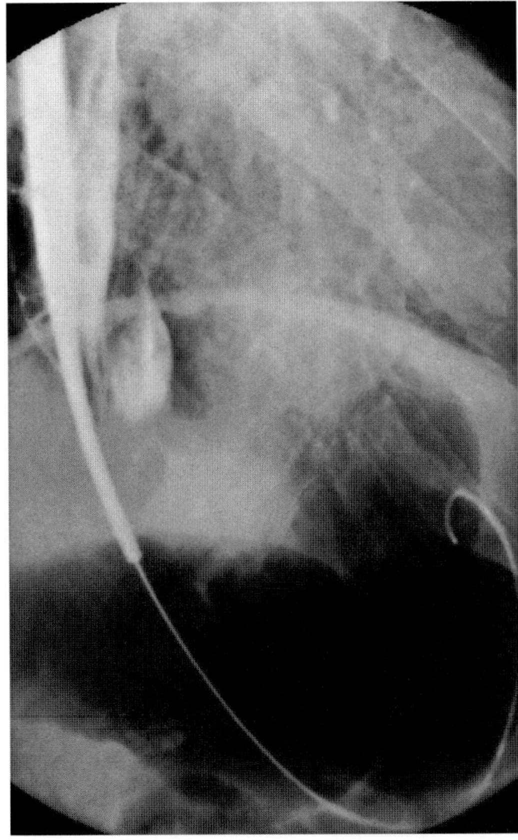

Figure 27. Traversal of a distal esophageal adenocarcinoma by the dilator and introducing sheath over an Amplatz wire.

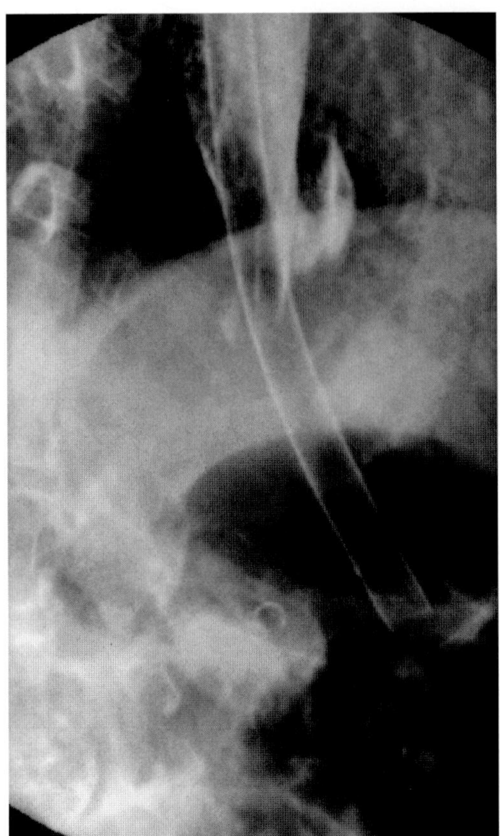

Figure 28. Introducer sheath in place, ready for stent placement.

Our technique is to traverse the lesion under fluoroscopic guidance using a pre-shaped 6.5-F angiographic catheter (Torcon, Cook) and a Bentson guide wire (Cook). An 0.038-inch Amplatz Super Stiff wire (Medi-Tech, Watertown, MA) is then placed, over which the dilator and introducing sheath are passed into the stomach **(Fig. 27)**. Dilation of the lesion prior to stent placement is required in some cases and should usually be done when using an Ultraflex stent. When using one of the stents with more expansile force, we pre-dilate the lesion with a 15-mm-diameter angioplasty balloon only if the stricture is extremely tight and we have trouble passing the introducing sheath. If the stent remains narrow after deployment, it can be dilated with a balloon at that point.

Stent Delivery

The technique of stent placement depends on the device used. The majority of our patients have been treated with the Cook Esophageal Z-stent and we will briefly describe its use as an example of how stents are placed. The stent is placed through a delivery sheath which is introduced over an angiographic guide wire using a large dilator **(Fig. 28)**. Two radiolucent markers on the dilator can be used to center the sheath at the level of the desired stent position.

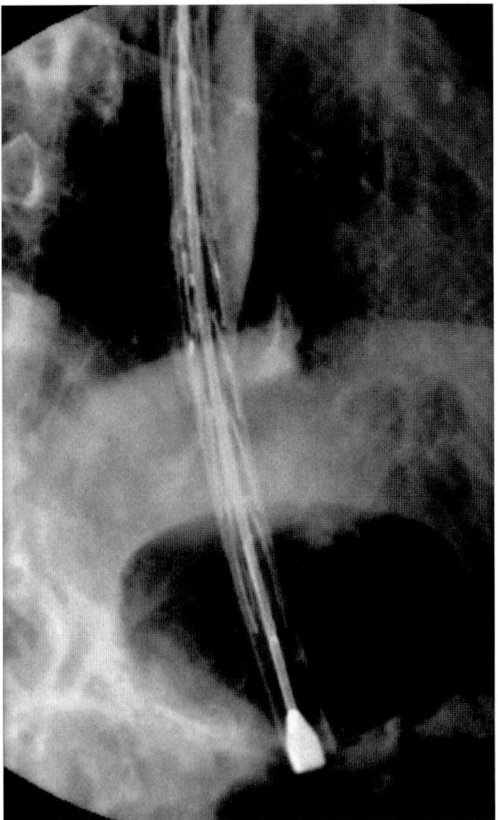

Figure 29. Placement of the Cook Esophageal Z-stent through the introducing sheath. The stent is pulled into place attached to a metal cannula at its leading edge.

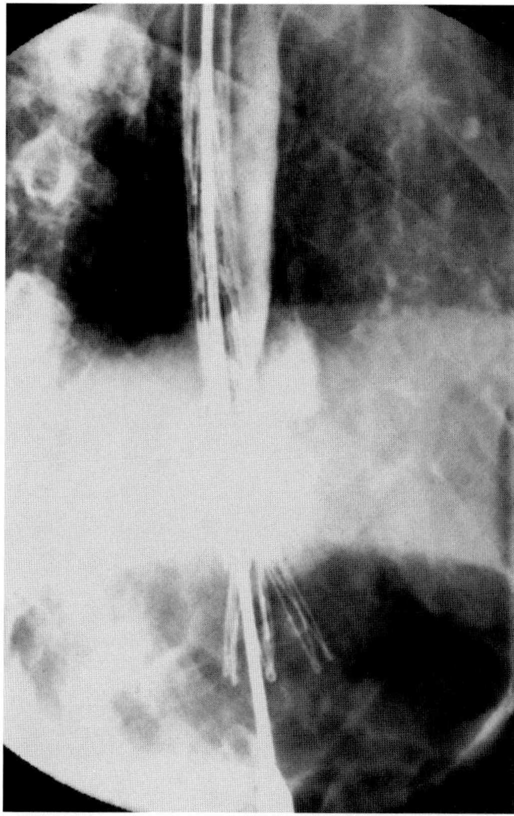

Figure 30. Partial deployment of the Z-stent with use of an unsheathing motion. The stent is held in place by the metal cannula while the sheath is smoothly withdrawn.

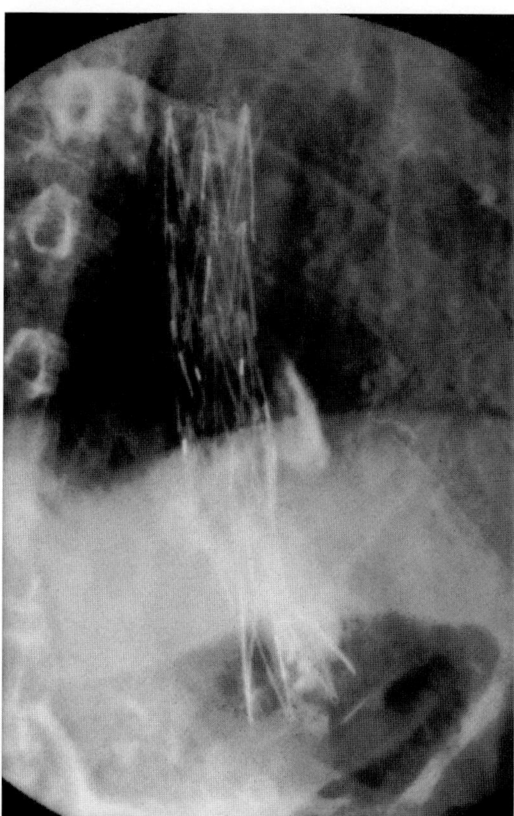

Figure 31. Final position of the deployed Z-stent across the stricture after the cannula has been removed.

Stent lengths are selected so that the proximal and distal ends extend beyond the esophageal stricture by at least 2 cm at each end. The stent is attached to the delivery system at the front of the leading body by a loop of thread that runs through a central metal cannula to the back of the delivery apparatus. The delivery system is introduced through the delivery sheath **(Fig. 28)** and across the lesion **(Fig. 29)**. The stent is deployed by withdrawing the outer sheath while holding the stent in position using the central cannula **(Figs. 30, 31)**. Finally, the stent is released from the metal cannula by cutting the loop of thread and removing it from the back of the delivery apparatus.

Postprocedure Recommendations

All patients have a follow-up esophagram immediately after stent placement. Esophagrams are also obtained when patients develop recurrent symptoms. All patients with distal esophageal stents that cross the esophagogastric junction are placed on a proton pump inhibitor to decrease reflux esophagitis, because reflux into the esophagus occurs without impediment with a stent in this location. Patients are also advised to remain upright for 2–3 hours following meals, and to increase their diet slowly over a 4-day period from liquids to soft foods and sometimes to a normal diet, as tolerated.

Results

Self-expanding esophageal stents have proven to be both safe and effective for the treatment of both MEO and REF. Comparison of published series on expandable stents with earlier series on rigid endoprostheses have suggested that metallic stents may be superior. To date only one randomized comparison has been reported. Knyrim et al compared the Wallstent to rigid endoprostheses and found that while both were effective in relieving obstruction, the complication rate was significantly lower with the expandable metallic stent.[38]

Results For MEO

For MEO the immediate technical and clinical success rates with metallic endoprostheses approach 100%, regardless of the stent used.[28–30,39–50] Immediate complications are rare with metallic endoprostheses. Stent dislodgement or incomplete stent opening account for most failures (<5%). Successfully placed stents are almost universally effective in relieving dysphagia (95%). Comorbid factors account for most cases of persistent symptoms following successful stent placement. For example, continued dysphagia after stent placement can be caused by decreased esophageal motility from extensive tumor infiltration of the esophagus that produces an achalasia-like situation.

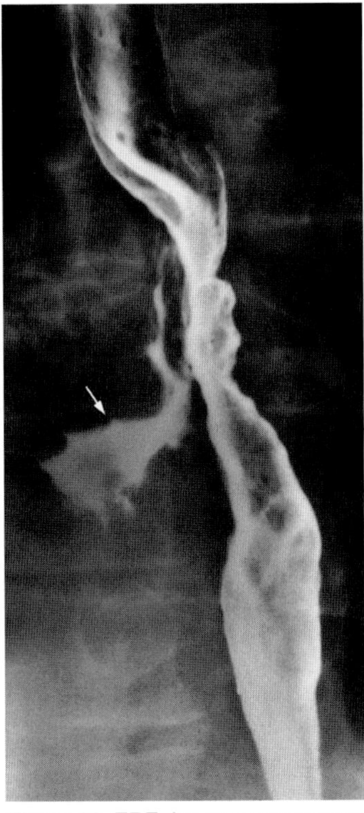

Figure 32. ERF due to squamous cell carcinoma of the esophagus, with opacification of the right mainstem bronchus (arrow) on barium swallow. Note the associated esophageal stricture at the site of the ERF.

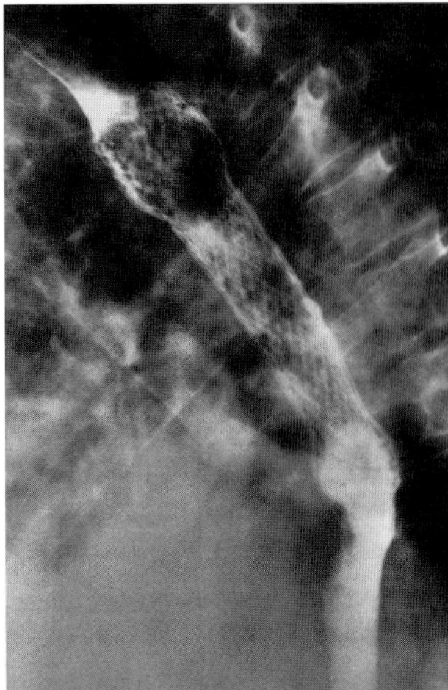

Figure 33. Same patient as in Figure 32. Successful sealing of the ERF with a Wallstent covered endoprosthesis. Barium swallow demonstrates exclusion of the fistulous track.

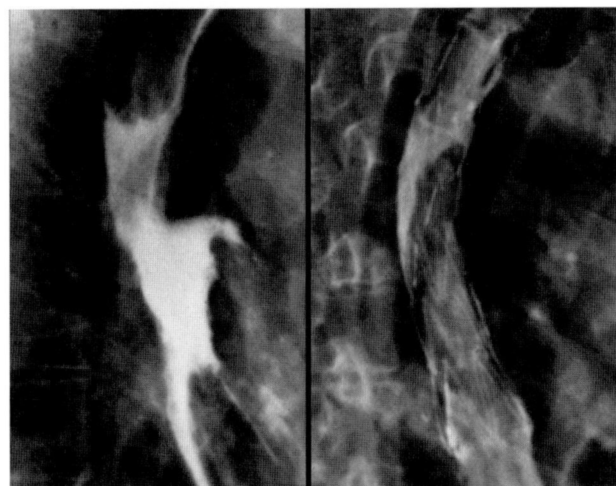

Figure 34. Barium swallow before stent placement in a patient with an ERF. Note the lack of a stenosis at the site of the fistula. After GRZ stent placement, there is transient sealing of the fistula.

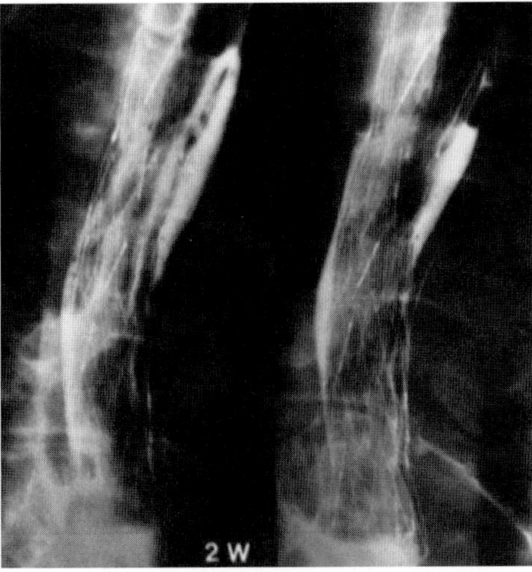

Figure 35. Same patient as in Figure 34. Two-week follow-up esophagram demonstrates leakage around the stent into the left mainstem bronchus.

Results for ERF

Endoprosthetic treatment of ERF and EPF requires a covered stent to seal the fistula. Both the Wallstent **(Figs. 32, 33)** and Z-stent have been used successfully. The presence or absence of an associated stricture at the site of an ERF is a major factor limiting effective palliation. If a stricture is not present, placement of a covered stent will most likely be unsuccessful due to continued leakage of secretions around the stent and into the fistulous track **(Figs. 34, 35)**. However, if a stricture is present, the fistula can almost always be sealed.

Clinical Follow-up

Recurrent dysphagia is seen in 5%–20% of patients after metallic endoprosthesis placement. Dysphagia can be caused by stent migration, tumor ingrowth, tumor overgrowth, or food impaction. Tumor overgrowth and food impaction occur rarely with both covered and noncovered stents. Tumor ingrowth occurs only with noncovered stents such as the Ultraflex **(Fig. 36)**. The incidence has been reported to be as high as 67% and is related to the duration of patient survival. When it leads to recurrent dysphagia (<20% of patients) it can be treated by placing another stent or using endoscopic laser treatments to restore patency.

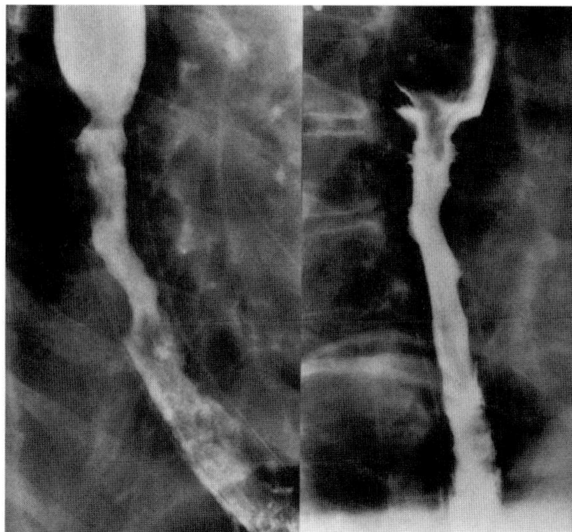

Figure 36. Barium swallow demonstrates recurrent obstruction of the distal esophagus due to tumor ingrowth in a noncovered Ultraflex stent, causing a stricture.

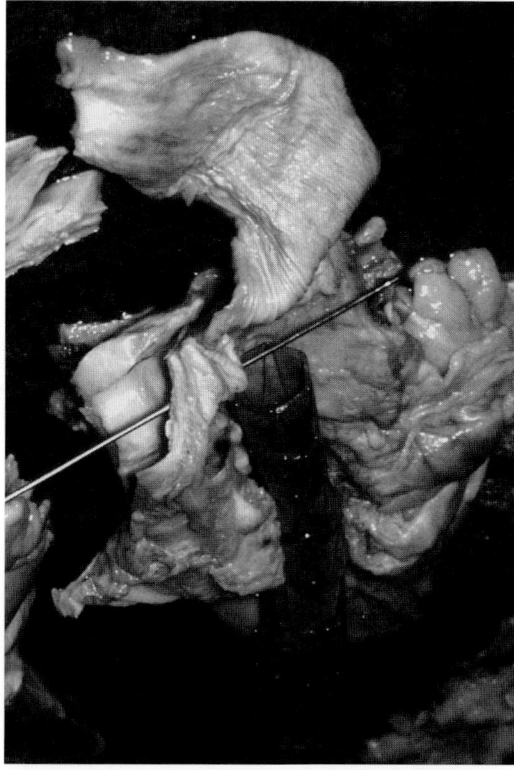

Figure 37. Pathologic specimen after esophageal stent placement demonstrates an aortoesophageal fistula that resulted in massive lethal bleeding. The fistula was shown to be due to tumor invasion of the aorta, not to the indwelling stent. The metal probe traverses the aortoesophageal fistula.

Complications

Food impaction in metallic endoprostheses is rare because they all have relatively large lumens (≥18 mm). When food does become impacted, it is easily cleared by passing an occlusion balloon down through the esophagus under fluoroscopic guidance. Tumor overgrowth is also rare but can lead to obstruction above or below the stent. It is best treated by placing an additional stent in the involved portion of the esophagus. Stent migration is seen in 10%–20% of patients and is more common with covered stents. Surprisingly, stent migration rarely leads to any complications other than recurrent dysphagia. For example, no cases have been reported of bowel perforation or obstruction caused by a migrating stent.

One persistent disadvantage of current covered stents has been the development of substantial chest discomfort after placement. Covered stents tend to be flared at the ends (usually ≥25 mm) to seal fistulas. In addition, all current covered stents are substantially stiffer than noncovered expandable metallic stents. These two facts likely account for the increased chest discomfort associated with the use of covered stents. Chest discomfort is usually transient but can necessitate management with narcotic analgesia, which is usually very effective in patients with chronic pain.

The most severe complication seen after stent placement is exsanguinatory upper gastrointestinal hemorrhage. The exact etiology of gastrointestinal bleeding after placement of esophageal stents remains unclear. A statistically significant association with prior radiation and chemotherapy has been reported.[43,50] On the other hand, 5%–8% of patients with untreated esophageal malignancy develop upper gastrointestinal bleeding. Severe bleeding may represent the natural progression of the underlying malignancy rather than a complication of stent placement **(Fig. 37)**. However, the overall palliative benefit of the expandable metallic stents outweighs the potential morbidity and mortality when compared to other treatment options.

Summary

Covered expandable metallic stents are an effective method of palliating both malignant dysphagia and the complications of ERF. Placement of an expandable metallic esophageal stent is a safe and inexpensive outpatient procedure that results in a significant improvement in the quality of life for patients with MEO and ERF. Stent placement should be considered the primary therapy in patients with unresectable esophageal malignancy.

References

1. Quint LE, Whyte RI, Kazerooni EA, et al. Stenosis of the central airways: evaluation by using helical CT with multiplanar reconstructions. Radiology 1995; 194:871–877.

2. Uchida BT, Putnam JS, Rösch J. Modifications of Gianturco expandable wire stents. AJR 1988; 150:1185–1187.

3. Petersen BD, Uchida BT, Barton RE, Keller FS, Rösch J. Gianturco-Rösch Z stents in tracheobronchial stenoses. J Vasc Interv Radiol 1995; 6:925–931.

4. Tojo T, Iioka S, Kitamura S, et al. Management of malignant tracheobronchial stenosis with metal stents and Dumon stents. Ann Thorac Surg 1996; 61:1074–1078.

5. Rousseau H, Dahan M, Lauque D, et al. Self-expandable prostheses in the tracheobronchial tree. Radiology 1993; 188:199–203.

6. Irving JD, Goldstraw P. Tracheobronchial stents. Semin Intervent Radiol 1991; 8(4):295–304.

7. Tsang V, Williams A, Goldstraw P. Sequential Silastic and expandable metal stenting for tracheobronchial strictures. Ann Thorac Surg 1992; 53:856–860.

8. Bousamra M, Tweddell JS, Wells RG, et al. Wire stent for tracheomalacia in a 5-year-old girl. Ann Thorac Surg 1996; 61:1239–1240.

9. Becker H, Wagner B, Lierman D, et al. Stenting of central airways. In: Lierman D, ed. Stents: state of the art and future developments. Polyscience Publications, Inc., 1995; 249–255.

10. Rousseau H, Carre P, Joffre F, et al. Self-expanding stents in the management of tracheobronchial stenosis. In: Cope C, ed. Current techniques in interventional radiology. Philadelphia: Current Medicine, 1994; 144–154.

11. Nashef S, Dromer C, Velly JF, Labrousse L, Couraud L. Expanding wire stents in benign tracheobronchial disease: indications and complications. Ann Thorac Surg 1992; 54:937–940.

12. Maynar M, Lopez L, Gorriz E, Reyes R, Pulido-Duque JM, Castaneda-Zuniga WR. Massive brachiocephalic artery bleeding due to a Gianturco tracheal stent. J Vasc Interv Radiol 4(2):289–291.

13. Montgomery W. T-tube tracheal stent. Arch Otolaryng 1965; 82:320–321.

14. Bolliger CT, Probst R, Tschopp K, Soler M, Perruchoud AP. Silicone stents in the management of inoperable tracheobronchial stenoses. Chest 1993; 104:1653–1659.

15. Carre P, Rousseau H, Lombart L, et al. Balloon dilatation and self-expanding metal Wallstent insertion. Chest 1994; 105:343–348.

16. Carre P, Rousseau H, Dahan M, et al. Therapeutic management of posttransplant bronchial stenosis by balloon dilatation and self-expandable metallic Wallstent insertion. Transplant Proc 1994; 26:253.

17. Brichon PY, Blanc-Jouvan F, Rousseau H, et al. Endovascular stents for bronchial stenosis after lung transplantation. Transplant Proc 1992; 24(6):2656–2659.

18. Luomanen RK, Watson WL. Autopsy finding. In: Watson WL, ed. Lung cancer: a study of five thousand Memorial Hospital cases. St. Louis: C.V. Mosby Company, 1968; 504–510.

19. Nomori H, Kobayashi R, Kodera K, Morinaga S, Ogawa K. Indications for an expandable metallic stent for tracheobronchial stenosis. Ann Thorac Surg 1993; 56:1324–1328.

20. Kishi K, Kobayashi H, Suruda T, et al. Treatment of malignant tracheobronchial stenosis by Dacron mesh-covered Z-stents. Cardiovasc Intervent Radiol 1994 17:33–35.

21. George PJ, Irving JD, Khaghani A, Dick R. Role of the Gianturco expandable metal stent in the management of tracheobronchial obstruction. Cardiovasc Intervent Radiol 1992; 15:375–381.

22. Wallace MJ, Charnsangavej C, Ogawa K, et al. Tracheobronchial tree: expandable metallic stents used in experimental and clinical applications. Work in progress. Radiology 1986; 158:309–312.

23. Varela A, Maynar M, Irving D, et al. Use of Gianturco self-expanding stents in the tracheobronchial tree. Ann Thorac Surg 1990; 49:806–809.

24. Sawada S, Tanigawa N, Kobayashi M, Furui S, Ohta Y. Malignant tracheobronchial obstructive lesions: treatment with Gianturco expandable metallic stents. Radiology 1993; 188:205–208.

25. Boyce HW Jr. Palliation of advanced esophageal cancer. Semin Oncol 1984; 11(2):186–195.

26. Watson A. Surgery for carcinoma of the oesophagus. Postgrad Med J 1988; 64:860–864.

27. Ogilvie AL, Dronfield MW, Fercuson R, Atkinson M. Palliative intubation of oesophagogastric neoplasms at fiberoptic endoscopy. Gut 1982; 23:1060–1067.

28. McClean GK, Cooper GS, Hartz WH, Burke DR, Meranze SG. Radiologically guided balloon dilation of gastrointestinal strictures. Radiology 1987; 165:35–40.

29. Johnsen A, Jensen LI, Mauritzen K. Balloon dilatation of esophageal strictures in children. Pediatr Radiol 1986; 16:388–391.

30. Starck E, Paolucci V, Herzer M, Crummy AB. Esophageal stenosis: treatment with balloon catheters. Radiology 1984; 153:637–640.

31. Postlethwait RW. Complications and deaths after operations for esophageal carcinoma. J Thorac Cardiovasc Surg 1983; 85:827–831.

32. Albertsson M, Ewers SB, Widmark H, Hambraeus G, Lillo-Gil R, Ranstam J. Evaluation of the palliative effect of radiotherapy for esophageal carcinoma. Acta Oncol 1989; 28:267–270.

33. Fleischer D, Sivak MV Jr. Endoscopic Nd:YAG laser therapy as palliation for esophagogastric cancer. Gastroenterology 1985; 89:827–831.

34. Rutgeerts P, Vantrappen G, Broeckaert L, et al. Palliative Nd:YAG laser therapy for cancer of the esophagus and gastroesophageal junction: impact on the quality of remaining life. Gastrointest Endoscopy 1988; 34(2):87–90.

35. Fleischer D. Endoscopic laser therapy for esophageal cancer: present status with emphasis on past and future. Lasers Surg Med 1989; 9:6–16.

36. Murray FE, Bowers GJ, Birkett DH, Cave DR. Palliative laser therapy of advanced esophageal carcinoma: an alternative perspective. Am J Gastroenterol 1988; 83(8):816–819.

37. Loizou LA, Grigg D, Atkinson M, Robertson C, Bown SG. A prospective comparison of laser therapy and intubation in endoscopic palliation for malignant dysphagia. Gastroenterology 1991; 100:1303–1310.

38. Knyrim K, Wagner HJ, Bethge N, Keymling M, Vakil N. A controlled trial of an expansile metal stent for palliation of esophageal obstruction due to inoperable cancer. N Engl J Med 1993; 329:1302–1307.

39. Wagner HJ, Stinner B, Schwerk WB, Hoppe M, Klose KJ. Nitinol prostheses for the treatment of inoperable malignant esophageal obstruction. J Vasc Interv Radiol 1994; 5:899–904.

40. Song HY, Do YS, Han YM, et al. Covered, expandable esophageal metallic stent tubes: experiences in 119 patients. Radiology 1994; 193:689–695.

41. Song HY, Choi KC, Kwon HC, Yang DH, Cho BH, Lee ST. Esophageal strictures: treatment with a new design of modified Gianturco stent. Work in progress. Radiology 1992; 184:729–734.

42. Watkinson AF, Ellul J, Entwisle K, Mason RC, Adam A. Esophageal carcinoma: initial results of palliative treatment with covered self-expanding endoprostheses. Radiology 1995; 195:821–827.

43. Saxon RR, Barton RE, Katon RM, et al. Treatment of malignant esophageal obstructions with covered metallic Z-stents: long-term results in 52 patients. J Vasc Interv Radiol 1995; 6:747–754.

44. Saxon RR, Barton RE, Katon R, et al. Treatment of malignant esophagorespiratory fistulas with silicone-covered metallic Z-stents. J Vasc Interv Radiol 1995: 6:237–242.

45. Payne WS. Surgical management of reflux-induced oesophageal stenoses: results in 101 patients. Br J Surg 1984; 71:971–973.

46. Benedict EB. Peptic stenosis of the esophagus: a study of 233 patients treated with bougienage, surgery, or both. Am J Dig Dis 1966; 11:761–770.

47. Miyayama S, Matsui O, Kadoya M, et al. Malignant esophageal stricture and fistula: palliative treatment with polyurethane-covered Gianturco stent. J Vasc Interv Radiol 1995; 6:243–248.

48. Randall GM, Jensen DM. Diagnosis and management of bleeding from upper gastrointestinal neoplasms. Gastrointest Endosc Clin North Am 1991; 1:401–427.

49. Cwikiel W, Stridbeck H, Tranberg KG, et al. Malignant esophageal strictures: treatment with a self-expanding Nitinol stent. Radiology 1993; 187:661–665.

50. Kinsman KJ, DeGregorio BT, Katon RM, et al. Prior radiation and chemotherapy increase the risk of life-threatening complications after insertion of metallic stents for esophagogastric malignancy. Gastrointest Endosc 1996; 43:196–203.

TUTORIAL 18
DIAGNOSTIC IMAGING OF URINARY TRACT OBSTRUCTION

Philip J. Kenney, M.D.

Introduction

The subjects addressed in this tutorial include:

1. Definition of obstructive uropathy
2. Pathophysiology of acute and chronic obstruction
3. Urography of acute and chronic obstruction
4. Role of urography in obstruction
5. Sonography in obstruction
6. Computed tomography scanning in obstruction
7. Nuclear medicine in obstruction
8. Magnetic resonance imaging in obstruction.

Urinary tract obstruction is a common urologic problem that demands prompt and accurate diagnosis and intervention to avoid permanent damage to the kidney. Knowledge of the underlying pathophysiology of obstruction helps in interpreting the resultant imaging features, and provides a foundation for evaluating the strengths and weaknesses of the various imaging methods available.

For diagnosis and treatment of urinary tract obstruction three key questions must be answered: Is there in fact obstruction? What is the site of obstruction? What is the cause of the obstruction? If all three questions cannot be answered with one diagnostic test, appropriate additional testing must be performed. The interventional radiologist must answer two other questions: Is the kidney salvageable? If so, what is the best approach for intervention? It may be best to treat the cause of the obstruction primarily; it may be best to relieve the obstruction by diversion; intervention from above or below the obstruction may be considered; surgical intervention may be best in some circumstances.

Diagnosis of urinary tract obstruction is not always straightforward. Nonobstructive processes may simulate the findings of obstruction. No single imaging procedure is infallible. This chapter will discuss the key diagnostic features of imaging of obstruction, primarily intravenous urography (IVU), sonography, and computed tomography (CT) scanning, with limited discussion of nuclear medicine techniques and magnetic resonance (MR) imaging. Discussion is focused on upper urinary tract obstruction—primarily ureteral obstruction and consequent changes in the kidney. Bladder outlet and urethral obstruction will not be addressed directly.

Causes of Nonobstructive Dilatation
• Postobstructive atrophy including old hydronephrosis of pregnancy • Extrarenal pelvis • Congenital megacalyces • Papillary necrosis • Reflux nephropathy • Acute infection (pyelonephritis) • Infrequent voiding • Diuretic state Water intoxication Diabetes insipidus • Neurogenic bladder • Prune belly syndrome

Figure 1.

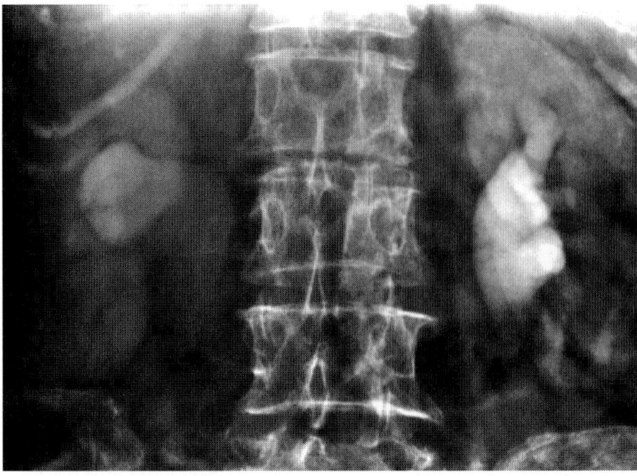

Figure 2. Urogram in an 82-year-old woman shows bilateral renal pelvic and calyceal dilatation.

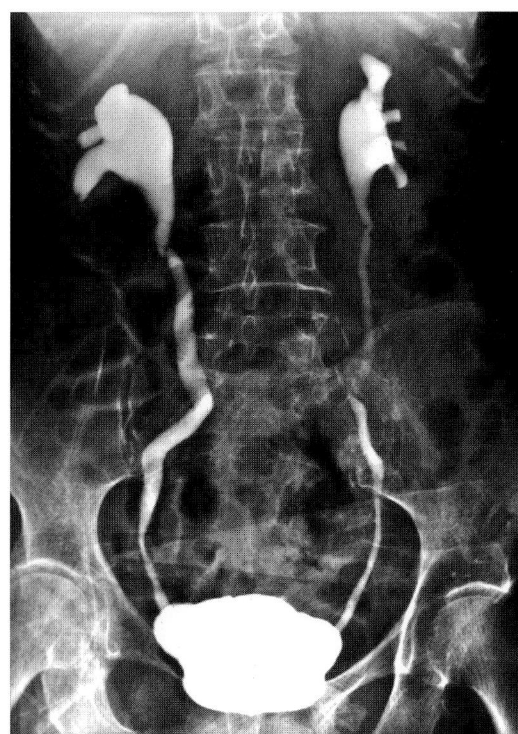

Figure 3. Same patient as in Figure 2. Voiding cystourethrogram shows reflux but no obstruction, suggesting a diagnosis of vesicoureteral reflux.

Obstructive Uropathy: Definitions

The term hydronephrosis is often considered to be synonymous with obstruction, but in common usage, hydronephrosis merely indicates dilatation of the collecting system, or pyelocaliectasis. Various nonobstructive causes can give rise to dilatation **(Figs. 1–7)**. The concept of urinary obstruction is somewhat subtle: complete obstruction virtually never exists; obstruction is partial to some degree, with the effect dependent on the rate of urine production. A low-grade obstruction may cause no problem except in high-flow states (just as a highway may only be congested during rush hour). Thus, the effect of a certain degree of obstruction can be different at different times. It is therefore very difficult to grade the degree of obstruction with imaging—a long-standing low-grade obstruction may look the same as a high-grade obstruction of short duration.

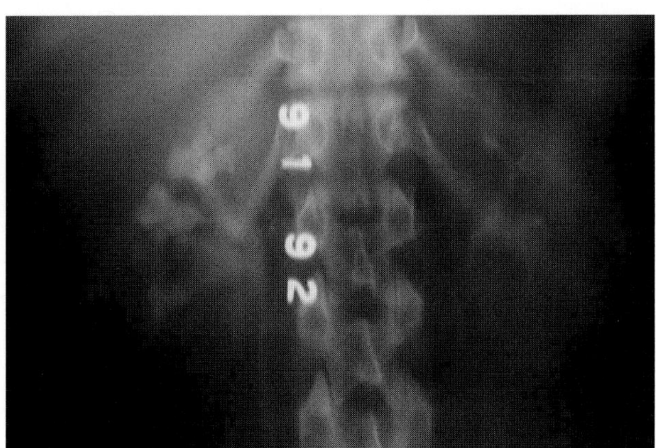

Figure 4. Early tomogram in an asymptomatic 21-year-old renal transplant donor shows a normal nephrogram and symmetric calyceal opacification bilaterally.

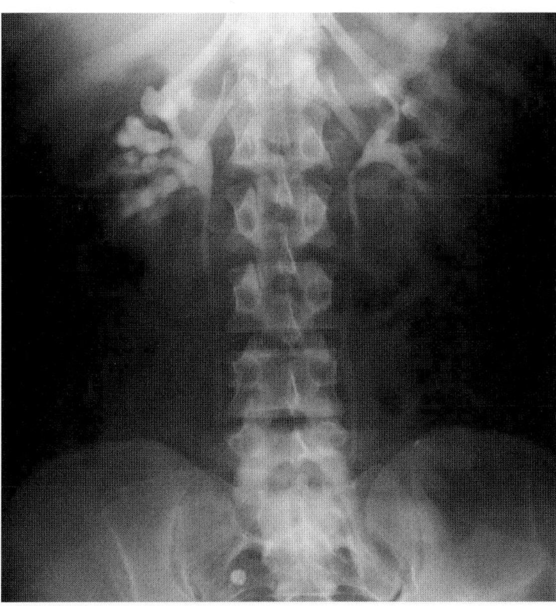

Figure 5. 15-minute film following the early tomogram in Figure 4 shows symmetric excretion with moderate right caliectasis. Renal function parameters, arteriography, and radionuclide nephrography were normal. The dilatation is due to congenital megacalyces.

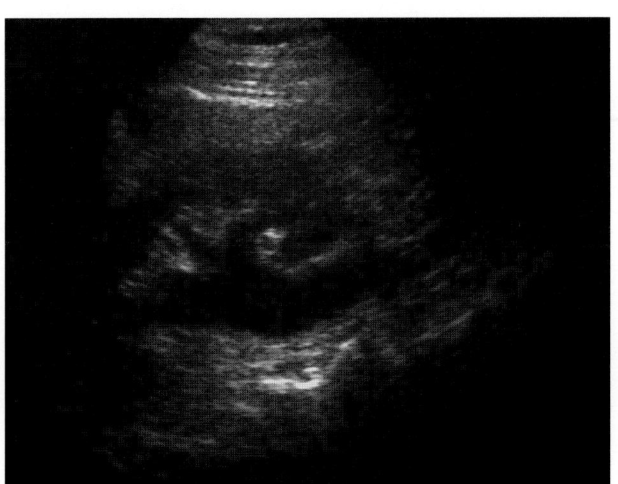

Figure 6. Nonobstructive dilatation in a 51-year-old man with neurogenic bladder. Longitudinal sonogram of the right kidney shows moderate pyelocaliectasis.

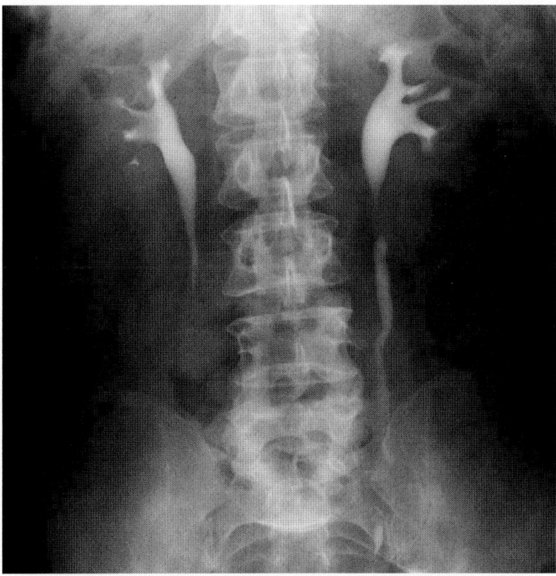

Figure 7. IVU following the sonogram in Figure 6 shows prompt symmetric excretion into capacious collecting systems; calyceal blunting is absent. Radionuclide scans and retrograde pyelograms were normal. The patient is presumed to have nonobstructive dilatation due to neurogenic bladder.

Classification of Obstructive Uropathy	
Mechanical	***Functional***
Congenital	Deficient emptying
Calculi	Vesicoureteral reflux
Clot, foreign body	Neurogenic bladder
Tumor	Bladder sphincter dyssynergia
Intrinsic, extrinsic	Diuretic state
Inflammatory	Water intoxication
Traumatic	Diabetes insipidus
Iatrogenic	

Figure 8.

Obstruction may be defined as a condition that reduces the rate of urine drainage below that of urine production, or in which pressure must be elevated to maintain urine drainage at the rate of production. Note that the latter definition implies that there may be compensated obstruction, which may only be detected by evaluating functional para-meters, or by reassessing periodically. Finally, while obstruction may be due to a mechanical lesion (one that results in a narrowing or compression), functional impairment of urine drainage in effect causes obstruction according to the above definitions **(Fig. 8)**.

Acute Obstruction: Physiology

Urine production is the result of renal blood flow (RBF), glomerular filtration (GF), tubular secretion, and tubular resorption. Urine passes by nephronic pressure, gravity, and ureteral peristalsis. Upper tract emptying is affected by bladder emptying—if the bladder cannot be emptied back pressure is eventually exerted on the upper tract even if the kidneys and ureters are intrinsically intact. With high-grade acute obstruction the pressure proximal to the obstruction increases as much as 50–70 mm Hg.

Peristalsis initially increases then diminishes and eventually fails when the pressure is so high the ureteral walls can no longer coapt. A standing column of urine then forms in the ureter to the point of the obstruction. RBF transiently increases, but with continued obstruction begins to fall. GF persists but filtration pressure is reduced because of the increased pelvic pressure. If the obstruction is not relieved, RBF, GF, and urine production continue to decline, largely due to vasoconstriction. In this manner, pelvic pressure returns to normal within several days to weeks.

Chronic Obstruction: Physiology and Pathology

Persistent obstruction results in destruction of renal parenchyma due to ischemia rather than elevated pressure. The kidney is affected overall but the medulla is more severely affected than the cortex. The changes of early acute obstruction are largely functional, but with chronic obstruction anatomic changes are seen, such as dilatation of the calyces, atrophy of papillae, and diffuse, smooth cortical thinning.

Factors Affecting Obstructive Atrophy

- Completeness of obstruction
- Duration of obstruction
- Anatomy of kidney
  Intrarenal versus extrarenal pelvis
- Urine production rate
- Infection
- Coexistent vascular disease

Figure 9.

Radiology of Obstructive Atrophy

- Loss of substance of renal papillae
- Symmetric thinning of renal parenchyma
- Dilatation of collecting system
  Degree of dilatation not equal to the degree of obstruction!!
- Difference in size from normal (usually smaller, may be larger)
- Decreased urine excretion

Figure 10.

Several factors, including the degree and duration of obstruction, determine the severity of the renal damage **(Fig. 9)**. A long-standing high-grade obstruction will cause the most damage; however, a high-grade obstruction of short duration may cause less damage than a long-standing low-grade obstruction. The amount of damage may also be modified by the anatomy of the kidney—an extrarenal pelvis can dilate, reducing the effect on the kidney. If the rate of urine production is high, the damage may be more severe. Coexistent vascular disease or superimposed infection results in more damage than would be seen with the same degree of obstruction alone. These factors account in part for the difficulty in determining the degree of obstruction.

If a poorly functioning kidney with a low rate of urine production becomes obstructed, little dilatation may be seen despite a high-grade obstruction. A very high-grade obstruction may cause less severe dilatation than a long-standing lower-grade obstruction, because the renal function and urine production will be less severely reduced in the latter situation. As a result, the degree of obstruction cannot be predicted accurately solely from the degree of dilatation seen on imaging studies.

Urography of Chronic Obstruction

The IVU findings of chronic obstruction match well with the pathologic anatomy described above **(Fig. 10)**.[1] Chronic obstruction results in loss of substance of the renal papillae, symmetric thinning of the renal parenchyma (with a smooth cortical surface), dilatation of the collecting system, and diminished urine excretion, usually evident as diminished excretion of contrast material. The obstructed kidney usually has a different size than the contralateral normal kidney. It is most often small and smooth, although it may be larger from normal if the hydronephrosis is very voluminous. Occasionally, it may be normal in size.

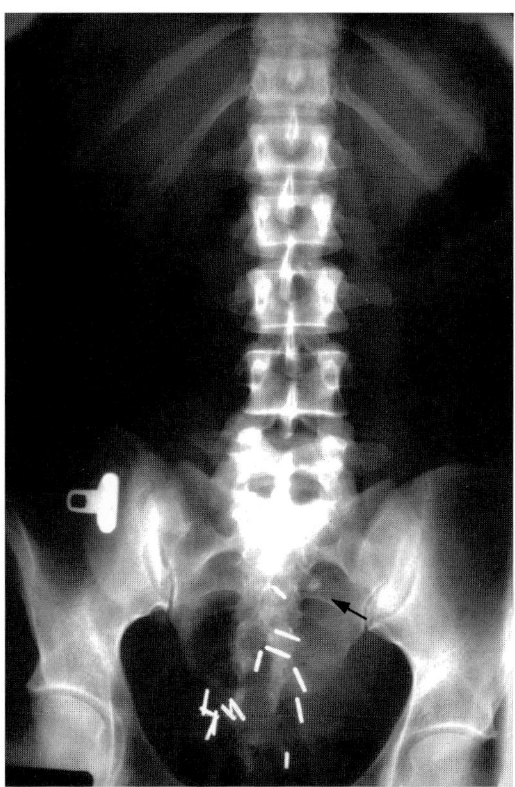

Figure 11. Scout radiograph in a 45-year-old with a history of hyperparathyroidism and colectomy for ulcerative colitis shows calcification overlying the left sacral ala (arrow).

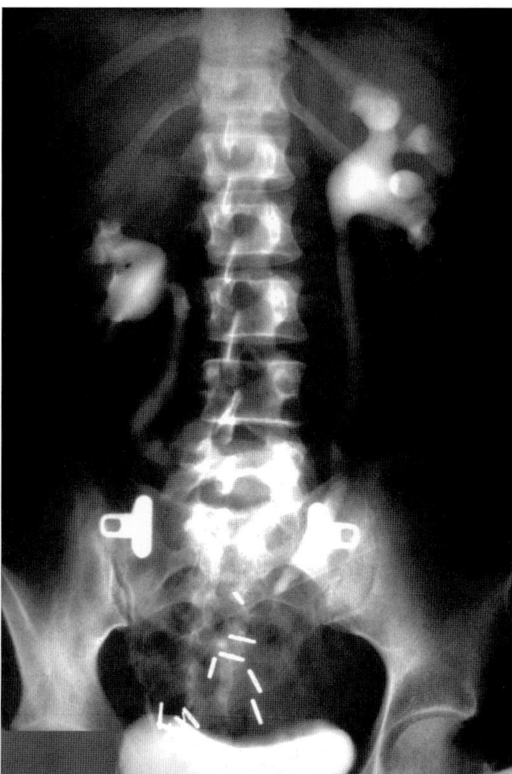

Figure 12. Same patient as in Figure 11. IVU shows distention of the renal pelvis and ureters bilaterally.

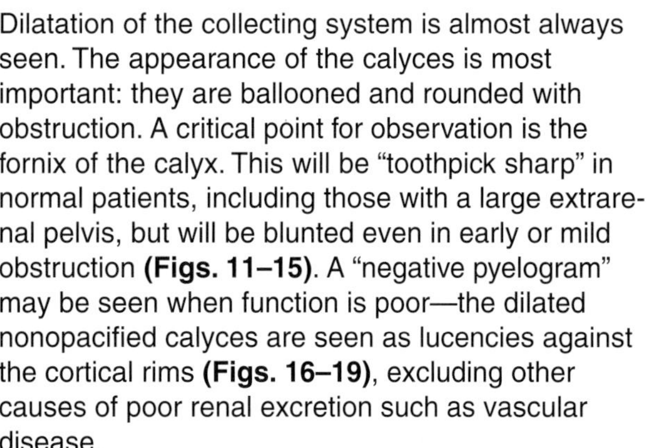

Dilatation of the collecting system is almost always seen. The appearance of the calyces is most important: they are ballooned and rounded with obstruction. A critical point for observation is the fornix of the calyx. This will be "toothpick sharp" in normal patients, including those with a large extrarenal pelvis, but will be blunted even in early or mild obstruction **(Figs. 11–15)**. A "negative pyelogram" may be seen when function is poor—the dilated nonopacified calyces are seen as lucencies against the cortical rims **(Figs. 16–19)**, excluding other causes of poor renal excretion such as vascular disease.

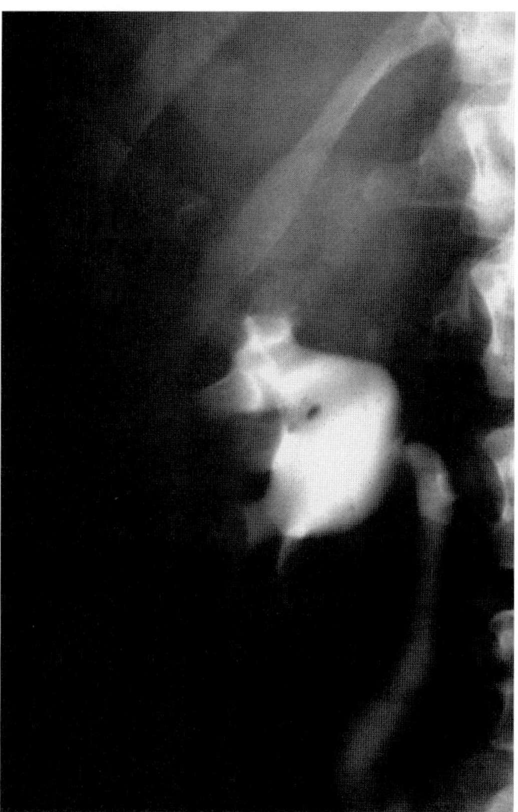

Figure 13. Same patient as in Figure 11. Fornices of the calyces on the right are sharp.

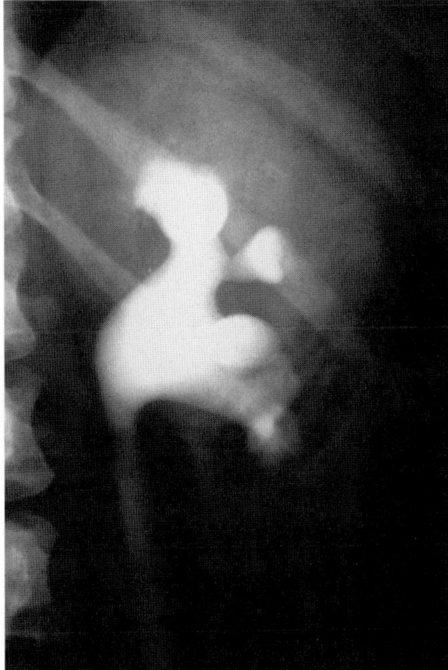

Figure 14. Same patient as in Figure 11. The left collecting system shows caliectasis with blunted fornices.

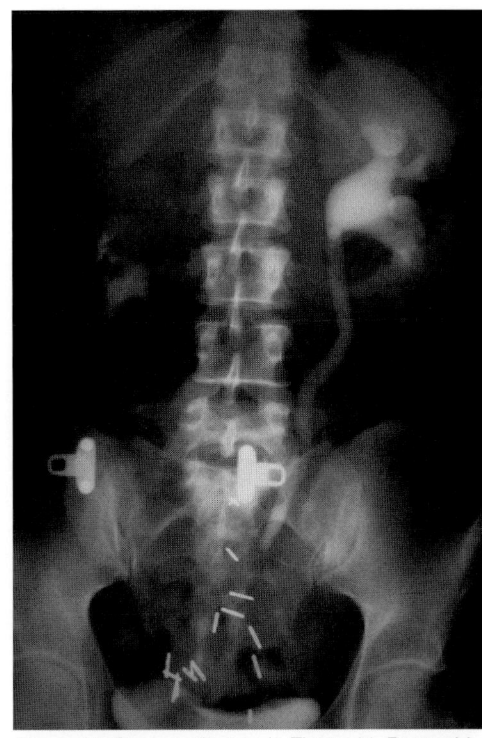

Figure 15. Same patient as in Figure 11. Post-void radiograph demonstrates persistent columning of the left ureter due to the calculus with normal drainage on the right.

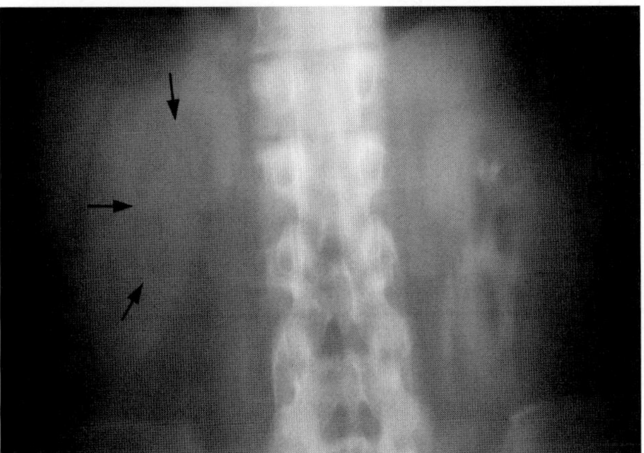

Figure 16. Chronic obstruction in an 85-year-old man with right-sided pain. An early tomogram shows no filling of the calyces on the right; the nephrogram is virtually normal compared to the left. A "negative pyelogram" is seen due to lucent dilated calyces (arrows).

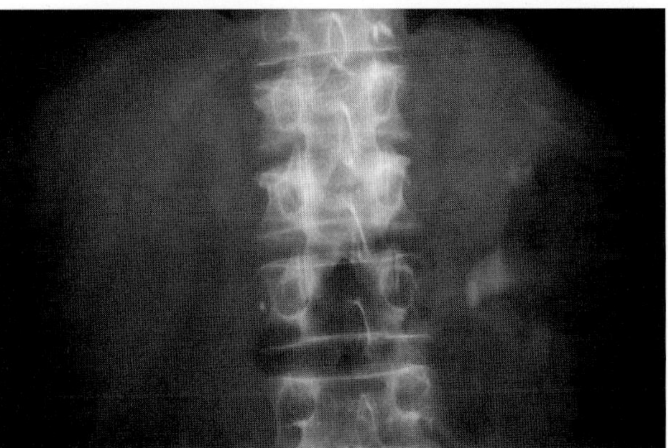

Figure 17. Same patient as in Figure 16. Five-minute film shows delayed pelvic filling on the right; the nephrogram is not increasing in density.

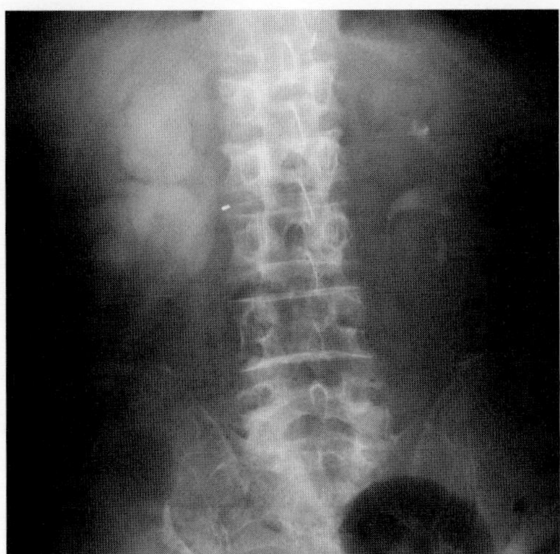

Figure 18. Same patient as in Figure 16. Twelve-hour film after the initial film shows filling of the dilated pelvis and calyces.

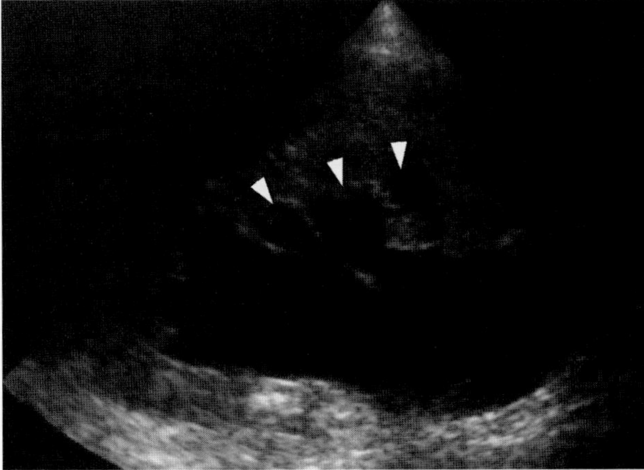

Figure 19. Same patient as in Figure 16. Sonogram of the right kidney also shows hydronephrosis. The calyces (arrowheads) communicate with the dilated pelvis. The patient was diagnosed with a ureteral stricture.

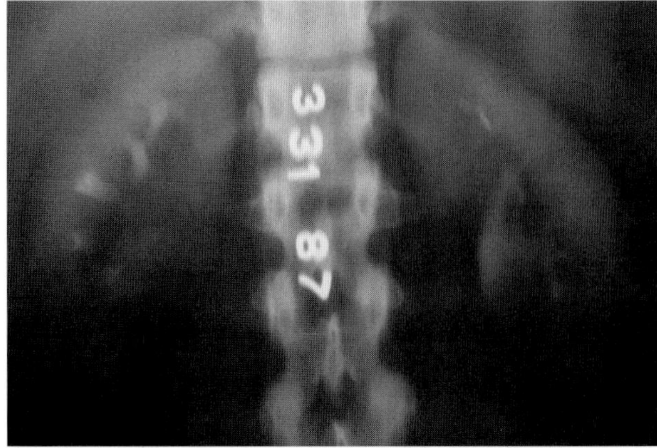

Figure 20. Chronic low-grade obstruction in a 31-year-old woman with intermittent right flank pain. An early tomogram shows normal and symmetric nephrograms and renal size bilaterally, but delayed filling of the right pelvis is noted.

Note that with chronic obstruction the nephrogram is usually normal to faint (because of reduced GF), but a hyperdense "obstructive nephrogram" is not seen **(Figs. 20–22)**.

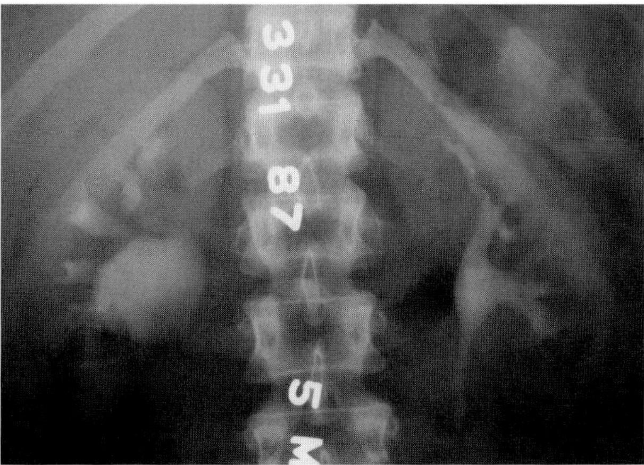

Figure 21. Same patient as in Figure 20. At 5 minutes, pyelocaliectasis persists on the right with no ureteral filling.

The key diagnostic features are parenchymal thinning, dilatation of the calyces, and loss of renal function. Cases of nonobstructive dilatation may seem to show obstruction on IVU, particularly in cases of postobstructive atrophy, bladder outlet obstruction, or congenital megacalyces. In general, however, significant obstruction can be excluded if the time of collecting system opacification is symmetric compared to the normal side, and if drainage of the upper tract can be seen on delayed post-voiding views. If enough renal function remains to opacify the ureter, persistent dilatation to the point of obstruction will be present. However, IVU often does not demonstrate this adequately.

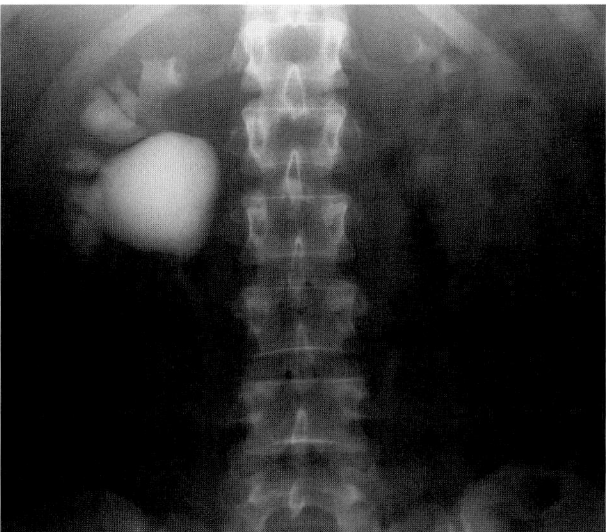

Figure 22. Same patient as in Figure 20. Delayed film shows lack of drainage on the right and mild cortical thinning, suggesting a diagnosis of ureteropelvic junction obstruction.

Urography of Acute Obstruction

The IVU findings of acute obstruction are very different from those of chronic obstruction. Minimal if any dilatation of the collecting system is seen. The primary findings are alterations in the pattern of contrast material excretion due to the physiologic changes. The immediate nephrogram may be slightly diminished as a result of the decreased filtration pressure, but an increasingly dense "obstructive nephrogram" is soon seen, although the nephrogram itself is not delayed. The nephrogram may have a striated appearance **(Figs. 23–26)**, resulting from the sluggish passage of opacified urine through the tubules, with increased resorption of fluid (in an attempt to reduce the pressure) that causes hyperconcentration in the collecting ducts. Ureteral peristalsis has usually failed, so opacification of the collecting system and ureter is slow, resulting in delayed visualization of the calyces, pelvis, and ureter compared to the nonobstructed contralateral side.

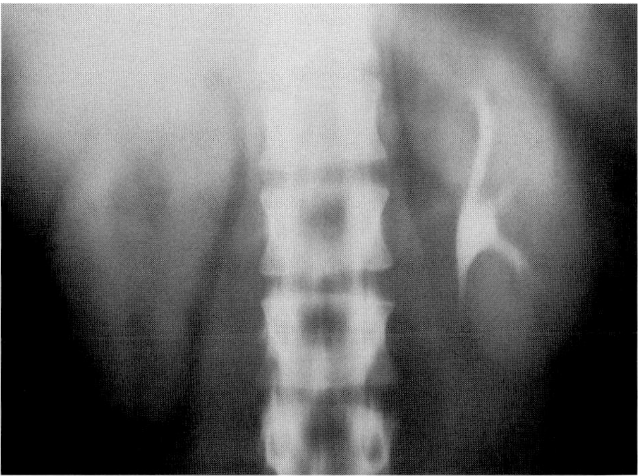

Figure 23. Acute obstruction in a young man with the sudden onset of flank pain. An immediate tomogram shows delayed calyceal filling on the right.

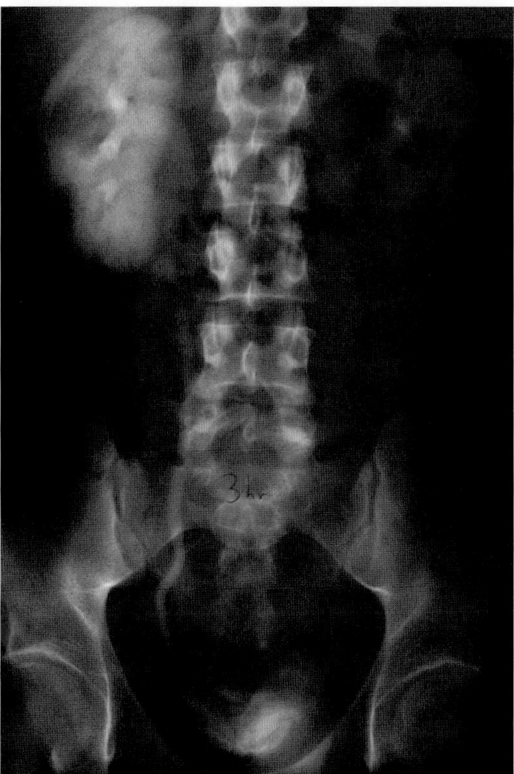

Figure 25. Same patient as in Figure 23. With further delay, columning of the ureter is seen to the level of a calculus.

Causes of Increasingly Dense Nephrogram

- Acute extrarenal obstruction
- Systemic hypotension
- Main renal artery stenosis
- Intratubular blockade
  Tamm-Horsfall protein, uric acid, multiple myeloma
- Acute tubular necrosis (rare)
- Renal vein thrombosis (only acute)

Figure 27.

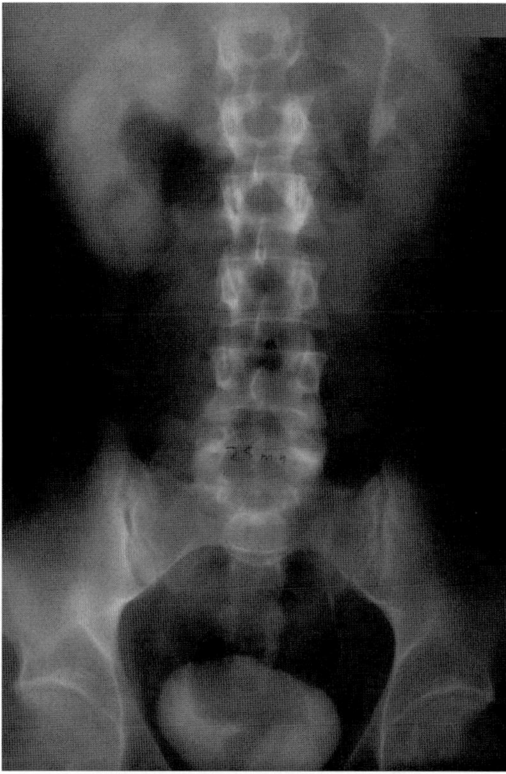

Figure 24. Same patient as in Figure 23. Delayed view shows a persistent, increasingly dense nephrogram.

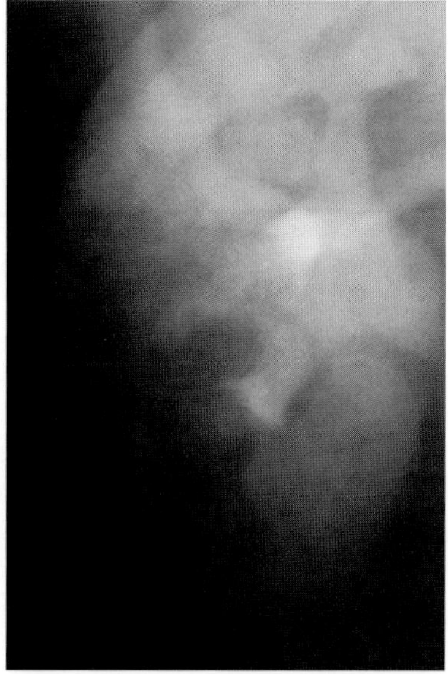

Figure 26. Same patient as in Figure 23. Note the striated appearance of the dense nephrogram and minimal caliectasis.

When an increasingly dense nephrogram is seen in a patient with acute flank pain, acute ureteral obstruction is most likely present, although some other conditions can cause this nephrographic pattern **(Fig. 27)**. The ureter will opacify eventually, permitting detection of the location and cause of obstruction, but this may take hours. Pyelosinus extravasation is seen in 5% of patients with acute obstruction.[2]

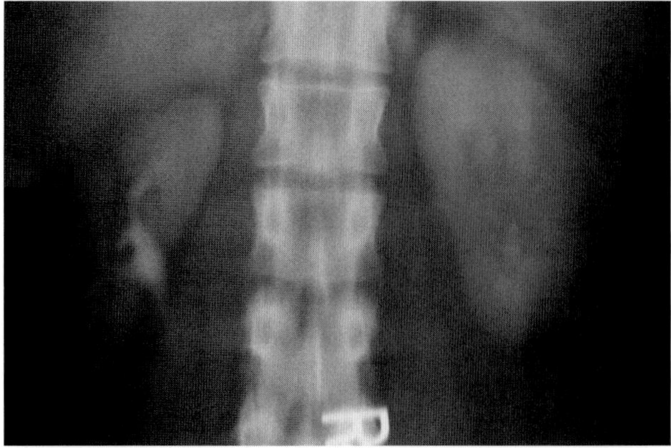

Figure 28. Acute obstruction in a 32-year-old with the acute onset of left-sided colicky pain and hematuria. An early tomogram shows delayed calyceal filling on the left and a dense nephrogram.

If the pelvic pressure rises high enough, the forniceal angle becomes disrupted, permitting leakage of urine into the renal sinus (pyelosinus backflow). This leakage may outline the ureter **(Figs. 28–30)**, and may be picked up by lymphatics (pyelolymphatic backflow) or veins (pyelovenous backflow). This phenomenon actually protects the system by reducing the pressure above the obstruction. It does not appear to inhibit the passage of stones, and may in fact improve it, as ureteral peristalsis may be restored. As long as the obstruction is relieved, this extravasation does not lead to harmful sequelae.

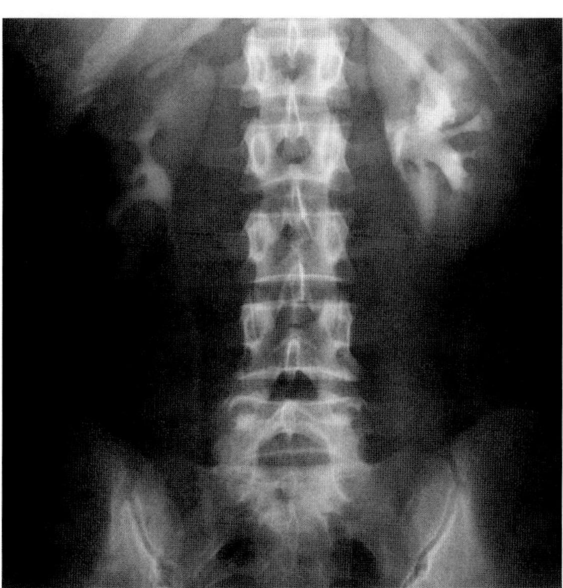

Figure 29. Same patient as in Figure 28. 10-minute film shows an increasingly dense nephrogram with some calyceal filling.

Role of Urography

IVU has certain advantages in the evaluation of obstructive uropathy. It is relatively inexpensive, widely available at all hours, and can usually identify acute or chronic obstruction. However, it does expose the patient to both radiation and iodinated contrast material. Visualization of the collecting system and ureter depends on renal function. Therefore, with chronic obstruction, the site and cause of the obstruction may not be determined, even if hydronephrosis is detected. It is sometimes difficult to determine on IVU whether a kidney is poorly functioning due to obstruction or other disease **(Figs. 31–33)**. Salvageability of the kidney is not easily predicted by IVU. Very thin parenchyma (<1 cm) and the absence of excretion would weigh against salvageability, while prompt visualization and normal parenchymal thickness (2.5–3.5 cm) are good signs.

IVU may be most cost-effective in assessing acute obstruction, particularly renal colic in patients with suspected calculi. Because IVU can show functional changes, most cases of significant obstruction will be detected. Most calculi are radiopaque, and the location and size of the stone can usually be determined, leading to appropriate management of the patient. However, IVU may be indeterminate in patients with ureteral calculi that cause minimal or no obstruction.

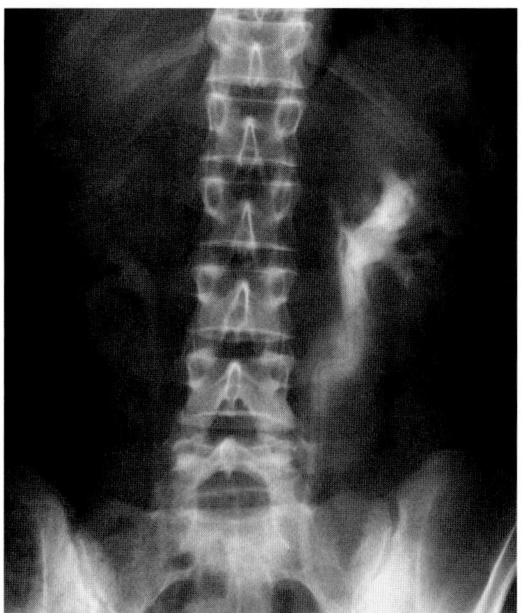

Figure 30. Same patient as in Figure 28. Delayed film reveals extravasation of contrast material into the renal sinus tracking outside the ureter, suggesting a diagnosis of acute obstruction due to ureteral calculus with spontaneous extravasation.

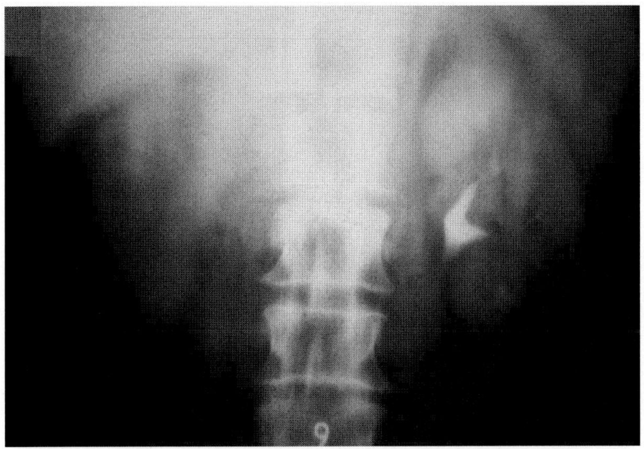

Figure 31. False-positive IVU in a 52-year-old man with right flank pain and hematuria. The urogram shows a persistent nephrogram on the right with delayed calyceal filling; the study seemed to indicate probable obstruction.

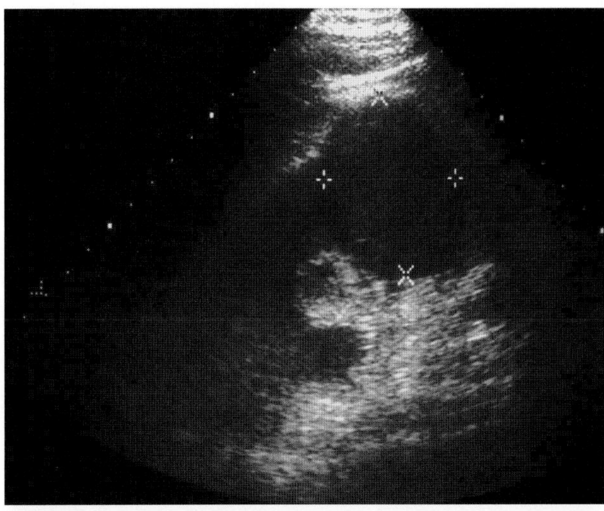

Figure 32. Same patient as in Figure 31. Sonogram shows a solid mass but no hydronephrosis.

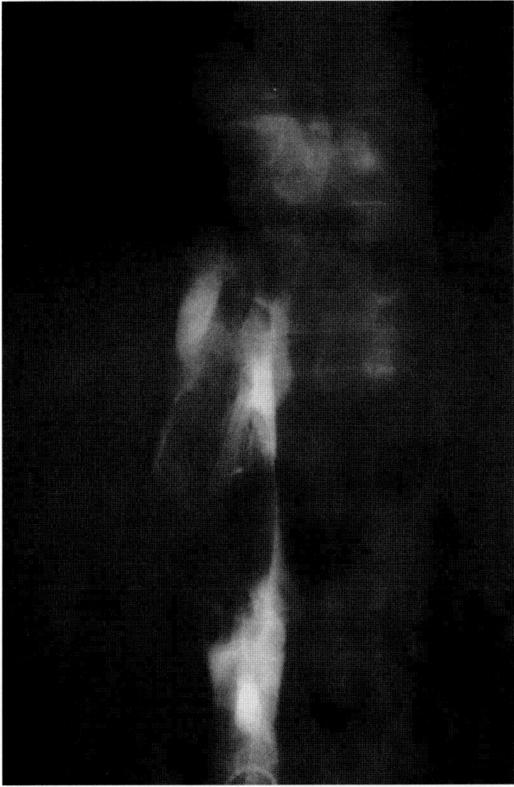

Figure 33. Same patient as in Figure 31. Inferior vena cavogram demonstrates tumor thrombosis extending into the renal vein. The patient was ultimately diagnosed with renal carcinoma with renal vein and caval extension.

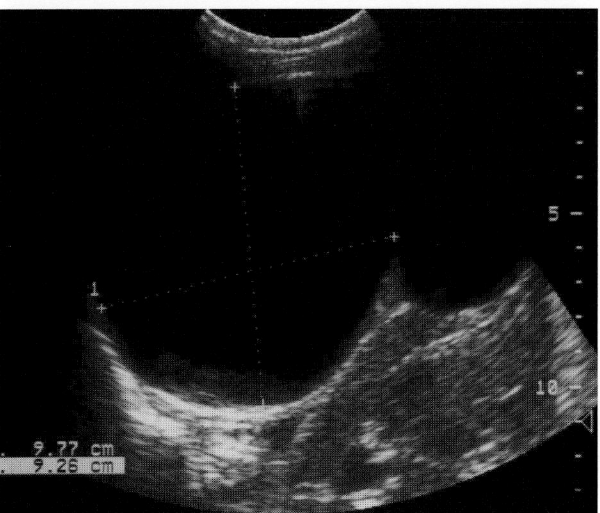

Figure 34. Chronic obstruction in a 25-year-old pregnant woman with proteinuria. A longitudinal sonogram of the right kidney shows marked hydronephrosis and cortical thinning; the ureter was not dilated. The patient was believed to have congenital ureteropelvic junction obstruction.

Sonography of Obstructive Uropathy

Ultrasound (US) is an extremely useful diagnostic tool for evaluating urinary tract obstruction. It can detect dilatation of the collecting system without the use of contrast material **(Fig. 34)**. Any separation (fluid filling) of the pelvis raises the possibility of obstruction, because the pelvis will be empty in a normal patient who is not in a diuretic state. US has been shown to be 98% sensitive for detecting hydronephrosis in patients with azotemia.[3] US can therefore distinguish obstruction from other causes of renal failure. Renal length and parenchymal thickness can be accurately measured and followed with US. The US grading of pyelocaliectasis into mild, moderate, and severe does appear to correlate fairly well with urographic appearances.[2]

Causes of Sonographic False Positives for Obstruction	
Extrarenal pelvis	Vesicoureteral reflux
Full bladder	Postobstructive dilatation
Renal blood vessels	Congenital megacalyces
Diuretic state	Papillary necrosis
Multiple cortical cysts	Chronic pyelonephritis
Multiple parapelvic cysts	Prune belly syndrome
Multicystic dysplasia	Acute infection (pyelonephritis)

Figure 35.

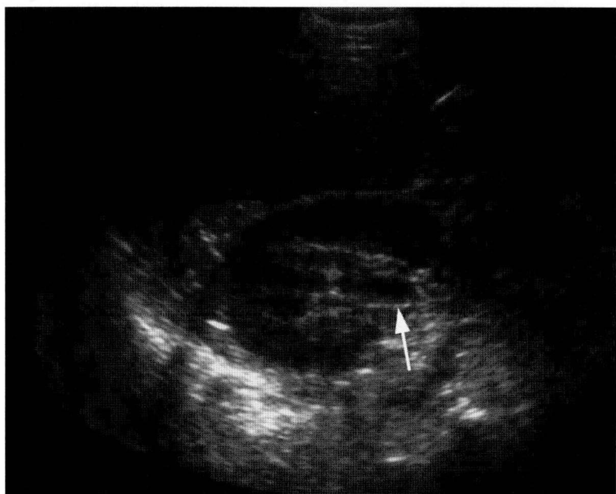

Figure 36. Transverse view of the right kidney shows possible dilatation of the pelvis (arrow).

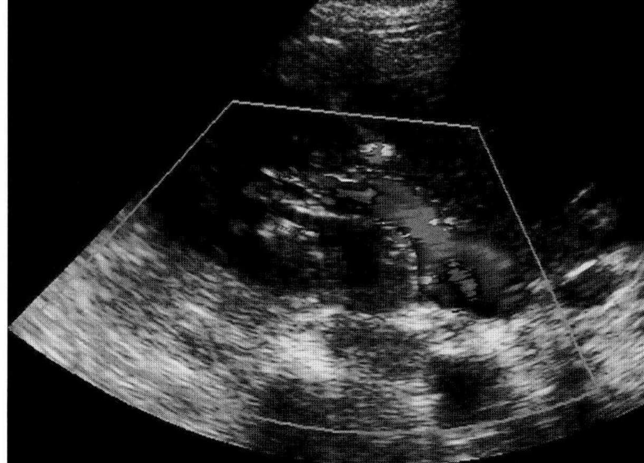

Figure 37. Same patient as in Figure 36. Color Doppler view reveals that the apparent "pelvis" is the distended renal vein.

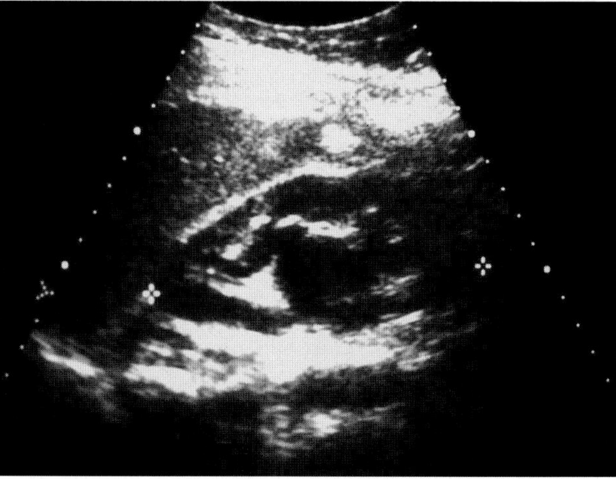

Figure 38. False-positive sonogram in a 40-year-old woman with left flank pain. A central fluid-filled structure is thought to be hydronephrosis.

However, reliance on the primary finding of dilatation of the collecting system results in inaccuracies. The high sensitivity of US is achieved at the expense of poor specificity; false-positive rates of up to 26% have been reported.[2] Numerous causes of sonographic false positives for hydronephrosis can be found **(Fig. 35)**, most notably nonobstructive dilatation of the collecting system and cystic lesions **(Figs. 36–41)**. Because the degree of dilatation does not correlate with the degree of obstruction, US is not good at indicating the severity of obstruction; in particular, high-grade obstruction with minimal dilatation may be missed.

While US is usually able to indicate the presence of obstruction, the etiology cannot often be elucidated **(Figs. 42–44)**. Calculi may be seen if they lie in the pelvis, or in the very proximal or very distal ureter, where the bladder acts as a sonographic window **(Figs. 45–52)**. However, calculi or other obstructive lesions affecting the mid ureter are usually obscured by bone and gas, especially in adults. US can indicate the likelihood of obstruction, but some other study is needed to answer the key questions.

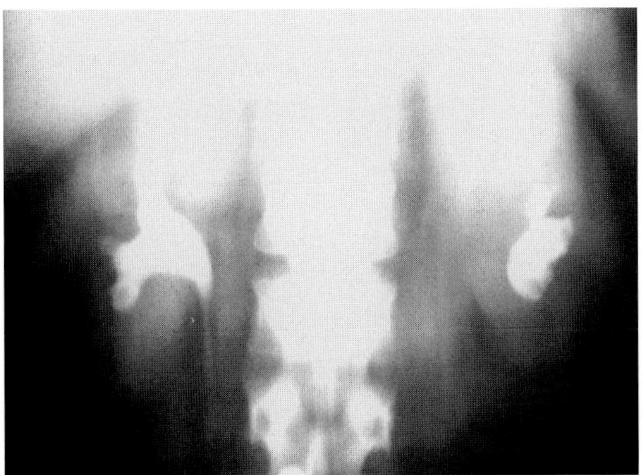

Figure 39. Same patient as in Figure 38. Urogram shows compression of the left renal pelvis by an extrinsic mass.

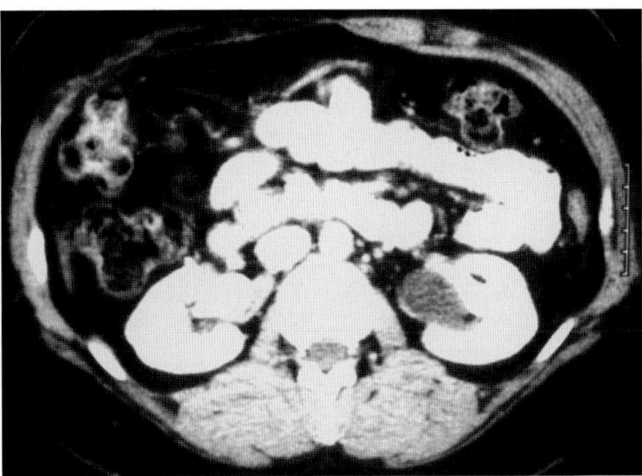

Figure 40. Same patient as in Figure 38. CT scan reveals a parapelvic cyst.

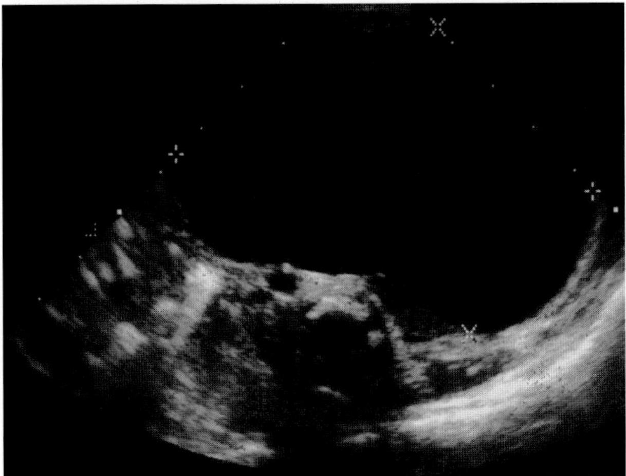

Figure 41. False-positive sonogram in a neonate with a palpable left flank mass. Sonogram of the left renal bed shows an ovoid fluid-filled structure with no clearly seen renal parenchyma; this was thought to be severe ureteropelvic junction obstruction and was diagnosed at surgery as multicystic dysplastic kidney.

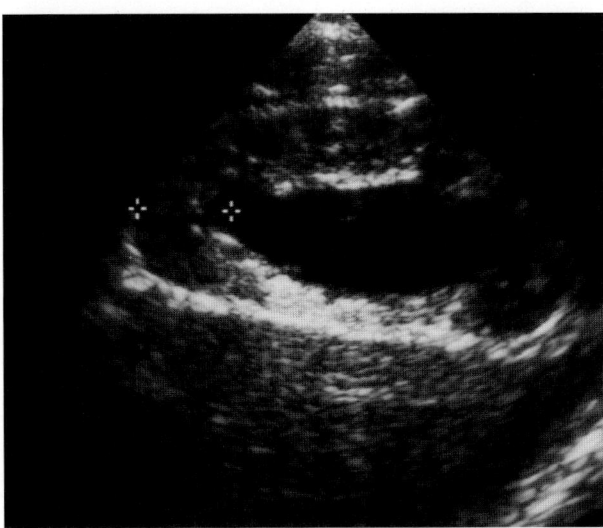

Figure 42. Chronic obstruction in a 1-year-old boy. A sonogram shows marked right hydronephrosis. The cortex measures 11 mm.

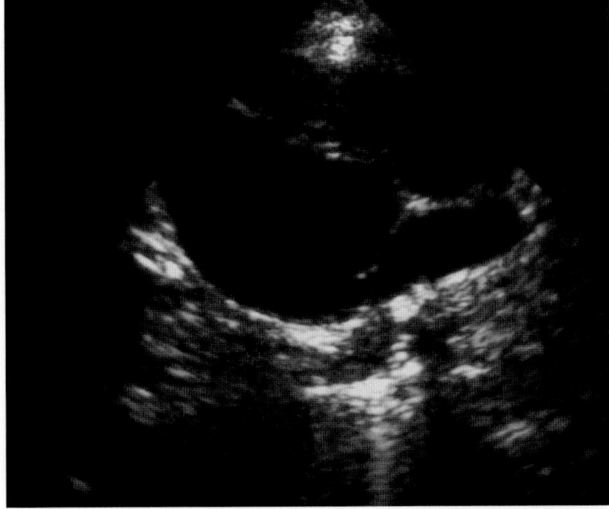

Figure 43. Same patient as in Figure 42. The proximal ureter is dilated but the obstructing lesion is obscure.

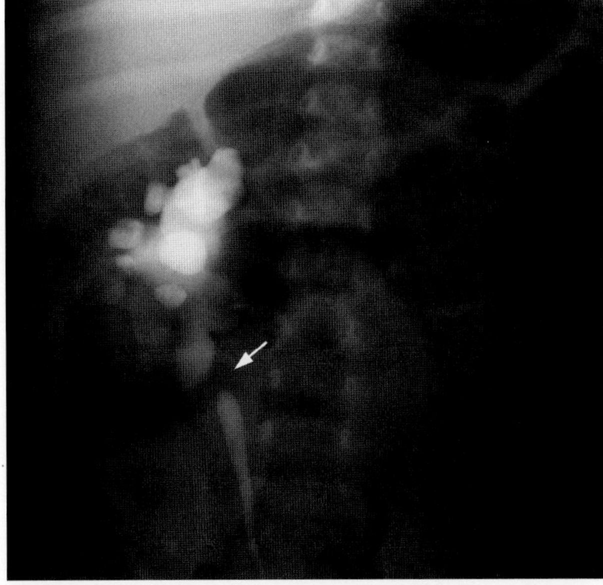

Figure 44. Same patient as in Figure 42. Retrograde pyelogram demonstrates a congenital ureteral stricture (arrow).

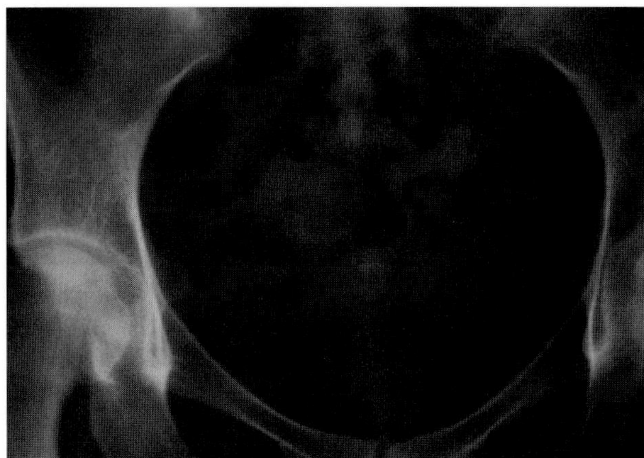

Figure 45. Minimal obstruction in a 24-year-old woman with intermittent pain and hematuria. The scout film shows no definite calculus.

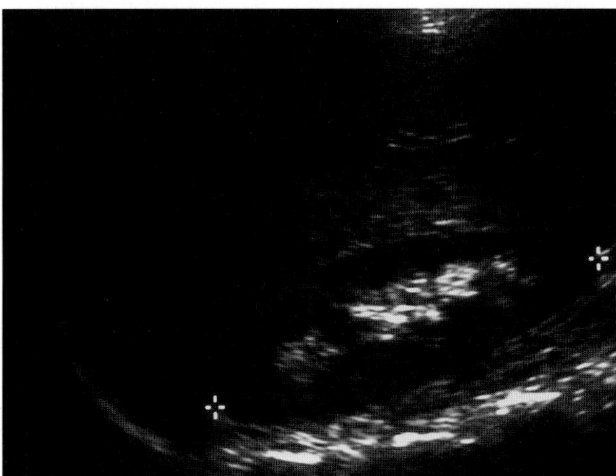

Figure 47. Same patient as in Figure 45. Sonogram of the right kidney is normal.

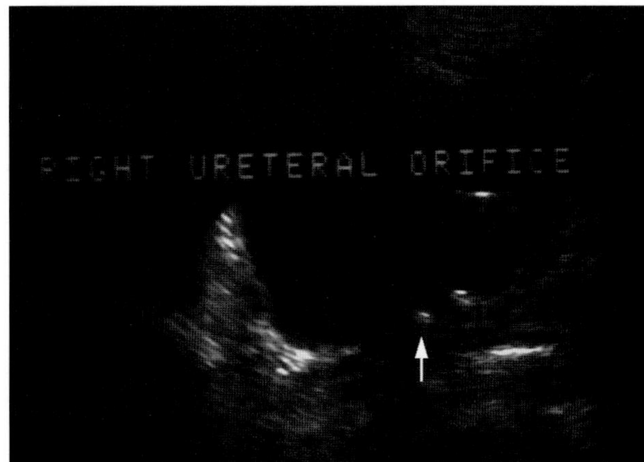

Figure 49. Same patient as in Figure 45. Sonogram of the bladder shows a right ureteral calculus (arrow).

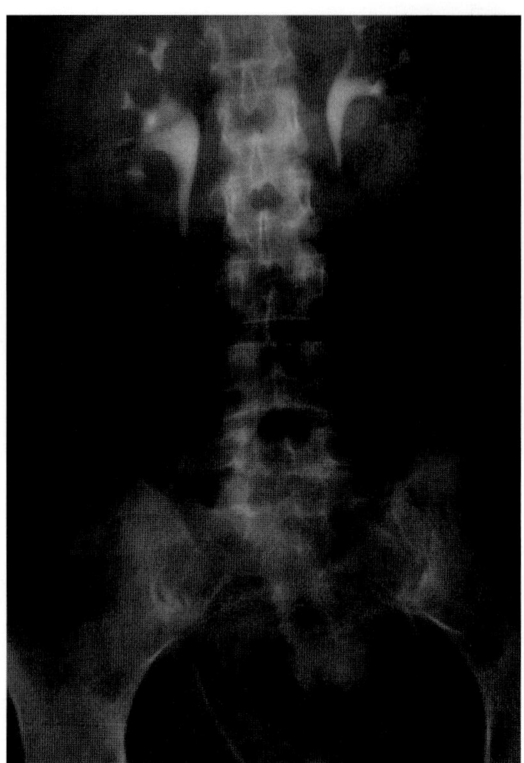

Figure 46. Same patient as in Figure 45. The IVU shows no significant obstruction.

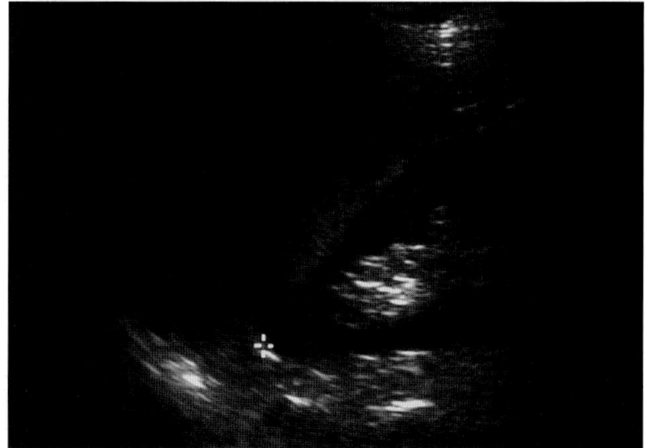

Figure 48. Same patient as in Figure 45. Sonogram of the left kidney is normal.

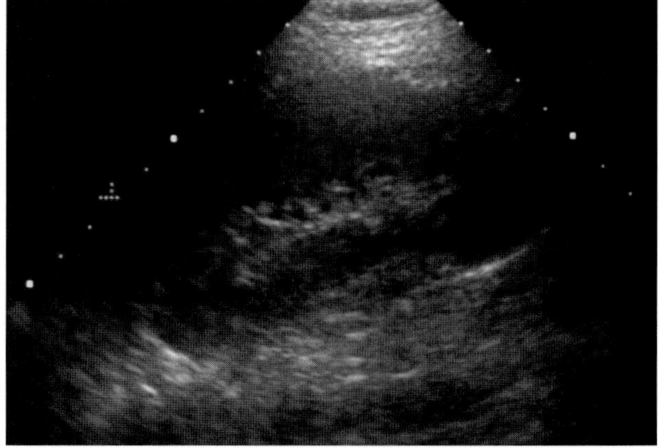

Figure 50. Acute obstruction in a 35-year-old woman with the acute onset of right lower quadrant pain. The left kidney is normal on sonography.

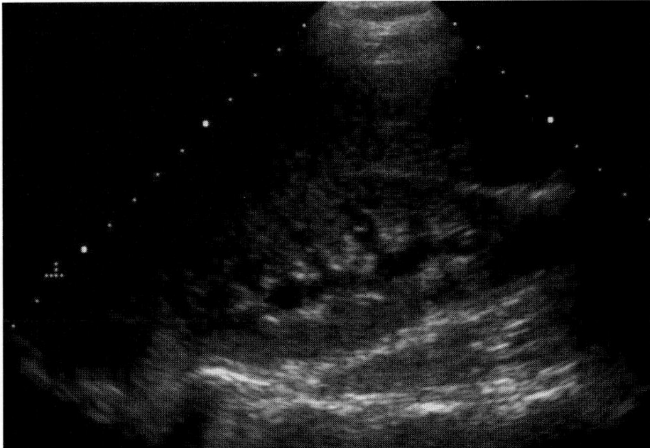

Figure 51. Same patient as in Figure 50. The right kidney shows moderate pyelocaliectasis.

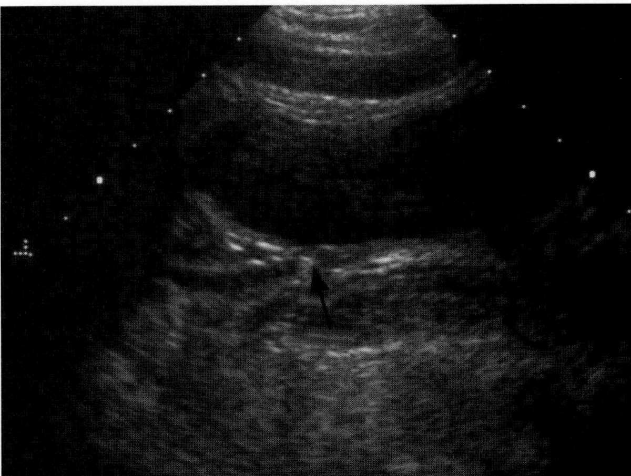

Figure 52. Same patient as in Figure 50. Longitudinal sonogram through the bladder shows a right ureterovesical junction calculus (arrow).

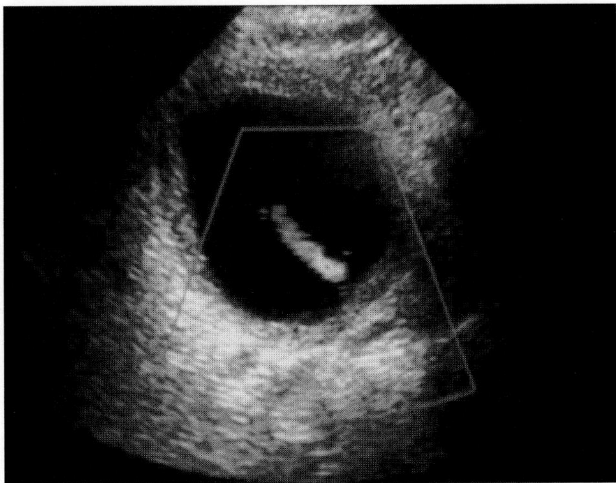

Figure 53. Transverse sonogram with color Doppler demonstrates a normal left ureteral jet.

Doppler Sonography of Ureteral Jets

The use of color Doppler US permits visualization of ureteral jets **(Fig. 53)**. The bolus of urine carried to the bladder by normal ureteral peristalsis causes an intermittent rush of urine that has a slightly different specific gravity compared to the static urine residing in the bladder. A "jet" of color flow is seen due to the velocity and specific gravity differences.[4,5]

Evaluation of these ureteral jets may be used as a diagnostic tool, because obstruction will reduce or eliminate the jet. The frequency of ureteral jets depends on the state of hydration; in one study the interval between jets varied from 2 to 150 seconds. A better parameter may be symmetry—the frequency should be nearly the same on both sides if normal, with the ratio between 1.0 and 1.2.[4] With use of these criteria, in a study of 17 normal patients and 26 patients with obstructing ureteral calculi, US identified all the normal patients correctly; absent or abnormal jets were seen in 16 patients with obstruction, but 10 of the obstructed patients had normal jets.[6]

Ureteral jets as diagnostic findings lack both sensitivity and specificity. With low-grade, partial obstruction, urine still passes the lesion—for instance, a stone—therefore, the jet may be normal. A false-negative rate of 21% for US was found in patients with partial obstruction due to calculi.[7] Conversely, a ureteral jet may be diminished or absent because of nonobstructive abnormalities, such as lack of urine production due to a vascular insult or infection of the kidney.

Resistive Index in Obstructive Uropathy

With Doppler technique, US can assess the vascular status of the kidney. Because obstruction alters RBF, assessment of the blood flow can help identify patients with obstruction. In particular, obstructive and nonobstructive pyelocaliectasis can be differentiated. Acute obstruction creates increased vascular resistance in the kidney, which is normally a low-resistance vascular bed with much diastolic flow. This can be shown by the resistive index (RI) (RI=peak systolic velocity minus end diastolic velocity divided by peak systolic velocity). Several studies have shown the RI to be less than 0.60 in normal kidneys.[8–10] Conversely, the RI in kidneys with acute obstruction has been shown to be over 0.70.[8,10]

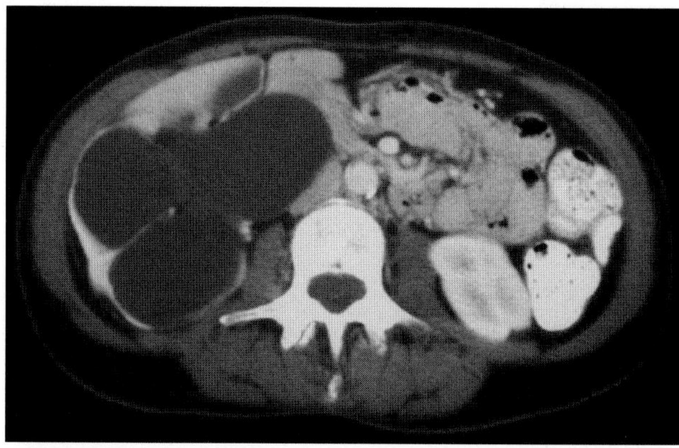

Figure 54. Chronic obstruction in an asymptomatic 61-year-old woman with a palpable right abdominal mass. Contrast-enhanced CT scan shows marked hydronephrosis with cortical thinning. The right ureter was not dilated. The patient was presumed to have congenital ureteropelvic junction obstruction.

In some studies the RI has been fairly accurate—92% sensitivity, 88% specificity—in detecting acute obstruction.[8] The RI was also found to be useful in distinguishing obstructive from nonobstructive dilatation in children (positive predictive value 95%, negative predictive value 100%).[10] However, in studies that included several patients with low-grade obstruction, accuracy was not as good; overall sensitivity of 52% was reported in a group of 33 patients with acute obstruction.[9] An animal model demonstrated no consistent change in RI in rabbits with partial obstruction.[11] In an attempt to enhance the detection of partial obstruction using the RI, some investigators have repeated measurement after injection of a diuretic. This did improve the accuracy, increasing sensitivity to 88% and specificity to 97%.[12]

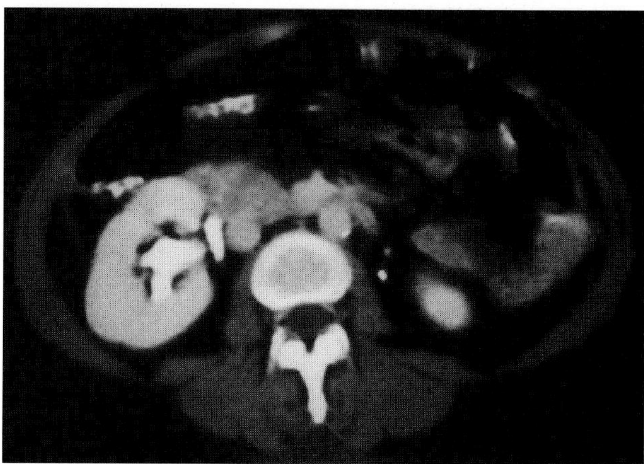

Figure 55. Extrinsic obstruction in a 38-year-old man with intermittent right flank pain. Contrast-enhanced CT scan shows mild pyelocaliectasis.

Role of Sonography

The advantages of US in evaluating obstructive uropathy include its relatively low cost, wide availability, and noninvasiveness. Because it does not expose the patient to radiation or iodinated contrast material, it is especially useful in children, pregnant women, and patients with renal insufficiency or other risk factors that preclude the use of contrast material. US is highly sensitive for the detection of obstruction, especially if the obstruction is high grade or of more than several days duration. US is particularly useful in chronic obstruction, since hydronephrosis is nearly always seen, and other methods such as urography are of limited use.

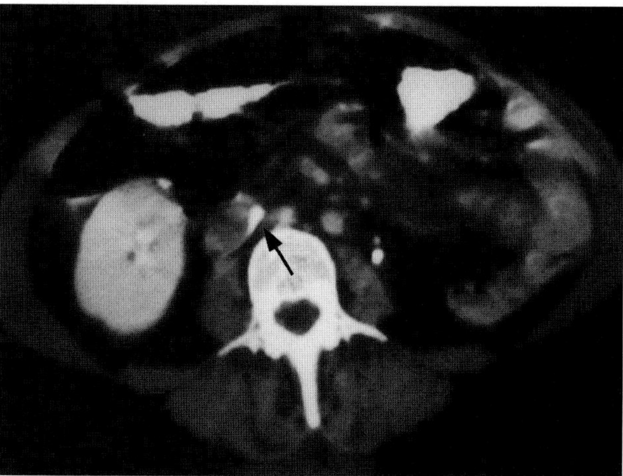

Figure 56. Same patient as in Figure 55. More inferiorly, the right ureter (arrow) courses posterior to the inferior vena cava.

The greatest disadvantages of US are its high rate of false positives and its low sensitivity for acute or low-grade obstruction. In acute obstruction, detectable caliectasis may not yet have developed. While the use of ureteral jets and RI may improve detection of acute obstruction without caliectasis, these parameters may be falsely negative with low-grade obstruction. The utility of the RI is also limited by two other factors: with long-standing obstruction, RBF diminishes and the RI may return to the normal range. More investigation is needed into this. More importantly, other disorders, such as transplant rejection, acute tubular necrosis, or infection, can also elevate the RI, resulting in potential confusion. Finally, the cause of obstruction often remains obscure on US, and salvageability of the kidney is difficult to assess, although the cortical thickness can be measured.

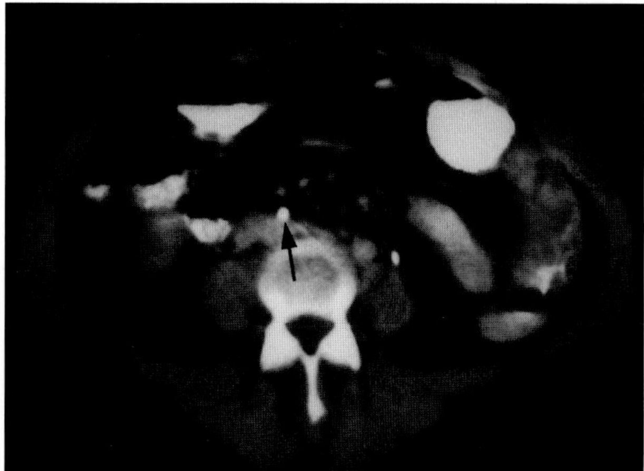

Figure 57. Same patient as in Figure 55. Further inferiorly, the right ureter (arrow) lies very medial. The patient was diagnosed with retrocaval ureter with low-grade chronic obstruction.

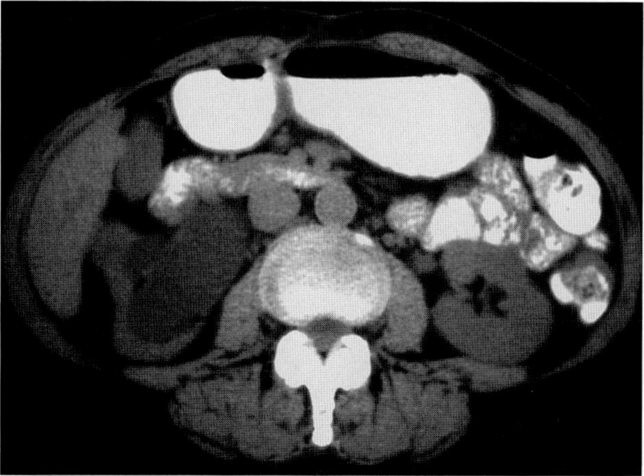

Figure 58. Extrinsic obstruction in a 54-year-old woman with a history of prior resection of colon carcinoma. Noncontrast CT scan shows marked right hydronephrosis.

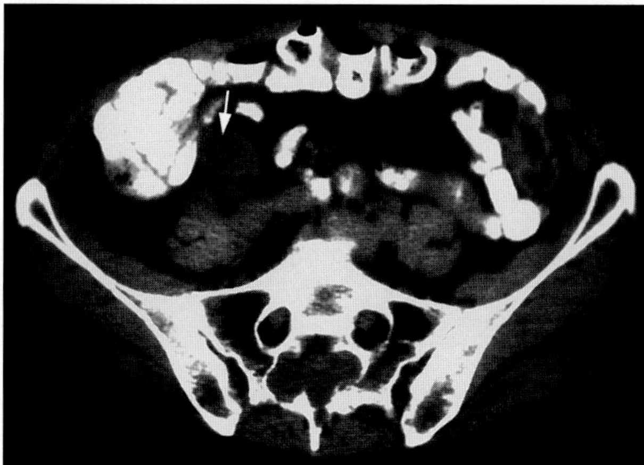

Figure 59. Same patient as in Figure 58. The nonopacified dilated right ureter can be seen easily (arrow).

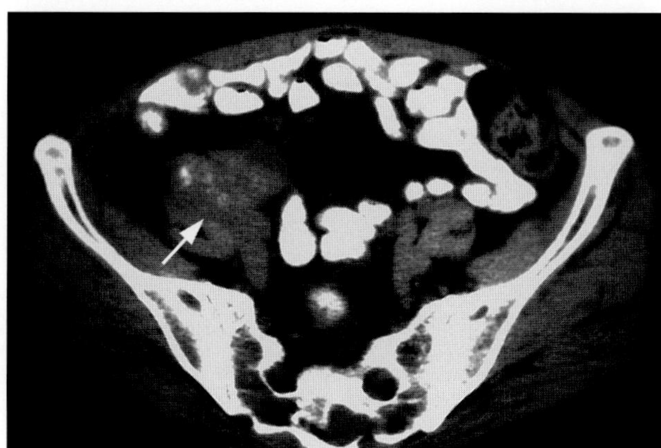

Figure 60. Same patient as in Figure 58. The dilated ureter leads to a calcified soft-tissue mass representing metastatic colon carcinoma (arrow).

CT Evaluation of Obstructive Uropathy

CT can be a very powerful noninvasive imaging tool for investigation of suspected urinary tract obstruction. It can show both anatomic changes and changes in the excretion of contrast material; it reveals not only all parts of the urinary tract but also all adjacent structures. Some modification of technique may be needed in patients with obstructive uropathy. If noncontrast views are not obtained, calculi may be missed because they can be obscured by contrast material. Delayed views may help to document the point of obstruction by allowing time for contrast material to fill dilated ureters. Reformatting may help to demonstrate the location of the lesion more graphically.

The anatomic changes of chronic obstruction are readily seen even on noncontrast CT scans: thinning of the renal parenchyma and dilatation of the collecting system and ureter **(Figs. 54)**. The nonopacified ureter can be followed to the point of obstruction even on noncontrast images. CT scanning is particularly useful when function is very poor, and it permits differentiation of intrinsic from extrinsic causes of obstruction **(Figs. 55–60)**. Abnormal excretion can be seen with the use of contrast material.

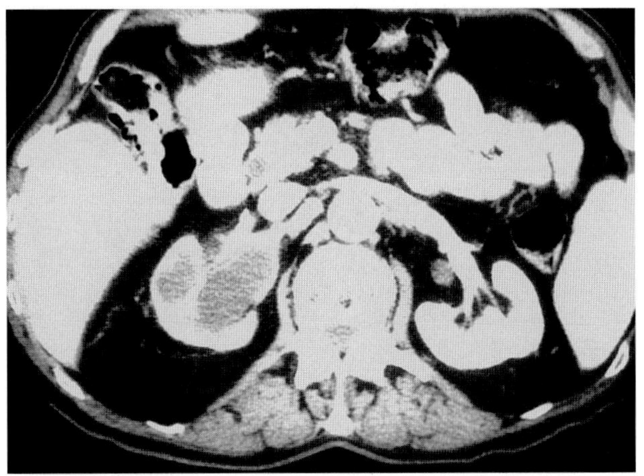

Figure 61. Intrinsic obstruction in a 72-year-old man with hematuria. The right kidney showed poor excretion on IVU. Contrast-enhanced CT scan demonstrates right hydronephrosis with marked cortical thinning indicating chronic obstruction.

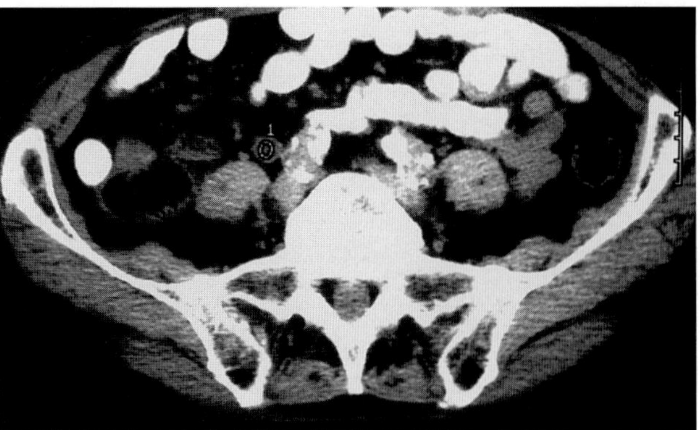

Figure 62. Same patient as in Figure 61. More inferiorly, the dilated ureter is of water density (3 HU).

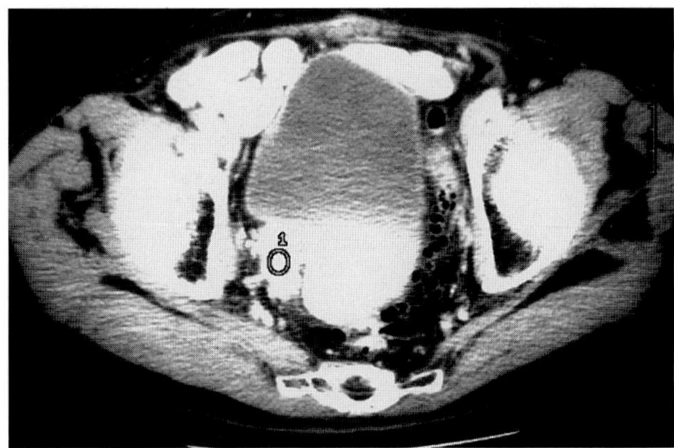

Figure 63. Same patient as in Figure 61. Further inferiorly, an intrinsic lesion within the ureter measured 30 HU pre-contrast (77 HU post-contrast).

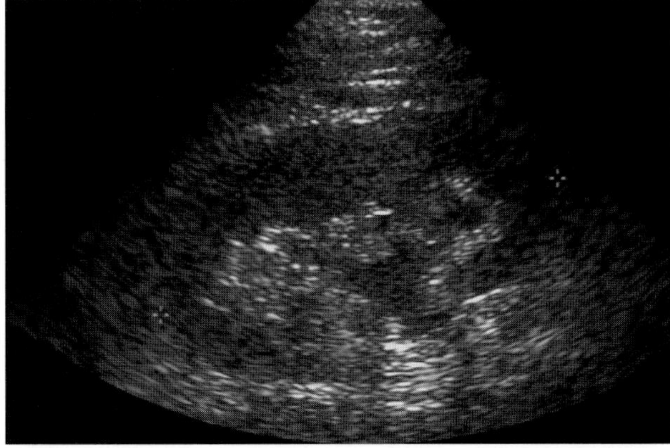

Figure 64. Acute obstruction in a 48-year-old man with the acute onset of left flank pain. Longitudinal sonogram of the left kidney shows mild pyelocaliectasis. RI was 0.75.

Because of its sensitivity to density, CT scanning can distinguish calculi, including radiolucent calculi, from tumors or blood clots **(Figs. 61–68)**. All calculi (even urate calculi) are over 100 Hounsfield units (HU) and appear white at standard window and level settings.[13] Ureteral tumors measure 30–40 HU on noncontrast images and enhance, whereas clots do not enhance. CT scanning is probably not very effective at determining salvageability of a kidney, although renal parenchymal thickness can be measured.

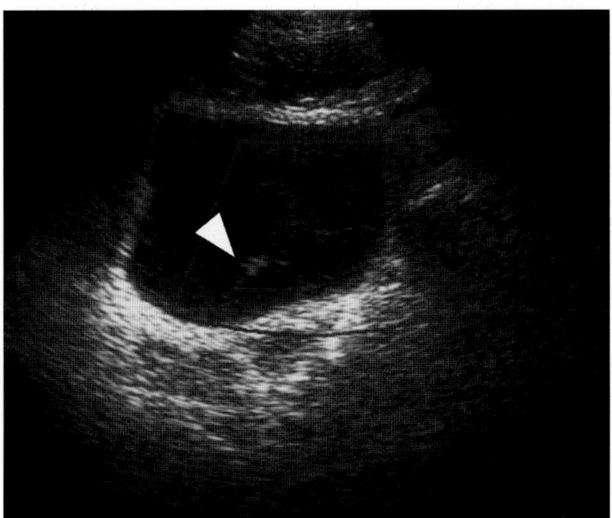

Figure 65. Same patient as in Figure 64. Transverse view of the bladder shows a right ureteral jet (arrowhead); no left jets were observed.

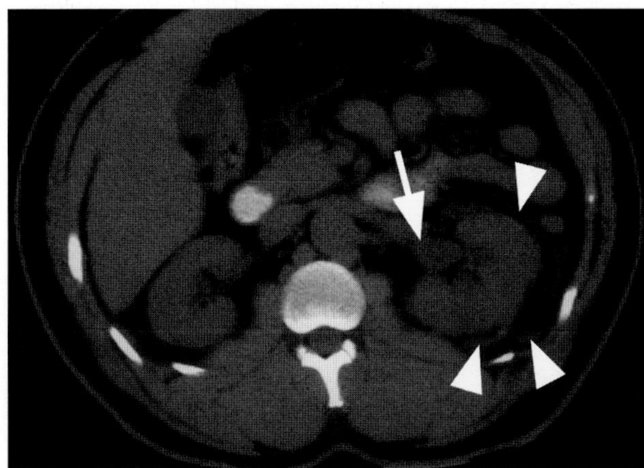

Figure 66. Same patient as in Figure 64. Noncontrast CT scan shows mild pyelocaliectasis (arrow) with perirenal stranding (arrowheads).

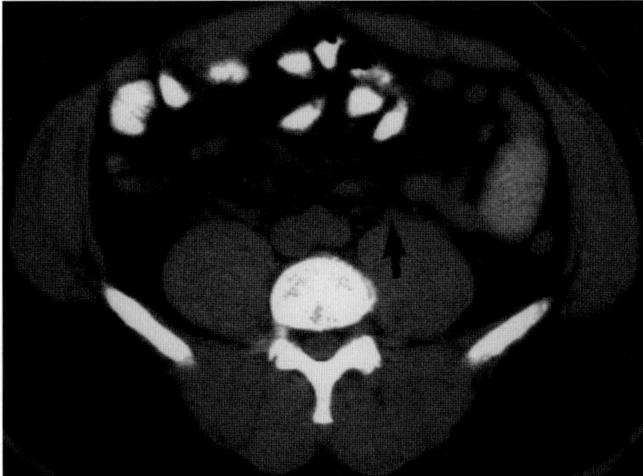

Figure 67. Same patient as in Figure 64. The nonopacified left ureter (arrow) can be followed on sequential images.

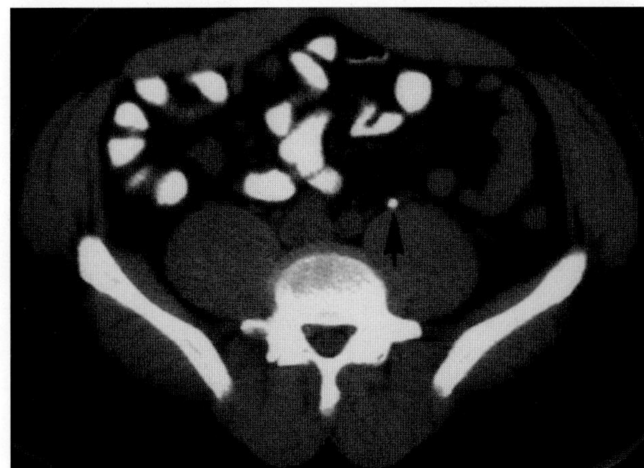

Figure 68. Same patient as in Figure 64. At a level just inferior to that shown in Figure 67, a calculus (arrow) is present in the left ureter.

CT of Acute Obstruction

CT scanning has not traditionally been used to evaluate acute obstruction. However, recent work shows that spiral CT scanning performed without intravenous or oral contrast material (therefore a rapid, low-cost procedure) is accurate in detecting or excluding ureteral calculi in patients with suspected renal colic. In one study of 210 patients, CT scanning detected 100 of the 104 patients with ureteral calculi and correctly excluded calculi in 103 of the 106 patients without calculi, for 97% sensitivity and 96% specificity.[14] In addition , CT scanning detected other abnormalities—adnexal disease, appendicitis, diverticulitis—in 31 patients who did not have stones. The ability to detect nonurinary disease is a strong advantage of CT over IVU.

The primary CT sign of ureteral calculus in this clinical setting is mild dilatation of the ureter with a dense ureteral filling defect (reformatting may help to display this). Ancillary signs can be helpful and can help avoid false positives from pelvic phleboliths or calcified lymph nodes. Distinguishing findings include the presence of a thin rim of soft tissue around the ureteral calculus (representing the ureteral wall; phleboliths do not have this). Patients with acute obstruction commonly have visible perirenal stranding that represents edema or even extravasation of urine.

Role of CT

In summary, CT scanning has distinct advantages in evaluating obstruction. It can take advantage of intravenous contrast material but is not dependent on it. It is especially useful in evaluating patients who have chronic obstruction with poor renal function. It is especially powerful at detecting the etiology of the obstruction, including disease extrinsic to the urinary tract. Patients with a history of malignant disease who have possible obstruction are well evaluated by CT scanning because it not only detects obstruction but can define the full extent of the tumor.

CT scanning is accurate and may be cost-effective in evaluating possible acute obstruction. However, proper technique must be used. Potential pitfalls include mistaking parapelvic cysts for hydronephrosis on noncontrast images and failing to detect calculi on contrast-enhanced images. The greatest limitation of CT scanning is its higher cost over IVU and US. If it can be done at lower cost, it might become useful as an initial study. Further investigation is needed, particularly comparison of CT with US imaging.

Nuclear Medicine Techniques

A full discussion of radionuclide imaging techniques is not possible in this tutorial. Nevertheless, some mention of the use of nuclear medicine in evaluating obstructive uropathy is warranted. Radionuclide imaging is specifically directed at assessing functional changes, because significant obstruction can be defined as that which results in functional alteration. The ability to assess function also is useful in evaluating salvageability of the kidney.

Radionuclide techniques allow quantitative assessment of several parameters of renal function, including estimation of GF and RBF, or effective renal plasma flow (ERPF). The percentage of function provided by each kidney can be calculated. With rigorous consistent technique, nuclear studies are reproducible and comparable as well as quantitative, allowing for sequential evaluation over time to follow the status of renal function. Sequential evaluation may be useful because significant obstruction can be expected to result in loss of renal function over time; the absence of such deterioration can indicate the lack of significant obstruction, or at least imply that intervention is not indicated. Diuretic renography, in which a diuretic agent is injected after a radionuclide tracer has reached the kidney, has been shown to be very useful in assessing urinary obstruction.

Factors Affecting Radionuclide Nephrography
• Renal function Nephrogram poor if GF rate <10–20 mL/min • Hydration Poor diuresis if dehydrated • Pharmaceutical Filtered versus filtered and secreted • Time of diuretic injection • Pelvis, ureter, bladder distensibility • Placement of region of interest, background

Figure 69.

The arrival and disappearance of the tracer is calculated and compared to the contralateral side. This challenges low-grade partial obstruction, allowing better detection and identification of nonobstructive dilatations. Radionuclide methods are also very useful in predicting salvageability of the kidney. If baseline (while still obstructed) renal function parameters (eg, ERPF, percent split renal function) are very low, the likelihood of salvage is low. In equivocal cases, the best predictor may be performance of the nuclear study both before and after the obstruction has been relieved by nephrostomy. If renal function fails to improve, the kidney can be considered unsalvageable.

Limitations of Nuclear Techniques

Although nuclear techniques are valuable and generally more sensitive than other imaging procedures, they are not infallible. Several factors affect the reliability of nuclear renal scans in evaluating suspected obstruction **(Fig. 69)**. Some residual renal function is needed; if uptake of the radionuclide is very poor, then diuresis will not result in a curve that shows prompt washout. If the rate of GF is less than 10–20 mL/min, an abnormal study cannot be considered reliable (although a normal study in such a situation probably does exclude obstruction). If renal function is very poor, background activity actually causes the renal function to be overestimated, because it represents a significant percentage of counts from the region of interest over the kidney.

The state of hydration is also important because dehydrated patients may not respond adequately to the diuretic. Technical factors that must be addressed include the choice and dose of radiopharmaceutical, proper imaging and calculation, timing of the diuretic injection, and correct choice of regions of interest. Errors or variation in these factors may result in spurious calculations or variations from one examination to another. A very distensile pelvis or ureter may result in spurious results calculated from a region of interest over the kidney; they may allow washout from the kidney itself, despite downstream obstruction.

MR Imaging of Obstruction

At present MR imaging has little if any cost-effective role in evaluating urinary tract obstruction, but it does have potential and may play a larger role in the future. MR imaging not only has the ability to image the urinary tract and adjacent structures like CT scanning, it also has the potential to evaluate excretion patterns and functional parameters. In addition, MR does not require exposure of the patient to radiation or iodinated contrast material.

Experience with MR imaging of obstruction is limited. MR imaging can clearly show dilated ureters, either with standard imaging or with use of extremely heavily T2-weighted fast imaging (MR urography).[15] The site of obstruction and an obstructing mass may be seen. In particular, MR imaging can be useful in evaluating pelvic tumors (eg, cervical carcinoma) with ureteral obstruction. Whether MR imaging has the resolution to detect small lesions, including small calculi, and whether it can distinguish obstructive from nonobstructive dilatation is unclear. Further study will be needed, including assessment of functional studies such as time-intensity curves of the kidneys (compared to each other) following intravenous gadolinium diethylenetetramine pentaacetic acid.

References

1. Hodson CJ, Craven JD. The radiology of obstructive atrophy of the kidney. Clin Radiol 1966; 17:305–320.

2. Talner LB. Urinary obstruction. In: Pollack HM, ed. Clinical urography. Philadelphia: W.B. Saunders Company, 1990; 1535–1628.

3. Talner LB, Scheible W, Ellenbogen PH, Beck CH, Gosink BB. How accurate is ultrasonography in detecting hydronephrosis in azotemic patients? Urol Radiol 1981; 3:1–6.

4. Cox IH, Erickson SJ, Foley WD, Dewire DM. Ureteric jets: evaluation of normal flow dynamics with color Doppler sonography. AJR 1992; 158:1051–1055.

5. Baker SM, Middleton WD. Color Doppler sonography of ureteral jets in normal volunteers: importance of the relative specific gravity of urine in the ureter and bladder. AJR 1992; 159:773–775.

6. Burge HJ, Middleton WD, McClennan BL, Hildebolt CF. Ureteral jets in healthy subjects and in patients with unilateral ureteral calculi: comparison with color Doppler US. Radiology 1991; 180:437–442.

7. Deyoe LA, Cronan JJ, Breslaw BH, Ridlen MS. New techniques of ultrasound and color Doppler in the prospective evaluation of acute renal obstruction—do they replace the intravenous urogram? Abdom Imaging 1995; 20:58–63.

8. Platt JF, Rubin JM, Ellis JH. Acute renal obstruction: evaluation with intrarenal duplex Doppler and conventional US. Radiology 1993; 186:685–688.

9. Chen JH, Pu YS, Liu SP, Chiu TY. Renal hemodynamics in patients with obstructive uropathy evaluated by duplex Doppler sonography. J Urol 1993; 150:18–21.

10. Kessler RM, Quevedo H, Lankau CA, et al. Obstructive versus nonobstructive dilatation of the renal collecting system in children: distinction with duplex sonography. AJR 1993; 160:353–357.

11. Coley BD, Arellano RS, Talner LB, Baker KB, Peterson T, Mattrey RF. Renal resistive index in experimental partial and complete ureteral obstruction. Acad Radiol 1995; 2:373–378.

12. Mallek R, Bankier AA, Etele-Hainz A, Kletter K, Mostbeck GH. Distinction between obstructive and nonobstructive hydronephrosis: value of diuresis duplex Doppler sonography. AJR 1996; 166:113–117.

13. Parienty RA, Ducellier R, Pradel J, Lubrano JM, Coquille F, Richard F. Diagnostic value of CT numbers in pelvocalyceal filling defects. Radiology 1982; 145:743–747.

14. Smith RC, Verga M, McCarthy S, Rosenfield AT. Diagnosis of acute flank pain: value of unenhanced helical CT. AJR 1996; 166:97–101.

15. Rothpearl A, Frager D, Subramanian A, et al. MR urography: technique and application. Radiology 1995; 194:125–130.

TUTORIAL 19
PERCUTANEOUS NEPHROSTOMY

Nilesh H. Patel, M.D., and
Allen J. Meglin, M.D.

Introduction

The subjects addressed in this tutorial include:
1. Indications for percutaneous nephrostomy
2. Anatomic considerations for percutaneous nephrostomy
3. Technical considerations for percutaneous nephrostomy
4. Step-by-step approach to percutaneous nephrostomy
5. Patient care and nephrostomy drainage catheter management.

The technique of percutaneous nephrostomy (PCN) was first described by Goodwin et al in 1955.[1] Over the years the technique has been refined and has become the mainstay in genitourinary interventions. Performed by both radiologists and urologists, the technical success rate of PCN is 95%–98% in obstructed, dilated systems and 85%–90% in nonobstructed systems or complex stone cases.[2]

Indications For PCN

PCN is performed when external drainage of the renal collecting system is desired. External drainage can be used to treat nondilated obstructive uropathy or pyeloureteral obstruction causing hydro- or pyonephrosis. PCN can divert urine from the renal collecting system in order to heal leaks and fistulas, and to decompress renal and perirenal fluid collections such as infected cysts, abscesses, and urinomas. PCN provides a track for inserting devices for stone retrieval, foreign body retrieval, biopsies, stricture dilation, and antegrade ureteral stent placement. The track can also be used to infuse antibiotics, chemotherapeutic agents, or drugs for dissolving stones.[3] PCN allows access for urodynamic studies, removal of endoprostheses/stents, endoluminal ultrasound, percutaneous endoscopy, and endopyelotomy. PCN aids in the management of complications of transplanted kidneys—obstructions and leaks—and can be performed to relieve urinary tract obstruction in pregnancy.

Preprocedure Preparation

As with any interventional procedure, all clinical data should be reviewed, including the patient's chart, the physical examination findings, pertinent laboratory values (hematocrit, platelet count, prothrombin time, partial thromboplastin time, blood urea nitrogen, creatinine, white blood cell count and differential, urinalysis, urine culture), and prior imaging studies (intravenous pyelogram, computed tomography [CT] scan, sonogram, magnetic resonance images). The only relative contraindication to PCN is bleeding diathesis. Abnormal coagulation factors should be corrected or at least optimized. If the urinary system is infected, appropriate antibiotic therapy should be instituted prior to performing PCN.[4] The use of prophylactic antibiotics is controversial. We administer intravenously either ampicillin, gentamicin, or ceftriaxone, beginning about 1 hour prior to the PCN procedure.

All patients should have an intravenous (IV) line in place for sedation and analgesics. PCN can usually be performed with local anesthesia and IV analgesics (fentanyl, morphine, etc). General anesthesia is required in children and may be required in complicated or uncooperative patients. Epidural or general anesthesia is used for percutaneous nephrolithotomy and nephrolithotripsy. Continuous monitoring of the patient's electrocardiogram, heart rate, blood pressure, and oxygen saturation is required.

Anatomy

The route of access (lower, mid, or upper pole) and method of access (fluoroscopy, ultrasound, or CT) to the renal collecting system will be guided by an understanding of anatomy and the goal of therapy.

The kidneys are retroperitoneal organs lying on each side of the vertebral column between the 12th thoracic and 2nd or 3rd lumbar vertebrae. The longitudinal axis of the kidney parallels the psoas muscle and the lordotic curvature of the lumbar spine **(Figs. 1, 2)**. Consequently, the upper pole is more posteriorly located than the lower pole. Since the kidney rests over the edge of the psoas muscle, it is tilted 30 degrees posterior to the coronal plane of the body, with the result that its lateral margin is more posteriorly positioned than the medial edge **(Fig. 3)**.[5]

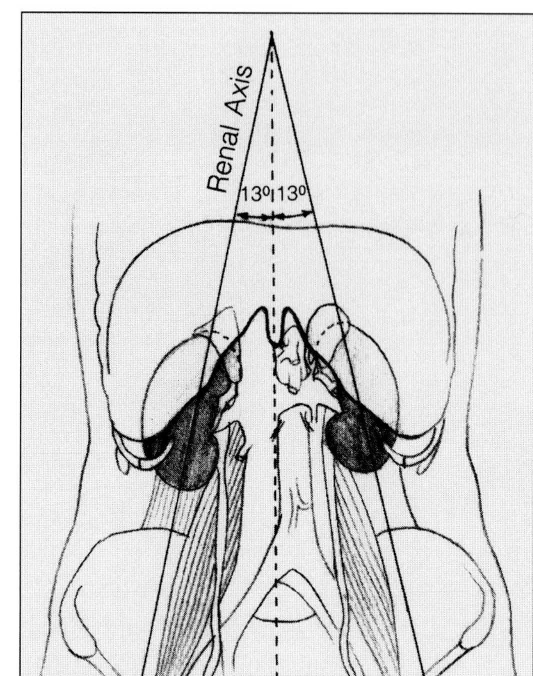

Figure 1. Renal longitudinal axis in the coronal plane.

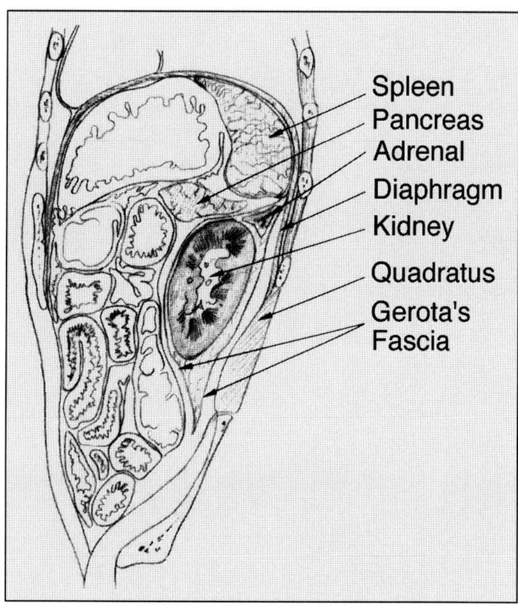

Figure 2. Renal longitudinal axis in the sagittal plane.

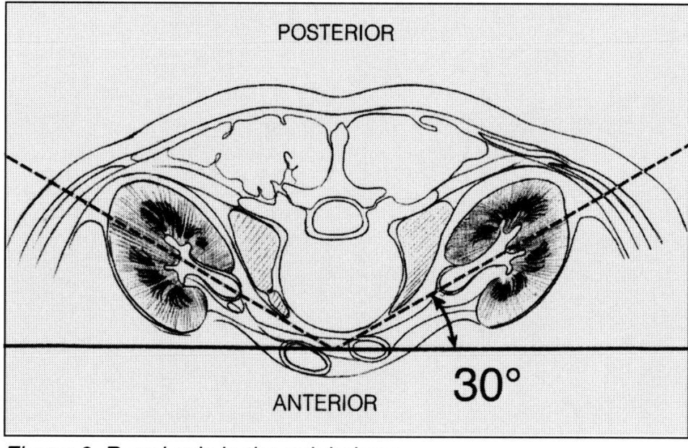

Figure 3. Renal axis in the axial plane.

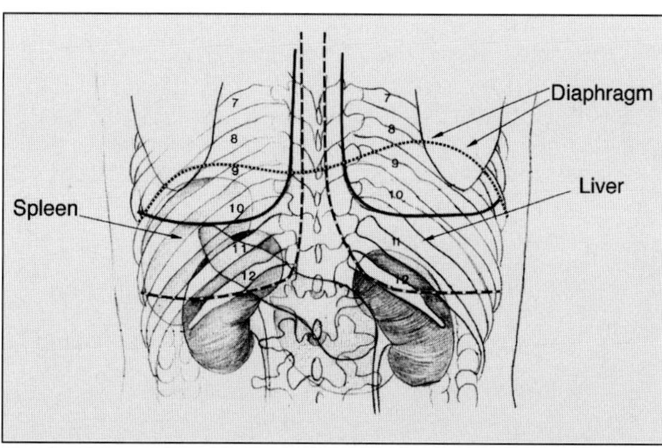

Figure 4. Posterior view of the abdomen depicts the relationship of the pleural space, liver, and spleen to the ribs and intercostal spaces.

Supracostal Approach to the Kidney

11th–12th Intercostal Space

Expiration

- Little risk to spleen and liver
- Lung in needle path in 29% of cases on the right and 14% on the left

Inspiration

- Lung in needle path in most patients (80%+)

10th–11th Intercostal Space

- Lung in needle path in most patients (85%–90%), regardless of respiration
- Spleen in needle path in 33% of cases

Figure 5.

Posteriorly, the 12th rib crosses the kidney at a 45-degree angle. The lower half of the left kidney extends below the pleural reflection, while the lower two thirds of the right kidney is below this reflection **(Fig. 4)**. Therefore, a supracostal approach may be complicated either by a pneumothorax, due to puncture of the lung, or by a hydrothorax, due to dissection of fluid along the nephrostomy track into the pleural space. **Figure 5** shows some of the pitfalls of a supracostal approach. If supracostal access is desired, these complications can be minimized with the use of lateral fluoroscopy to choose an intercostal entry point that will avoid puncturing the lung. Other risks of supracostal access are pain due to irritation of the intercostal nerve and periosteum from rubbing of the drainage tube with respiration, and significant bleeding caused by laceration of the intercostal vessels.

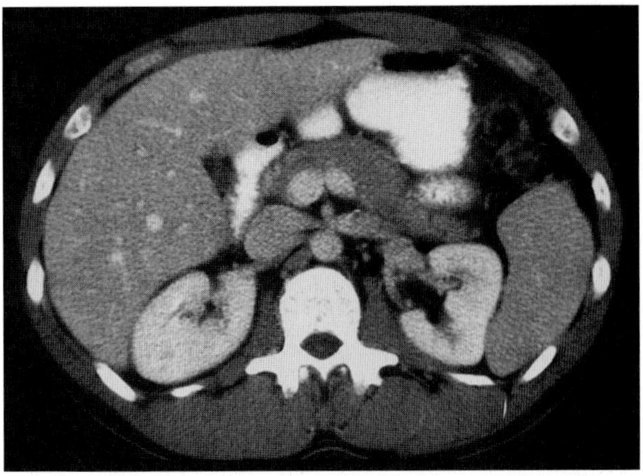

Figure 6. Axial CT slice through the upper poles of the kidneys. The spleen and liver abut the posterior lateral margin of the kidneys, necessitating a paraspinal route for percutaneous needle access to the renal collecting system.

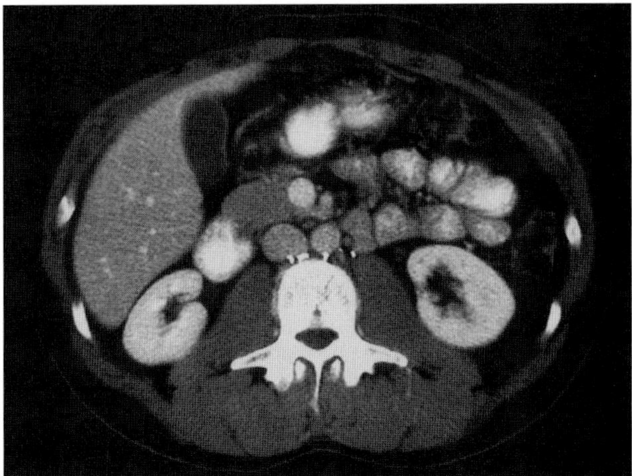

Figure 7. Axial CT slice through the lower poles of the kidneys. Just lateral to the paraspinal muscles is an ideal percutaneous needle entry site into the renal collecting system.

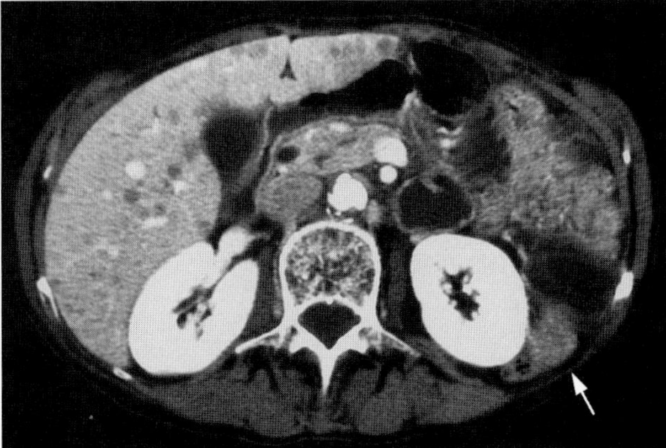

Figure 8. Axial CT slice through the mid pole of the kidneys. Colon is interposed between the left kidney and posterior abdominal wall (arrow).

Near the upper pole of the kidneys, the liver and spleen are quite medial **(Fig. 6)**. Therefore, to avoid injury when accessing an upper pole calyx, a more medial entry point through the paraspinal muscles is required. Near the mid and lower poles of the kidneys, the liver and spleen are more laterally placed **(Fig. 7)**, so a lateral entry just at the edge of the paraspinal muscles is desired. In up to 10% of cases, the colon may be interposed between the kidney and the posterior abdominal wall **(Fig. 8)**.[6]

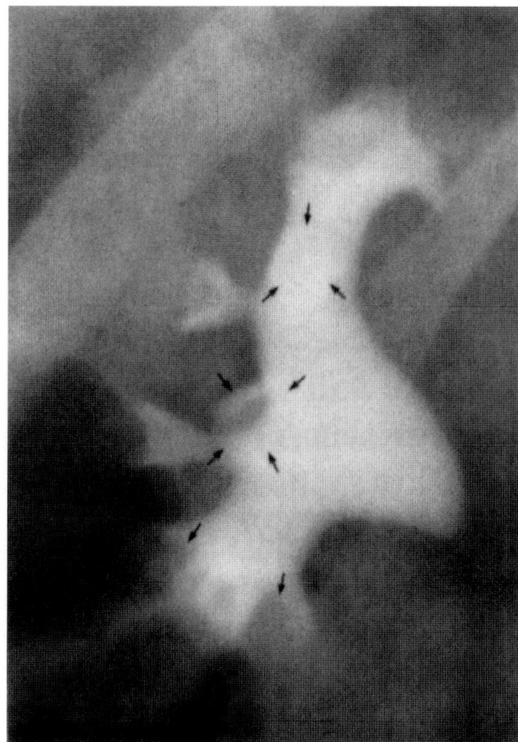

Figure 9. Orientation of calyces. In the anteroposterior view, note the typical en face profile of posterior calyces (arrows).

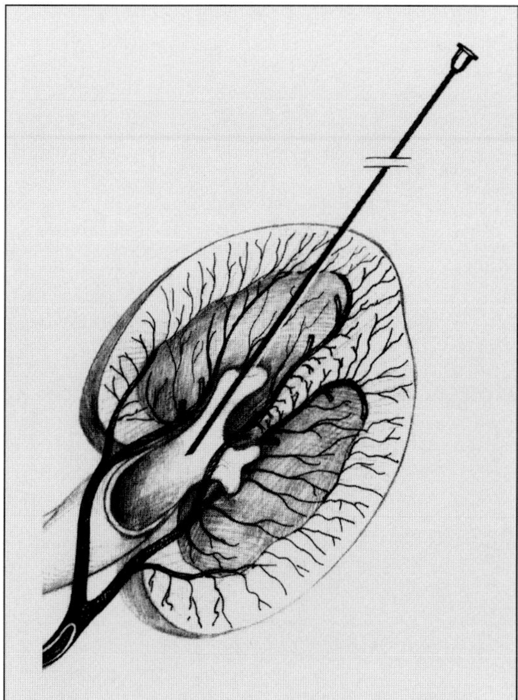

Figure 10. Cross section of the kidney delineates Brödel's avascular zone and the ideal needle access path to a posterior calyx.

The fetal kidney has 14 independent lobes, 7 anterior and 7 posterior. After the 28th week of gestation, fusion of these lobes occurs to various degrees, resulting in a reduction in the number of calyces and papillae.[6] The calyces fuse to a greater degree than the papillae, with subsequent formation of a compound calyx which may drain two or more papillae. The posterior angulation of the kidney on the psoas muscle edge results in more lateral positioning of the anterior calyces and more medial positioning of the posterior calyces. Therefore, on an intravenous pyelogram, the posterior calyces are located medially and are seen en face, whereas the anterior calyces are located laterally and seen en profile **(Fig. 9)**. Compound calyces tend to have a midline position in the kidney and are usually more common in the upper and lower poles.

Brödel first described the segmental distribution of the renal artery.[7] The main renal artery divides into anterior and posterior branches. The segmental arteries lie deep in the kidney and run close to the infundibula within the hilar area. The anterior segmental arteries supply the anterior and posterior surfaces of the anterior calyces and the anterior surface of the posterior calyces. The posterior segmental artery supplies the posterior aspect and, rarely, the anterior surface of the posterior calyces.[8] This plane of arterial division is relatively avascular **(Fig. 10)**. The interlobar arteries, which supply blood to the papillae, can cross the infundibula.[9]

Procedure

Informed consent should detail the benefits, risks, and complications of the procedure, as well as alternative therapies. After informed consent is obtained, the patient is placed on the angiographic table in a prone or prone-oblique position with the operative side elevated 20–30 degrees. The choice depends on physician preference and patient comfort. The flank and back on the operative side are prepared and draped in a sterile fashion.

An 18- to 21-gauge needle can be used for access. Based on our review of anatomy, the skin entry site should be 2–3 cm below the 12th rib, just lateral to the edge of the paraspinal muscles. The needle should pass through Brödel's avascular zone into a middle or lower pole posterior calyx. This technique will minimize access-related complications. A middle pole calyx access further facilitates easy antegrade access to the ureter for ureteral interventions or antegrade ureteral stent placement.

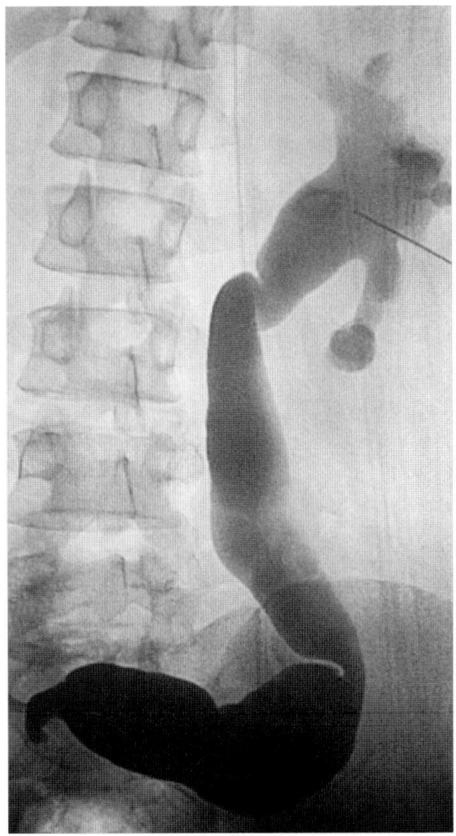

Figure 11. A 30-year-old man with a history of prune belly syndrome presents with chills, fever, and symptoms of urinary obstruction. An antegrade pyelogram obtained prior to percutaneous nephrostomy demonstrates distal ureteral obstruction with proximal dilatation.

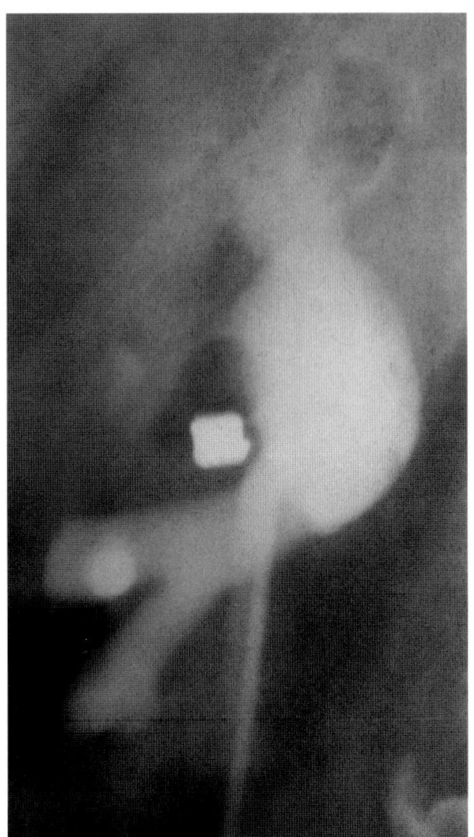

Figure 12. Use of antegrade contrast-gas nephrostogram. Anteroposterior view of the needle accessing a gas-filled posterior calyx.

Posterior calyceal access may be guided by fluoroscopy or real-time ultrasound. The fluoroscopic method requires opacification of the renal collecting system either by IV administration of contrast material in a nondilated system, or direct percutaneous instillation of contrast material and gas (CO_2 or air) into the renal pelvis in a dilated system. In the latter case, a 15-cm, 21-gauge needle is introduced percutaneously into the renal pelvis, which has been outlined on the skin by ultrasound **(Fig. 11)**. A volume of urine greater than the volume of contrast material and gas to be instilled is removed. This safeguards against overdistention of the obstructed system and the risk of septicemia. The gas will outline the nondependent posterior calyces **(Figs. 12, 13)**. We routinely send an aspirated urine sample for culture.

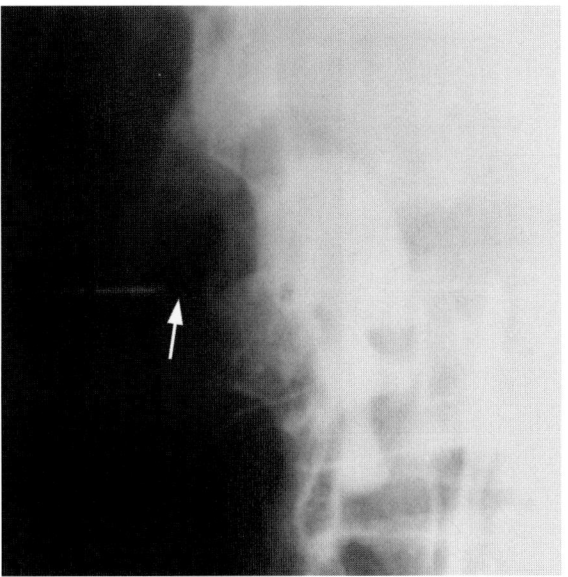

Figure 13. Use of antegrade contrast-gas nephrostogram. Lateral view of the needle (arrow) accessing a gas-filled posterior calyx.

Once a posterior calyx is localized, a fine needle percutaneous access set (eg, Neff or Jeffrey set, or Cope introduction system, [Cook, Bloomington, IN]) is used to access the kidney. These sets include a 15-cm, 21-gauge needle, an introducer catheter, and an 0.018-inch platinum-tipped Cope mandril guide wire. Our step-by-step method is as follows.

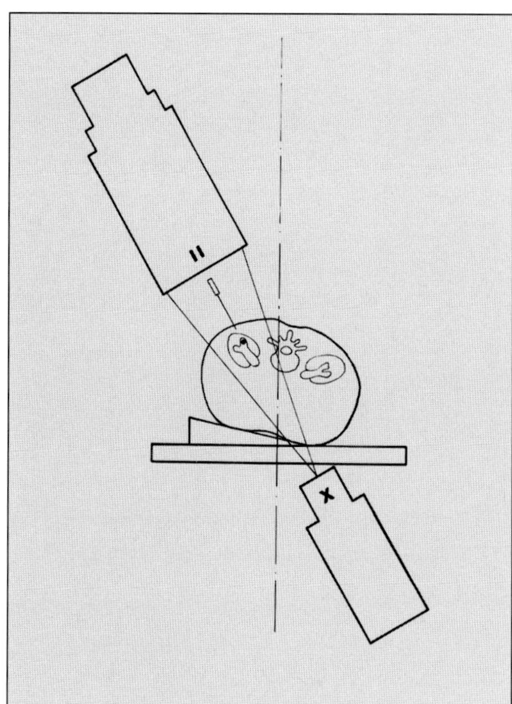

Figure 14. Use of multidirectional C-arm fluoroscopy to guide needle access of a posterior calyx (black dot). The C-arm has been rotated so that the x-ray beam is parallel to the needle.

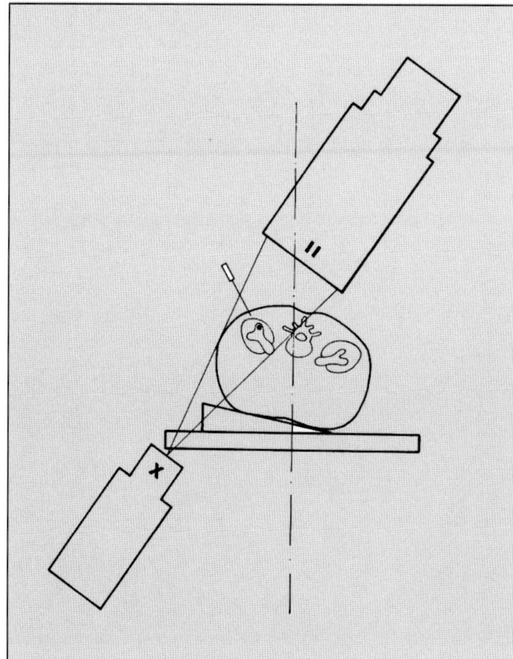

Figure 15. Use of multidirectional C-arm fluoroscopy to guide needle access of a posterior calyx (black dot). The C-arm has been rotated so that the x-ray beam is perpendicular to the needle.

1. The skin entry site and intended needle path are infiltrated with 1% lidocaine. A small skin incision is made at the entry site and the needle is advanced under fluoroscopic or ultrasound guidance toward the desired posterior calyx during suspended mid inspiration. With the fluoroscopic method, the needle is advanced incrementally. Tangential angulation of the x-ray tube between needle advancements will help guide the needle through a direct path into the intended posterior calyx **(Figs. 14, 15)**. In our experience, a 15-cm, 19- or 20-gauge needle is easier to see and guide under real-time ultrasound.
2. Once the needle tip is in the collecting system, reflux of urine should be seen. If not, a 10-mL syringe attached to flexible tubing is attached to the needle. With gentle aspiration the needle is slowly withdrawn until urine is aspirated. Once urine is aspirated, a test injection of contrast material is made for confirmation. An 0.018-inch platinum-tipped Cope mandril guide wire is advanced through the needle into the posterior calyx. It is then manipulated through the infundibulum and into the renal pelvis.
3. The introducer catheter is advanced over the 0.018-inch guide wire and its tip is positioned in the renal pelvis. The wire is exchanged for a stiff guide wire (eg, Rosen [Cook], Amplatz [Medi-Tech, Boston Scientific Corporation, Watertown, MA]).
4. Before track dilation is undertaken, the size of the nephrostomy tube must be chosen. We choose the size based on the initial urine aspirate. If it is clear, we use an 8.5-F locking Cope loop drainage catheter. If the urine is cloudy and contains sediment or purulent material which would clog the tube, we use a 10.2-F locking Cope loop drainage catheter. Track dilation is accomplished by passing dilators of increasing size over the guide wire. If necessary, the track should be dilated to one or two French sizes larger than the size of the drainage catheter to be placed.
5. The drainage catheter-stiffener assembly is advanced over the guide wire. Once the stiffener tip is in the renal parenchyma, the drainage catheter is pushed off the stiffener and advanced into the renal pelvis. To avoid hemorrhage from vessel injury, the stiffener should not be pushed beyond the renal parenchyma into the collecting system.

6. Once the side-holes of the drainage catheter are in the renal pelvis, the wire is withdrawn into the drainage catheter. Pulling on the string and gently rotating the shaft of the drainage catheter clockwise aids in the formation of the Cope loop. Once the loop is formed, the trocar and guide wire are removed and contrast material injected to confirm positioning **(Fig. 16)**. The string is then locked in place according to the manufacturer's guidelines for the device. The tube can be secured to the patient's skin with various skin fixation devices (Molnar disc, Tru-Fix, etc). We favor a simple suture around the drainage catheter, followed by sterile gauze and bio-occlusive dressings.

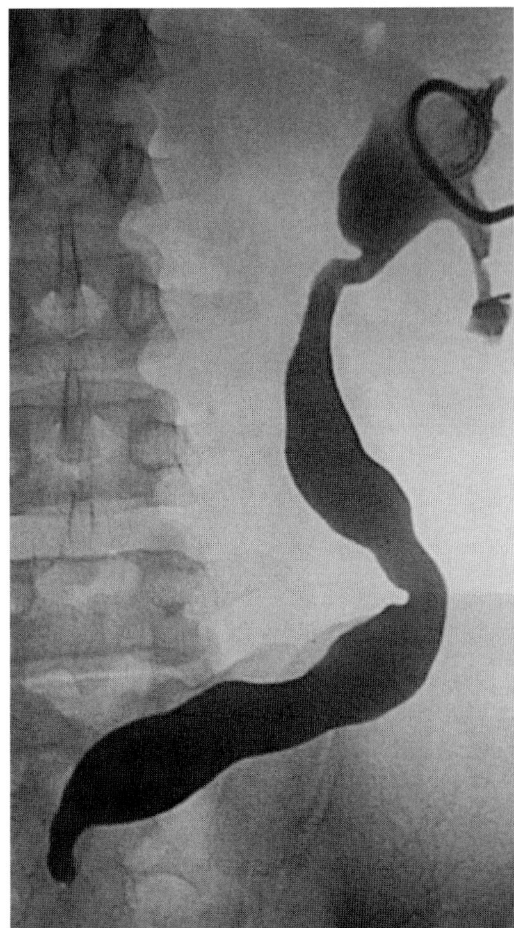

Figure 16. Final placement of an 8.5-F locking Cope loop drainage catheter in this 30-year-old man with urinary obstruction. Note that the access will easily facilitate future antegrade catheterization of the ureter.

The choice of calyceal access for pelvocaliceal stone(s) extraction requires a combined Interventional Radiology and Urology approach.[10] It is imperative that both services review the pertinent imaging modalities and plan the access route jointly in order to ensure successful stone(s) removal. For a more thorough discussion of percutaneous techniques for managing renal stone disease, **see Tutorial 22: Renal and Ureteral Calculi**.

Special Cases

1. Transplant kidney. Patients are placed in the supine position and access is gained through the anterior abdominal wall. An upper or middle portion anterior calyx should be accessed, thereby avoiding injury to the vascular pedicle and facilitating antegrade access to the ureter. Preprocedural axial imaging is highly recommended to delineate this anatomy.
2. Horseshoe kidney. Due to the unusual axis of the kidney, the renal artery and vein may be situated superficial to the renal parenchyma from a posterior approach. Cross-sectional imaging to determine which calyx and the best skin-to-calyx track is recommended. Either an anterior abdominal wall or retroperitoneal, posterior approach can be used. The posterior approach may require a more lateral track to avoid the medially located renal artery and vein.
3. Duplex kidney. In duplex kidneys, the upper moiety becomes obstructed and the lower moiety has reflux. Therefore, drainage of the obstructed upper moiety collecting system requires a more medial skin puncture at the 10th-11th or 11th-12th intercostal space to access an upper pole posterior calyx and avoid injury to the spleen or liver. However, an added risk of pleural and adrenal damage exists.

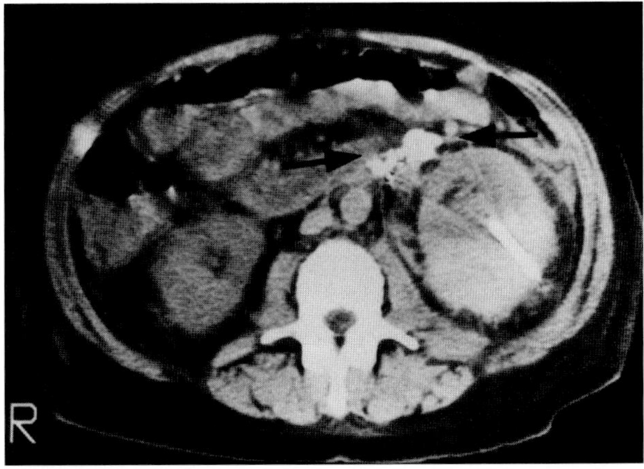

Figure 17. Large subcapsular hematoma from a left nephrostomy (arrows).

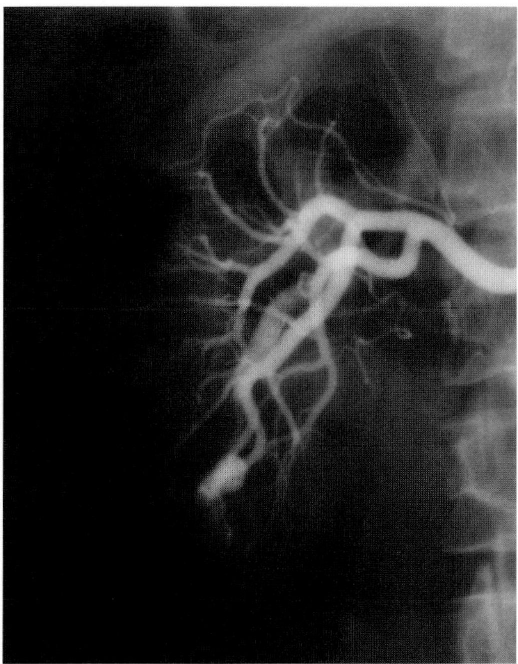

Figure 18. Pseudoaneurysm with an arteriovenous communication from a previous percutaneous nephrostomy.

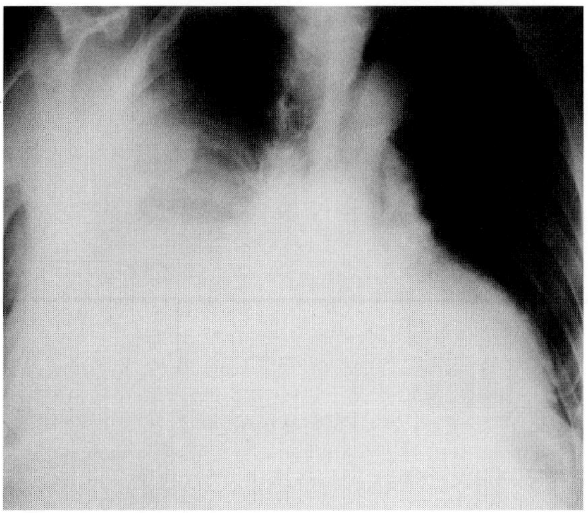

Figure 19. Large right hydrothorax due to a supracostal access for percutaneous nephrolithotripsy.

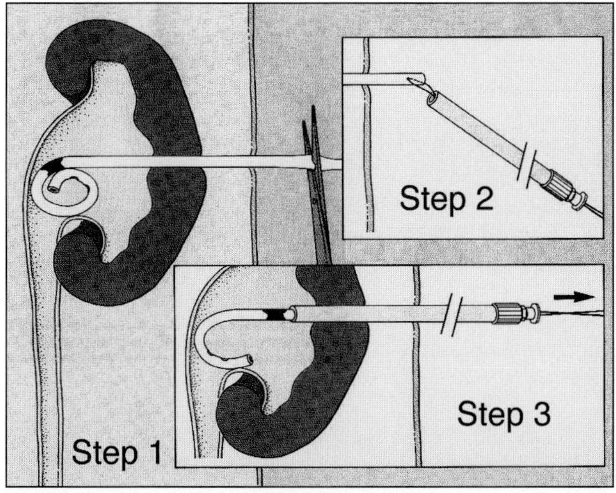

Figure 20. Removal of an occluded nephrostomy drainage catheter.

Complications

The mortality rate with PCN is 0.2%, compared to the mortality of surgical nephrostomy of 6%. The overall rate of major complications is about 4%–6% and includes massive hemorrhage requiring surgery or transcatheter embolization (1%), pneumothorax or hydrothorax (1%), death due to hemorrhage (<2%), and rarely, peritonitis **(Figs. 17–19)**. The overall rate of minor complications is about 10%–28% and includes microscopic hematuria, gross hematuria which clears in 24–48 hours, perirenal bleeding (rare), clinically unsuspected retroperitoneal hematoma (13%), urine extravasation (<2%), and infection (1.4%–21%). Catheter-related problems (dislodgement, obstruction, malposition) occur in about 12% of cases.

Accidental dislodgement of a drainage catheter is not uncommon. Generally, the track may be cannulated successfully within 72 hours of dislodgement. Contrast material is injected through flexible extension tubing, whose distal end abuts the skin site of the track, to confirm track communication and opacification of the renal collecting system. We prefer to use a short, angled catheter and an angled hydrophilic wire to traverse the track and pass into the renal collecting system. Once the catheter is verified to be in the collecting system by injection of contrast material, an 0.035-inch Rosen guide wire is introduced and the angled catheter exchanged for a nephrostomy drainage catheter.

The drainage catheter may become occluded by encrustations, so it is important to instruct the patient to contact the interventionalist immediately if signs or symptoms (poor drainage, sepsis, etc) of an obstructed drainage catheter are apparent.

A partially occluded drainage catheter can be easily exchanged for a new catheter over a guide wire. A completely obstructed drainage catheter presents more of a problem. Forceful irrigation of the catheter is not recommended; instead, the hub and locking mechanism of the drainage catheter should be cut off **(Fig. 20)**. Then a 2.0 silk suture is sewn through the cut end of the catheter and passed through a peel-away Teflon sheath. The sheath should be the same size or one French size larger than the existing drainage catheter. With gentle tension on the suture, the peel-away sheath is advanced over the drainage catheter until its tip is within the renal collecting system. The drainage catheter is removed and an 0.035-inch Rosen guide wire is advanced through the peel-away sheath and coiled in the renal collecting system. A new drainage catheter can then be introduced over the guide wire and the peel-away sheath removed.

Postprocedure Management and Tube Care

The patient's vital signs should be checked every 30 minutes for 4 hours after the procedure, then every 1 hour for 4 hours. The patient should be maintained at bedrest for 4 hours or until hematuria begins to clear.

If clots are present in the pelvocaliceal system after PCN, forward flush with 5 mL of bacteriostatic normal saline followed by aspiration should be performed every 4 hours. Blood-tinged urine may be seen up to 48 hours after PCN. If gross hematuria persists, the catheter position should be checked. Renal arteriography with embolization of a bleeding branch may be necessary. If the serum hematocrit falls in the absence of gross hematuria, a CT scan should be performed to exclude a retroperitoneal hematoma. Bleeding or leakage of urine around the drainage catheter may be tamponaded by upsizing the tube.

If no complications arise, the patient can be discharged 24 hours after PCN. Many centers now perform nephrostomy on an outpatient basis. The patient is instructed to: 1) empty the drainage bag frequently, using sterile technique; 2) apply clean dressings over the tube insertion site daily; and 3) take no tub baths and protect the skin entry site from getting wet while bathing. The patient is advised to contact Interventional Radiology if discharge or breakdown of the skin around the catheter is apparent, if leakage of urine soaks the dressing around the catheter, or if the catheter position changes or the catheter has been pulled out.

For patients who require long-term urinary diversion, the catheter should be checked every 6 to 8 weeks and changed every 3 to 4 months.

Unlike other drainage procedures, PCN does not require that a mature track develop before the nephrostomy drainage catheter is removed.[11] The tube may be removed once adequate antegrade urine flow is re-established. This may require internal ureteral stent placement or surgical diversion. A stent may be placed antegrade through the PCN track by an interventionalist or retrograde through the bladder by a urologist.

References

1. Goodwin WE, Casey WC, Woolf W. Percutaneous trocar (needle) nephrostomy in hydronephrosis. JAMA 1955; 157:891.

2. Castaneda-Zuniga WR, Brady TM, Thomas R, et al. Percutaneous uroradiologic techniques. In: Casteneda - Zuniga WR, ed. Interventional radiology. 3rd edition. Baltimore: Williams and Wilkins, 1997.

3. Banner MP, Ramchandani P, Pollack HM. Interventional procedures in the upper urinary tract. Cardiovasc Intervent Radiol 1991; 14(5):267–284.

4. Reznek RH, Talner LB. Percutaneous nephrostomy. Radiol Clin North Am 1984; 22(2):393–406.

5. Coleman CC, Castaneda-Zuniga WR, et al. A systemic approach to puncture site selection for percutaneous urinary tract stone removal. Semin Intervent Radiol 1984; 1.

6. Hodson J. The lobar structure of the kidney. Br J Urol 1972; 44:246–261.

7. Brodel M. The intrinsic blood vessels of the kidney and ureter. Johns Hopkins Hosp Bull 118:10, I1901.

8. Vordermark JS. Segmental anatomy of the kidney. Urology 1981; 17:521–531.

9. Graves FT. Arterial anatomy of the kidney. Bristol, England: John Wright and Sons, Ltd., 1971.

10. Bush WH, Brannen GE, et al. Access techniques for successful percutaneous nephrostolithotomy. Appl Radiol 1985.

11. Roven SJ, Rosen RJ. Percutaneous nephrostomy and maintenance of nephrostomy drainage. Urology 1984; 23:25–28.

TUTORIAL 20
URODYNAMIC MEASUREMENT: THE WHITAKER TEST

Robert T. Andrews, M.D., and
Anthony C. Venbrux, M.D.

Introduction

The subjects addressed in this tutorial include:

1. Definition of urinary manometry
2. Techniques for performing the Whitaker test
3. How to interpret the results of a Whitaker test
4. Pitfalls and complications of the Whitaker test.

It is well documented that the radiographic and sonographic appearance of the urinary collecting system does not always correlate with its function.[1,2] Hydroureteronephrosis can be present without ureteral obstruction in cases of reflux, previous obstruction, congenital megacalyx or megaureter, or during periods of diuresis. Similarly, high-grade outflow obstruction can exist without causing hydroureteronephrosis, as in cases of renal failure, dehydration, or urinary tract encasement by benign or malignant disease.[3] Even physiological imaging studies using radioisotopes and Lasix can over- and underestimate the degree of obstruction, especially when renal function is poor.[4,5]

Dynamic urinary manometry, also known as the Whitaker test, is indicated when the question of obstruction exists and the results of noninvasive imaging studies are inconclusive or contradictory.[6] The Whitaker test provides a direct measurement of the pressure gradient between the upper urinary tracts and the urinary bladder during the percutaneous infusion of dilute contrast material.[7–11] By simultaneously measuring the pressures in the renal pelvis and urinary bladder directly, a pressure gradient can be calculated by subtracting the renal pelvic pressure from the urinary bladder pressure. An elevation of the pressure gradient is seen with obstruction at any level between the renal calyces and the bladder. Results are independent of renal function, and are not affected by bladder outlet obstruction or neurogenic bladder.

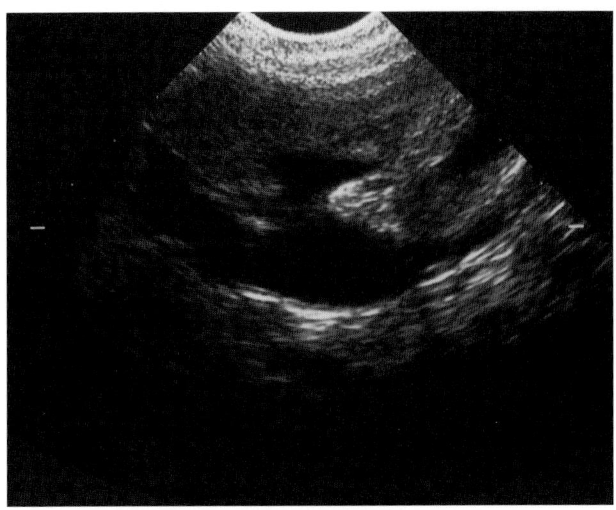

Figure 1. Sonogram shows hydronephrosis.

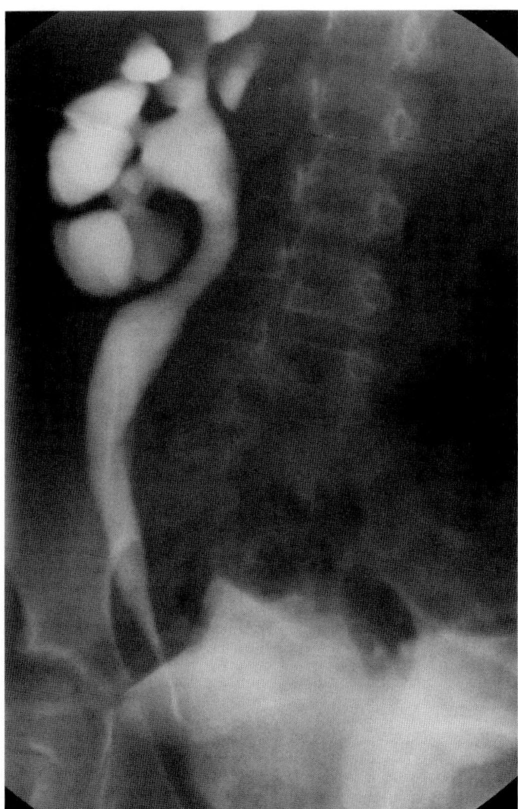

Figure 2. Spot film obtained during a Whitaker test, with caliectasis and proximal ureterectasis.

The limitations of anatomic imaging to evaluate urinary tract obstruction can be overcome by using physiologic data.[12,13] For example, this young woman was born with a cloaca and had persistent hydronephrosis following bladder reconstruction **(Fig. 1)**. An antegrade pyelogram obtained during her Whitaker test **(Fig. 2)** confirms the presence of hydronephrosis with proximal hydroureter due to diffuse distal ureteral stenosis. Despite the marked anatomic abnormalities, the maximal upper tract pressure was 25 cm H_2O, with a maximal gradient of 11.5 cm H_2O. These results are in the normal range and suggest that the physiologic function of the urinary tract was normal despite the abnormal anatomic appearance.[10,11] The patient did well without additional treatment, confirming this assessment.

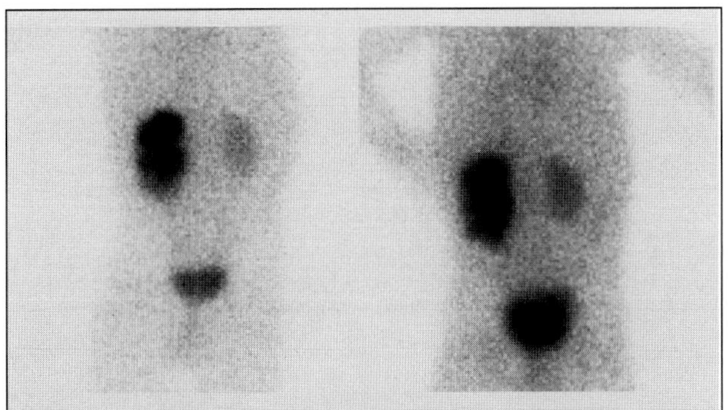

Figure 3. Lasix-enhanced technetium-99 DTPA acid renal scan suggests left renal obstruction (posterior view).

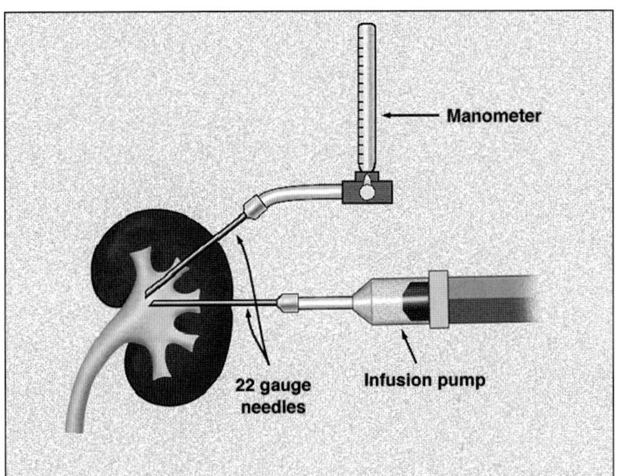

Figure 5. Basic configuration for a urinary Whitaker test.

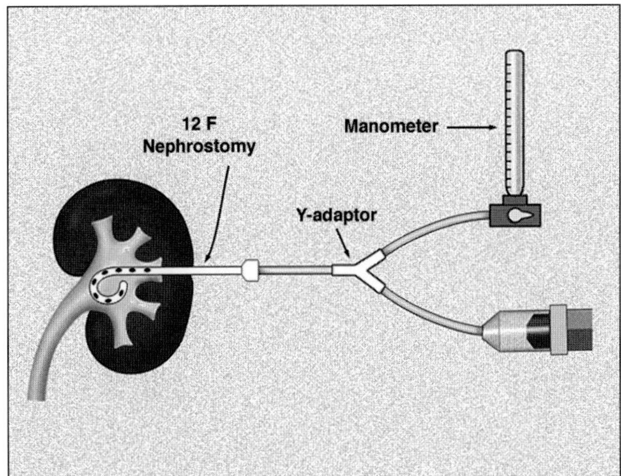

Figure 6. A nephrostomy tube can be used both for infusion and for measuring renal pelvis pressures by using a "Y" adapter.

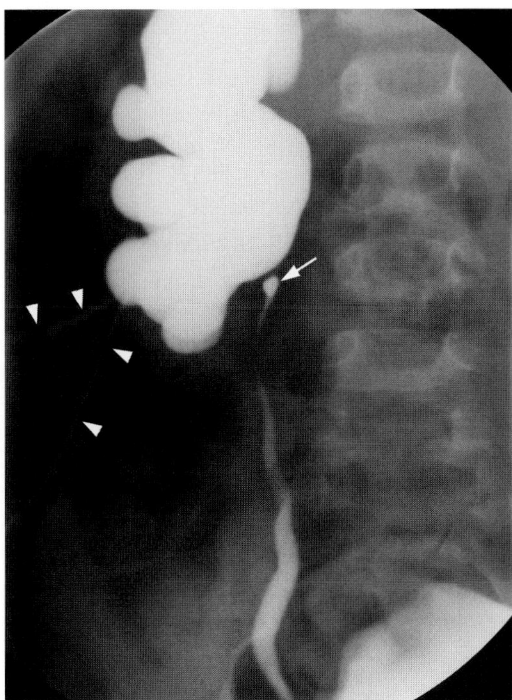

Figure 4. Spot film obtained during a Whitaker test, with hydronephrosis and a UPJ stenosis (arrow). Arrowheads point to the needles used for pressure measurements and fluid instillation.

Another example is the patient shown in **Figure 3**, who was asymptomatic after surgical repair of a congenital ureteropelvic junction (UPJ) obstruction. The postoperative nuclear renogram with use of technetium-99 diethylene-triamine pentaacetic acid (DTPA) and Lasix shows minimal drainage from the left renal calyces and pelvis. This finding was considered indicative of ureteral obstruction. Images from a Whitaker test **(Fig. 4)** demonstrate a focal stricture at the UPJ repair site. Nonetheless, pressure measurements revealed a maximal upper tract pressure of 22 cm H_2O and a urinary bladder pressure of 12 cm H_2O, giving a maximal gradient of 10 cm H_2O. These results are normal, and the patient did not require further treatment.

In general, the Whitaker test is performed by placing a "skinny needle" into the renal pelvis for infusion and pressure measurement. Pressure in the renal pelvis is compared to that in the urinary bladder as measured through a Foley catheter **(Fig. 5)**. If a nephrostomy drainage catheter is already in place, it can be used instead of the needle for instillation and measurement of the renal pelvic pressures **(Fig. 6)**. If the patient has had a cystectomy, the Foley catheter can be placed into the ileal loop or similar neobladder.

Patient Preparation

The patient is screened for coagulopathy and urinary tract infection, both of which are relative contraindications to performing the test. After informed consent is obtained, antibiotics and a mild sedative are administered. A Foley catheter or similar device is placed into the urinary bladder (or equivalent) and connected to the manometer or pressure transducer through a three-way stopcock **(Fig. 7)**.

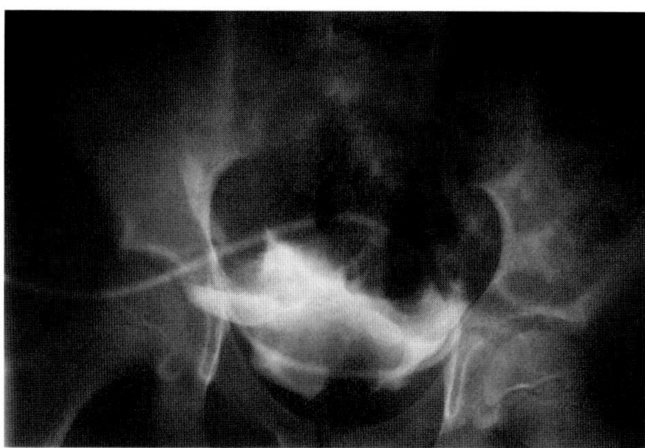

Figure 7. The catheter is located in a neobladder (suprapubic approach). This can be used to measure pressures below the ureter.

The renal collecting system is entered percutaneously, with use of a 21- or 22-gauge (skinny) needle. If only one needle is placed, the infusion will have to be stopped periodically so that pressure measurements can be taken. If two needles are placed, or a nephrostomy catheter at least 12 F in size is used, infusion and measurement can be performed simultaneously **(Fig. 8)**.[14] The upper tract access is connected to an infusion pump and a manometer or transducer through stopcocks.

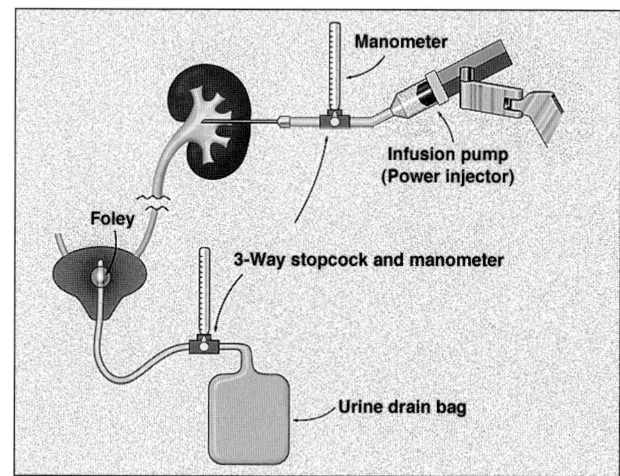

Figure 8. Modifications to the basic Whitaker test permit simultaneous infusion and pressure measurement.

Procedure

A 1:1 mixture of contrast material and saline is infused into the collecting system at a constant rate. In his original work, Whitaker used a rate of 10 mL/min (5 mL/min in children). At our institution 15 mL/min (10 mL/min in children) is used, which gives equivalent results in less time.

Pressures within the renal collecting system and bladder are measured continuously for 10 minutes (if the two-needle technique is used), or intermittently after total infusion volumes of 25, 50, 75, 100, 125, and 150 mL. Absolute and gradient pressures are recorded, where the gradient pressure equals the collecting system pressure minus the bladder pressure.

Intermittent fluoroscopy is used to evaluate for structural abnormalities and the degree of distention, with spot films being taken as necessary. The procedure is terminated if the patient experiences significant pain.

Study Interpretation[10,11]

1. A gradient of 0–14 cm H_2O is normal and indicates no significant obstruction. (It should be noted that others have advocated using a pressure gradient of 10 or 12 cm H_2O as the upper limit of normal.)[15]
2. A gradient of 15–20 cm H_2O is equivocal. In this case, the urinary tract can be further evaluated by repeating the study at a higher flow rate (usually 20 mL/min).
3. A gradient greater than 20 cm H_2O or an absolute renal pressure greater than 30 cm H_2O indicates a significant obstruction. If clinically indicated, the percutaneous access can be converted to a nephrostomy drainage catheter.

Endpoints

The Whitaker test is terminated if any of the following occur during the exam:

1. Pain or other evidence of a change in clinical condition.
2. Extravasation or backflow of contrast material.
3. Relative pressure gradient greater than 20 cm H_2O.
4. Absolute renal pressure greater than 30 cm H_2O, beyond which the risk of sepsis and renal injury increases significantly.
5. Successful infusion of 150 mL of fluid, with normal pressure gradients and no evidence of flank pain.

Endpoints 1–4 constitute a failed Whitaker test, while endpoint 5 suggests that no physiologically significant obstruction is present.

Potential Pitfalls and Complications

1. Underestimation of the gradient because of an underfilled renal collecting system. Massively dilated collecting systems should be completely filled with a 1:1 mixture of contrast material and saline before the timed infusion and measurement are begun.
2. Underestimation of the gradient because of an overfilled urinary bladder. During timed infusion, the urinary bladder should be allowed to drain to gravity.
3. Direct renal trauma during the percutaneous needle puncture. The procedure should only be performed by trained interventionalists using appropriate imaging guidance.
4. Renal trauma or induction of sepsis related to elevated upper tract pressure. As stated above, these complications are more likely if the absolute pressure is allowed to rise above 30 cm H_2O. Prophylactic antibiotic coverage is recommended.

Conclusion

The Whitaker test is a safe, albeit invasive, method of distinguishing between anatomic abnormalities of the urinary collecting system and true physiologic urinary tract obstruction. In the presence of gross anatomic abnormalities, clinical decision making is often best based upon the physiologic consequences of these abnormalities. Similar principles have been successfully applied to the biliary system **(see SCVIR Syllabus Volume III, *Biliary Interventions*)**.

References

1. Pfister RC, Papanicolaou N, Yoder IC. Diagnostic morphologic and urodynamic antegrade pyelography. Radiol Clin North Am 1986; 24(4):561–571.

2. Amis ES, Cronan JJ, Pfister RC, Yoder IC. Ultrasonic inaccuracies in diagnosing renal obstruction. Urology 1982; 19(1):101–105.

3. Rascoff JH, Golden RA, Spinowitz BS, Charytan C. Nondilated obstructive nephropathy. Arch Intern Med 1983; 143:696–698.

4. Spital A, Valvo JR, Segal AJ. Nondilated obstructive uropathy. Urology 1988; 31(6):478–482.

5. Maillet PJ, Pelle-Francoz D, Laville M, Gay F, Pinet A. Nondilated obstructive acute renal failure: diagnostic procedures and therapeutic management. Radiology 1986; 160:659–662.

6. O'Reilly PH. Nuclear medicine. In: O'Reilly PH, ed. Obstructive uropathy. Heidelberg: Springer-Verlag, 1986.

7. Hay AM, Norman WJ, Rice ML, Steventon RD. A comparison between diuresis renography and the Whitaker test in 64 kidneys. Br J Urol 1984; 56:561–564.

8. Senac MO, Miller JH, Stanley P. Evaluation of obstructive uropathy in children: radionuclide renography versus the Whitaker test. AJR 1984; 143:11–15.

9. O'Reilly PH. Diuresis renography 8 years later: an update. J Urol 1986; 136(3):993–999.

10. Whitaker RH. An evaluation of 170 diagnostic pressure flow studies of the urinary tract. J Urol 1979; 121:602–604.

11. Whitaker RH. Methods of assessing obstruction in dilated ureters. Br J Urol 1973; 45:15–22.

12. Jaffe RB, Middleton AW. Whitaker test: differentiation of obstructive from nonobstructive uropathy. AJR 1980; 134:9–15.

13. Barbaric Z. Principles of genitourinary radiology. 2nd edition. New York: Thieme Medical Publishers, 1994; 25–27.

14. Amis ES, Pfister RC, Newhouse JH. Resistances of various renal instruments used in ureteral perfusion. Radiology 1982; 143:267–268.

15. Personal communication with Scott Trerotola, M.D.

TUTORIAL 21
PERCUTANEOUS URETERAL STENTS

Mark W. Wilson, M.D.

Introduction

The subjects addressed in this tutorial include:

1. Indications for percutaneous ureteral stent placement
2. Types of percutaneous ureteral stents available
3. Techniques of percutaneous ureteral stent placement
4. Technical difficulties, pitfalls, and complications of percutaneous ureteral stent insertion
5. Management of patients with percutaneously placed ureteral stents.

Interventional radiology currently plays an important role in the management of urologic disorders. This is well demonstrated by the increasing frequency with which percutaneous ureteral stent placement is performed in both renal transplant and non-transplant patients.

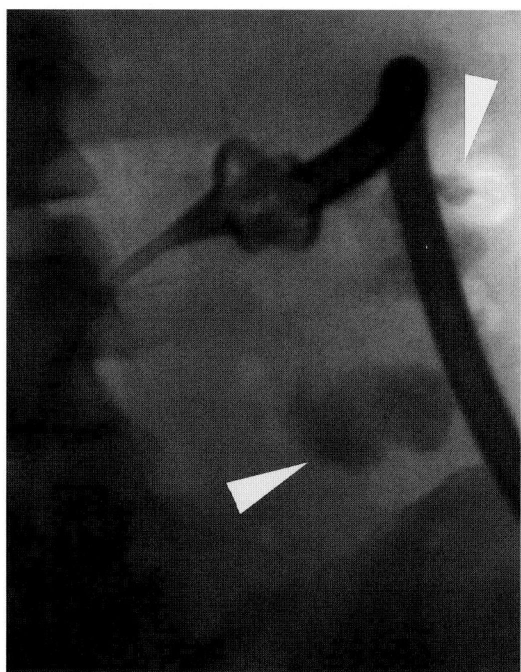

Figure 1. A locking Malecot nephroureteral stent is in place after percutaneous endoscopic nephrolithotomy. Several retained calculi are present in mid and lower calyces (arrowheads).

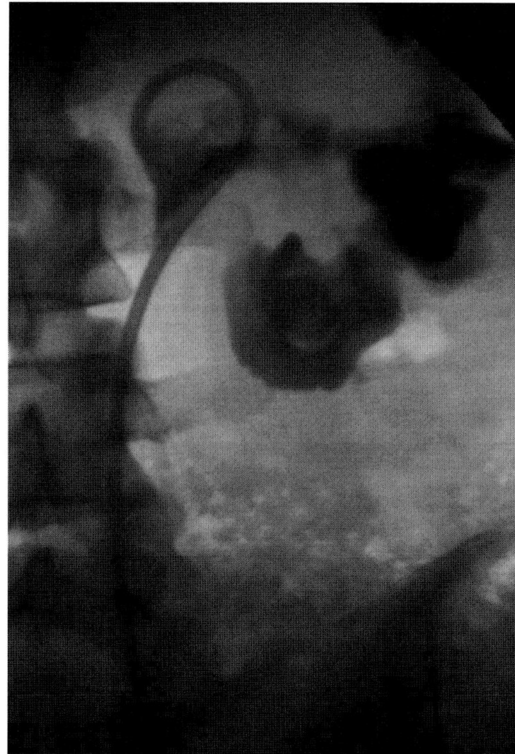

Figure 2. Same patient as in Figure 1. The nephroureteral stent was replaced with an antegrade double-J ureteral stent. The proximal loop of the stent decompresses the renal pelvis, while the distal loop drains into the bladder.

Indications

The work-up of abnormal renal function, flank pain, or urinary tract infection usually involves an assessment for ureteral obstruction. The causes of native ureteral obstruction can be intrinsic, intraluminal, or extrinsic. Intrinsic and intraluminal causes include calculi **(Figs. 1–3)**; epithelial tumors (transitional cell or squamous cell carcinoma); congenital ureteropelvic junction (UPJ) obstruction **(Figs. 4, 5)**; congenital ureterovesical junction (UVJ) obstruction; infectious processes such as tuberculosis and schistosomiasis; anastomotic strictures (eg, ureteroileostomy anastomosis); and blood clots.

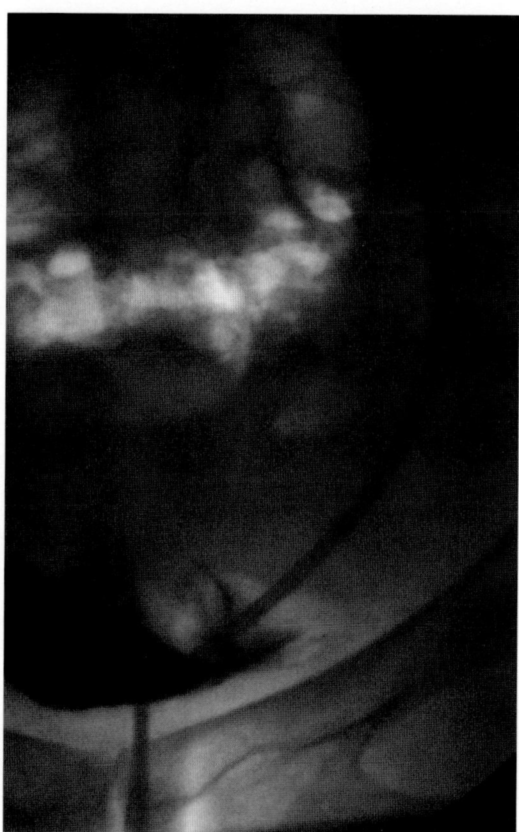

Figure 3. Same patient as in Figure 1 showing the distal loop of the double-J stent.

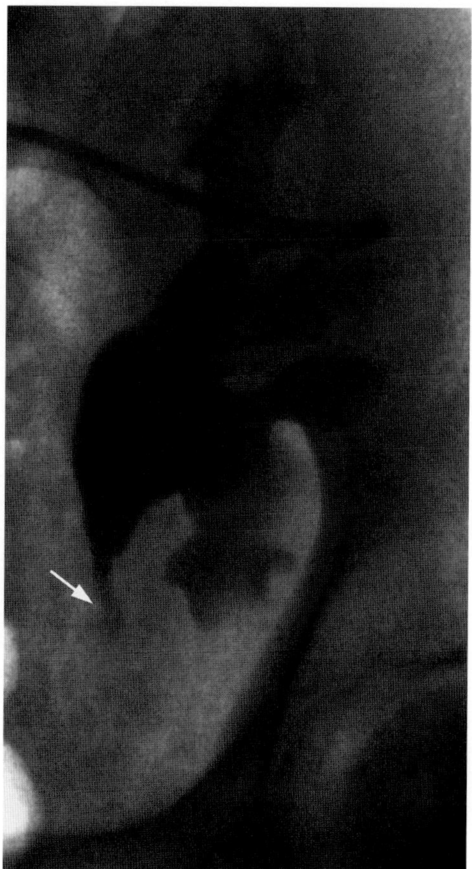

Figure 4. Renal transplant patient with a high-grade UPJ stricture (arrow).

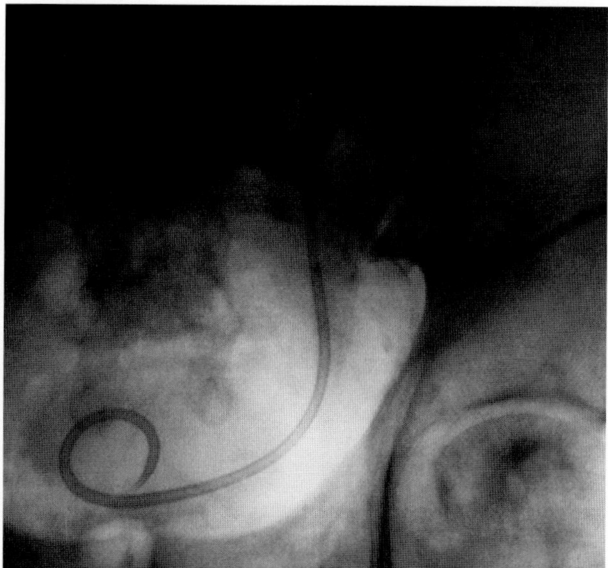

Figure 5. Same patient as in Figure 4. The UPJ stricture was traversed successfully, permitting placement of an 8-F double-J ureteral stent.

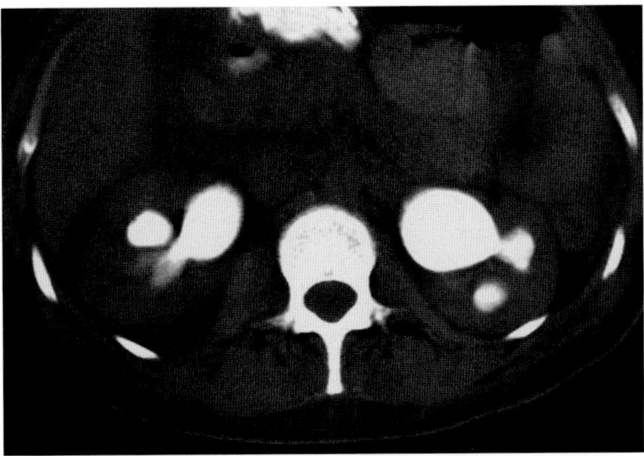

Figure 6. CT scan shows marked bilateral hydronephrosis in a female patient who has recently undergone gynecologic surgery.

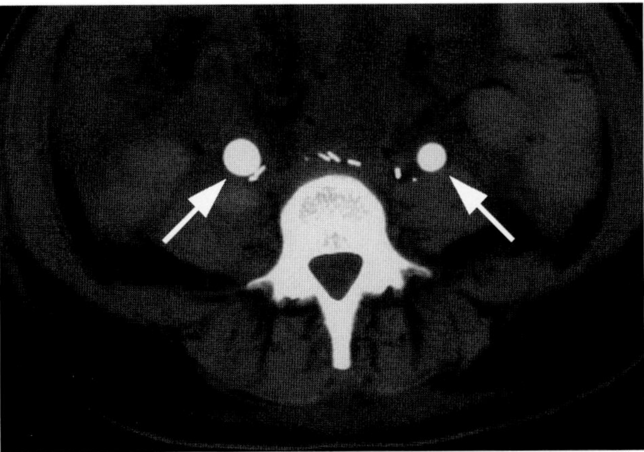

Figure 7. Same patient as in Figure 6. Lower cut from the CT scan shows marked bilateral hydroureter (arrows).

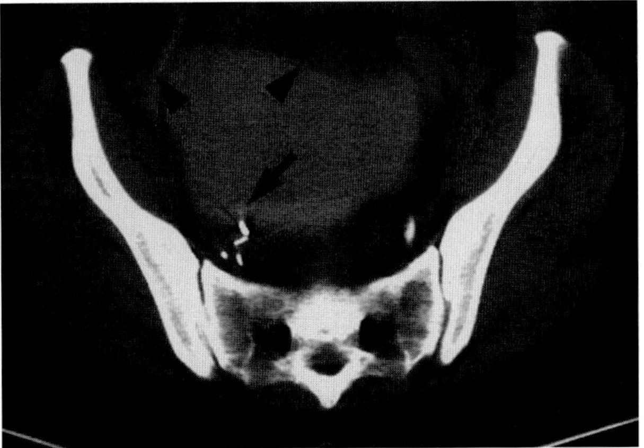

Figure 8. Same patient as in Figure 6. The right ureter (arrow) terminates at the level of the presacral surgical clips. Free fluid is also present (arrowheads).

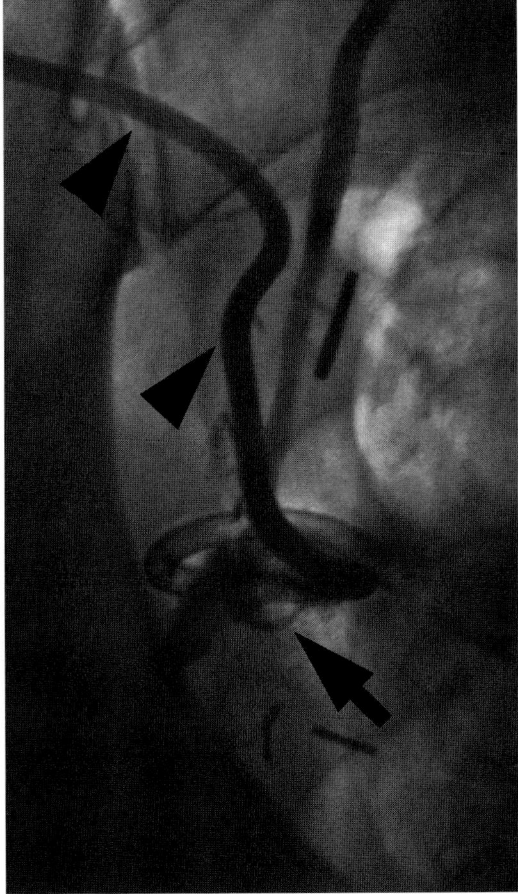

Figure 9. Same patient as in Figure 6.Antegrade pyelography demonstrates the right ureter to be completely transected (arrow). Wires and catheters could not be passed across the site of injury. Extravasated contrast material flows readily through the previously placed urinoma drain (arrowheads).

Extrinsic causes of ureteral obstruction include lymphadenopathy; lymphocele; urinoma; prostate carcinoma; gynecologic disorders such as malignancies, pelvic inflammatory disease, and endometriosis; trauma (iatrogenic and noniatrogenic) **(Figs. 6–9)**; Crohn's disease; pelvic abscesses; retroperitoneal fibrosis; iliac artery aneurysms; and pregnancy. The purpose of ureteral stent placement is to bypass the obstructed or leaking segment of the ureter, thereby allowing antegrade flow of urine and reestablishing physiologic renal function.

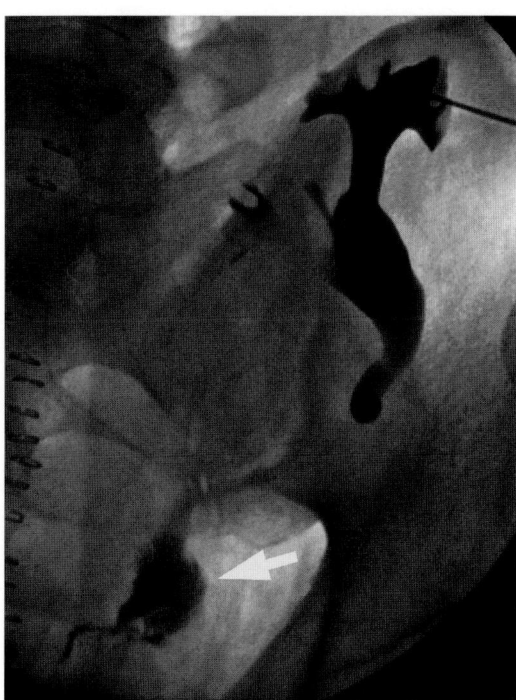

Figure 10. Antegrade pyelogram in a renal transplant patient demonstrates a ureterovesical anastomotic leak (arrow).

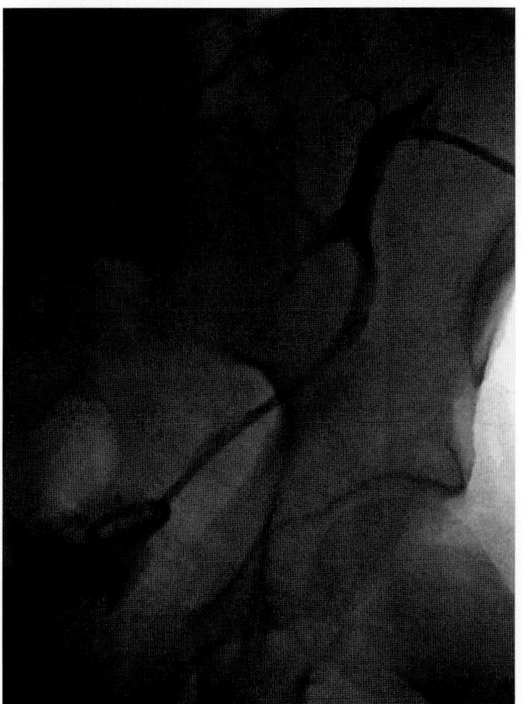

Figure 11. Same patient as in Figure 10. Nephroureterostomy tube check demonstrates healing of the leak site after 6 weeks of conservative management with placement of a ureteral stent and concomitant urinary diversion.

In the renal transplant patient with deteriorating renal function, the major diagnostic issue is whether the declining function is due to obstruction or rejection. The widely used technique of submucosal tunneling at the ureteroneocystostomy has a 1%–5% complication rate, with the two major complications being obstruction and leakage.[1]

Transplant ureteral obstruction usually occurs at the UVJ. Causes include ureteral ischemia, kinking, calculi, post-inflammatory stricture, blood clot, mucosal edema, or extrinsic compression by a urinoma or lymphocele. Graft rejection may also be associated with ureteral obstruction;[1] therefore, the diagnosis of one does not completely exclude the other.

Transplant ureteral leaks most commonly occur at the ureteroneocystostomy and are often secondary to technical problems **(Figs. 10, 11)**. Leaks can occur at other sites along the ureter and renal pelvis, with ischemia and/or rejection frequently implicated.

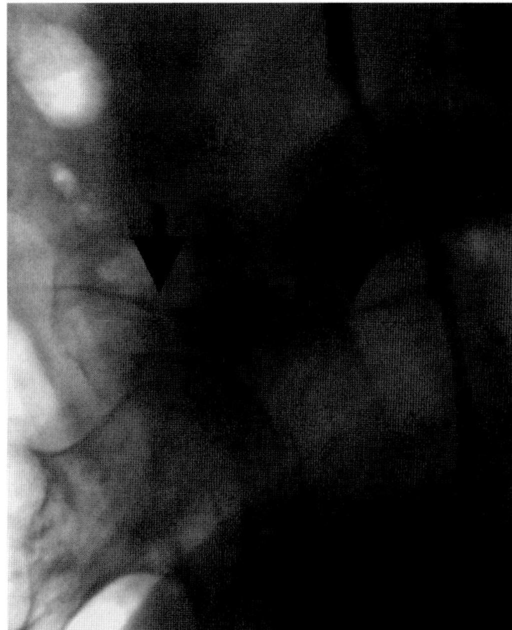

Figure 12. Distal ureterocutaneous fistula (arrows) complicating surgery for cervical carcinoma. Contrast material has been injected through a newly placed nephroureteral stent.

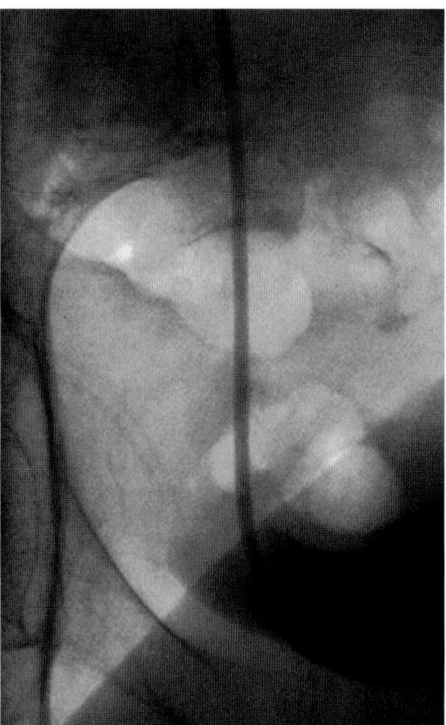

Figure 13. Same patient as in Figure 12. The ureterocutaneous fistula has healed after conservative treatment with a ureteral stent for 4 months.

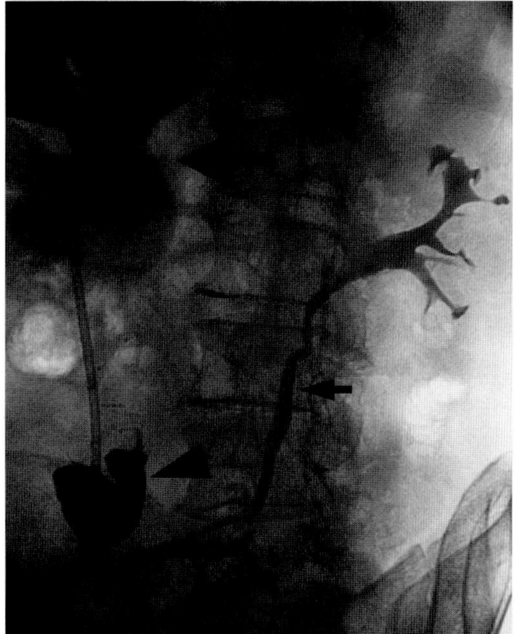

Figure 14. Patient with bilateral ureteroileostomies after bladder resection for transitional cell carcinoma, complicated by right-sided ureteroileostomy stricture. The right-sided nephroureteral stent is obstructed, with secondary hydronephrosis (large arrow). The ileal loop (arrowhead) was opacified with contrast material to demonstrate the orifice of the left ureter, which was successfully catheterized and opacified prior to stent placement for preoperative localization (small arrows).

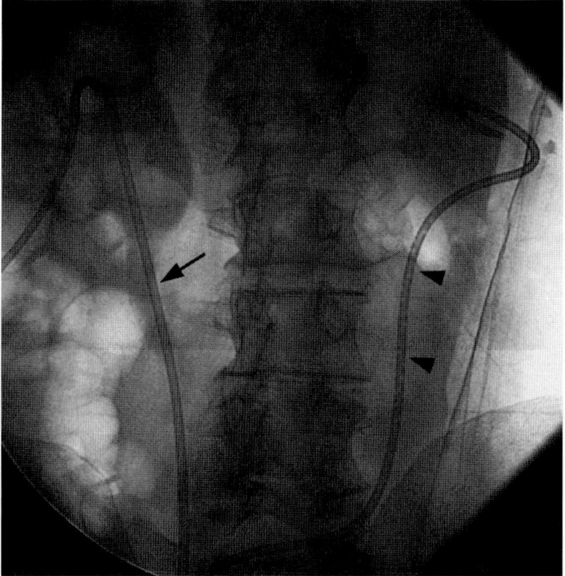

Figure 15. Same patient as in Figure 14. The obstructed right-sided nephroureteral stent was exchanged over a wire for a new 10-F nephroureteral stent (arrow). A left ureteral stent (arrowheads) was placed in retrograde fashion to aid in intraoperative localization for a right-to-left ureteroureterostomy.

Ureteral stent placement can be performed to treat both native and transplant ureteral obstruction and leakage. Indications for ureteral stent placement include ureteral obstruction (benign and malignant), ureteral leaks (traumatic, postoperative), ureteral fistulas (malignant, inflammatory) **(Figs. 12, 13)**, and preoperatively for ureteral surgery **(Figs. 14, 15)** or extracorporeal shock wave lithotripsy.

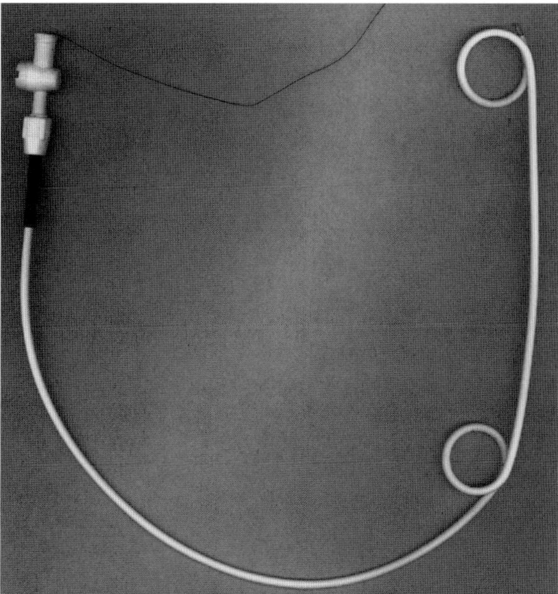

Figure 16. Renal transplant 8-F, 10-cm nephroureterostomy stent (Medi-Tech, Boston Scientific Corporation, Watertown, MA) with a non-tapered distal end.

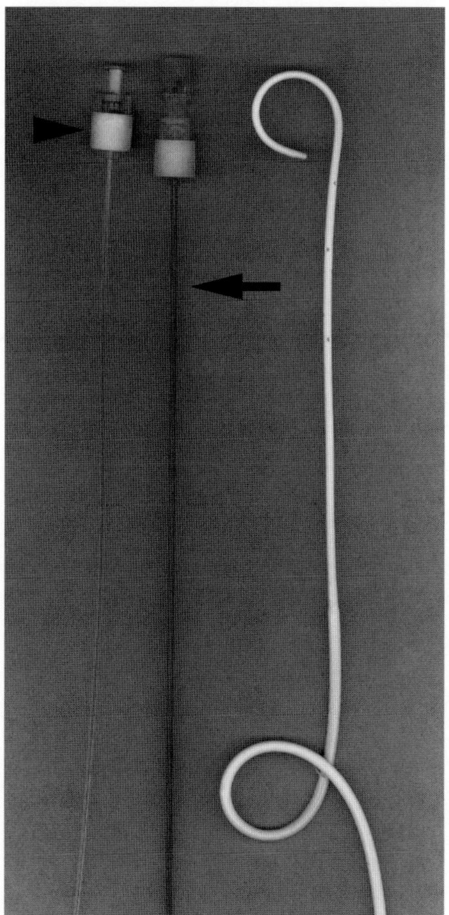

Figure 17. The Cope nephroureterostomy stent (Cook, Bloomington, IN) has a tapered distal end. As with most types of nephroureteral stents, this stent is inserted with the aid of a flexible (arrowhead) or rigid (arrow) stiffening cannula.

In most situations, stents can be placed both from the percutaneous antegrade approach or from a retrograde approach under cystoscopic guidance;[2] the method chosen is usually at the discretion of the referring physician. In many practices, cystoscopic retrograde stent placement is the initial approach because it is believed to be less invasive and to carry a decreased risk of renal parenchymal damage. When the ureteral orifice cannot be cannulated or is obstructed or obscured by tumor or blood clot, antegrade stent placement is preferred. There are circumstances where these anatomic or pathologic factors favor antegrade stent insertion with a combined approach.[3,4] If a nephrostomy tube is already in place, antegrade stent placement is usually the most expedient method.

Types of Ureteral Stents

The nephroureterostomy stent (also called nephroureterostomy tube, nephroureteral stent, or universal stent) and the double-J stent (or double pigtail stent) are the designs most commonly used for both transplant and native kidneys. The stents range in length from 22 to 32 cm for native ureters and 10 to 15 cm for transplant ureters.

The nephroureteral stent is essentially a nephrostomy tube combined with a ureteral stent **(Fig. 16)**. Loops are formed in the urinary bladder and renal pelvis to secure the stent while the externalized portion provides access for tube checks and exchanges over a guide wire. The external portion can be capped to facilitate internal drainage of urine across the ureter. Nephroureteral stents range in size from 8 to 10.2 F. In some models the distal portion is tapered to 6 or 7 F **(Fig. 17)**.

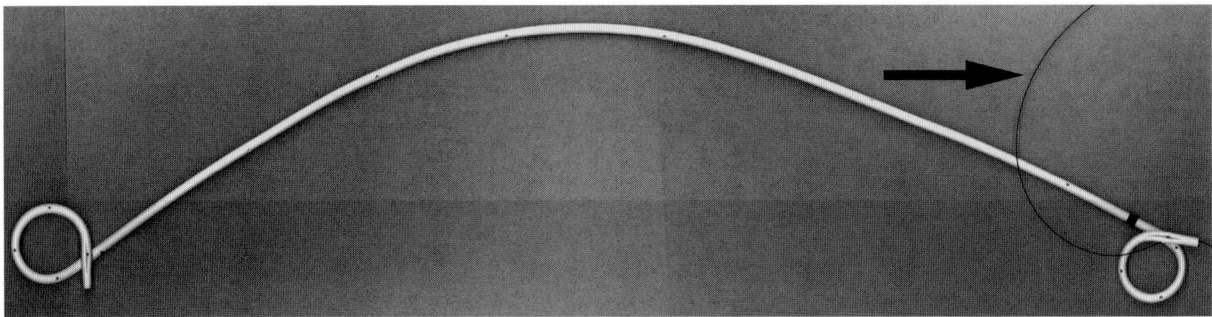

Figure 18. Standard double-J ureteral stent. Note the proximal suture loop (arrow), which aids in stent positioning at the time of deployment.

The double-J stent is completely internalized within the ureter **(Fig. 18)**. Like the nephroureteral stent, it is stabilized by loops in both the bladder and renal pelvis. Double-J stents typically range in size from 6 to 10 F. Larger (8–10 F) caliber stents are often placed percutaneously because they provide the greater mechanical strength needed for percutaneous insertion. Some models have a suture loop near the proximal end to facilitate stent repositioning after deployment (Druy Universal Length Stent [Cook], Medi-Tech Ureteral Stent [Medi-Tech]). The Druy Universal Length Stent has multiple proximal and distal loops that allow a single stent to be adjusted to fit a range of ureteral lengths (22–32 cm).

Other stent configurations are available for specialized applications. Stents composed of a large-bore proximal drainage catheter (up to 30 F), with or without a Malecot tip, tapering to an 8- to 8.5-F ureteral stent are useful for track maintenance and urine drainage after percutaneous nephrolithotomy **(Fig. 19)**.

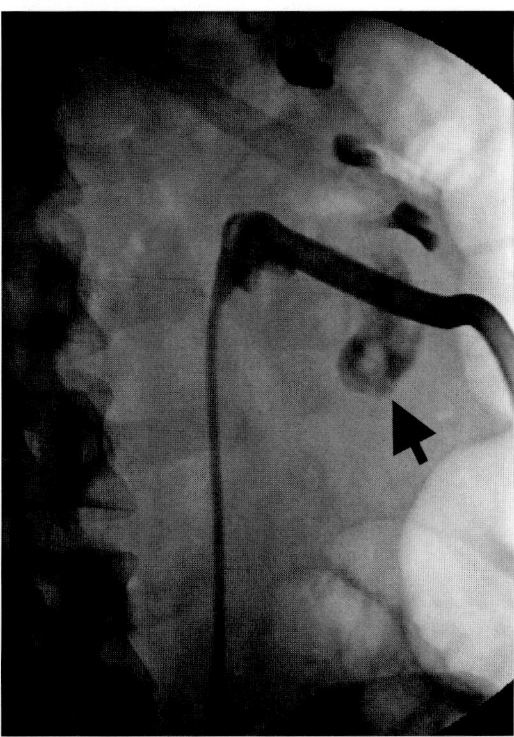

Figure 19. Large-bore nephroureteral stent with Malecot fixation and a distal ureteral stent, placed after endoscopic stone extraction. A retained calculus is present in a lower pole calyx (arrow).

Ureteral Stent Materials

Stent materials become an important consideration in the settings of tight strictures, where the coefficient of friction is a factor, and long-term ureteral stent placement, where biocompatibility becomes a factor. Polyurethane stents have the advantages of good radiopacity, stiffness, and high flow rates. These stents, however, appear to have higher rates of encrustation, brittleness, and fracture over the long term. While Silastic stents are more resistant to encrustation and are well tolerated, their high coefficient of friction can make placement problematic.[5]

Cormio et al studied eight double-J stent brands placed in pigs for 6 weeks.[6] They found that silicone and hydrophilically coated stents induced less urothelial inflammation and destruction when compared to certain brands of polyurethane stents. Hydrophilically coated stents were also less prone to encrustation than silicone stents over the long term.

Recent investigations into the viability of metallic endoprostheses such as the Wallstent (Schneider, Minneapolis, MN) in the treatment of benign and malignant obstructions have shown them to be easy to insert and usually well tolerated by patients.[7,8] Despite the large internal lumen of the metallic stents, any clear advantage over plastic stents has yet to be demonstrated. A recent study of metallic stents in normal canine ureters demonstrated failure of incorporation at 6 months and a submucosal inflammatory/fibrotic response that may limit their long-term patency.[9]

Technique

Patient Preparation

The degree of patient preparation varies according to whether a nephrostomy tube is already in place. Preprocedural coagulation and platelet studies are always performed. Appropriate blood products should be transfused to correct any coagulopathy, especially when the coagulation profile is greater than 1.4–1.5 times control and platelet count less than 50,000.

A first or second generation cephalosporin is administered prophylactically prior to the procedure, with modifications made for patients at risk for bacterial endocarditis. Antibiotics are continued for at least 24 hours after the procedure.

After the patient is placed in a prone or semiprone position and low-dose supplemental oxygen is administered, conscious sedation and analgesia are initiated.

Traversing and Measuring the Ureter

Nephrostomy access and antegrade pyelography to identify the level of the obstruction, leak, or fistula are essential prerequisites to percutaneous antegrade stent placement. Further diagnostic information may also be obtained from these studies, such as an unsuspected leak and compressive urinoma in the clinical setting of obstruction. If the significance of a stenosis is questionable on the antegrade pyelogram, a Whitaker test can be performed using the same nephrostomy access **(See Tutorial 20)**.

Entry into a mid or upper calyx provides the best trajectory for ureteral catheterization and stent placement, although antegrade stents can be easily placed from a lower pole puncture, especially with the use of stiff guide wires. The choice of the entry calyx must be governed by the ease of ureteral accessibility versus the greater risk of pleural transgression with an upper pole or intercostal route. Once access into the collecting system has been obtained, a 7- or 8-F check-flow sheath can be inserted, replacing any existing nephrostomy tube. Placing a safety wire through this sheath into the renal pelvis is an option at this point. A torquable, hydrophilic guide wire inserted through a straight or preshaped catheter is useful for traversing tight strictures. The wire and catheter are advanced into the bladder.

The length of the ureter must be determined prior to stent placement. Once a catheter has been advanced into the bladder, an 0.035-inch standard guide wire is inserted through the catheter down to the center of the bladder. The proximal end of the wire is bent at the hub of the catheter. The distal end of the wire is then withdrawn into the renal pelvis, and the proximal end again bent at the catheter hub. The distance between the bends in the wire approximates the length of the ureter. This measured distance is also the desired distance between the proximal and distal loops of the double-J stent or nephroureterostomy tube, and an appropriately sized stent should be selected for insertion.

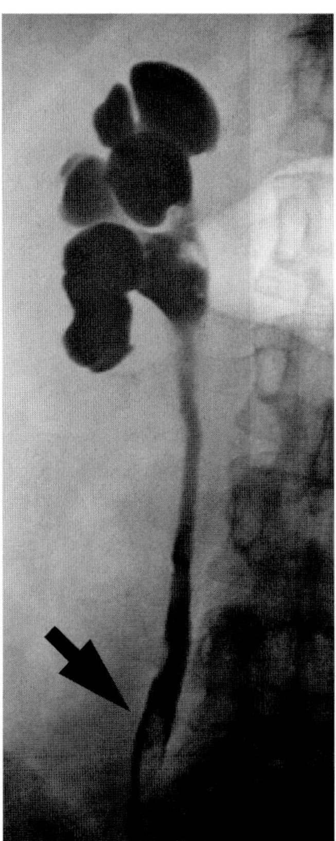

Figure 20. Retrograde catheterization of the right ureter under fluoroscopic guidance demonstrates ureteral obstruction due to blood clot (arrow).

Nephroureterostomy Stent Placement

After the torquable or measuring wire has been exchanged for an extra-stiff guide wire, dilation of any strictures can usually be performed with a balloon catheter inserted over the stiff wire. The check-flow sheath is then removed and the nephroureterostomy tube inserted over the extra-stiff wire. A peel-away sheath is optional at this point. The distal pigtail is positioned in the urinary bladder and formed by removal of the wire. The wire is then removed completely, allowing the proximal loop to be formed in the renal pelvis by pulling on the drawstring. A segment of the stent is left protruding from the flank to drain externally. After 24 hours the tube can be capped to allow antegrade internal drainage, barring any signs of infection or other complication.

Double-J Stent Placement

Double-J stents come fitted over a stiff straightening catheter. After antegrade placement of an extra-stiff guide wire through the ureter and into the bladder, a peel-away sheath is inserted over the wire and into the renal pelvis. This stent-straightener assembly is inserted over the wire and the distal end positioned in the bladder. As the wire and stiffener are withdrawn, the distal loop of the stent forms in the bladder. As the wire and stiffener are further withdrawn, the proximal loop forms in the renal pelvis. A suture looped through the proximal portion of some brands of stents aids in positioning the proximal loop of the stent properly in the renal pelvis. A wire is reinserted through the peel-away sheath, the sheath is removed, and an 8- or 10-F nephrostomy tube is inserted into the renal pelvis. Alternatively, without the use of a peel-away sheath, the wire is reinserted through the pusher or a nephrostomy tube is used as the pusher for the ureteral stent. If there are no complications, the nephrostomy tube is capped after 24 hours to test for successful drainage through the double-J stent. If the patient does well, a nephrostogram is performed and the nephrostomy tube removed after 2 to 3 days.

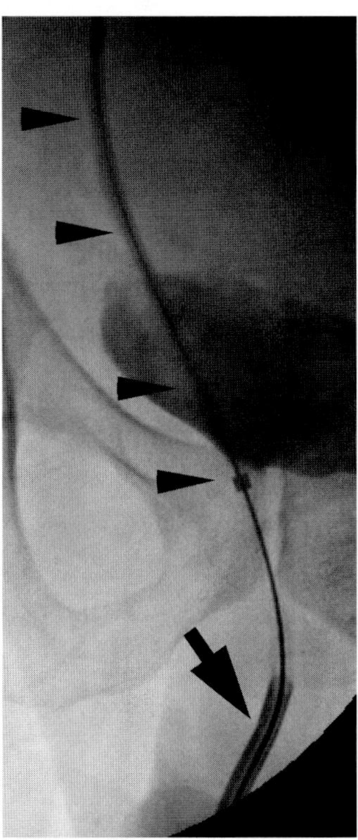

Figure 21. Same patient as in Figure 20. Retrograde advancement of a double-J ureteral stent (arrowheads) up the right ureter (over a wire) via a sheath introduced through the urethra (arrow).

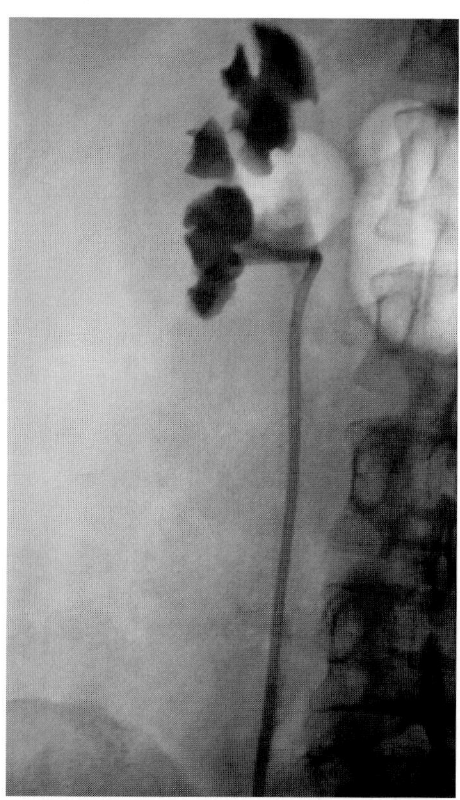

Figure 22. Same patient as in Figure 20. Final position of the double-J stent with the proximal loop in the renal pelvis.

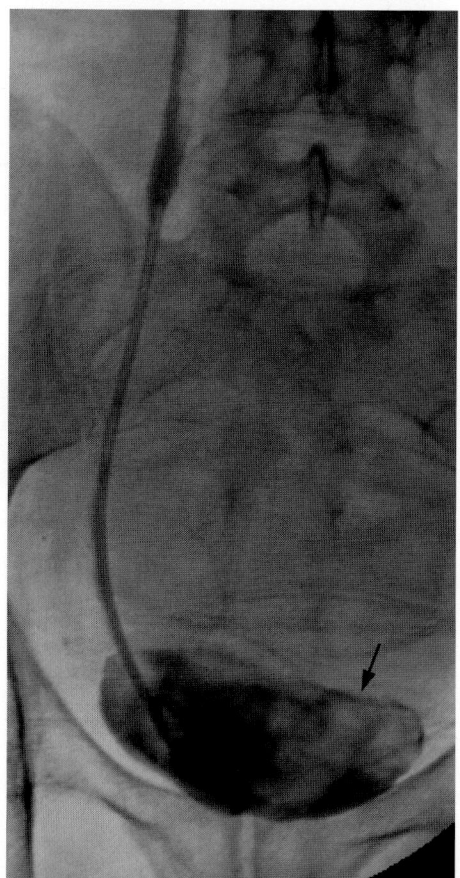

Figure 23. Same patient as in Figure 20. The distal loop is in the bladder, with decompression of the collecting system (note the blood clot in the bladder, arrow).

Occasionally, it may be necessary or advantageous to place a retrograde double-J stent with use of imaging-guided techniques.[4,10] This may be accomplished by probing the region of the bladder trigone for the ureteral orifice with a short curved catheter and guide wire introduced through a Foley catheter. Filling the bladder with dilute iodinated contrast material and adjusting the angulation of the image intensifier may also help to demonstrate the UVJ projecting above the bladder, which can then be gently probed and cannulated with a wire. Once a wire is negotiated up into the ureter, the double-J stent is inserted over the wire **(Figs. 20–23)**. **(See Teaching File Case 38)**.

Technical Difficulties and Complications

Barring complete ligation or clipping of the ureter, even the tightest of obstructions can usually be traversed by a guide wire with patience and ingenuity (torquable, hydrophilic wires are useful). However, delivery of the stent over the wire may not be possible. Use of a check-flow or peel-away sheath combined with an extra-stiff guide wire and access via a mid or upper calyx are helpful in transmitting force longitudinally down the ureter and reducing redundancy.[11]

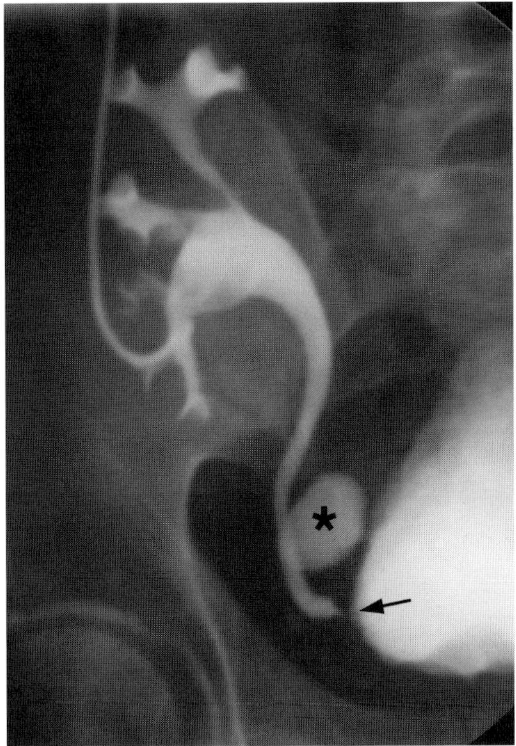

Figure 24. High-grade ureterovesical anastomotic stricture in a renal transplant patient (arrow). A bladder diverticulum (asterisk) is an incidental finding.

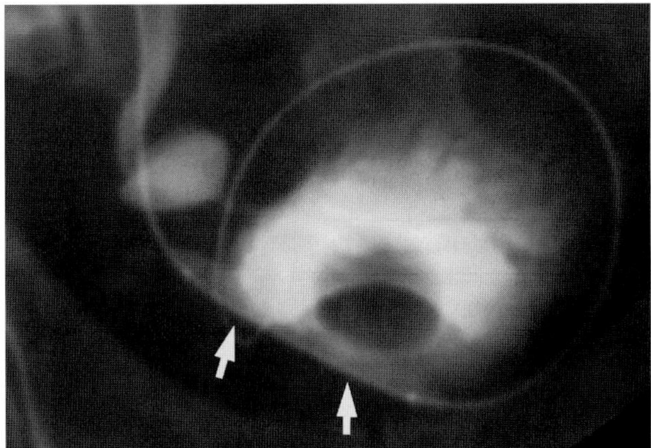

Figure 25. Same patient as in Figure 24. The UVJ stricture is traversed and successfully dilated with a 4-mm-diameter balloon (arrows).

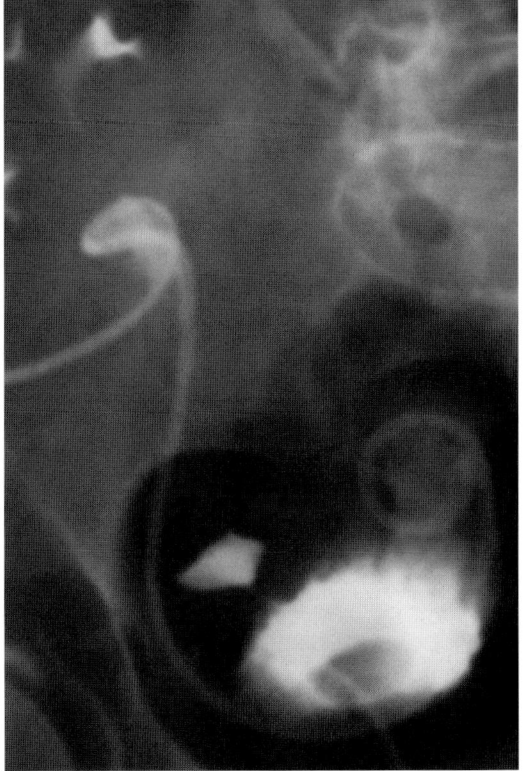

Figure 26. Same patient as in Figure 24. Final placement of an 8-F nephroureterostomy stent across the UVJ stricture, resulting in decompression of the transplant renal pelvis.

A balloon catheter will usually cross the stricture and can be used to dilate the narrowing prior to stent insertion **(Figs. 24–26)**. Asch et al have described a pull-through technique in which the antegrade wire is snared from below by a transurethral loop snare in the urinary bladder.[3] Control of both ends of the wire reduces ureteral redundancy and facilitates crossing of tight stenoses. The hydrophilic Glidex coating (Medi-Tech) on some ureteral stents helps overcome friction at tight strictures.

Tortuous ureters may impede stent insertion at the UPJ, UVJ, or along the ureter itself. Decompression by nephrostomy drainage for a few days helps reduce the ureteral redundancy produced by the obstruction. Decompression allows the ureter to resume a more normal course which facilitates ureteral stent insertion. Negotiation of a tortuous ureter with a catheter and torquable hydrophilic wire followed by exchange for an extra-stiff wire also helps to straighten the ureter.[11] Care should be taken to avoid overdistending the ureter with contrast material as inadvertent ureteral perforations or false passages may fill the retroperitoneum with contrast material, making further fluoroscopic visualization more difficult.

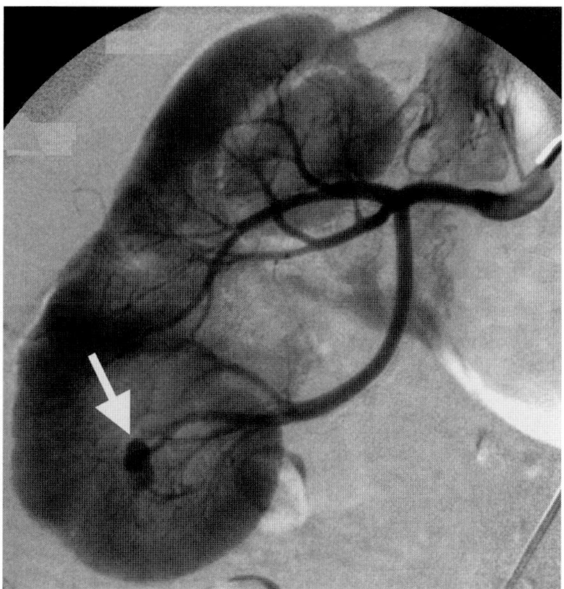

Figure 27. Selective renal arteriogram demonstrates a lower pole renal artery branch false aneurysm secondary to prior ureteral stent placement (arrow).

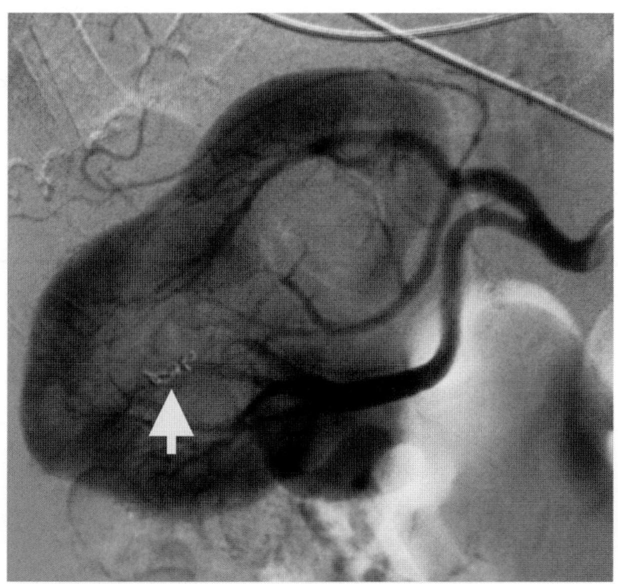

Figure 28. Same patient as in Figure 27. Successful transcatheter embolization of the lower pole branch pseudoaneurysm with microcoils (arrow).

Malpositioning of internalized stents usually occurs when the guide wire and pusher are removed prematurely, resulting in deployment of the proximal loop in the proximal ureter. This problem is often readily solved by pulling up on the suture that is looped through the proximal portion of some stent models. If the model does not have this suture loop, the loop has already been removed, or pulling on the loop is ineffective, then snaring the proximal portion of the stent with a loop-snare or stone basket allows it to be pulled up into the renal pelvis.[12]

Renovascular injury is a potential complication of any percutaneous urologic procedure. Severe bleeding from the percutaneous track, unremitting hematuria, and severe or symptomatic drops in hematocrit all warrant immediate resuscitation (with transfusions as needed) and emergent arteriography to identify a bleeding site. Pseudoaneurysms, small arteriovenous fistulas, and small foci of extravasation can usually be managed by transcatheter embolization with good results and limited risk in skilled hands **(Figs. 27, 28)**. Additionally, if ureteral stents are left in place for a prolonged period of time or if the patient has Crohn's disease or has undergone radiation therapy, then the stent can erode into the iliac vessels.

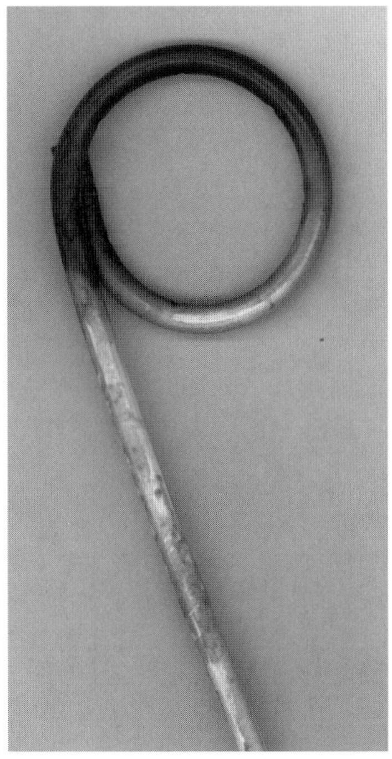

Figure 29. A double-J stent, just exchanged after 4 months, demonstrates a typical degree of material degradation.

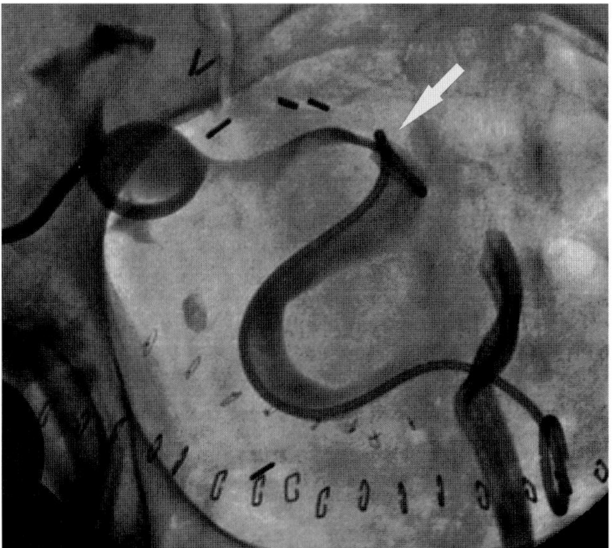

Figure 30. Nonfunctioning double-J stent which has retracted back into the proximal ureter (arrow).

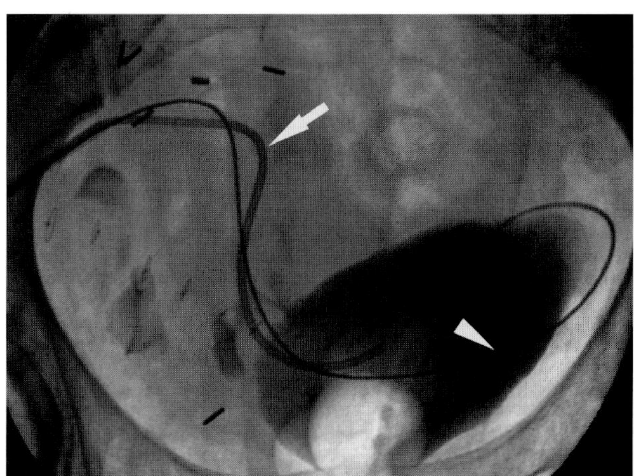

Figure 31. Same patient as in Figure 30. The double-J stent (arrow) is engaged with an Amplatz Gooseneck snare (Microvena, White Bear Lake, MN) and withdrawn through a 6-F sheath. A safety wire is left in place to preserve access (arrowhead).

Management

Given the inevitable occurrence of stent encrustation and material degradation **(Fig. 29)**, double-J stents must be changed either cystoscopically (with general or epidural anesthesia) or fluoroscopically (by recreating percutaneous nephrostomy access and snaring the stent) every 3 to 6 months **(Figs. 30–32)**.[13,14] For this reason, some patients and clinicians prefer nephroureterostomy stents, which make for an easier exchange. At our institution these are changed every 6 to 8 weeks. Because of the stent's external portion, an increased risk of infection exists, especially in transplant patients. In fact, some patients are placed on long-term oral antibiotics to minimize the risk of infection introduced through the external portion of the stent.

The processes of stent encrustation and degradation are accelerated in ureteroileostomy patients due to the presence of intestinal secretions **(Fig. 33)**. Consequently, more frequent stent changes may be necessary.

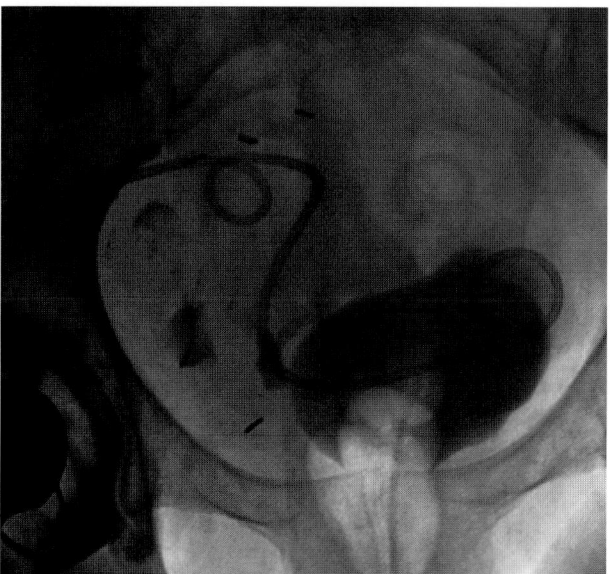

Figure 32. Same patient as in Figure 30 . The 6-F sheath is removed and a nephroureteral stent inserted over the safety wire, with effective decompression of the collecting system at the completion of the procedure.

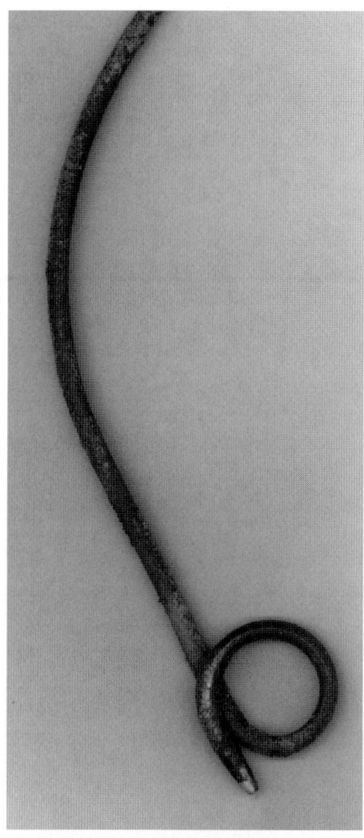

Figure 33. Distal portion of a nephroureteral stent which has been within an ileal loop for almost 3 months. Note the extensive degradation and encrustation (compare to Figure 29).

An alternative to the standard fluoroscopic and cystoscopic techniques is the retrograde snare-removal of double-J stents with retrograde fluoroscopic replacement, all through a transurethral catheter. Wetton et al successfully performed this procedure on an outpatient basis on 27 stents in 15 patients.[10] Local anesthesia, antibiotic prophylaxis, and intravenous sedation were given. The procedure was well tolerated by all patients in the series, with no serious complications. More recently, de Baere et al had a 97% success rate with this technique on 165 stents.[15] The cost savings using this approach are readily apparent.

Patients with ureteral stents must be aggressively worked up if flank pain, fever, renal dysfunction, or pyuria develops. Particularly in the transplant patient, prompt evaluation is essential to prevent damage to the graft. Ultrasound with Doppler techniques can rule out obstruction. If a nephroureteral stent is present, a tube check can be performed to evaluate for stent patency (being careful not to overdistend the pelvocaliceal system and precipitate sepsis). The nephroureteral stent can be exchanged for a new stent if it is obstructed, or for a temporary nephrostomy tube during treatment of urosepsis if necessary. Obstructed double-J stents can be exchanged from a retrograde (usually cystoscopic) approach or by obtaining new nephrostomy access for snaring and removal of the stent from above. As with nephroureterostomy stents, a temporary nephrostomy tube should be placed during treatment of urosepsis, if present, prior to insertion of a new double-J stent.

References

1. Hunter DW, Castaneda-Zuniga WR, Coleman CC, Herrera M, Amplatz K. Percutaneous techniques in the management of urological complications in renal transplant patients. Radiology 1983; 148:407–412.

2. Kenny B, Lynch N, Hurley GD. Antegrade stenting of malignant ureteral strictures. Eur Radiol 1995; 5:623–625.

3. Asch MR, Jaffer NM. Antegrade placement of a ureteric stent by a pull-through technique. Can Assoc Radiol J 1995; 46:465–467.

4. Huang TY, Perkins T, Mader G. Retrograde placement of internal double-J ureteral stents by using cystographic guidance. AJR 1994; 163:371–372.

5. Castaneda-Zuniga WR, Brady TM, Thomas R, Castaneda F, Letourneau JG, Hulbert JC. Interventional uroradiology in interventional radiology. 3rd edition. Baltimore: Williams & Wilkins, 1997; 1071–1073.

6. Cormio L, Talja M, Koivusalo A, et al. Biocompatibility of various indwelling double-J stents. J Urol 1995; 153:494–496.

7. Pollak JS, Rosenblatt MM, Egglin TK, Dickey KW, Glickman M. Treatment of ureteral obstructions with the Wallstent endoprosthesis: preliminary results. J Vasc Interv Radiol 1995; 6:417–425.

8. Lugmayr HF, Pauer W. Wallstents for the treatment of extrinsic malignant ureteral obstruction: midterm results. Radiology 1996; 198:105–108.

9. Thijssen AM, Millward SF, Mai KT. Ureteral response to the placement of metallic stents: an animal model. J Urol 1994; 151:268–270.

10. Wetton CW, Gedroyc WM. Retrograde radiological retrieval and replacement of double-J ureteric stents. Clin Radiol 1995; 50:562–565.

11. Lu DS, Papanicolaou N, Girard M, Lee MJ, Yoder IC. Percutaneous internal ureteral stent placement: review of technical issues and solutions in 50 consecutive cases. Clin Radiol 1994; 49:256–261.

12. Patel U, Kellett MJ. Misplaced double-J ureteric stent: technique for repositioning using the Nitinol “Gooseneck” snare. Clin Radiol 1994; 49:333–336.

13. Isaacson S, Pugash RA. Use of a variation of loop snare for manipulation of ureteral stents. AJR 1996; 166:1169–1171.

14. Breen DJ, Cowan NC. Fluoroscopically guided retrieval of ureteric stents. Clin Radiol 1995; 50:860–863.

15. de Baere T, Denys A, Pappas P, Challier E, Roche A. Ureteral stents: exchange under fluoroscopic control as an effective alternative to cystoscopy. Radiology 1994; 190:887–889.

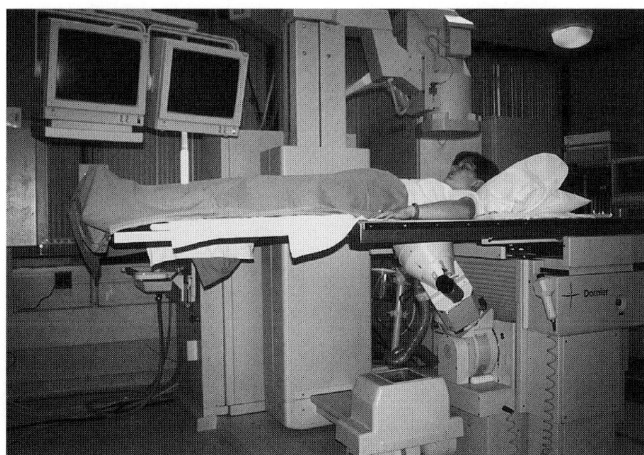

Figure 1. Third generation multifunctional extracorporeal shock wave lithotripter.

TUTORIAL 22
RENAL AND URETERAL CALCULI

Allen J. Meglin, M.D., and Pierce B. Irby, M.D.

Introduction

The subjects addressed in this tutorial include:

1. Indications for percutaneous nephrolithotomy of renal and ureteral calculi
2. Indications for extracorporeal shock wave lithotripsy
3. Techniques of percutaneous nephrolithotomy
4. Indications, contraindications, and outcome analysis for percutaneous nephrolithotomy and extracorporeal shock wave lithotripsy stone procedures
5. Complications of percutaneous nephrolithotomy.

Interest in the skills and techniques associated with percutaneous renal interventions is coming full circle since the introduction of these procedures almost two decades ago.[1] As percutaneous surgery reached maturity in the early 1980s, another emerging technology, extracorporeal shock wave lithotripsy (ESWL) (Dornier Medical Systems, Inc., Kennesaw, GA), was introduced.[2] This latter form of minimally invasive surgery revolutionized the treatment of urinary stone disease, severely limiting the use of the more invasive percutaneous procedures **(Fig. 1)**.

After a decade of experience, the limitations of ESWL have become apparent, particularly in the treatment of large-burden upper tract stone disease, infected stones, inferior calyceal stones, and other complex situations where internal drainage of the collecting system is suboptimal. Percutaneous nephrolithotomy (PNL) is enjoying a resurgence in these cases **(Figs. 2–5)**.[3]

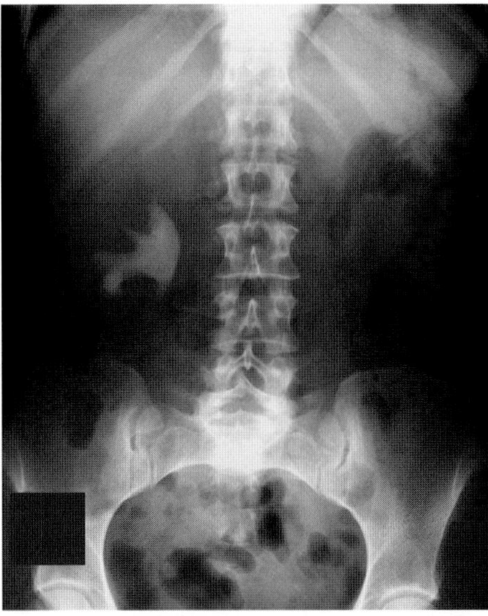

Figure 2. Kidneys, ureter, bladder (KUB) study demonstrates a complete right staghorn calculus in a 42-year-old woman with recurrent urinary tract infections.

The application of percutaneous techniques for intrarenal surgery has broadened beyond the treatment of stone disease in recent years.[4] The placement of percutaneous nephrostomy tubes for obstructive uropathy is now routine **(Figs. 6, 7)**. Management of ureteropelvic junction (UPJ) obstruction by antegrade endopyelotomy has become common, with success rates approaching those of open pyeloplasty in the most experienced centers.[5,6] While seldom performed, and rightly so, there is growing expertise in the percutaneous excision of upper tract tumors in selected patients. Percutaneous ablation of calyceal diverticula is now commonly used to manage these vexing abnormalities.[7,8–10]

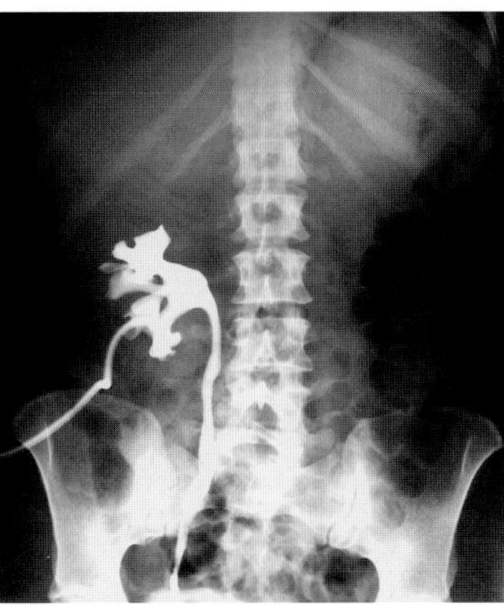

Figure 3. Same patient as in Figure 2. Nephrostogram following PNL through a lower pole posterior calyceal access.

Urologic laparoscopy has emerged in the past 5 years, initially fueling great expectations for this new endosurgical field **(Figs. 8–10)**. To date, advanced urologic laparoscopic techniques have not made a significant impact on the treatment of stone disease.

Establishing access for percutaneous interventions is the first and most critical step in the procedure. When possible, this step should be planned and performed by radiologists in conjunction with urologists to ensure appropriate access position for subsequent stages of the intervention. Clear communication between the two specialists is mandatory. This tutorial describes the principles and techniques of gaining access to the intrarenal collecting system under both typical and exceptional circumstances.

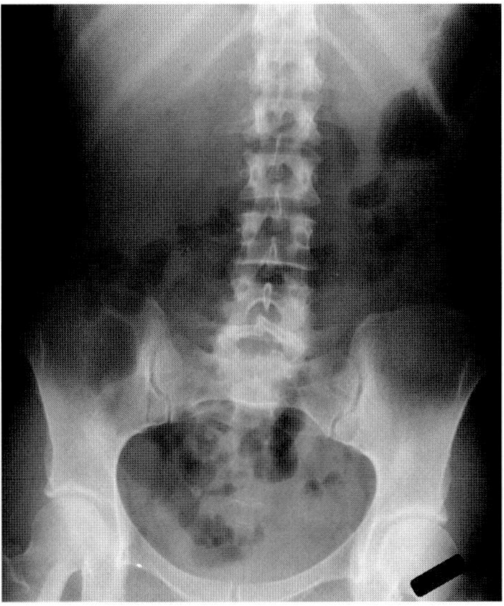

Figure 4. Same patient as in Figure 2. Postoperative KUB confirms no residual fragments.

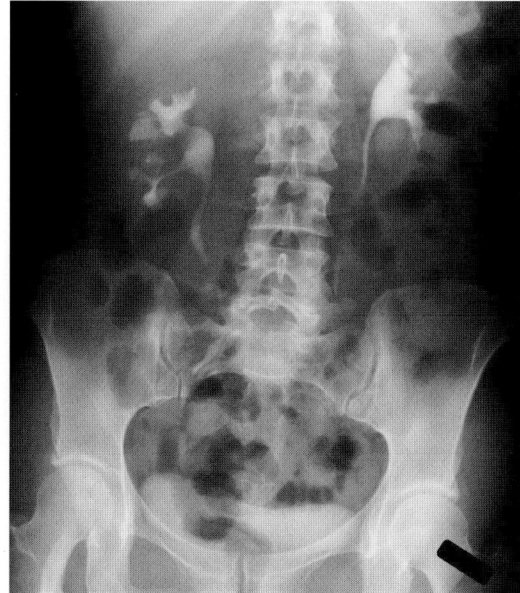

Figure 5. Same patient as in Figure 2. Follow-up intravenous pyelogram (IVP) after 3 months.

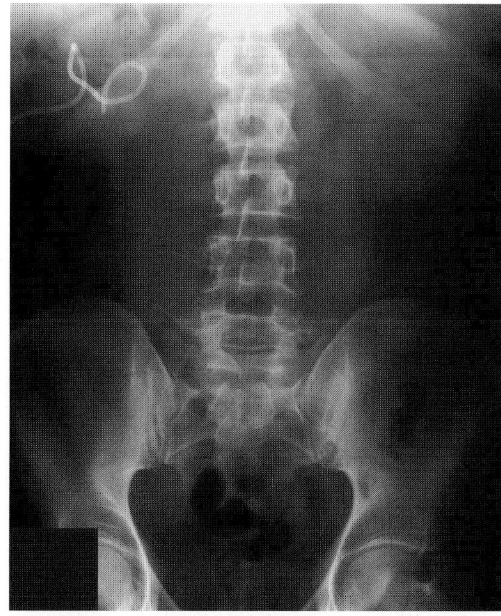

Figure 6. KUB following percutaneous nephrostomy for an obstructing radiolucent right mid ureteral stone in a 48-year-old man.

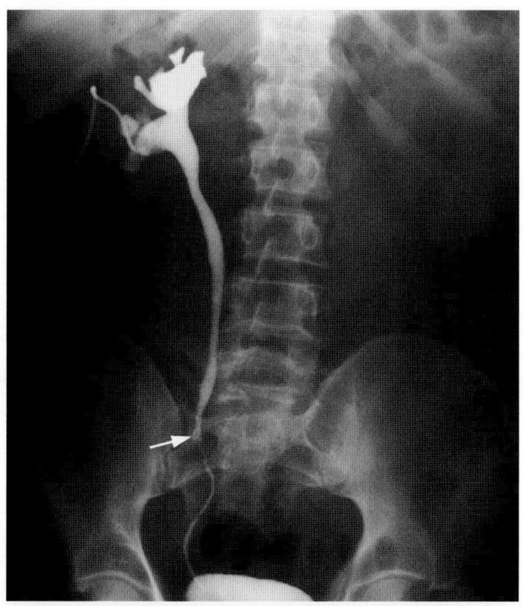

Figure 7. Same patient as in Figure 6. Nephrostogram demonstrates an impacted uric acid stone (arrow).

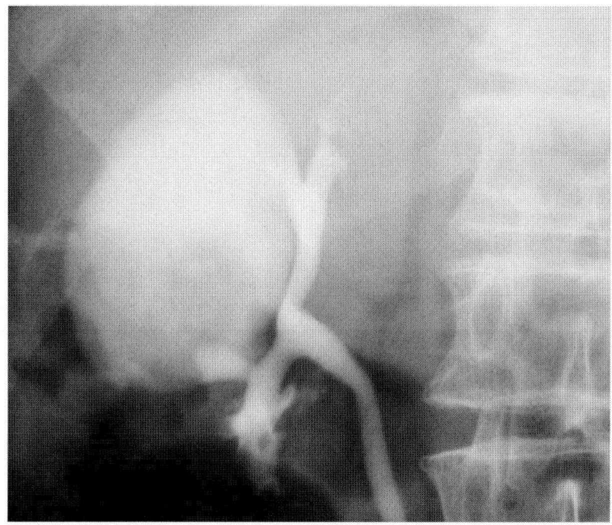

Figure 8. Retrograde pyelogram with a large right interpolar calyceal diverticulum in a 63-year-old man with flank pain.

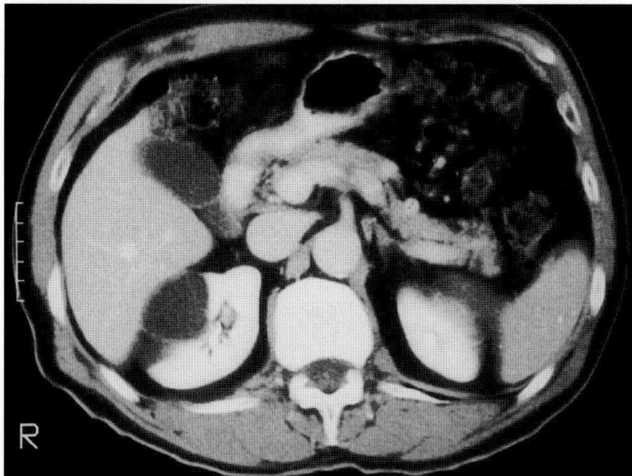

Figure 9. Same patient as in Figure 8. Noncontrast computed tomography (CT) scan demonstrates the anterior location of the diverticulum, which is not amenable to percutaneous approach.

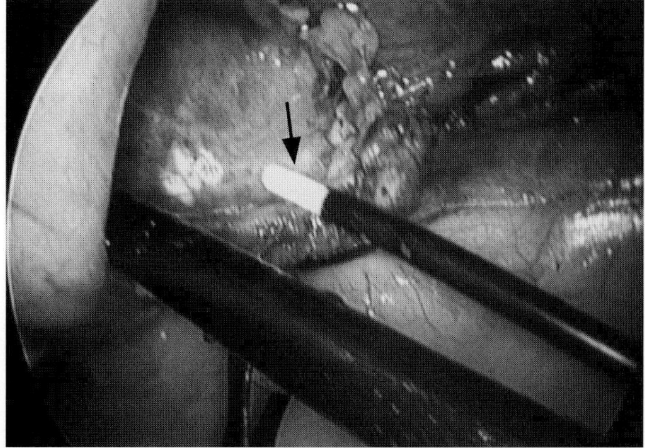

Figure 10. Same patient as in Figure 8. Laparoscopic unroofing and ablation of the diverticulum ostium using an argon beam coagulator (arrow).

Indications for Percutaneous Intervention

1. Large-burden stones greater than 2.5 cm in diameter, which are typically not amenable to ESWL **(Fig. 11)**.[7]
2. Lower pole stones, especially those larger than 1.0 cm in diameter; the stone-free rate after ESWL in these cases is only 50% **(Fig. 12)**.
3. ESWL failures, particularly in cases where the stones are extremely hard, such as those of composed of calcium oxalate monohydrate and cystine.
4. Patients who are inappropriate for ESWL due to body habitus, obesity, deformities, congenital anomalies, vascular aneurysms, and ureteral obstruction. Percutaneous access may be required in some cases to perform antegrade ureteroscopy and stone manipulation and extraction.

Contraindications

Coagulopathy, untreated urinary tract infection, and morbid obesity such that instrumentation length is inadequate are all contraindications to percutaneous intervention.

Technique

Nephrostomy access obtained in a single setting followed by surgery decreases both patient anxiety and the risk of tube dislodgement. No outcome advantage is gained for staged procedures in the hands of an experienced interventional/surgical team unless complications develop. We advocate a single setting for all percutaneous interventions except in the rare cases when rapid tamponade due to unexpected hemorrhage or drainage due to unexpected infection arises.

Before the procedure is begun, a Foley catheter is placed in the bladder and a ureteral occlusion balloon catheter is secured to it **(Figs. 13–15)**. The ureteral occlusion balloon catheter is placed retrograde into the ureter to permit instillation of contrast material into the collecting system and to create hydronephrosis for ease of access **(Figs. 16–18)**. Time can be saved if the urologist places the catheter in the interventional suite using flexible cystoscopy with the patient in the supine or prone position. Methylene blue dye mixed with dilute contrast material can be instilled via the ureteral occlusion catheter to confirm needle access into the collecting system at the time of percutaneous nephrostomy, as blue-colored fluid will be aspirated through the access needle.

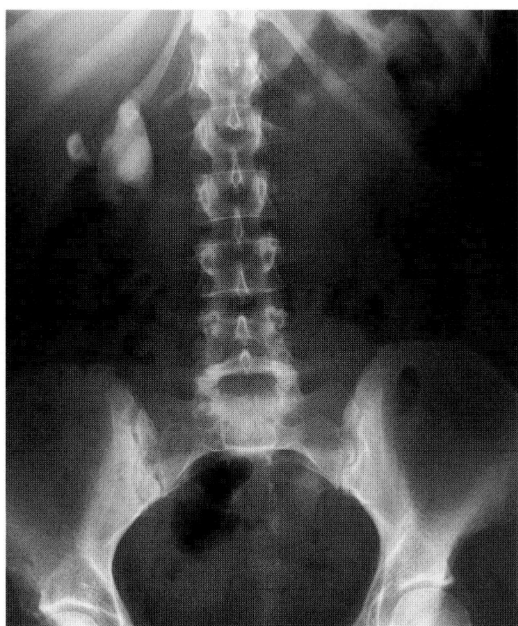

Figure 11. Staghorn calculus, too large for ESWL.

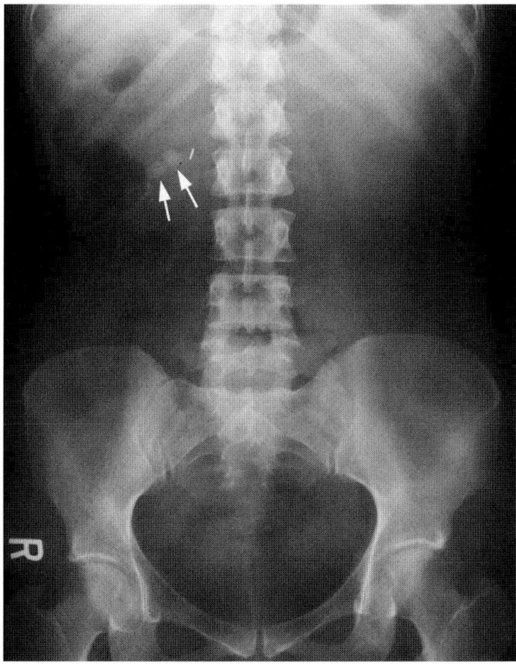

Figure 12. Lower pole calyceal stones greater than 1 cm in diameter (arrows).

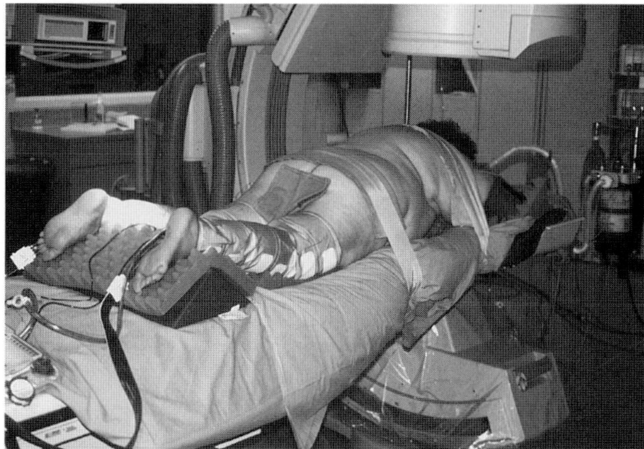

Figure 13. Prone patient positioning for PNL.

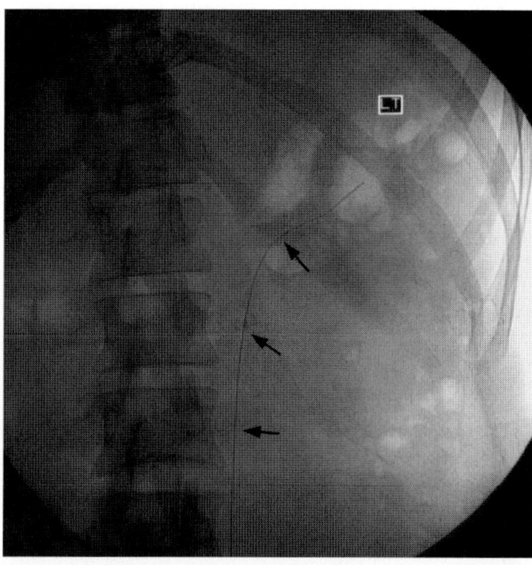

Figure 14. 35-year-old man with adult polycystic kidney disease and a 5-cm radiolucent left pelvic stone. Flexible cystoscopy was used to place an 0.025-inch guide wire into the renal pelvis with the patient in the supine position (arrows).

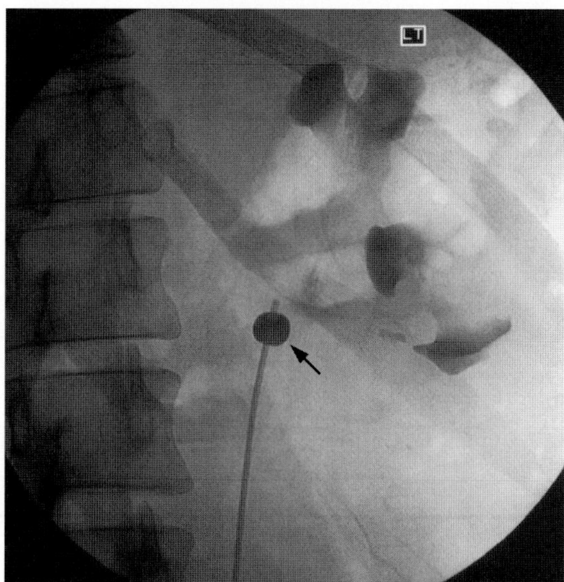

Figure 15. Same patient as in Figure 14. Ureteral occlusion balloon catheter (6 F) passed over a wire (arrow). Patient in the supine position.

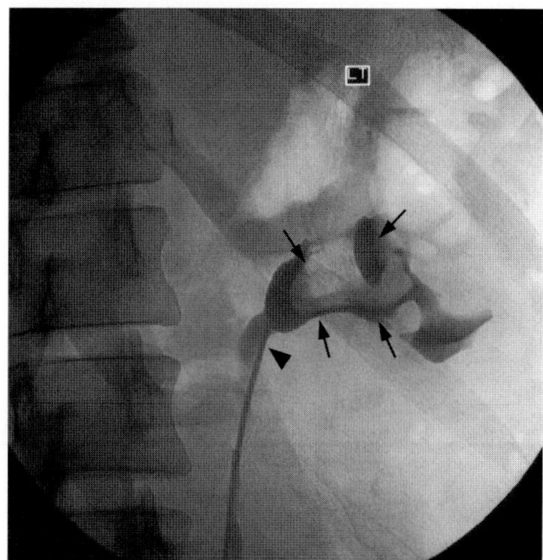

Figure 16. Same patient as in Figure 14. Supine retrograde contrast study shows the stone as a filling defect (arrows). The occlusion balloon is inflated (arrowhead).

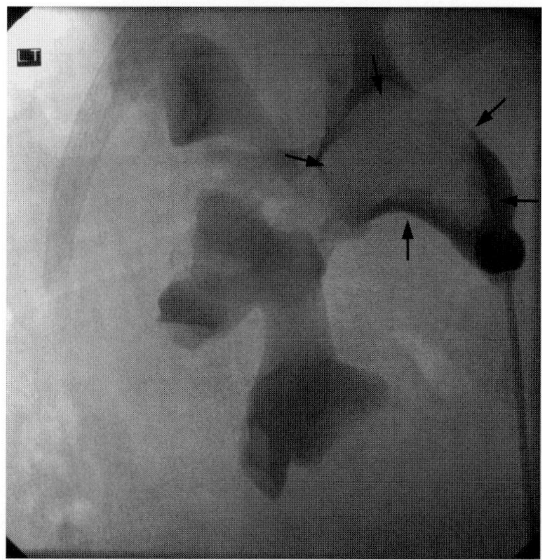

Figure 17. Same patient as in Figure 14, repositioned in the prone position. The balloon is inflated, occluding the UPJ. Contrast shows the stone as a filling defect (arrows).

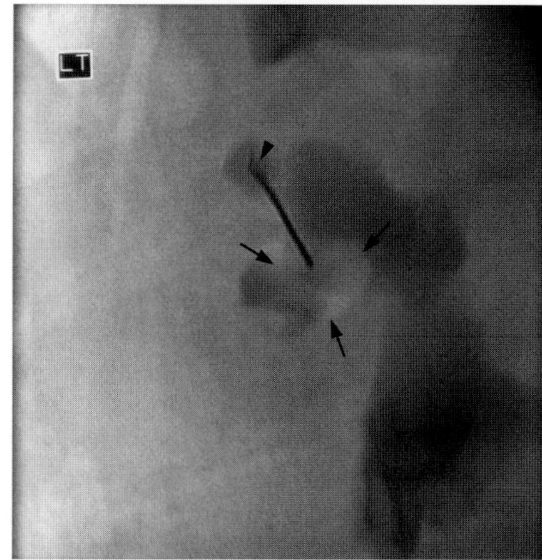

Figure 18. Same patient as in Figure 14, prone position. Hydronephrosis created by retrograde instillation of dilute contrast material and gas. The needle (arrowhead) is directed at a posterior air-filled calyx (arrows).

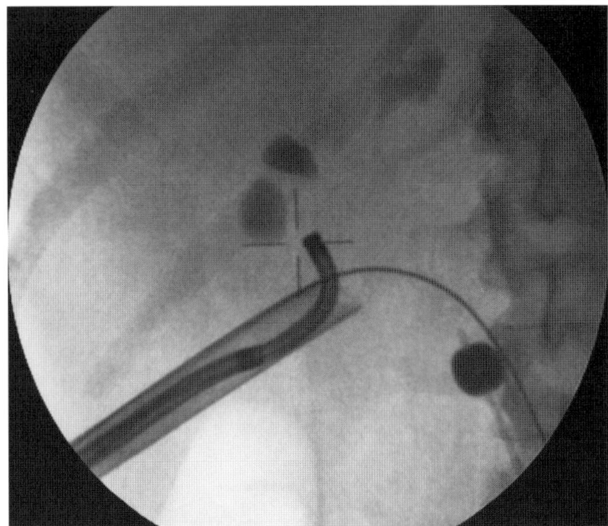

Figure 19. Same patient as in Figure 12. An inferior calyx was entered but this access site did not permit the flexible nephroscope to reach the stones. Patient in the supine position.

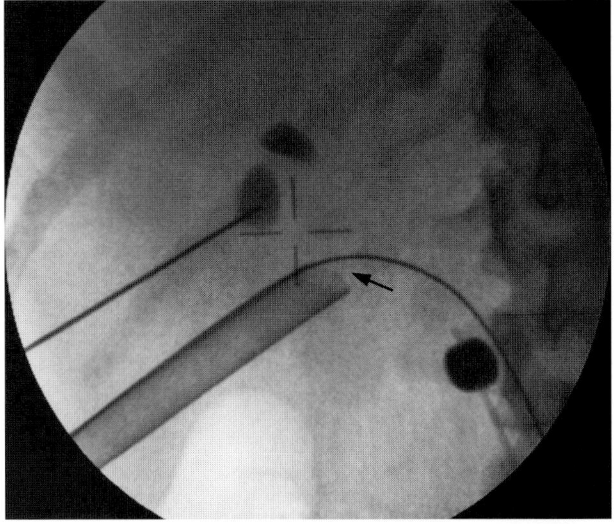

Figure 20. A separate, supracostal access site was required to treat the calyceal stones (arrow). Patient in the supine position.

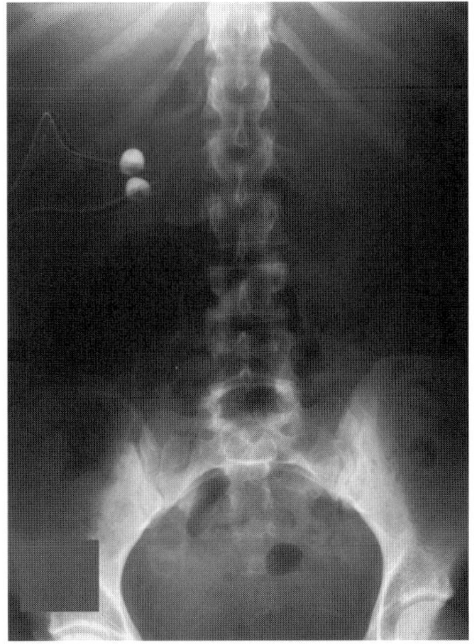

Figure 21. At the conclusion of the procedure in Figure 20, Foley catheters are placed in both tracks.

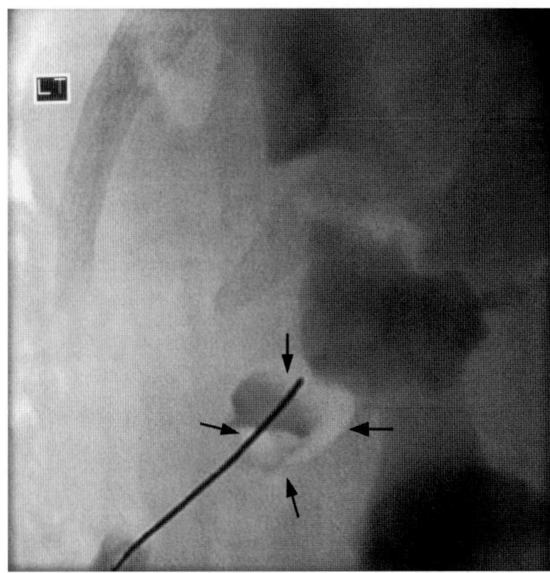

Figure 22. Same patient as in Figure 14. Multiplanar complex angulation allows the fluoroscopy beam to align with the Jeffrey needle ("down-the-barrel"). The calyx filled with gas in the prone position identifies a posterior, inferior pole location for the best approach to the collecting system (arrows). Off-axis angulation shows the needle in profile.

The ideal approach to the renal collecting system for stone disease targets a posterior, inferior pole calyx **(Figs. 19)**.[8] Although this will vary with each patient, in the majority of cases such access will ultimately permit the introduction of a rigid or flexible nephroscope capable of reaching and manipulating most, if not all, of the collecting system. For large-burden staghorn calculi with multiple branched shapes or multiple stones in separate calyces, multiple access tracks may be necessary and should be planned **(Figs. 20, 21)**. If antegrade ureteroscopy is planned, an upper pole or interpolar calyceal puncture access may provide the greatest mechanical advantage.

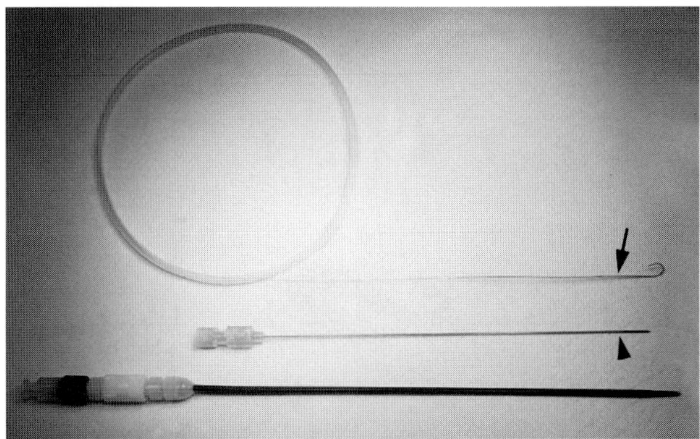

Figure 23. Jeffrey needle exchange set with an 0.18-inch "steerable" J-tip stainless steel wire (arrow), 21-gauge two-piece puncture needle (arrowhead), and fascial dilator with a 6-F introducer sheath for passage of a second safety wire.

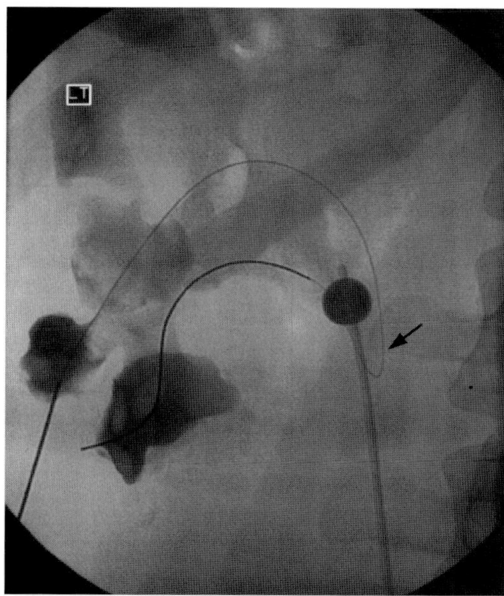

Figure 24. Jeffrey wire manipulated down the ureter (arrow) past the occlusion balloon. Patient in the prone position.

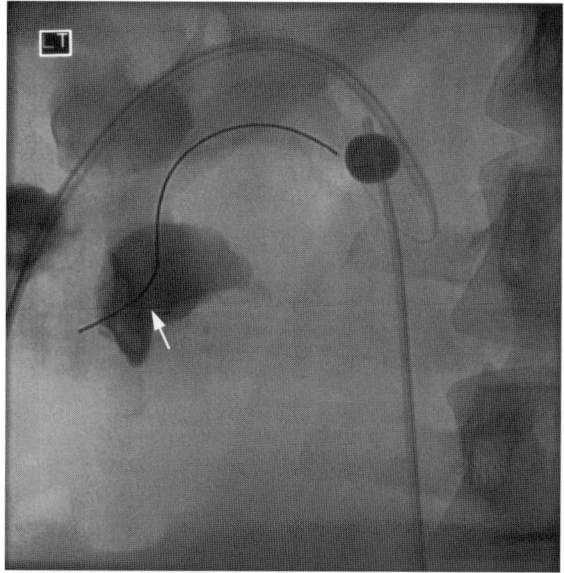

Figure 25. Dilator and sheath passed over the wire beyond the UPJ. Note the wire tip in the lower pole anterior calyx (arrow). Patient in the prone position.

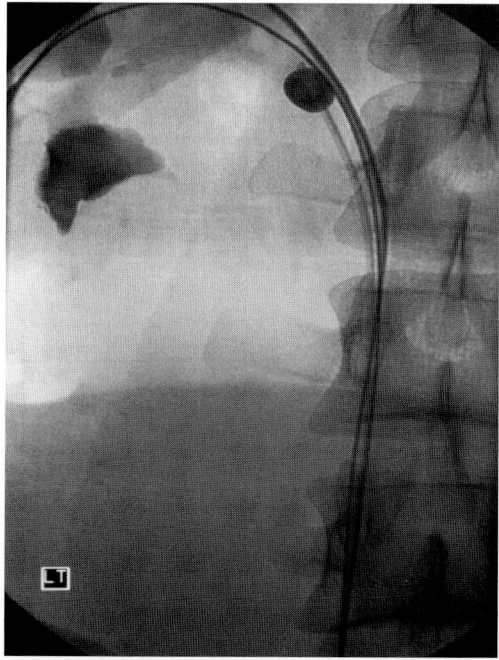

Figure 26. Jeffrey wire exchanged for working and safety 0.038-inch Teflon J-tip guide wires passed down the ureter.

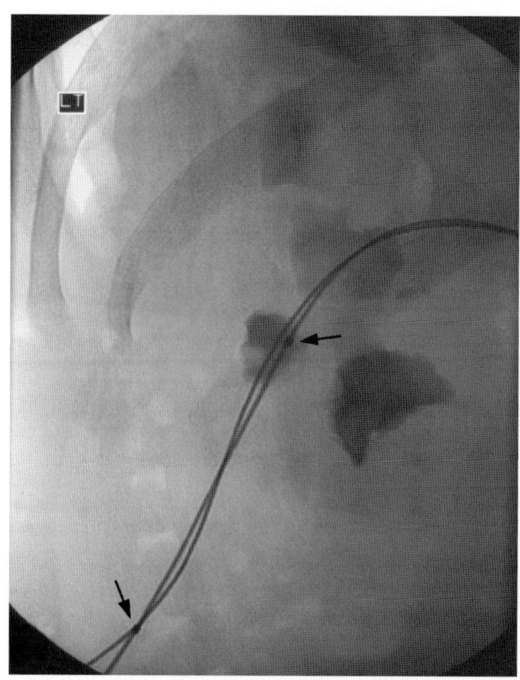

Figure 27. Olbert nephrostomy track balloon dilator (7 F), passed over a working wire into the target calyx (radiopaque markers at arrows show balloon length).

Needle puncture access into the targeted calyx can be performed relatively safely using a two-piece 21-gauge needle **(Figs. 22–27)**. Retrograde instillation of gas may fill posterior calyces in the prone position to aid in distinguishing posterior from anterior calyces.[9] In our practice, room air in small quantities has been used for this purpose. The risk of air embolus requires constant monitoring of the volume and pressure of gas used. Continuous fluoroscopic guidance is requisite when infusing room air or CO_2. Some authors advocate the use of CO_2 rather than room air as it is known to be safe when introduced into the vascular system outside the intracranial circulation.[10] Working and safety guide wires are manipulated down the ureter to ensure secure access when possible.

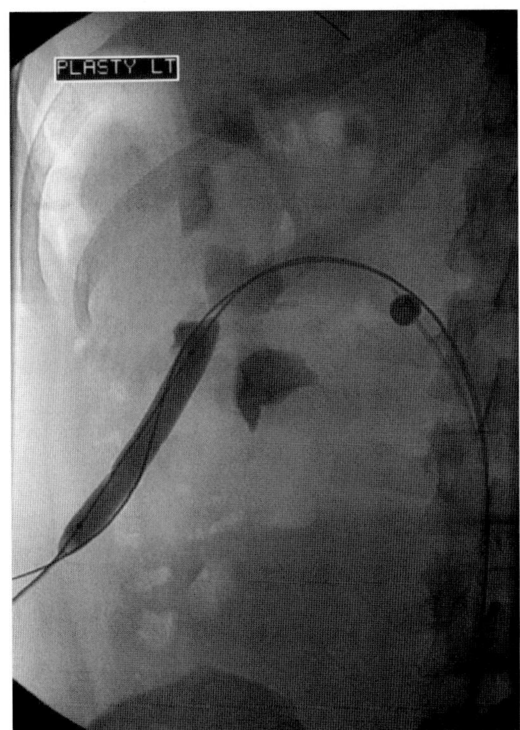

Figure 28. Balloon is inflated to dilate the track to 10 mm (30 F).

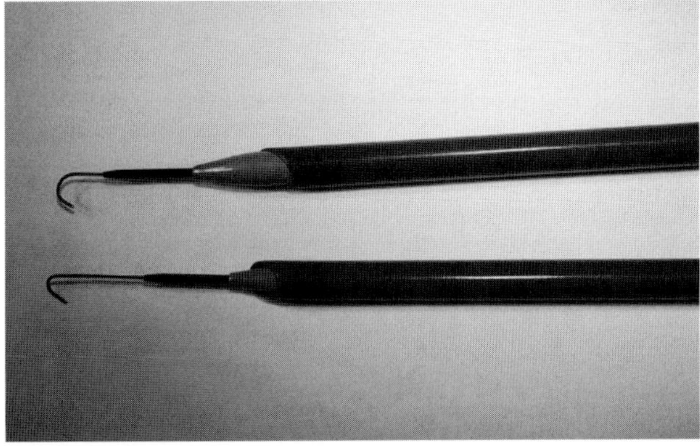

Figure 30. Amplatz renal dilators and sheath set.

The nephrostomy track is then dilated with a 10-mm (30-F) balloon dilator. Forward pressure on the balloon is necessary because it may back out of the track as it is inflated **(Figs. 28, 29)**. Additionally, the balloon must be positioned precisely in the renal parenchyma and not the calyceal infundibulum as infundibular rupture will cause bleeding and extravasation of contrast material, which can obscure the field of view.

Alternatively, rigid sequential Amplatz dilators can be used, but these are more traumatic than balloon dilation.[6] Sufficient space must exist in the collecting system for the tapered nose of the Amplatz dilators to rest. Otherwise, renal tissue may be sheared off during the process, causing severe hemorrhage **(Figs. 30–32)**.[6]

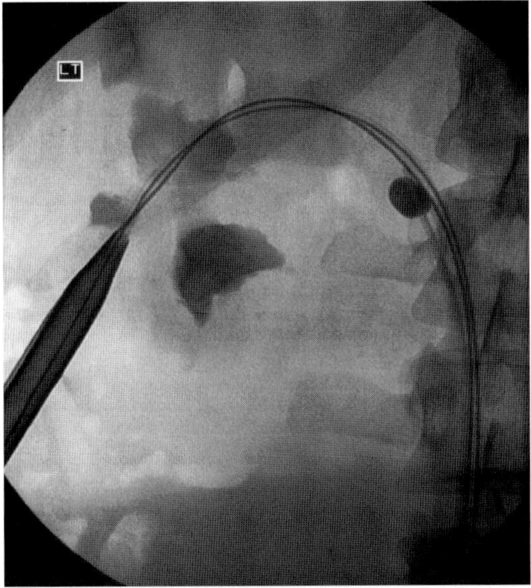

Figure 29. After balloon dilation, angioplasty dilators are sequentially placed with the resultant 30-F sheath as the endpoint.

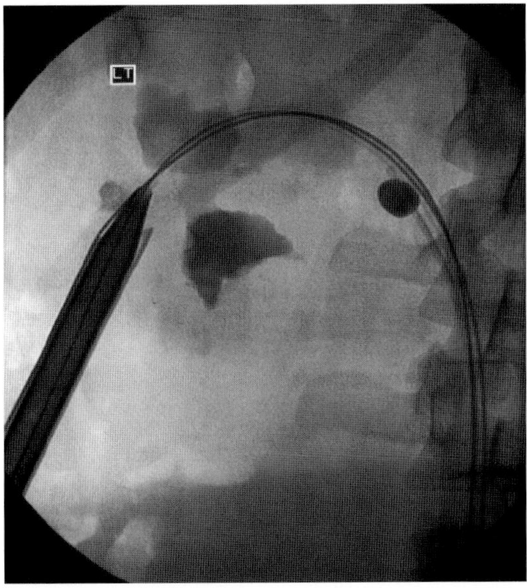

Figure 31. 30-F Amplatz dilator (tip only) passed into the lower pole. With the dilator tip barely in the calyx, sheath advancement is unsafe. The rigid sheath could shear off part of the papilla. The dilator tip must be well within the calyx.

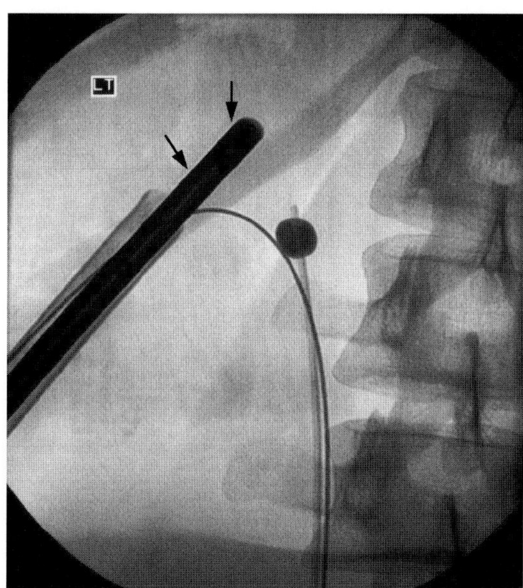

Figure 32. Sheath in the lower pole with a rigid nephroscope (arrows) in the sheath.

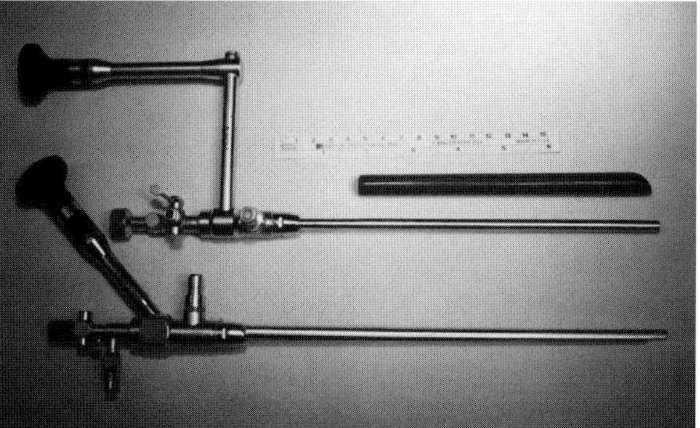

Figure 33. Standard and long rigid nephroscopes with a 30-F Amplatz sheath.

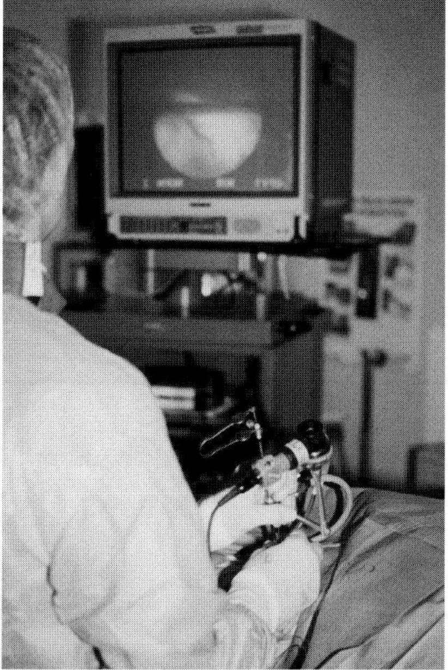

Figure 34. Use of a video camera enhances vision, efficiency, safety, and team participation.

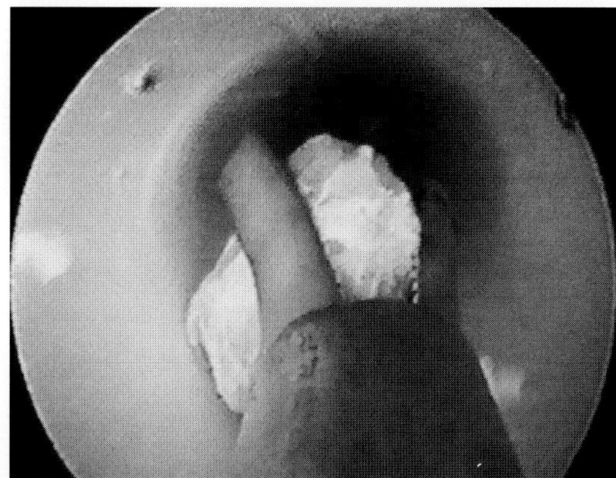

Figure 35. Stones smaller than 10 mm in diameter are removed intact with graspers through the Amplatz sheath.

The open Amplatz sheath is the most desirable access sheath because it provides a low-pressure system for subsequent nephroscopy, thereby preventing the complications of high-pressure irrigant flow (extravasation, intravasation, bacteremia). The rigid nephroscope is inserted into the 30-F sheath. A video camera is used routinely for improved visualization and for teaching. It also provides better operating room communication, helps maintain team interest, and protects the surgeon from contaminated fluids, blood, and lithotripsy aerosols **(Figs. 33, 34)**.

The most important juncture comes next—determining whether or not the scope is in the collecting system. Even experienced operators can easily become disoriented. Clues to correct positioning are the characteristic appearance of the epithelial lining of the collecting system and stone material. Irrigation instillation must be kept to a minimum until proper scope location has been positively confirmed. When stone material is identified, large stones and fragments less than 10 mm in size are removed through the sheath with rigid graspers **(Fig. 35)**.[10–12] Stones too large to pass through the sheath are fragmented with ultrasonic or electrohydraulic lithotripsy.

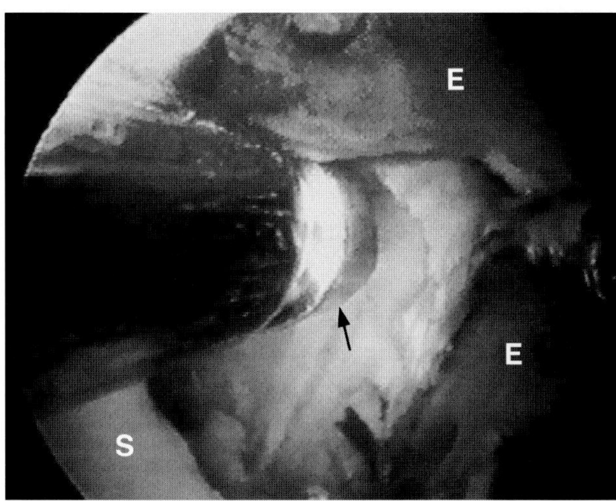

Figure 36. Smooth epithelium (E) of the collecting system is noted at the top and lower right. An ultrasonic lithotrite probe is engaged against a large stone for pulverization (arrow). An Amplatz sheath (S) tip at the left of the probe is placed against the stone.

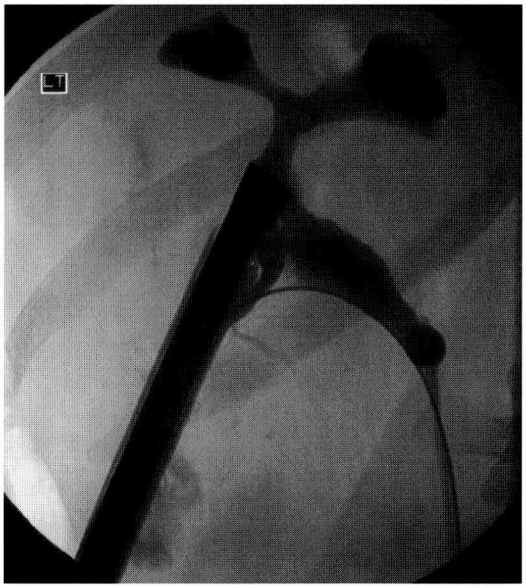

This probe vibrates using ultrasound or spark gap shock wave energy and has an oscillating burr tip that can bore a hole in the hardest of stones **(Fig. 36)**.

Irrigation cools the probe tip while suction through the hollow probe tip removes particulate material like a vacuum cleaner. The stones break along cleavage planes and fragments are removed by graspers. Following removal of all stone material with the rigid nephroscope, residual fragments and stones are located by flexible nephroscopy. All calyces of the collecting system must be meticulously inspected **(Fig. 37)**. Residual fragments can be flushed out, basketed, or fragmented further with a flexible electrohydraulic lithotripsy probe as small as 1.9 F (0.6 mm). The occlusion balloon prevents fragments from escaping down the ureter to cause obstruction. Unless a large amount of bleeding impedes visualization, the operation continues until all stone material is removed.[4]

Figure 37. Nephroscope advanced through the sheath into the pelvis following ultrasonic lithotripsy and stone removal. Inspection of the upper pole infundibulum and calyces with a rigid nephroscope.

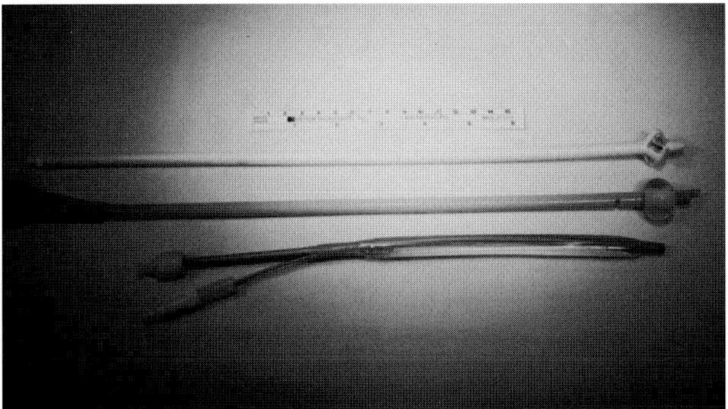

Figure 38. Nephrostomy tubes. Malecot (top); Foley balloon catheter with the distal tip shortened (middle); and Kaye nephrostomy track tamponade balloon catheter (bottom).

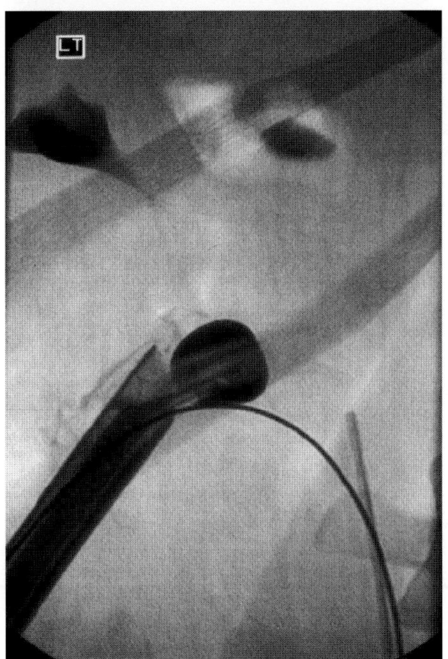

Figure 39. A 22-F Foley balloon catheter is passed through the sheath into the renal pelvis. 3 mL of contrast material is then injected into the balloon.

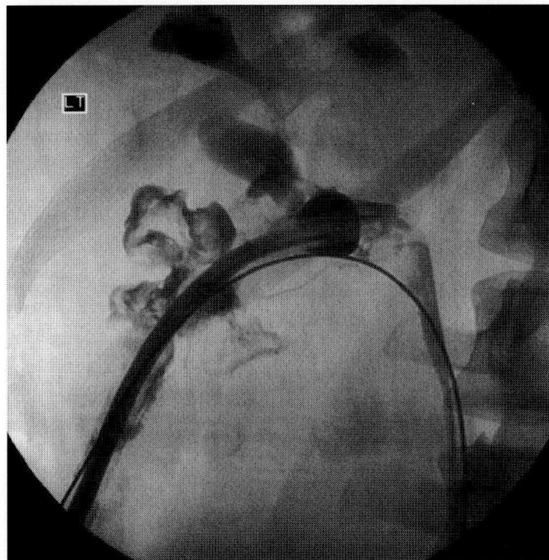

Figure 40. The sheath has been removed and the ureteral occlusion balloon has been deflated. The nephrostogram confirms tube position. The safety wire remains in place until the patient is ready for transport.

When the operation is finished, a large-caliber nephrostomy tube (24 F if possible) is placed for adequate drainage of urine, blood, and any residual stone sediment. This may be of the Malecot type (with or without re-entry ureteral extension) which can be passed over a guide wire. Alternatively, a balloon catheter (Foley type) with 2–3 mL of contrast material inflated in the renal pelvis can be used. A postprocedure nephrostogram confirms placement of this tube **(Figs. 38–40)**.

When the Amplatz sheath is removed and the tamponade effect is lost, there may be significant bleeding from the track around the nephrostomy tube and through the tube.[13] If bleeding does not stop immediately after occlusion of the tube and placement of a pressure dressing about the tube, the nephrostomy tube should be replaced with a nephrostomy track tamponade balloon catheter (Kaye catheter).[14] This will tamponade the renal parenchyma and track and can be left in place for up to 48 hours if necessary to control bleeding while draining the collecting system. The tamponade balloon catheter should always be readily available in the operating suite during PNL.

Technical Hints

1. Study the anatomy of the preoperative intravenous pyelogram or CT scan to plan the approach to the collecting system. CT scanning with and without contrast material is useful to confirm the anterior versus posterior location of calyceal stones. In extremely obese patients, CT scanning will determine the distance from the skin to the stone and collecting system. When this distance is greater than 16 cm, special extra-long instruments (nephroscopes, sheaths, graspers) should be used **(Fig. 41)**.
2. Use dilute contrast material for retrograde instillation to avoid obscuring the stone. The guide wire serves as an important landmark when locating the renal pelvis and ureter. Retrograde instillation of methylene blue dye during subsequent nephroscopy can also help find the renal pelvis and UPJ. As above, the blue-colored urothelium can be helpful in ensuring correct scope location.
3. Ensure adequate sedation. General anesthesia is preferred, although epidural or continuous spinal techniques may be acceptable for circumstances where general anesthesia is contraindicated (obesity, pulmonary disease).
4. Use fluoroscopic equipment that has multiplanar capability.
5. Renal ultrasound with a needle guide is a useful adjunct that will minimize radiation exposure in many cases. It is less helpful in obese patients or when the patient does not have hydronephrosis **(Fig. 42)**.
6. Ensure that appropriate preoperative intravenous antibiotics are administered based on the urine culture. With a history of infected stones, it is especially important to have 24-hour prophylaxis with good tissue levels regardless of the preoperative urine culture results. Cultures may be sterile, but stone fragmentation with bacterial release and subsequent bacterial infection may initiate life-threatening sepsis.
7. Proper positioning of the prone patient with padding is extremely important to prevent pressure sores and nerve palsies. The chest should be supported by rolled towels wrapped with egg-crate foam. Axillary rolls support the brachial plexus from stretch injury. The elbows and shoulders should not be extended beyond 90 degrees. The medial humeral condyle and ulnar nerve should be well padded. The kneecaps and ankles should be padded with the legs flexed. Pneumatic compression pumps should be applied to the calves.

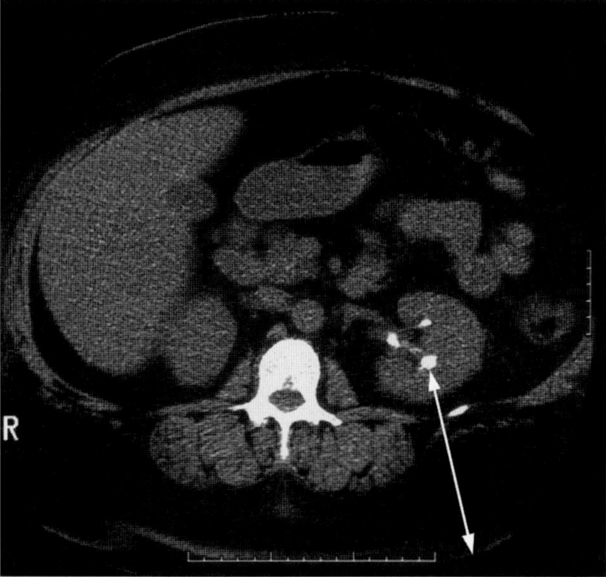

Figure 41. CT scan shows a staghorn calculus in a morbidly obese 49-year-old woman. The depth from the skin to the posterior, inferior calyx under the 12th rib is 12 cm (arrows).

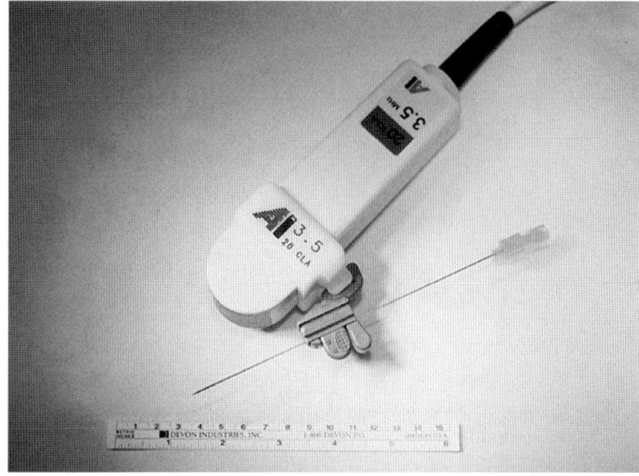

Figure 42. 3.5 MHz ultrasound transducer with needle guide for a 21-gauge puncture needle.

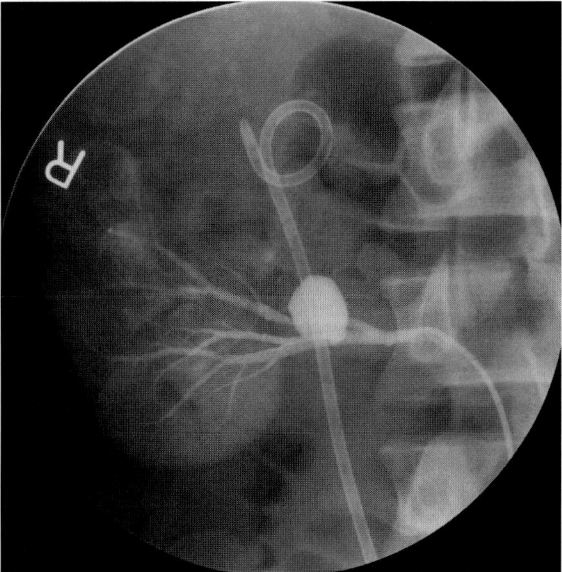

Figure 43. Pseudoaneurysm of a right inferior pole accessory renal artery following percutaneous endopyelotomy and persistent hemorrhage in a 19-year-old man with recurrent UPJ obstruction. A double-J ureteral stent is in place.

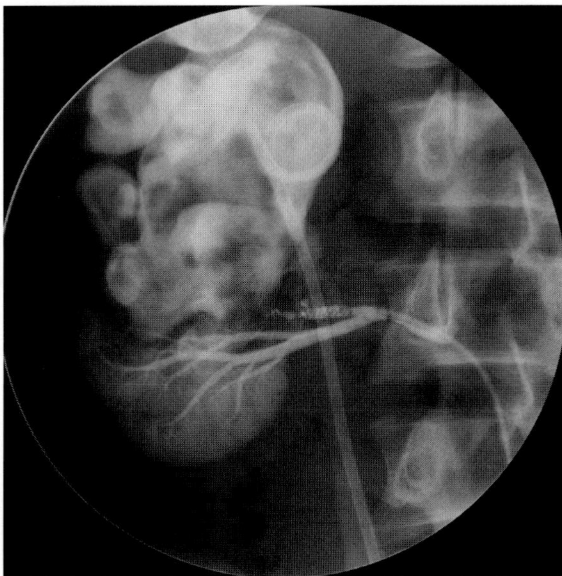

Figure 44. Selective metallic coil embolization of a segmental renal vessel with resolution of the hemorrhage.

8. Although infracostal PNL access is preferred, occasionally upper pole access cannot be accomplished simply with severe cranial angulation. In this circumstance, an intercostal access track may be required. With this access, there are higher risks of splenic and liver injury, and preprocedural axial imaging as well as intraprocedural sonographic or CT guidance are helpful. By definition, intercostal access means the pleura will be crossed and fluoroscopic evaluation at a minimum for pneumothorax is requisite.[13] Follow-up evaluation for hydrothorax (from infusate), empyema (if infected stones are being treated), and hemothorax (if there is significant procedural hemorrhage) also must be considered if an intercostal approach is used.

Outcome

Stone-free rates following PNL depend on the size, location and anatomic complexity of the stone disease. Solitary renal pelvis stones have the highest stone-free rates, approaching 95%.[15] For partial and complete staghorn stones, stone-free rates depend on the burden of stone, complexity of renal calyceal anatomy, the extent of meticulous flexible nephroscopy or multiple access tracks used, and the use of adjunctive techniques such as ESWL and/or irrigation with dissolution agents during the same hospitalization. Rates as high 85% can be obtained in these difficult cases.[9] These rates are far superior to ESWL (30%–50% stone-free after multiple treatments) and can be equaled only by the most expert surgeons with open nephrolithotomy.[9]

Complications

Injury to adjacent viscera (colon, spleen, duodenum) has been reported as a result of access misadventures.[16,17] Fortunately, most of these can be avoided with scrupulous technique and attention to these structures during fluoroscopic- and especially ultrasound-guided access. As mentioned earlier, an intercostal approach increases these risks. For upper pole access, review of preoperative CT scans will show the anatomic relationships between neighboring organs and will confirm the best retroperitoneal window approach to the kidney.[18]

Punctures lateral to the posterior axillary line have an increased risk of injury to the colon. This error may first be noticed at the end of the case when a nephrostogram demonstrates extravasation of contrast material into the colon. This complication can be managed by pulling the nephrostomy tip back into the colon for controlled colostomy drainage for a day or so.

Medial perforation of the renal pelvis can occur due to access or stone manipulation during nephroscopic lithotripsy. Vascular pedicle injury, though uncommon, can occur if excessive medial and anterior forces are used during access or track dilation.[3] This devastating complication can be avoided with careful technique. Embolotherapeutic techniques may be life-saving in this situation **(Figs. 43, 44)**. Pneumothorax can occur in up to 10%–15% of supracostal access tracks.[17]

Hydrothorax and hemothorax can result from excessive irrigation during the procedure. The need for postoperative transfusion for PNL has arisen in approximately 3%–4% of cases in our experience, but we still offer the patient the opportunity for autologous blood donation.[19]

Conclusion

PNL is one of the most rewarding procedures available, both for the patient and the radiologist or urologist. With this form of minimally invasive surgery, disabling renal or ureteral stones can usually be removed in a single setting.[20,21] Hospitalization is typically 5 days or less and complete recovery is commonly within 1–2 weeks. Appropriate access placement with meticulous technique is the key to avoiding complications.

The procedure requires radiographic, interventional, and endoscopic equipment. Close collaboration between the radiologist and urologist is also critical and has been extremely fruitful at our institution. High success rates make this an extremely cost-effective and preferred procedural choice for properly selected patients.

References

1. Segura JW, Patterson DE, LeRoy AJ, et al. Percutaneous removal of kidney stones: review of 1,000 cases. J Urol 1985; 134:1077–1081.

2. Atala A, Steinbock GS. Extracorporeal shock wave lithotripsy of renal calculi. Am J Surg 1989; 157:350–358.

3. Crowley AR, Smith AD. Percutaneous ultrasonic lithotripsy: a simplified treatment for renal stones. Postgrad Med 1986; 79:57–64.

4. Spirnak JP. Retrograde percutaneous access technique. Probl Urol 1992; 6:23–35.

5. Callaway TW, Lingardh G, Basata S, Sylven M. Percutaneous nephrolithotomy in children. J Urol 1992; 148:1067.

6. Segura JW, Preminger GM, Assimos DG, et al. Nephrolithiasis Clinical Guidelines Panel summary report on the management of staghorn calculi. J Urol 1994; 151:1648–1651.

7. Hulbert JC, Reddy PK, Hunter DW, Castaneda-Zuniga W, Amplatz K, Lange PH. Percutaneous techniques for the management of caliceal diverticula containing calculi. J Urol 1986; 135:225–227.

8. Lingeman JE, Siegel YI, Steele B, Nyhuis AW, Woods JR. Management of lower pole nephrolithiasis: a critical analysis. J Urol 1994; 151:663–667.

9. Kadir S, ed. Current practice of interventional radiology. St. Louis: Mosby Year Book, 1991.

10. Hawkins IF. Carbon dioxide digital subtraction arteriography. AJR 1982; 139:19–24.

11. Mindell HJ, Cochran ST. Current perspectives in the diagnosis and treatment of urinary stone disease. AJR 1994; 163:1314–1315.

12. Jones DJ. Kellett MJ, Wickham JE. Percutaneous nephrolithotomy and the solitary kidney. J Urol 1991; 145:477–480.

13. Lang EK. Percutaneous nephrostolithotomy and lithotripsy: a multi-institutional survey of complications. Radiology 1987; 162:25–30.

14. Smith AD. Controversies in endourology. Philadelphia: W.B. Saunders Company, 1995.

15. Streem SB. Long-term incidence and risk factors for recurrent stones following percutaneous nephrostolithotomy or percutaneous nephrostolithotomy/extracorporeal shock wave lithotripsy for infection-related calculi. J Urol 1995; 153:584–587.

16. Appel R, Musmanno MC, Knight JG. Nephrocolic fistula complicating percutaneous nephrostolithotomy. J Urol 1988; 140:1007–1008.

17. Picus D, Weyman PJ, Clayman RV, McClennan BL. Intercostal space nephrostomy for percutaneous stone removal. AJR 1986; 147:393–397.

18. Jones DJ. Wickham JE, Kellett MJ. Percutaneous nephrolithotomy for calculi in horseshoe kidneys. J Urol 1991; 145:481–483.

19. Stoller ML, Wolf JS Jr, St. Lezin MA. Estimated blood loss and transfusion rates associated with percutaneous nephrolithotomy. J Urol 1994; 152:1977–1981.

20. Lingeman JE, Woods J, Toth PD, Evan AP, McAteer JA. The role of lithotripsy and its side effects. J Urol 1989; 141:793–797.

21. Kavoussi LR, Albala DM, Basler JW, Apte A, Clayman RV. Percutaneous management of urolithiasis during pregnancy. J Urol 1992; 148:1069–1071.

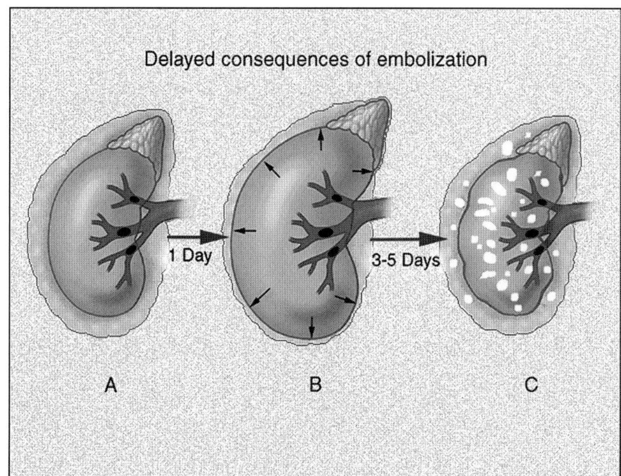

Figure 1. Drawing of surgical ligation around the proximal renal artery.

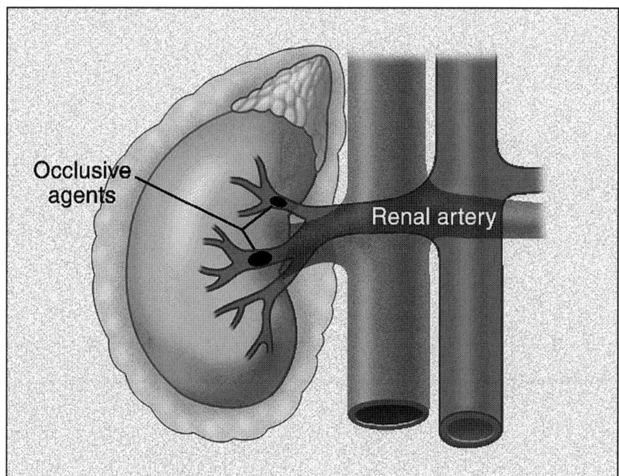

Figure 2. Drawing of embolized kidney with occlusion of segmental renal arteries.

TUTORIAL 23
RENAL EMBOLIZATION

Allen J. Meglin, M.D.

Introduction

The subjects addressed in this tutorial include:
1. General principles of embolotherapy
2. Embolotherapy as it applies to the kidney
3. Contraindications to renal embolization
4. Outcome expectations for renal embolization.

General Considerations

Principles of Embolotherapy

Embolotherapy is generally performed to decrease blood flow to a particular vascular bed. It can be done preoperatively to decrease potential blood loss during surgery, to decrease organ engorgement prior to venous ligation, to infarct an organ and shrink or devitalize it prior to resection, or, in the case of endocrine tumors, to decrease the physiologic consequences of tissue palpation during surgery (ie, release of active hormones) **(Fig. 1)**.

Embolotherapy can also be performed in the acute setting to decrease ongoing blood loss (ie, post-traumatic), to palliate symptoms (such as pain), or to decrease physiologic effects caused by the target organ (such as hypertension in the case of increased renin production).[1]

In some cases, organ damage caused by embolotherapy with consequent tissue devitalization may release antigens, initiating an immunologic response to the tumor.[1] Some surgeons report that the edema caused by tissue devitalization can also help in the separation of fascial planes and thereby speed the process of tumor removal.[1] Additionally, segmental renal artery embolization can be performed to preserve normal renal parenchyma while devitalizing abnormal renal tissue. In vessels too small to treat with percutaneous transluminal angioplasty or in pediatric patients, this can be an effective treatment of renovascular hypertension **(Fig. 2)**.[2]

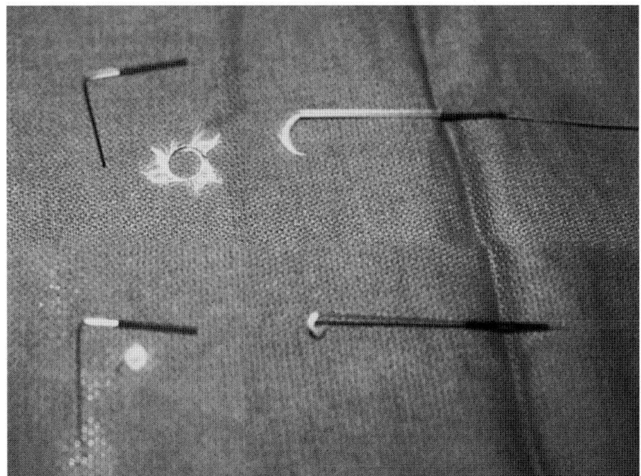

Figure 3. Coils being deployed from the metal casing.

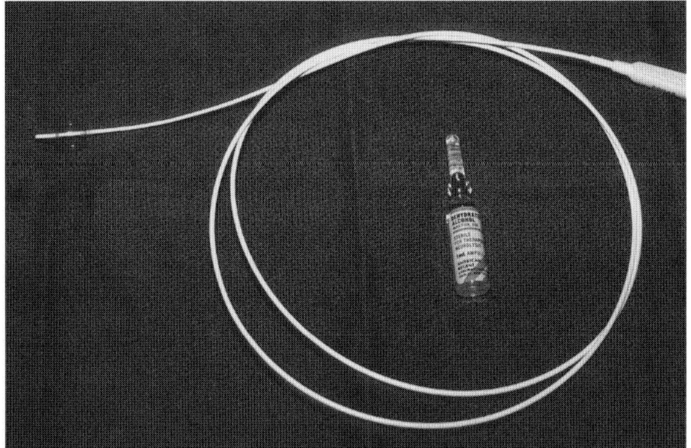

Figure 5. Occlusion balloon and absolute alcohol.

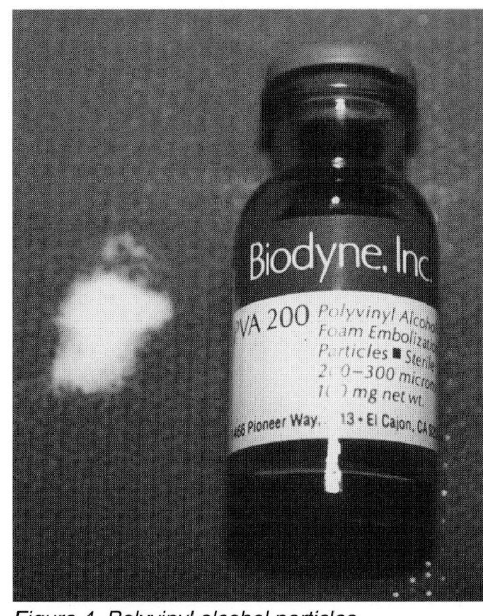

Figure 4. Polyvinyl alcohol particles.

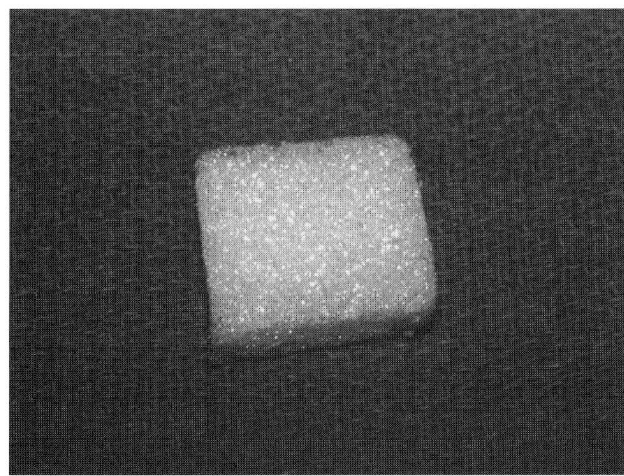

Figure 6. Gelfoam block.

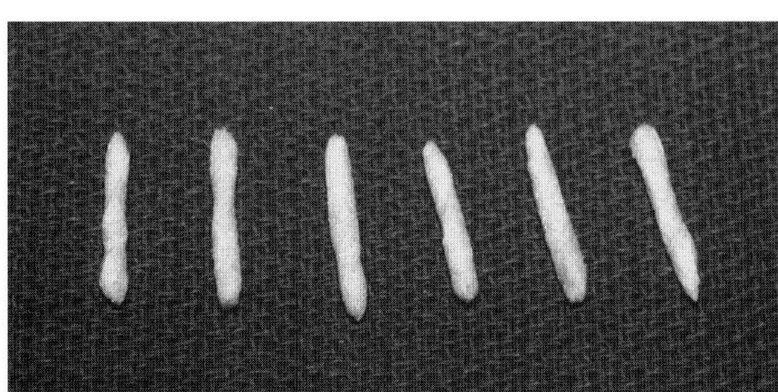

Figure 7. Gelfoam torpedoes.

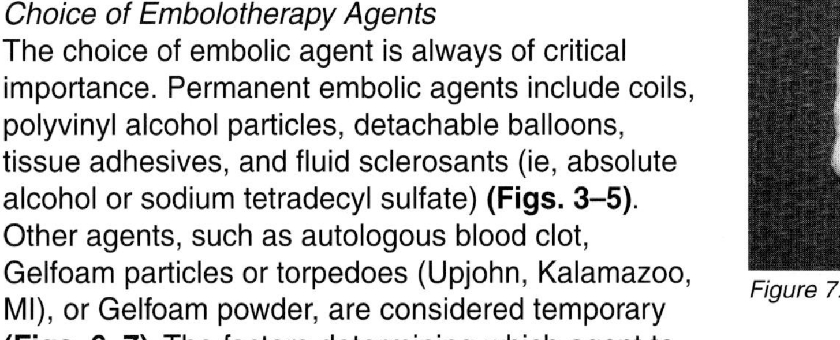

Choice of Embolotherapy Agents

The choice of embolic agent is always of critical importance. Permanent embolic agents include coils, polyvinyl alcohol particles, detachable balloons, tissue adhesives, and fluid sclerosants (ie, absolute alcohol or sodium tetradecyl sulfate) **(Figs. 3–5)**. Other agents, such as autologous blood clot, Gelfoam particles or torpedoes (Upjohn, Kalamazoo, MI), or Gelfoam powder, are considered temporary **(Figs. 6, 7)**. The factors determining which agent to use have been covered in the **SCVIR Syllabus Volume VI, *Thoracic and Visceral Vascular Interventions*.**[3] However, if nephrectomy is planned, nonpermanent agents provide a higher margin of safety in the event of inadvertent non-target embolization.

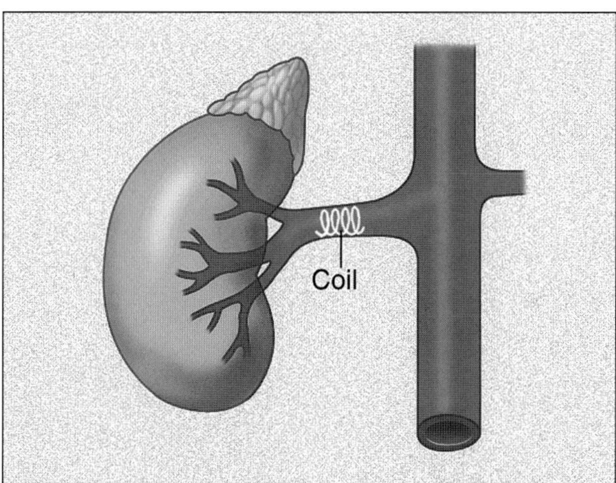

Figure 8. Coil in the proximal renal artery: the analog to surgical ligation.

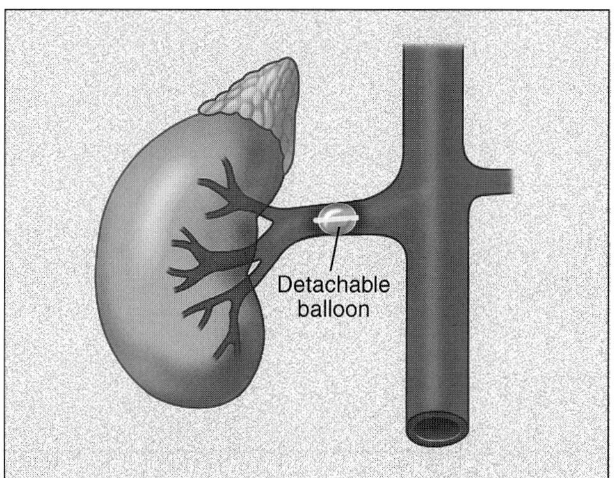

Figure 9. Detachable balloon in the proximal renal artery.

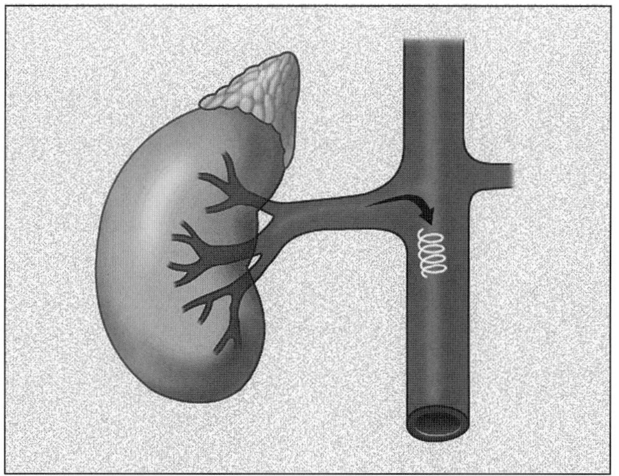
Figure 10. Coil manipulated out of the proximal renal artery and into the aorta with consequent inadvertent embolization.

In general, temporary agents are the best choice when the aim of embolotherapy is short-term occlusion. Cases in which short-term occlusion is desirable include preoperative embolization or in the setting of acute hemorrhage in which the goal is to supplement natural hemostatic mechanisms.

Although many physicians prefer to use absolute alcohol preoperatively, this treatment can be very painful and is best done when the patient will have the nephrectomy immediately after the embolization. Additionally, since it is a liquid agent, inadvertent flow of the alcohol either by reflux into the aorta or by collaterals to radiculomedullary arteries of the spinal cord can occur, leading to paralysis. In a similar fashion, alcohol embolization has also led to colonic and testicular infarction.

The size of the embolic agent is also important. Larger agents cause proximal occlusions, while smaller agents cause occlusions more distally in the vascular bed. The larger agents (ie, coils, detachable balloons) can be seen as analogs to proximal surgical ligation **(Figs. 8, 9)**.

Coils are different from surgical ligation, however, because they can be dislodged at surgery during organ manipulation. In the case of nephrectomy, this can result in inadvertent embolization **(Fig. 10)**. Prenephrectomy embolization with smaller, more distally acting agents is recommended.[4]

Postembolization Syndrome

- Fever
- Elevated white count
- Pain
- Soft-tissue gas

Figure 11.

Postembolization Syndrome

A final aspect of embolotherapy that must be considered is the postembolization syndrome (PES). Successful embolotherapy causes devascularization of the target tissue **(Fig. 11)**. The resultant tissue necrosis has several consequences. There is often pain that begins anywhere from immediately after the procedure to 3 to 5 days later. Tissue swelling, fever, and elevated white blood cell count may occur. Soft-tissue gas may be seen on plain film or other imaging modalities. This constellation of findings may be difficult to differentiate from infection, and sometimes it is best to treat the patient for both. Pretreatment with steroids and antibiotics can often minimize the effects of PES. The severity of the PES is often correlated with the amount of tissue infarcted; the larger the volume of tissue embolized, the greater the likelihood of PES.

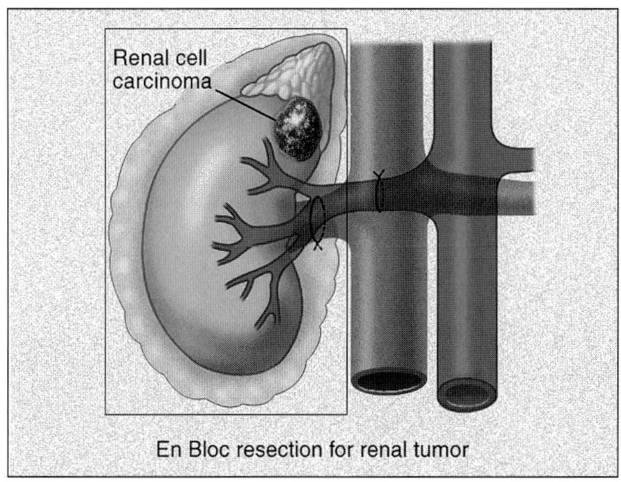

Figure 12. Surgical ligation of the kidney with en bloc devitalization.

Considerations Specific to Renal Embolization

The term renal embolization actually encompasses embolization of the kidney, adrenal gland, and nearby structures (including tumor thrombus) **(Fig. 12)**. These other structures are included in the target area of embolization because they are included in the en-bloc resection performed during nephrectomy. Renal embolization is not always performed with the intent of surgical extirpation, however.

In some practices, 50% or more of renal embolotherapy procedures are performed for definitive treatment of post-traumatic hemorrhage. In our practice, if the bleeding source can be identified by selective catheterization, both the technical and clinical success rates approach 100%. We have had no complications using Gelfoam and coils **(Figs. 13–16)**. In cancer referral centers, however, the bulk of the renal bed may be embolized as a preoperative adjunct. In renal dialysis, renal transplant, or nephrology referral centers, renal embolization may largely be performed to treat medical conditions such as refractory proteinuria or hematuria when other forms of nephron mass devitalization (nonsteroidal anti-inflammatory administration, surgical nephrectomy) are undesirable.[5]

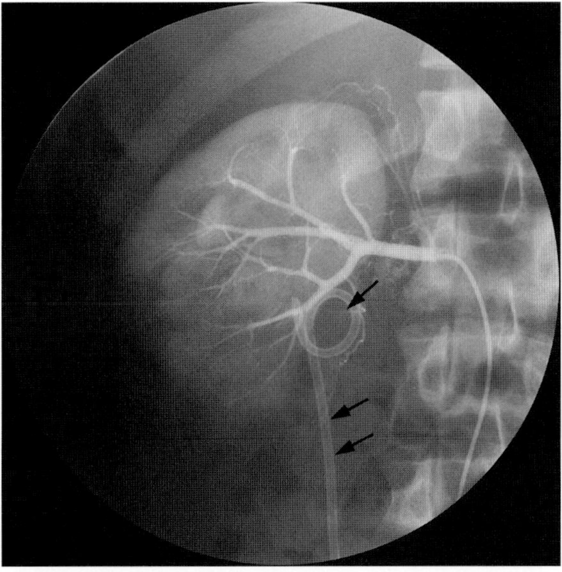

Figure 13. A patient with multiple renal arteries shows normal renal arteriogram of an upper pole branch. A ureteral stent is in place (arrows).

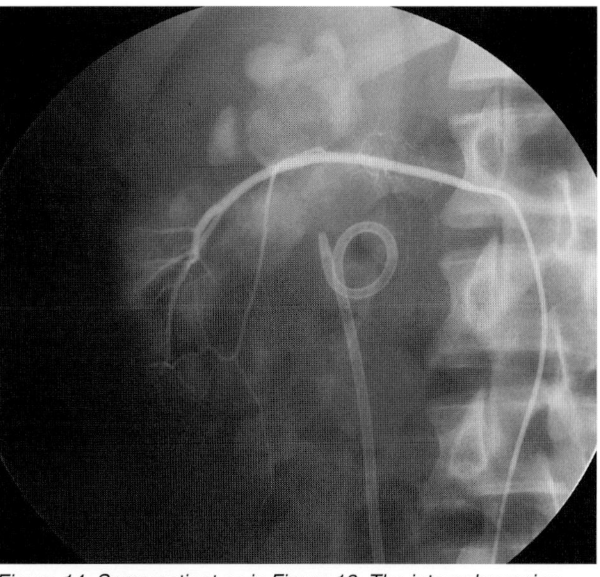

Figure 14. Same patient as in Figure 13. The interpolar region segmental artery is also normal.

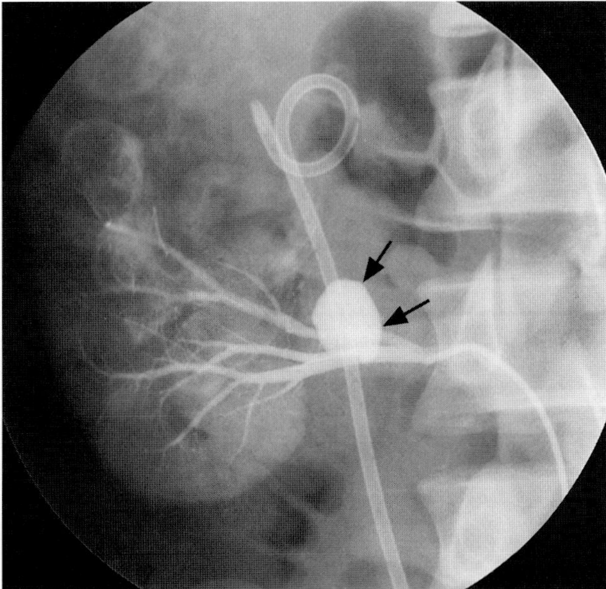

Figure 15. Same patient as in Figure 13. A lower pole branch artery is lacerated, with flow of contrast material and blood into the collecting system. The collection of contrast material represents an immature pseudoaneurysm (arrows).

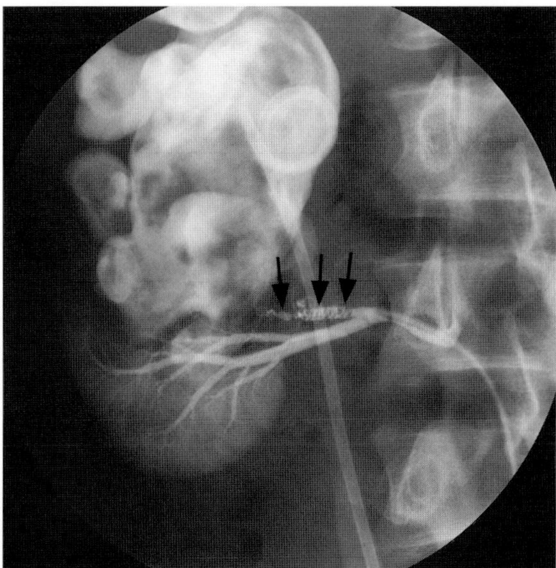

Figure 16. Same patient as in Figure 13. Coil embolization (arrows) distal and proximal to the vessel laceration with nonvisualization of the pseudoaneurysm. The vessel laceration occurred at the time of retrograde endopyelotomy. Note contrast material in the renal collecting system.

There are several considerations specific to embolotherapy in the renal vascular bed. The net goal of the embolization will determine the choice of embolic agents, the timing of the embolization, and the technique used.

	Definitive Treatment	*Palliation*	*Preoperative or Nephrectomy*
Indication	Arteriovenous fistula Arteriovenous malformation Post-traumatic hemorrhage Renal-induced hypertension Renal-induced endocrine abnormality	Renal cell carcinoma Transitional cell carcinoma Cystic renal disease	Renal cell carcinoma Transitional cell carcinoma
Agents	Sclerosing agents Coils Gelfoam Balloons Polyvinyl alcohol Tissue adhesives (above in combination)	Sclerosing agents Permanent embolic agents Particulate agents Tissue adhesives Coils (above in combination)	Gelfoam Sclerosing agents
Location	Central renal artery and distally	Distal to main renal artery (may be converted to nephrectomy)	Distal to main renal artery
Adjunctive therapy	Analgesics Anti-inflammatories	Analgesics Anti-inflammatories	Analgesics

Renal Embolization

Figure 17.

It is best to divide the goals of renal embolization into three categories: definitive treatment, palliation, and preoperative treatment prior to nephrectomy.[6] The indications, agents, location of embolization, and adjunctive therapies can be listed and compared by treatment goal **(Fig. 17)**. In the case of renal artery pseudoaneurysms, renal or adrenal hemorrhage due to trauma, postoperative aneurysms, or arteriovenous fistulas, embolotherapy is often the definitive treatment **(Figs. 18–21)**.[5]

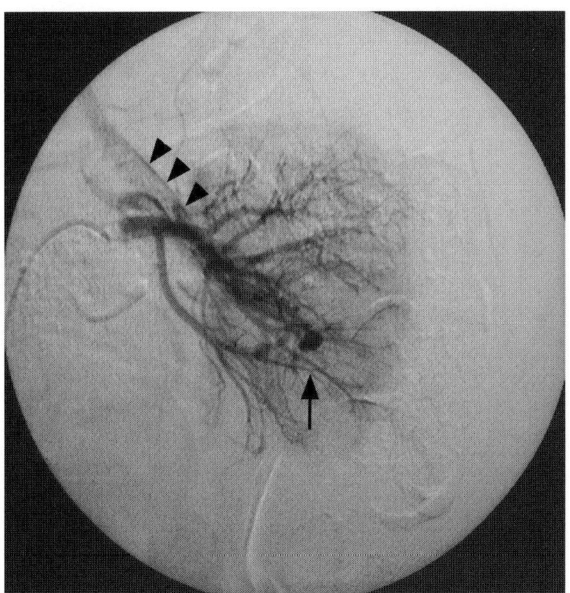

Figure 18. Arterial phase of a selective renal arteriogram shows a post-traumatic (renal biopsy) small intrarenal pseudoaneurysm (arrow) and early draining vein (arrowheads) indicating an arteriovenous fistula.

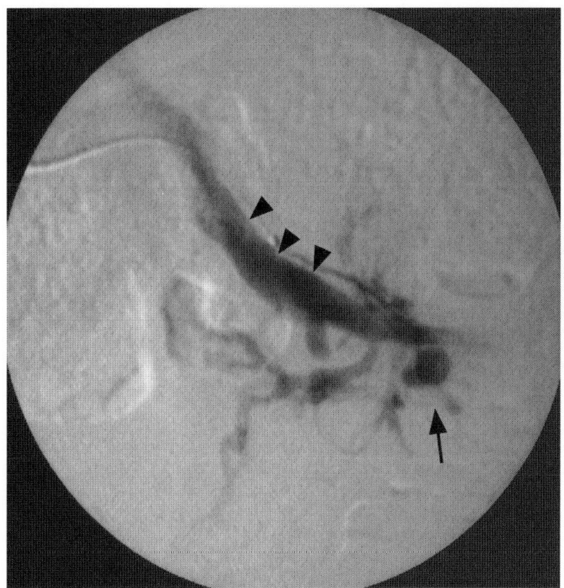

Figure 19. Same patient as in Figure 18. Direct injection into the segmental renal artery shows fistulous communication with the renal vein. Arrow shows the pseudoaneurysm. Arrowheads show the early draining vein.

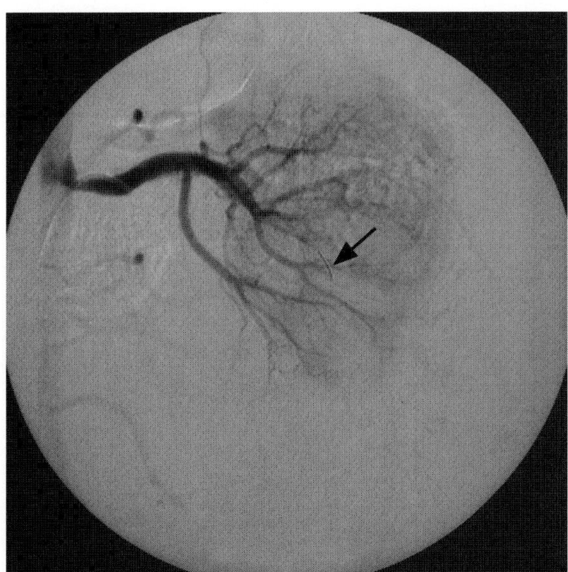

Figure 20. Same patient as in Figure 18. Microcatheter with tip in the feeding vessel of the pseudoaneurysm (arrow).

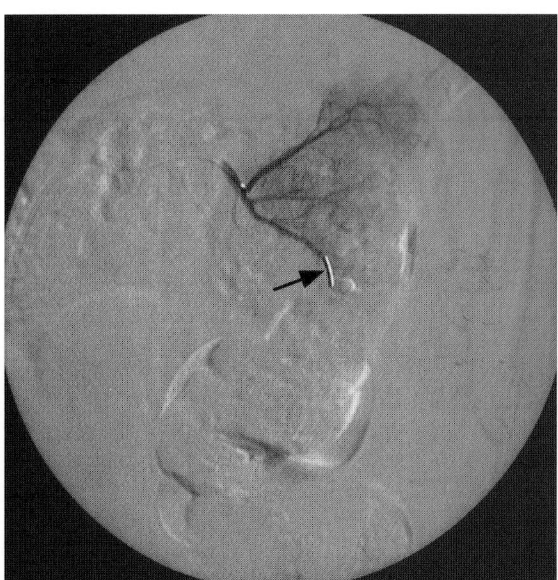

Figure 21. Same patient as in Figure 18. Single platinum coil placed into the feeding vessel (arrow).

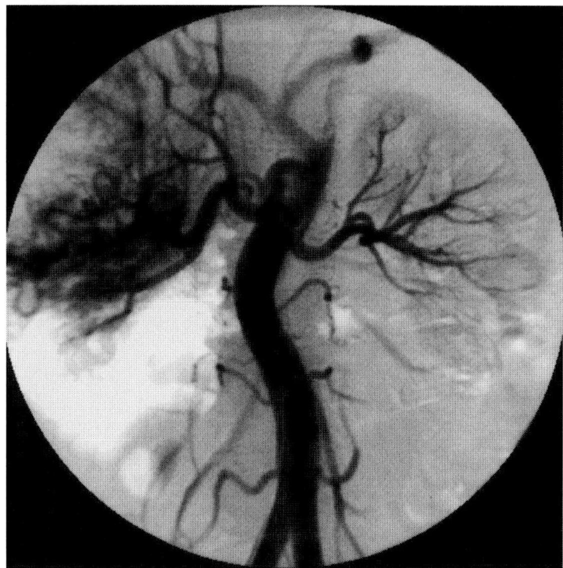

Figure 22. Large renal cell carcinoma preoperatively embolized with Gelfoam. Flush aortogram shows hypervascular right renal cell carcinoma replacing much of the kidney.

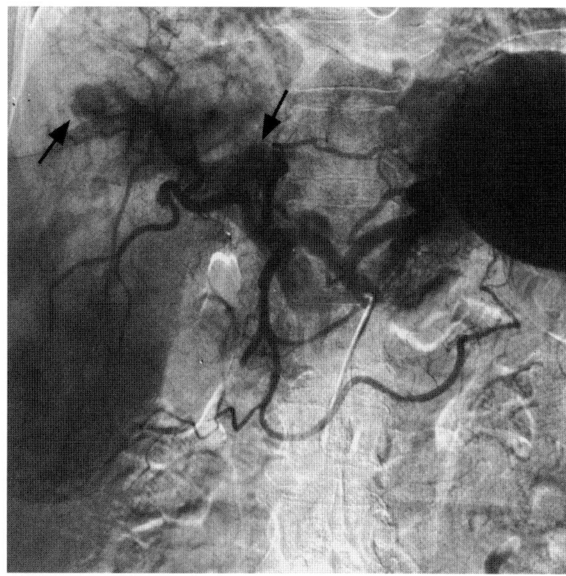

Figure 23. Selective celiac injection to evaluate for parasitization of mesenteric vessels by renal cell carcinoma. Several hepatic hemangiomas are identified (arrows) which could be mistaken for hypervascular metastases. No celiac artery supply to the tumor was evident.

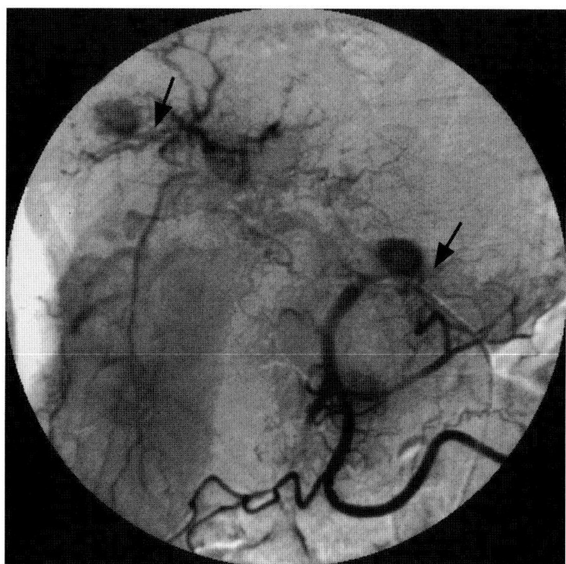

Figure 24. Selective gastroduodenal injection again shows liver hemangiomas (arrows). Metastases often have other abnormal vascular characteristics such as pooling, tortuous feeding vessels, arteriovenous shunting, and early draining veins.

In patients who are not surgical candidates, decreasing the size of the tumor mass can help palliate pain or symptoms caused by mass effect upon adjacent structures **(Figs. 22–26)**. However, it must be remembered that the larger the tumor burden infarcted, the more likely PES will occur.[5] The goal of palliative therapy is to decrease the symptomatology, so the tumor often will not be completely infarcted. To minimize the risks of PES, multiple embolotherapy sessions separated over time may be required.[7]

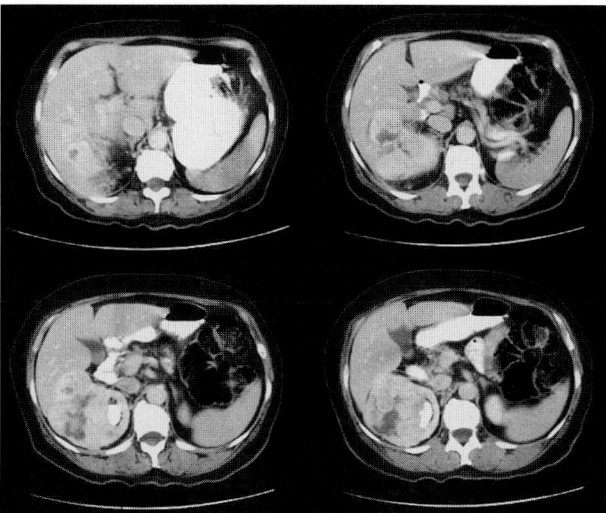

Figure 25. Computed tomography (CT) images show renal tumor extending up to, but not into the liver. Sonography showed a clear cleavage plane between the liver and perirenal tissues. Renal cell carcinoma almost never metastasizes to the liver.

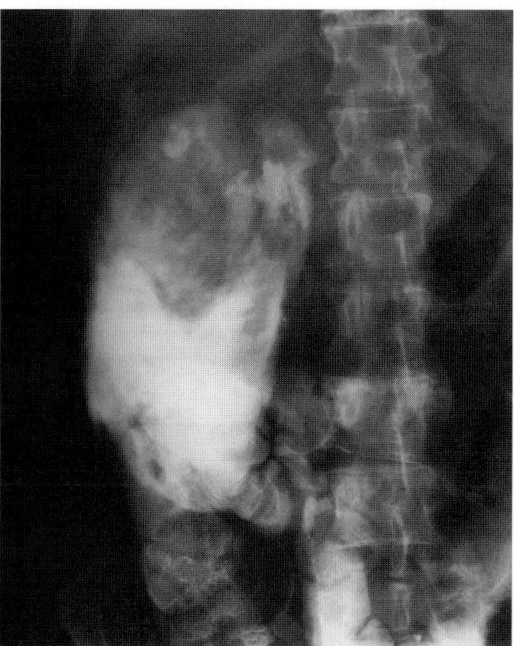

Figure 26. Plain film shows the kidney 20 minutes after embolization with a Gelfoam/contrast material mixture. Notice that the contrast material does not wash out of the kidney because there is no significant arterial inflow. The renal staining is from the embolization mixture.

In the case of prenephrectomy embolization, the arteriogram takes on special importance.[8,9] Some surgeons think that careful preoperative evaluation of the renal vein for variant anatomy is beneficial. Delayed images showing the collecting system (intravenous pyelogram phase) in relation to the tumor and feeding vessels are often helpful in planning for nephrectomy or partial nephrectomy.

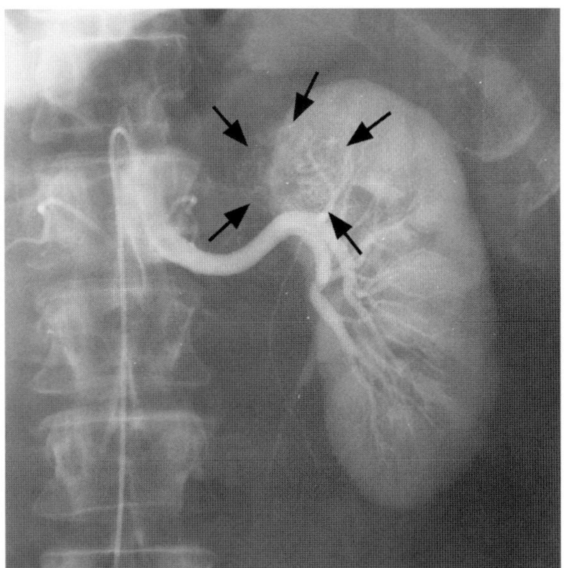

Figure 27. Arterial phase of selective renal arteriogram. Note the exophytic hypervascular mass in the upper pole of the left kidney (arrows) representing a renal cell carcinoma.

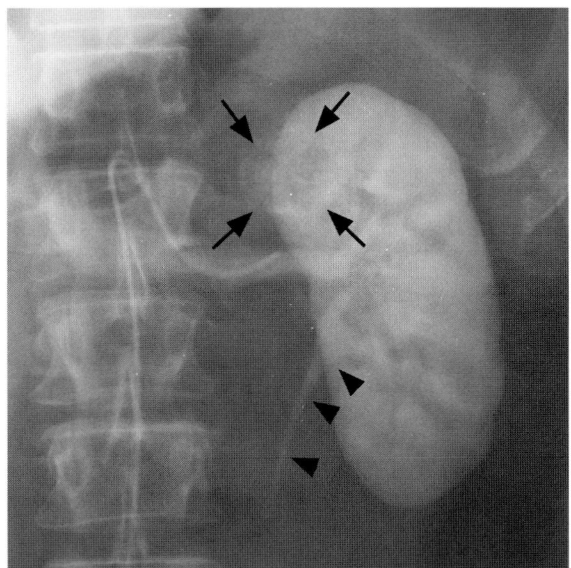

Figure 28. Same patient as in Figure 27. Venous phase of the selective renal arteriogram shows a hypervascular mass (arrows). Also note the collecting system (arrowheads). Late venous phase arteriograms that show the collecting system are particularly useful to surgeons planning a partial nephrectomy.

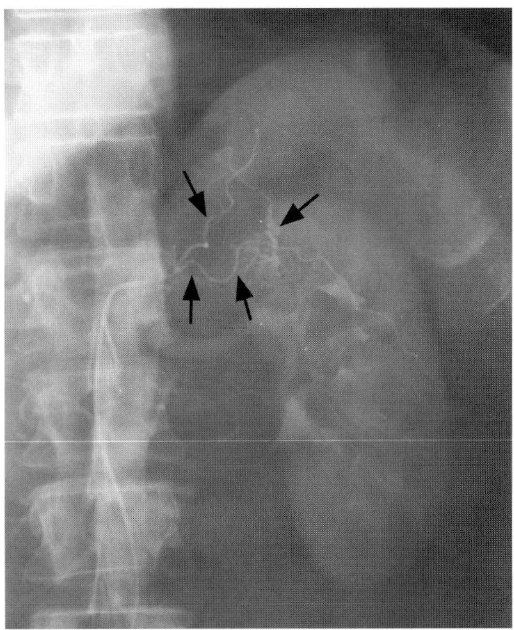

Figure 29. Same patient as in Figure 27. Branches of the intercostal and adrenal arteries (arrows) have been parasitized and now feed the upper pole renal cell carcinoma.

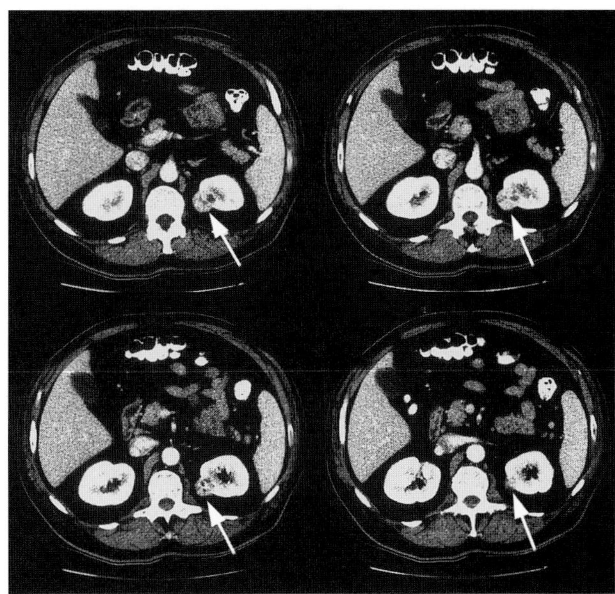

Figure 30. Same patient as in Figure 27. CT scan of the upper pole mass (arrows).

Additionally, evaluation for parasitization of other vessels (mesenteric and lumbar) by the tumor is important **(Figs. 27–30)**.[10] Given these considerations, some interventionalists advocate a two-step arteriographic approach to the expected nephrectomy case. That is, planning arteriography would be performed initially, with therapeutic intervention performed at a separate encounter.

In cases where partial nephrectomy is planned, embolization can be limited to segmental vessels.[11,12] It is sometimes uncertain whether embolotherapy will be the definitive treatment or simply an adjunctive, preoperative therapy. Cases such as these are best done with the surgical team available and in close communication. In any case, careful preoperative evaluation of the contralateral kidney for renal artery stenosis, presence of another functioning kidney, and simultaneous renal tumors is essential.[6,7,13]

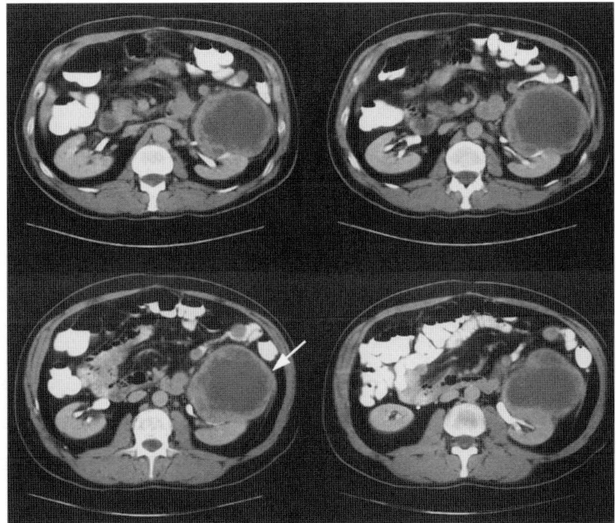

Figure 31. Contrast-enhanced CT scan shows a large renal cell carcinoma. Note the relatively low density center, likely an area of tumor or necrosis (arrow).

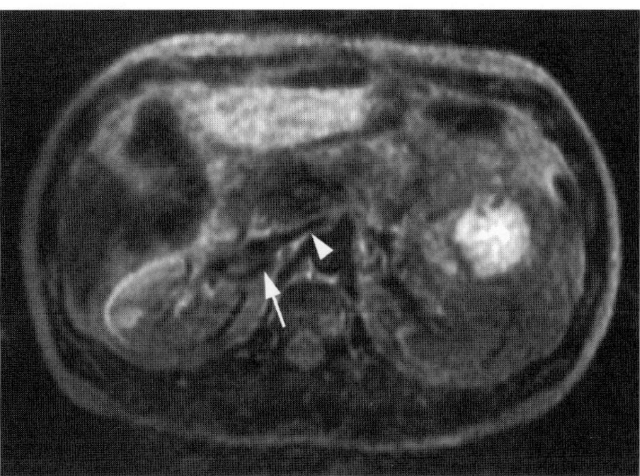

Figure 32. Magnetic resonance (MR) image (TR=2000, TE=80) of the left kidney with renal cell carcinoma. No tumor thrombus is seen in the renal vein (arrow) or inferior vena cava (arrowhead).

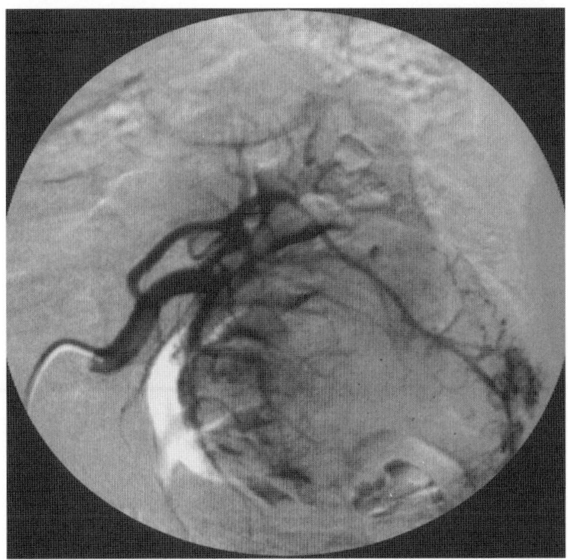

Figure 33. Same patient as in Figure 31. Early arterial phase of a selective renal injection reveals the hypervascular nature of the tumor.

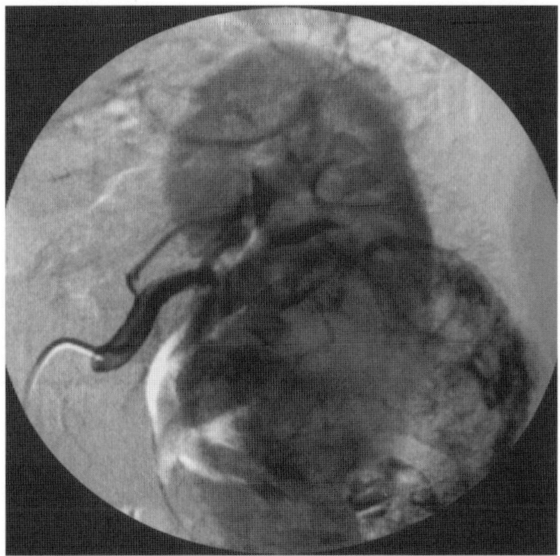

Figure 34. Same patient as in Figure 31. Capillary and early venous phase shows a hypervascular tumor rim with a hypovascular center. This correlates well with CT and MR findings.

The timing of embolotherapy is also important if the endpoint is surgical nephrectomy.[1,4,6–8,10] At our institution the surgeons prefer to go directly from the angiography suite to the operating room. This approach limits scheduling flexibility but has the advantages of decreased patient discomfort and a lower risk of postembolization syndrome. Craven et al have suggested that separating the embolization and the surgical dates has potential benefits.[4] They think that tumor and tumor thrombus shrinkage make surgical intervention easier. Tissue necrosis **(Figs. 31–38)** may also result in antigenic release from the tumor, eliciting an immunologic response which may decrease the risk of tumor recurrence.[1,4,8]

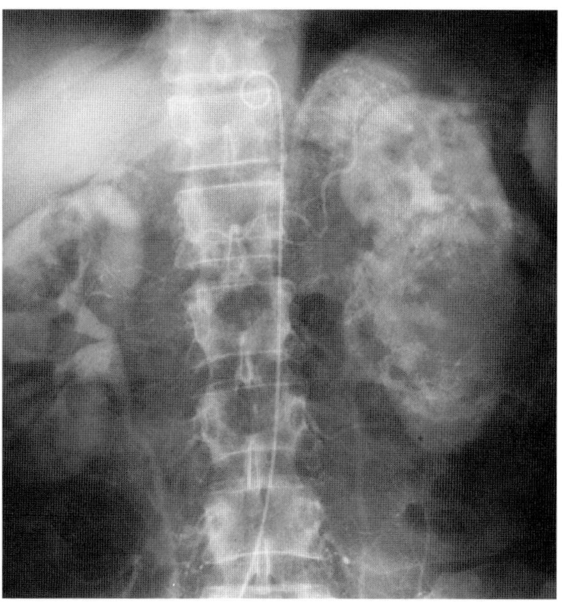

Figure 35. Delayed phase from a flush aortogram shows the relationship of the tumor to the renal parenchyma, renal pelvis, and ureter.

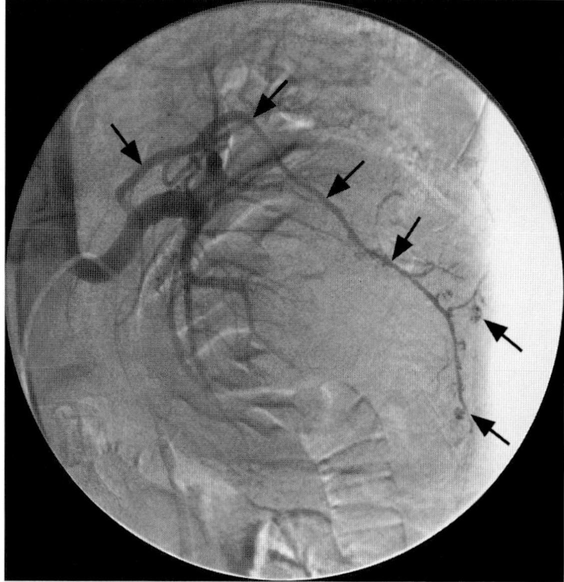

Figure 36. Selective renal arteriogram shows recruitment of adrenal and capsular vessels (arrows) to supply the hypervascular renal cell carcinoma.

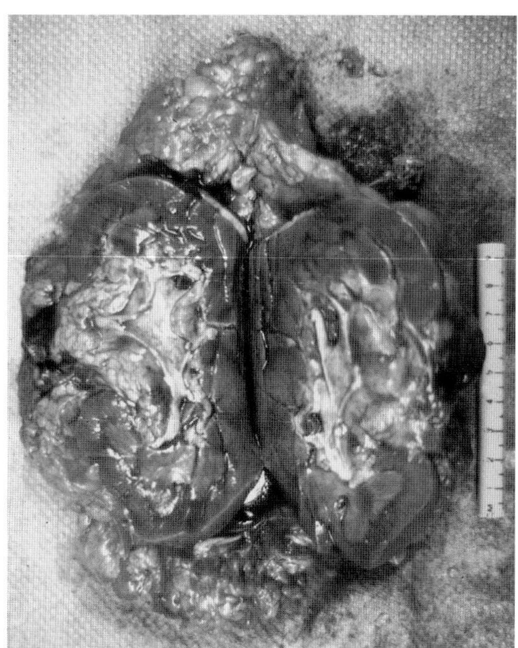

Figure 37. Gross anatomic photograph of renal cell carcinoma after nephrectomy.

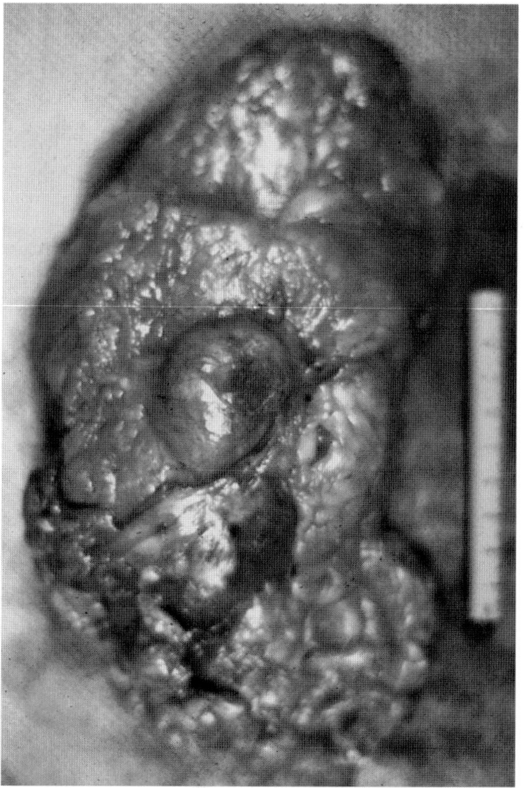

Figure 38. Gross anatomic photograph of renal cell carcinoma after nephrectomy.

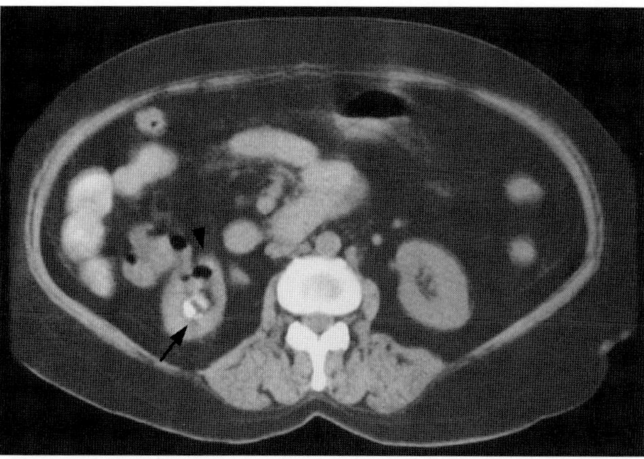

Figure 39. Noncontrast CT scan shows a stone in the renal pelvis and air (arrowhead) in the collecting system and kidney (arrow). The patient has emphysematous pyelonephritis. No instrumentation of the urinary bladder or ureteral tract was performed prior to the CT scan.

Contraindications

There are relatively few contraindications to prenephrectomy embolization, but these include: pyelonephritis, contralateral renal artery stenosis, contralateral renal metastasis, and hypovascular tumor **(Fig. 39).**[6,7]

Outcome

While there is disagreement regarding the effect of prenephrectomy renal embolization on survival, most surgeons agree that the intraoperative blood loss during nephrectomy is significantly decreased.[1,4,10] Craven et al also found improved survival in patients with higher grade tumors who underwent preoperative embolization.[4] Clearly, when embolotherapy spares the patient a surgical procedure the risk is reduced. When used as a surgical adjunct, it may speed up the process of renal extirpation by increasing perinephric edema, making fascial plane separation easier.[1,4,8,10]

Conclusion

In cases where it is performed as a definitive treatment (ie, post-traumatic hemorrhage, renal hypertension, arteriovenous fistula) renal embolotherapy is beneficial. Embolotherapy can also be palliative or performed as an adjunct to surgical intervention. While there are risks to percutaneous intervention (bleeding, contrast material allergy, inadvertent embolization) these are significantly lower than for surgery. The surgical alternative is often total nephrectomy, and significant preservation of nephron mass can be achieved in many cases if percutaneous therapy alone is employed.[3,6,7,11,12] In most cases, embolotherapy can be performed during a short hospital stay with a rapid postprocedural recovery time.

References

1. McLean GK, Meranze SG. Embolization techniques in the urinary tract. Urol Clin North Am 1985; 12:743–754.

2. Teigen CL, Mitchell SE, Venbrux AC, Christenson MJ, McLean RH. Segmental renal artery embolization for treatment of pediatric renovascular hypertension. J Vasc Interv Radiol 1992; 3:111–117.

3. Haskal Z, Kerlan RK, Trerotola SO, eds. Thoracic and Visceral Vascular Interventions. Reston, VA: Society of Cardiovascular and Interventional Radiology, 1996.

4. Craven WM, Redmond PL, Kumpe DA, Durham JD, Wettlaufer JN. Planned delayed nephrectomy after ethanol embolization of renal carcinoma. J Urol 1991; 146:704–708.

5. Peregrin JH, Zabka J, Stribrna J, Boruvka V, Martinek V. Long-term control of hypertension and the predictive value of peripheral plasma renin activity after ablation of end stage kidneys with a new embolic agent. Cardiovasc Intervent Radiol 1993; 16:355–360.

6. Wojtowycz M. Handbook of interventional radiology and angiography. 2nd edition. St. Louis: Mosby Year Book, 1995.

7. Kadir S. Current practice of interventional radiology. St. Louis: Mosby Year Book, 1991.

8. Fischedick AR, Peters PE, Kleinhans G, Pfeifer E. Preoperative renal tumor embolization. Acta Radiol 1987; 28:303–306.

9. Jafri SZ, Ellwood RA, Amendola MA, Farah J. Therapeutic angioinfarction of renal carcinoma: CT follow-up. J Comput Assist Tomogr 1989; 13(3):443–447.

10. Konchanin RP, Cho KJ, Grossman HB. Preoperative devascularization of advanced renal adenocarcinoma using a sclerosing agent. J Urol 1987; 137:199–201.

11. Beaujeux R, Saussine C, al-Fakir A, et al. Superselective endovascular treatment of renal vascular lesions. J Urol 1995; 153:14–17.

12. Heyns CF, van Vollenhoven P. Increasing role of angiography and segmental artery embolization in the management of renal stab wounds. J Urol 1992; 147:1231–1234.

13. Eastham JA, Wilson TG, Larsen DW, Ahlering TE. Angiographic embolization of renal stab wounds. J Urol 1992; 148:268–270.

Endnotes

Figures 14–18 courtesy of William Miller, M.D., Columbus, OH.

Figures 39 and 40 courtesy of Dennis Peppas, M.D.

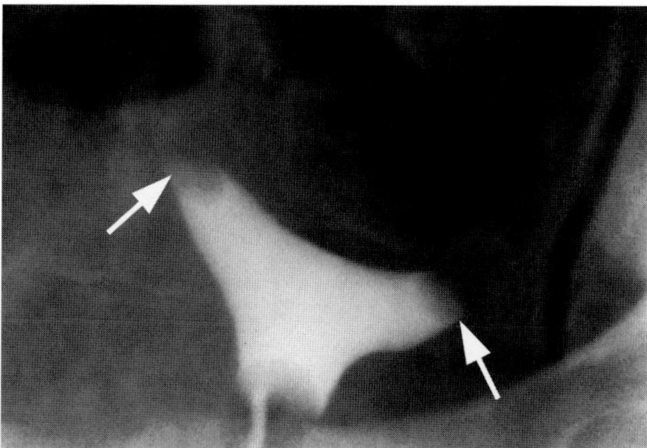

Figure 1. Normal "early filling" film of the uterus. Arrows indicate air bubbles in the cornua bilaterally.

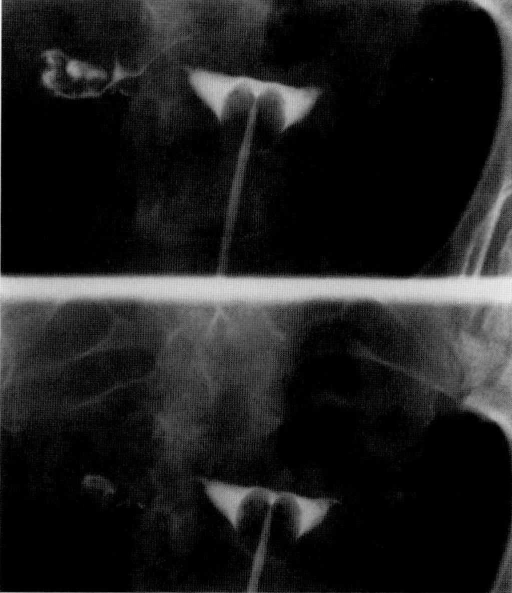

Figure 2. Opacification of normal fallopian tubes.

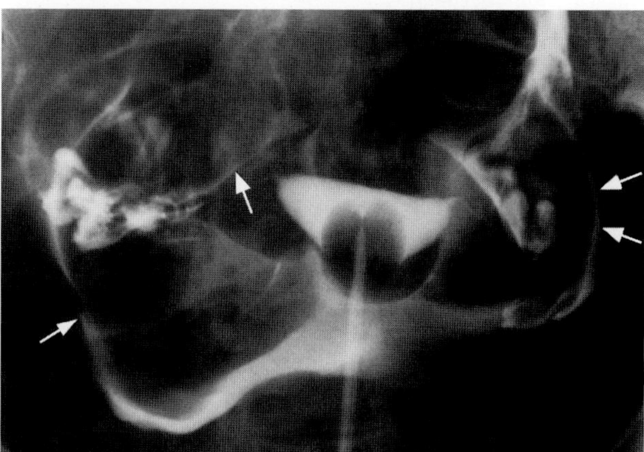

Figure 3. HSG demonstrates intraperitoneal spilling of contrast material. The contrast material outlines loops of bowel (arrows).

TUTORIAL 24 HYSTEROSALPINGOGRAPHY

Vincent D. McCormick, M.D.

Introduction

The subjects addressed in this tutorial include:

1. Indications for hysterosalpingography
2. Technique for performing hysterosalpingography
3. Normal and variant anatomy
4. Common fallopian tube abnormalities
5. Common congenital and acquired uterine abnormalities.

Hysterosalpingography remains the primary imaging modality for the assessment of infertility and should be performed early in the diagnostic evaluation. Additional indications for HSG include evaluation of patients who have had repeated abortions, and postoperative evaluation after myomectomy. HSG complements the sonographic evaluation of uterine myomas and depicts the morphology of congenital malformations. Supplemental imaging of anomalies with magnetic resonance (MR) and/or ultrasound imaging serves to clarify the anatomy of complex or confusing cases. Contraindications to HSG include recent uterine or tubal surgery, acute pelvic inflammatory disease (PID), active bleeding, and pregnancy.[1]

Technique

Most radiologists use the balloon catheter technique. An 8-F catheter is filled with contrast material before the cervix is cannulated to avoid introducing air, which might simulate pathologic abnormalities. After the catheter has been positioned in the endometrial cavity or endocervical canal, 5–8 mL of water- soluble contrast material are injected under fluoroscopic control. Placing an endometrial cavity catheter under mild tension forms a seal over the internal os, thus preventing reflux of contrast material around the catheter into the vagina.

The initial anteroposterior (AP) spot film is obtained after the injection of contrast material when the uterine cavity is opacified but before the fallopian tubes have filled **(Fig. 1)**. This early phase film detects small filling defects that could be obscured on later films when the uterus is more densely opacified. After injection of additional contrast material, oblique views are obtained to display the fallopian tubes **(Fig. 2)**, following which another AP film should confirm peritoneal spilling and tubal patency by demonstrating contrast material outlining loops of bowel **(Fig. 3)**. A prone drainage film, obtained 5–10 minutes after the catheter has been removed, helps detect loculated collections due to peritubal adhesions.[2]

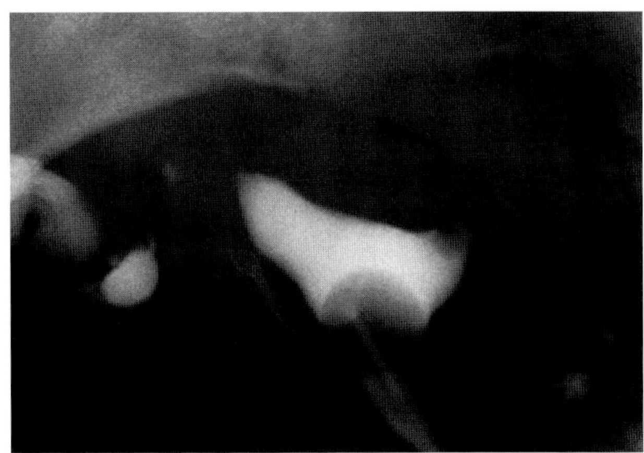

Figure 4. Balloon catheter inflated in the endometrial cavity.

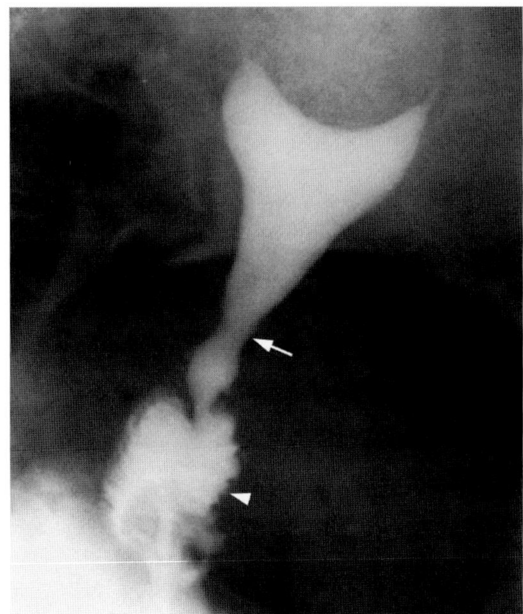

Figure 5. Balloon catheter in the cervix. The lower uterine segment (arrow) and the cervix (arrowhead) are both seen.

Lack of tubal filling may be due to obstruction secondary to prior infection or previous surgery, cornual spasm, inadequate injection of contrast material, and mucus plugging. Maintaining constant pressure on the syringe (without causing undue patient discomfort) or reinjecting contrast material may result in tubal opacification. Alternatively, placing the patient in the prone position for several minutes and re-opacifying the uterus may distinguish between true obstruction and transient non-filling.

When the balloon catheter is inflated in the endometrial cavity the cervix is not opacified; the balloon may also partially obscure the uterine anatomy **(Fig. 4)**. Deflating the balloon at the end of the examination will usually opacify the lower uterine segment and cervix sufficiently that spot films display the anatomy satisfactorily. On the other hand, inflation of the balloon in the endocervical canal allows satisfactory evaluation of the endometrial cavity and cervix **(Fig. 5)**.

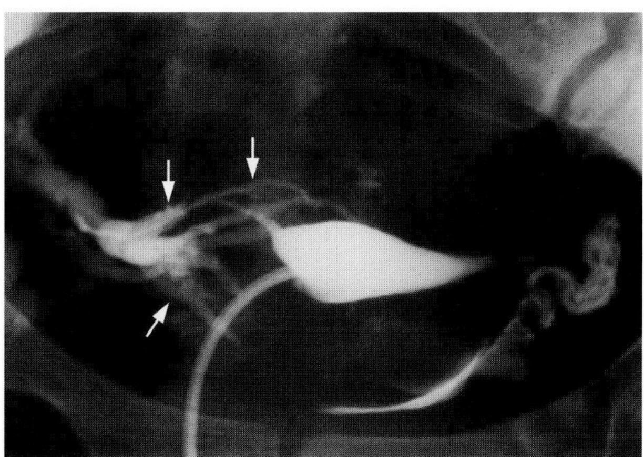

Figure 6. Venous intravasation, with venous opacification (arrows). Note spillage of contrast material outlining loops of bowel, confirming left tubal patency.

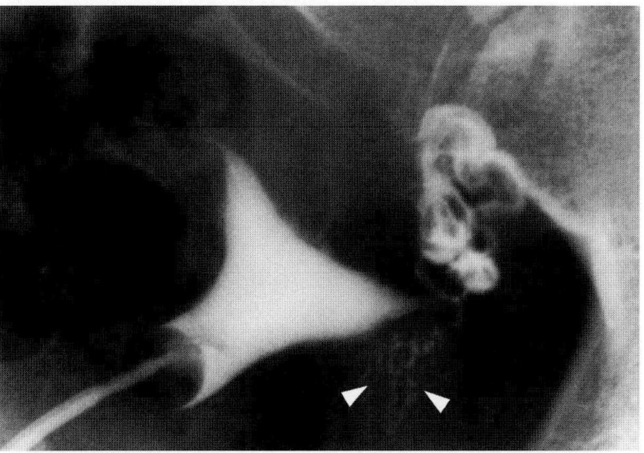

Figure 7. Lymphatic intravasation, with lymphatic opacification (arrowheads).

Difficulty cannulating the cervix may be encountered if cervical stenosis is present. Rigid balloon catheters and a plastic cannula system have been developed which may facilitate cannulation of the cervix in these patients.[3,4] Another option is to place a vessel dilator of suitable caliber (4–7 F) in the cervical canal, thereby occluding the canal and permitting injection of contrast material to achieve satisfactory opacification of the uterus and tubes.

Complications related to HSG are uncommon. The patient may experience minor, transient discomfort from distention of the uterine cavity and tubes. Reactions to the contrast material can occur, but postprocedure infection and uterotubal injury are rare. Venous or lymphatic intravasation of contrast material may result from excessive injection pressure. Venous opacification is transitory **(Fig. 6)**, whereas the fine, reticular lymphatics may remain visible for a longer time **(Fig. 7)**. The appearance of the uterine fundus in **Figure 7** is indistinct, another manifestation of intravasation. Tubal disease, synechiae (intrauterine adhesions), submucous myomas, and uterine anomalies may predispose to intravasation.

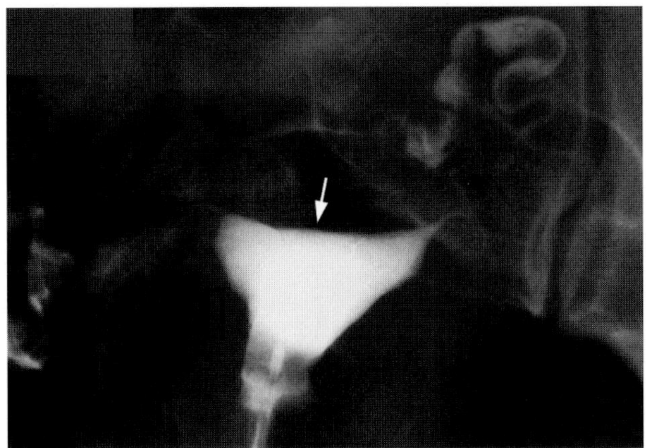

Figure 8. Normal contour of the uterine fundus (arrow).

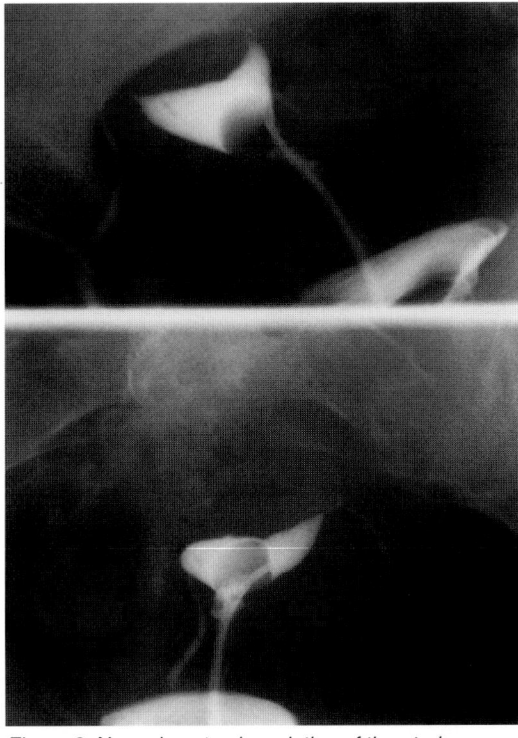

Figure 9. Normal anatomic variation of the uterine fundus.

Anatomy

The normal uterine cavity has a triangular configuration and a smooth contour on HSG. The fundus is usually straight **(Fig. 8)** but may also be slightly convex or concave **(Fig. 9)**. Arcuate uterus is a minor fusion anomaly in which the fundal concavity is accentuated; it is considered a normal variant **(Fig. 10)**. When the concavity is pronounced, it may simulate the appearance of a bicornuate uterus. Conversely, a fundal myoma presenting as a small filling defect may simulate the appearance of an arcuate uterus. Ultrasound or MR imaging can be performed to distinguish these conditions.

Fine unilateral or bilateral linear lucencies may cross the base of the cornu, a normal variant termed the cornual ring **(Fig. 11)**. The uterus is normally anteflexed and when this angulation is accentuated, the typical triangular configuration on the AP film is no longer apparent **(Fig. 12)**. Oblique views demonstrate the normal uterine outline and confirm that the uterus is anteflexed **(Fig. 13)**.

The normal cervix is 3–5 cm in length, has a serrated margin due to longitudinal ridges of the mucosa (plicae palmatae), and tapers to its narrowest point at the internal os **(Fig. 14)**. The fallopian tubes are 10–12 cm in length and are divided into four parts: the interstitial or intramural portion is in the muscular wall of the uterus at the cornu; the isthmic segment is the narrow, elongated portion; the ampulla is the wide, undulating, distal portion of the tube; and the terminal, fimbriated aspect surrounds the tubal ostium, which communicates with the peritoneal cavity **(Fig. 15)**.

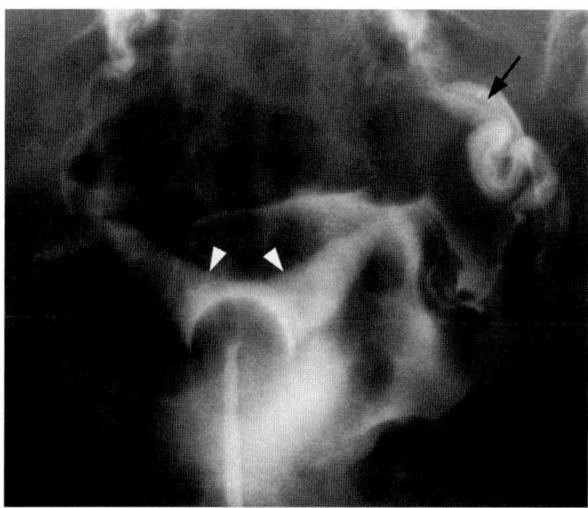

Figure 10. HSG shows an arcuate uterus, with accentuation of the fundal concavity (arrowheads). The curvilinear lucency in the ampulla of the left fallopian tube represents a normal rugal or luminal fold (arrow).

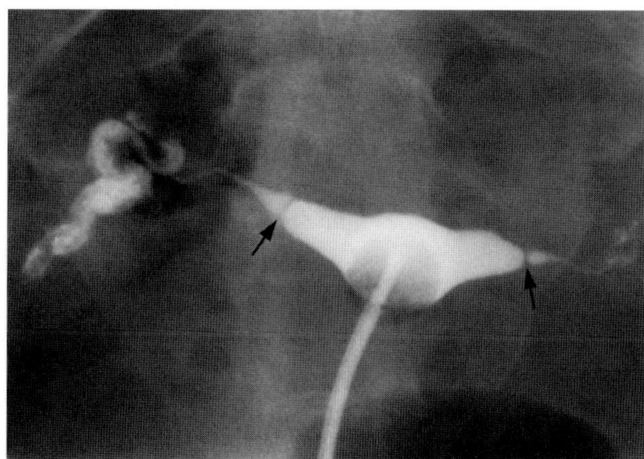

Figure 11. Cornual rings (arrows) are another normal anatomic variant.

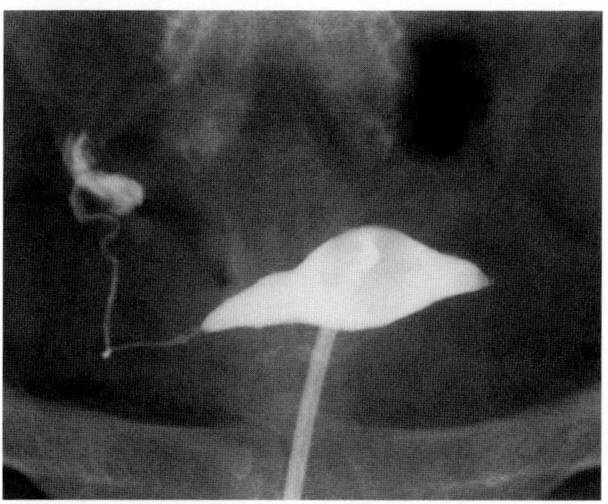

Figure 12. AP HSG shows the appearance of an anteflexed uterus.

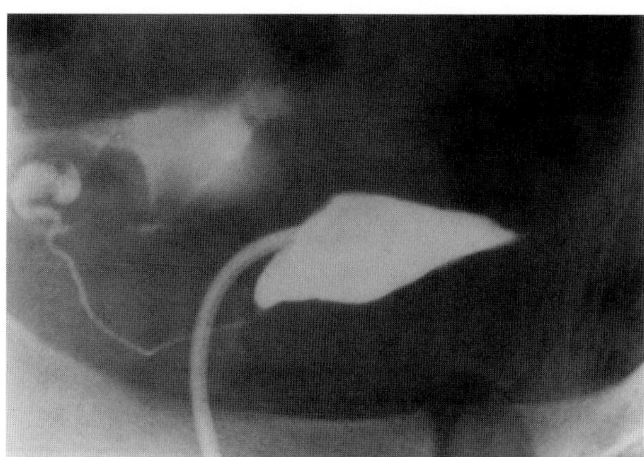

Figure 13. Oblique HSG more accurately demonstrates that the uterus is anteflexed.

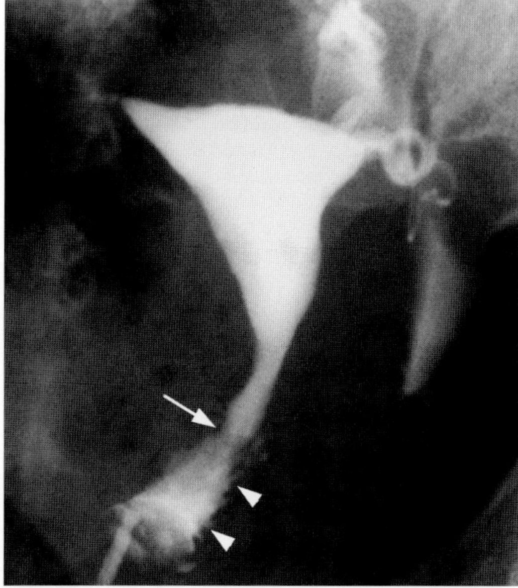

Figure 14. Normal cervical anatomy, with the characteristic serrated margin (arrowheads) and the internal os (arrow).

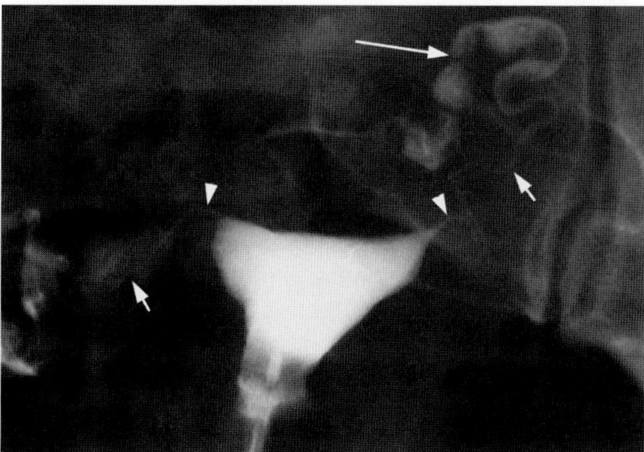

Figure 15. Fallopian tube anatomy, with the intramural portion seen at the cornu (arrowheads), the elongated isthmic segment (short arrows), and the distal ampulla (long arrow).

Fallopian Tube Abnormalities

Obstruction of the interstitial portion of the tube is usually secondary to infection or endometriosis, whereas tubal ligation and salpingectomy account for most cases of isthmic obstruction. Bulbous enlargement characteristically occurs at the termination of the ligated tube **(Fig. 16)**. Hydrosalpinx due to ampullary obstruction is most frequently related to prior infection that results in scarring and occlusion of the ostium of the ampulla. The thin-walled, distensible ampullary segment is preferentially dilated, whereas dilatation of the muscular, relatively thick-walled isthmic portion is rare **(Fig. 17)**.

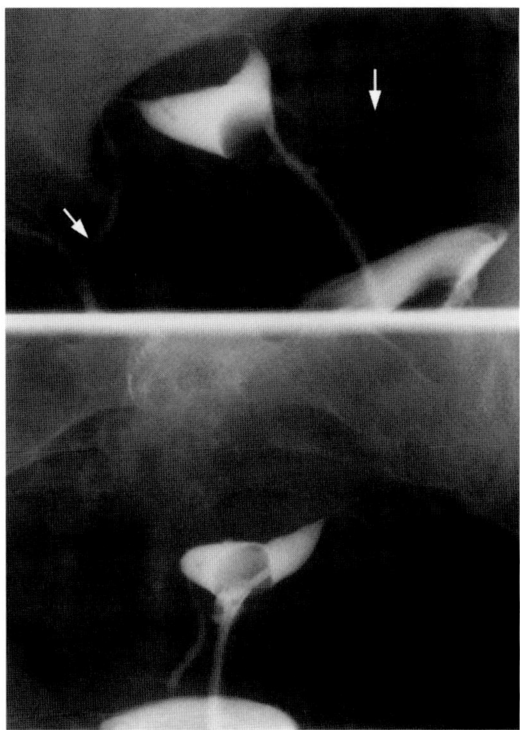

Figure 16. Tubal ligation. Arrows indicate the termination of the ligated tube.

Hydrosalpinx and obstruction may be bilateral **(Fig. 18)** or unilateral, with a normal, patent contralateral fallopian tube **(Fig. 19)**. Peritubal adhesions are frequently associated with hydrosalpinx and obstruction. Adhesions are manifested on HSG as crowding or "clumping" of the ampulla, with loculation of contrast material adjacent to the fimbriated aspect of the tube instead of the normal dispersion of contrast material from patent tubes which should outline loops of bowel **(Fig. 20)**.[5]

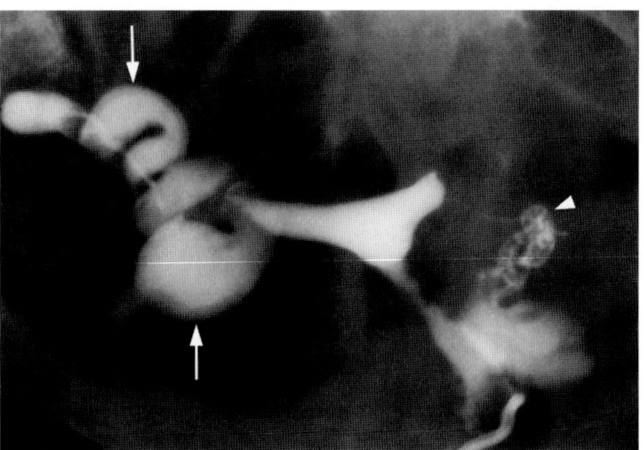

Figure 17. An AP film in a patient with a history of PID demonstrates moderately severe dilatation of the right tube with effacement of the rugal folds (arrows). Multiple small nodular filling defects in the left ampulla reflect the presence of ongoing or prior inflammatory disease (arrowhead).

Salpingitis isthmica nodosa (SIN) is an uncommon condition (4% in one large HSG series) of uncertain origin; it occurs bilaterally in 50% of cases. SIN is often associated with PID, infertility (30%), and ectopic pregnancy (10%).[6] The HSG appearance of SIN is characteristic: multiple 1–2-mm diverticular collections of contrast material arise from the isthmic portion of the tube, often accompanied by tubal obstruction **(Fig. 21)**. Tuberculous salpingitis may have an appearance on HSG similar to that of SIN.

Uterine Abnormalities

Filling defects within the uterine cavity may be due to polyps, submucosal myomas, air bubbles, synechiae (adhesions), blood clot, endometrial hyperplasia, and endometrial carcinoma. Exposing a film early in the filling phase ensures that small or subtle abnormalities will not be obscured by a densely opacified uterine cavity later in the examination. Small (5–10 mm) polypoid/curvilinear filling defects in the endometrial canal may be seen normally throughout the menstrual cycle **(Figs. 22, 23)**. Hysteroscopic and histologic evaluation has confirmed that these defects are usually not associated with a specific endometrial abnormality.[7] HSG cannot reliably detect endometrial hyperplasia.

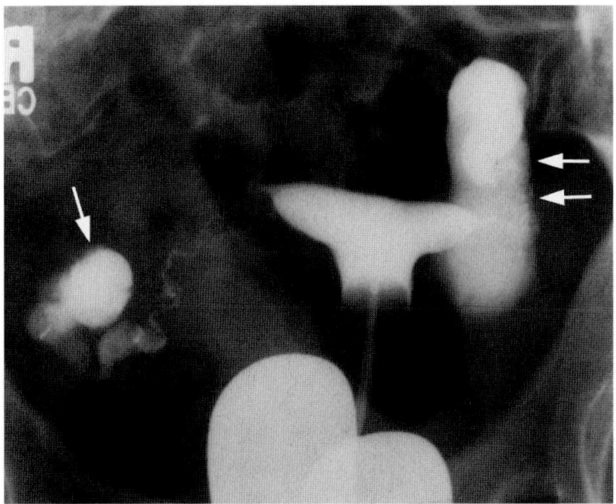

Figure 18. Bilateral hydrosalpinx (arrows).

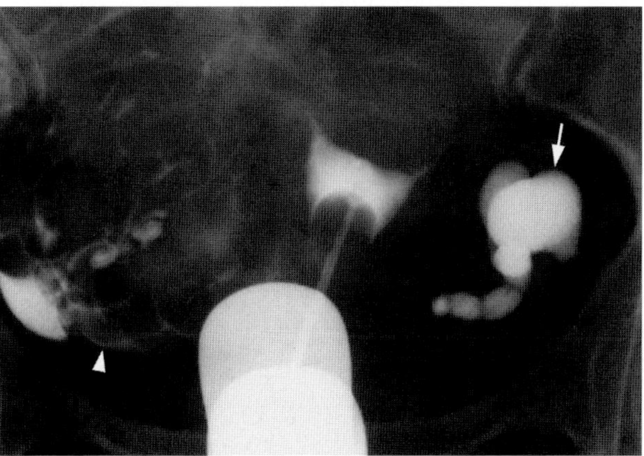

Figure 19. Left-sided hydrosalpinx (arrow). The contralateral tube is normal (arrowhead).

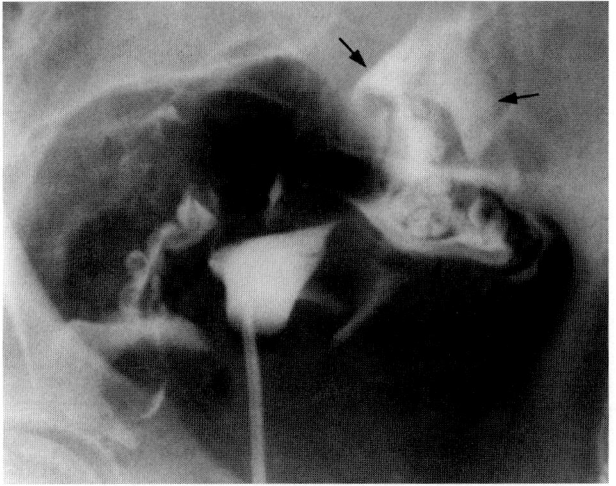

Figure 20. Peritubal adhesions (arrows).

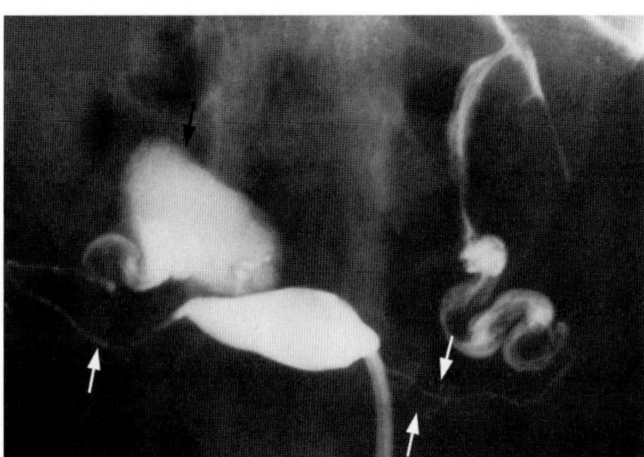

Figure 21. SIN with diverticular collections of contrast material (white arrows). Loculation of contrast material due to right-sided peritubal adhesions is also evident (black arrow).

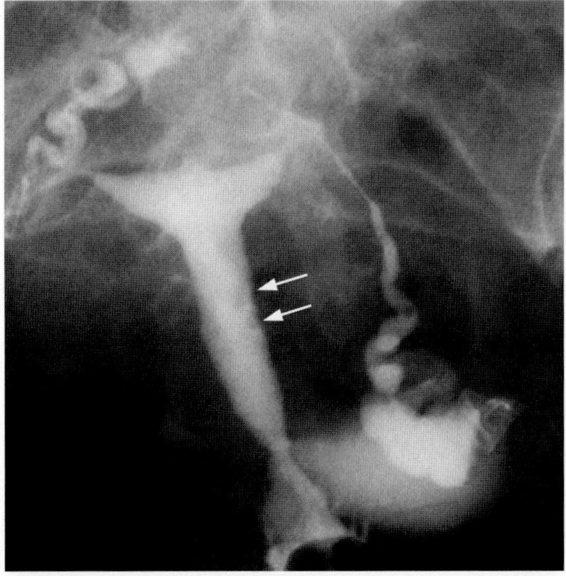

Figure 22. Endometrial "polyps" (arrows).

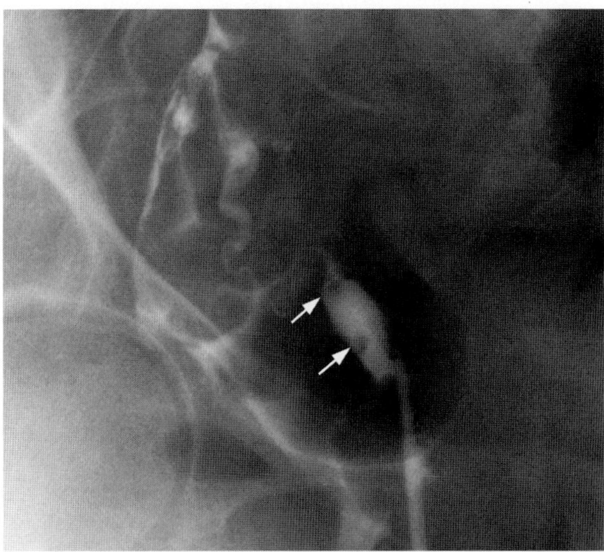

Figure 23. Endometrial filling defects (arrows).

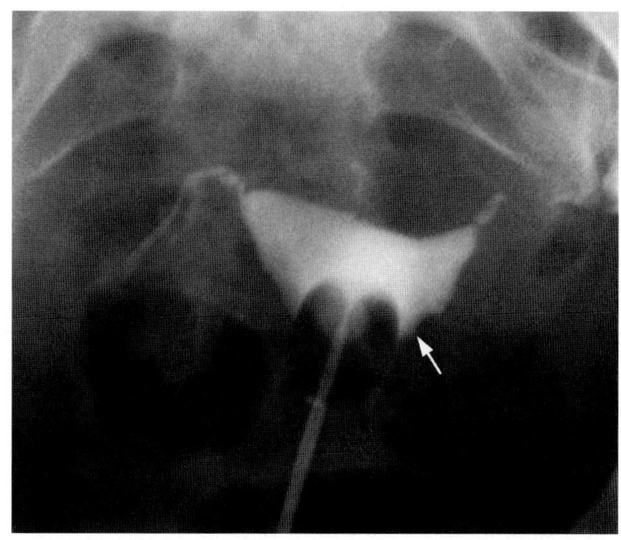

Figure 24. Submucosal myoma (arrow).

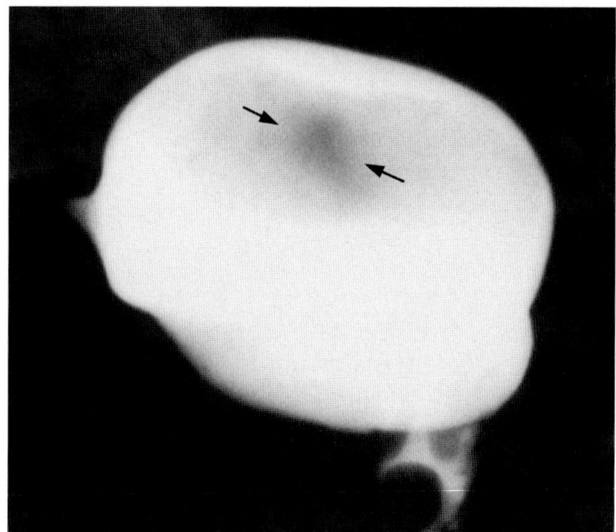

Figure 25. Fundal myoma causing a filling defect in the uterine fundus (arrows).

Uterine myomas are very common, especially in women over 35 years of age. Although submucosal myomas are less common than intramural and subserosal fibroids, they are often symptomatic because of their location **(Fig. 24)**. Intramural and subserosal myomas often can not be seen on HSG, but when they become large they can distort the endometrial cavity, resulting in a bizarre appearance. A filling defect in the uterine fundus **(Fig. 25)** is due in this case to a large intramural myoma which gives a capacious, globular appearance to the endometrial cavity. **Figure 26** shows a huge intramural fibroid which compresses and elongates the uterine cavity.

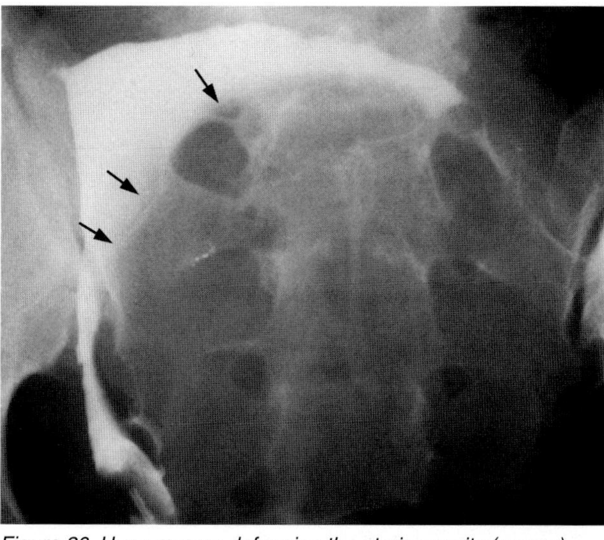

Figure 26. Huge myoma deforming the uterine cavity (arrows).

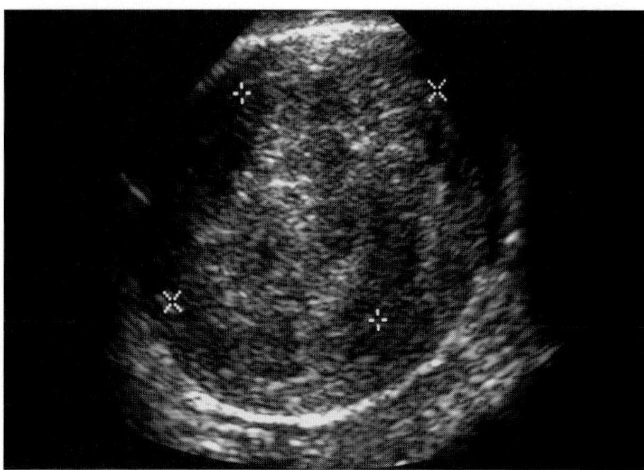

Figure 27. Endovaginal sonogram reveals a large myoma.

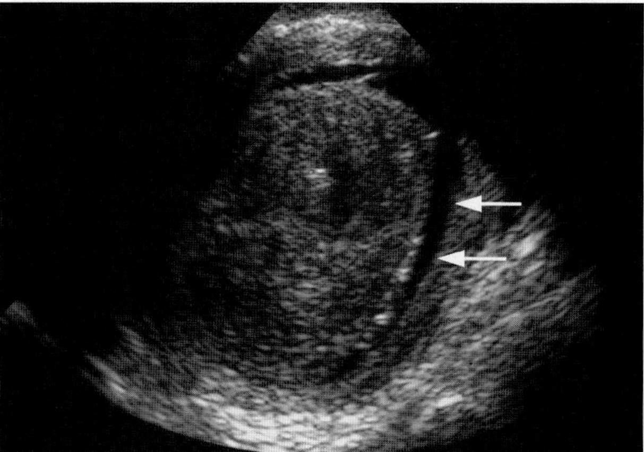

Figure 28. Sonohysterogram shows the myoma to better advantage. Note saline (arrows).

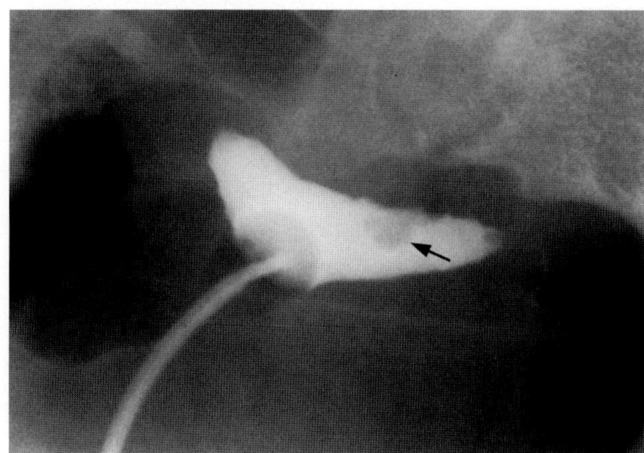

Figure 29. Endometrial polyp (arrow).

Sonohysterography involves the instillation of sterile saline into the endometrial cavity via an HSG catheter; the procedure is monitored with endovaginal scanning. Sonohysterosalpingography facilitates the differentiation of intraluminal, endometrial, and submucosal abnormalities.[8] In particular, the size and location of myomas can be delineated. In **Figure 27**, cursors outline an apparent large myoma on an endovaginal sonogram prior to saline instillation. After saline injection, a repeat scan displays the size and configuration of the myoma **(Fig. 28)**. Postoperative HSG may be used to demonstrate residual fibroids or postoperative complications such as synechiae or diverticula.

A filling defect in the fundus proved to be a polyp in this case **(Fig. 29)**. However, hysteroscopy may be necessary to differentiate polyps and/or endometrial hyperplasia from other benign masses and from endometrial carcinoma. HSG is usually performed to evaluate infertility; because endometrial carcinoma is most common after the age of fifty, it is rarely demonstrated on hysterosalpingograms.

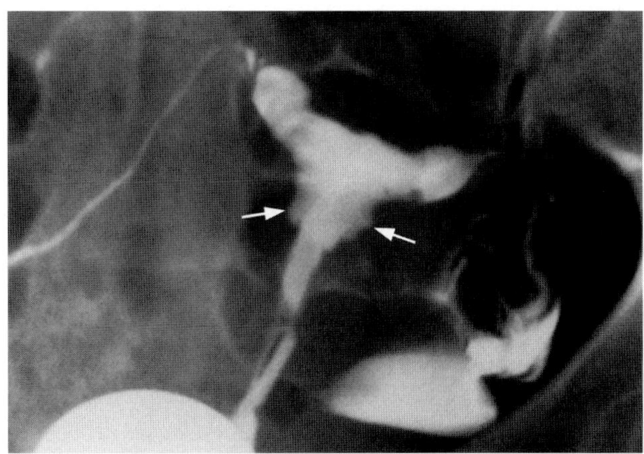

Figure 30. Adenomyosis indicated by the presence of small opacified cystic spaces (arrows).

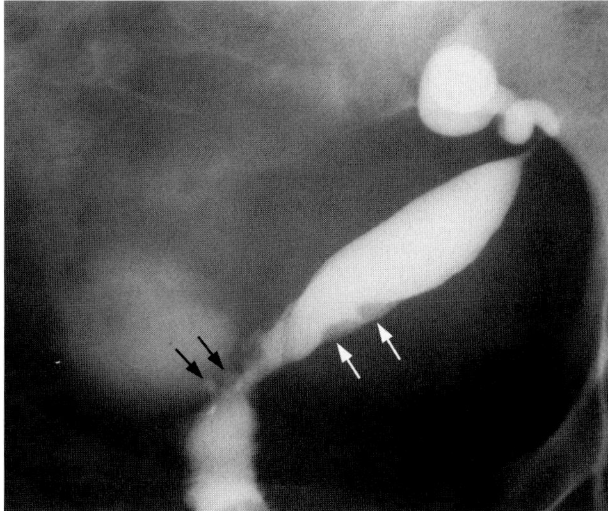

Figure 31. "Uterine cavities" (white arrows) in the lower portion of the uterus or near the cervical isthmus are a normal anatomic variant. Also, note polypoid filling defects in the body of the uterus (black arrows) and an obstructed left tube.

Adenomyosis is caused by the presence of endometrium deep within the myometrium. This disease infrequently manifests itself on HSG as contrast-filled cystic spaces smaller than 5 mm in diameter **(Fig. 30)**. MR imaging is much more sensitive for detecting adenomyosis and is the preferred imaging modality for this disease.

Small cavities in the lower uterine segment or near the cervical isthmus **(Fig. 31)** are usually due to cystic dilatation of glands, not adenomyosis.[9] As such they are of no clinical significance.

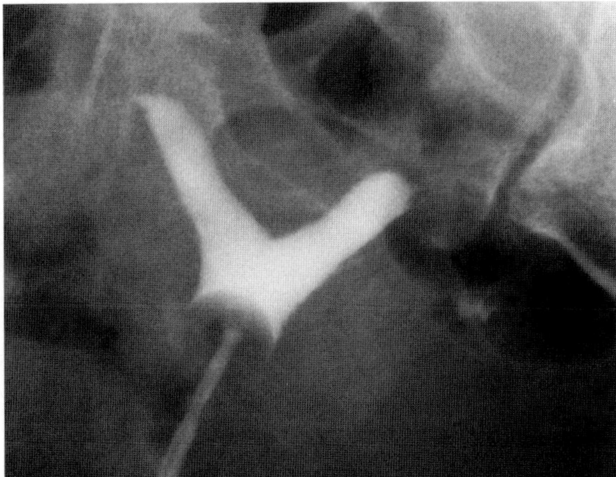

Figure 32. Bicornuate uterus.

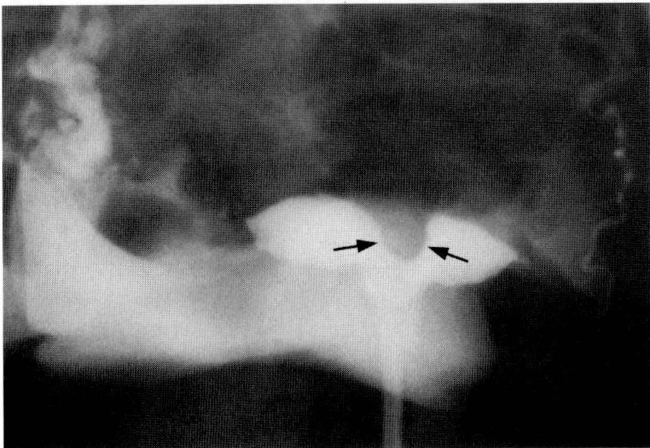

Figure 33. Septate uterus. Arrows indicate the horns, which subtend a relatively acute angle.

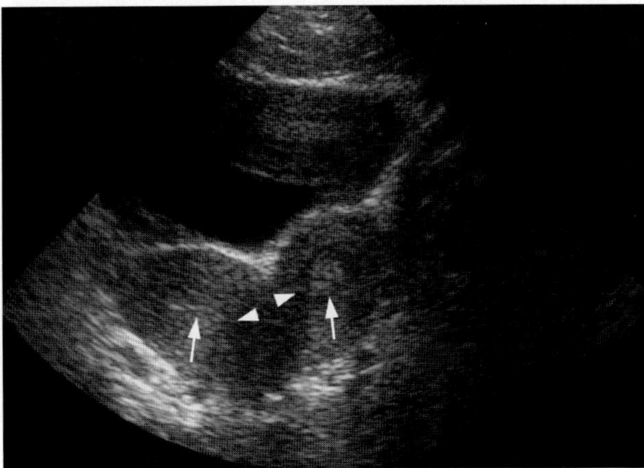

Figure 34. Sonogram demonstrates a bicornuate uterus. Two endometrial cavities are present (arrows). The septum between the cavities is a full-thickness myometrium (arrowheads).

Congenital Uterine Anomalies

While congenital anomalies can contribute to infertility, they are frequently detected incidentally and are not related to the patient's presenting complaint. Embryologically, the uterus originates from the paired Müllerian ducts, and most malformations are due to partial failure of fusion of these ducts (bicornuate uterus and uterus didelphys) or failure of resorption of the normal embryonic midline fusion of the ducts (septate uterus). The uterine septum in the latter condition may be complete or incomplete. Unicornuate uterus results from incomplete development of one of the Müllerian ducts. Urinary tract abnormalities (renal agenesis, ectopic kidney) frequently accompany uterine anomalies.

HSG can differentiate between the most common anomalies, bicornuate and septate uterus. However, diagnostic accuracy in distinguishing these conditions on the basis of HSG and clinical evaluation alone was only 62% in one series. Combining sonographic and HSG findings increases the accuracy rate to 90%.[10] Two separate cavities are displayed in both malformations. Widely divergent horns are seen in bicornuate uterus **(Fig. 32)**, whereas the angle between the horns in septate uterus is more acute **(Fig. 33)**. When the angle between the two cavities is less than 75 degrees, a confident diagnosis of septate uterus can be made. If the angle between the horns exceeds 105 degrees, bicornuate uterus is likely present but sonographic confirmation is recommended.[11]

When the uterine horns subtend angles between 75 and 105 degrees, either malformation may be present. In addition, combined bicornuate/septum anomalies also occur. Sonography and/or MR imaging is necessary in order to make the diagnosis in these complex, often confusing cases.[12] Making the distinction between bicornuate uterus and septate uterus is important because the latter is associated with multiple second trimester abortions but is relatively easy to correct surgically. Correction of bicornuate uterus requires a major surgical procedure, and these patients are usually offered the option of a pregnancy trial before undergoing surgical repair.

Sonography depicts two endometrial cavities in both anomalies **(Fig. 34)**. The cavities are separated by normal full-thickness myometrium in bicornuate uterus, whereas they are more closely apposed in septate uterus, being separated only by a thin septum.

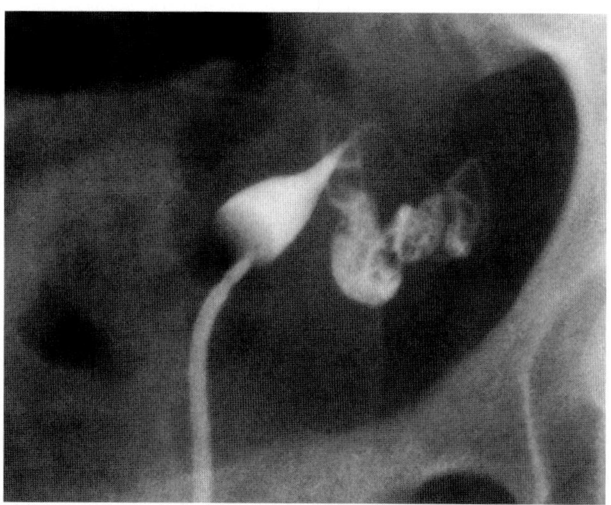

Figure 35. Simulation of a unicornuate uterus due to incorrect catheter positioning.

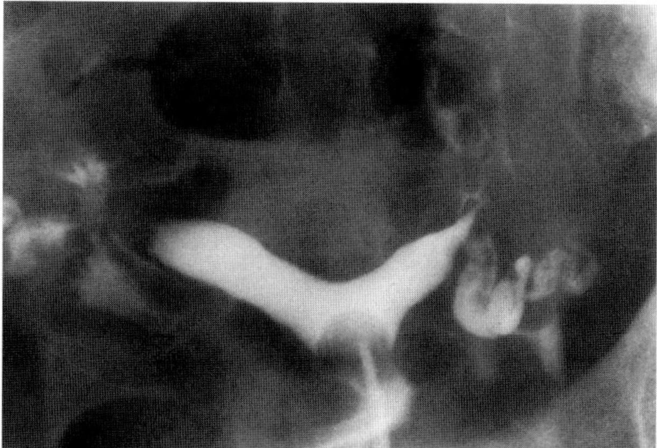

Figure 36. Bicornuate uterus.

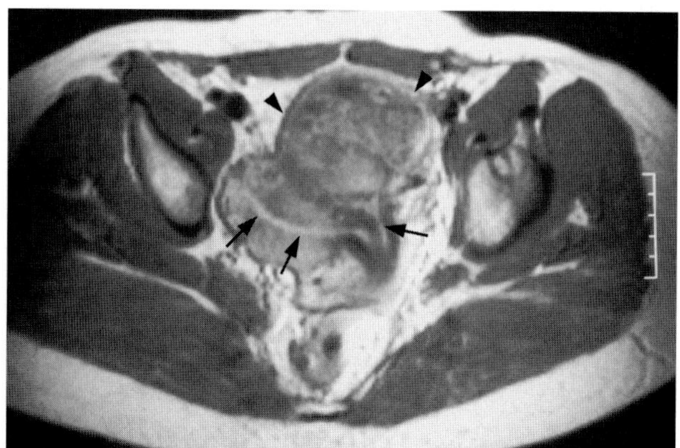

Figure 37. MR image of a bicornuate uterus displays two endometrial cavities (arrows) and a myoma arising from the left horn (arrowheads).

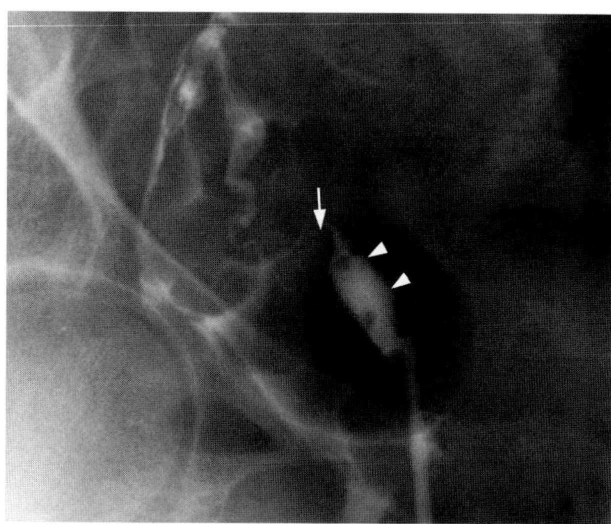

Figure 38. Unicornuate uterus. Arrowheads indicate the location of the missing horn. The tube arises from the upper pole of the opacified horn (arrow).

Inadvertent catheterization of one horn of a bicornuate uterus may simulate a unicornuate uterus **(Fig. 35)**. Retracting the balloon catheter into the lower uterine segment or cervix and reinjecting contrast material will accurately display the anatomy of the duplication anomaly **(Figs. 36, 37)**.

Unicornuate uterus is a rare anomaly which may be accompanied by an absent, rudimentary, or obstructed horn **(Fig. 38)**. Origination of the tube from the upper pole of the opacified horn is typical. The obstructed or rudimentary horn is not demonstrated on HSG but may be detected by MR imaging. In uterus didelphys, duplication of the uterus and cervix is associated with septation or duplication of the vagina **(Fig. 39)**.

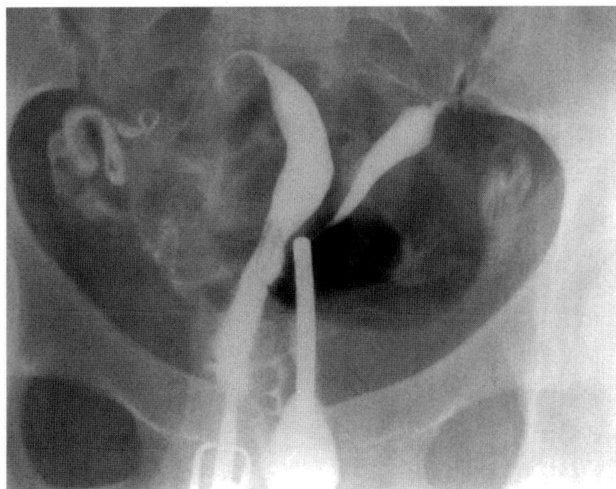

Figure 39. Uterus didelphys.

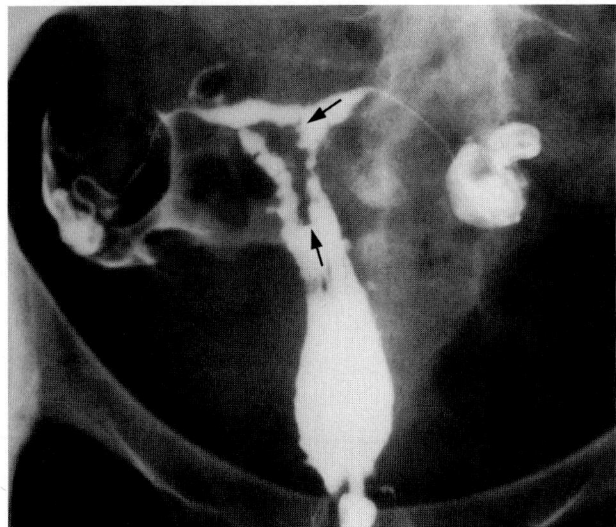

Figure 40. Uterine synechiae (arrows).

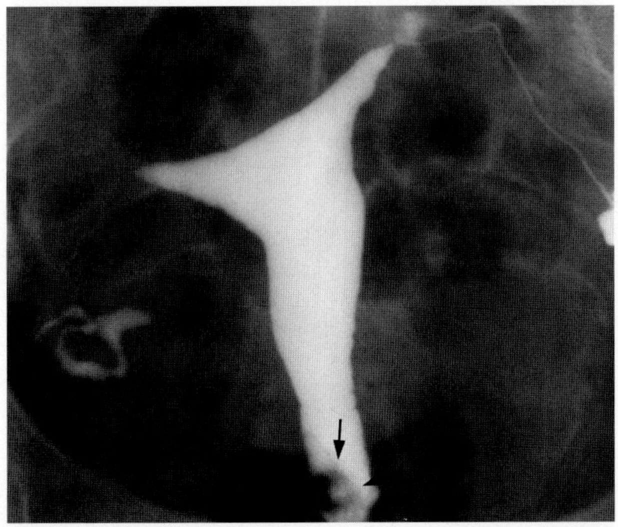

Figure 41. Uterine synechiae (arrows).

Miscellaneous

Synechiae (intrauterine adhesions) are usually caused by endometrial trauma, almost always after a post partum dilation and curettage or uterine infection. Endometritis may be a contributing factor. Adhesions occur in all parts of the uterus and are seen on imaging as single or multiple irregular, serpiginous, and angular filling defects of the uterine cavity **(Figs. 40, 41)**.[13] If severe, significant deformity and contraction of the endometrial cavity develop and when the cornua are involved, infertility often ensues.

In utero exposure to diethylstilbestrol results in developmental and morphologic abnormalities. The uterus is hypoplastic with a small irregular cavity presenting the classic "T-shaped" configuration on HSG.[14]

References

1. Ott DJ, Fayez JA. Hysterosalpingography: a text and atlas. Baltimore: Urban & Schwarzenberg, 1990.

2. Yoder IC, Hall DA. Hysterosalpingography in the 1990s. AJR 1991; 157:675–683.

3. Sholkoff SD. Balloon hysterosalpingography catheter. AJR 1987; 149:995–996.

4. Margolin FR. A new cannula for hysterosalpingography. AJR 1988; 151:729–730.

5. Karasick S, Goldfarb AF. Peritubal adhesions in infertile women: diagnosis with hysterosalpingography. AJR 1989; 152:777–779.

6. Creasy JL, Clark RL, Cuttino JT, Groff TR. Salpingitis isthmica nodosa: radiologic and clinical correlates. Radiology 1985; 154:597–600.

7. Slezak P, Tillinger KG. Hysterographic evidence of polypoid filling defects in the uterine cavity. Radiology 1975; 115:79–83.

8. Cullinan JA, Fleischer AC, Kepple DM, Arnold AL. Sonohysterography: a technique for endometrial evaluation. Radiographics 1995; 15:501–514.

9. Slezak P, Tillinger KG. The incidence and clinical importance of hysterographic evidence of cavities in the uterine wall. Radiology 1976; 118:581–586.

10. Reuter KL, Daly DC, Cohen SM. Septate versus bicornuate uteri: errors in imaging diagnosis. Radiology 1989; 172:749–752.

11. Hall DA, Yoder IC. Ultrasound evaluation of the uterus. In: Callen P. Ultrasonography in obstetrics and gynecology. Philadelphia: W.B. Saunders Company, 1994; 593.

12. Pellerito JS, McCarthy AM, Doyle MB, Glickman MG, DeCherney AH. Diagnosis of uterine anomalies: relative accuracy of MR imaging, endovaginal sonography, and hysterosalpingography. Radiology 1992; 183:795–800.

13. Krysiewicz S. Infertility in women: diagnostic evaluation with hysterosalpingography and other imaging techniques. AJR 1992; 159:253–261.

14. Hunt RB, Siegler AM. Hysterosalpingography: techniques and interpretation. Chicago: Year Book Medical Publishers, 1990.

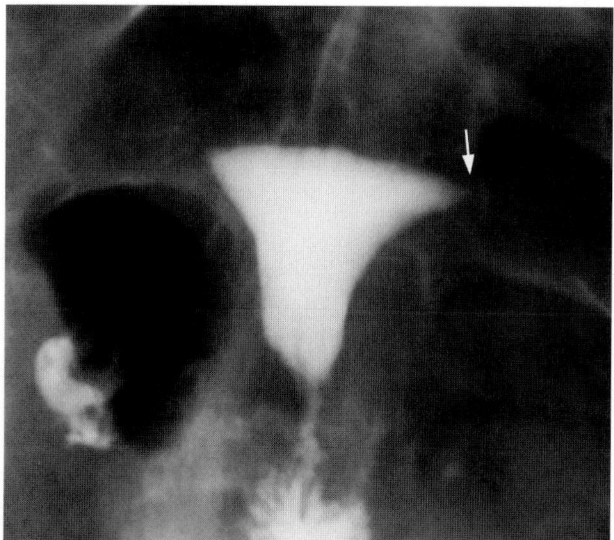

Figure 1. Hysterosalpingogram suggests left proximal tubal obstruction (arrow).

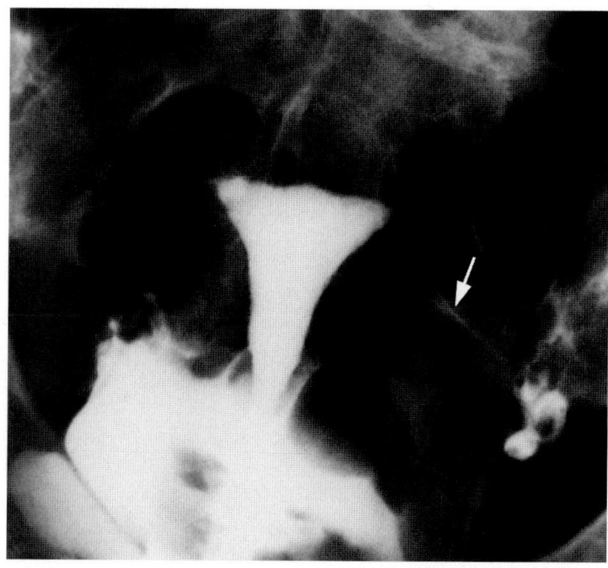

Figure 2. Same patient as in Figure 1. Placing the patient prone results in filling of the left fallopian tube (arrow).

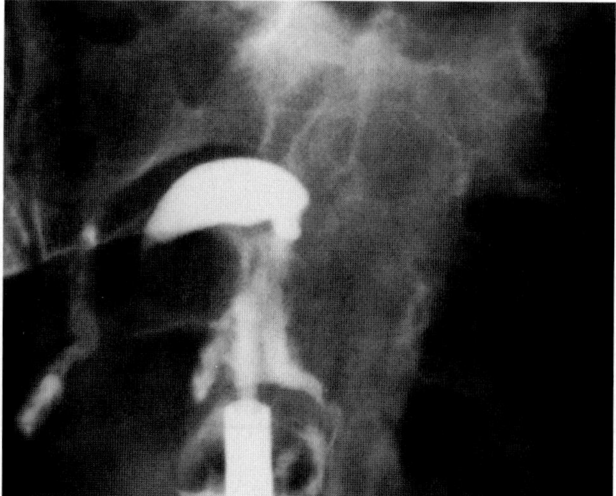

Figure 3. Hysterosalpingogram suggests left proximal tubal obstruction.

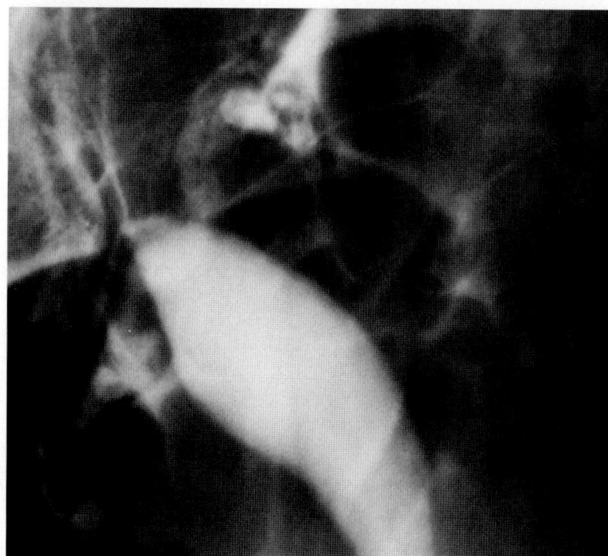

Figure 4. Same patient as in Figure 3. Placing traction on the uterus demonstrates the typical shape of a unicornuate uterus with congenital absence of the left tube.

TUTORIAL 25 FALLOPIAN TUBE RECANALIZATION

Amy Thurmond, M.D.

Introduction

The subjects addressed in this tutorial include:

1. Technique of fallopian tube recanalization
2. Complications of fallopian tube recanalization
3. Results of fallopian tube recanalization.

Proximal Tubal Obstruction

A large number of pathologic conditions can affect the proximal tube and cause infertility. Inspissated debris, inflammation, and fibrosis are the leading causes. Tubal "spasm" **(Figs. 1, 2)**, and unicornuate uterus **(Figs. 3, 4)** can mimic tubal occlusion; therefore, an adequately performed diagnostic hysterosalpingogram (HSG) is mandatory.

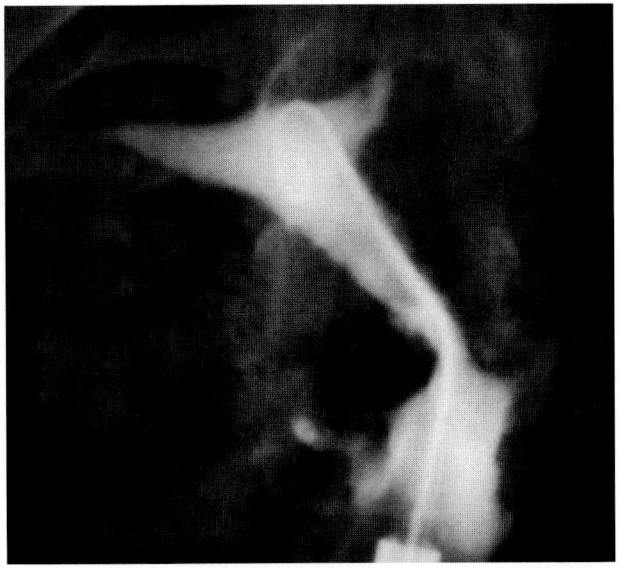

Figure 5. Pushing on the fundus of the uterus with the guide wire, as in this case, causes pain and bleeding.

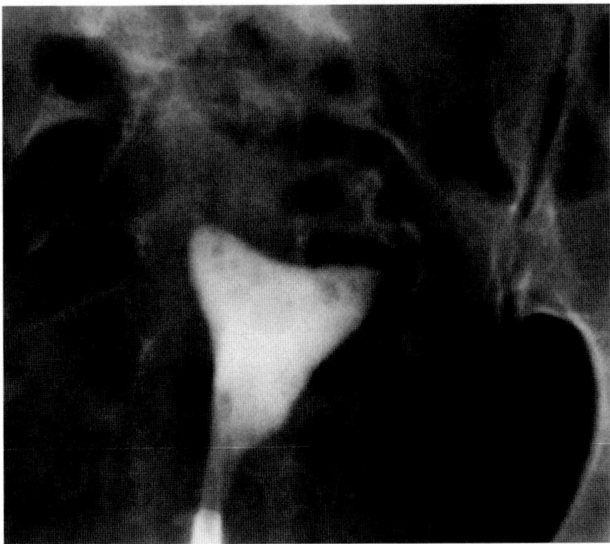

Figure 6. Right ostial salpingogram confirms tubal occlusion.

Uterine Technique

A variety of instruments and techniques for fluoroscopic fallopian tube catheterization, selective salpingography, and recanalization have been described.[1–4] The procedure is performed during the follicular phase of the menstrual cycle, with sterile technique and antibiotic prophylaxis. The early portion of the menstrual cycle is chosen to ensure that the procedure does not disrupt a pregnancy. A conventional HSG with dilute water-soluble contrast material is performed initially, which localizes the uterine cornua without obscuring the catheters. A 5.5-F polyethylene catheter is advanced over 0.035-inch-diameter J and straight guide wires. Cramping and bleeding occur if the guide wire or catheter pushes against the uterine fundus **(Fig. 5)**. Minimal discomfort is felt if the 5.5-F catheter is efficiently wedged in the uterine cornu.

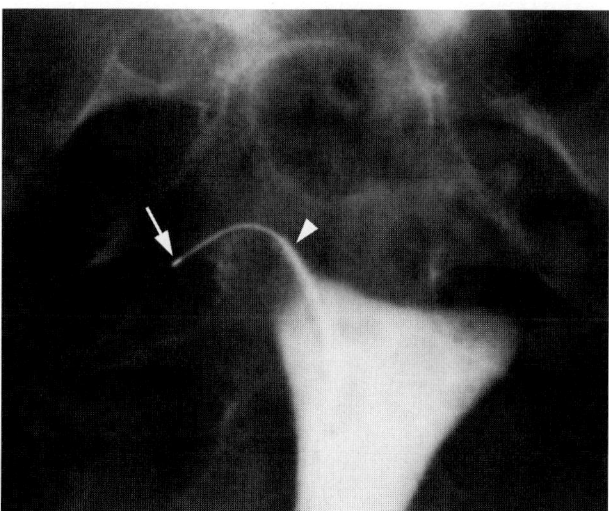

Figure 7. Same patient as in Figure 6. Right tubal recanalization with a flexible platinum-tipped wire (arrow) inserted coaxially through a 5.5-F catheter (arrowhead).

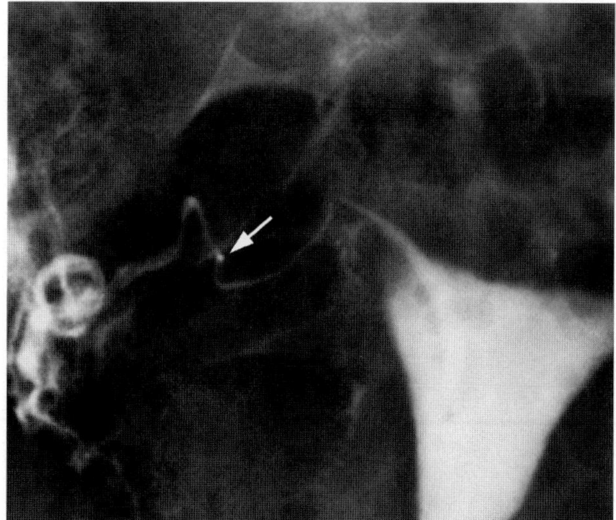

Figure 8. Same patient as in Figure 6. Right intratubal salpingogram obtained through the 3-F catheter (arrow) after successful passage of the wire demonstrates patency with intraperitoneal spilling of injected contrast material.

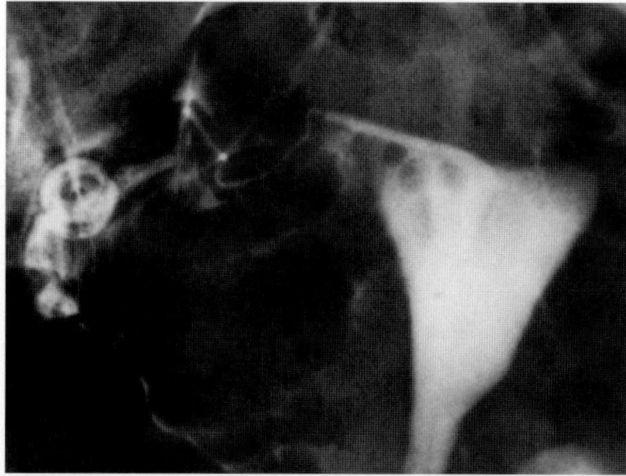

Figure 9. Same patient as in Figure 6. Completion right ostial salpingogram obtained through the 5.5 catheter after recanalization confirms patency with intraperitoneal spilling of contrast material.

Tubal Technique

After direct injection into the tubal ostium to confirm obstruction (ostial salpingogram), an 0.015-inch guide wire with a flexible platinum tip and 3-F Teflon catheter (Cook, Bloomington, IN) are advanced together through the 5.5-F catheter into the fallopian tube, and an attempt is made to recanalize the obstruction with gentle probing movements of the guide wire **(Figs. 6–9)**.

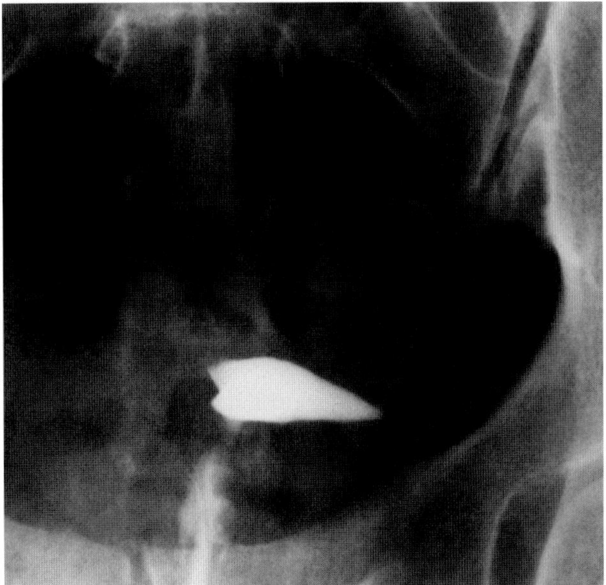
Figure 10. Initial HSG demonstrates blocked tubes and an anteflexed uterus.

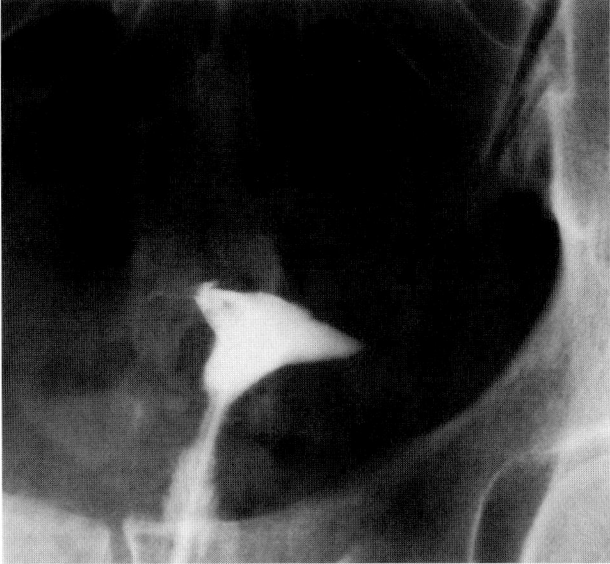
Figure 11. Same patient as in Figure 10. Placing traction on the uterus straightens it and aids catheterization.

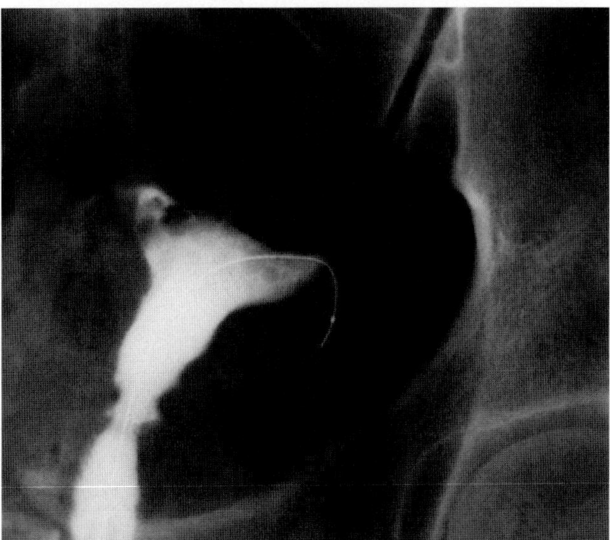
Figure 12. Same patient as in Figure 10. The tube forms an acute angle with the uterine cavity, so a softer, tapered guide wire and catheter should be used.

Advanced Tubal Technique

If an acute angulation is present in the tube at the site of the obstruction, or if the obstruction is in the isthmic portion of the tube, a softer tapered guide wire and catheter are used (Taper guide wire and Tracker-18 catheter, Target Therapeutics, Fremont, CA) **(Figs. 10, 11)**. When the guide wire passes the obstruction, the guide wire is removed and contrast material injected through the 3-F catheter to obtain an intratubal salpingogram **(Fig. 12)**. Once the recanalization is completed, the 3-F catheter is removed and contrast material injected through the 5.5-F catheter, which is still wedged in the tubal ostium, to better delineate the tube and visualize the site of recanalization **(Fig. 13)**.

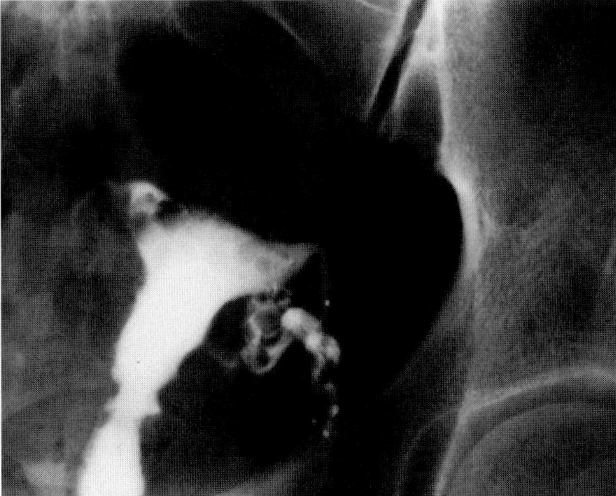
Figure 13. Same patient as in Figure 10. Follow-up ostial salpingogram through the 5.5-F catheter demonstrates tubal patency after successful recanalization.

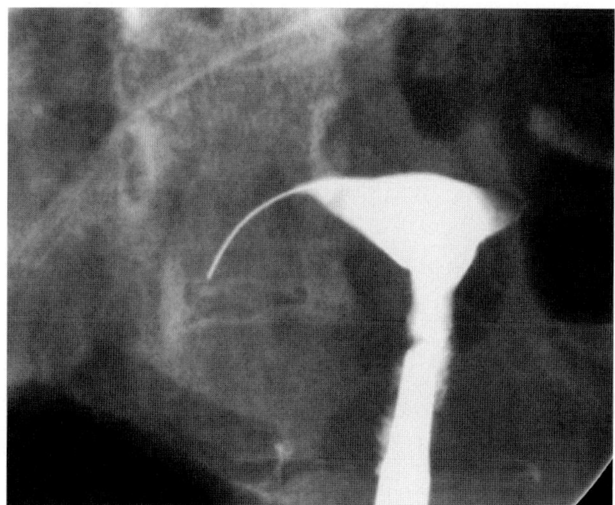

Figure 14. Attempt at recanalization with the wire in the expected portion of the mid fallopian tube.

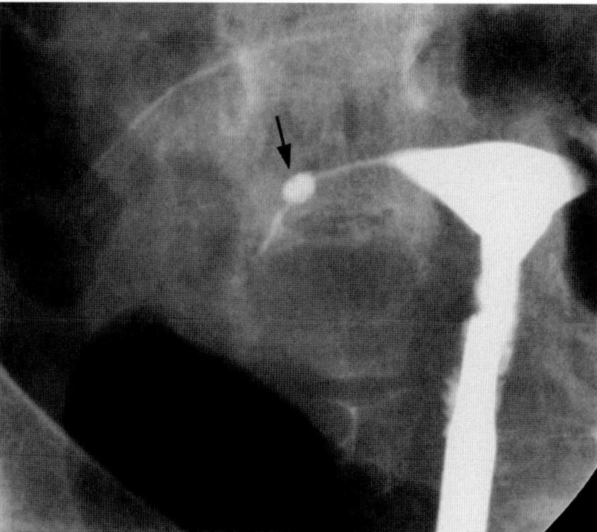

Figure 15. Same patient as in Figure 14. Intratubal salpingogram demonstrates a small perforation induced by the guide wire (arrow).

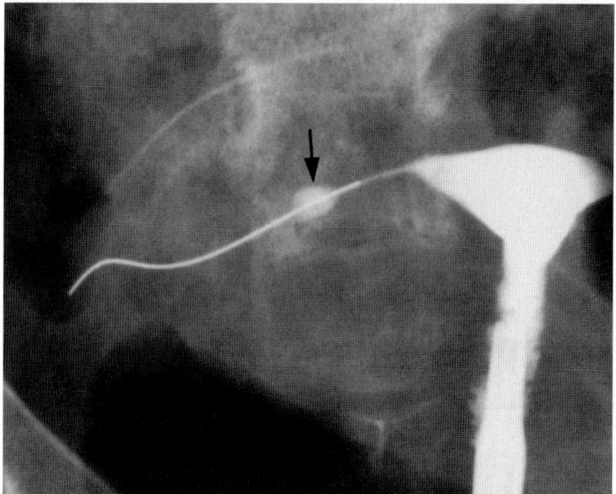

Figure 16. Same patient as in Figure 14. Because normal tube is visible beyond the site of perforation (arrow), the guide wire is carefully advanced again into the distal tube and recanalization is again attempted.

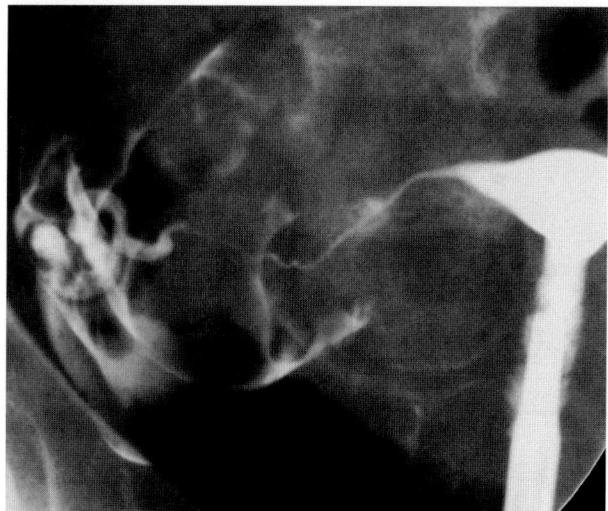

Figure 17. Same patient as in Figure 14. Intratubal salpingogram demonstrates successful recanalization.

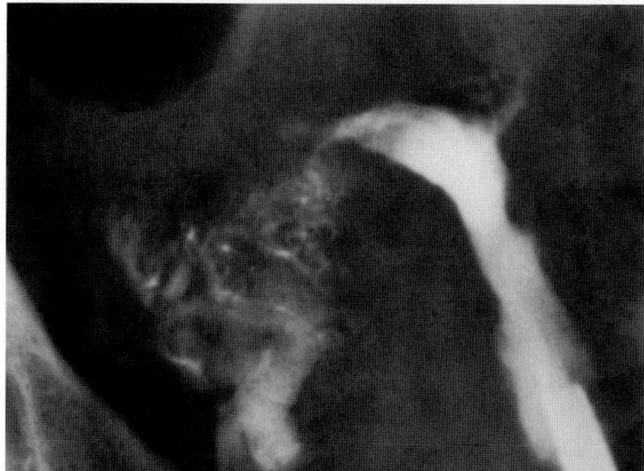

Figure 18. Intratubal salpingogram in a different patient following attempted tubal recanalization demonstrates filling of pelvic veins only. No further attempts were made to recanalize the right tube.

Complications

Mild uterine cramping and vaginal bleeding usually occur with fallopian tube catheterization. Perforation occurs in about 2% of tubes and has not required additional monitoring or treatment **(Figs. 14–18)**.[5,6] The radiation dose to the ovaries during fluoroscopic catheterization is less than 1 rad (10 Gy).[7] This is in the same range as the radiation dose delivered during a barium enema or an intravenous pyelogram.

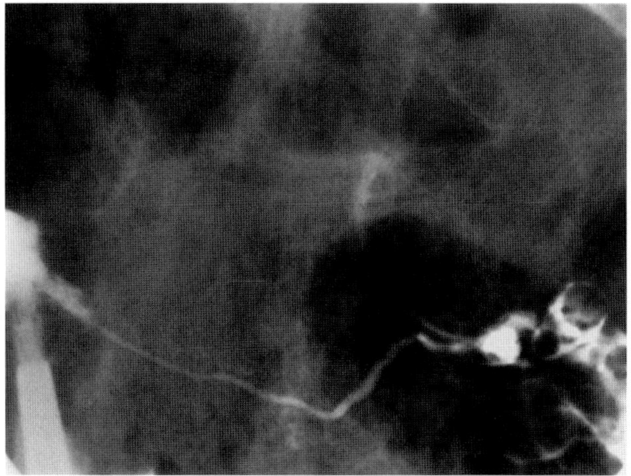

Figure 19. Same patient as in Figure 18. Successful recanalization of the occluded left tube. The patient conceived shortly afterward.

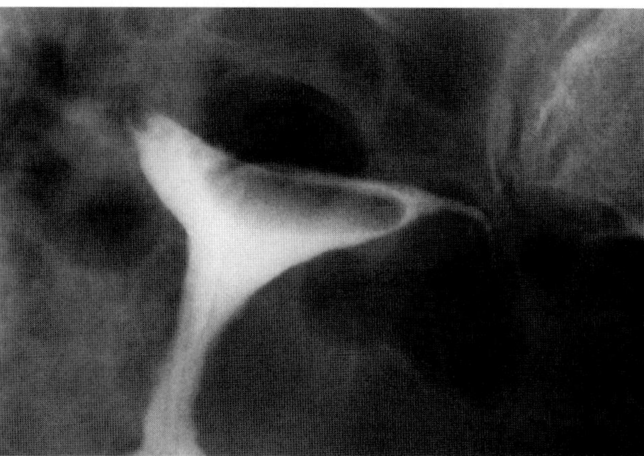

Figure 20. Left ostial salpingogram via a 5.5-F catheter confirms tubal occlusion.

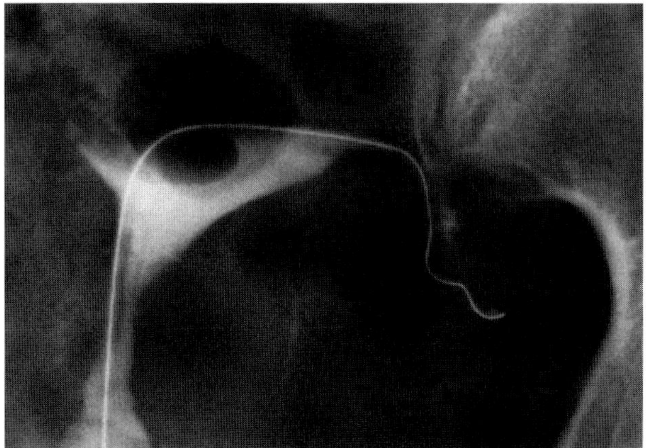

Figure 21. Same patient as in Figure 20. Recanalization using an 0.015-inch guide wire.

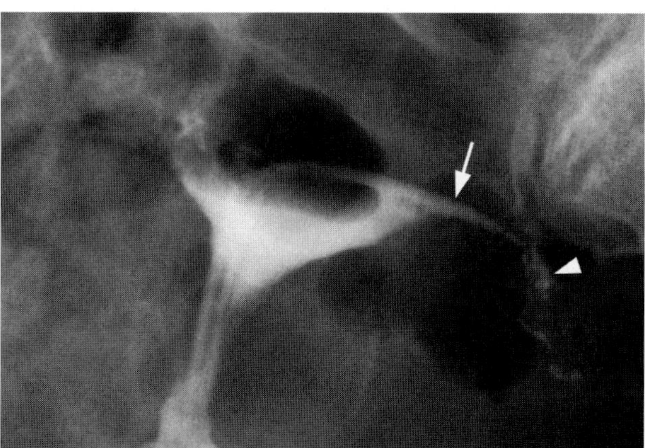

Figure 22. Same patient as in Figure 20. Intratubal salpingogram demonstrates salpingitis isthmica nodosa (arrow) and a second, more distal obstruction (arrowhead).

Diagnostic Results

Fluoroscopic fallopian tube catheterization improves tubal diagnosis. The ability to establish proximal tubal patency is 80%–85%. Approximately one third of patients who undergo successful fluoroscopic fallopian tube recanalization for unilateral or bilateral proximal tubal obstruction have normal-appearing tubes after the procedure **(Fig. 19)**. Another third have patent tubes; however, the appearance of the tubes and the peritoneal spill suggest peritubal adhesions. Of the remaining patients, approximately 10% have patency with a small dilatation at the site of the obstruction, approximately 10% have patency with salpingitis isthmica nodosa (SIN) **(Figs. 20–23)**, and approximately 10% have proximal patency but distal occlusion with hydrosalpinx **(Figs. 24–26)**.[8]

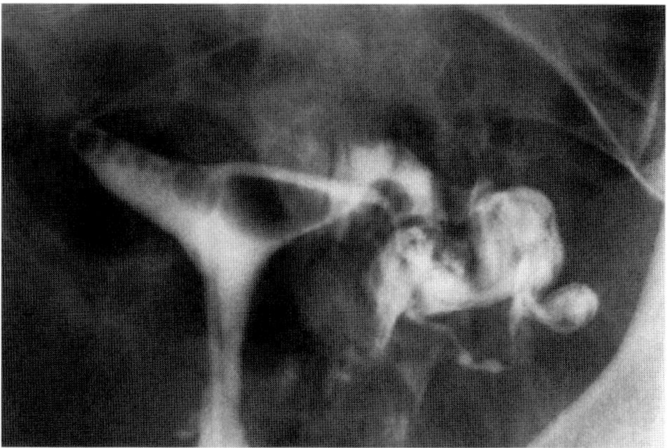

Figure 23. Same patient as in Figure 20. The guide wire was carefully advanced through the diseased segment, and recanalization was achieved.

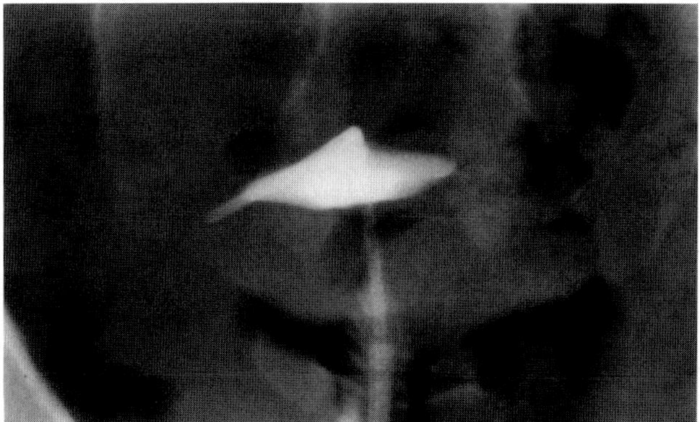

Figure 24. Right ostial salpingogram with a 5.5-F catheter.

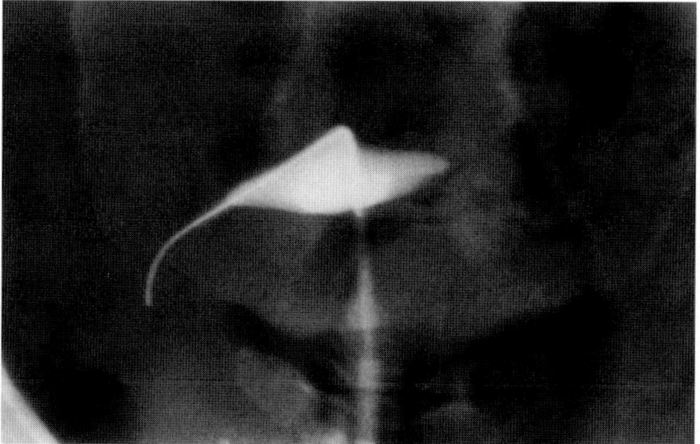

Figure 25. Same patient as in Figure 24. Recanalization using a guide wire.

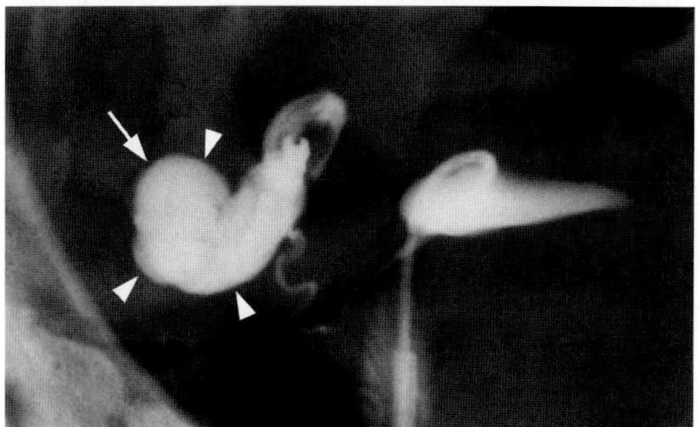

Figure 26. Same patient as in Figure 24. Intratubal salpingogram demonstrates distal tubal disease (arrow) and a hydrosalpinx (arrowheads).

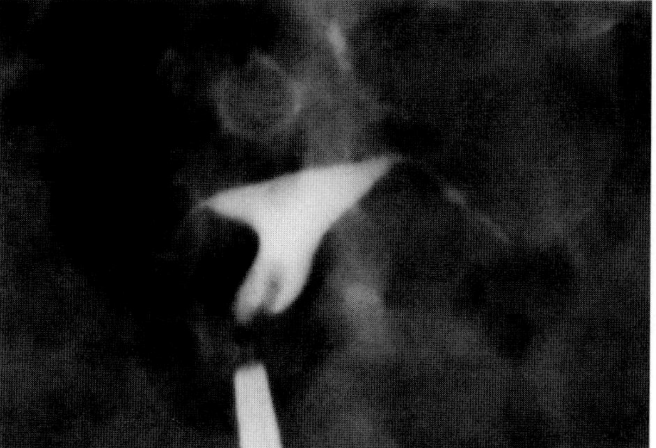

Figure 27. This woman was advised to have in vitro fertilization after laparoscopy and two hysterosalpingograms confirmed bilateral proximal tubal occlusion.

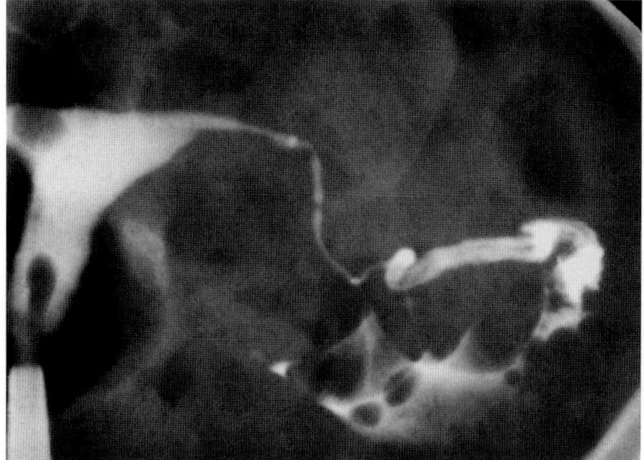

Figure 28. Same patient as in Figure 27. Left catheter recanalization was successful.

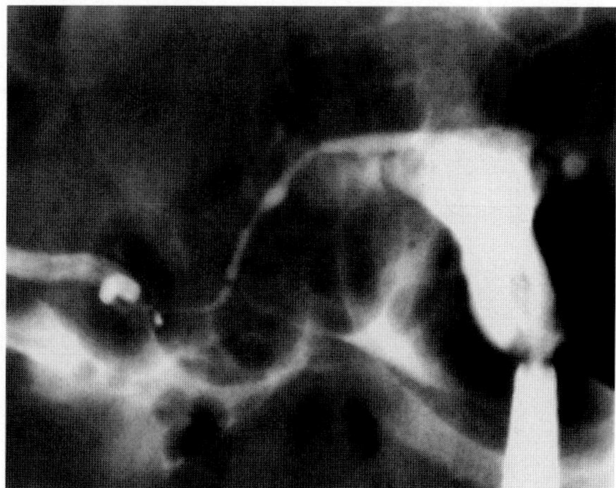

Figure 29. Same patient as in Figure 27. Right catheter recanalization was successful, and the patient conceived the next month.

Therapeutic Results

Most investigators now agree that tubal catheterization is also a treatment for infertility. This is more difficult to prove, however, because of the many clinical variables involved in achieving pregnancy.[9] In one study, 20 patients with isolated proximal tubal obstruction recommended for tubal microsurgery or in vitro fertilization underwent catheter recanalization instead. Recanalization of one or both tubes was successful in 95% of cases. One year after the procedure, 58% of the women had conceived without receiving any other therapy, and all pregnancies were intrauterine **(Figs. 27–29)**.

In a more heterogeneous group that includes women with SIN and other tubal or pelvic disease, a lower recanalization rate can be expected **(Figs. 30, 31)**. The lower short-term intrauterine pregnancy rate is in the 20%–30% range, with an approximately 3% tubal pregnancy rate.[5,6,10]

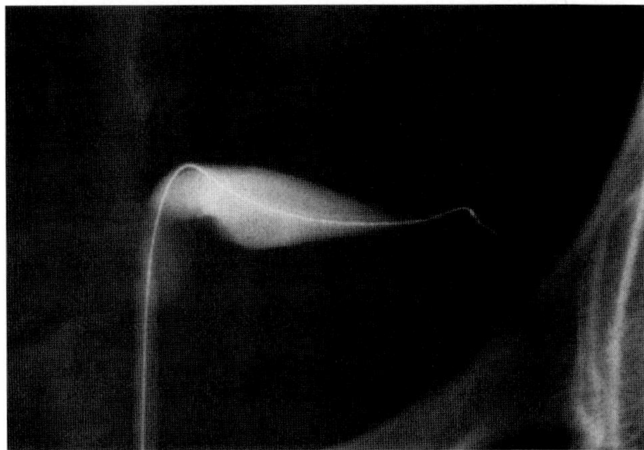

Figure 30. Attempt to recanalize the left tube.

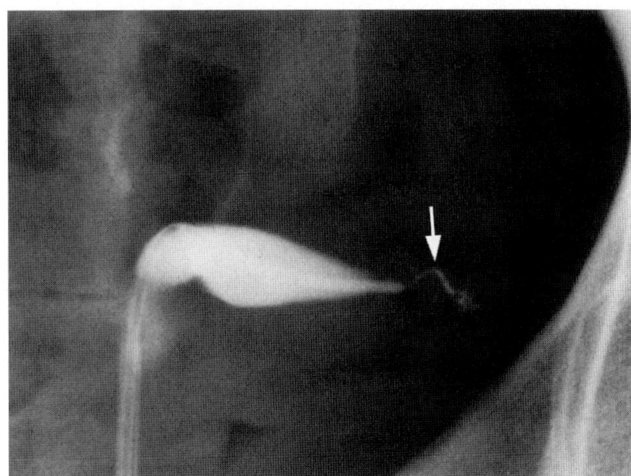

Figure 31. Same patient as in Figure 30. Follow-up intratubal salpingogram demonstrates severe SIN (arrow), and recanalization was not achieved.

References

1. Thurmond AS, Uchida BT, Rösch J. Device for hysterosalpingography and fallopian tube catheterization. Radiology 1990; 174:571–572.

2. Thurmond AS, Rösch J. Fallopian tubes: improved technique for catheterization. Radiology 1990; 174:572–573.

3. LaBerge JM, Ponec DJ, Gordon RL. Fallopian tube catheterization: modified fluoroscopic technique. Radiology 1990; 176:283–284.

4. Meyerovitz MF. Hysterosalpingography and fallopian tube cannulation: use of a double-balloon introducing catheter. Radiology 1991; 181:901–902.

5. Thurmond AS, Rösch J. Nonsurgical fallopian tube recanalization for treatment of infertility. Radiology 1990;174:371–374.

6. Kumpe DA, Zwerdlinger SC, Rothbarth LJ, Durham JD, Albrecht BH. Proximal fallopian tube occlusion: diagnosis and treatment with transcervical fallopian tube catheterization. Radiology 1990; 177:183–187.

7. Hedgpeth PL, Thurmond AS, Fry R, Schmidgall JR, Rösch J. Radiographic fallopian tube recanalization: absorbed ovarian radiation dose. Radiology 1991; 180:121–122.

8. Thurmond AS, Rösch J, Patton PE, Burry KA, Novy M. Fluoroscopic transcervical fallopian tube catheterization for diagnosis and treatment of female infertility caused by tubal obstruction. Radiographics 1988; 8:621–640.

9. Thurmond AS. Pregnancies after selective salpingography and tubal recanalization. Radiology 1994; 190:11–13.

10. Thurmond AS, Burry KA, Novy MJ. Salpingitis isthmica nodosa: results of transcervical fluoroscopic catheter recanalization. Fertil Steril 1995; 63:715–722.

TUTORIAL 26
PERCUTANEOUS BONE BIOPSIES

William Clark, M.D., and
Georges Y. El-Khoury, M.D.

Introduction

The subjects addressed in this tutorial include:

1. Types of bone biopsies
2. Indications for percutaneous biopsy
3. Risks and contraindications
4. Types of biopsy needles
5. Vertebral biopsy
6. Pelvic and sacral biopsy
7. Biopsy of the appendicular skeleton.

Despite advancing imaging technology, the definitive diagnosis of bone tumors requires bone biopsy to obtain tissue for cytologic or histologic examination. The decision to perform a biopsy is guided by clinical and radiographic findings. In most cases the safest and least expensive technique for obtaining tissue for diagnosis is a percutaneous needle biopsy. This can be guided by computed tomography (CT) scanning or fluoroscopy. Percutaneous needle biopsy is also used to obtain bacteriologic samples in cases of infection.

Types of Bone Biopsies

Bone biopsies can be broadly classified into open biopsies and percutaneous needle biopsies. Open biopsy is the surgical excision of a piece of bone. Percutaneous needle biopsy uses radiographic guidance to obtain a cellular aspirate or a core sample of bone. The advantages of the percutaneous technique are the avoidance of a general anesthetic, diminished morbidity, and lower cost. It can also be performed on an outpatient basis. Its principal disadvantage is reduced size and quality of the tissue sample as compared to open biopsy. However, percutaneous needle biopsy provides sufficient material for cytologic or histologic diagnosis in most cases of bone tumor.

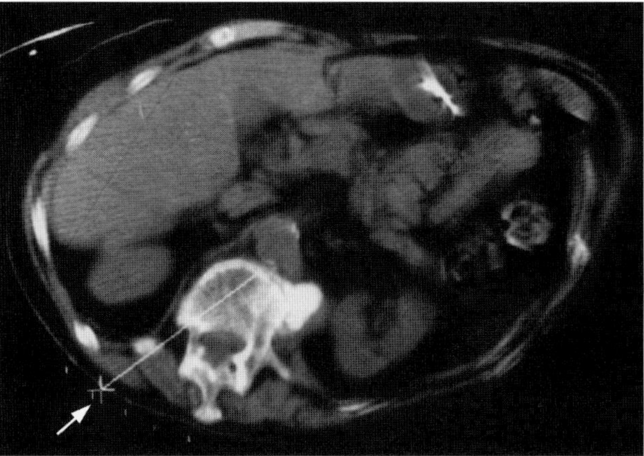

Figure 1. Pre-biopsy CT plan. Note the skin markers (arrow), which help define the needle entry point.

Indications for Percutaneous Biopsy

Common indications for percutaneous bone biopsy are:

1. Suspected bone metastasis (with or without known primary tumor)
2. Suspected primary bone malignancy
3. Recurrent tumor
4. Suspected round cell tumor
5. Infectious lesion
6. Vertebral compression fractures (to exclude underlying tumor)
7. Spine or deep pelvic biopsy, as these locations are more amenable to percutaneous rather than open biopsy.

Percutaneous needle biopsy has been shown to have high accuracy rates for both primary and secondary bone malignancy.[1]

Risks and Contraindications

The risks of bone needle biopsy depend upon the anatomic location, and include infection, bleeding, nerve or spinal cord damage, and pneumothorax. The principal contraindication to percutaneous needle biopsy is bleeding diathesis. The risk of bleeding relates directly to the gauge of the needle and is of particular concern with core biopsies and trephine needles, which are larger gauge needles. Contraindications to trephine biopsy are platelet count <50,000/mm^3 and abnormal coagulation studies. Aspirin or other anti-inflammatory medications should be discontinued for several days prior to biopsy. It is important to note that metastases from renal cell carcinoma are particularly prone to hemorrhage.

Planning the Biopsy

All biopsies of possibly malignant lesions should be planned in conjunction with the tumor surgeon. Curative tumor resection includes resection of the needle path and any compartments contaminated by it. A cytopathologist should be in attendance for all aspiration biopsies. Sedation with intravenous morphine and/or midazolam is useful, especially if the patient is very anxious or if the biopsy is likely to be painful. Depending on the local anatomy, a safe needle path that avoids vital structures should be chosen. The needle path can be mapped and measured on CT scans **(Fig. 1)**. Aspiration biopsy is usually performed first and the adequacy of the sample assessed by the cytopathologist. Several passes can be made. If a diagnostic aspirate is not obtained, core biopsy may be required.

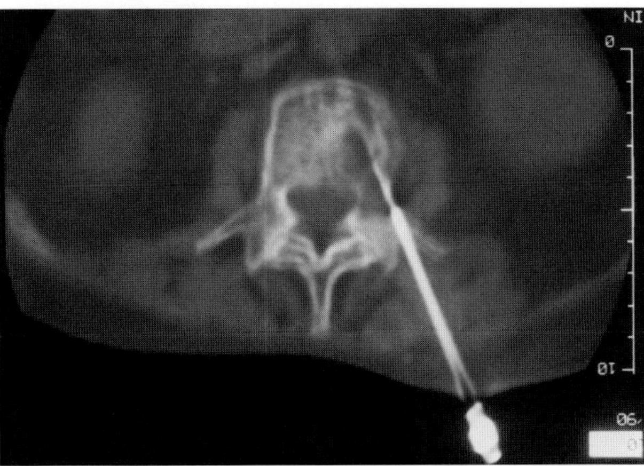

Figure 2. Coaxial biopsy of a vertebral body with use of an outer trephine and an inner 22-gauge aspiration needle.

Types of Aspiration Needles

Aspiration needles range from 18 to 25 gauge. The needle comprises an outer sheath and a central stylet. Following insertion into the lesion, the stylet is removed and cellular material aspirated through the lumen of the needle. The most commonly used and cheapest needle is a 22-gauge spinal needle or, if a longer needle is required, a 20- or 22-gauge Chiba needle. These needles are adequate for soft-tissue masses or lytic lesions with cortical destruction. If the cortex is intact, a cutting needle may be required to transgress it. A non-trephine cutting needle (such as a Franseen needle) can be used to aspirate directly or to provide a coaxial sheath for an aspiration needle. Trephine needles can also be used for coaxial aspiration biopsies **(Fig. 2)**.

Trephine Needles

Trephine needles are used to penetrate intact cortical bone and to sample sclerotic lesions. These needles are typically 12–14 gauge and have a serrated or smooth cutting edge with which to transgress cortical bone. After cortical penetration, the needle can be aspirated directly, which may yield a fragmented sample of cortical and medullary bone. The fragmentation of the specimen is a limitation of trephine specimens. The trephine needle can also be used as an outer sheath for coaxial aspiration or core biopsy. The latter involves the coaxial use of a soft-tissue core biopsy needle such as a "Tru-cut" or "biopsy-gun." This technique can be used to obtain a "soft-tissue" core of the medullary space. By angling the trephine needle, several aspiration or core specimens can be obtained.

Core Biopsy Needles

Soft-tissue core biopsy needles are extremely useful for sampling nonsclerotic bone tumors. These core needles will not penetrate bone cortex but can be used directly when the cortex is destroyed or there is a soft-tissue mass. When the cortex is intact, a coaxial technique is useful for sampling the bone medulla. This approach uses a trephine needle to breach the cortex then act as an outer sheath for the soft-tissue core needle. In this way, discrete tissue specimens are obtained, which have advantages over the fragmented specimens obtained with trephine needles alone. Commonly used soft-tissue core needles for bone biopsy are the Tru-Cut and biopsy-gun needles. Useful sizes are 14–18 gauge.

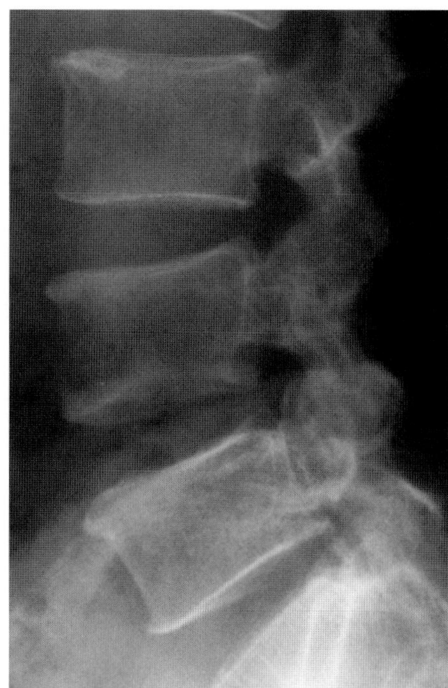

Figure 3. Lateral radiograph of the lumbar spine in an elderly man. Anterior cortical destruction of the L4 vertebral body is seen.

Vertebral Biopsy

The vertebral column is a common site for bone malignancy, particularly metastatic disease. Metastases typically seed in the pedicles and vertebral bodies. Vertebral biopsy should be planned in conjunction with the tumor surgeon. Not all vertebral lesions are suitable for percutaneous needle biopsy. Expansile cystic tumors such as aneurysmal bone cysts or giant cell tumors are poor candidates for needle biopsy. Extreme caution should attend biopsy of possible renal cell carcinoma metastases. These are prone to severe hemorrhage which could compromise the contents of the spinal canal. Vertebral biopsy can be performed with either CT or fluoroscopic guidance. CT guidance is generally preferable and engenders more confidence in needle placement within the lesion.

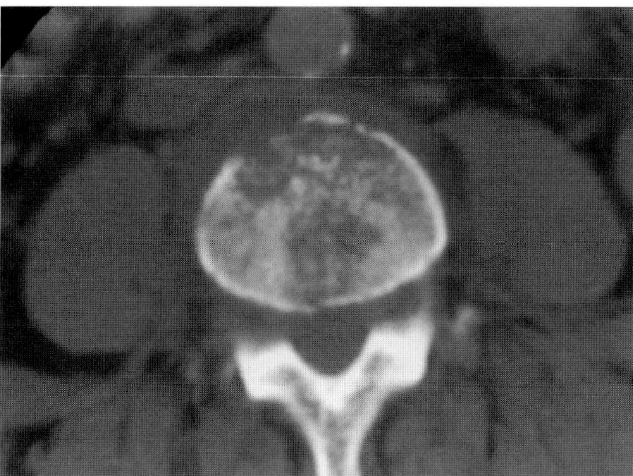

Figure 4. Same patient as in Figure 3. CT scanning confirms the anterior cortical destruction.

Lumbar Spine Biopsy

Needle biopsy is performed in the CT scanner with the patient lying prone and is done from either a posterolateral or transpedicular approach. The posterolateral approach uses a starting point 6–8 cm lateral to midline, angling the needle 45 degrees from sagittal, to enter the vertebral body directly **(Figs. 3–5)**. This approach is also used for paraspinal masses. The transpedicular technique uses a parasagittal needle path through the pedicles into the posterior vertebral body **(Figs. 6–8)**. With cautious technique this is a safe route, and can be used with either CT or fluoroscopic guidance. The transpedicular approach is also less likely to damage spinal nerve roots.

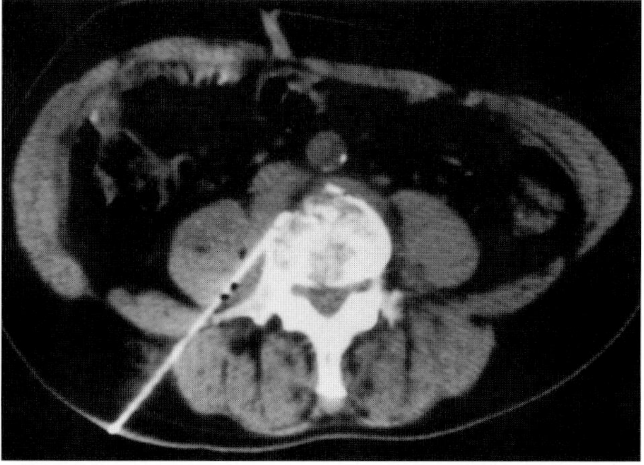

Figure 5. Fine needle aspiration biopsy with a 20-gauge Franseen needle performed from a posterolateral approach. Cytology was positive for metastatic carcinoma.

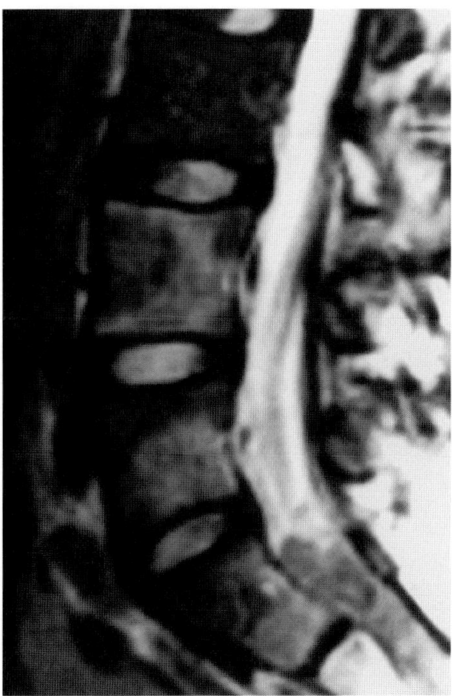

Figure 6. T2-weighted, sagittal magnetic resonance image of the lumbar spine in a 23-year-old woman with Hodgkin's disease shows abnormal signal of the vertebral bodies and a soft-tissue mass in the sacral spinal canal.

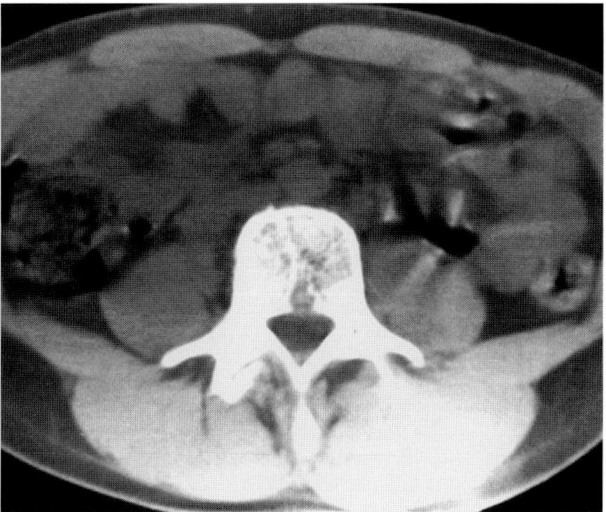

Figure 7. Same patient as in Figure 6. A 20-gauge Franseen needle was used for transpedicular fine needle aspiration of the L4 vertebra.

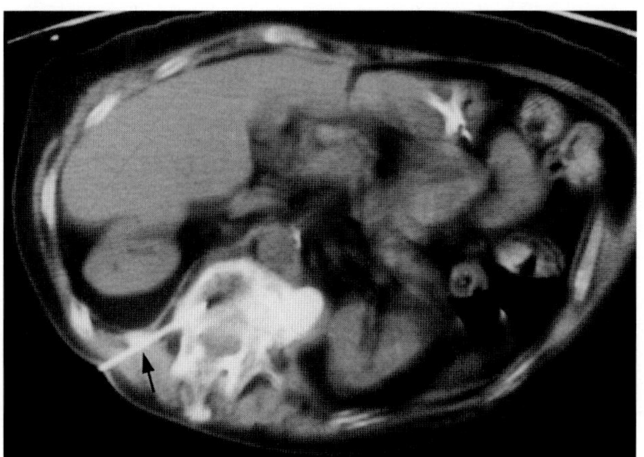

Figure 9. Aspiration biopsy of the T10 vertebral body with an 18-gauge Franseen needle (arrow) and posterolateral approach. Cytology revealed metastatic carcinoma.

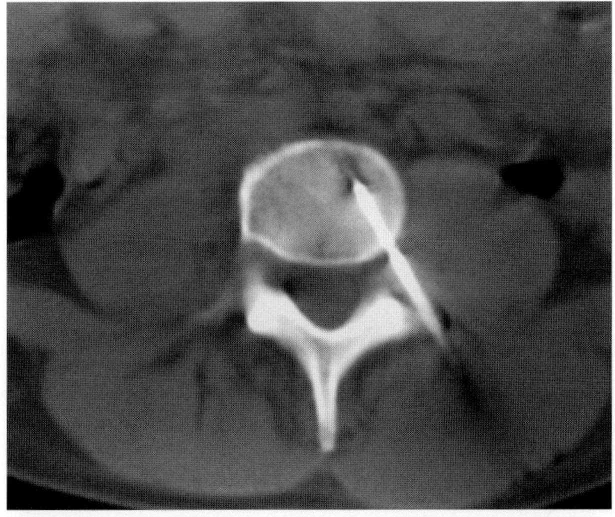

Figure 8. Same patient as in Figure 6. Cytologic sample from the fine needle aspiration was inadequate so a trephine biopsy was performed. A similar needle path was chosen but the trephine needle is seen below the pedicle, adjacent to the left L4-L5 neural foramen. This position places the left L4 nerve root at risk and could be avoided by a more sagittal approach and more frequent scans to check needle position. The histopathology confirmed Hodgkin's disease in the bones.

After the approach for vertebral biopsy has been decided on, a needle must be chosen. If the cortex is destroyed, aspiration or soft-tissue core needles can be used directly. If the cortex is intact but diffusely osteoporotic, a 20-gauge aspiration needle can usually penetrate directly to the medulla. When the cortex is intact and not osteoporotic, a bone cutting needle must be used. The cutting needle can be a non-trephine type (such as an 18-gauge Franseen needle) or a larger gauge trephine needle (such as a 12-gauge Ackerman needle). A smaller gauge needle can then be used in a coaxial manner for aspiration or core biopsy **(Fig. 9)**.

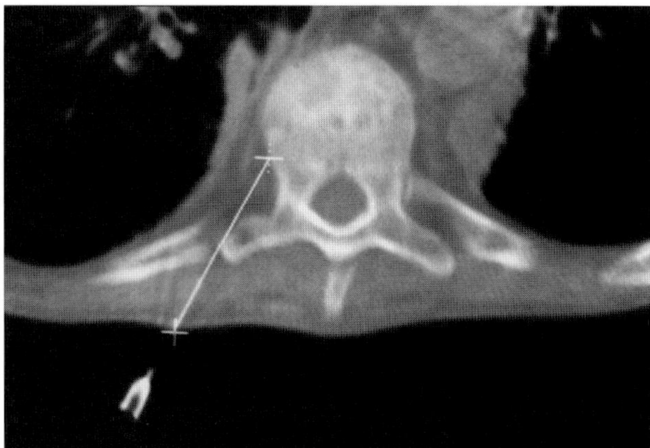

Figure 10. CT image from the mid thoracic spine. A mixed lytic and sclerotic lesion is present in the anterior vertebral body. A transcostovertebral approach for biopsy has been mapped out, between the neck of the rib and the lateral aspect of the transverse process. A 25-gauge local anesthetic needle marks the skin entry point.

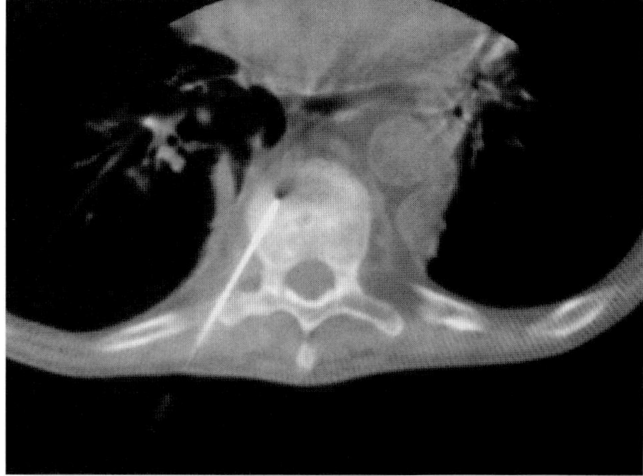

Figure 11. Same patient as in Figure 10. Transcostovertebral biopsy performed with a 20-gauge Franseen needle.

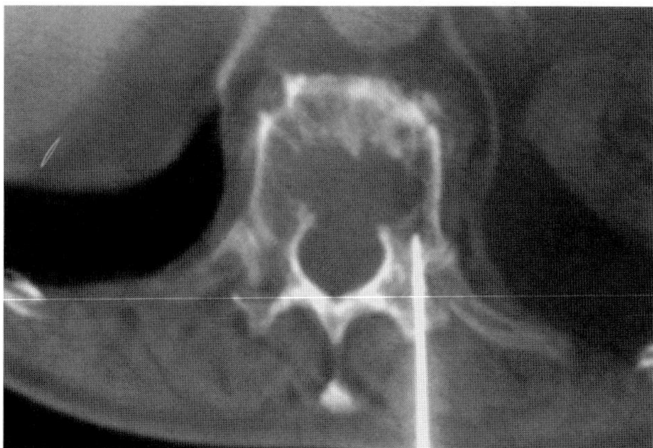

Figure 12. Transpedicular biopsy of the T11 vertebral body. The posterior cortex was breached with an 18-gauge Franseen needle.

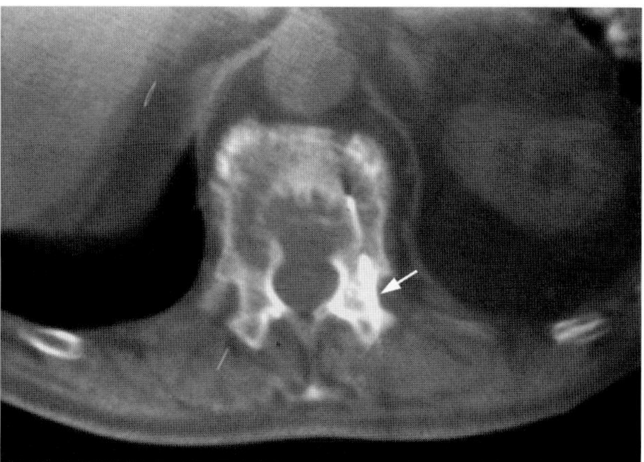

Figure 13. Same patient as in Figure 12. A 22-gauge Chiba needle was passed through this outer sheath for fine needle aspiration. Note the sagittal course of the needle (arrow).

Thoracic Spine Biopsy

Biopsy of the thoracic spine can be done from three different approaches:

1. Paraspinal biopsy of an extraosseous soft-tissue mass
2. Posterolateral (transcostovertebral) approach
3. Transpedicular approach.

A paravertebral soft-tissue mass can be aspirated with a fine needle passed between the ribs, transverse processes, and pleura. For vertebral body biopsy, either a posterolateral or transpedicular approach is used. The posterolateral approach starts more medially in the thoracic than the lumbar spine in order to avoid the pleura. The needle passes between the transverse process and the neck of the rib (transcostovertebral) and penetrates the anterior pedicle before entering the vertebral body.

The transcostovertebral approach is suitable for paraspinal and peripheral vertebral body lesions **(Figs. 10, 11)**. However, most vertebral body lesions are more readily biopsied via a transpedicular approach. This technique is particularly useful for lesions in the central vertebral body **(Figs. 12, 13)**. Of course, the proximity of the spinal canal makes meticulous technique imperative. The advantages of the transpedicular approach include: 1) lower risk of pneumothorax and spinal nerve damage compared to a paraspinal or transcostovertebral approach; 2) bleeding and tumor seeding are contained within the vertebral body; and 3) a larger volume of the vertebral body can be accessed from the transpedicular route than other approaches.

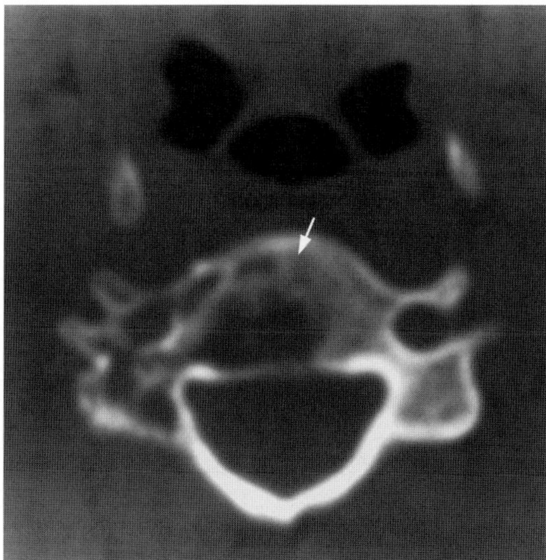

Figure 14. CT scan of the C5 vertebra. The patient is a 25-year-old man with the presenting complaint of neck pain. Lytic foci are present in the left lateral mass and the central vertebral body (arrow).

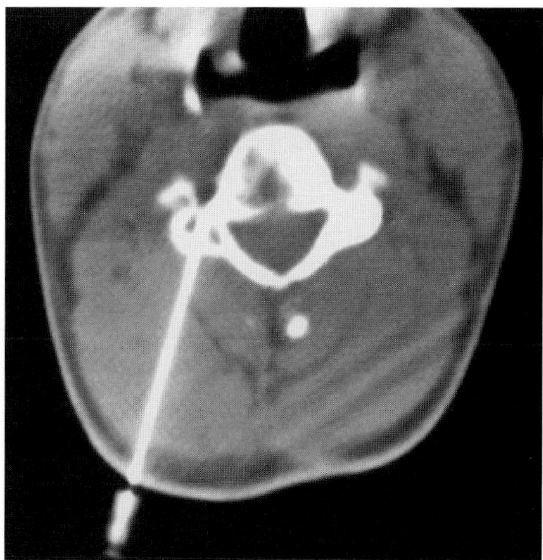

Figure 15. Same patient as in Figure 14. Biopsy of the left lateral mass of the C5 vertebra. An 18-gauge Franseen needle and posterolateral approach were used. Note the proximity of the vertebral artery. Cytology revealed a round cell tumor, consistent with Ewing's sarcoma.

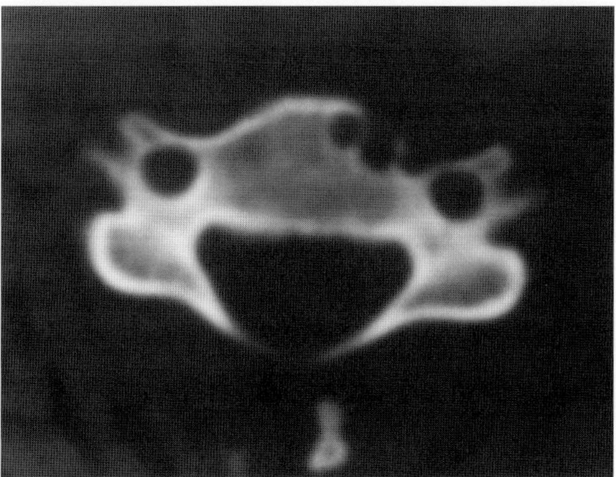

Figure 16. CT scan of the C5 vertebra. The patient is a 39-year-old woman with a presenting complaint of neck pain. Note the bubbly, lytic lesion in the anterolateral vertebral body on the left.

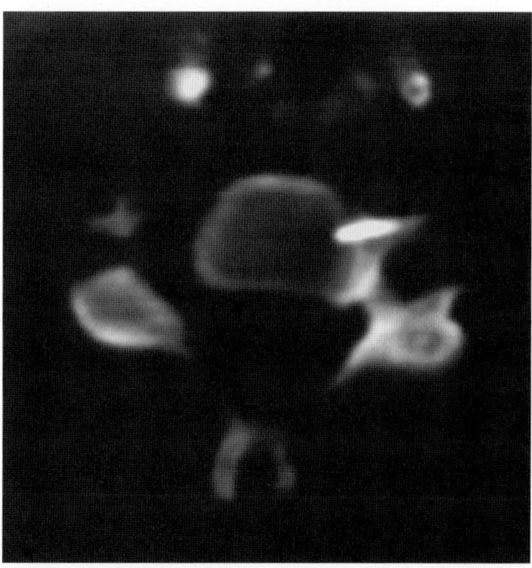

Figure 17. Same patient as in Figure 16. Needle biopsy performed with a 20-gauge Franseen needle. A small core of tissue was obtained, and chordoma was diagnosed histologically.

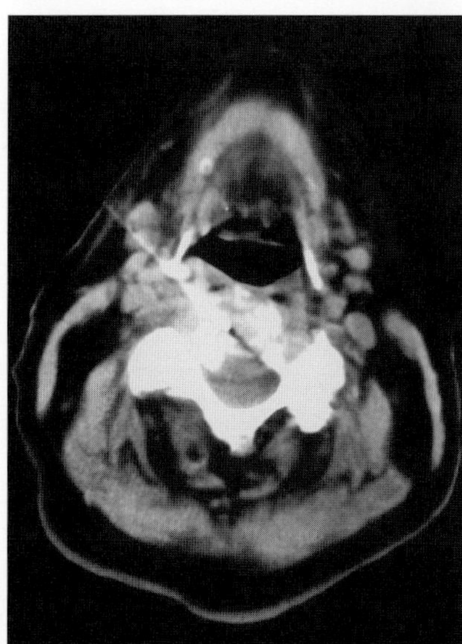

Figure 18. Fine needle aspiration biopsy of a destructive lesion of the C3 vertebral body. Note the proximity of the needle to the jugular vein, hyoid bone, and hypopharynx. Cytology revealed metastatic carcinoma. There was no known primary tumor.

Cervical Spine Biopsy

Cervical vertebral lesions are technically more difficult to biopsy than their lumbar and thoracic counterparts. The biopsy route is determined on a contrast-enhanced CT study to avoid puncturing the cervical vessels and hypopharynx. Lesions in the C4 to C7 vertebral bodies are sampled from an anterolateral approach with the patient lying supine **(Figs. 14–17)**. The needle path is typically at 45 degrees to the sagittal plane but individually tailored to avoid major structures. The C2 vertebral body is usually biopsied from a transpedicular approach (with the patient supine). Either an anterolateral or transpedicular approach can be used to biopsy the C3 vertebral body **(Fig. 18)**.

Brugieres et al reviewed a series of 12 CT-guided percutaneous cervical spine biopsies.[2] They used a coaxial trephine method with the following steps:
1. 18-gauge puncture down to bone (avoiding major structures)
2. Position confirmed by CT scanning
3. Guide wire introduced down to bone
4. Needle exchanged over the wire for a trephine needle
5. Repeat samples by angling the trephine needle
6. Coaxial fine needle aspirate in three cases.

A correct diagnosis was made in 11 of the 12 cases. Three patients had transient recurrent laryngeal nerve palsy, presumably due to local anesthetic, which resolved within 24 hours. There were no other complications.

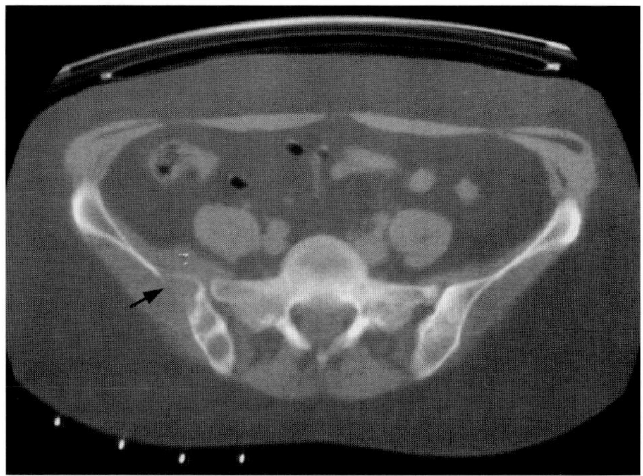

Figure 19. CT scan of the pelvis. A lytic lesion is present in the right iliac wing, with cortical destruction (arrow). Skin markers over the buttock are used to calculate the needle entry point for CT-guided bone biopsy.

Pelvis and Sacrum

Pelvic biopsies are normally performed with use of CT guidance **(Figs. 19, 20)**. The sacrum and posterior pelvis are usually approached from the posterior with the patient lying prone. It is important to avoid the sacral spinal canal and sacral foramina in order to prevent injury to the sacral nerves. The approach to lesions elsewhere in the pelvis should be tailored according to local anatomy. The same principles which guide the choice of needle apply equally to the pelvis. Purely lytic lesions and extraosseous soft-tissue masses can be biopsied with fine aspiration needles or soft-tissue core needles. If the cortex is intact, a trephine needle may be required to breach it. In this circumstance, a coaxial technique is useful if the lesion is lytic.

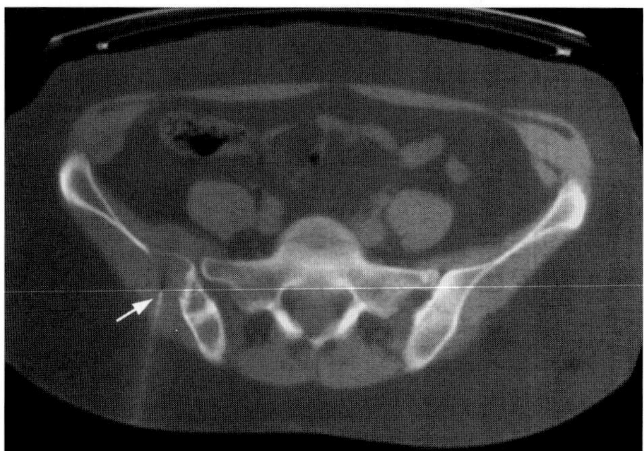

Figure 20. Fine needle aspiration of the iliac bone. Biopsy was performed with a 22-gauge spinal needle (arrow).

Appendicular Skeleton

The appendicular skeleton lends itself to both fluoroscopic and CT-guided biopsies. The former is useful when the lesion is visible on radiographs or involves the bone extensively. Major vessels and nerves should be avoided, so a knowledge of local anatomy is required. The anatomic compartment through which the needle passes must be planned in conjunction with the tumor surgeon. The skin should be marked with a permanent marker in case the surgeon needs to excise the needle track. The choice of needle is again based on principles described previously. If the cortex is intact, a trephine needle is usually necessary. If a trephine needle is used, then coaxial technique (with a fine aspiration needle or a soft-tissue core biopsy needle) is often useful.

Figures 21–25 show examples of biopsies of the appendicular skeleton.

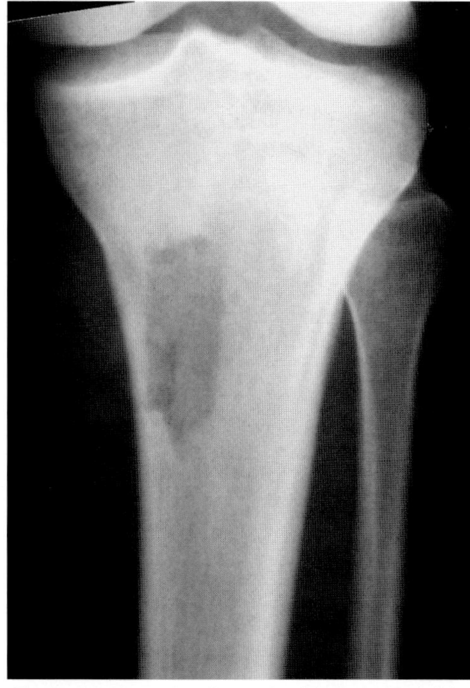

Figure 21. Frontal radiograph of the proximal tibia in a young man. There is well-circumscribed bone destruction in the proximal tibial diametaphysis.

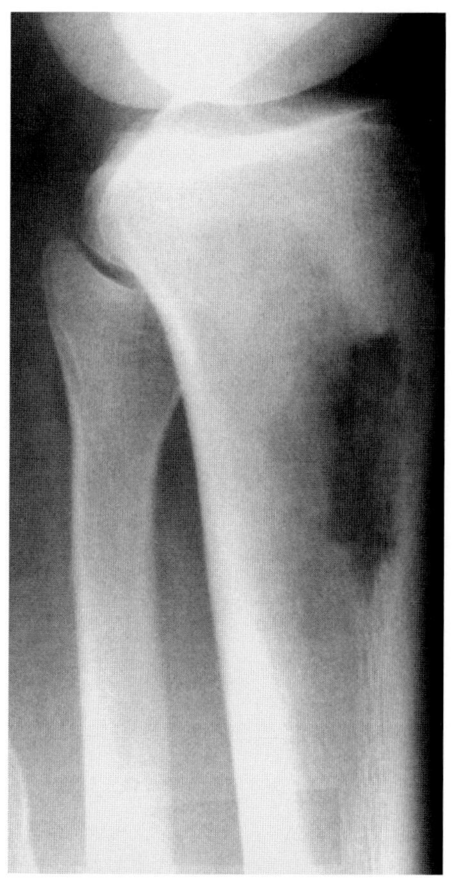

Figure 22. Same patient as in Figure 21. Lateral radiograph of the proximal tibia.

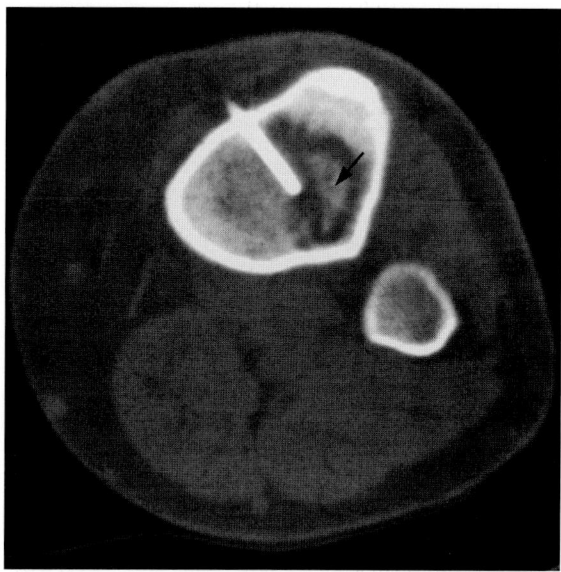

Figure 23. Trephine biopsy performed under CT guidance with use of an Ackerman needle. Pus was aspirated and the culture grew Staphylococcus aureus. Note the sequestrum—a classic finding in osteomyelitis (arrow).

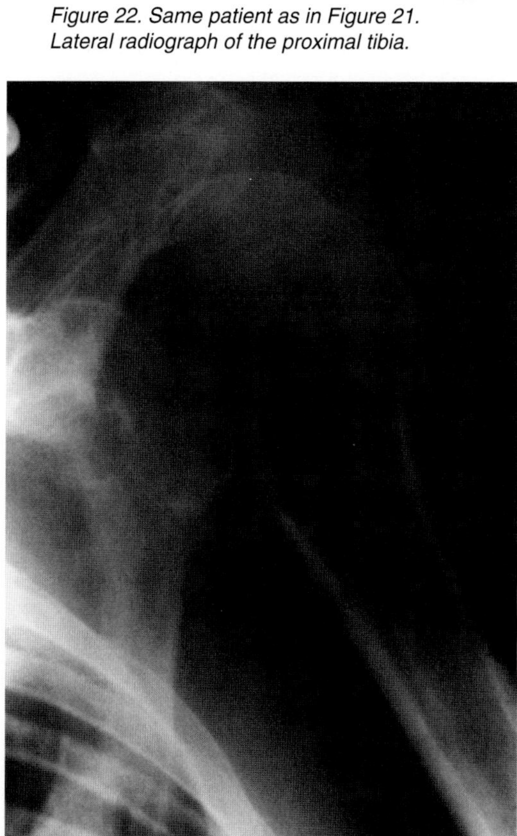

Figure 24. Radiograph of the left shoulder in a 70-year-old man with known carcinoma of the prostate. A lytic lesion with a pathologic fracture of the humerus is present.

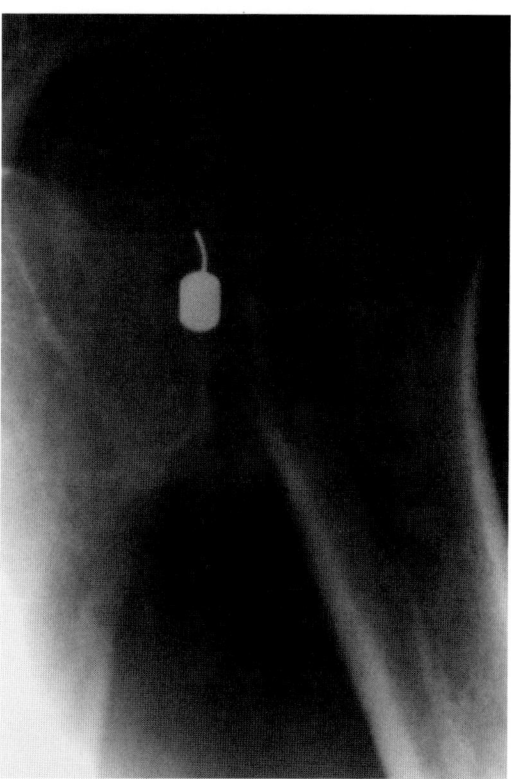

Figure 25. Fine needle biopsy with a 22-gauge spinal needle. Cytology showed the lesion to be a metastasis from a second primary tumor arising in the lung.

References

1. Stoker DJ, Kissin MK. Percutaneous vertebral biopsy: a review of 135 cases. Clin Radiol 1985; 569–577.

2. Brugieres P, Gaston A, Voison MC, Ricolfi F, Chakir N. CT-guided percutaneous biopsy of the cervical spine: a series of 12 cases. Neuroradiology 1992; 34:358–360.

TUTORIAL 27 MUSCULOSKELETAL SPINAL INTERVENTION

William Clark, M.D., and Georges Y. El-Khoury, M.D.

Introduction

The subjects addressed in this tutorial include:

1. Epidural steroid injection
2. Facet injection
3. Lumbar and sacral nerve block
4. Diskography
5. Sacroiliac joint injection.

Epidural Injections

Injection of corticosteroids and saline relieves pain in many patients with low back pain or sciatica. The steroid is thought to exert its anti-inflammatory effect upon inflamed nerve roots as they transgress the epidural space. The technique is particularly efficacious in patients who have acute inflammation of the spinal nerve due to disk disease. Studies have shown that radiographic guidance increases the likelihood of depositing the steroid into the correct compartment—the sacral epidural space.[1] The procedure is therefore best performed by radiologists using fluoroscopic guidance. In cases of acute agonizing pain, a local anesthetic agent such as bupivacaine can be added to the injection mixture.

Spinal Epidural Anatomy

The spinal epidural space extends from the foramen magnum to the sacral hiatus. It separates the dura mater of the thecal sac from the periosteum of the spinal canal. It contains fat, loose areolar tissue, and an epidural venous plexus, and gives transit to the exiting spinal nerve roots covered by their respective dural sheaths. The inferior margin of the thecal sac is usually located at or above the inferior margin of the S2 vertebral body. To avoid intrathecal injection, the ideal location for the needle tip is at the inferior margin of S3.

The Sacral Hiatus
The sacral hiatus which is used to enter the sacral epidural space is a defect in the dorsal cortex of the sacrum and is located at the S5 level. On surface anatomy, this corresponds to the superior margin of the natal cleft. It is bordered on either side by the sacral cornua and superiorly by the inferior margin of the median sacral crest. It is the sacral cornua on either side and the median sacral crest above that are easier to palpate than the bony defect itself. The sacral hiatus provides a window for entry into the sacral epidural space.

Plica Mediana Dorsalis
The plica mediana dorsalis is an incomplete septum separating the right and left sides of the epidural space **(Fig. 1)**. It is rarely intact, but if so, will act as a midline mechanical barrier between the two sides. In this rare circumstance each side may require separate injections, depending upon the localization of the symptoms.

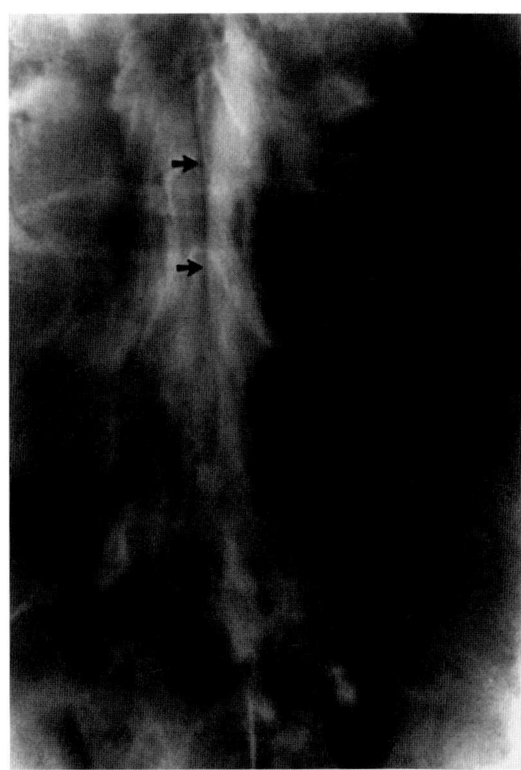

Figure 1. Frontal projection of a lumbosacral epidurogram. Note the incomplete plica mediana dorsalis (arrows).

Indications for Epidural Injection
Tumor and infection should always be excluded as causes for low back pain before epidural injection is contemplated. With these entities excluded, most patients with low back pain or sciatica respond favorably to epidural steroid injection. The majority of patients have either a disk protrusion or spinal canal stenosis. Patients with disk protrusion have a better response rate because their nerve roots are more likely to be inflamed. However, it is difficult to predict which patients will respond well on the basis of radiographic findings. After all, the radiographic abnormality may not correspond to the patient's clinical presentation. Any patient with significant chronic low back pain or sciatica is a potential candidate for epidural steroid injection.

Risks of Epidural Injection
The major risks associated with epidural steroid injection are infection, arachnoiditis, and bleeding.

Infection—epidural abscess or osteomyelitis—is the main risk, and scrupulous sterile technique is required to prevent this. The risk of arachnoiditis arises if corticosteroids are injected into the thecal sac; this complication can be prevented by correct needle position. The risk of bleeding from the epidural venous plexus is minimal unless the patient has a bleeding diathesis. Overall, the risk of a correctly performed epidural steroid injection is very small. There are the additional risks of postural hypotension and lower limb numbness if epidural local anesthetic is used.

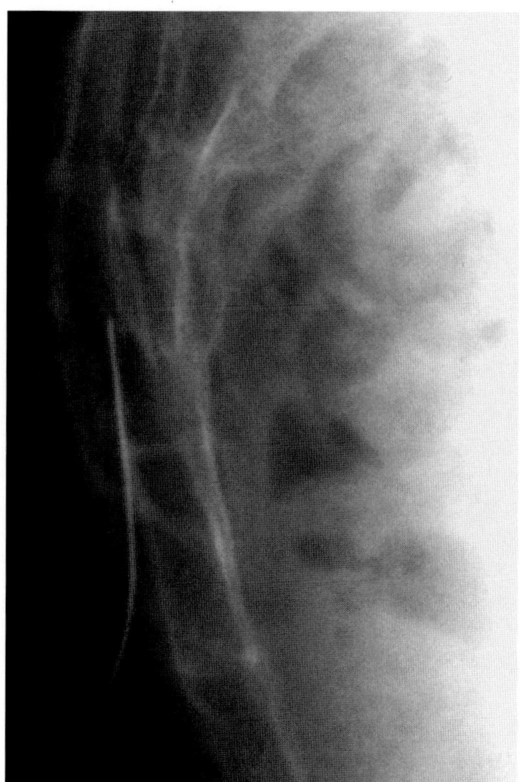

Figure 2. True lateral projection of the sacrum with a 22-gauge spinal needle in the sacral spinal canal. The needle tip is at the inferior margin of S3.

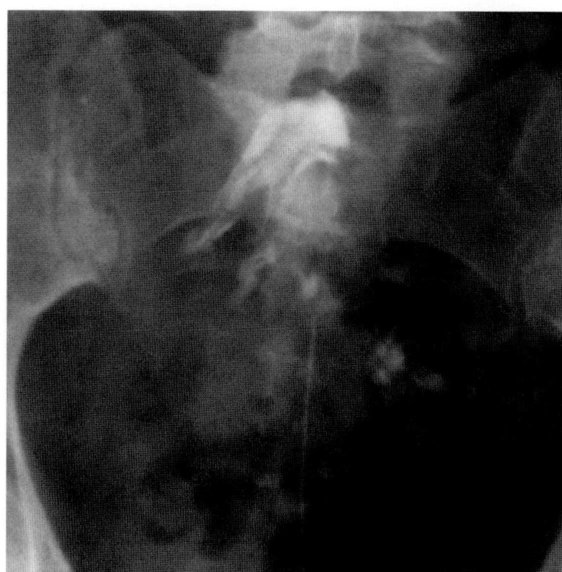

Figure 3. Epidurogram shows contrast outlining the sacral nerve roots. Note the midline position of the needle (arrow), which must be between the sacral foramina in the frontal projection.

Contraindications

Contraindications to sacral epidural steroid injection include tumor or infection as the cause of pain, pilonidal sinus, infected skin over the sacral hiatus, and bleeding disorders. Contrast material allergy is not a contraindication because epidural injection can be performed without the use of contrast material to confirm position.

Technique

If magnetic resonance (MR) or myelogram images are available, they should be examined for the inferior level of the thecal sac, for sacral Tarlov cysts, and for sacral bony anomalies. Informed consent should be obtained. With the patient lying prone on the fluoroscopy table, the sacral hiatus is palpated and marked with a skin marker. Gauze swabs can be placed between the cheeks of the buttocks to prevent irritating antiseptic solution from reaching the perineum. Povidone-iodine and then alcohol solutions are used to sterilize the skin prior to draping with an aperture drape. The skin and subcutaneous tissues down to the periosteum are anesthetized with 1% lidocaine. With use of sterile technique, a 22-gauge spinal needle is introduced into the sacral hiatus at an angle of approximately 45 degrees to the horizontal. After the sacral hiatus is penetrated, the needle is maneuvered into a more horizontal position and pushed into the sacral spinal canal.

The needle is rotated as it is advanced into the sacral spinal canal to prevent the bevel from entering the bone of the sacrum. Both frontal and lateral projections should be used to check the position of the needle. It is crucial to obtain a true lateral projection when checking needle position **(Fig. 2)**. At this point, the patient should be asked to cough and the needle hub checked for cerebrospinal fluid. An injection of 2–4 mL of nonionic contrast material confirms the epidural position. Look for the typical "Christmas tree" pattern of epidural contrast which may outline sacral nerve roots **(Fig. 3)**. Once correct needle position has been confirmed, the epidural space is injected with 3 mL (18 mg) betamethasone followed by 3 to 6 mL normal saline. The saline acts in a mechanical fashion to propel the steroid superiorly into the lower lumbar spine where the critical pathology is usually located. In the setting of acutely distressing pain, bupivacaine can be added to the saline (one part 0.25% bupivacaine to three parts normal saline). However, the addition of bupivacaine is rarely necessary.

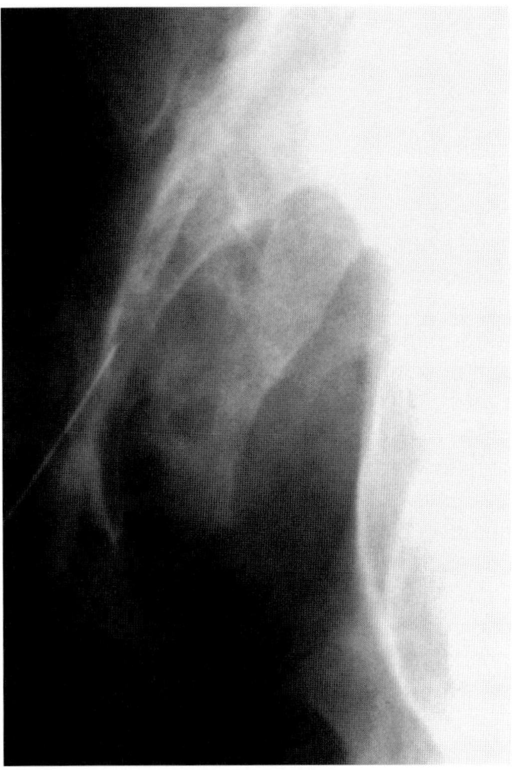

Figure 4. Spinal needle incorrectly positioned in the posterior paraspinal muscles. The lateral projection is somewhat oblique, which does not permit accurate assessment of needle position.

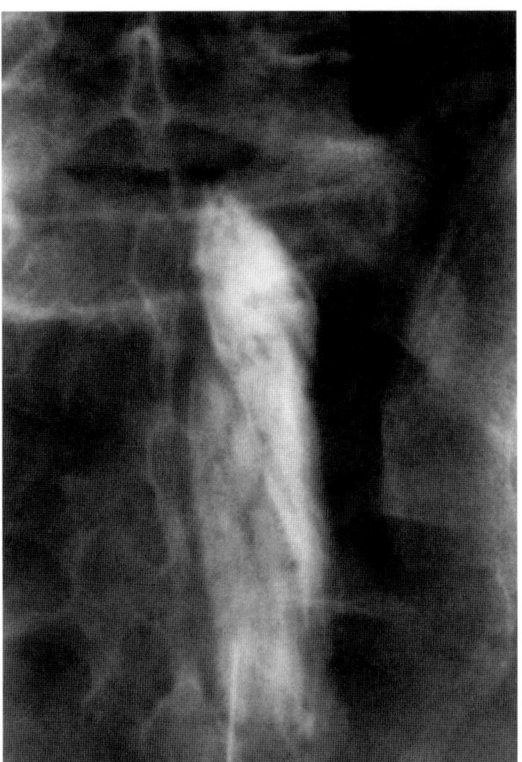

Figure 5. Same patient as in Figure 4. Spinal needle incorrectly positioned in the posterior paraspinal muscles. In this case, contrast material forms a featureless clump, with none of the characteristics of an epidurogram.

The most common incorrect needle location is in the paraspinal muscles posterior to the sacrum **(Figs. 4–7)**. As stated earlier, to avoid this complication it is crucial to obtain a true lateral projection to evaluate needle position prior to injection of contrast material. The needle may also penetrate osteoporotic bone with minimal resistance. If embedded in bone, it produces pain and resistance on injection. The needle can penetrate the anterior cortex and enter the rectum, in which case it must be discarded and fresh sterile technique used. Incorrect needle tip position within the sacral spinal canal includes sacral nerve root sheath (only a single nerve sheath fills), epidural vein, sacral Tarlov cyst, and thecal sac. In the former two cases, the needle tip should be repositioned until an adequate contrast epidurogram is obtained **(Fig. 8)**. In the latter two situations (Tarlov cyst or thecal sac), the procedure should be terminated and rescheduled for several days later **(Fig. 9)**. Inspection of MR or myelographic images (when available) is useful to avoid this complication.

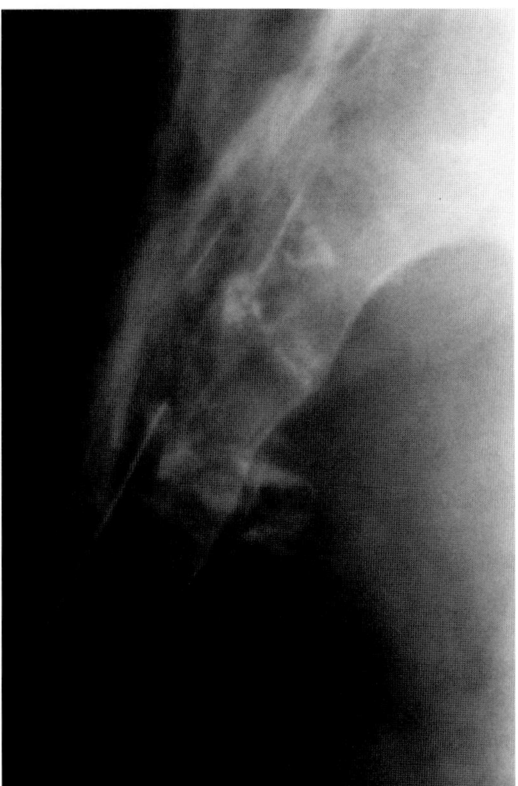

Figure 6. Same patient as in Figure 4. After needle repositioning, the lateral projection now confirms an epidural position.

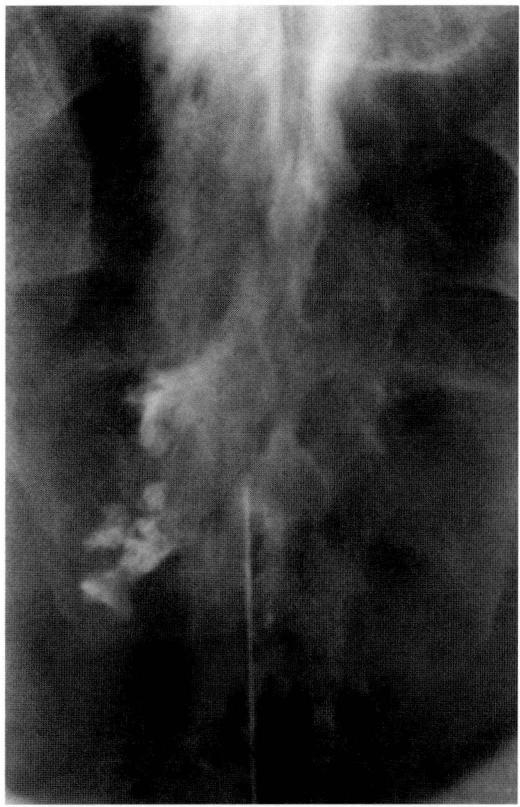

Figure 7. Same patient as in Figure 4. After needle repositioning, the epidurogram is now satisfactory.

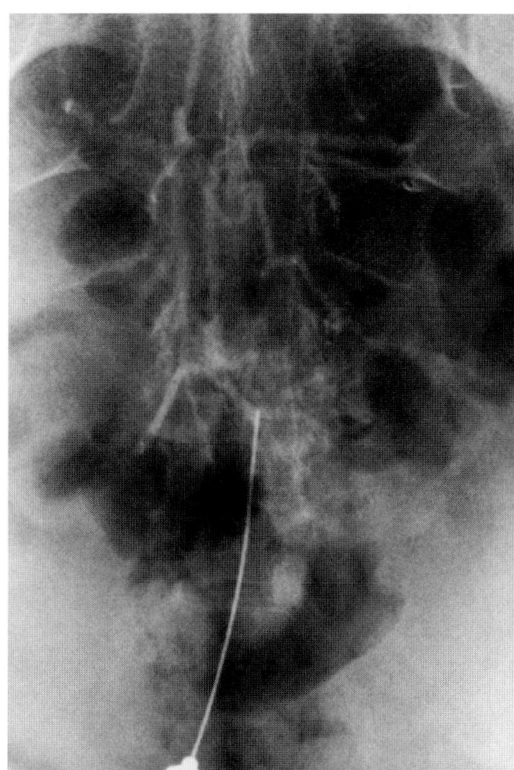

Figure 8. Epidural venogram shows contrast material filling the sacral epidural venous plexus. Frontal and lateral fluoroscopy confirmed the needle position within the sacral spinal canal. The needle was advanced 5 mm, and an adequate epidurogram was obtained prior to injection of betamethasone and saline.

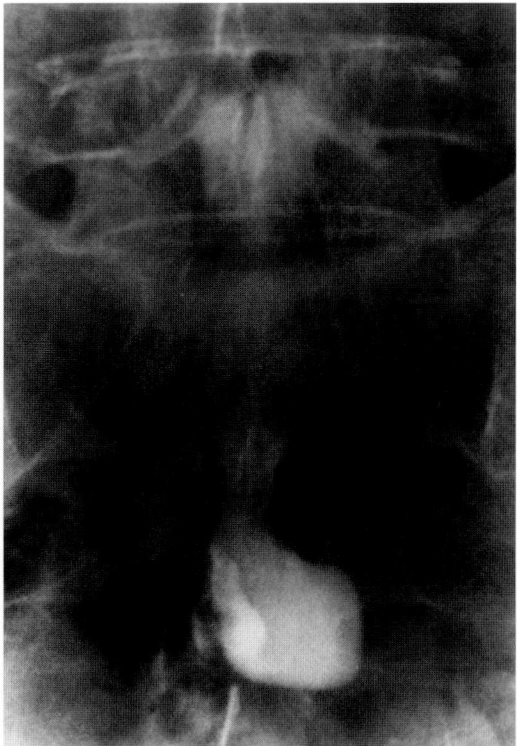

Figure 9. Contrast material fills a sacral Tarlov cyst. Contrast material is also present in the thecal sac. The tip of the needle is at the S3 level.

Postprocedure Advice

The patient should be advised not to expect any improvement for at least 48 hours. Pain relief after this time may last for weeks, months, or occasionally, years. Unless epidural bupivacaine has been given, the patient can be discharged directly. Routine monitoring of blood pressure and pulse rate should be recorded prior to discharge to exclude vasovagal episodes. Follow-up instructions should include a description of the symptoms of infection, as this is the most common significant complication. If epidural bupivacaine has been administered, observation for at least 1 hour is necessary, with blood pressure and pulse rate recorded every 15 minutes during this time. The patient can be discharged after 1 hour if these readings remain stable.

Facet Injection

The contribution of the zygapophyseal joint to low back pain is often unclear. The term "facet syndrome" was coined to describe pain thought to originate in these joints. This was really a diagnosis of exclusion, when no other cause of pain could be identified. In fact, the only way to establish the diagnosis is to inject local anesthetic into the facet joint and observe for symptomatic relief. For patients with nonspecific low back pain, facet injections are a good diagnostic method, allowing exclusion of the lumbar facet syndrome. More prolonged pain relief in patients with proven facet pain can be effected by injecting a corticosteroid and a longer acting local anesthetic. Facet injections are largely confined to the lumbar spine, but are occasionally done in the cervical and thoracic spine.

Patient Selection

Patient selection for facet injection is problematic because no clear clinical distinction is made between diskogenic and zygapophyseal pain. Schwartzer et al prospectively studied 176 patients with low back pain who were treated with facet injection of a local anesthetic.[2] They concluded that no specific clinical features were predictive of a good response to facet injection, and they questioned the existence of a clinically definable "facet syndrome." If this is the case, then any patient with chronic, unexplained, unrelieved low back pain and osteoarthritic facet joints is a potential candidate for facet injection. Facet injection may also be an option in patients who derive no relief from epidural corticosteroid injection.

Mechanism of Action

The mode of action of facet joint injections is controversial. If the facet joint itself is indeed the cause of pain, then the intra-articular effect of local anesthetic and corticosteroid on an inflamed and painful synovium may bring about pain relief. However, there is usually periarticular seepage of the active components which may act upon the dorsal ramus of the nerve root or enter the neural foramen or spinal epidural space. One school of thought believes that a periarticular injection is as likely to mediate pain relief as an intra-articular facet injection. In any case, the facet injection is not likely to provide analgesia unless the facet joint demonstrates some abnormality on radiographic images.

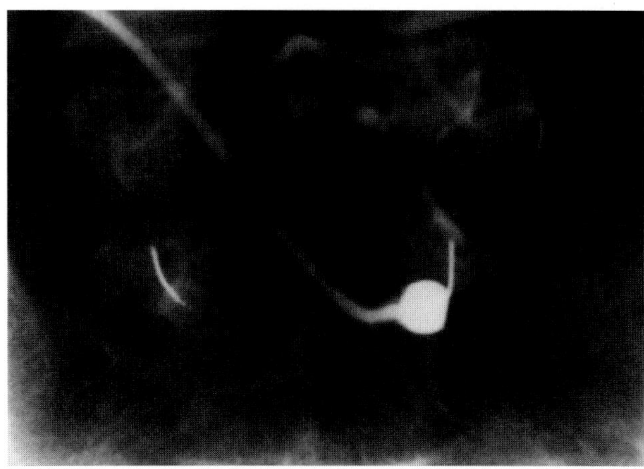

Figure 10. Bilateral L5-S1 facet injections into the inferior recesses. An intra-articular position has been confirmed with contrast on the right. Note that the joint line is not visualized in the frontal projection. The inferior recess is located at the inferior margin of the inferior facet of L5.

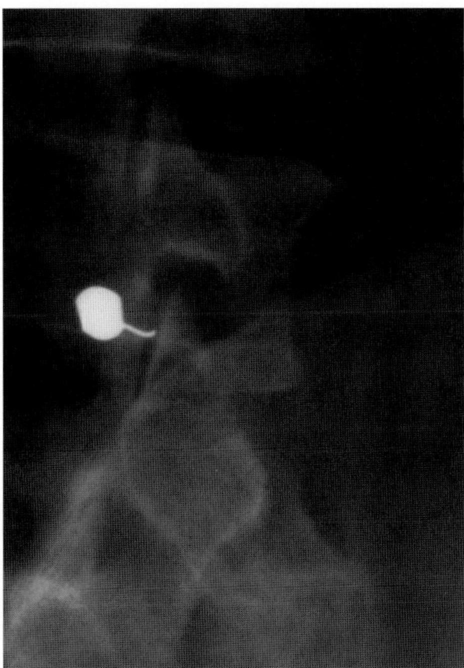

Figure 11. Puncture straight down the line of the joint in an oblique projection. The needle has passed directly into the joint space.

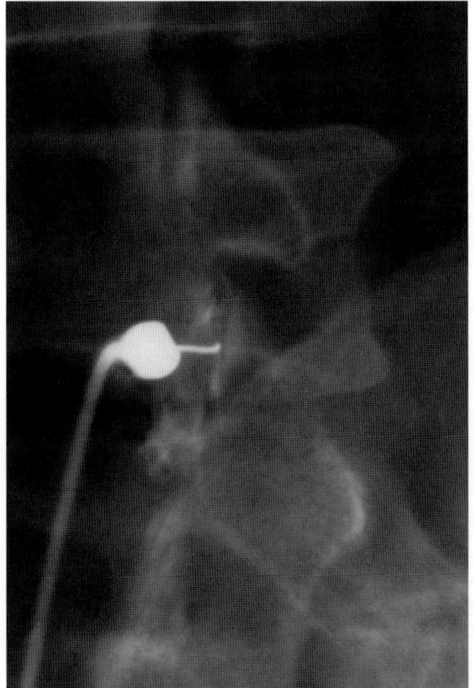

Figure 12. Same patient as in Figure 11. On the right L5-S1 arthrogram, intra-articular position is confirmed with contrast. Note the contrast material filling the inferior recess.

Indications for Facet Injection

The indications for facet injection include 1) chronic low back pain of possible zygapophyseal joint origin; 2) chronic pain with previous favorable response to facet injection; 3) pars interarticularis defects; and 4) aspiration of synovial cysts. Defects in the pars interarticularis usually communicate with adjacent ipsilateral facet joints. Injection of the facet joints is technically the simplest means of injecting the pars defect for the purpose of diagnosis (ie, to determine how much pain it contributes) or therapy. Injections of pars defects are most easily accomplished by injecting the closest facet joint. Needle aspiration of the facet joint has also been used to decompress synovial cysts in the spinal canal.

Technique

When viewed in the axial plane, the lumbar facet joints are curved structures. The posterior lip of the facet joint is sagittal in the upper lumbar spine and oriented in a posterolateral plane in the lower lumbar spine and lumbosacral junction. Each facet joint has inferior and superior expansions, called the inferior and superior recesses, respectively. The inferior recess is the more capacious.

To perform facet injection, the patient is first laid prone on a fluoroscopy table. With use of fluoroscopy the position of puncture is marked with a skin marker. Following instillation of local anesthetic, a 22-gauge spinal needle is introduced with use of sterile technique. The two common approaches to facet injection are 1) puncture the presumed position of the inferior recess (posteroanterior [PA] projection); or 2) puncture directly down the line of the joint (oblique projection).

The inferior recess lies adjacent to the inferomedial corner of the inferior facet. Even if the joint line is not visualized, a puncture in this position has a good chance of entering the joint space **(Fig. 10)**. The needle is introduced directly from a PA approach with the patient prone. If the joint space is not visualized in this position, the patient can be rolled ipsilateral side up after the needle has been inserted. The position of the needle tip with respect to the joint line can thus be determined. The needle tip should be at the inferior margin of the joint in this projection. If it is not, the needle should be repositioned. This approach is particularly useful at the L4-L5 and L5-S1 levels.

The alternative is to aim directly down the line of the joint. In the upper lumbar spine, this can be accomplished with direct PA puncture. However at L4-L5 and L5-S1 levels (the most common sites for injection), fluoroscopy in an oblique sagittal plane is usually required; this makes the puncture more difficult technically. This is less problematic if the table has a C-arm. Because the facet joint is an obliquely curving structure, the minimal obliquity in which the joint space is seen is usually that which runs tangent to the posterior lip **(Figs. 11, 12)**. Marginal osteophytes are another barrier to success with this approach. In any case, intra-articular positioning is confirmed with injection of 0.5 mL contrast material; then 0.5 mL (3 mg) betamethasone and 1.5 mL 0.25% bupivacaine are injected. However, this can rupture the joint, which has a capacity of 1–1.5 mL. If osteophytosis precludes an intra-articular position, a para-articular position for injection is acceptable.

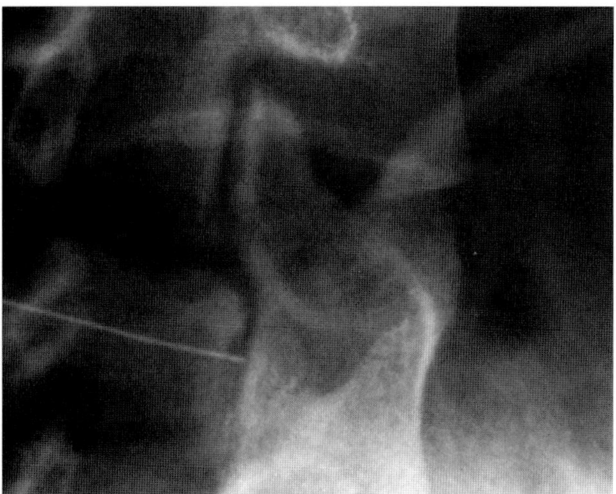

Figure 13. Oblique projection of the right L5-S1 facet shows a defect in the pars interarticularis. A 22-gauge spinal needle has been passed from a posteromedial approach with its tip in the line of the joint.

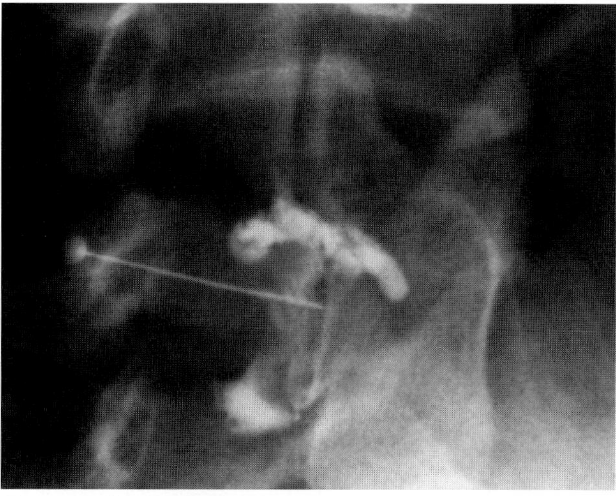

Figure 14. Same patient as in Figure 13. Injection of contrast material demonstrates communication of the facet joint with the pars defect. Contrast material is filling the inferior recess.

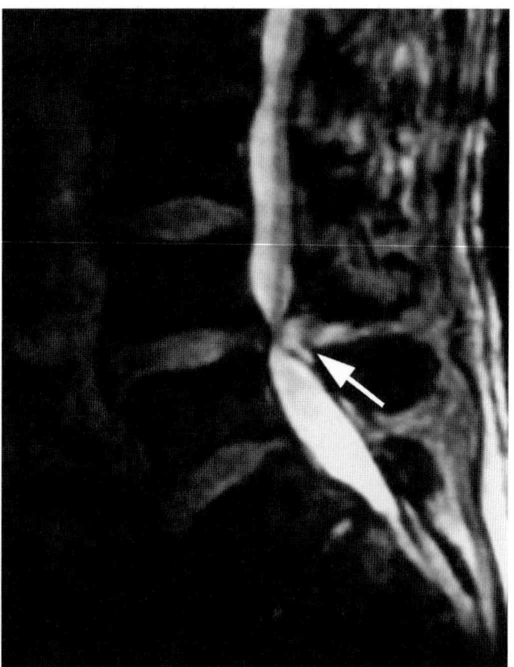

Figure 15. Sagittal, T2-weighted MR image of the lumbar spine in an elderly patient with clinical spinal canal stenosis. A posterior mass lesion (arrow) is present in the spinal canal at the L4-L5 level. The lesion has high signal and is adjacent to the facet joint.

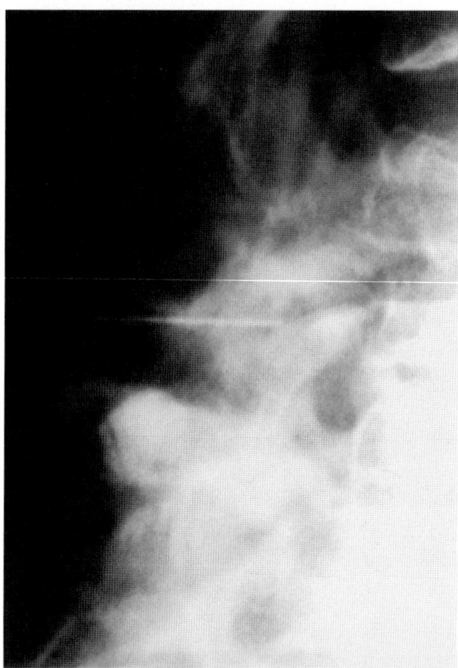

Figure 16. Same patient as in Figure 15. Facet needle placement, L4-L5. This synovial cyst was aspirated with a 20-gauge spinal needle. The patient derived symptomatic relief.

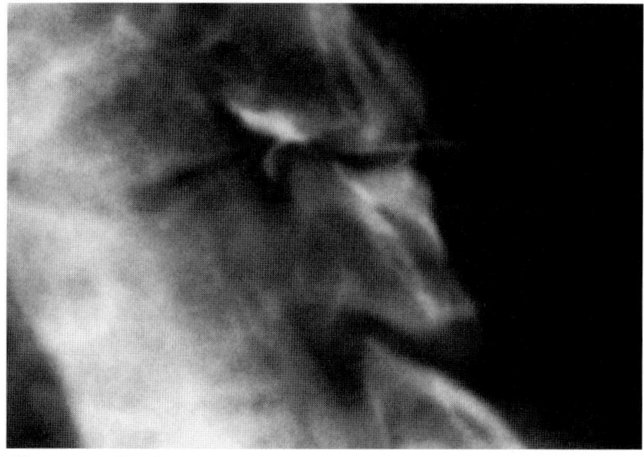

Figure 17. C3-C4 facet injection in a 42-year-old woman with persistent neck pain.

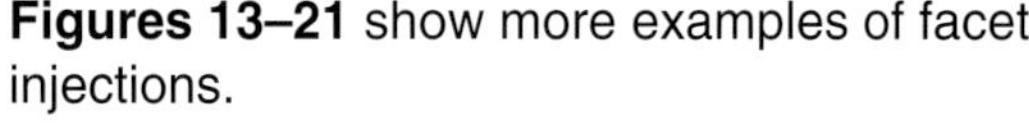

Figures 13–21 show more examples of facet injections.

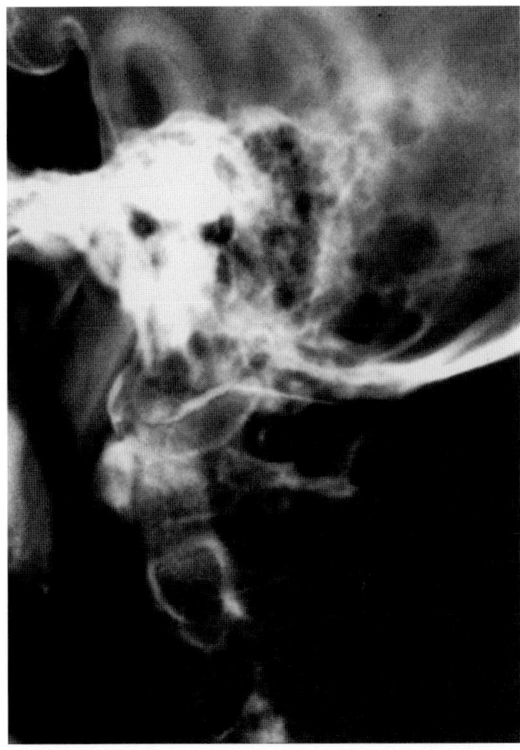

Figure 18. Lateral projection of an atlanto-occipital joint injection in a 56-year-old with post-traumatic neck pain and torticollis.

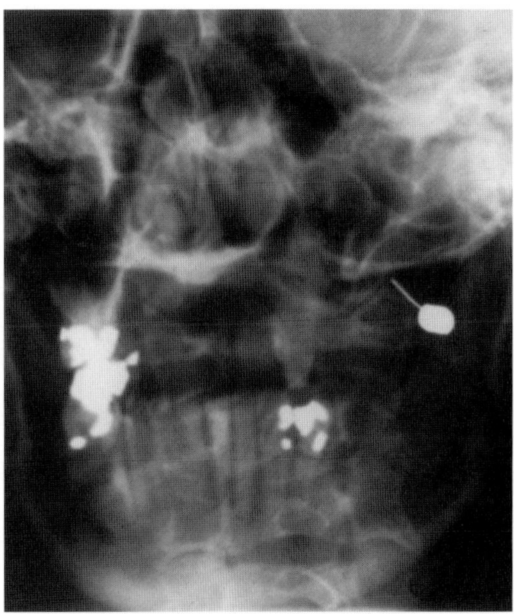

Figure 19. Same patient as in Figure 19. Frontal projection of an atlanto-occipital joint injection.

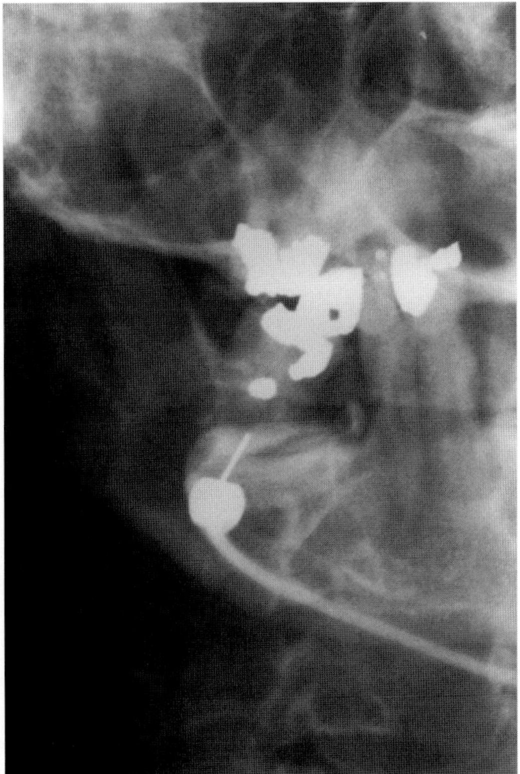

Figure 20. Frontal projection of a C1-C2 facet injection. Note the sagittal approach of the needle.

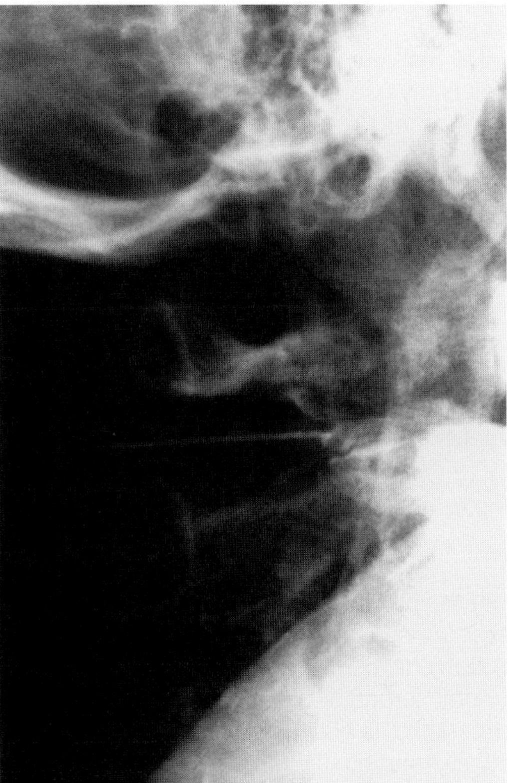

Figure 21. Lateral projection of a C1-C2 facet injection. Note the sagittal approach of the needle.

Lumbar Nerve Blocks

Anatomy

The lumbar nerve roots arise just above the conus medullaris, which is normally located between T12 and L2. The nerve roots descend in the thecal sac before passing inferolaterally into the dural nerve root sleeves to exit the spinal canal under the pedicle. Under the pedicle, the dorsal root gives rise to the dorsal root ganglion and then combines with the ventral root to form the spinal nerve. The nerve root sleeve fuses with the spinal nerve to become its perineurium. The spinal nerve is 1–7-mm long before it divides into the dorsal and ventral rami. The dorsal ramus is directed posteriorly to supply paraspinal muscles. The ventral ramus passes anteriorly, laterally, and inferiorly at the side of the vertebral body and disk. Most injections of the "spinal nerve" adjacent to the intervertebral foramen are really injections of the ventral ramus.

Indications

Indications for lumbar nerve block may be either diagnostic or therapeutic. Diagnostic block with 1% lidocaine can determine the spinal nerve level which is causing sciatica. This may be useful in the setting of surgical planning when imaging findings and symptoms are contradictory; in multilevel pathology, to define the symptomatic level; and for recurrent postoperative pain. Therapeutic lumbar nerve blocks using bupivacaine and corticosteroid may relieve sciatica when surgery is not contemplated and epidural corticosteroid injection gives no relief. This is particularly useful for lateral disk protrusions.

Technique

Analgesia and sedation may be needed if the patient has acute, severe pain. The level chosen for injection depends on imaging studies or the patient's clinical symptoms. The patient lies prone on a fluoroscopy table with biplanar C-arm capability. The C-arm is rotated in two planes until superior and inferior end-plates are seen end-on and the superior facet projects halfway between the sides of the vertebral body. In this projection the pedicle should appear as an oval. Following antiseptic skin washing and instillation of a local anesthetic, a 20-gauge spinal or Chiba needle is introduced in the axis of fluoroscopy, aiming for a point 3 mm inferior to the pedicle.

When the needle tip encounters the spinal nerve (or ventral ramus) the patient will experience pain. The patient should be asked if the sensation is a reproduction of the typical sciatic pain. Nonionic contrast material (1–2 mL) is injected and the perineural spread of contrast material, which should outline the ventral ramus, is observed. If the patient cries out when the injection is started, the needle should be withdrawn 1–2 mm; it was probably within the substance of the nerve. For diagnostic purposes, 2 mL of 1% lidocaine can be injected. For therapeutic purposes, a combination of 1.5 mL 0.25% bupivacaine and 1–1.5 mL betamethasone may be used. After the procedure, the patient should be asked to quantify the degree of symptomatic relief on a scoring or percentage basis.

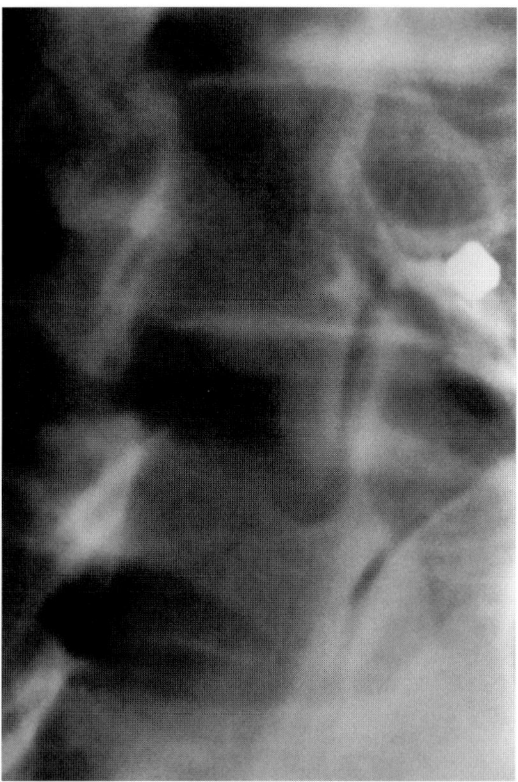

Figure 22. Right L4 nerve sheath injection. The fluoroscope has been obliquely oriented tangent to the vertebral end-plates in order to project the superior facet midway between the two sides of the vertebral body. A 22-gauge needle has been aimed for a point 3 mm inferior to the pedicle. Note the contrast material adopting the tubular shape of the nerve sheath.

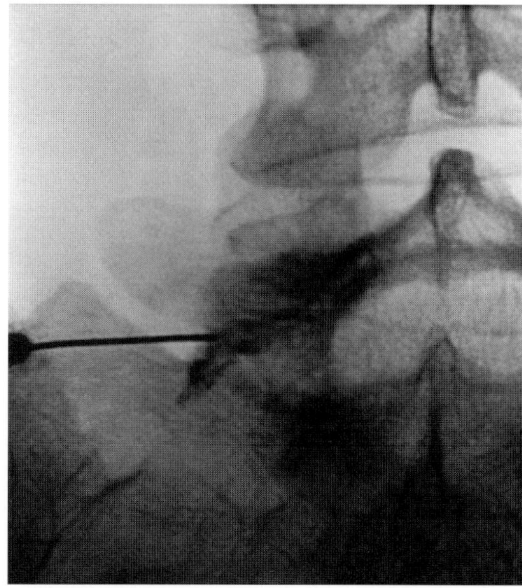

Figure 23. Frontal projection of a left L5 nerve sheath injection. Note the tubular pattern of contrast as it outlines the ventral ramus of the spinal nerve. This is the ideal contrast pattern to confirm needle position in the nerve sheath.

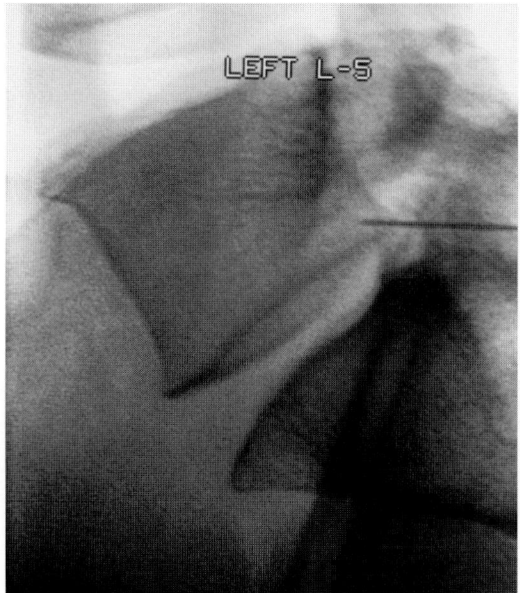

Figure 24. Same patient as in Figure 23. Lateral projection of the needle position.

Examples of lumbar nerve block injections are shown in **Figures 22–24**.

Sacral Nerve Block

Injection of the S1 nerve root requires a different technique. The C-arm should be angled cephalad until the dorsal and ventral sacral foramina overlap. A 22-gauge spinal needle is then introduced into the first dorsal sacral foramen. Once the needle is within the foramen, the C-arm is rotated laterally. The needle tip is passed through the ventral foramen, 1 to 3 mm beyond the anterior cortex of the sacrum. This is in the vicinity of the S1 ventral ramus, although the nerve may run away from the needle as there is no structure to pin it against (as in the case of lumbar nerve roots). After the needle has been passed, contrast material is injected under frontal fluoroscopy, and the typical perineural spread with a central filling defect is observed **(Fig. 25)**. Once a perineural position has been confirmed, local anesthetic is injected, with or without corticosteroid depending on the indication.

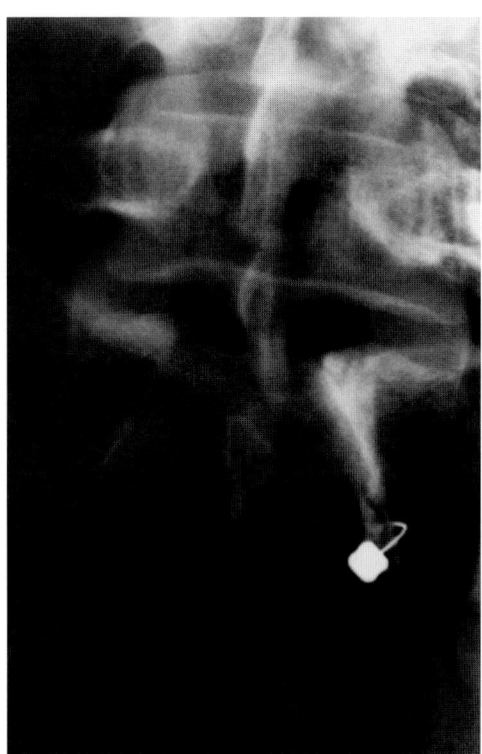

Figure 25. Right S1 nerve sheath injection. The needle was passed through the right first posterior then anterior sacral foramina. Contrast material has been injected with fluoroscopy in the frontal projection. Note the contrast outlining the right S1 nerve as far proximally as the epidural space.

Diskography

Diskography is a diagnostic test that aims to assess intervertebral disks as a cause of chronic low back pain. The procedure is usually performed in a preoperative setting to determine the possible efficacy of spinal fusion at this level. Contrast material is injected into an intervertebral disk in order to reproduce diskogenic pain. It has been suggested that, in some patients, low back pain radiating to the lower extremities may arise from within the disk itself. In these cases, the radiating lower limb pain may be referred from the disk and be unrelated to direct nerve root compression. Increasing the tension within the disk by intradiskal injection of contrast material theoretically may reproduce this diskogenic pain.

The unique diagnostic information provided by diskography is reproduction of diskogenic pain. In judging the clinical utility of diskography, two questions must be answered: Does the pain relate causally to the patient's symptoms? Does the procedure help predict the results from spinal fusion? These questions have not been answered adequately by prospective, randomized clinical trials. Until they are answered, the role of diskography in the management of low back pain will remain unclear.

Clinical Indications

The place of diskography in the assessment of low back pain remains a contentious issue. However, possible indications for diskography include: 1) to diagnose internal disk derangement; 2) as a last resort to exclude a diskogenic cause for pain when all other tests are negative; 3) to determine the symptomatic level when multilevel disk pathology is present; and 4) prior to chemonucleolysis.

Complications

The major risk of diskography is of disk infection. The incidence of diskitis has been reported as between 1% and 3%. With careful technique it should be closer to 1%. This risk can be reduced by the administration of prophylactic antibiotics or the addition of antibiotics to the injected material.

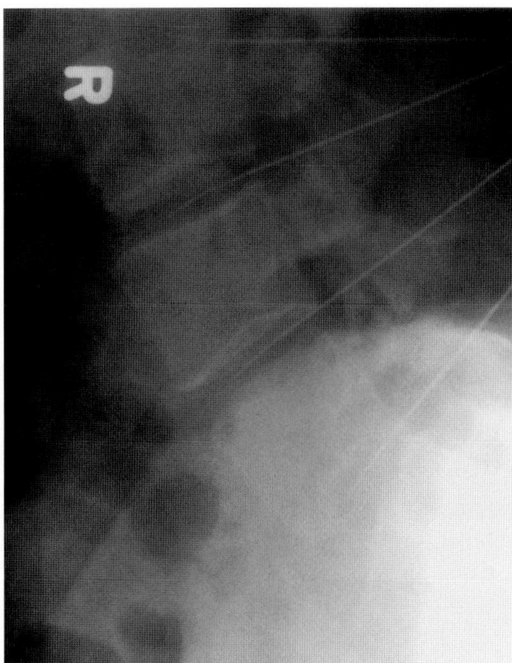

Figure 26. Lateral projection of diskography of the lower four lumbar disks. A coaxial technique has been used. A 20-gauge sheath has been passed to the edge of the disk and a 25-gauge needle has been passed centrally to penetrate the disk. The needle tip projects in the central third of the disks.

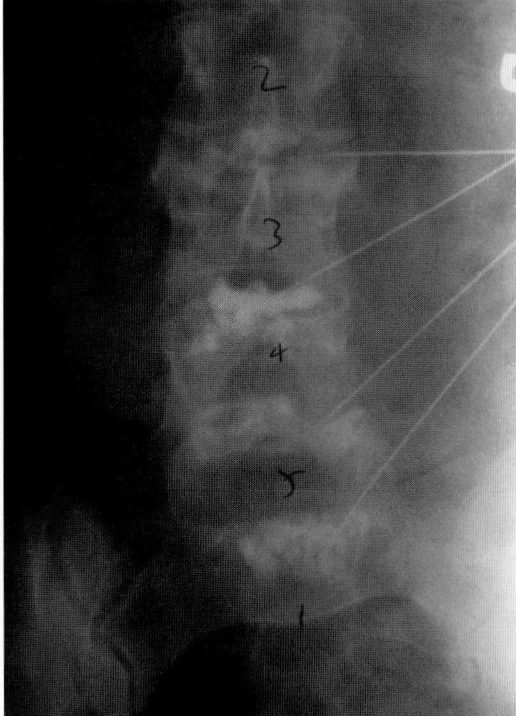

Figure 27. Frontal projection of diskography of the lower four lumbar disks. Contrast material is seen within the disks.

Technique

Lumbar diskography is an outpatient procedure performed with the patient lying prone on a biplane fluoroscopy table. Light sedation with benzodiazepine and narcotic makes the procedure more comfortable. The C-arm should be rotated obliquely in a craniocaudal plane until tangent to the adjacent vertebral end-plates. It should then be rotated 30 to 60 degrees so that the superior facet is projected midway between the sides of the vertebral body. Antiseptic skin wash, sterile technique, and local anesthetic should be used. A 15–20-cm needle is introduced in the axis of imaging, aiming for a point midway between vertebral end-plates and slightly anterior to the superior facet. Either a 20-gauge needle for direct disk puncture or a coaxial technique, with use of an outer 18-gauge sheath and an inner 22-gauge needle, may be used.

Needle tip position within the middle third of the disk should be confirmed on frontal and lateral imaging **(Figs. 26, 27)**. The L5-S1 level is the most technically challenging. A longer needle (usually 20 cm) and a more oblique path are necessary. A coaxial technique with use of 18-gauge and 22-gauge needles is recommended. The 18-gauge needle is introduced as far as the disk margin. A 45-degree curve should be imparted to the 22-gauge inner needle so that it enters the disk in the axial plane. If multiple levels are to be injected, all needles should be positioned prior to the first injection to facilitate comparison of the pain induced by each injection. At each level, 1.5–2 mL of contrast material are injected until the patient feels pain or resistance is noted.

Interpretation

The essential information elicited by this test is the pain induced by injection. The patient must be questioned carefully during the procedure regarding the character and severity (ranked 1 to 10) of the pain experienced. It is particularly important to ascertain whether or not the procedure reproduced the patient's typical pattern of pain.

Other considerations in interpretation are:

1. Injected volume—normal range is 1–1.5 mL before pain or resistance arises. More is abnormal.
2. Resistance to injection—a firm end point is normal.
3. Disk morphology—routinely assessed on a post-diskogram CT scan.

CT diskography is performed to ascertain that the injection is intranuclear. Although structural disk abnormalities can be demonstrated, these are of secondary interest. However, the diskogram should only be considered positive when the typical pain provocation correlates with a pathologic disk pattern.

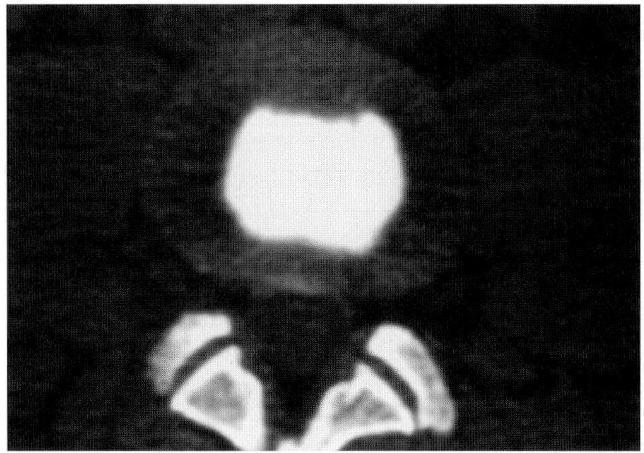

Figure 28. Normal diskogram. Contrast is confined to the nucleus pulposis.

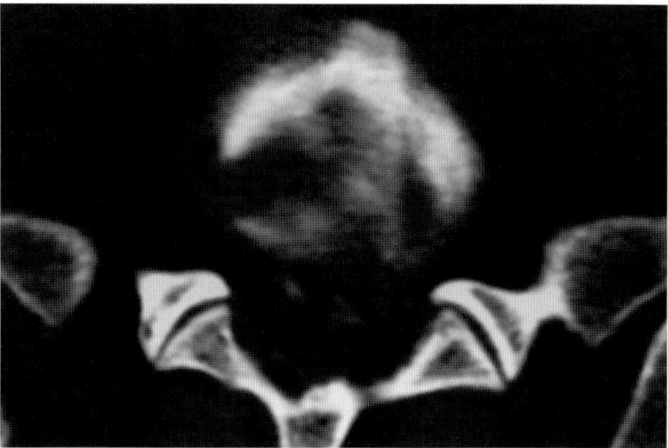

Figure 29. Internal disk derangement.

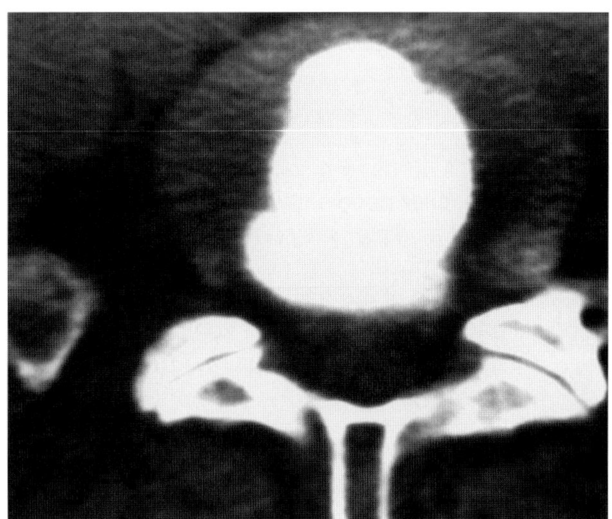

Figure 30. Annular tear and diffuse disk bulge.

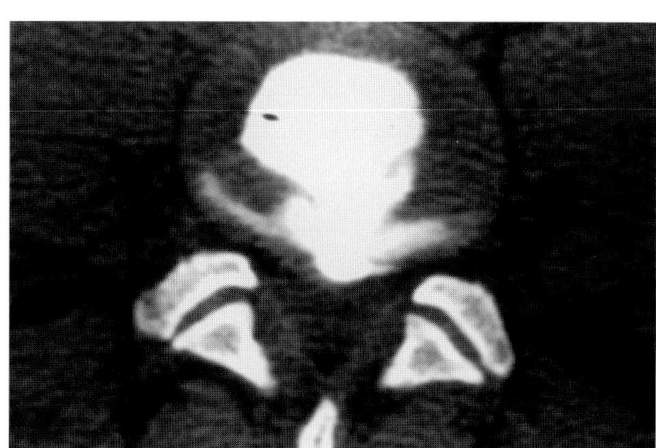

Figure 31. Annular tear with posterocentral disk protrusion.

Figures 28–31 illustrate common diskogram patterns.

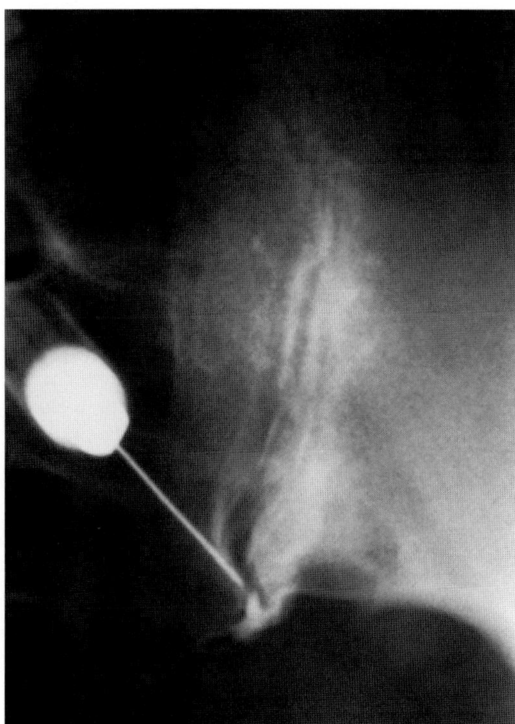

Figure 32. Frontal projection of a right SI joint injection. The 22-gauge spinal needle has been introduced from a posteromedial approach, starting 3.8 cm from the midline and aiming for the inferior 1 cm of the joint. Intra-articular position has been confirmed with an injection of contrast material.

Cervical Diskography

The place of cervical diskography is less widely accepted than that of lumbar diskography. This is a technically more difficult procedure than lumbar diskography and bears a higher risk of complication. Shinomaya et al reported the results of diskography in 148 patients, including 72 patients with chronic neck pain and 76 patients with neurologic symptoms but no significant neck pain.[3] Of the patients in the symptomatic neck pain group, 65% had their pain reproduced. Of the control group (neurologic symptoms only), 50% complained of induced neck pain. The authors therefore concluded that cervical diskography is unreliable for determining symptomatic disk levels.

Sacroiliac Joint Injection

Aspiration of the sacroiliac (SI) joint is indicated when septic arthritis is suspected. This condition is most common in infants and intravenous drug users. In the setting of painful SI arthropathies, pain relief can be effected by injection of local anesthetic into the SI joint. This procedure can be performed with either CT or fluoroscopic guidance, depending on operator preference.

Anatomy

The SI joint is a synovial joint. The joint surfaces are irregularly shaped, with the interconnecting bones fitting snugly. As a consequence, the fluoroscopic appearance of the joint space is of several sets of line pairs, depending upon which undulations of the joint parallel the x-ray beam. It is difficult to determine which of these line pairs (if any) represent the posterior margin of the SI joint. This anatomic feature can make fluoroscopic needle insertion into the SI joint difficult. Where necessary, this problem can be overcome with CT guidance, although CT assistance lacks the maneuverability of fluoroscopic guidance.

Technique

The patient lies prone. With use of CT guidance, the inferior half of the joint is scanned and the most accessible site punctured. With use of fluoroscopic guidance, the needle is directed toward the inferior 1 cm of the SI joint. The skin is then punctured 3.5–4 cm from the midline, with the needle directed anterolaterally toward the inferior SI joint until it contacts bone. If more than one line pair represents the inferior joint line, the most medial often represents the posterior joint surface. With the needle in place it may help to use a slightly more oblique projection (ipsilateral side down) to better visualize the posterior joint margin. Intra-articular position should be confirmed with an 0.5–1 mL injection of contrast material **(Fig. 32)**. A mixture of 0.5 mL (3 mg) betamethasone and 1.5 mL 0.25% bupivacaine is then injected into the SI joint.

References

1. Renfrew DL, Moore TE, Kathol MH, el-Khoury GY, Lemke JH, Walker CW. Correct placement of epidural steroid injections: fluoroscopic guidance and contrast administration. Am J Neuroradiol 1991; 12:1003–1007.

2. Schwarzer AC, Aprill CN, Derby R, Fortin J, Kine G, Bogduk N. Clinical features of patients with pain stemming from the lumbar zygapophysial joints. Is the lumbar facet syndrome a clinical entity? Spine 1994; 19:1132–1137.

3. Shinomiya K, Nakao K, Shindoh S, et al. Evaluation of cervical diskography in pain origin and provocation. J Spinal Disord 1993; 6:422–426.

Selected Readings

Babu NV, Titus VT, Chittaranjan S, Abraham G, Prem H, Korula RJ. Computed tomographically guided biopsy of the spine. Spine 1994; 19:2436–2442.

Bowman SJ, Wedderburn L, Whaley A, Grahame R, Newman S. Outcome assessment after epidural corticosteroid injection for low back pain and sciatica. Spine 1993; 18:1345–1350.

Brugieres P, Gaston A, Heran F, Voisin MC, Marsault C. Percutaneous biopsies of the thoracic spine under CT guidance: transcostovertebral approach. J Comput Assist Tomogr 1990; 14:446–448.

Brugieres P, Gaston A, Voisin MC, Ricolfi F, Chakir N. CT-guided percutaneous biopsy of the cervical spine: a series of 12 cases. Neuroradiology 1992; 358–360.

Bush K, Hillier S. A controlled study of caudal epidural injections of triamcinolone plus procaine for the management of intractable sciatica. Spine 1991; 16:572–575.

Dooley JF, McBroom RJ, Taguchi T, Macnab I. Nerve root infiltration in the diagnosis of radicular pain. Spine 1988; 13:79–83.

el-Khoury GY, Ehara S, Weinstein JN, Montgomery WJ, Kathol MH. Epidural steroid injection: a procedure ideally performed with fluoroscopic control. Radiology 1988; 168:554–557.

el-Khoury GY, Renfrew DL, Walker CW. Interventional musculoskeletal radiology. Curr Probl Diagn Radiol 1994; 23(5):161–203.

el-Khoury GY, Terepka RH, Mickelson MR, Rainville KL, Zaleski MS. Fine needle aspiration biopsy of bone. J Bone Joint Surg Am 1983; 65:522–525.

Greenspan A, Amparo EG, Gorczyca DP, Montesano PX. Is there a role for diskography in the era of magnetic resonance imaging? Prospective correlation and quantitative analysis of computed tomography-diskography, magnetic resonance imaging, and surgical findings. J Spinal Disord 1992; 5:26–31.

Jelinek JS, Kransdorf MJ, Gray R, Aboulafia AJ, Malawer MM. Percutaneous transpedicular biopsy of vertebral body lesions. Spine 1996; 21:2035–2040.

Logan PM, Connell DG, O'Connell JX, Munk PL, Janzen DL. Image-guided percutaneous biopsy of musculoskeletal tumors: an algorithm for selection of specific biopsy techniques. AJR 1996; 166:137–141.

Maldague B, Mathurin P, Malghem J. Facet joint arthrography in lumbar spondylolysis. Radiology 1981; 140:29–36.

Moran R, O'Connell D, Walsh MG. The diagnostic value of facet joint injections. Spine 1988; 13:1407–1410.

Schweitzer ME, Deely DM. Percutaneous biopsy of osteolytic lesions: use of a biopsy gun. Radiology 1993; 189:615–616.

Schweitzer ME, Gannon FH, Deely DM, O'Hara BJ, Juneja V. Percutaneous skeletal aspiration and core biopsy: complementary techniques. AJR 1996; 166:415–418.

Stoker DJ, Kissin CM. Percutaneous vertebral biopsy: a review of 135 cases. Clin Radiol 1985; 569–577.

Stanley D, McLaren MI, Euinton HA, Getty CJ. A prospective study of nerve root infiltration in the diagnosis of sciatica: a comparison with radiculography, computed tomography, and operative findings. Spine 1990; 15:540–543.

Stringham DR, Hadjipavlou A, Dzioba RB, Lander P. Percutaneous transpedicular biopsy of the spine. Spine 1994; 19:1985–1991.

White LM, Schweitzer ME, Deely DM. Coaxial percutaneous needle biopsy of osteolytic lesions with intact cortical bone. AJR 1996; 166:143–144.

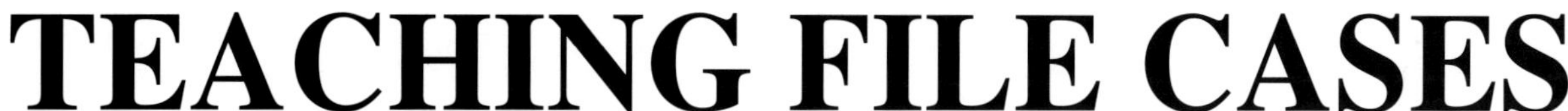

TEACHING FILE CASES

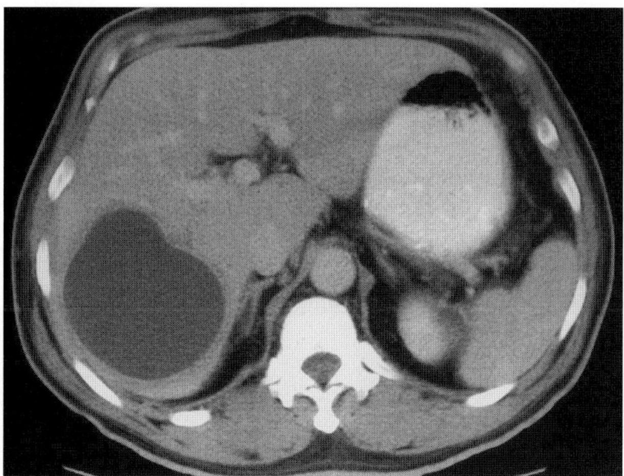

Figure 1. CT scan through the right lobe of the liver.

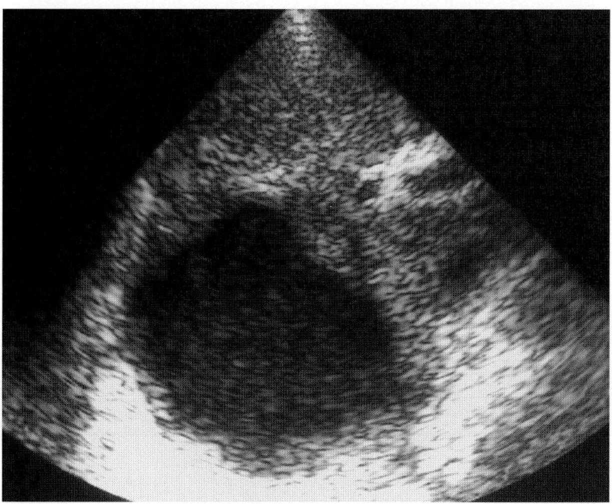

Figure 2. Longitudinal sonogram of the right lobe of the liver.

TEACHING FILE CASE 1

Siobhan Dumbleton, M.D.

History

A 62-year-old recent Vietnamese immigrant was admitted to the hospital with right upper quadrant pain. A computed tomography (CT) scan and a sonogram were obtained **(Figs. 1, 2)**.

What is your diagnosis?

Radiographic Findings

On the CT scan a 9-cm nonenhancing, homogeneous cystic lesion with a thin hypodense rim representing adjacent compressed hepatic parenchyma is identified in the right lobe of the liver in a subdiaphragmatic position **(Fig. 3)**. The ultrasound (US) examination confirms the juxtadiaphragmatic location and demonstrates diffuse low-level echoes in an otherwise cystic lesion **(Fig. 4)**.

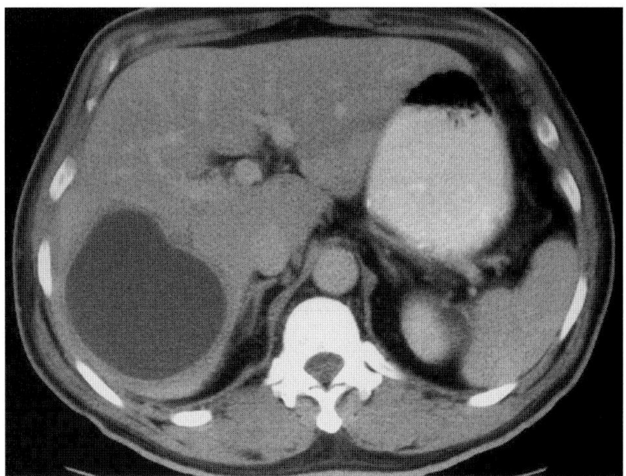

Figure 3. CT scan demonstrates a 9-cm cystic lesion in the right lobe of the liver adjacent to the liver capsule and surrounded by a thin hypodense rim.

Diagnosis

Amebic liver abscess.

How would you manage this patient?

Management

Amebic titers were positive but because of the size of the lesion, the patient's associated medical problems, and the risk of rupture, the decision was made to drain the abscess percutaneously under US guidance. Approximately 100 mL of thick, reddish material (the so-called "anchovy paste") was obtained and a drainage catheter was left in place for several days, until only minimal daily drainage was present. The catheter was removed.

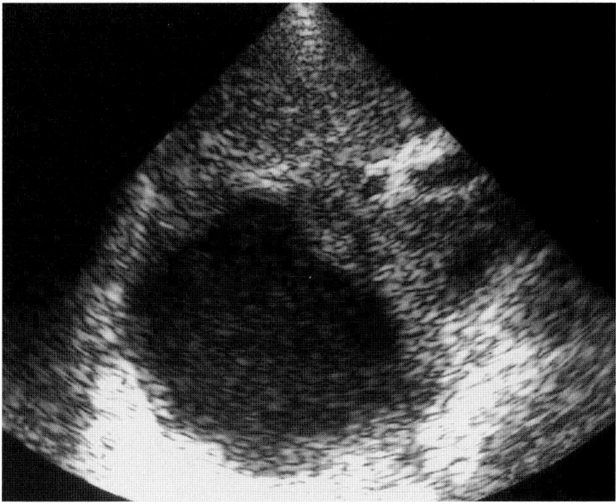

Figure 4. Longitudinal US demonstrates homogeneous low-level echoes in the cyst, which is in a subdiaphragmatic position.

Discussion

Intestinal amebiasis is caused by the protozoan *Entamoeba histolytica*. Although the organism is endemic to the United States, most cases are associated with travel abroad to areas with poor sanitation or found in immigrants from those same areas. Up to 10% of the world's population may be infected, but only 10% of those infected will show clinical symptoms, usually intestinal manifestations such as diarrhea. The most common extraintestinal complication is liver abscess, which affects up to 9% of all patients with intestinal amebiasis.

E. histolytica is introduced into the body when the cysts are ingested, usually through contaminated water. The cysts pass through the stomach to reach the intestine, where the outer layer of the cyst is dissolved enzymatically and the trophozoites is released. The trophozoites invade the intestinal mucosa, especially in the colon, sometimes causing ulceration and diarrhea. The organisms can enter the mesenteric venules where they are carried to the liver. They lodge in distal portal vein branches where they produce inflammation and subsequent vascular thrombosis with associated hepatic infarction. These areas of infarction and hepatic destruction may coalesce to produce an abscess.

The clinical picture of an amebic abscess is variable, with right upper quadrant/epigastric pain and tender hepatomegaly being the predominant manifestations. Up to 2% of cases are reported to rupture, and the rupture can occur into the peritoneal space, the pleural space, or into the pericardium. The mortality rate from rupture may reach as high as 42%, with the highest mortality rate associated with pericardial rupture. Indications that an abscess may rupture include: abscess diameter greater than 5–10 cm; enlarging abscess; and left lobe abscess.

Diagnosis is made on the basis of a space-occupying lesion within the liver and strongly positive serology (>1:512 titer on indirect hemagglutination). US, CT, magnetic resonance (MR) imaging, or nuclear medicine scans may be used to identify the liver lesion. On sonograms, a round- or oval-shaped lesion may be seen which is hypoechoic to the liver parenchyma, has homogeneous low-level echoes throughout, demonstrates acoustic enhancement with through transmission, and is contiguous to the liver capsule or diaphragm. On CT scans, the abscess usually appears as a solitary hypodense lesion of variable shape and may demonstrate internal trabeculae and nodular borders. MR imaging demonstrates increased enhancement of the capsule. This finding differentiates amebic abscesses from liver cysts. Nuclear medicine studies may also be used to identify a space-occupying lesion within the liver.

Most amebic abscesses occur within the right lobe of the liver, probably because of portal flow dynamics. It has been postulated that the right lobe is preferentially affected because the dominant flow of blood comes from the superior mesenteric vein into the right lobe and from the splenic vein to the left lobe. Since most cases of hepatic amebic abscess are consequent to intestinal infection, seeding will occur via the portal vein.

Treatment

Although catheter drainage of pyogenic liver abscesses is an accepted means of treatment, amebic abscesses are primarily treated with amebicidal drugs such as metronidazole, and more than 90% of cases will respond to medical therapy alone. Percutaneous catheter drainage is reserved for patients who do not respond to amebicidal therapy, who have very large abscesses, or who develop bacterial superinfection and have a significant risk of rupture. With percutaneous drainage the typical “anchovy paste” may be aspirated. The organism *E. histolytica* is not usually identified in aspirates because it exists at the junction of necrotic and viable liver. Currently, surgery is reserved for those cases in which the abscess has ruptured.

Selected Readings

Barreda R, Ros PR. Diagnostic imaging of liver abscess. Crit Rev Diagn Imaging 1992; 33:29–58.

Nordestgaard AG, Stapleford L, Worthen N, Bongard FS, Klein SR. Contemporary management of amebic liver abscess. Am Surg 1992; 58:315–320.

Ralls P, Colletti PM, Quinn MF, Halls J. Sonographic findings in hepatic amebic abscess. Radiology 1982; 145:123–126.

Saraswat VA, Agarwal DK, Baijal SS, et al. Percutaneous catheter drainage of amebic liver abscess. Clin Radiol 1992; 45:187–189.

Van Allan RJ, Katz MD, Johnson MB, Laine LA, Liu Y, Ralls PW. Uncomplicated amebic liver abscess: prospective evaluation of percutaneous therapeutic aspiration. Radiology 1992; 183:827–830.

Endnote

Figures courtesy of Jeet Sandhu, M.D., University of North Carolina School of Medicine.

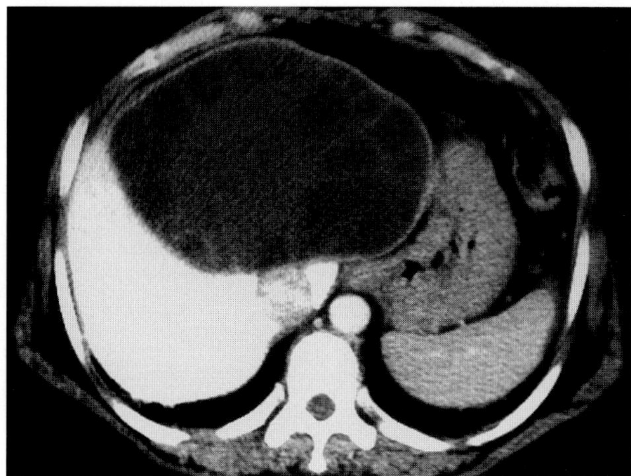

Figure 1. Image from the CT portogram.

TEACHING FILE CASE 2

Siobhan Dumbleton, M.D.

History

A 58-year-old Russian immigrant came to the hospital with abdominal bloating. A computed tomography (CT) scan was obtained. An image from a CT portogram is shown **(Fig. 1)**.

What is your diagnosis?

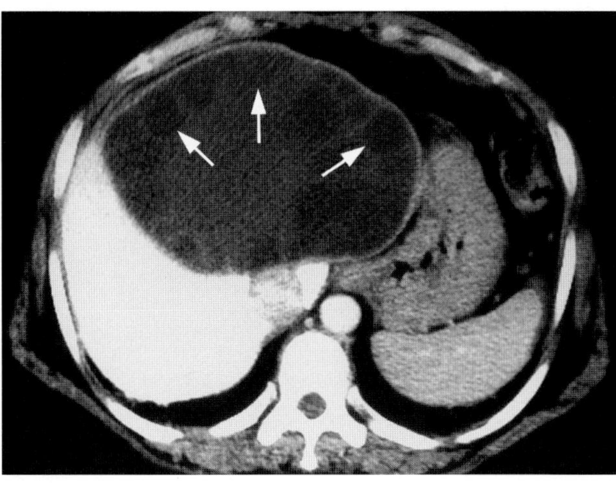

Figure 2. CT portogram shows a 12-cm mass in the left lobe of the liver composed of central soft-tissue material surrounded by multiple low-density daughter cysts along the periphery (arrows).

Radiographic Findings

A solitary 12-cm mass is noted in the left lobe of the liver with a central area of soft tissue surrounded by multiple low-density cystic spaces **(Fig. 2)**. No other lesions were noted in the liver, and the remainder of the abdominal CT scan was normal. An ultrasound-guided biopsy of the mass was performed which demonstrated scoleces compatible with *Echinococcus*.

Diagnosis

Hydatid disease of the liver.

How would you manage this patient?

Management

Given the complex nature of the lesion, the decision was made to perform surgical removal of the mass with a left hepatic lobe resection instead of pursuing percutaneous drainage and ethanol sclerosis. Despite a stormy postoperative course, the patient eventually recovered and was discharged in stable clinical condition without clinical symptoms.

Discussion

The organ most often affected by hydatid disease is the liver, with the lung being the second most commonly affected organ. This condition represents infection from the larval stage of *Echinococcus granulosa*. A more invasive form of the disease, manifested by diffuse infiltration of tissues and direct extension of the larvae through the duodenum, is due to infection by *Echinococcus multilocularis*. *E. vogeli* is a rare cause of hydatid infection.

E. granulosa is a tapeworm that lives in the intestine of the definitive host. Eggs are excreted in the feces where they are ingested by the intermediate vectors. *E. granulosa* infection is endemic to cattle- and sheep-raising regions throughout the world, especially the Mediterranean basin and the Soviet republics. Two forms exist—the sylvan form and the pastoral form. Although the infection is caused by the same organism, the two forms have different hosts and intermediate vectors. The more common form is the pastoral form, where the dog is the host and sheep or cattle are infected. In the sylvan form, the wolf or fox is the host and becomes infected by feeding on deer and elk. The sylvan form is found in northern climates such as Canada and Alaska.

The infection is acquired by eating food contaminated with feces that contains the eggs of the organism or by coming into contact with infected dogs which may carry the eggs in their fur. The larvae are released within the duodenum after the external shell of the egg is lysed. The larvae subsequently penetrate the intestinal wall and reach the liver via the portal circulation. The larvae embed themselves in the liver and can grow there. If the larvae pass through the liver, they may reach the pulmonary bed and from there enter the systemic circulation, thereby producing infection in almost any organ within the body. Although the primary infection is usually acquired during childhood, patients do not experience symptoms for 20 to 30 years, when the cyst has become large enough to induce symptoms. Consequently, most of the patient's symptoms are due to mass effect from the large cysts.

Many patients may be asymptomatic when the cysts are discovered. Symptoms that may occur include vague right upper abdominal and/or epigastric pain and hepatomegaly. A palpable mass may be found in up to 87% of patients. The cyst may rupture into the biliary or bronchial tree. Free rupture into the pleural or peritoneal spaces may also occur. Superinfection with bacteria occurs in 20% of cases. Anaphylaxis may theoretically result from the highly antigenic cyst contents, but this has not been borne out in clinical practice.

Serologic evaluation establishes the diagnosis in 80% of cases by detecting immunoglobulin G antibodies (which indicates exposure). High levels of immunoglobulin M and immunoglobulin A antibodies are seen during active infection. Definitive diagnosis may require biopsy.

Histologically, the cyst wall contains three layers. The pericyst is formed by condensed, indurated liver tissue which may incorporate adjacent vascular structures and biliary radicles. The intermediate layer is amorphous, gelatinous, acellular material derived from the parasite and is the exocyst. The inner germinal layer (endocyst) is the only layer which contains the living parasite. It produces the cyst fluid, scoleces, and daughter cysts. A fine layer composed of scoleces and brood capsules may be detected in the cyst and is known as hydatid sand.

On plain radiographs, 20%–30% of hydatid cysts may be calcified. Gharbi et al described five sonographic appearances of the hydatid cyst:

Type 1 lesions are the most common. They are purely cystic and hydatid sand is often present. These lesions are best suited for percutaneous therapy.

Type 2 lesions occur when the intermediate layer splits from the pericyst, producing a floating membrane. This appearance is virtually pathognomonic of a hydatid cyst.

Type 3 lesions are multiseptated cysts with multiple peripheral daughter cysts and echogenic or soft-tissue-density material between the cysts. This appearance was present in the current case and is also highly characteristic of echinococcal cysts.

Type 4 lesions represent complex heterogeneous masses. This appearance may result from superinfection.

Type 5 lesions are the least common form with lesional or wall calcification that represents the death of the parasite. As a result, a hyperechoic wall or increased dense echogenicity may be seen in the lesion.

CT scans demonstrate unilocular and/or multilocular cystic masses with a thin high-attenuation rim which usually does not enhance. The cyst may appear multilocular secondary to daughter cysts. As with ultrasound, a floating membrane may be seen.

Treatment

Scolecidal therapy with agents such as albendazole and mebendazole is inadequate as a sole means of treatment. Therefore, management has typically involved surgery with radical hepatic resection or more conservative therapy with cyst resection and removal of the germinal layer. The recurrence rate is as high as 30% despite surgical intervention. Percutaneous catheter drainage with the instillation of ethanol or hypertonic saline had previously been reserved for recurrent lesions or patients who are not surgical candidates because of the fear of anaphylactic shock or seeding secondary to intraperitoneal spillage during percutaneous drainage. However, several series have reported successful percutaneous treatment of hydatid cysts in combination with scolecidal drugs without significant anaphylactic reactions. To minimize the risk of intraperitoneal spillage, a transhepatic route should be used and percutaneous therapy reserved for the less complex cysts.

Selected Readings

Acunas B, Rozanes I, Celik L, et al. Purely cystic hydatid disease of the liver: treatment with percutaneous aspiration and injection of hypertonic saline. Radiology 1992; 182:541–543.

Bonakdarpour A. Echinococcus disease: report of 112 cases from Iran and a review of 611 cases from the United States. AJR 1967; 99:660–667.

Gharbi HA, Hassine W, Brauner MW, Dupuch K. Ultrasound examination of the hydatid liver. Radiology 1981; 139:459–463.

Giorgio A, Tarantino L, Francica G, et al. Unilocular hydatid liver cysts: treatment with US-guided, double percutaneous aspiration and ethanol injection. Radiology 1992; 184:705–710.

Jha R, Lyons EA, Levi CS. US case of the day. Hydatid cyst (*Echinococcus granulosus*) in the right lobe of the liver. Radiographics 1994; 14:455–458.

Lupetin AR, Dash N. Intrahepatic rupture of hydatid cyst: MR findings. AJR 1988; 151:491–492.

Mentes A. Hydatid liver disease: a perspective in treatment. Dig Dis 1994; 12:150–160.

Sayek I, Yalin R, Sanac Y. Surgical treatment of hydatid disease of the liver. Arch Surg 1980; 115:847–850.

Suwan Z. Sonographic findings in hydatid disease of the liver: comparison with other imaging methods. Ann Trop Med Parasitol 1995; 89:261–269.

Endnote

Figures courtesy of Jeet Sandhu, M.D., University of North Carolina School of Medicine.

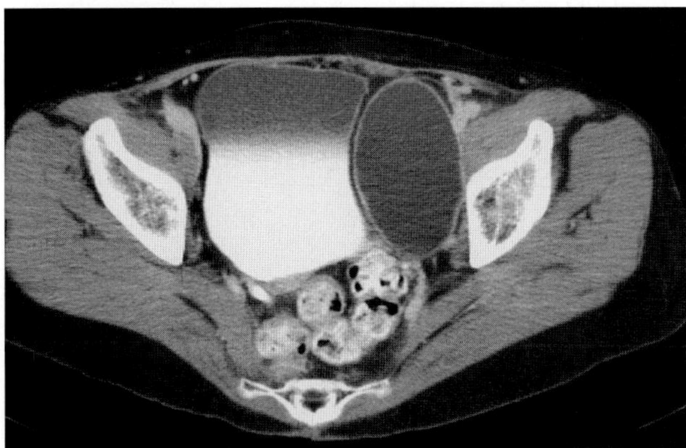

Figure 1. CT scan of the abdomen and pelvis with oral and intravenous contrast material.

TEACHING FILE CASE 3

Mark L. Lukens, M.D., and
Allen J. Meglin, M.D.

History

A 56-year-old woman with a history of endometrial carcinoma and prior total abdominal hysterectomy with bilateral salpingo-oophorectomy came to the hospital 21 days after her surgery with left lower quadrant pain. A computed tomography (CT) scan was obtained with oral and intravenous contrast material **(Fig. 1)**.

What is your diagnosis?

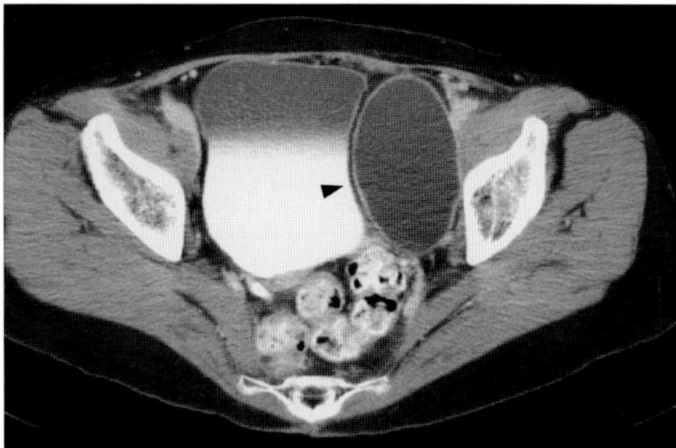

Figure 2. CT scan shows a well-defined fluid collection in the left lower quadrant. Note compression of the adjacent bladder by the fluid collection (arrowhead).

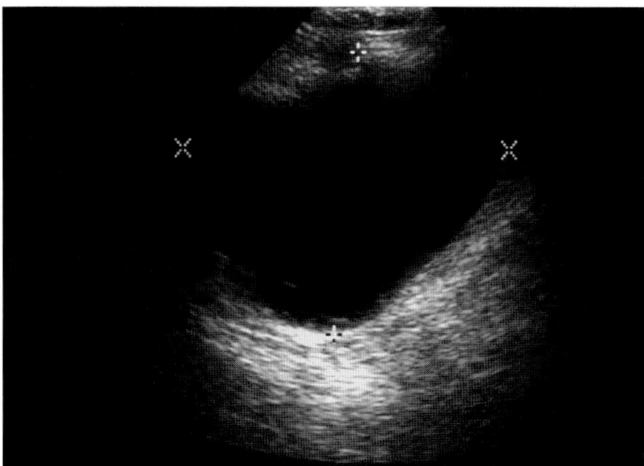

Figure 3. Transabdominal sonogram shows a large hypoechoic mass in the left lower quadrant.

Radiographic Findings

The CT scan shows a well-defined fluid collection with a Hounsfield unit value of 1 **(Fig. 2)**.

Preliminary Diagnosis

Postoperative fluid collection.

How would you manage this patient?

Management

The differential diagnosis includes lymphocele, urinoma, hematoma, seroma, and abscess. Initial sonographic evaluation was performed from a transabdominal approach **(Fig. 3)**. A trocar type, all-purpose drainage catheter was placed into the fluid collection under sonographic guidance, and 105 mL of turbid whitish-colored fluid were removed.

Laboratory analysis of the fluid demonstrated creatinine levels approaching those of serum, consistent with a lymphocele. After 1 week of persistent drainage, a more definitive solution was sought. A sinogram demonstrated a smooth, well-decompressed cavity **(Fig. 4)**. Approximately 10 mL of povidone-iodine solution was instilled into the cavity and left in place for 90 minutes **(Fig. 5)**. During that time, the patient was placed in the supine, prone, left lateral decubitus, and right lateral decubitus positions for equal periods of time.

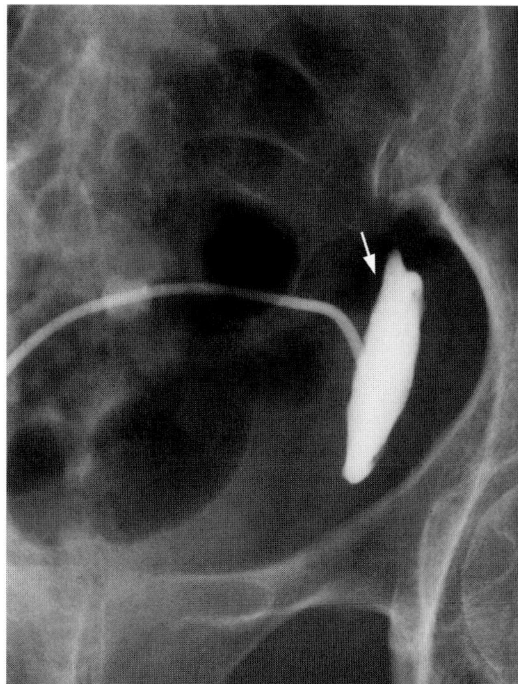

Figure 4. Sinogram shows a well-decompressed cavity with smooth walls and no communication with adjacent structures (arrow).

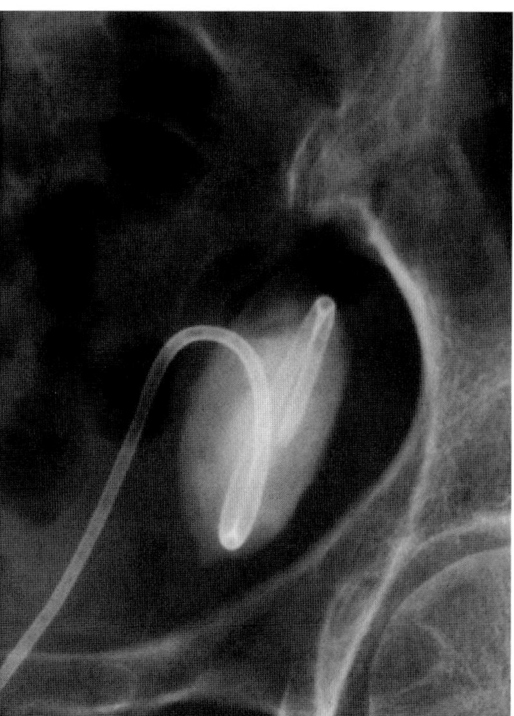

Figure 5. Radiograph obtained during sclerosis shows the mildly radiopaque nature of povidone-iodine solution.

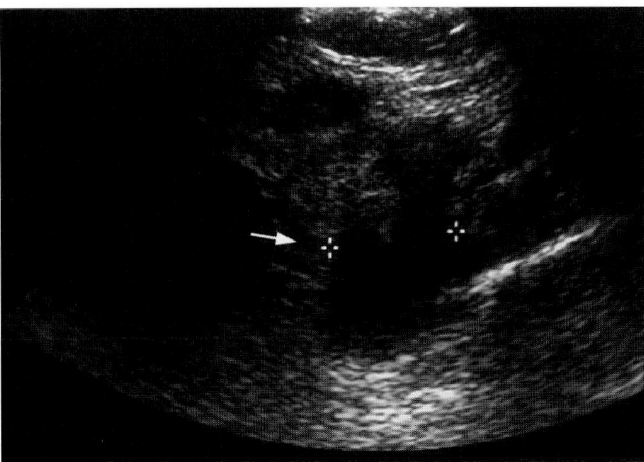

Figure 6. A small, irregular fluid collection was noted on sonography following sclerosant therapy (arrow).

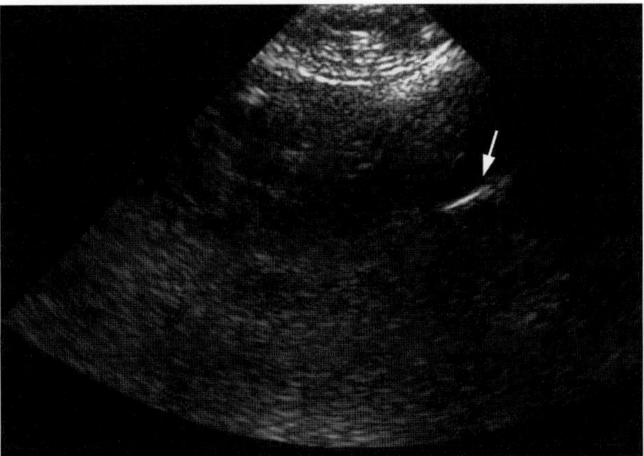

Figure 7. Sonography performed 1 week after drainage shows no residual fluid collection. Note the echogenic catheter within the collapsed cavity (arrow).

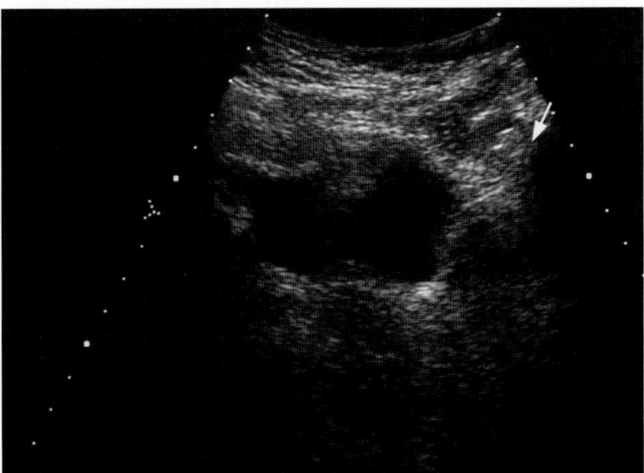

Figure 8. Transverse pelvic sonogram shows no fluid collection 5 weeks after sclerosant therapy. Arrow shows the area of the previous lymphocele.

The povidone-iodine solution was then removed and the catheter was reattached to a suction grenade. Sonograms at 2 and 5 days after sclerosis showed only minimal residual fluid collection **(Fig. 6)**. Seven days after sclerosis, the drainage had become negligible and the sonogram showed no evidence of residual fluid collection **(Fig. 7)**. The catheter was subsequently removed. Five weeks after the original sclerosis, a sonogram showed no evidence of fluid collection, consistent with complete resolution of the lymphocele **(Fig. 8)**.

Final Diagnosis

Post-hysterectomy lymphocele.

Discussion

Leakage of lymph following renal transplantation and pelvic surgery is a well-known complication. If the leak persists without encapsulation, it may be necessary to surgically ligate the weeping lymphatics. Encapsulation of the leak results in a lymphocele. In the past, surgical correction consisted of marsupialization of the fluid collection to the peritoneal cavity where the fluid can be resorbed. Alternatively, the collections can be drained percutaneously. Single aspiration results in a 50% cure rate, and similar results were noted with a 3-day aspiration technique. Following drainage, sclerosis can be performed with one of many agents (ethanol, tetracycline, and povidone-iodine), but povidone-iodine is used the most. This simple percutaneous technique can result in resolution of the lymphocele without the need for surgical marsupialization and its inherent risks.

Selected Readings

Akhan O, Cekirge S, Ozmen M, Besim A. Percutaneous transcatheter ethanol sclerotherapy of postoperative pelvic lymphoceles. Cardiovasc Intervent Radiol 1992; 15:224–227.

Burgos FJ, Teruel JL, Mayayo T, et al. Diagnosis and management of lymphoceles after renal transplantation. Br J Urol 1988; 61:289–293.

Cohan RH, Saeed M, Schwab SJ, Perlmutt LM, Dunnick NR. Povidone-iodine sclerosis of pelvic lymphoceles: a prospective study. Urol Radiol 1988; 10:203–206.

Crummy AB, McDermott JC. Percutaneous management of lymphoceles. In: Kadir S, ed. Current practice of interventional radiology. St. Louis: Mosby Year Book, 1991.

Dodd GD, Rutledge F, Wallace S. Postoperative pelvic lymphocysts. AJR 1970; 108:312–323.

Gilliland JD, Spies JB, Brown SB, Yrizarry JM, Greenwood LH. Lymphoceles: percutaneous treatment with povidone-iodine sclerosis. Radiology 1989; 171:227–229.

Greenberg BM, Perloff LJ, Grossman RA, Naji A, Barker CF. Treatment of lymphocele in renal allograft recipients. Arch Surg 1985; 120:501–504.

Lorimer WS III, Glassford DM, Sarles HE, Remmers AR Jr, Fish JC. Lymphocele: a significant complication following renal transplantation. Lymphology 1975; 8:20–23.

Shokeir AA, el-Diasty TA, Ghoneim MA. Percutaneous treatment of lymphocele in renal transplant recipients. J Endourol 1993; 7:481–485.

Teruel JL, Escobar EM, Quereda C, Mayayo T, Ortuno J. A simple and safe method for management of lymphocele after renal transplantation. J Urol 1983; 130:1058–1059.

vanSonnenberg E, Wittich GR, Casola G, et al. Lymphoceles: imaging characteristics and percutaneous management. Radiology 1986; 161:593–596.

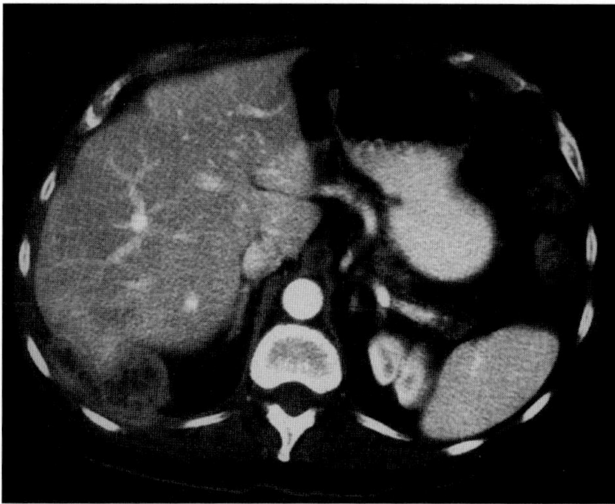

Figure 1. Abdominal CT scan, upper image.

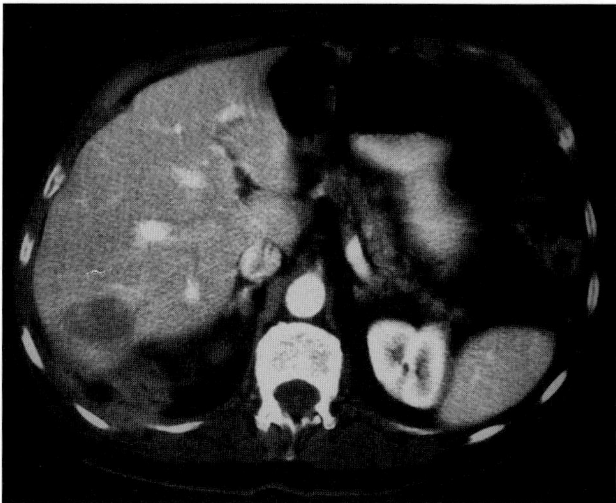

Figure 2. Abdominal CT scan, lower image.

TEACHING FILE CASE 4

J. Mark McKinney, M.D.

History

An 80-year-old man came to the hospital with complaints of right upper quadrant abdominal pain and a low-grade fever. Laboratory analysis revealed leukocytosis. He had undergone laparoscopic cholecystectomy 3 months earlier. A computed tomography (CT) scan of the abdomen was obtained **(Figs. 1, 2)**.

What is your diagnosis?

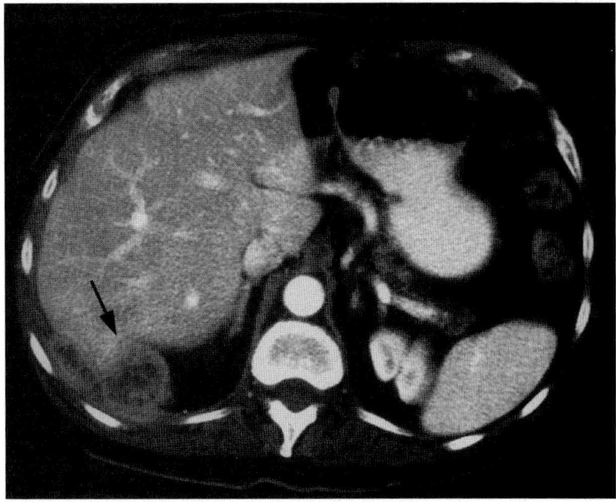

Figure 3. Abdominal CT scan demonstrates a complex fluid collection in the subhepatic space (arrow).

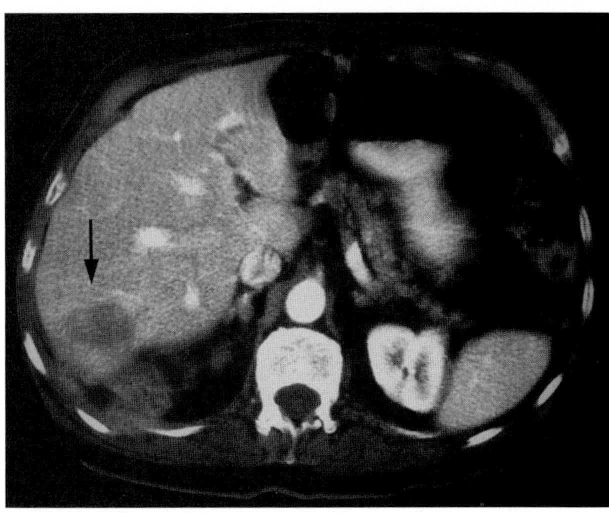

Figure 4. Abdominal CT scan shows intrahepatic involvement (arrow).

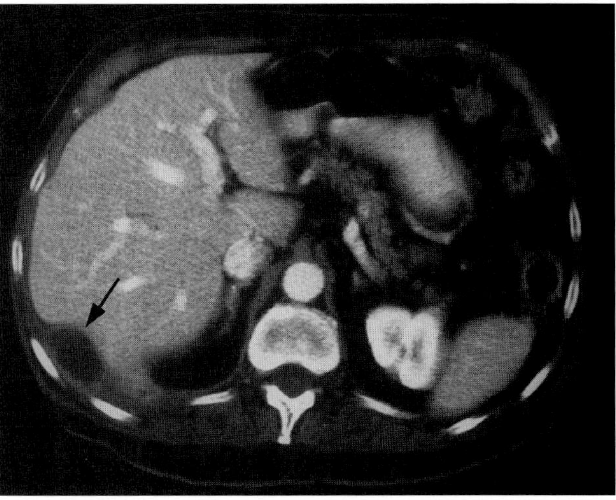

Figure 5. Abdominal CT scan obtained 5 months later reveals a residual small loculated subhepatic abscess (arrow).

Radiographic Findings

The CT images **(Figs. 3, 4)** demonstrate a complex fluid collection with both intra- and extrahepatic involvement of the posterior margin of the right lobe of the liver. CT-guided needle aspiration of this collection yielded infected material.

Diagnosis

Subhepatic abscess following laparoscopic cholecystectomy.

What are the treatment options?

Management

Percutaneous drainage using interventional radiology techniques is an effective method of treating subhepatic abscesses. This patient, however, underwent open surgical drainage via a posterior approach. At surgery multiple gallstones were found in the subhepatic collection. Five months after surgical drainage, the patient returned because of a persistent draining sinus track exiting his right posterior flank. A repeat CT scan **(Fig. 5)** showed a small residual subhepatic abscess. Interventional Radiology was consulted to place a drainage catheter into the collection through the existing sinus track.

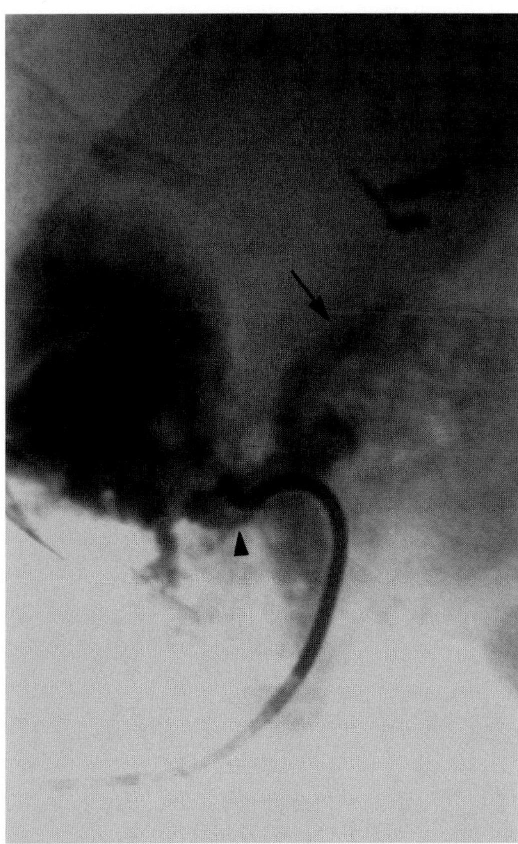

Figure 6. A hook-shaped angiographic visceral catheter was reformed in a blind pocket (arrow) and pulled back into the drainage track (arrowhead).

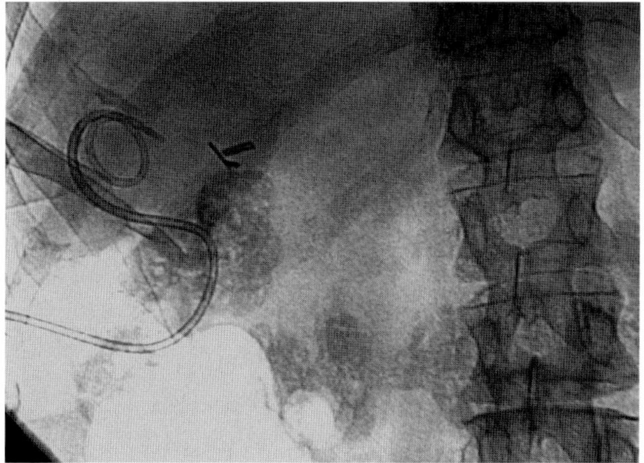

Figure 7. Drainage catheter extending through the tortuous sinus track into the subhepatic abscess.

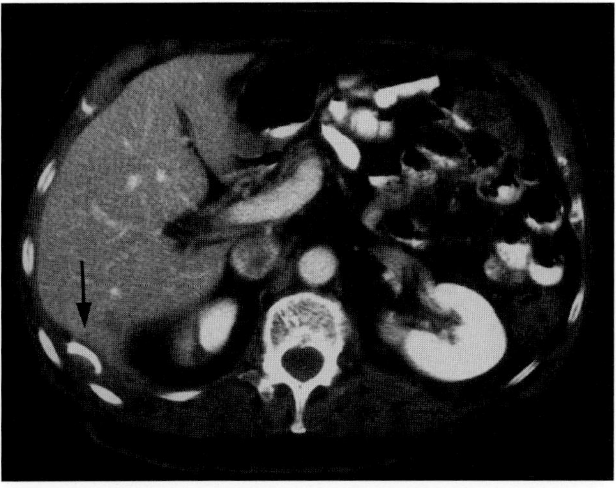

Figure 8. Catheter in the collapsed subhepatic cavity (arrow).

Multiple attempts to traverse the sinus track were unsuccessful because of a sharply angulated reversal of the track in the posterior soft tissues. An angiographic visceral catheter was then reformed in a blind pocket and pulled back into the angulated drainage track **(Fig. 6)**. The catheter was exchanged for an 8.5-F drain over a stiff wire **(Fig. 7)**. The cavity was gently irrigated with sterile saline. Follow-up CT scanning 1 day later revealed that the drainage catheter had collapsed the abscess cavity and was well positioned **(Fig. 8)**. The catheter was removed after 10 days, and the abscess did not recur.

Discussion

Subhepatic collections are a well-recognized complication of open or laparoscopic cholecystectomy. Most resolve spontaneously and represent noninfected bilomas or hematomas. However, secondary infection can occur, especially if stones are left behind at surgery that can serve as a nidus for infection. If clinical evidence of infection is equivocal, diagnostic needle aspiration can help determine if catheter drainage is required.

Percutaneous drainage of this subhepatic abscess prevented additional surgical procedures and obviated the need for hospitalization. As in this case, sinus tracks are often tortuous and poorly developed. Selecting catheters and wires of the appropriate shapes is very important to negotiating the track successfully. The use of an existing sinus track prevents contamination of adjacent noninfected tissues and possible spread of the abscess. Once the abscess cavity has collapsed and there is no evidence of communication with other viscera, the catheter can be removed and the sinus track will close spontaneously.

Selected Readings

Elboim CM, Goldman L, Hann L, Palestrant AM, Silen W. Significance of postcholecystectomy subhepatic fluid collections. Ann Surg 1983; 198:137–141.

Gervais DA, Gazelle GS, Lu DS, Han PF, Mueller PR. Percutaneous transpulmonary CT-guided liver biopsy: a safe and technically easy approach for lesions located near the diaphragm. AJR 1996; 167:482–483.

Nuñez D, Becerra JL, Martin LC. Subhepatic collections complicating laparoscopic cholecystectomy: percutaneous management. Abdom Imaging 1994; 19:248–250.

Society of Cardiovascular and Interventional Radiology Standards of Practices Committee. Quality improvement guidelines for adult percutaneous abscess and fluid drainage. J Vasc Interv Radiol 1995; 6:68–70.

vanSonnenberg E, Casola G, Wittich GR, et al. The role of interventional radiology for complications of cholecystectomy. Surgery 1990; 107:632–638.

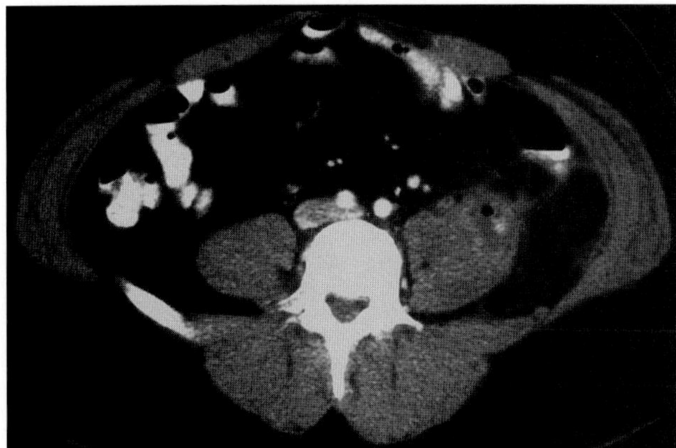

Figure 1. Supine abdominal CT scan.

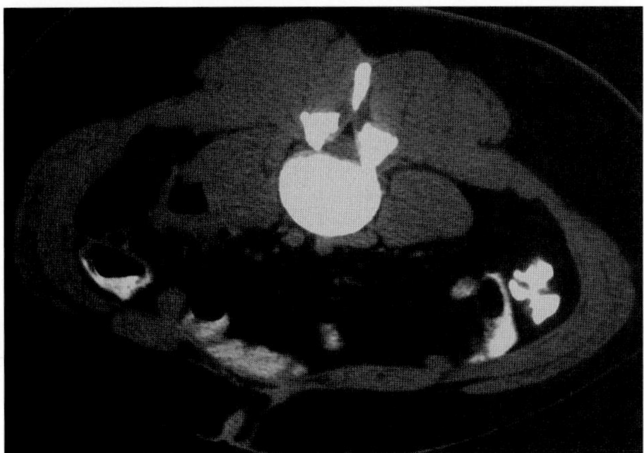

Figure 2. Prone abdominal CT scan.

TEACHING FILE CASE 5

J. Mark McKinney, M.D., and David E. Panzer, M.D.

History

The patient is a 31-year-old man with left lower quadrant abdominal pain that worsens when he moves his left leg. He has had fevers to 101° F. A computed tomography (CT) scan of the abdomen was obtained **(Figs. 1, 2)**.

What is your diagnosis?

Radiographic Findings
The CT scan of the abdomen reveals a mixed-attenuation fluid and gas collection on the left psoas muscle with a faint track extending to the descending colon **(Fig. 3)**. The prone scan demonstrates gas in the psoas cavity **(Fig. 4)**.

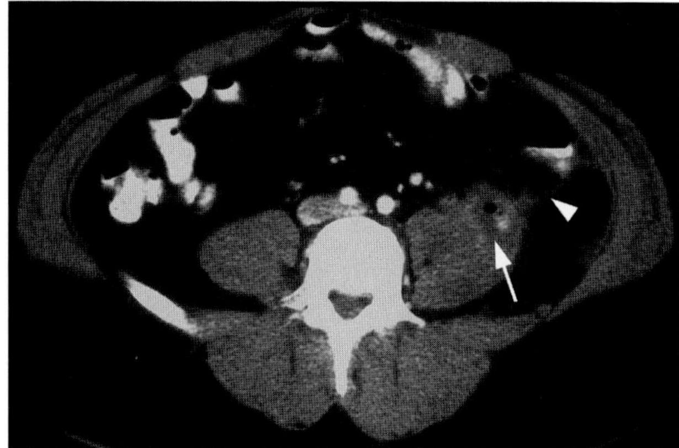

Figure 3. CT scan of the abdomen demonstrates a mixed-attenuation fluid and gas collection involving the left psoas muscle (arrow). Note the track to the colon (arrowhead).

Diagnosis
Secondary psoas abscess that communicates with the colon.

Management
An 18-gauge needle was advanced directly into the psoas abscess **(Fig. 5)**. An 0.035-inch wire was then coiled in the cavity **(Fig. 6)**. The track was dilated to 8-F size, and an 8.5-F locking loop drainage catheter was placed **(Fig. 7)**. A follow-up sinogram revealed the track that communicates with the descending colon **(Fig. 8)**.

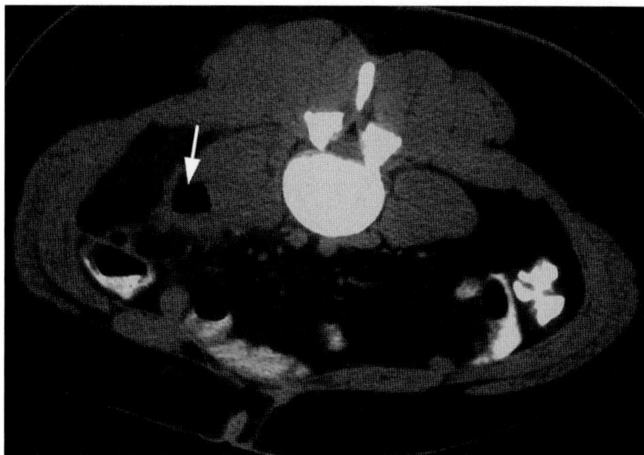

Figure 4. Prone CT scan shows that gas (arrow) has entered the left psoas abscess from the descending colon.

The abscess was drained percutaneously from a posterolateral approach. This approach avoids possible injury to the small intestines or colon. CT imaging is often the best modality for diagnosis and drainage guidance, but ultrasound may also be used. The radiologist's function is not only to place the catheter, but to follow the patient closely and manage the catheter as appropriate.

Discussion
Psoas abscesses have many different etiologies. Psoas muscles are susceptible to both hematogenous spread of bacteria (ie, as with tropical pyomyositis), as well as direct extension from an adjacent infectious process, such as discitis. Urinomas from ureteral injury can also cause large fluid collections in the psoas muscles. Classically, diverticular abscesses, which occur most frequently in the sigmoid colon, are thought of as being confined in the sigmoid mesocolon. However, diverticular abscesses can extend to involve continuous structures including the abdominal wall, vagina, bladder, thigh, flank, and the psoas muscle. In this case, the fistulous track identified on the CT examination as well as further filling of the abscess cavity with air indicates that the psoas abscess originates from the colon and is compatible with a diverticular abscess. The follow-up sinogram confirms the origin of the abscess from the colon since the fistula filled the colon.

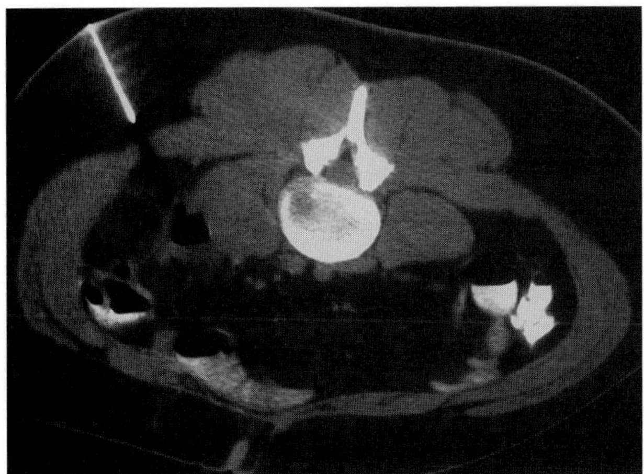

Figure 5. Access needle directed toward the psoas abscess with CT guidance.

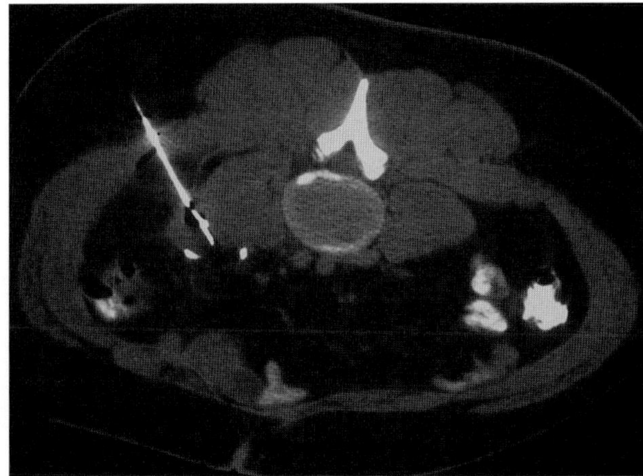

Figure 6. Wire placed through the needle and coiled in the abscess.

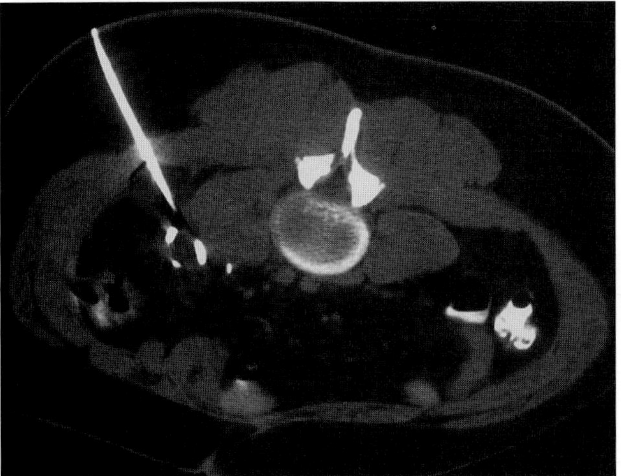

Figure 7. 8.5-F drain in the abscess cavity.

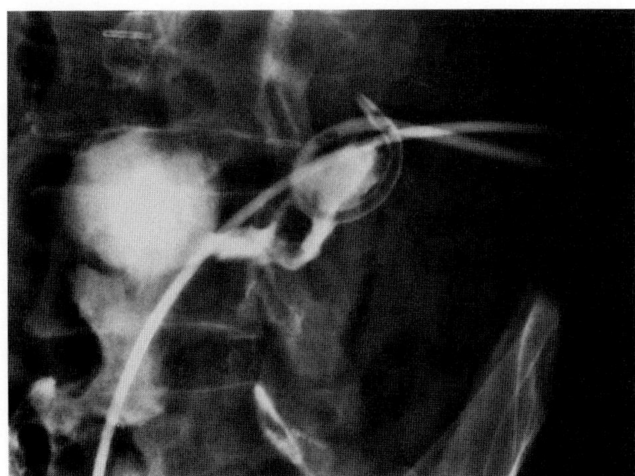

Figure 8. Follow-up sinogram demonstrates communication with the descending colon.

Diverticular disease is the most common colonic disease encountered in developed countries and is secondary to a low-residue diet. With low-residue dehydrated stools, increased intracolonic pressures are generated during defecation. Because of these high intracolonic pressures, the mucosa and submucosa protrude through areas of greatest wall weakness, which is where the vasa recta penetrate the colonic wall. Poor emptying of these diverticula causes stool or other material to become lodged in the diverticulum, resulting in inflammatory changes which may lead to perforation of the diverticulum and a clinical syndrome of acute diverticulitis.

The incidence of diverticulosis increases with age. Approximately 5% of the population will have diverticula at the age of 40, while over 50% of the population will have diverticula by age 80. It is estimated that 20% of patients with diverticulosis will develop diverticulitis during their lifetime. The vast majority of these cases will be managed medically with intravenous antibiotics. One to two percent of cases will require surgical or radiologic intervention.

The hallmark of diverticulitis is inflammation of the diverticulum with subsequent perforation at the apex of the diverticulum. In most cases, limited pericolonic inflammatory changes occur secondary to the perforation which resolve with conservative treatment and intravenous antibiotics. With a more significant perforation, a diverticular abscess can develop and rarely, frank fecal contamination of the peritoneum can occur. Because of the lower incidence of diverticula in the younger population, diverticulitis may not be a primary clinical diagnostic consideration; therefore, adequate evaluation and treatment may be delayed, resulting in a more severe clinical presentation. Studies have also noted that the clinical presentation is more severe in the younger age group and the need for intervention is greater in this patient population.

If an adequate approach to a drainable abscess is present, percutaneous drainage should be the initial intervention. In many cases, even if a diverticular fistula is identified, the fistula may heal with prolonged catheter drainage alone, obviating the need for surgery. Even in those cases where surgical resection is to be performed, initial drainage of the diverticular abscess can convert a multistage surgical procedure into a single-stage operation. Success rates of 50%–90% have been noted for percutaneous management of diverticular abscesses with or without fistulas. In this case, because of the relatively large fistulous communication from the colon to the cavity, the decision was made to proceed with surgical resection after the acute abscess had been treated. The clinical management of patients with diverticular abscesses can be improved significantly with percutaneous drainage techniques.

Selected Readings

Jacobs JE, Birnbaum BA. CT of inflammatory disease of the colon. Semin Ultrasound CT MR 1995; 16:91–101.

McAuliffe W, Clarke G. The diagnosis and treatment of psoas abscess: a 12-year review. Aust N Z J Surg 1994; 64: 413–417.

Santaella RO, Fishman EK, Lipsett PA. Primary versus secondary iliopsoas abscess: presentation, microbiology, and treatment. Arch Surg 1995; 130:1309–1313.

Society of Cardiovascular and Interventional Radiology Standards of Practices Committee. Quality improvement guidelines for adult percutaneous abscess and fluid drainage. J Vasc Interv Radiol 1995; 6:68–70.

Vignati PV, Welch JP, Cohen JL. Long-term management of diverticulitis in young patients. Dis Colon Rectum 1995; 38:627–629.

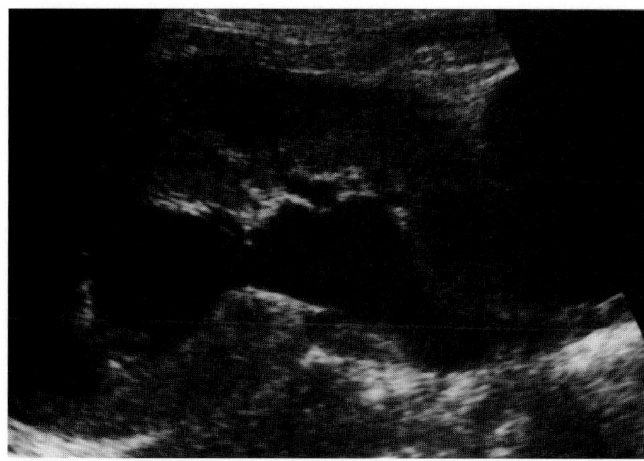

Figure 1. Sonogram of a transplant kidney.

TEACHING FILE CASE 6

Rajiv Sawhney, M.D.

History

A 53-year-old man came to the hospital with lower abdominal and pelvic pain and fullness 5 weeks after a renal transplant. Physical examination revealed discomfort on palpation of the left lower quadrant. The patient was afebrile and his white blood cell count and serum creatinine were not elevated. Sonography was performed **(Fig. 1)**.

What is your diagnosis?

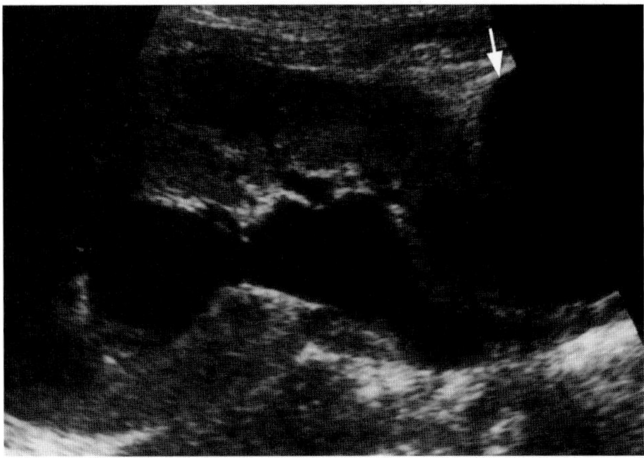

Figure 2. Sonogram shows a lymphocele (arrow) compressing the ureter and causing hydronephrosis in a transplant kidney.

Radiographic Findings

An image from a sonographic study **(Fig. 2)** shows hydronephrosis within the transplant kidney caused by mass effect on the ureter by a fluid collection.

Diagnosis

Postoperative lymphocele causing hydronephrosis.

How would you manage this patient?

Management

The abnormal fluid collection was drained percutaneously with ultrasound-guided placement of a drainage catheter **(Fig. 3)**. The fluid was straw-colored and a sample was sent for Gram stain, culture, and chemistry (urea and creatinine) analysis. The patient was placed on prophylactic antibiotics. The patient returned after 3 days for a sinogram study through the tube **(Fig. 4)**. No fistulous connections were identified. Given the clinical history, the appearance of the fluid, and urea and creatinine values which approximated those of serum, the fluid collection was presumed to represent a lymphocele.

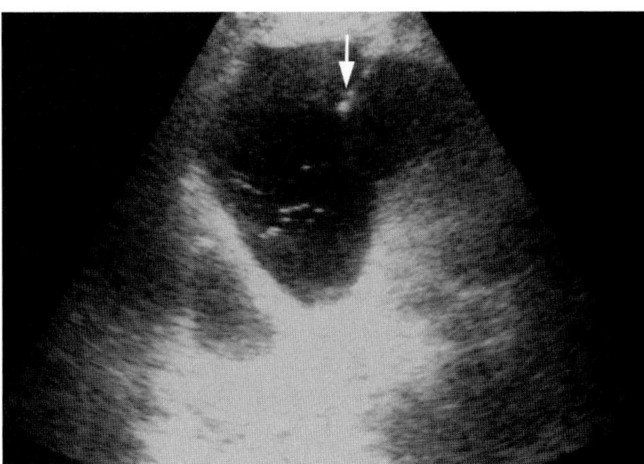

Figure 3. Sonogram shows a needle (arrow) in the lymphocele during ultrasound-guided drainage.

Because lymphoceles usually have prolonged drainage, repeated sessions of percutaneous sclerosis with absolute alcohol were performed. A volume of absolute alcohol approximating one quarter to one half the initial volume of fluid aspirated from the collection was instilled into the lymphocele cavity. Alcohol was retained in the cavity for 30 minutes and then aspirated. The sclerosis sessions were repeated two times per day, three times per week. The catheter was removed when the patient's symptoms resolved and the drainage output decreased to less than 10 mL for 3 days. The duration of percutaneous drainage and sclerosis was 32 days.

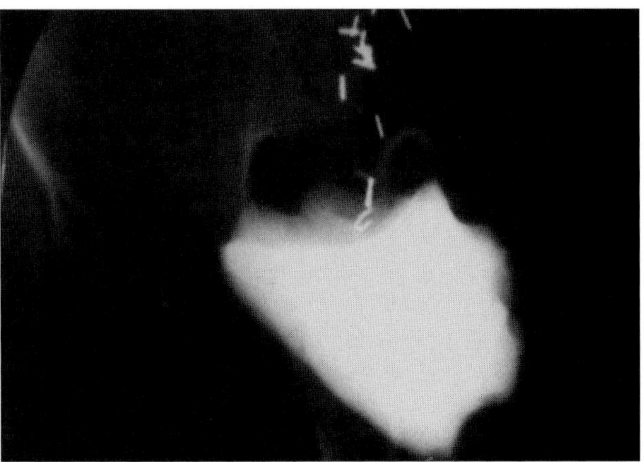

Figure 4. Sinogram obtained before sclerosis shows no fistulous communication.

A follow-up sonogram performed 9 weeks after catheter removal showed no evidence of reaccumulation and no hydronephrosis **(Fig. 5)**. The patient was followed in the Interventional Radiology clinic for 1 year after catheter removal, and no signs or symptoms of recurrence were evident.

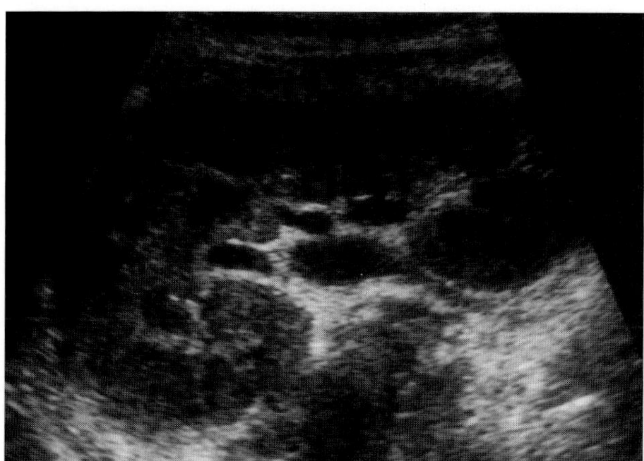

Figure 5. Repeat sonogram obtained 9 weeks after catheter removal shows no recurrence and no hydronephrosis.

Discussion

Fluid collections in the postoperative period can result from a wide variety of etiologies including seromas, urinomas, hematomas, abscesses, and lymphoceles. It is important to review the patient's clinical status and categorize the aspirated fluid to differentiate these possibilities. Hematomas will yield old blood, while abscesses will have turbid fluid and the patient may have signs of infection. A urinoma will show an elevated creatinine in the aspirated fluid relative to the serum creatinine. Fluid from seromas and lymphoceles will be clear and straw-colored like fluid from urinomas but will not have an elevated creatinine. Seromas should not have protracted drainage while lymphoceles will.

Lymphoceles result from injury to the lymphatic channels during surgery and can occur in up to 30% of radical pelvic node dissections and in 20% of renal transplants. Although most are asymptomatic and can resorb, up to 7% will cause symptoms including pain and distention or symptoms referable to compression of adjacent structures. Hydronephrosis from compression of the ureter can occur, as in this case, as can deep venous thrombosis from compression of the iliac or femoral vessels.

Although surgical drainage or marsupialization can have success rates of 90%, they carry with them the risks of surgery. As a result, percutaneous drainage and treatment have become accepted as less invasive means of treating lymphoceles. Percutaneous drainage of lymphoceles is successful but reaccumulation of lymphatic fluid and protracted drainage are expected. In addition, recurrence can follow catheter removal after simple drainage. Sclerosing agents such as tetracycline, alcohol, povidone-iodine, and ampicillin have been used in the hope that they will obliterate the injured lymphatic channels that maintain persistent fluid output and cause recurrence. The use of sclerosing agents with routine catheter drainage of postoperative lymphoceles has increased cure rates from approximately 50%–80% to 80%–100%. Unless the injured lymphatic channels are obliterated with a sclerosant, reaccumulation of the fluid can be expected and a simple aspiration or drainage will not suffice to cure the patient.

The treatment of lymphoceles by percutaneous drainage and sclerosis has been shown to be safe and effective and should be considered instead of surgical treatment. Sterile technique and prophylactic antibiotics are essential to prevent infection. Adequate lymphocele drainage, catheter changes as needed, repeated sclerosis sessions, and adherence to catheter removal criteria assist in preventing recurrence.

Selected Readings

Akhan O, Cekirge S, Ozmen M, Besim A. Percutaneous transcatheter ethanol sclerotherapy of postoperative pelvic lymphoceles. Cardiovasc Intervent Radiol 1992; 15:224–227.

Cohan RH, Saeed M, Schwab SJ, Perlmutt LM, Dunnick NR. Povidone-iodine sclerosis of pelvic lymphoceles: a prospective study. Urol Radiol 1988; 10:203–206.

Conte M, Panici B, Guariglia L, Scambia G, Greggi S, Mancuso S. Pelvic lymphocele following radical para-aortic and pelvic lymphadenectomy for cervical carcinoma: incidence rate and percutaneous management. Obstet Gynecol 1990; 76:268–271.

Gilliland JD, Spies JB, Brown SB, Yrizarry JM, Greenwood LH. Lymphoceles: percutaneous treatment with povidone-iodine sclerosis. Radiology 1989; 171:227–229.

Sawhney R, D'Agostino HB, Zinck S, et al. Treatment of postoperative lymphoceles with percutaneous drainage and alcohol sclerotherapy. J Vasc Interv Radiol 1996; 7:241–245.

Schurawitzki H, Karnel F, Mostbeck G, Langle F, Watschinger B, Hubsch P. Radiologic therapy of symptomatic lymphoceles following kidney transplantation. Rofo Fortschr Geb Rontgenstr Neuen Bildgeb Verfahr 1990; 152:71–75.

Shokeir AA, el-Diasty TA, Ghoneim MA. Percutaneous treatment of lymphocele in renal transplant recipients. J Endourol 1993; 7:481–485.

vanSonnenberg E, Wittich GR, Casola G, et al. Lymphoceles: imaging characteristics and percutaneous management. Radiology 1986; 161:593–596.

White M, Mueller PR, Ferrucci JT, et al. Percutaneous drainage of postoperative abdominal pelvic lymphoceles. AJR 1985; 145:1065–1069.

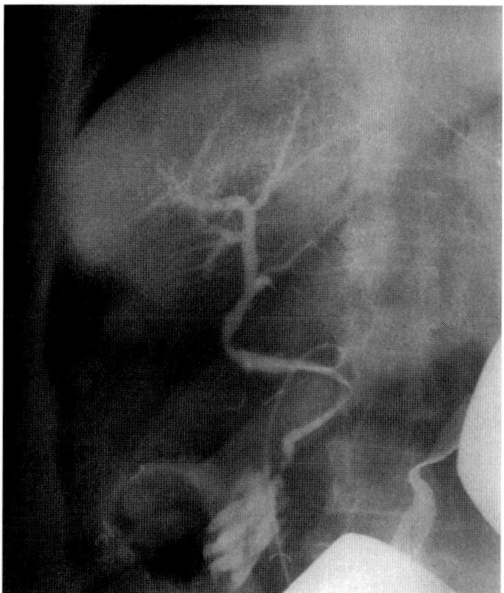

Figure 1. Intraoperative cholangiogram.

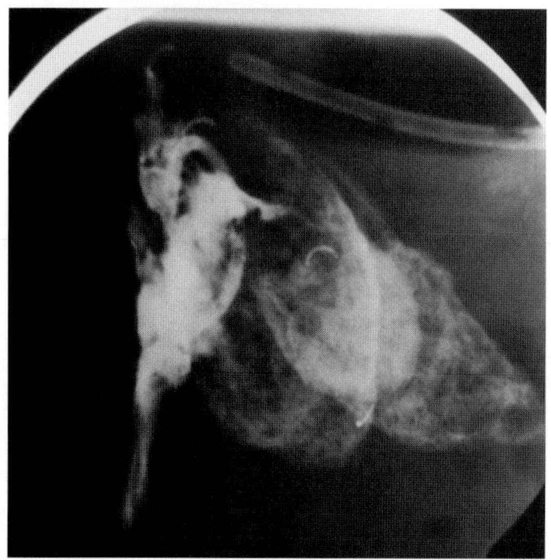

Figure 2. Percutaneous drainage.

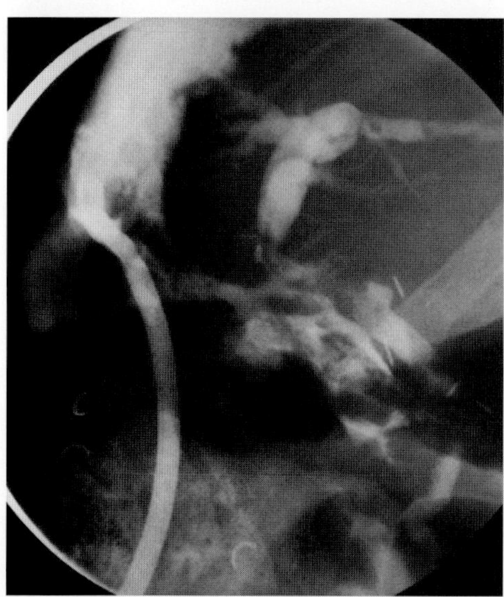

Figure 3. Catheter check/abscessogram.

TEACHING FILE CASE 7

Jeffrey P. Houston, M.D., and Jeffrey S. Pollak, M.D.

History

The patient is a 61-year-old man who underwent a right lobe liver resection for metastatic colon carcinoma. **Figure 1** shows the intraoperative cholangiogram. The patient did well in the immediate postoperative period but developed fevers about 3 weeks later. An ultrasound examination demonstrated a 5-cm x 5-cm x 3-cm complex perihepatic collection. Percutaneous drainage was performed **(Fig. 2)**. The patient continued to have persistent bilious drainage and returned 1 week after the initial drainage for a catheter check and abscessogram **(Fig. 3)**.

What is your diagnosis?

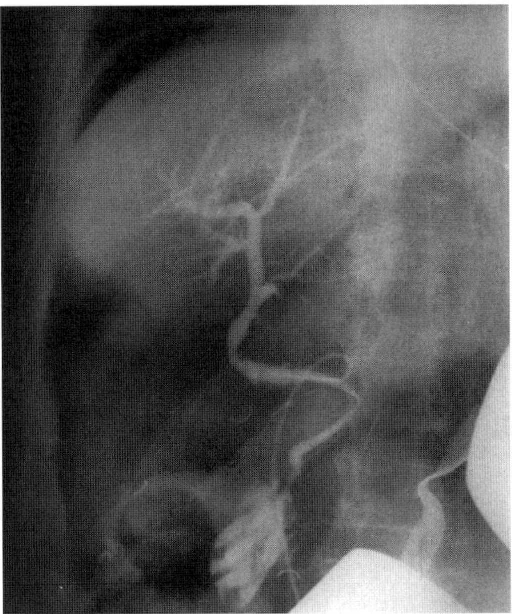

Figure 4. Intraoperative cholangiogram shows patent biliary ducts with no strictures or leaks. Surgical biliary drain and pneumoperitoneum are noted.

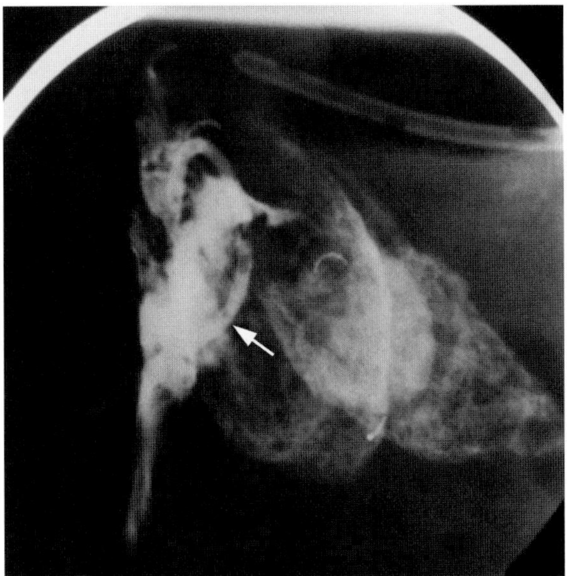

Figure 5. Abscessogram shows the percutaneous pigtail drainage catheter (arrow) within the contrast-filled perihepatic cavity. No communication to the biliary tract is demonstrated.

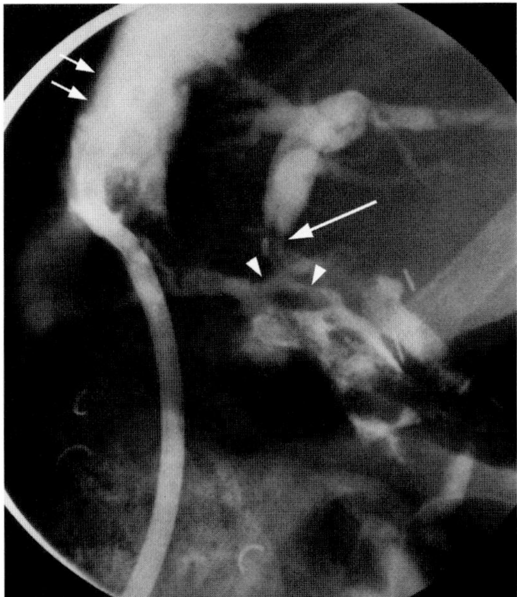

Figure 6. Catheter check/abscessogram shows a new subphrenic collection (arrows), a complex fistula to the common hepatic duct (arrowheads), and a suggestion of common hepatic duct stricture (long arrow).

Radiographic Findings

The intraoperative cholangiogram **(Fig. 4)** demonstrates patent intra- and extrahepatic bile ducts with no evidence of leak or stricture. Percutaneous aspiration and drainage of the complex right upper quadrant collection yielded thick yellow fluid. No fistulous communications are demonstrated on the abscessogram at this time **(Fig. 5)**.

The catheter check and abscessogram demonstrate a new subphrenic collection, a complex fistula to the common hepatic duct, and a suggestion of common hepatic duct stricture **(Fig. 6)**.

Diagnoses

1. Infected biloma (postoperative).
2. Recurrent biloma with extrahepatic biliary fistula.
3. Common hepatic duct stricture.

How would you manage this patient?

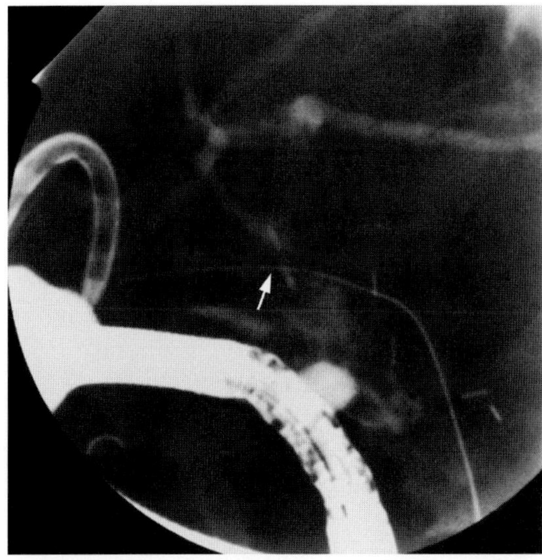

Figure 7. Imaging during ERCP shows the wire exiting the fistulous track (arrow).

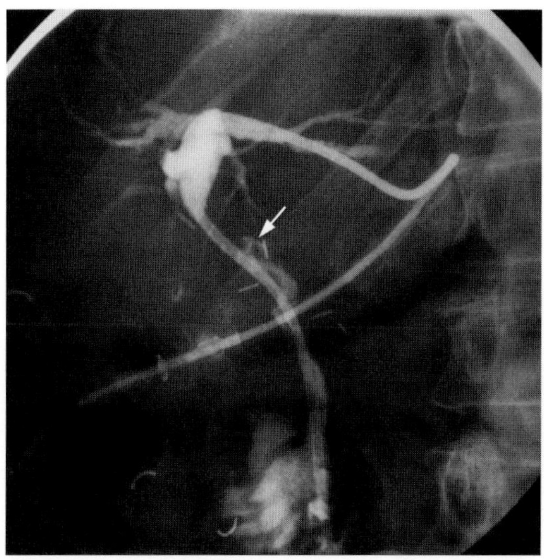

Figure 8. Left PTC and internal/external biliary catheter placement. Injection of contrast material through the biliary catheter only partially fills the complex fistula (arrow), indicating diversion of bile flow.

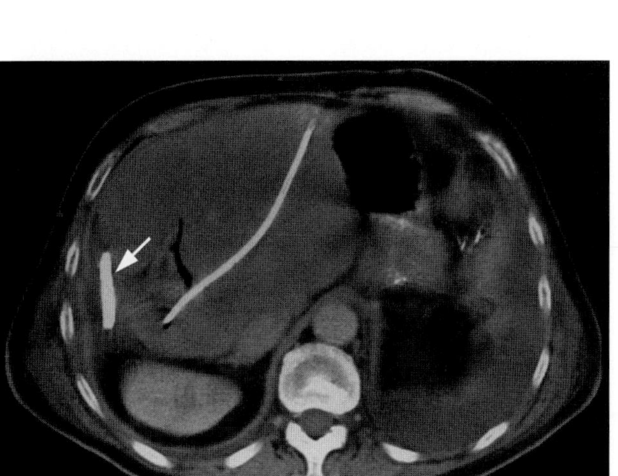

Figure 9. Abdominal CT scan shows the pigtail drainage catheter in the collapsed perihepatic collection (arrow). The percutaneous biliary catheter drain is in place. Pleural effusions and pneumobilia are noted.

Management

Biliary catheter drainage and placement is indicated where there is persistent communication of a biloma with the extrahepatic biliary tree. This patient continued to have significant biloma drainage 10 days after the catheter check, so endoscopic retrograde cholangiopancreatography (ERCP) was performed with attempts to access the central ducts for endoprosthesis placement. Despite multiple passes, attempts to advance past the complex fistula were unsuccessful because the wire preferentially exited the multiple tracts **(Fig. 7)**. Left percutaneous transhepatic cholangiography (PTC) and biliary catheter drainage with an internal/external catheter were performed the following day **(Fig. 8)**. The patient thereafter had decreased biloma drainage and a computed tomography (CT) scan obtained 4 days later showed no significant perihepatic collection **(Fig. 9)**.

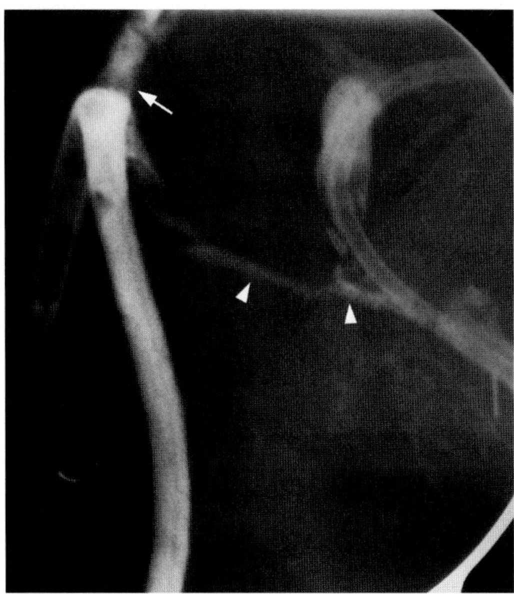

Figure 10. Catheter check and abscessogram show a decreased perihepatic cavity (arrow) and a residual simple fistula (arrowheads).

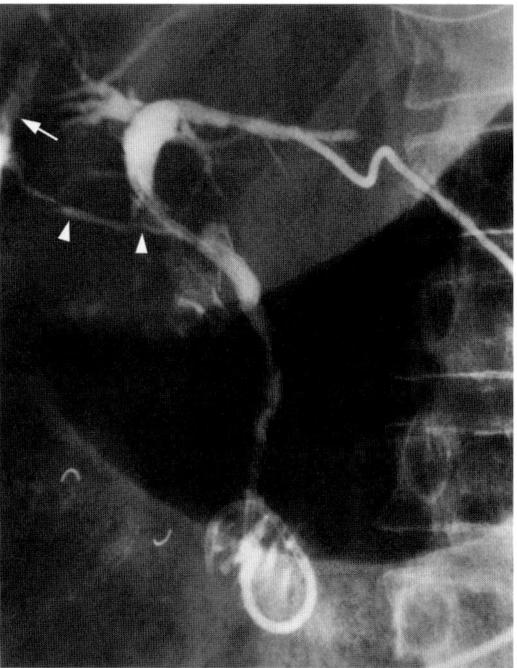

Figure 11. Catheter check and abscessogram show a decreased perihepatic cavity (arrow) and a residual simple fistula (arrowheads).

A follow-up catheter check and abscessogram 1 week later showed a significantly decreased collection and a simple fistula **(Figs. 10, 11)**. Drainage stopped completely 8 days after the catheter check, and the biloma catheter was removed before the patient was discharged home. A pull-back cholangiogram at 1-month follow-up showed no residual fistula and a severe common hepatic duct stricture **(Fig. 12)**. The patient eventually had the stricture percutaneously dilated, and, although he required prolonged catheter stent placement, he did well with this system for over a year until his sudden death from a presumed cardiac event.

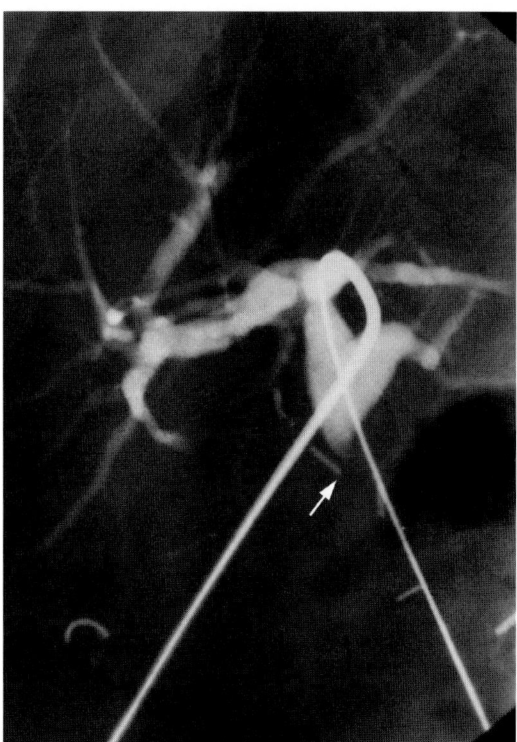

Figure 12. Pull-back cholangiogram shows no residual fistula and a severe common hepatic duct stricture (arrow).

Discussion

Bilomas are localized collections of bile that can be intraparenchymal, subcapsular, or subhepatic in location and can occur as the result of severe liver trauma or complications of hepatobiliary procedures. Bilomas associated with extrahepatic duct injuries may present challenging management issues whether they result from trauma or from complications of hepatobiliary interventions. The classic surgical management of extrahepatic duct injuries is primary reanastomosis or biliary-enteric anastomosis. However, given the technical difficulties of exploring (or re-exploring) the inflamed periportal region, as well as the often critical condition of patients in this population, there is increasing interest in minimally invasive techniques that obviate surgical therapy.

Percutaneous aspiration and drainage under ultrasound-CT guidance fulfills both a diagnostic and therapeutic role in the initial management of bilomas. Injection of contrast material into the biloma cavity is performed to assess communication with the biliary tree. While a biloma may resolve if its fistulous track closes spontaneously, a collection will always recur in the presence of a persistent biliary fistula (especially with a concomitant common duct stricture) **(Fig. 6)**. In delineating the biliary anatomy and demonstrating fistulas and associated duct strictures, PTC serves as the template for percutaneous biliary drainage (PTBD) and catheter stent placement. PTBD and catheter stent placement decompress the biliary system, divert bile flow, and promote fistula closure **(Fig. 8)**. Sequential catheter checks provide radiographic demonstration of biloma cavity resolution and fistula healing. As demonstrated in this case, even complex fistulas will close over time with appropriate percutaneous catheter drainage **(Figs. 10–12)**. Biloma catheter drainage should only be discontinued when there is clinical evidence and/or radiographic documentation of fistula closure. In patients with associated common duct strictures, percutaneous cholangioplasty and prolonged catheter drainage may be performed in attempts to eliminate the need for surgical biliary reconstruction. In those patients requiring definitive surgery, percutaneous biliary drainage allows time for the patient's clinical condition to stabilize and the periportal inflammation to resolve. Moreover, percutaneous catheter placement is surgically advantageous in these patients because the stent provides a technical landmark in an often scarred periportal region.

Selected Readings

Branum G, Schmitt C, Baillie J, et al. Management of major biliary complications after laparoscopic cholecystectomy. Ann Surg 1993; 217(5):532–540.

Fernandez MP, Murphy FB. Hepatic biopsies and fluid drainages. Radiol Clin North Am 1991; 29(6):1311–1328.

Horattas MC, Lewis RD, Fenton AH, Awender HM. Modern concepts in nonsurgical management of traumatic biliary fistulas. J Trauma 1994; 36(2):186–189.

Howdieshell TR, Purvis J, Bates WB, Teeslink CR. Biloma and biliary fistula following hepatorrhaphy for liver trauma: incidence, natural history, and management. Am Surg 1995; 61(2):165–168.

Jurkovich GJ, Hoyt DB, Moore FA, et al. Portal triad injuries. J Trauma 1995; 39(3):426–434.

Kaufman SL. Percutaneous management of operative biliary trauma and fistulas. In: Kadir S, ed. Current practice of interventional radiology. St. Louis: Mosby Year Book, 1991.

Kaufman SL, Kadir S, Mitchell SE, et al. Percutaneous transhepatic biliary drainage for bile leaks and fistulas. AJR 1985; 144:1055–1058.

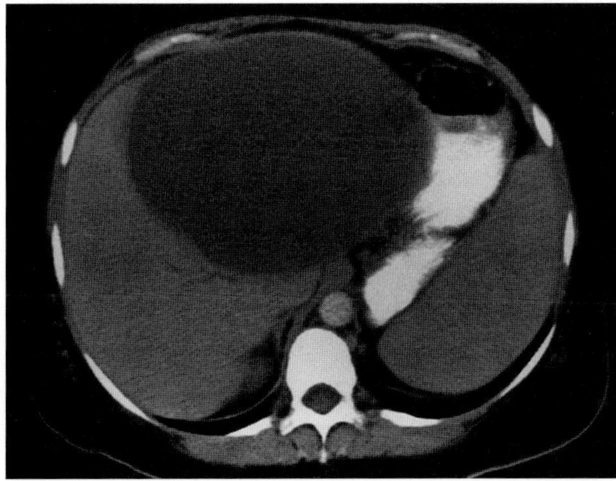

Figure 1. Contrast-enhanced CT scan.

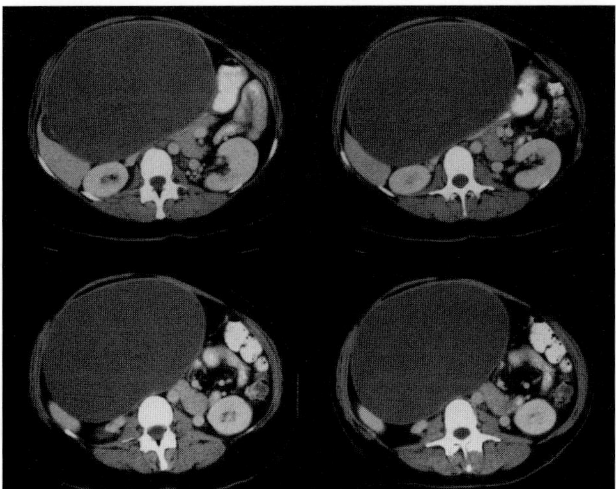

Figure 2. Four lower images from a contrast-enhanced CT scan.

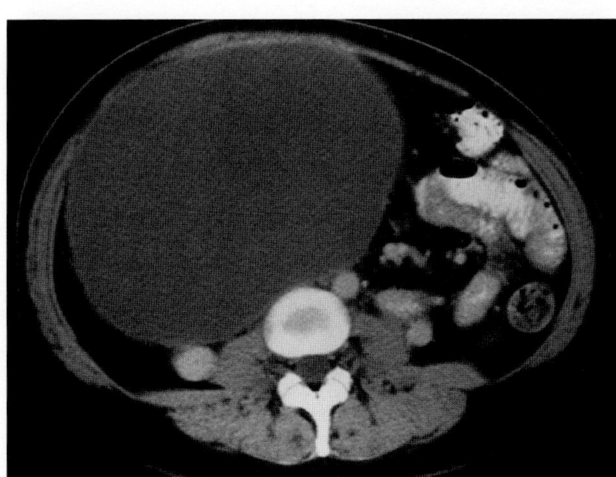

Figure 3. Low abdominal image from a contrast-enhanced CT scan.

TEACHING FILE CASE 8

Jeffrey S. Pollak, M.D.

History

A 42-year-old woman came to the hospital with progressive, worsening upper abdominal discomfort and mild left lower extremity edema. Other than an umbilical hernia repair 2 years earlier and hepatitis A infection 12 years earlier, she had no significant past medical history. Physical examination revealed a midline abdominal mass. Laboratory studies were unremarkable except for mild anemia and minimal elevation of her aspartate and alanine transaminases. A computed tomography (CT) scan was obtained **(Figs. 1–3)**.

What is your diagnosis?

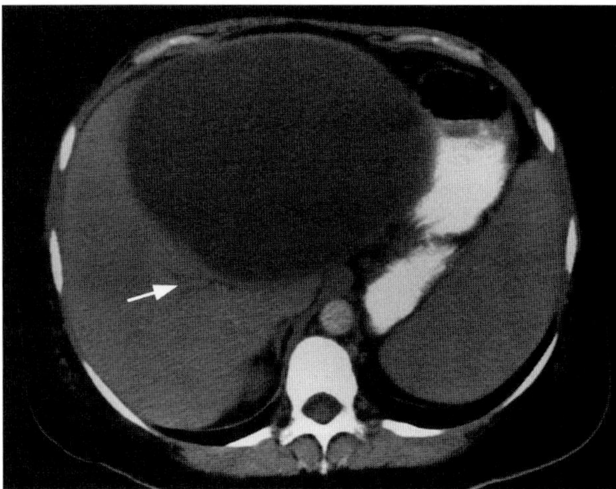

Figure 4. Large, simple cyst originating in the left lobe of the liver, with mild right intrahepatic bile duct dilatation (arrow).

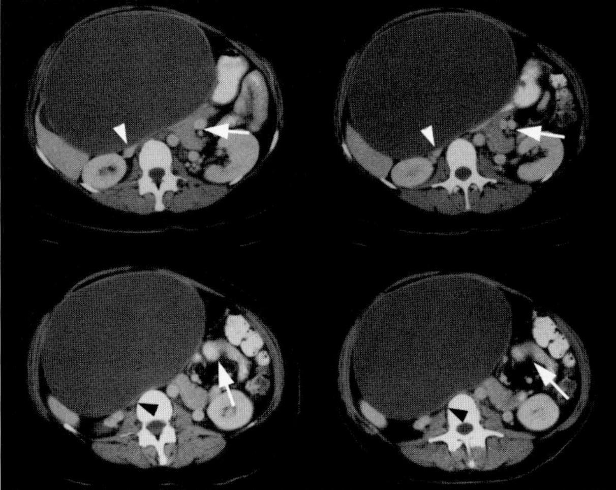

Figure 5. Displacement of the inferior vena cava at the level of the renal vein to the right and posterior (white arrowheads) while the infrarenal cava is completely effaced (black arrowheads at its expected location). Retroperitoneal collateral veins are present. The pancreas and superior mesenteric artery and vein are displaced to the left (arrows).

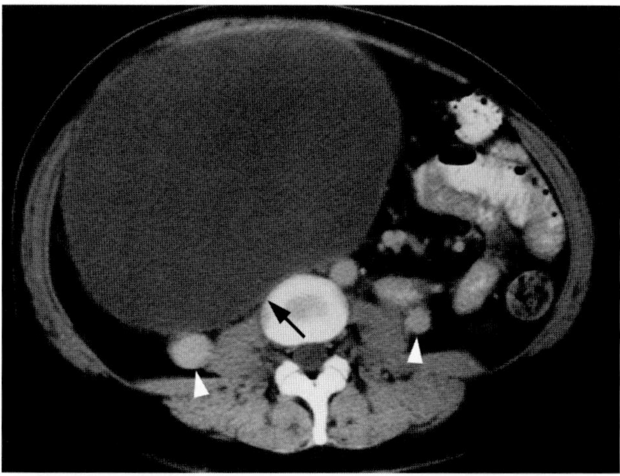

Figure 6. Low abdominal CT image shows complete effacement of the infrarenal inferior vena cava (arrow at its expected location) and retroperitoneal collaterals lateral to the psoas muscles (arrowheads).

Radiographic Findings

The CT scan shows a single, large simple-appearing cyst emanating from the left lobe of the liver **(Fig. 4)** and extending down to the low abdomen **(Figs. 5, 6)**. It has a thin rim and its contents are homogeneous and of low (water density) attenuation. Mild right intrahepatic bile duct dilatation is present **(Fig. 4)**.The inferior vena cava is displaced to the right and posteriorly at the renal level **(Fig. 5)**, while the infrarenal inferior vena cava is completely effaced **(Figs. 5, 6)**. Enlarged retroperitoneal venous collaterals are present lateral to the psoas muscles. The pancreas and superior mesenteric vessels are displaced to the left **(Fig. 5)**.

Diagnosis

Symptomatic simple congenital hepatic cyst.

How would you manage this patient?

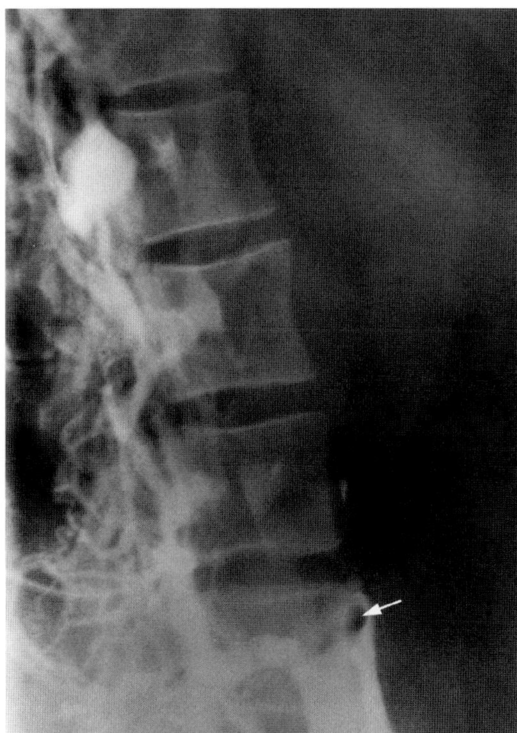

Figure 7. Filling defect representing thrombus in the low inferior vena cava (arrow), below the region of compression. Numerous retroperitoneal collaterals are present.

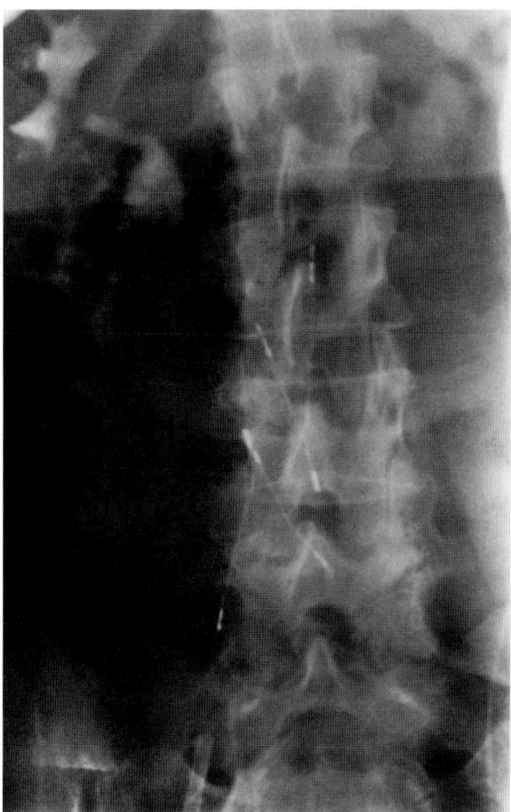

Figure 8. Bird's Nest Filter in the compressed region of the infrarenal inferior vena cava, above the thrombus.

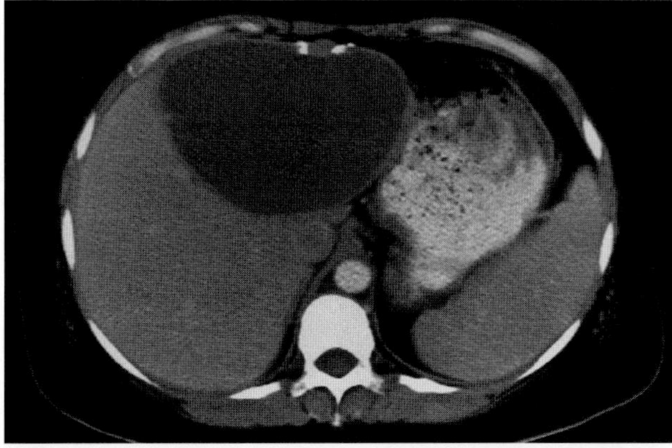

Figure 9. CT scan shows significant reduction in cyst size 3 months after surgery.

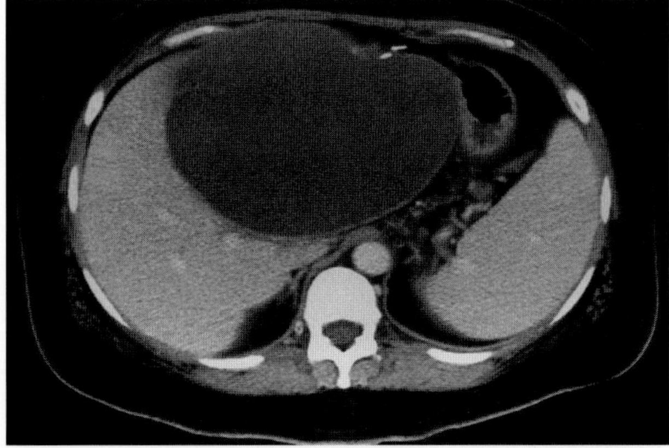

Figure 10. CT scan shows marked enlargement in cyst size 1 year after surgery.

Management

Prior to the surgical marsupialization, the patient underwent transfemoral venography to assess for thrombus in the static venous segments below the compressed vena cava because the CT scan was inconclusive for thrombus in this region. Indeed, a filling defect was identified in the low inferior vena cava **(Fig. 7)**. A Bird's Nest Filter (Cook, Bloomington, IN) was placed from a jugular venous approach into the compressed infrarenal inferior vena cava above the thrombus to prevent embolization after cyst decompression **(Fig. 8)**. The patient underwent laparoscopic drainage and marsupialization of the cyst 4 days later. The cyst appeared much smaller on a CT scan obtained 3 months later **(Fig. 9)**, but the patient returned 1 year later with recurrent abdominal discomfort and marked enlargement of the cyst remnant **(Fig. 10)**.

How could this patient be managed now?

Management: Transcatheter Cyst Alcohol Sclerotherapy

This time, the patient underwent transcatheter alcohol sclerotherapy. Under ultrasound guidance, a window to the cyst was located along the right mid axillary line **(Fig. 11)**. The window traversed a small portion of hepatic parenchyma yet avoided vascular structures and the gallbladder. An 8-F drainage catheter was placed into the cyst with use of standard techniques, and 1,400 mL of serous, brown-colored fluid was removed. Subsequently, 400 mL of contrast material was injected and the patient was asked to roll 360 degrees **(Figs. 12, 13)**. The contrast material was entirely contained by the cyst, with no fistula to the biliary tree, the peritoneum, or the blood stream.

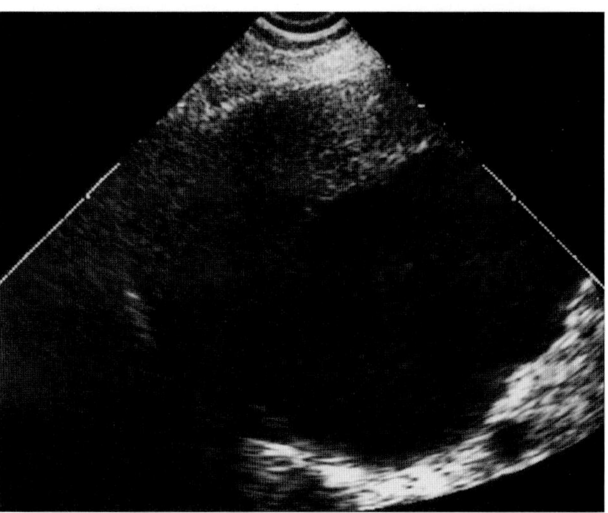

Figure 11. Ultrasound shows a route to the cyst traversing several centimeters of the liver.

After draining the contrast material, 50 mL of 1% lidocaine was instilled for 10 minutes, with the patient spending time in different positions. The lidocaine was then drained and 250 mL of absolute alcohol was injected. The alcohol was retained for 30 minutes, during which time the patient spent several minutes each in the supine, prone, and right and left lateral decubitus positions. The catheter was left to external drainage and the patient was sent home. She returned for three more instillations of alcohol over the next week, after which the drainage was scant. **Figure 14** shows the reduced size of the cyst prior to the fourth treatment. The tube was clamped at that time. A CT scan obtained several days later **(Fig. 15)** showed marked reduction in the cyst size. The drain was removed and the patient remained asymptomatic at 18 months follow-up. In fact, an ultrasound at that time showed no remnant of the cyst. Cytology of the fluid showed red blood cells but no malignant cells. A culture was negative.

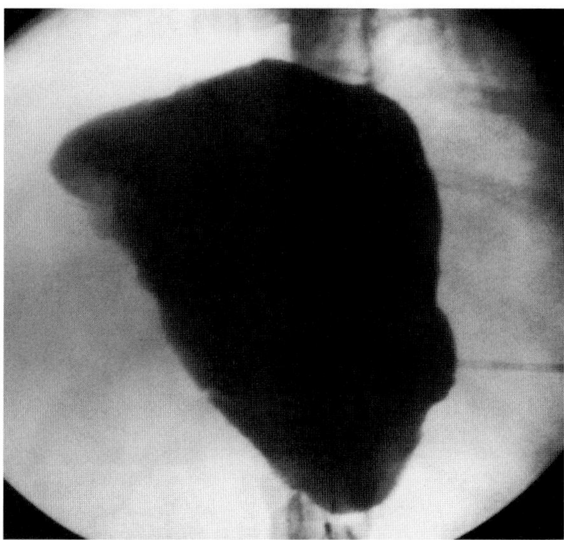

Figure 12. Prone view of the contrast cystogram. No communication to other structures can be seen.

Discussion

Congenital hepatic cysts are believed to arise from developmental defects in the formation of bile ducts. Congenital cysts result from dilatation of these biliary microhamartomas. Histologically, they contain cuboidal bile duct epithelium with secretory capabilities, which accounts for the fluid in the simple cysts. These cysts are found in approximately 2.5% of cross-sectional studies, although the incidence of symptomatic cysts is far less—16.8% of all cysts in a surgically diagnosed series were symptomatic. They appear to be more common in women and may be single or multiple. Multiple hepatic cysts may be associated with autosomal dominant polycystic kidney disease and von Hippel-Lindau disease.

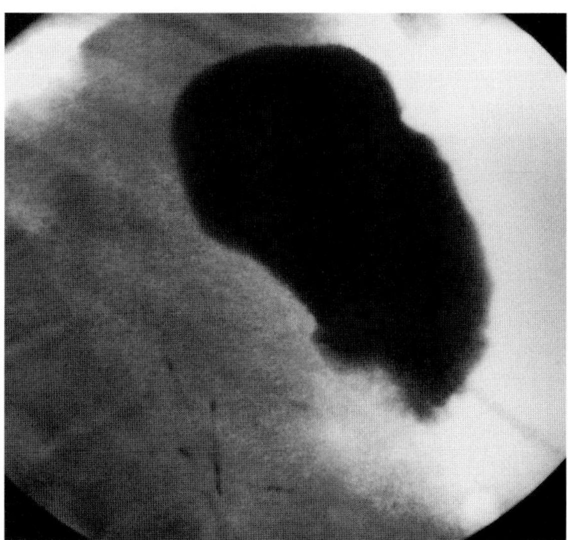

Figure 13. Left-side-down view of the contrast cystogram. Again, no communication to other structures can be seen.

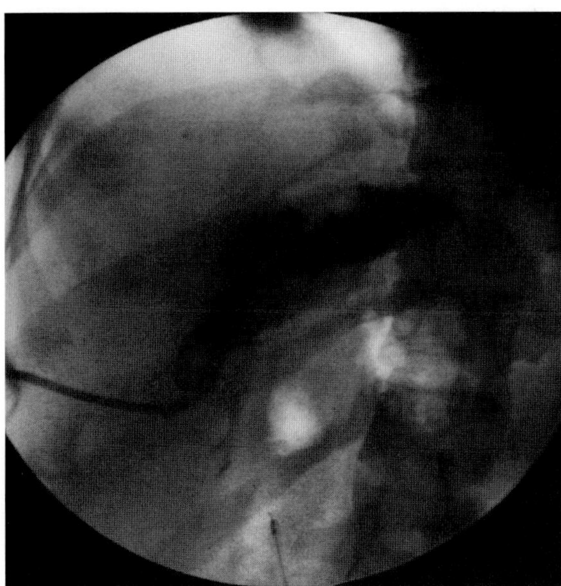

Figure 14. Reduced cyst size on a contrast study prior to the fourth session of alcohol sclerotherapy.

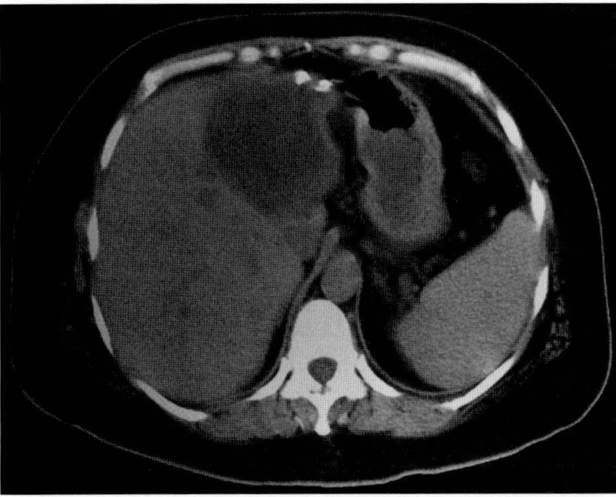

Figure 15. CT scan several days after clamping the drain shows marked reduction in the size of the cyst.

The diagnosis of a simple cyst depends on the characteristic findings on cross-sectional studies: imperceptibly thin walls, anechoic with enhanced through-transmission on ultrasonography, and homogeneous water-density attenuation with no mural enhancement on CT scanning. Echinococcal cysts, amebic cysts, and abscesses occasionally have a similar appearance, although laboratory tests and the clinical picture are usually revealing. More characteristic findings of hydatid disease are detached membranes, mural calcification, multiseptation, and daughter cysts. Abscesses generally have attenuation greater than water density and have enhancing walls. The other major differential diagnoses are hematoma, biliary cystadenoma, and cystic or necrotic metastatic tumors. This patient had no history of trauma or tumor.

Symptoms generally arise in adults rather than children because of the slow rate of cyst growth. Clinical effects appear to be related to pressure within the cyst, pressure on surrounding structures, or hepatomegaly. Because the hepatic parenchyma is preserved and remains normal, even large cysts only rarely result in liver failure or hepatic decompensation. More common symptoms are the presence of an abdominal mass, abdominal distention, and abdominal discomfort or pain, although other manifestations include jaundice from biliary obstruction, early satiety from bowel compression, weight loss, respiratory compromise, portal hypertension leading to esophageal varices and bleeding, and cyst infection, which can be lethal. Compression of the inferior vena cava or hepatic veins (with Budd-Chiari syndrome) is an unusual but serious complication and may be accompanied by thrombosis, as in this case.

Surgical options for treating symptomatic cysts include fenestration, unroofing, cyst resection, partial liver resection, marsupialization to the peritoneum, drainage to a Roux-en-Y jejunal loop, and even transplantation. However, there is a very high incidence of cyst recurrence despite repeated surgical interventions because the secretory epithelium of the cyst is still present. Percutaneous treatment should be considered the primary modality for symptomatic simple hepatic cysts, with catheter drainage and sclerosis as the primary techniques. These offer the advantages of being minimally invasive and easily repeated for persistent, recurrent, or newly symptomatic cysts. Additionally, percutaneous therapy can be done on an outpatient basis. Alternative percutaneous treatments include needle aspiration and catheter drainage without sclerotherapy. Although these options may reduce the cyst size, the cyst will recur because the epithelial lining of the cyst has not been addressed.

Access to the cyst can be obtained under ultrasound or CT guidance, and choosing a route through a small portion of the liver reduces the risk of inadvertent spillage into the peritoneum of the cyst contents or fluids instilled into the cyst. Simple cyst aspiration has been shown to be ineffective, with nearly uniform reaccumulation and a high incidence of recurrent symptoms. Consequently, sclerosis with various agents has been proposed. Most commonly, 95% alcohol or absolute alcohol has been used, although other agents that have been proposed or tried are tetracycline, minocycline chloride, doxycycline, formaldehyde, and Pantopaque (Lafayette Pharmaceutical, Inc., Lafayette, IN).

Technique

Before the sclerosant is given, contrast material is injected and the patient rolled 360 degrees to assess for communication to other structures, such as the biliary tract, peritoneal cavity, or blood stream. A communication is a contraindication to therapy because of the risks of sclerosing cholangitis, peritonitis, thrombosis, and cardiac toxicity. After the contrast material is removed, lidocaine is instilled and retained for approximately 10 minutes, after which the sclerosing agent is administered. Most series using alcohol report instillation of as little as 10 mL to as much as one half the volume removed, usually retaining the fluid for 20 to 30 minutes. Leaving a drainage catheter in place facilitates the multiple instillations that are often needed, especially in large cysts; however, before placing a drain, it should be ascertained that the drain will not be degraded by the sclerosant. More than one instillation can be given on the first day and repeat sessions can be done every 1–3 days. A drop in catheter drainage to scant amounts is the end point of therapy and suggests a good prognosis. A follow-up imaging study can be obtained several days after clamping the tube to evaluate for reaccumulation while a route for further therapy remains in place, or a study can be done several weeks after removing the tube.

Excellent results have also been obtained with single-session sclerotherapy. The cyst is assessed in the routine fashion. Absolute alcohol in a volume of one third the cyst volume (maximum of 100 mL of alcohol) is administered and allowed to contact all surfaces of the cyst for 20 minutes. This procedure is repeated twice for cysts smaller than 400 mL and three times for larger cysts. After the final instillation, the catheter is removed and after appropriate monitoring, the patient is discharged home. Single-session sclerotherapy has had a reported response rate of 97%.

Sclerotherapy is successful in reducing cyst size significantly and alleviating or improving symptoms in 78%–100% of cases. Factors that limit the effectiveness of sclerotherapy include the presence of a bleeding disorder contraindicating cyst puncture, numerous cysts with no dominant one(s) clearly responsible for the clinical manifestations, a cystic tumor masquerading as a simple cyst, insufficient dwell time for the sclerosant, insufficient sclerosant volume (permitting the agent to be diluted by residual cyst fluid), and an inadequate number of sclerosis sessions. Communication of the cyst with other internal structures appears to be quite rare.

Complications

Complications arise from the procedure to access the cyst or from the effects of the sclerosant. Pain during the instillation of alcohol is common and presumably caused by pericatheter leakage to the peritoneum. It usually subsides within several minutes after the injection is stopped and appears to be reduced by prior instillation of lidocaine. If pain limits the administration of a sufficient volume of alcohol despite an unremarkable contrast cystogram, switching to another agent may be helpful. Less common adverse events are a low-grade fever, hemorrhage into the cyst, mild intoxication, pneumothorax, pleural effusion, and secondary cyst infection.

Selected Readings

Andersson R, Jeppsson B, Lunderquist A, Bengmark S. Alcohol sclerotherapy of nonparasitic cysts of the liver. Br J Surg 1989; 76:254–255

Bean WJ, Rodan BA. Hepatic cysts: treatment with alcohol. AJR 1985; 144:237–241.

Kairaluoma MI, Leinonen A, Stahlberg M, Paivansalo M, Kiviniemi H, Siniluoto T. Percutaneous aspiration and alcohol sclerotherapy for symptomatic hepatic cysts: an alternative to surgical intervention. Ann Surg 1989; 210:208–215.

Newman KD, Torres VE, Rakela J, Nagorney DM. Treatment of highly symptomatic polycystic liver disease. Preliminary experience with a combined hepatic resection-fenestration procedure. Ann Surg 1990; 212:30–37.

Saini S, Mueller PR, Ferrucci JT Jr, Simeone JF, Wittenberg J, Butch RJ. Percutaneous aspiration of hepatic cysts does not provide definitive therapy. AJR 1983; 141:559–560.

Simonetti G, Profili S, Sergiacomi GL, Meloni GB, Orlacchio A. Percutaneous treatment of hepatic cysts by aspiration and sclerotherapy. Cardiovasc Intervent Radiol 1993; 16:81–84.

Tikkakoski T, Mäkelä JT, Leinonen S, et al. Treatment of symptomatic congenital hepatic cysts with single-session percutaneous drainage and ethanol sclerosis: technique and outcome. J Vasc Interv Radiol 1996; 7:235–239.

Torres VE, Rastogi S, King BF, Stanson AW, Gross JB Jr, Nogorney DM. Hepatic venous outflow obstruction in autosomal dominant polycystic kidney disease. J Am Soc Nephrol 1994; 5:1186–1192.

vanSonnenberg E, Wroblicka JT, D'Agostino HB, et al. Symptomatic hepatic cysts: percutaneous drainage and sclerosis. Radiology 1994; 190:387–392.

Yaqoob M, Saffman C, Finn R, Carty AT. Inferior vena caval compression by hepatic cysts: an unusual complication of adult polycystic kidney disease. Nephron 1990; 54:89–91.

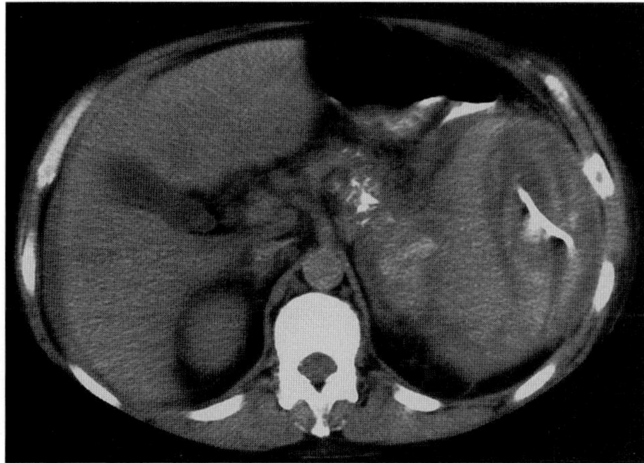

Figure 1. Noncontrast abdominal CT scan.

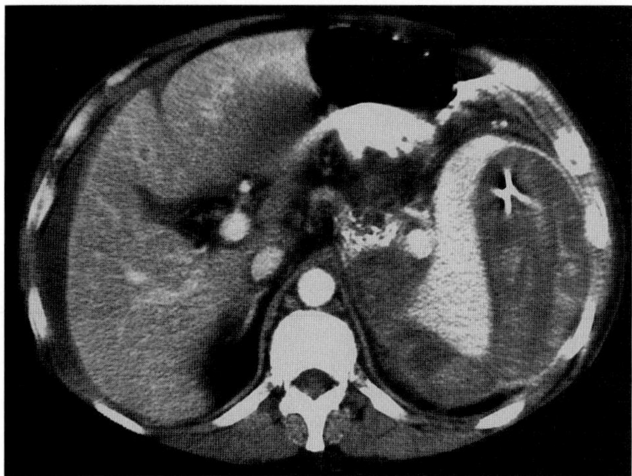

Figure 2. Contrast-enhanced abdominal CT scan.

TEACHING FILE CASE 9

Albert A. Nemcek, Jr., M.D., and Robert L. Vogelzang, M.D.

History

The referring medical service obtained noncontrast **(Fig. 1)** and contrast-enhanced **(Fig. 2)** computed tomography (CT) scans on a 52-year-old man with complicated pancreatitis. The patient had had a drain placed in a perisplenic collection, which drained culture-negative black fluid. The service states that the patient is doing worse, with persistent fevers and hypotension, and asks if there is "something else to drain."

What is your diagnosis?

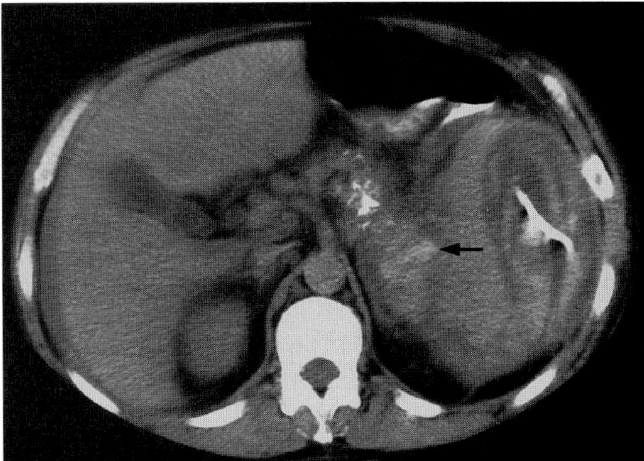

Figure 3. Noncontrast CT scan shows a mixed-attenuation collection in the left upper quadrant suggestive of hemorrhage. The tip of the drainage catheter is in the perisplenic fluid collection. Note the high-density structure just medial to the collection (arrow).

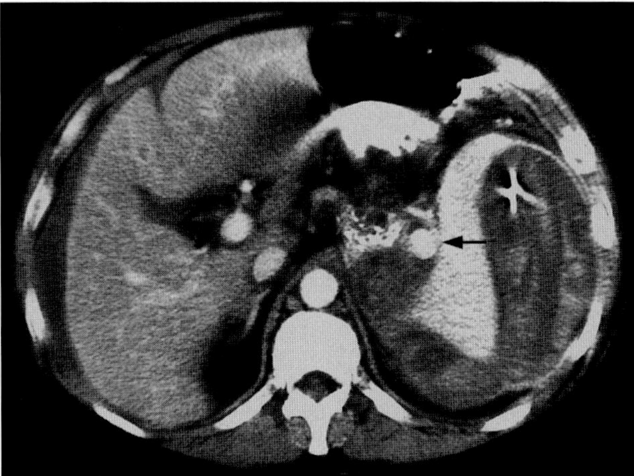

Figure 4. Contrast-enhanced CT scan shows enhancement of the pseudoaneurysm (arrow).

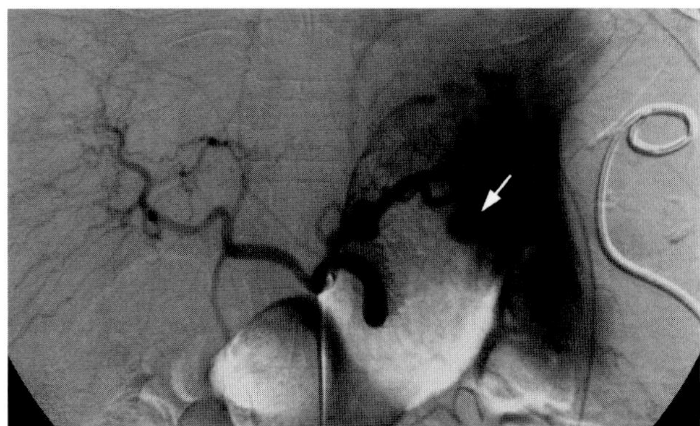

Figure 5. Selective celiac arteriogram shows a pseudoaneurysm (arrow).

Radiographic Findings

The CT scan shows a lateral perisplenic collection with heterogeneous density suggesting a hemorrhage within the collection. A rounded, relatively high density structure medial to the spleen shows contrast enhancement, is larger than adjacent blood vessels, and appears to be surrounded by hemorrhage **(Figs. 3, 4)**. The suspicion was raised that a pseudoaneurysm had developed as a consequence of pancreatitis, and visceral arteriography was recommended. Selective celiac **(Fig. 5)** and subselective splenic **(Fig. 6)** arteriography reveals a focal, round accumulation of contrast material arising from splenic artery branches. It begins to opacify as the splenic artery branches opacify, fills in with contrast material, and remains opacified on late films.

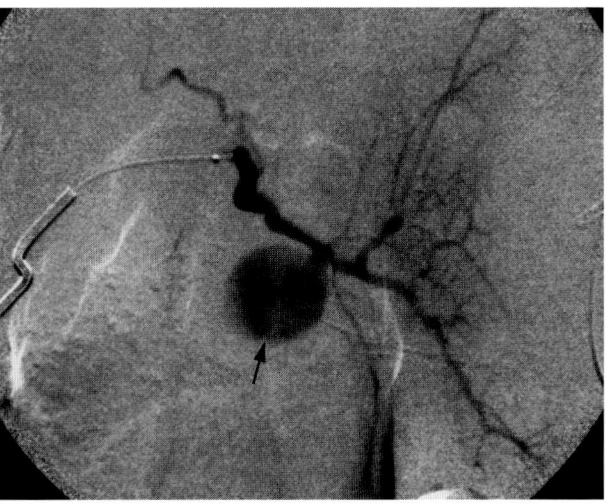

Figure 6. Subselective splenic branch arteriogram shows the pseudoaneurysm to better advantage (arrow).

Diagnosis

Splenic branch pseudoaneurysm.

What treatment would you recommend?

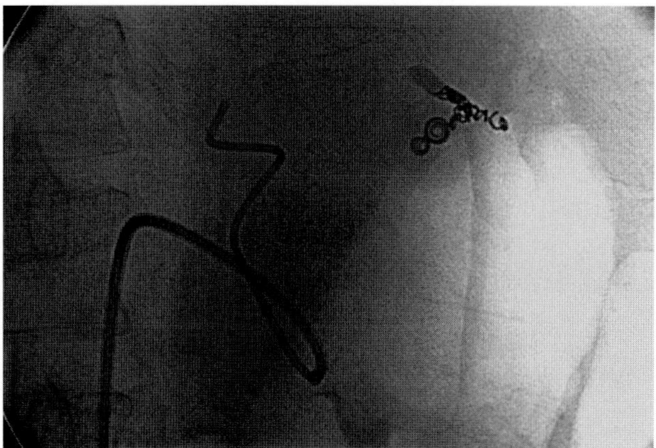

Figure 7. Spot film shows coils in the splenic artery branch.

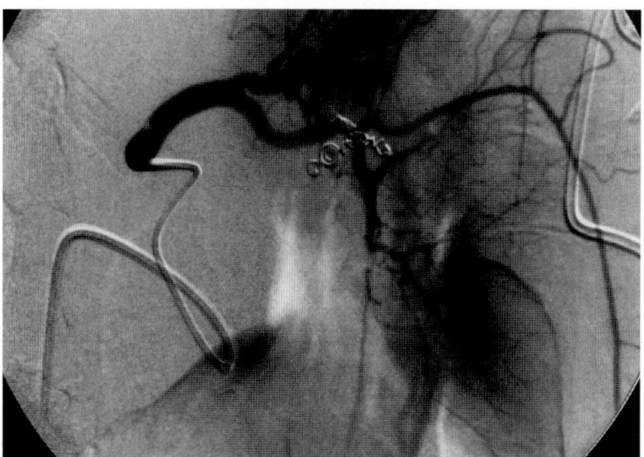

Figure 8. Postembolization splenic arteriogram. The pseudoaneurysm is no longer seen.

Management

Transcatheter embolization is generally the preferred therapy for this complication. In this case, a microcatheter was placed coaxially into the splenic arterial branch feeding the pseudoaneurysm. Several helical fibered microcoils were then placed, bridging and entering the neck of the pseudoaneurysm **(Fig. 7)**; postembolization arteriography shows no further opacification of the lesion **(Fig. 8)**. The patient's hemoglobin and hematocrit stabilized.

Discussion

Vascular lesions such as pseudoaneurysms are well-recognized complications of acute pancreatitis. They result from the digestive effect of pancreatic enzymes on the walls of peripancreatic blood vessels. Interventional radiologists should maintain a high level of suspicion for such lesions, not only because they may rupture if left untreated, but also because drainage of a "pancreatic fluid collection" complicated by a hemorrhagic lesion may unleash catastrophic bleeding. Suspicion for pseudoaneurysm may be based upon imaging studies (as in this case), endoscopic demonstration of bleeding from the pancreatic duct, or clinical data suggesting hemorrhage. Arteriography is the procedure of choice for demonstrating these pseudoaneurysms.

Treatment is mandatory because pseudoaneurysms may rupture and result in life-threatening hemorrhage. Therapeutic options include both surgical repair and transcatheter embolization. Transcatheter embolotherapy is generally preferred. If successful, it may obviate the need for any further therapy, and even if surgery is required for other reasons the procedure may help stabilize the patient and improve surgical risk.

Permanent agents such as metallic coils or detachable balloons should be used. Ideally, embolization should obliterate the pseudoaneurysm but leave the feeding vessel patent. In practice, however, this may prove difficult, and treatment consists of cutting off the pseudoaneurysm from its blood supply by placing embolic agents across its orifice.

A complication of embolization is infarction of organs supplied by the bleeding vessel; avoiding the use of small particulate or liquid agents and placing the embolic agents carefully can minimize this complication. Other potential complications include rupture of the pseudoaneurysm during arteriography, damage to selectively catheterized vessels, and other standard complications of arteriography such as puncture site hematoma or thrombosis.

Selected Readings

Boudghéne F, L'Herminé C, Bigot JM. Arterial complications of pancreatitis: diagnostic and therapeutic aspects in 104 cases. J Vasc Interv Radiol 1993; 4:551–558.

Lee MJ, Saini S, Geller SC, Warshaw AL, Mueller PR. Pancreatitis with pseudoaneurysm formation: a pitfall for the interventional radiologist. AJR 1991; 156:97–98.

Mauro MA, Jaques P. Transcatheter management of pseudoaneurysms complicating pancreatitis. J Vasc Interv Radiol 1991; 2:527–532.

Vujic I. Vascular complications of pancreatitis. Radiol Clin North Am 1989; 27:81–91.

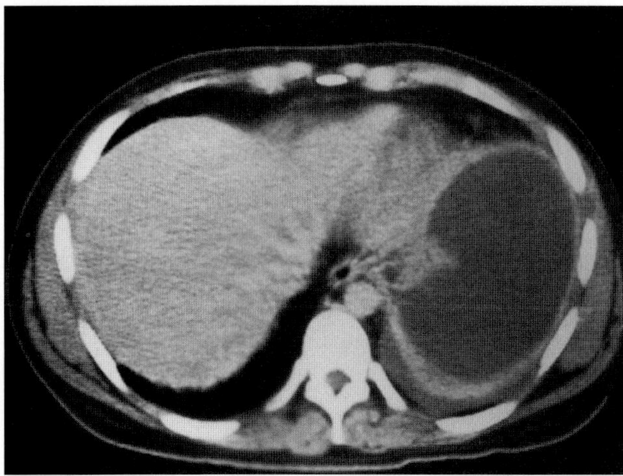

Figure 1. Postoperative abdominal computed tomography scan.

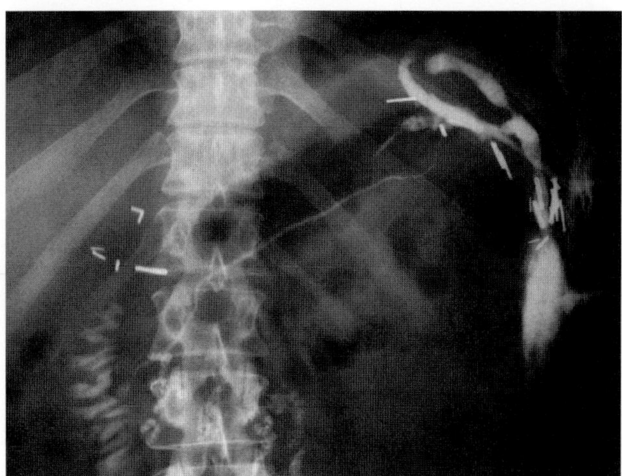

Figure 2. Tube check 6 weeks after drainage of a left upper quadrant fluid collection.

TEACHING FILE CASE 10

Albert A. Nemcek, Jr., M.D., and Robert L. Vogelzang, M.D.

History

An elderly man with a history of lymphoma developed a left upper quadrant fluid collection following splenectomy **(Fig. 1)**. This was drained because of pain and a suspicion of infection. After drainage, output from the catheter was more than 100 mL per day. A tube check was performed 6 weeks after the initial drainage **(Fig. 2)**.

What is your diagnosis?

Radiographic Findings

A fluid collection is present in the splenic bed **(Fig. 3)**. After drainage, the left upper quadrant cavity has diminished significantly in size. However, communication with the pancreatic duct is demonstrated **(Fig. 4)**. The duct shows no gross evidence of obstruction, and contrast material flows into the duodenum.

Diagnosis

Fistula from pseudocyst to the pancreatic duct.

How would you manage this patient?

Management

The management of pancreatic fistulas depends on several factors, including the site of communication; the status of the pancreatic duct, which can be evaluated by catheter sinograms or endoscopic retrograde cholangiopancreatography; the patient's overall clinical status, including nutritional status; the etiology of the fistula; and the amount of drainage. In this case, no evidence of antecedent or current pancreatitis was seen. The cause was presumably iatrogenic trauma to the pancreatic tail during surgery. The pancreatic duct appeared normal. The fistula was managed conservatively with continued catheter drainage and intermittent prophylactic tube changes. The tube output gradually decreased and finally ceased. About 1 year after the initial drainage, a repeat sinogram revealed no residual fistula **(Fig. 5)**. The catheter was removed and the patient had no recurrent fluid accumulation.

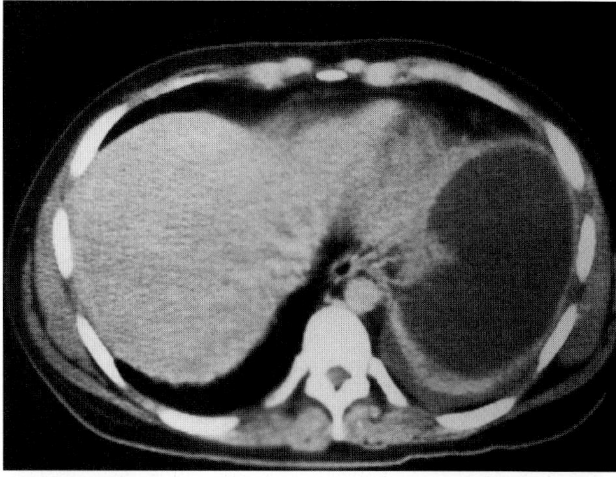

Figure 3. CT scan shows a large low-density collection in the left upper quadrant.

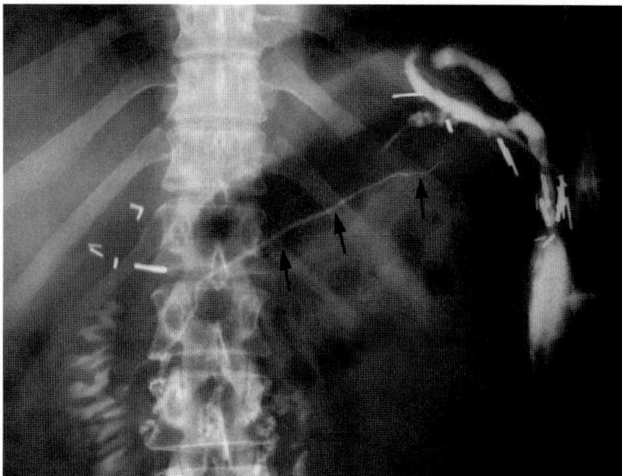

Figure 4. Catheter sinogram demonstrates a fistula to the pancreatic duct (arrows).

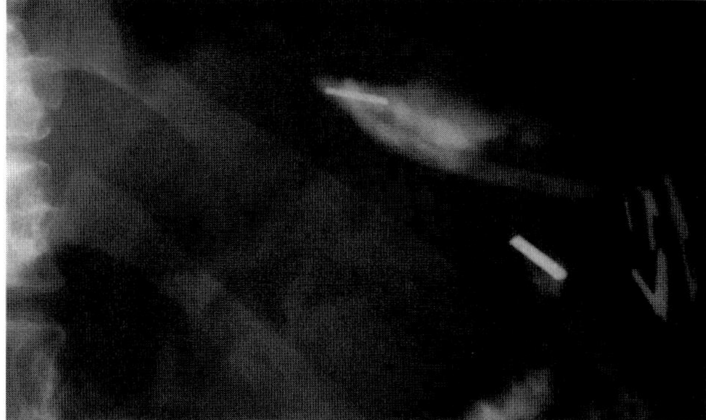

Figure 5. Catheter sinogram after prolonged drainage demonstrates closure of the fistula.

Discussion

Although it frequently cannot be demonstrated on initial imaging studies, communication between the pancreatic duct and an externally drained pancreatic fluid collection is common and readily seen on follow-up studies. Continued drainage is usually sufficient to treat these fistulas, and further complications generally do not develop. However, when a fistula is present prolonged drainage is usually required. Ultimate closure of the fistula depends on the factors discussed above and others. Factors which make closure unlikely include transection of the pancreatic duct, obstruction or significant narrowing of the duct, persistent inflammation or infection, poor patient nutrition, and high-dose steroid therapy. With a widely patent duct and no other complicating factors, the success rate of drainage is reported to exceed 90%.

Management of fistulas includes both optimization of drainage and treatment of underlying predisposing causes (by surgical, endoscopic, or radiologic methods). Pancreatic "rest," achieved by administering either a low-fat diet or total parenteral nutrition, may be helpful. Finally, octreotide, a synthetic somatostatin analog, may be given to reduce pancreatic exocrine function. Specifically, it decreases the secretion of secretin and cholecystokinin. It is administered by subcutaneous injection at doses of 100–500 mcg three times daily.

Selected Readings

D'Agostino HB, Fotoohi M, Aspron MM, Oglevie S, Kinney T, Rose S. Percutaneous drainage of pancreatic fluid collections. Semin Intervent Radiol 1996; 13:101–136.

Freeny PC. Percutaneous management of pancreatic fluid collections. Baillieres Clin Gastroenterol 1992; 6:259–272.

Freeny PC, Lewis GP, Traverso LW, Ryan JA. Infected pancreatic fluid collections: percutaneous catheter drainage. Radiology 1988; 167:435–441.

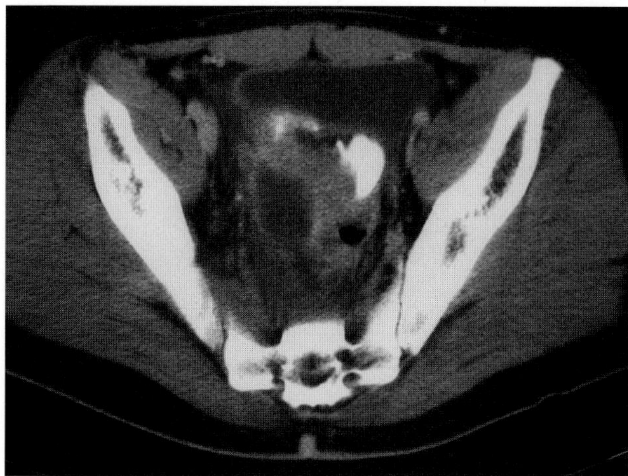

Figure 1. CT scan of pelvic abscess.

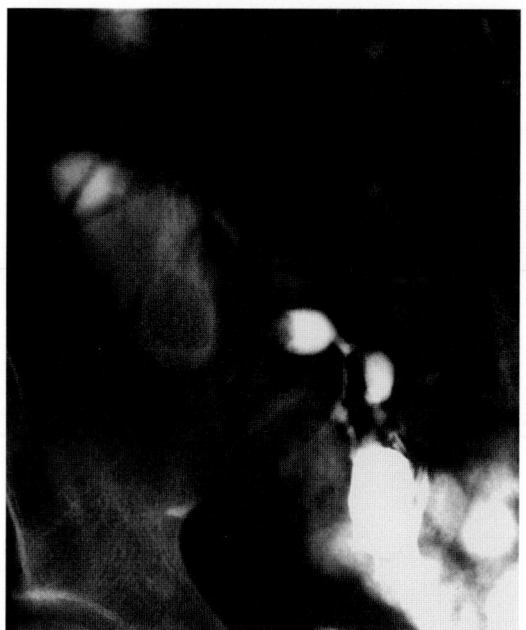

Figure 2. Tube check after transrectal pelvic abscess drainage.

TEACHING FILE CASE 11

Jeet Sandhu, M.D.

History

The patient is a 26-year-old man who underwent transrectal drainage of a pelvic abscess **(Fig. 1)** with placement of an 8-F Cope loop drainage catheter. Five days after initial catheter placement, a sinogram was obtained **(Fig. 2)**.

What is your diagnosis?

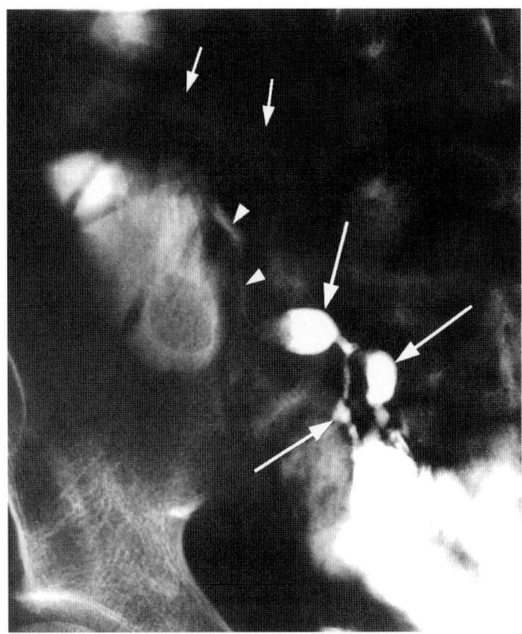

Figure 3. Tube sinogram shows fistulous communications (long arrows) to the appendix (arrowheads) with eventual filling of the cecum. The terminal ileum (arrows) is identified separate from the fistula and appendix.

Radiographic Findings

The tube check indicates that the cavity has resolved and is the same size as the Cope loop **(Fig. 3)**. However, a fistulous track to the appendix is present, with eventual entry of contrast material into the cecum. Oral contrast material from a prior computed tomography (CT) scan identifies the terminal ileum and confirms that the fistulous track is separate from it.

Diagnosis

Periappendiceal abscess with persistent fistula to the appendix.

How would you manage this patient?

Management

In most cases of appendiceal fistula, continued catheter drainage will allow the fistula to close spontaneously, after which an interval appendectomy can be performed if necessary. In this particular case, an appendectomy was performed after the tube check because the patient had a recurrent periappendiceal abscess.

Discussion

Periappendiceal abscesses occur in approximately 2%–16% of all cases of acute appendicitis. The most significant factor influencing the rate of perforation with subsequent abscess formation is patient delay in presenting to the hospital. Patients with appendiceal perforation waited two times longer before coming to the hospital than patients with inflamed appendices only.

Appendiceal perforation significantly complicates the surgical approach to appendicitis, resulting in significant surgical morbidity. The complication rate is 20%–35% when simultaneous surgical abscess drainage and appendectomy are performed. Not only is the appendectomy technically more difficult when an associated abscess is present, the rate of postoperative complications such as abscess recurrence, fecal fistulas, wound dehiscence, and infection is significantly higher.

Percutaneous catheter-based drainage of periappendiceal abscesses offers numerous advantages over initial surgical drainage of the abscess. If interval appendectomy is to be performed, initial percutaneous drainage permits a technically much simpler operation and reduces the postoperative complication rate by clearing the infected area prior to surgical intervention. Percutaneous drainage is successful in resolving periappendiceal abscesses in 90%–95% of cases. Percutaneous drainage also reduces hospital stays and subsequent costs compared to a two-stage surgical procedure.

The need for interval appendectomy remains controversial and is the subject of continuous debate. Many authors argue that once an appendiceal abscess has developed, the appendix itself has autolyzed and fragmented. In that case, interval appendectomy may not be necessary and percutaneous drainage as a sole treatment for the periappendiceal abscess would be sufficient. Several studies have followed patients for up to 3 years after appendiceal abscess drainage without interval appendectomy and have found no instances of recurrent appendicitis.

In patients suspected of having a perforated appendix, CT should be the imaging modality of choice because it can adequately distinguish between an appendiceal phlegmon and an appendiceal abscess. Appendiceal phlegmons are usually treated conservatively with intravenous antibiotics, while appendiceal abscesses can be approached with percutaneous drainage.

Initial access to the abscess should be achieved through the most direct route with no intervening structures. Ideally, this should be through the anterior or lateral abdominal wall, but if no safe access route exists, transrectal or transvaginal drainage can be performed. A catheter sinogram should be obtained 2 to 3 days after the initial drainage.

In up to 40% of cases of appendiceal abscess drainage, contrast material is seen to enter the cecum or appendix on the catheter sinogram, which is indicative of fistula. In almost all cases, this low-output fistula closes over time. Patients can be discharged from the hospital with the catheter in place and the catheter sinogram can be performed on an outpatient basis. Once output has diminished to less than 10 mL per day and no further evidence of fistulous communication is seen, the catheter can be removed and interval appendectomy performed if and when necessary.

Selected Readings

Flancbaum L, Nosher JL, Brolin RE. Percutaneous catheter drainage of abdominal abscesses associated with perforated viscus. Am Surg 1990; 56:52–56.

Jeffrey RB Jr, Tolentino CS, Federle MP, Laing FC. Percutaneous drainage of periappendiceal abscesses: review of 20 patients. AJR 1987; 149:59–62.

Nunez D, Huber JS, Yrizarry JM, Mendez G, Russell E. Nonsurgical drainage of appendiceal abscesses. AJR 1986; 146:587–589

Temple CL, Huchcroft SA, Temple WJ. The natural history of appendicitis in adults: a prospective study. Ann Surg 1995; 221:278–281.

vanSonnenberg E, Wittich GR, Casola G, et al. Periappendiceal abscesses: percutaneous drainage. Radiology 1987; 163:23–26.

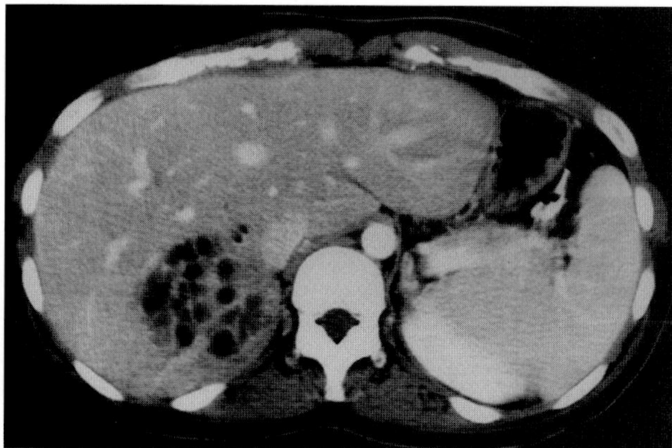

Figure 1. Contrast-enhanced abdominal CT scan with images through the liver.

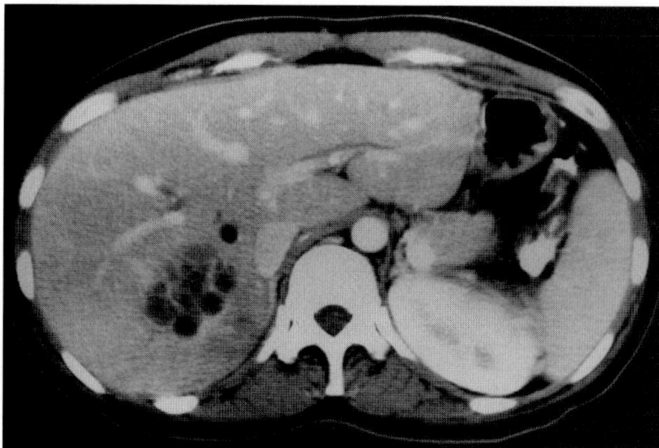

Figure 2. A more inferior contrast-enhanced CT scan.

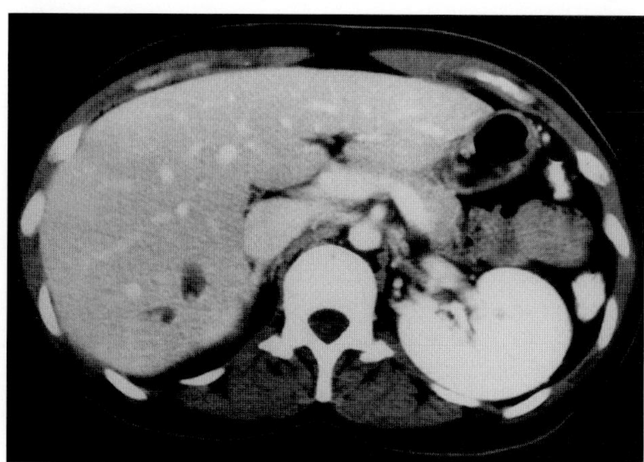

Figure 3. Contrast-enhanced abdominal CT scan.

TEACHING FILE CASE 12

Jeet Sandhu, M.D.

History

A 42-year-old woman came to the hospital with right upper quadrant pain and fevers. A computed tomography (CT) scan was obtained **(Figs. 1–3)**.

What is your diagnosis?

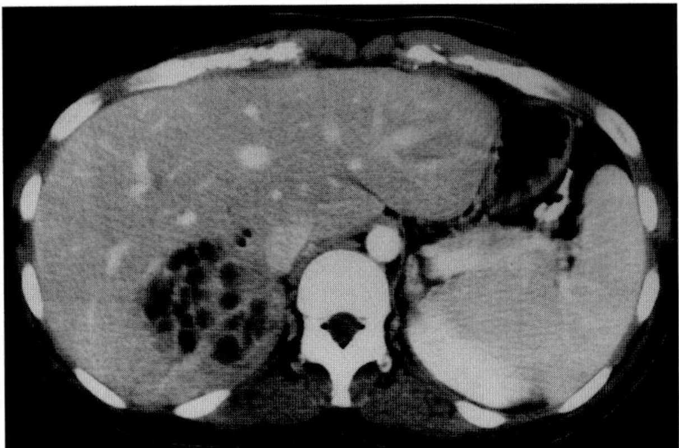

Figure 4. Multiseptated, multiloculated, low-density collection in the posterior segment of the right lobe of the liver.

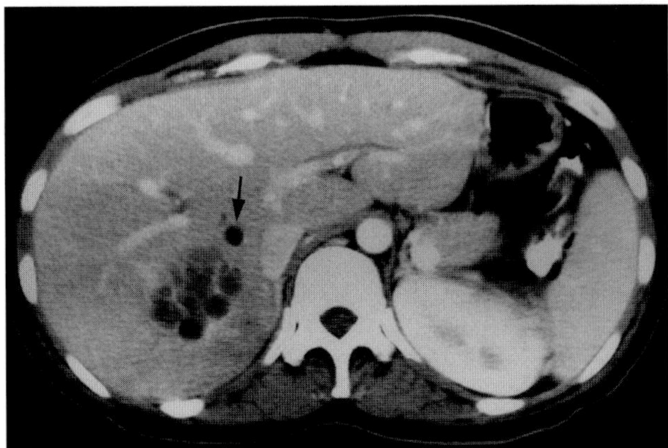

Figure 5. Inferior extent of the abscess. A separate 1-cm low-density collection (arrow) is actually a dilated bile duct.

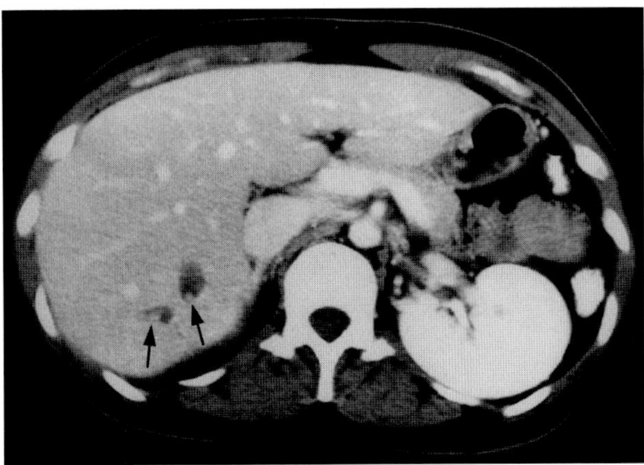

Figure 6. Two high-density areas are identified within the low-density bile ducts, compatible with intrahepatic stones (arrows).

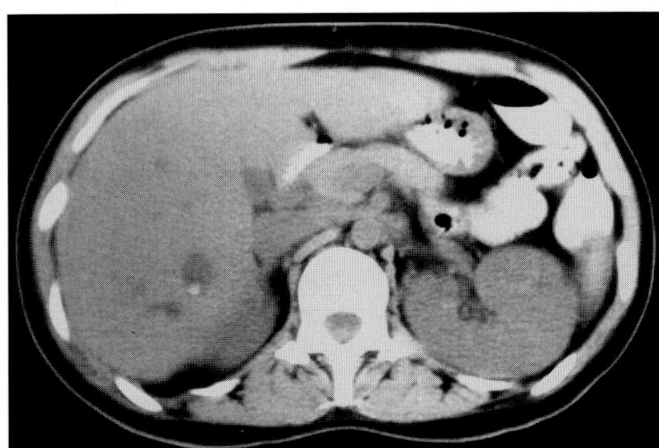

Figure 7. Noncontrast CT slice at the same level as in Figure 6 shows that the high-density areas within the bile ducts are stones and not enhancing structures such as blood vessels.

Radiographic Findings

A multiseptated low-density fluid collection is identified in the right lobe of the liver **(Fig. 4)**. **Figure 5** demonstrates the inferior extent of this collection with a separate 1-cm low-density area which is a dilated bile duct. Within the bile ducts are high-density foci **(Fig. 6)** which could be misinterpreted as vessels but were confirmed to be intrahepatic stones on a noncontrast CT scan **(Fig. 7)**.

Diagnosis

Pyogenic liver abscess secondary to biliary obstruction from biliary tract stricture with associated intrahepatic stones.

How would you manage this patient?

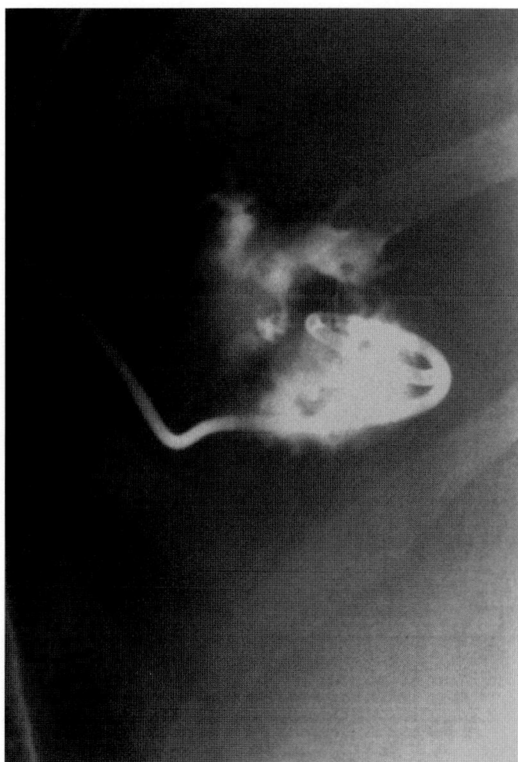

Figure 8. Injection of contrast material during percutaneous drainage of the liver abscess shows communication between the various cavities identified on the CT scan.

Management

Percutaneous transhepatic drainage of this abscess was performed. Although the CT appearance suggests the presence of multiple loculated collections and numerous septations within the abscess, these collections almost invariably communicate with each other and drainage with a single catheter will usually suffice **(Fig. 8)**.

To drain a multiseptated, multiloculated collection like this one, the catheter should be placed in the largest cavity possible. Preferably, the catheter should be in the inferior portion of the collection so that gravity drainage allows complete evacuation of the abscess. In this case, 40 mL of pus was removed, and the abscess cavity resolved with external drainage. After resolution of the abscess, endoscopic retrograde cholangiopancreatography showed multiple strictures and intrahepatic stones in the right lobe of the liver. Due to the large extent of the disease, the patient had a right hepatic lobectomy.

Discussion

Pyogenic hepatic abscess is a focal bacterial infection within the hepatic parenchyma. Untreated pyogenic liver abscesses carry almost a 100% mortality rate. The introduction of antibiotics and surgical drainage reduced the mortality rate to 28%. Despite the aggressive use of either fine needle aspiration (FNA) or tube drainage, the mortality rate still remains 15%–20%, mainly due to underlying disease such as malignancy.

The etiology of pyogenic liver abscesses can be divided into several categories based on the source of infection. Historically, the most common source of pyogenic liver abscesses was portal pyemia from an intraabdominal infectious source, most commonly appendicitis or diverticulitis. Rarely, other inflammatory conditions such as colitis can produce portal pyemia. In the initial series categorizing the etiologies of liver abscesses, appendicitis was the most common cause, secondary to portal pyemia or pylephlebitis. With more accurate clinical diagnosis, more aggressive surgical intervention, and the use of antibiotics, the incidence of liver abscesses from intraabdominal infectious sources has decreased dramatically.

Currently, the most common etiologies of hepatic abscess are cryptogenic or secondary to obstructive biliary tract disease. Depending on the series, cryptogenic abscesses account for 40%–45% of all cases of liver abscesses. Obstructive biliary disease from benign or malignant causes accounts for 40% of all cases. Other rare causes of hepatic abscess include bacteremia from indwelling arterial catheters, superinfection of cysts or necrotic tissue, and direct contamination of the liver from penetrating trauma.

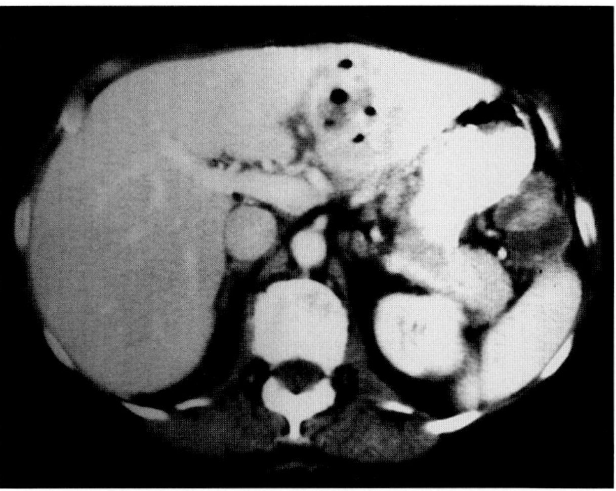

Figure 9. Contrast-enhanced abdominal CT scan shows a low-density fluid collection with multiple bubbles of gas in the left lobe of the liver.

Infection can also enter the liver from adjacent organs from direct continuous spread secondary to processes such as cholecystitis or peptic ulcer disease. For example, this patient presented with mid epigastric pain and a liver abscess with multiple bubbles of air identified in the left lobe of the liver **(Fig. 9)**. The patient improved after percutaneous drainage, but contrast material was noted to enter the duodenum on a tube sinogram **(Fig. 10)**. Subsequent upper endoscopy identified a perforated duodenal ulcer.

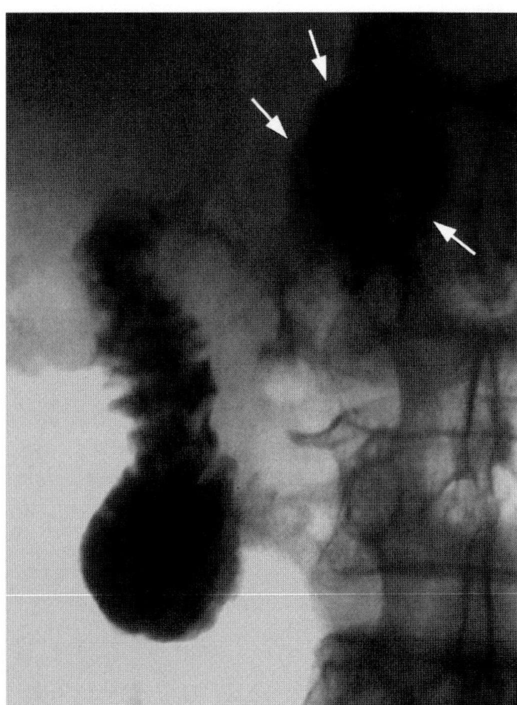

Figure 10. Injection of contrast material through the catheter that was placed into the left lobe liver abscess shows opacification of the cavity (arrows) with extension of contrast material into the duodenal bulb and down the duodenum, indicating the presence of a fistulous track to the duodenum.

Patients with hepatic abscesses classically present with right upper quadrant pain, fever, and an elevated white blood cell count. However, up to a quarter of patients may not be febrile. Other nonspecific presenting symptoms include malaise, myalgia, vomiting, nausea, anorexia, weight loss, or night sweats. The presence of an elevated bilirubin level or clinical jaundice suggests underlying biliary tract disease. In line with the nonspecific clinical features, up to a third of patients may have no abdominal pain.

Patients with diabetes seem to have a slightly higher risk of developing pyogenic liver abscesses. The incidence of hepatic abscesses may also be slightly higher in patients with a history of ethanol abuse, possibly secondary to an abnormal reticuloendothelial system.

Because hepatic abscesses can have an extremely variable appearance on imaging, other etiologies for cystic masses in the liver should be considered, including echinococcal cyst, cystic tumors of the liver, bilomas, or extrapancreatic pseudocyst. Necrotic neoplasms and metastases can occasionally mimic hepatic abscesses. If any question remains as to the etiology of the fluid collection, aspiration for cytologic and microbiologic analysis can be performed prior to definitive tube drainage.

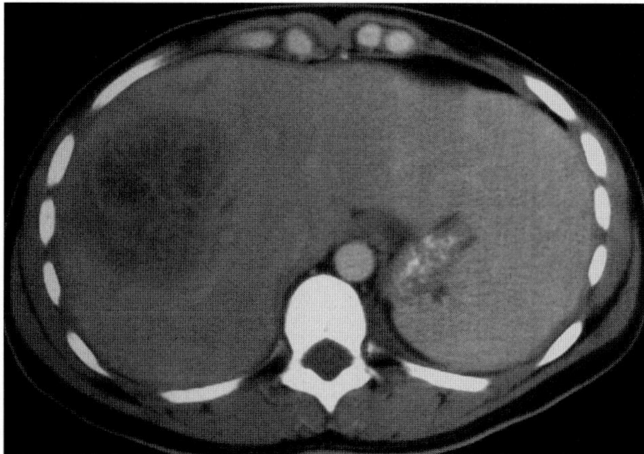

Figure 11. Typical multiseptated appearance of a pyogenic liver abscess with a surrounding low-density rim secondary to edematous liver parenchyma. The multiseptated appearance is likely due to coalescence of the small cluster of microabscesses.

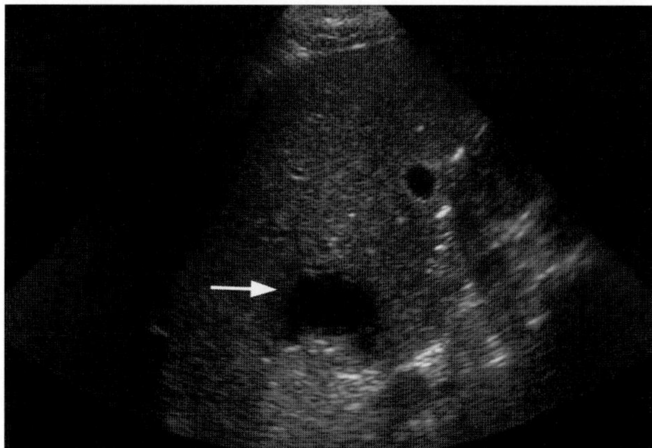

Figure 12. Unilocular fluid collection (arrow) in the liver with some echogenic material in the inferior portion of this fluid collection.

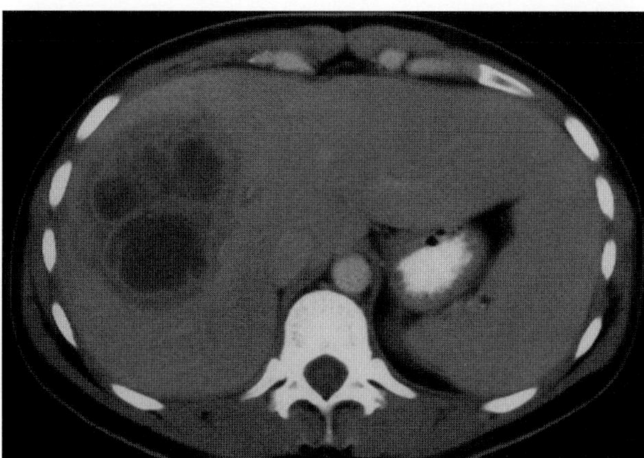

Figure 13. Larger coalescent liver abscess with thickened septa and irregular-sized fluid collections. A high-density enhancing rim is noted around the fluid collection with a low-density peripheral rim. This is the "double-target" sign, which is suggestive of pyogenic liver abscess.

Jeffrey et al have described the so-called "cluster" sign as relatively specific for small pyogenic liver abscesses. This consists of a cluster of small low-density areas that are contiguous with one another. Over time these low-density areas may enlarge and coalesce to form the more classic multiseptated appearance noted with larger hepatic abscesses **(Fig. 11)**. The septa are thicker and more irregular and the cavities are not of a uniform size as would be seen with an echinococcal cyst. Liver abscesses can also appear unilocular **(Fig. 12)**, but the presence of air or echogenic material within the abscess cavity distinguishes it from a simple cyst. Another appearance suggestive of an abscess is the "double-target" sign. Here, the low-density center with an enhancing rim is surrounded by a low-density peripheral rim which represents the compressed edematous hepatic parenchyma around the abscess **(Fig. 13)**. Multiple abscesses are seen in 50%–70% of patients, and 50% of these patients have involvement of both lobes of the liver.

The most common location for hepatic abscess is the right lobe of the liver. This is thought to be due to preferential blood flow from the superior mesenteric vein into the posterior portion of the right lobe of the liver. Because one etiology of hepatic abscess is portal pyemia from either an intraabdominal infection or transient bacteremia, and since the right lobe of the liver receives most of the superior mesenteric venous blood, it is not surprising that the right lobe is a more common location for hepatic abscesses.

If the abscess lies immediately underneath the diaphragm or in the peripheral subcapsular portion of the liver and the patient is from or has visited an area endemic for *Entamoeba histolytica*, an amebic abscess should be considered and appropriate serologic titers obtained before percutaneous drainage is performed. Enteric bacteria such as *Escherichia coli*, aerobic streptococci, and microaerophilic streptococci are commonly found in hepatic abscesses. Anaerobic bacteria may account for 45% of all hepatic abscesses. Consequently, cultures for anaerobic bacteria should be obtained whenever hepatic abscesses are aspirated or drained to ensure that appropriate antibiotic therapy is instituted.

The cause of hepatic abscess is usually readily apparent on abdominal CT or ultrasound images. However, as noted earlier, the incidence of hepatic abscesses for which no cause can be positively identified is relatively high. Some authors have recommended aggressive work-up of these patients with upper and lower endoscopy as well as exploratory laparotomy to determine the etiology. They argue that a very aggressive work-up will detect small tumors that will ultimately prove to be the cause of the hepatic abscess.

Other investigators have found that even with an aggressive work-up, no cause for the hepatic abscess can be determined in most cases. In an autopsy series of patients with cryptogenic hepatic abscess, no cause was found even at autopsy. The current state of our knowledge seems to suggest that patients in whom a discernible cause of the abscess cannot be identified probably do not need an intensive, aggressive work-up. Patients with cryptogenic liver abscesses may have some alteration or dysfunction in the reticuloendothelial system which provides inadequate clearing of bacteria from the liver compared to normal patients.

Controversy exists as to the best means of managing patients with hepatic abscesses. Percutaneous catheter-based drainage has been used most often to treat hepatic abscesses and has a success rate of over 90%. Repetitive FNA of the liver abscess without placement of a drainage catheter has had a near 100% success rate. Other investigators comparing FNA to percutaneous drainage have found a higher recurrence rate and a higher mortality rate with FNA. Although controversy persists, percutaneous drainage using standard Seldinger or trocar techniques is probably the best means of draining abscesses, especially larger ones with a multiseptated, multiloculated appearance. Rarely, septic shock can be induced by the drainage procedure, and the patient should always be given intravenous antibiotics beforehand. Unilocular abscesses smaller than 5 cm in diameter can likely be treated with simple aspiration **(Fig. 14)**.

Treatment with intravenous antibiotics alone may be appropriate for lesions smaller than 2 cm in diameter. For abscesses 2–5 cm in diameter, either FNA or catheter drainage can be performed. Surgical drainage should be reserved for patients with severe underlying biliary disease or in whom catheter drainage has failed. Causes for failure of catheter drainage include infected hematomas within the liver, necrotic tumors, or very thick, viscous fluid in the abscess cavities. Certain authors recommend surgery for multiple abscesses, but percutaneous drainage can be successful in such cases if a catheter is inserted into each abscess.

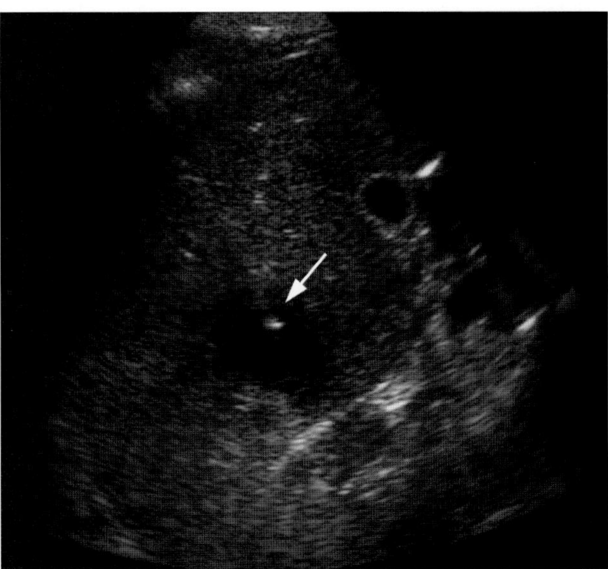

Figure 14. Needle aspiration of a unilocular liver abscess with the echogenic tip of the needle identified within the collection (arrow).

Selected Readings

Barreda R, Ros PR. Diagnostic imaging of liver abscess. Crit Rev Diagn Imag 1992; 33:29–58.

Bernardino ME, Berkman WA, Plemmons M, Sones PJ, Price RB, Casarella WJ. Percutaneous drainage of multiseptated hepatic abscess. J Comp Assist Tomogr 1984; 8:38–41.

Giorgio A, Tarantino L, Mariniello N, et al. Pyogenic liver abscesses: 13 years of experience in percutaneous needle aspiration with US guidance. Radiology 1995; 195:122–124.

Greenwood LH, Collins TL, Yrizarry JM. Percutaneous management of multiple liver abscesses. AJR 1982; 139:390–392.

Hashimoto L, Hermann R, Grundfest-Broniatowski S. Pyogenic hepatic abscess: results of current management. Am Surg 1995; 61:407–411.

Huang CJ, Pitt HA, Lipsett PA, et al. Pyogenic hepatic abscess: changing trends over 42 years. Ann Surg 1996; 223:600–609.

Jeffrey RB, Tolentino CS, Chang FC, Federle MP. CT of small pyogenic hepatic abscesses: the cluster sign. AJR 1988; 151:487–489.

Seeto RK, Rockey DC. Pyogenic liver abscess: changes in etiology, management, and outcome. Medicine 1996; 75:99–113.

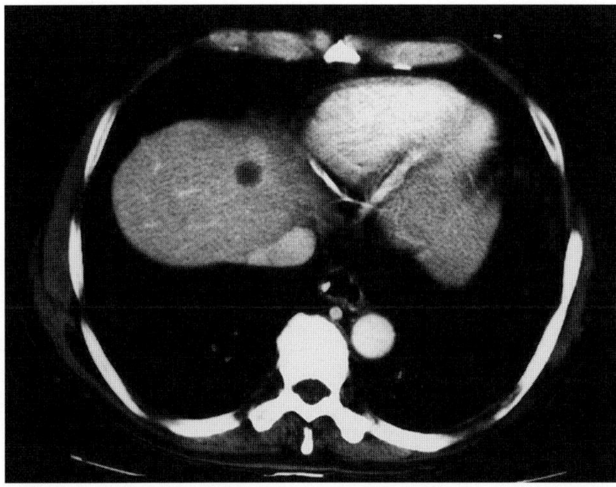

Figure 1. Contrast-enhanced CT scan of the liver.

TEACHING FILE CASE 13

Christine C. Esola, M.D., Shailendra Chopra, M.D., M.R.C.P., F.R.C.R., and Gerald D. Dodd III, M.D.

History

This 66-year-old man came to the hospital with jaundice, weight loss, nausea, and vomiting. His serum bilirubin was markedly elevated and his transaminases were mildly elevated. Sonography revealed extensive intra- and extrahepatic biliary ductal dilatation. On endoscopic retrograde cholangiopancreatography, a small mass was seen at the ampulla of Vater and brush biopsies were taken. The diagnosis was ampullary cholangiocarcinoma.

A computed tomography (CT) scan of the abdomen was obtained to evaluate for metastases **(Fig. 1)**.

What is your diagnosis?

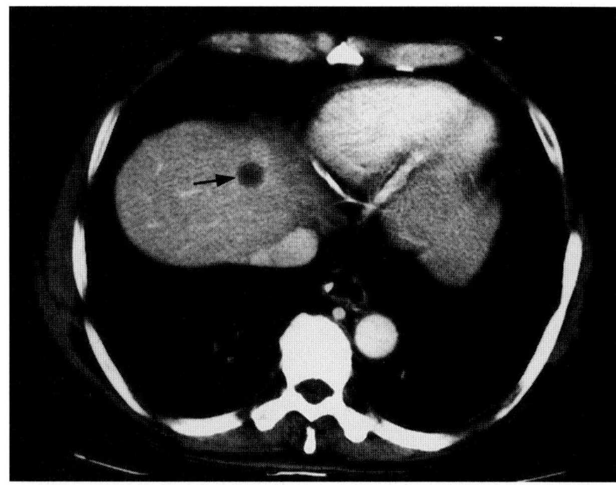

Figure 2. Contrast-enhanced CT scan shows the lesion (arrow) in the dome of the liver, surrounded by lung parenchyma and near the heart.

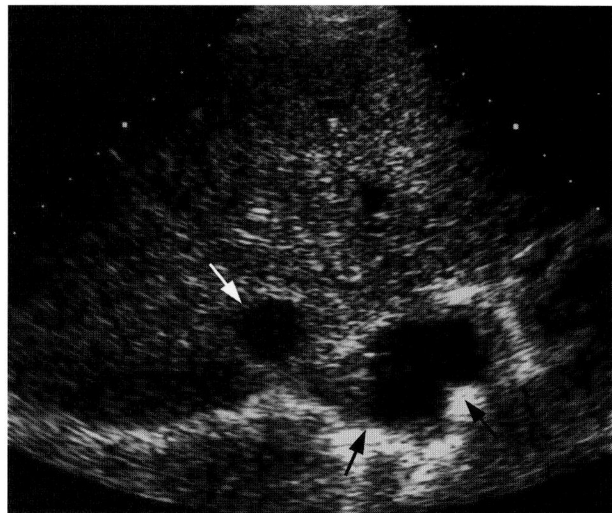

Figure 3. Sonography shows the lesion (white arrow) and its proximity to the heart (black arrows).

Radiographic Findings

The contrast-enhanced CT scan shows a 1.5-cm hypodense lesion in the dome of the liver **(Fig. 2)**. A noncontrast CT scan was not obtained. At this level, the liver is surrounded by pulmonary parenchyma and the lesion is in close proximity to the heart. Because of these findings and the risks they posed for CT-guided biopsy, a targeted sonogram of the liver lesion was obtained to evaluate whether the lesion was accessible to percutaneous biopsy under sonographic guidance **(Fig. 3)**. The lesion and its location relative to the heart are clearly seen via a subxiphoid approach.

Diagnosis

Probable metastatic liver lesion, precariously located for imaging-guided percutaneous biopsy.

How would you perform this biopsy?

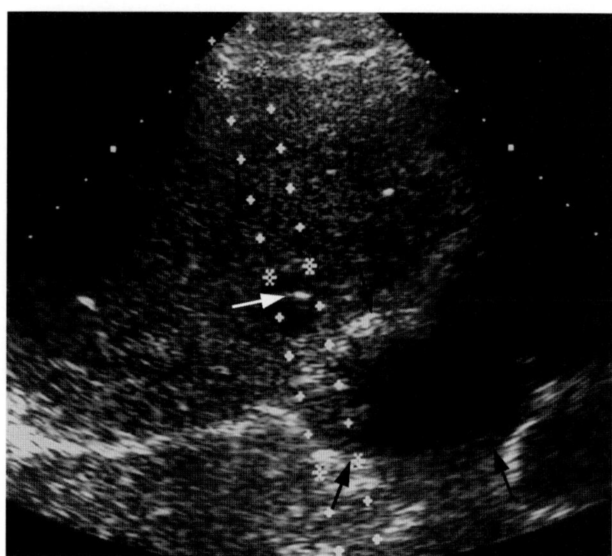

Figure 4. Sonography shows the hypoechoic lesion aligned in the needle guide track, the hyperechoic needle tip (white arrow) within the lesion, and the heart (black arrows).

Management

Sonographic guidance was used to perform a needle biopsy of the liver lesion through a needle guide, angling cephalad from a subxiphoid approach. Sonography shows the hypoechoic lesion within the path of the needle guide, the hyperechoic needle tip within the lesion, and the heart nearby **(Fig. 4)**. Two passes were made with a 20-gauge needle, and diagnostic tissue was obtained, confirming adenocarcinoma metastatic to the liver.

Sonography enabled the operator to maintain real-time visualization of both the needle and the lesion throughout the procedure. Such visualization was particularly reassuring in light of the close proximity of the lesion to the heart. Also, because the needle traversed only hepatic tissue and no lung parenchyma, the risk of pneumothorax was eliminated.

Discussion

If this lesion were adequately seen on unenhanced CT images, percutaneous biopsy with CT guidance could probably have been performed. In this case, two confounding factors make sonographic guidance a safer and more logical choice. The first of these is the risk of pneumothorax (up to 45% incidence on transthoracic biopsy of lung lesions) inherent in any procedure which requires transgression of pulmonary parenchyma. Sonography allows a subcostal approach to most liver lesions, including those in the dome. The subcostal approach eliminates the risk of pneumothorax and the risk of damage to intercostal vessels, both of which are considerations during performance of a biopsy via an intercostal route. Perhaps more compelling in this case is the short distance between the lesion and the heart. Visualization of the needle, the lesion, and the heart throughout the procedure allows the biopsy to be accomplished more quickly and with greater operator confidence.

Selected Readings

Dodd GD III, Esola CC, Memel DS, et al. Sonography: the undiscovered jewel of interventional radiology. Radiographics 1996; 16:1271–1288.

Kazerooni EA, Lim FT, Mikhail A, Martinez FJ. Risk of pneumothorax in CT-guided transthoracic needle aspiration biopsy of the lung. Radiology 1996; 198:371–375.

Reading CC, Charboneau JW, James EM, Hurt MR. Sonographically guided percutaneous biopsy of small (3 cm or less) masses. AJR 1988; 151:189–192.

Endnote

Figure 2 from Dodd GD III, Esola CC, Memel DS, et al. Sonography: the undiscovered jewel of interventional radiology. Radiographics 1996; 16:1271–1288. Used with permission.

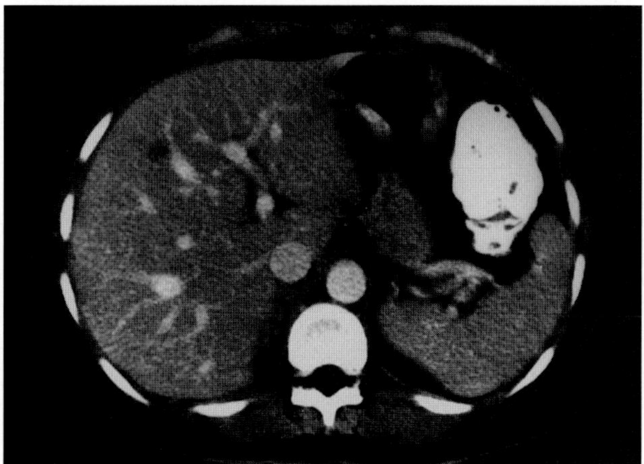

Figure 1. Contrast-enhanced CT scan of the liver.

TEACHING FILE CASE 14

Christine C. Esola, M.D., Shailendra Chopra, M.D., M.R.C.P., F.R.C.R., and Gerald D. Dodd III, M.D.

History

This 37-year-old woman came to the hospital with a 1-year history of tenesmus and hematochezia, and a 25-pound weight loss over the last several months. Colonoscopy revealed a large polypoid mass in the rectum which was confirmed at biopsy to be adenocarcinoma. A computed tomography (CT) scan of the abdomen was performed to evaluate for metastatic disease **(Fig. 1)**.

What is your diagnosis?

Radiographic Findings

On the contrast-enhanced CT scan **(Fig. 2)**, a small hypodense lesion is present in the anterior segment of the right hepatic lobe, immediately adjacent to the middle hepatic vein. No lesion was seen on the noncontrast CT scan.

Diagnosis

Small liver lesion suspicious for metastatic disease.

How would you manage this patient?

Management

A percutaneous biopsy of the lesion in the right hepatic lobe was requested prior to instituting therapy. Because this lesion was small, immediately adjacent to a large blood vessel, and not seen on the noncontrast CT scan, a targeted sonogram of the liver was obtained using landmarks from the CT scan. Gray-scale and color Doppler sonography were used to identify vascular structures known to be near the lesion. A careful search of the area revealed a very subtle hyperechoic lesion in the expected location adjacent to the middle hepatic vein **(Fig. 3)**. Percutaneous needle biopsy was performed under real-time sonographic guidance. Two passes were made with a 20-gauge needle, and a tissue sample adequate for diagnosis was obtained. Biopsy confirmed metastatic adenocarcinoma.

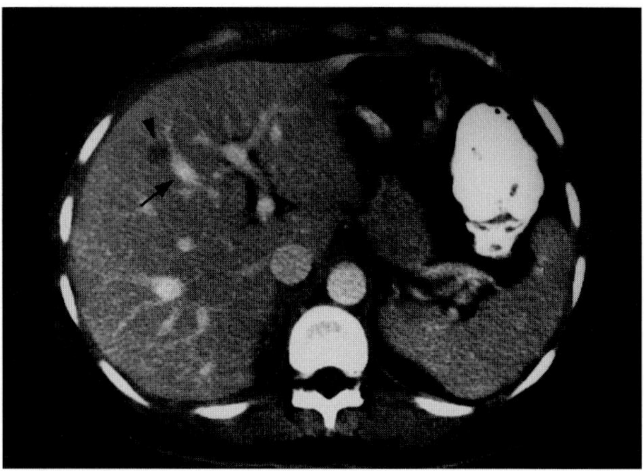

Figure 2. Contrast-enhanced CT scan shows a right lobe lesion (arrowhead) adjacent to the middle hepatic vein (arrow).

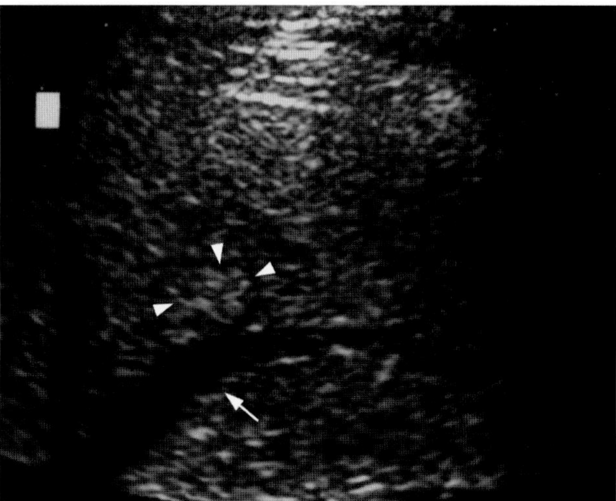

Figure 3. Sonogram shows a very subtle hyperechoic lesion (arrowheads) adjacent to the middle hepatic vein (arrow), corresponding to the abnormality seen on the CT scan.

Discussion

Although CT-guided biopsy of liver lesions is performed routinely, CT has limitations as a guidance modality. If a lesion is not visible on noncontrast CT scans, it is very difficult to maintain enhancement of the lesion for the time required to perform a biopsy. The respiratory variation inherent in CT scans may compound the risk and difficulty of a biopsy, particularly when a lesion is very small or is located near a significant structure. In most instances, liver lesions requiring biopsy can be seen on sonography. In difficult or subtle cases, a targeted sonogram with color Doppler can locate a lesion in relation to nearby vessels seen on the CT scan. The biopsy is performed with real-time visualization of the needle, the lesion, and surrounding structures. Because of this, the operator can be confident that the needle placement is safe and accurate and that the tissue obtained is from the lesion.

Selected Readings

Dodd GD III, Esola CC, Memel DS, et al. Sonography: the undiscovered jewel of interventional radiology. Radiographics 1996; 16:1271–1288.

Reading CC, Charboneau JW, James EM, Hurt MR. Sonographically guided percutaneous biopsy of small (3 cm or less) masses. AJR 1988; 151:189–192.

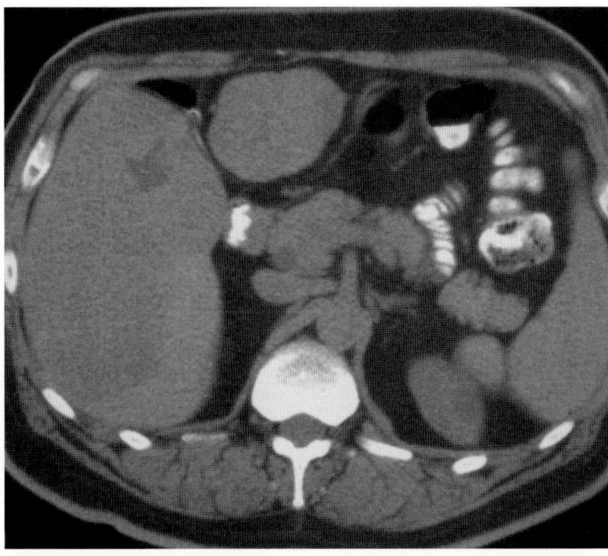

Figure 1. Axial noncontrast CT scan of the liver at the level of the superior mesenteric artery.

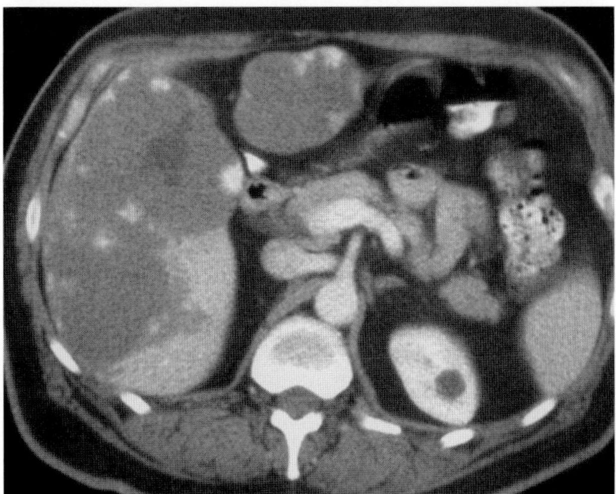

Figure 2. Contrast-enhanced CT scan at the same level as in Figure 1, obtained during the portal venous phase.

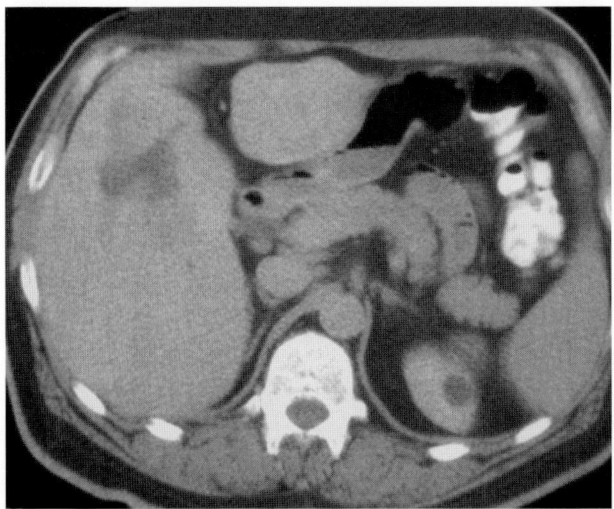

Figure 3. Five-minute delayed CT image obtained at the same level as in Figure 1.

TEACHING FILE CASE 15

Rendon Nelson, M.D., and Mark Berger, M.D.

History

A 64-year old woman with a history of colorectal cancer underwent computed tomography (CT) scanning as part of her staging evaluation **(Figs. 1–3)**. Non-contrast images, dynamic portal venous phase images and delayed images were obtained.

Would you biopsy these lesions and if so how?

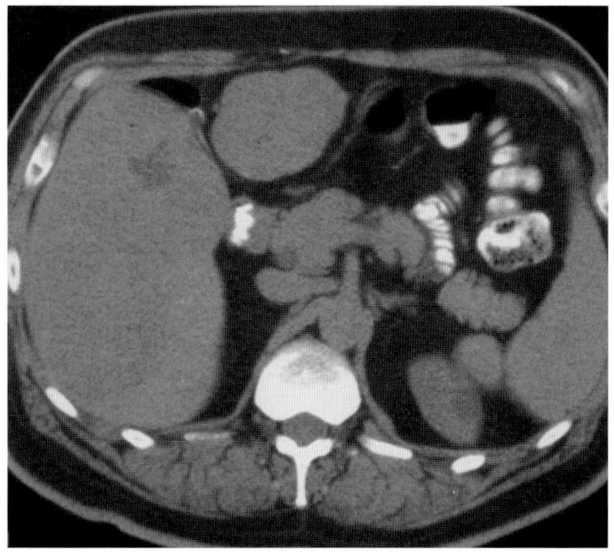

Figure 4. CT scan shows a large, well-circumscribed, slightly hypoattenuating mass involving nearly the entire right hepatic lobe, the anterior aspect of which is of lower attenuation. The density of the periphery of the lesion is similar to that of the aorta. A second smaller homogeneous lesion is present in the medial segment of the left hepatic lobe, also similar in attenuation to that of the aorta.

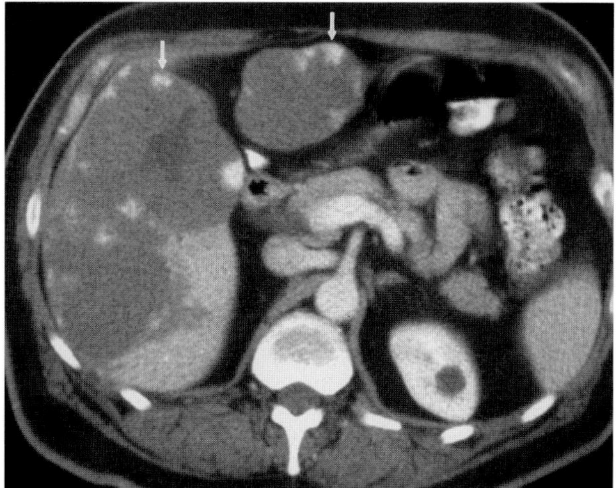

Figure 5. Peripheral nodular enhancement (arrows) of both lesions is seen during the portal venous phase of contrast enhancement.

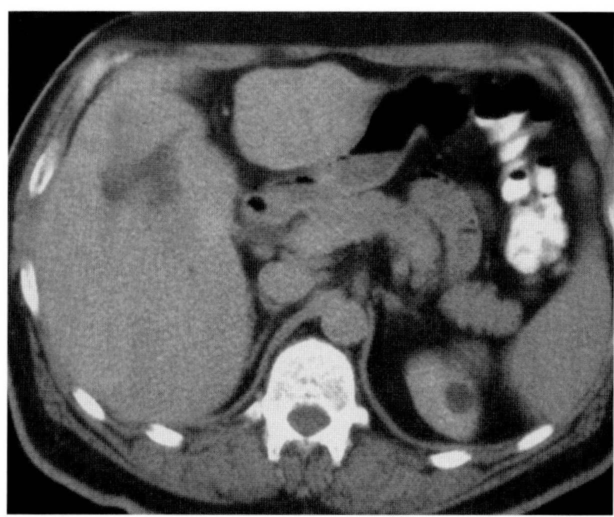

Figure 6. Delayed imaging at 5 minutes demonstrates progressive enhancement towards the center of both masses (centripetal). The central low-attenuation area in the right hepatic lobe mass has yet to enhance.

Radiographic Findings

The noncontrast CT scan of the liver demonstrates a well-circumscribed slightly low-attenuation mass in the right hepatic lobe, with a central stellate focus of even lower attenuation **(Fig. 4)**. The periphery of the mass is similar in attenuation to that of the aorta. A second smaller low-attenuation lesion is seen in the medial segment of the left hepatic lobe. A dynamic contrast-enhanced image during the portal venous phase shows peripheral, nodular “cotton wool” or “cloud-like” enhancement of both masses **(Fig. 5)**. The peripheral nodules have a similar attenuation to that of the aorta. Delayed images 5 minutes post-contrast show progressive fill-in of both masses from the periphery to the center of the lesion (centripetal) **(Fig. 6)**. The lower attenuation center of the right hepatic lobe mass has not yet enhanced.

Diagnosis

Cavernous hemangiomas, the larger one with a central scar. Because the imaging features of these lesions are classic for uncomplicated, benign cavernous hemangiomas, no further work-up or biopsy is warranted.

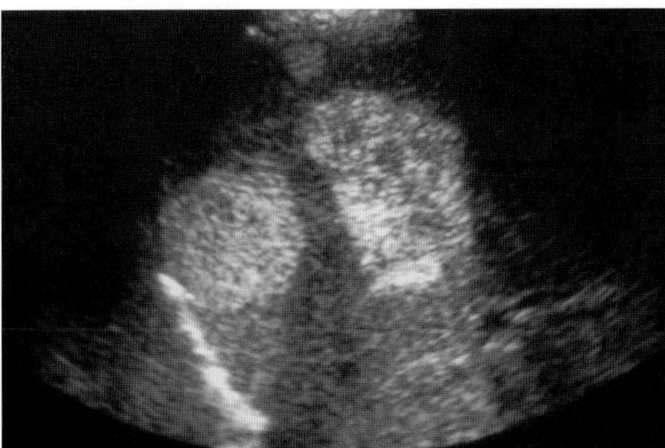

Figure 7. Ultrasound image of the mid right hepatic lobe shows well-defined, homogeneous, echogenic masses with posterior acoustical enhancement.

Management

Because of the classic findings for hemangioma, biopsy is not indicated in this patient. In many cases, however, the imaging features are not entirely classic, thus indicating the need for another correlative imaging study. The choice of subsequent imaging depends upon personal preference, equipment availability, and the size of the lesion. In general, for lesions larger than 2.5 cm, a technetium-99m labeled red blood cell study is probably the most reliable and cost effective. For smaller lesions, magnetic resonance (MR) imaging, with or without the use of a gadolinium chelate, is the most reliable. It is important to remember that larger lesions are more likely to develop internal hyaline scars (as in this case), and the presence of a scar often complicates the diagnosis because of its less than classic appearance with various imaging techniques.

Discussion

Cavernous hemangiomas are the most common benign liver tumor, found in 7.3% of patients at autopsy. These tumors may occur at any age, and 70%–95% of them are seen in women. They are usually solitary, but are multiple in up to 10% of cases. They are usually less than 3 cm in diameter and homogeneous, but can attain sizes of greater than 20 cm. When larger than 4 cm they are classified as "giant hemangiomas" and often have a central scar. Histologically, these tumors consist of blood-filled spaces lined by a single layer of endothelium and separated by fibrous septa. Hepatic hemangiomas are usually asymptomatic, although large tumors may result in liver enlargement and abdominal discomfort. Spontaneous hemorrhage may occur, but is infrequent.

The typical ultrasound findings include a homogeneous, hyperechoic mass with well-defined margins and posterior acoustic enhancement **(Fig. 7)**. A small hypoechoic focus may be seen centrally, but a hypoechoic collar, which is frequently seen with metastases, is notably absent. These typical findings may vary and are dependent on the appearance of the surrounding hepatic parenchyma. A liver with diffuse fatty infiltration or other chronic parenchymal diseases may make a hemangioma appear relatively isoechoic or even hypoechoic. Hemangiomas may also appear heterogeneous, secondary to the presence of a central scar, hemorrhage, or necrosis.

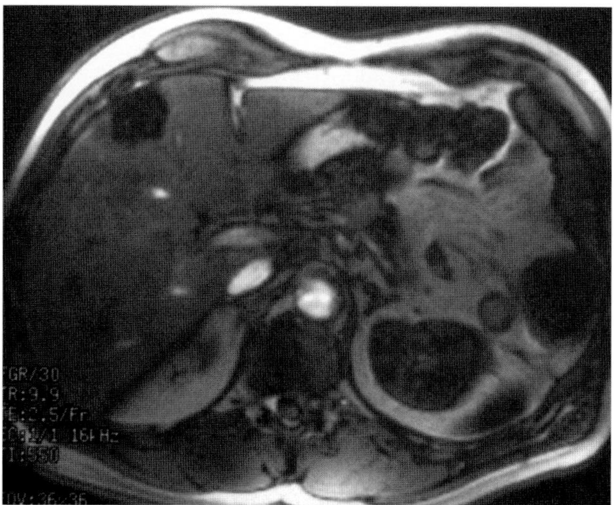

Figure 8. T1-weighted gradient echo image of the liver demonstrates a well-defined mass of decreased signal intensity in the right hepatic lobe.

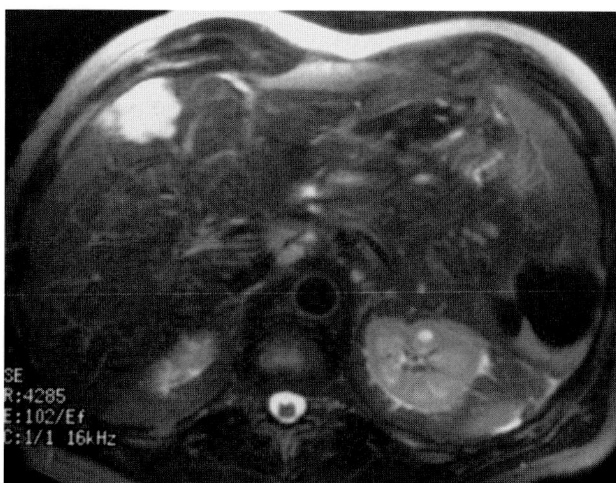

Figure 9. T2-weighted spin echo image shows this mass to be of markedly increased signal intensity, equal to that of cerebrospinal fluid.

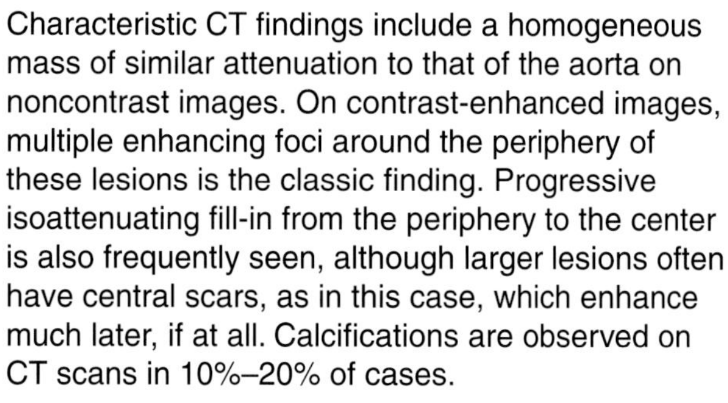

Characteristic CT findings include a homogeneous mass of similar attenuation to that of the aorta on noncontrast images. On contrast-enhanced images, multiple enhancing foci around the periphery of these lesions is the classic finding. Progressive isoattenuating fill-in from the periphery to the center is also frequently seen, although larger lesions often have central scars, as in this case, which enhance much later, if at all. Calcifications are observed on CT scans in 10%–20% of cases.

On MR images, cavernous hemangiomas, like malignant tumors, demonstrate long T1 and T2 characteristics. The lengthening of T2, however, is generally greater for hemangiomas (150 msec) than for malignant tumors (~80 msec). As a result, hemangiomas tend to be markedly hyperintense on T2-weighted images, similar to the signal intensity of water-containing substances such as cerebrospinal fluid. Low-signal-intensity areas within hemangiomas on T2-weighted images correlate with zones of fibrosis **(Figs. 8, 9)**. Gadolinium-enhanced images demonstrate a similar peripheral nodular enhancement pattern to that seen on CT scans **(Fig. 10)**. As noted earlier, MR imaging is the technique of choice for smaller lesions (<2.5 cm).

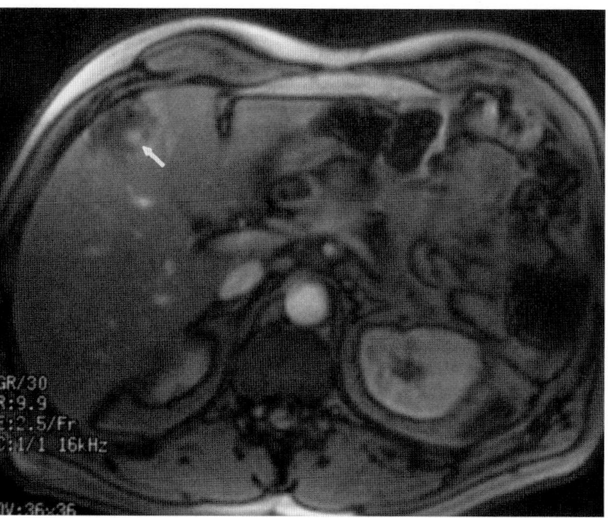

Figure 10. T1-weighted post-gadolinium dynamic imaging of this mass demonstrates peripheral nodular enhancement (arrow).

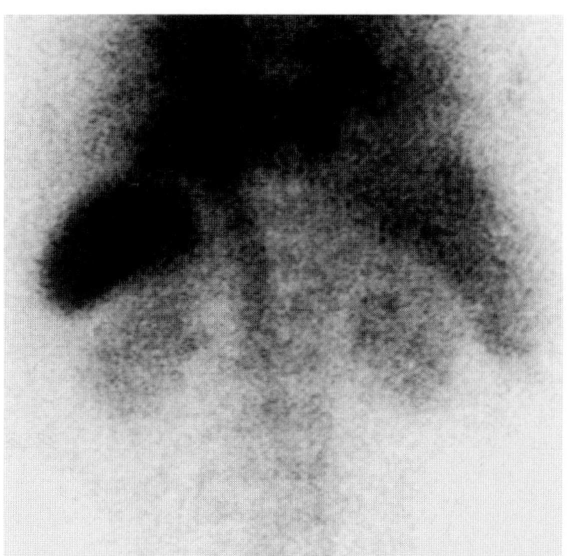

Figure 11. Technetium-99m red blood cell study. Posterior view of a coronal image of the abdomen taken shortly after injection of tracer. Homogeneous uptake is seen throughout the liver.

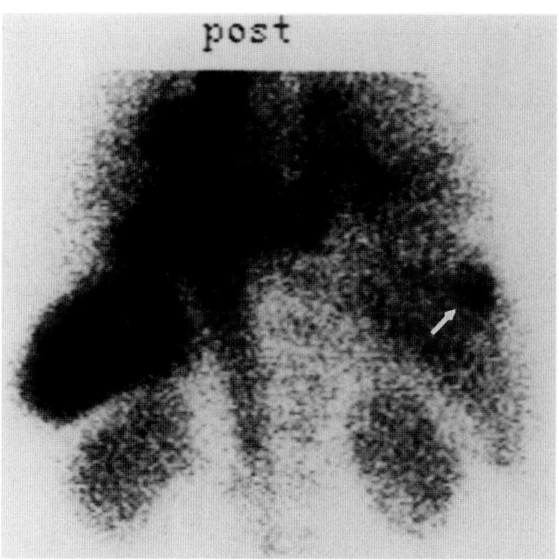

Figure 12. Blood pool image acquired 2 hours after injection of tracer. A focal area of relatively increased uptake is seen within the right hepatic lobe superiorly (arrow).

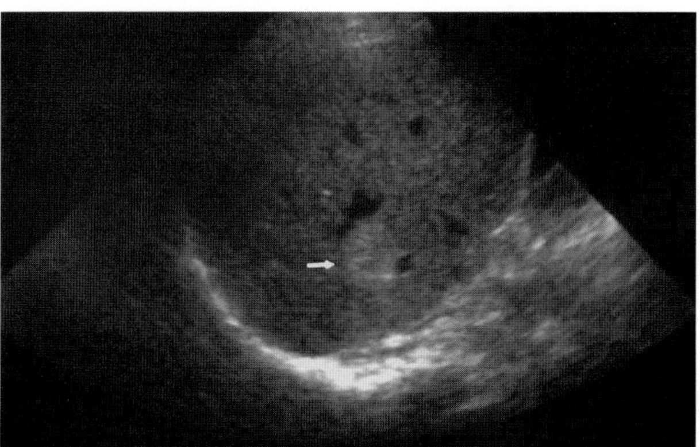

Figure 13. Ultrasound image of the right hepatic lobe shows a well-circumscribed, hypoechoic lesion (arrow) with slightly increased through-transmission.

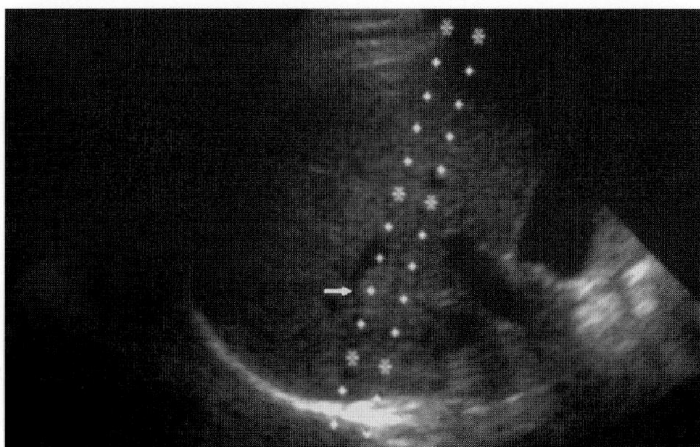

Figure 14. Ultrasound image in a similar plane as in Figure 13 with the lesion targeted in the needle guide (arrow).

Technetium-99m red blood cell scintigraphy classically shows decreased activity on early dynamic images and increased activity on delayed blood pool images **(Figs. 11, 12)**. Unlike dynamic imaging with CT or MR, scintigraphy rarely shows peripheral enhancement with progressive fill-in during the dynamic phase. Single photon emission CT imaging has been shown to be more sensitive than planar imaging for detecting hepatic cavernous hemangiomas, particularly lesions smaller than 3 cm. However, scintigraphy is the technique of choice for larger lesions ($\geq$2.5 cm), mainly because of its lower cost.

Percutaneous biopsy is reserved for those cases where the imaging findings are inconclusive. Due to the marked vascularity of hemangiomas, hemorrhage during needle biopsy is a potential complication, although the reported incidence is low. The risk of hemorrhage can be diminished by directing the needle into the lesion through a cuff of normal hepatic parenchyma **(Figs. 13, 14)**. This is particularly important with subcapsular lesions.

Since hemangiomas are benign, excision is performed only if the lesions cause persistent pain or are complicated by hemorrhage.

Selected Readings

Abrams RM, Bernbaum ER, Santos JS, Lipscon J. Angiographic features of cavernous hemangioma of the liver. Radiology 1969; 92:308–312.

Birnbaum BA, Weinreb JC, et al. Definitive diagnosis of hepatic hemangiomas: MR imaging versus Tc-99m-labeled red blood cell SPECT. Radiology 1990; 176:95–101.

Cronan JJ, Esparza AR, et al. Cavernous hemangioma of the liver: role of percutaneous biopsy. Radiology 1988; 166:135.

Freeny PC, Marks WM. Hepatic hemangioma: dynamic bolus CT. AJR 1986; 147:711–719.

Ishak KG, Rabin L. Benign tumors of the liver. Med Clin North Am 1975; 59:995–1013.

Nelson RC, Chezmar JL. Diagnostic approach to hepatic hemangiomas. Radiology 1990; 176:11–13.

Ros PR. Computed tomography pathologic correlations in hepatic tumors. Advances in hepatobiliary radiology. St. Lous: C.V. Mosby, 1990; 75–108.

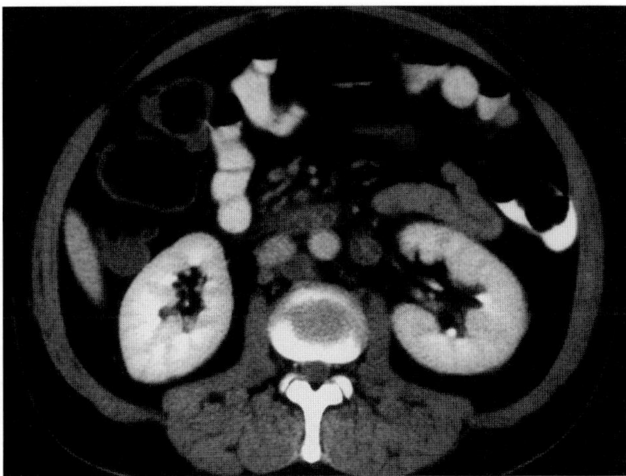

Figure 1. Axial contrast-enhanced CT scan at the level of the renal hilum.

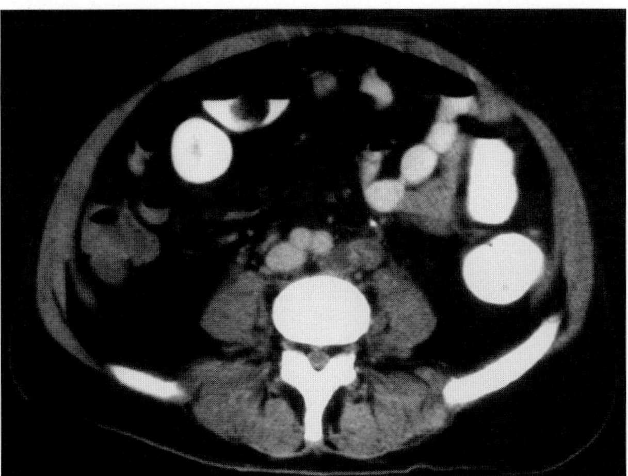

Figure 2. Axial contrast-enhanced CT scan at the level of the aortic bifurcation.

TEACHING FILE CASE 16

Mark W. Wilson, M.D.

History

A 47-year-old man with a history of acquired immunodeficiency syndrome (AIDS) came to the emergency department complaining of progressive abdominal pain and fever for the last 2 weeks. A computed tomography (CT) scan was obtained to evaluate the patient's symptoms **(Figs. 1, 2)**.

What is your diagnosis?

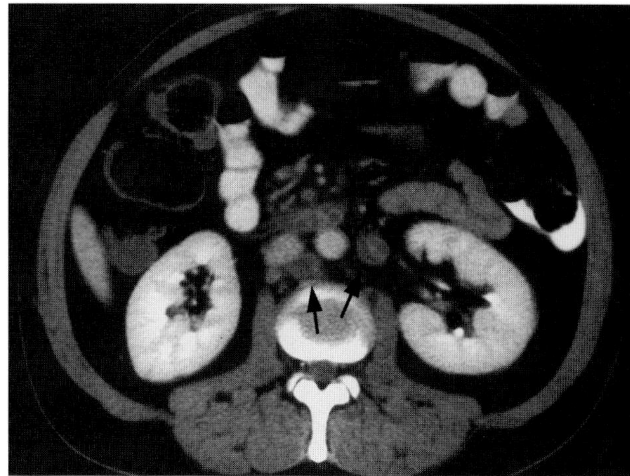

Figure 3. Enlarged (up to 2 cm) retroperitoneal lymph nodes at the renal hilar level demonstrate low attenuation on the CT scan (arrows).

Radiographic Findings

Selected images from the contrast-enhanced CT scan **(Figs. 3, 4)** demonstrate numerous enlarged retroperitoneal lymph nodes in a predominately aortocaval distribution. The lymph nodes measure up to 2 cm in diameter, with several demonstrating central low attenuation. There is no evidence of free fluid, bowel abnormalities, or other masses which could account for the patient's presentation.

Diagnosis

Retroperitoneal lymphadenopathy.

How would you manage this patient?

Management

Repeat CT scanning was performed with the patient in the prone position, and the enlarged lymph nodes were again localized. A nodal site was biopsied under CT guidance with the patient prone **(Figs. 5, 6)**. The biopsy was performed with a 22-gauge Chiba needle from a paraspinous approach. At laboratory analysis the biopsy specimens stained strongly positive for acid-fast bacilli. Culture results a few days later were positive for mycobacterium avium complex (MAC).

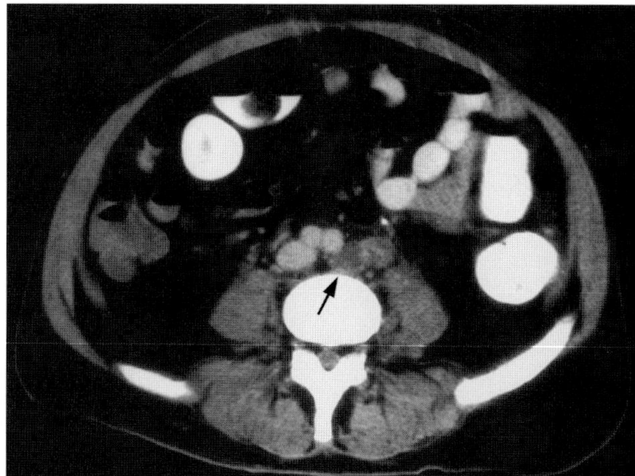

Figure 4. Enlarged retroperitoneal lymph nodes at the level of the aortic bifurcation (arrow).

Discussion

Benign and malignant intraabdominal pathologic processes can complicate AIDS. Four major processes are responsible for most cases of AIDS-related retroperitoneal lymphadenopathy:

1. Persistent generalized lymphoid hyperplasia (PGLH);
2. MAC;
3. AIDS-related non-Hodgkin's lymphoma (NHL);
4. Kaposi's sarcoma (KS).

PGLH and MAC are benign, while NHL and KS are malignant. Other benign and malignant nodal processes are possible (eg, metastatic adenocarcinoma, seminoma), but are less likely in the setting of AIDS.

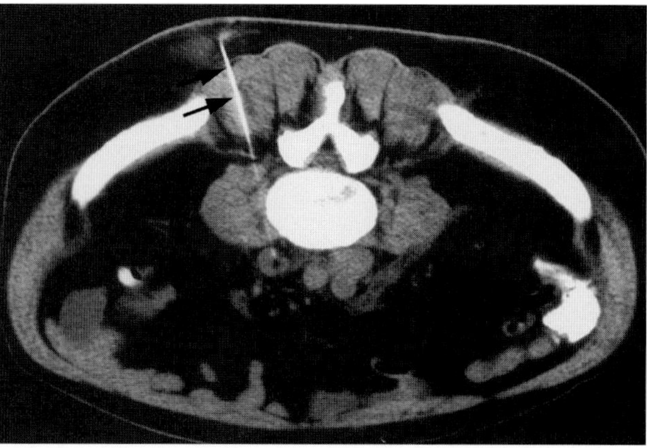

Figure 5. CT-guided fine-needle aspiration of an enlarged left retroperitoneal lymph node. The patient has been placed in the prone position. A 22-gauge Chiba needle is used for the biopsy, introduced via the left paraspinous approach (arrow).

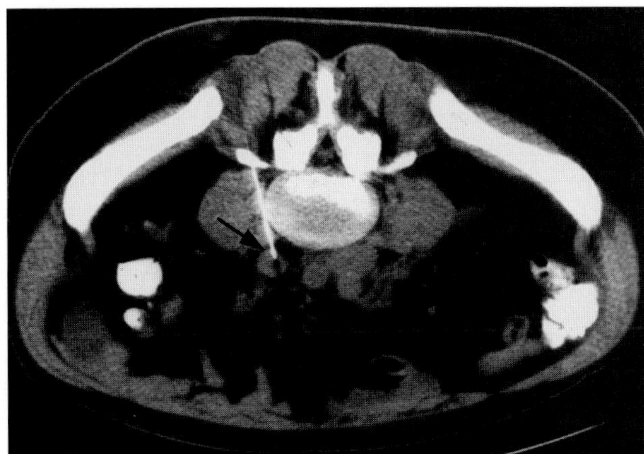

Figure 6. Slightly lower section from the biopsy in Figure 5 shows the needle tip in the lesion (arrow).

PGLH is characterized by multifocal mild lymph node enlargement (<1.5 cm) and splenomegaly. MAC, on the other hand, can involve the lung, reticuloendothelial system, liver, and bowel. Bulky retroperitoneal lymphadenopathy (>1.5 cm) is often present in this systemic process. AIDS-related NHL, like MAC, affects multiple organ systems, and also causes bulky retroperitoneal lymphadenopathy. KS can demonstrate bulky retroperitoneal lymphadenopathy as well as gastrointestinal tract and pulmonary involvement. Nearly all patients with advanced KS will have cutaneous manifestations as well.

All of these processes may present with a similar clinical picture that includes pain and fever. With the possible exception of PGLH, these diseases can be virtually indistinguishable on cross-sectional imaging studies. The presence of central low attenuation is nonspecific. Biopsy is needed to differentiate between these processes so that proper treatment can be instituted.

CT-guided fine-needle aspiration biopsy (FNAB) is currently the most effective method for obtaining retroperitoneal nodal specimens for cytologic and microbiologic analysis. CT guidance allows reproducible localization of nodal masses as well as localization of neighboring structures that need to be avoided. The location of the mass determines the approach. Retroperitoneal lymphadenopathy is usually accessible by the paraspinous approach, as demonstrated in this case. Multiple FNAB passes can be made in a single session. The procedure is best performed with a cytologist in attendance to confirm the adequacy of the specimen(s). Needles ranging in size from 20 to 22 gauge are most effective.

Diagnostic accuracy of FNAB of retroperitoneal lymph nodes ranges from 50% to over 90%. Special stains, specialized culture conditions, and advanced analysis techniques (eg, immunocytochemistry, lymphoid marker studies) all influence the diagnostic accuracy.

FNAB has few contraindications, but coagulopathy is a major one. Every attempt should be made to correct any coagulation abnormalities prior to biopsy. Complications are rare, but they include hemorrhage, bowel perforation, pneumothorax/hemothorax, and seeding of malignant cells.

Selected Readings

Chaisson RE. Mycobacterium avium complex and HIV. J Int Assoc Physicians AIDS Care 1995; 1:10–15.

Charboneau JW, Reading CC, Welch TJ. CT and sonographically guided needle biopsy: current techniques and new innovations. AJR 1990; 154:1–10.

Federle MP. A radiologist looks at AIDS: imaging evaluation based on symptom complexes. Radiology 1988; 166:553–562.

Martin-Bates E, Tanner A, Suvarna SK, Glazer G, Coleman DV. Use of fine needle aspiration cytology for investigating lymphadenopathy in HIV positive patients. J Clin Pathol 1993; 46:564–566.

Smith EH. Complications of percutaneous abdominal fine-needle biopsy. Radiology 1991; 178:253–258.

Steel BL, Schwartz MR, Ramzy I. Fine needle aspiration biopsy in the diagnosis of lymphadenopathy in 1,103 patients. Role, limitations, and analysis of diagnostic pitfalls. Acta Cytol 1995; 39:76–81.

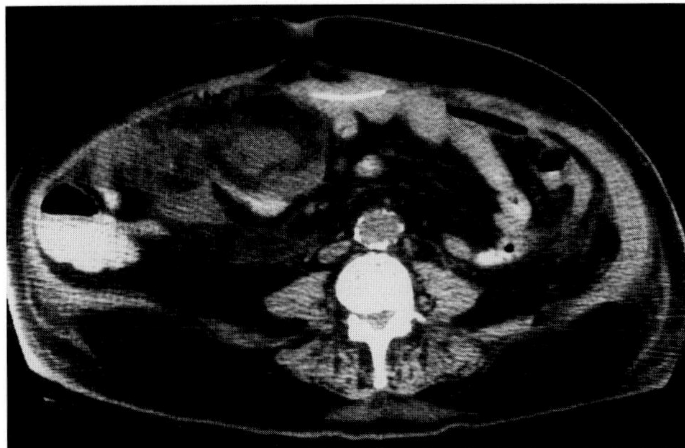

Figure 1. Axial contrast-enhanced CT scan through the lower abdomen.

TEACHING FILE CASE 17

Mark W. Wilson, M.D.

History

A 54-year-old man was admitted for an acute myocardial infarction. Three days after admission he developed diffuse abdominal pain, abdominal distention, and fever. A computed tomography (CT) scan was obtained **(Fig. 1)**.

What is your diagnosis?

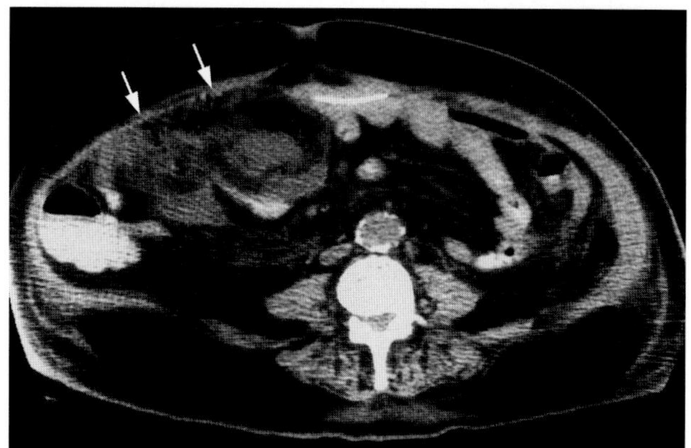

Figure 2. CT scan shows a focal, irregular fluid collection (arrows) adjacent to the ascending colon containing gas bubbles and the suggestion of an air-fluid level. These features are compatible with a diverticular abscess.

Radiographic Findings

Selected images from the contrast-enhanced CT scan **(Fig. 2)** demonstrate a focal, predominantly fluid-density collection adjacent to the ascending colon. The collection has gaseous components and the suggestion of an air-fluid level as well.

Diagnosis

Acute diverticular abscess.

How would you manage this patient?

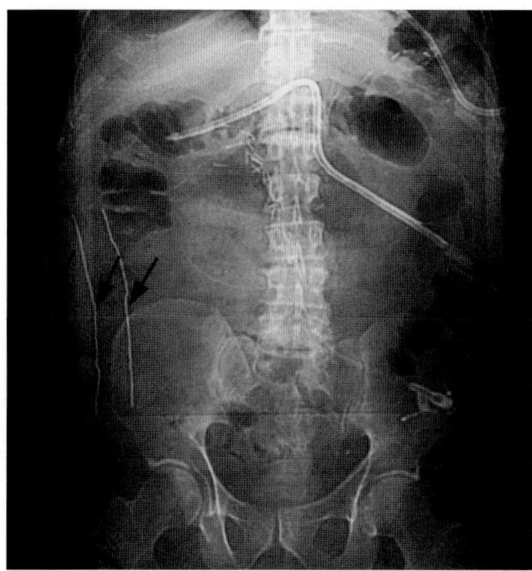

Figure 3. Localization of the abscess with metallic paper clips taped to the abdomen as reference markers (arrows).

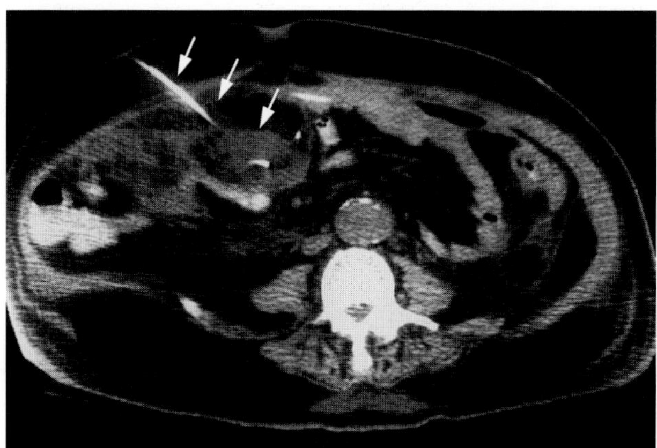

Figure 4. CT-guided percutaneous drainage. A guide wire has been passed into the largest component of the abscess (arrows).

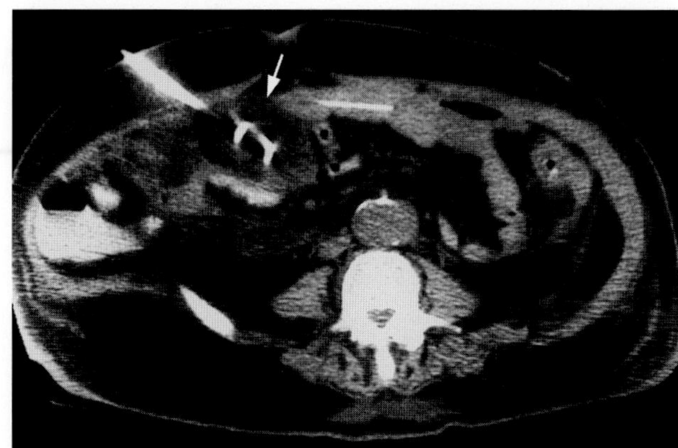

Figure 5. CT-guided percutaneous drainage. Final placement of the drainage catheter into the diverticular abscess (arrow).

Management

This patient had a known history of diverticulosis. He was believed to be a poor surgical candidate given his underlying ischemic heart disease. The collection was localized with metallic paper clips taped to the abdomen as reference markers **(Fig. 3)**. This permitted CT-guided insertion of a percutaneous drain into the collection **(Figs. 4, 5)**. The abscess was managed with percutaneous drainage and intravenous antibiotics alone. No fistula was ever demonstrated, and the drain was removed after 3 months without complication.

Discussion

Diverticular disease of the colon has numerous manifestations and complications. Inflammation (diverticulitis), hemorrhage, obstruction (usually a sequela of diverticulitis), and perforation are all possible. Perforation may result in diffuse peritonitis, or it may be contained, forming a diverticular abscess. In a patient with known diverticulosis, the presence of a focal pericolic collection with liquid, gaseous, and/or occasional phlegmonous components is compatible with a diverticular abscess. However, other entities, such as inflammatory bowel disease and perforation of an adenocarcinoma, must still be considered and excluded. The etiology of diverticular perforation is unclear, but ischemia, ulcerations, and foreign bodies have been associated with it.

Traditional surgical management of diverticulitis consists of a three-staged procedure involving drainage and proximal diverting colostomy, delayed segmental bowel resection, and delayed re-anastomosis. There is presently a trend toward initial CT-guided abscess drainage with broad-spectrum antibiotic coverage, followed by a single-staged partial colectomy and primary anastomosis. This treatment is successful in 50% to 90% of patients. A localized perforation without free fecal spillage can sometimes be managed with percutaneous drainage and antibiotics alone, particularly if the patient is a poor surgical candidate, as in this teaching file case. Percutaneous drainage should therefore be considered in all cases of diverticular abscess, as it may preclude the need for surgery.

Selected Readings

Neff CC, vanSonnenberg E, Casola G, et al. Diverticular abscesses: percutaneous drainage. Radiology 1987; 163:15–18.

Peoples JB, Vilk DR, Maguire JP, Elliott DW. Reassessment of primary resection of the perforated segment for severe colonic diverticulitis. Am J Surg 1990; 159:291–294.

Stabile BE, Puccio E, vanSonnenberg E, Neff CC. Preoperative percutaneous drainage of diverticular abscesses. Am J Surg 1990; 159:99–104.

Telford GL. Diverticular disease. In: Greenfield LJ, Mulholland MW, Oldham KT, Zelenock GB. Surgery: scientific principles and practice. Philadelphia: J.B. Lippincott, 1993.

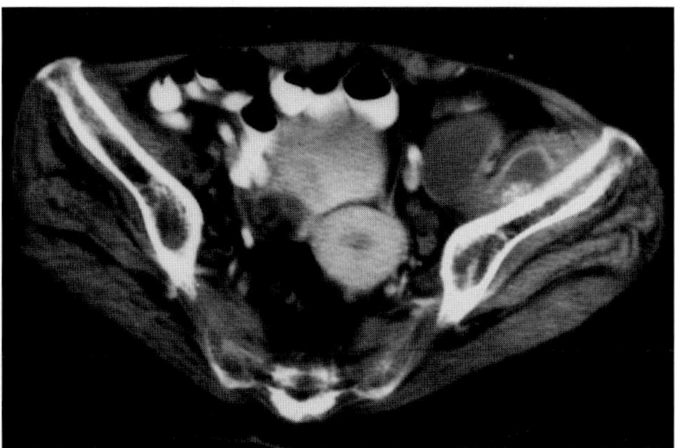

Figure 1. Axial pelvic CT scan at the level of the iliac fossa.

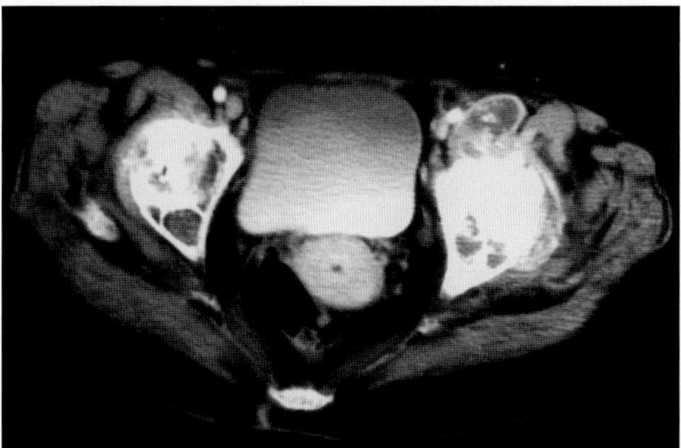

Figure 2. Axial CT scan at the upper acetabular level.

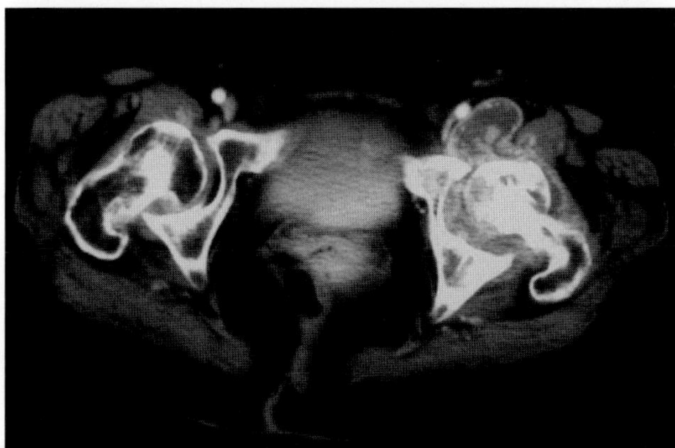

Figure 3. Axial CT scan through the hip joints.

TEACHING FILE CASE 18

Mark W. Wilson, M.D., and Robert K. Kerlan, Jr., M.D.

History

A 54-year-old woman was transferred from a nursing home with chronic pain and swelling involving the left hip. There was clinical suspicion of an insufficiency fracture. A computed tomography (CT) scan was obtained **(Figs. 1–3)**.

What is your diagnosis?

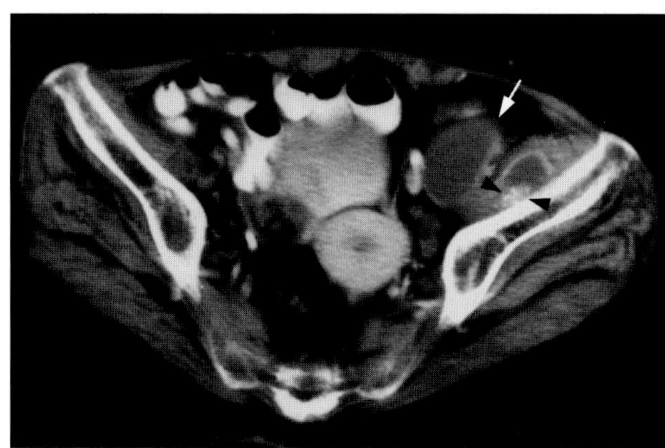

Figure 4. Multiloculated fluid collection involving the left iliopsoas muscle (arrow). Note the flocculent calcification adjacent to the ilium in the iliacus component of the collection (arrowheads). These findings are compatible with a tuberculous abscess.

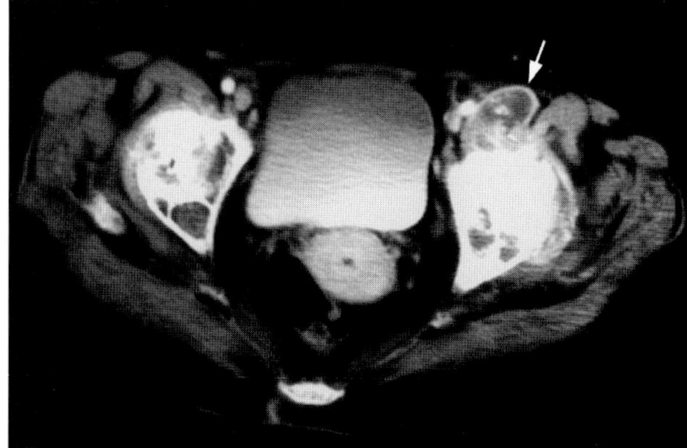

Figure 5. Iliopsoas abscess extending down to the superior portion of the acetabulum (arrow).

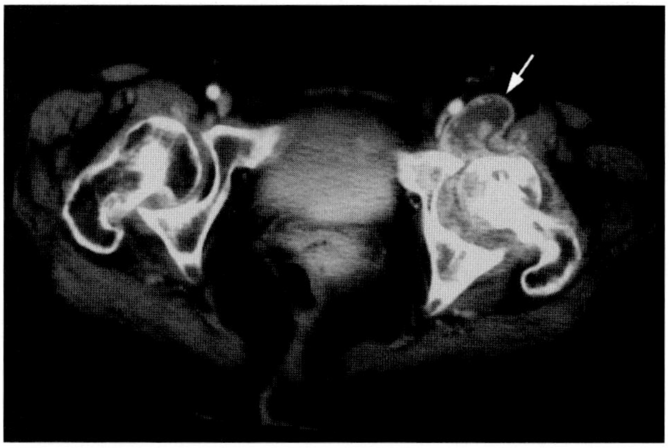

Figure 6. Iliopsoas abscess involving the left hip joint with associated fragmentation of the femoral head (arrow).

Radiographic Findings

Selected images from the contrast-enhanced CT scan **(Figs. 4–6)** demonstrate a multiloculated, fluid-density collection involving the left iliopsoas muscle and extending into the left hip joint. Associated fragmentation of the left femoral head is seen. Flocculent dense foci are present within the collection, compatible with calcification.

Diagnosis

Iliopsoas tuberculous ("cold") abscess with left hip tuberculous arthritis.

How would you manage this patient?

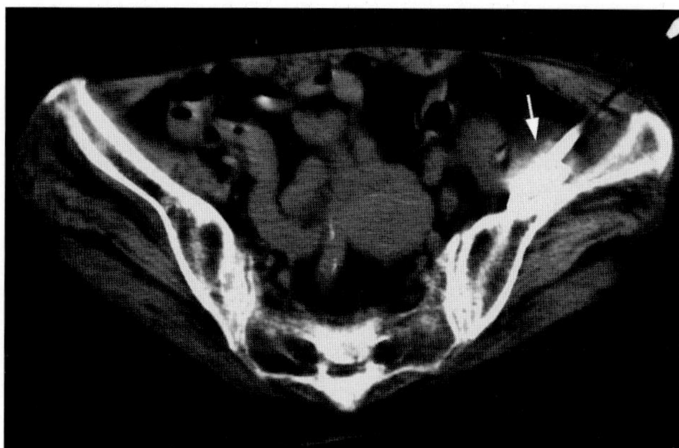

Figure 7. CT-guided insertion of an initial drainage catheter into the collection in the iliac fossa region (arrow).

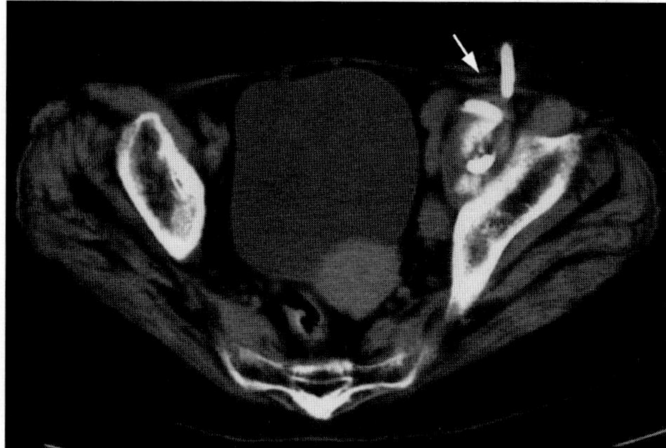

Figure 8. CT-guided insertion of the second drainage catheter into the supraacetabular portion of the collection (arrow).

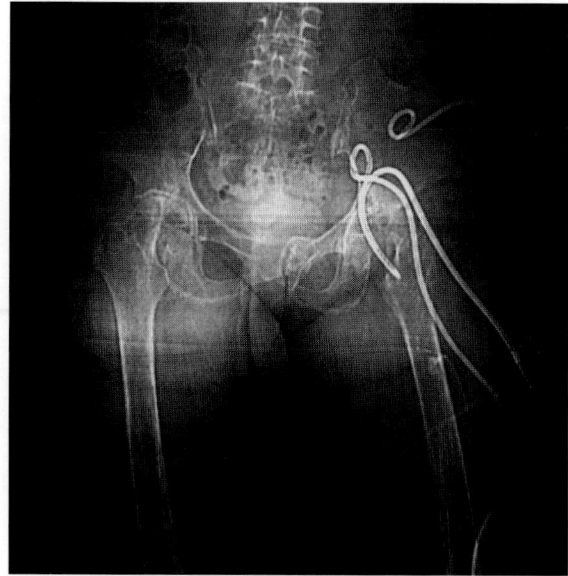

Figure 9. CT scout image demonstrates the final positions of the three iliopsoas abscess drains.

Management

Percutaneous drains were inserted into the collection under CT guidance **(Figs. 7–9)**. Three catheters were placed to drain the multiloculated collection from the iliac fossa to the level of the hip joint.

Repeat CT examination performed 2 weeks after drain insertion demonstrates a significant decrease in the iliac fossa and supraacetabular collections **(Figs. 10, 11)**. Hip joint involvement has increased, however, with progressive destruction of the femoral head **(Fig. 12)**.

Although the iliopsoas components responded well to triple-drug therapy and percutaneous drainage, progressive left hip involvement and femoral head destruction, associated with unremitting pain, necessitated open surgical debridement and resection of the femoral head.

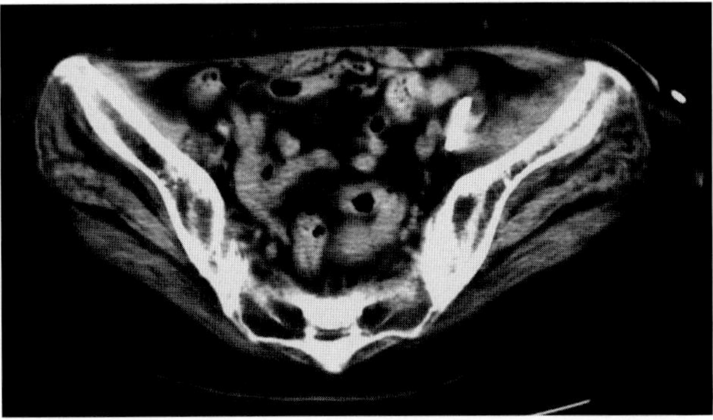

Figure 10. Axial CT image demonstrates a significant decrease in the size of the iliac fossa component of the abscess after 2 weeks of percutaneous drainage. (Compare to Figure 1.)

Discussion

This patient had a known history of tuberculosis (TB) which, it is suspected, was not treated completely. A fluid specimen from the collection stained strongly positive for acid-fast bacilli. Culture results a few days later confirmed *Mycobacterium tuberculosis.*

A primary iliopsoas tuberculous abscess is uncommon. The more likely scenario is seeding from some other focus of infection. Genitourinary TB, if treated inadequately, can be complicated by spread to the psoas muscle with abscess formation. Spinal TB (Pott's disease) can also spread to adjacent paraspinous and psoas muscles. The hip joint is a common site of tuberculous arthritis. The primary hip infection can conceivably spread to the iliopsoas muscle. Tuberculous adenitis tends to occur in the cervical nodes (termed scrofula); however, in approximately one third of cases it occurs in extracervical nodal sites. Retroperitoneal or pelvic tuberculous adenitis can possibly lead to a psoas or iliopsoas abscess, but there should be associated retroperitoneal or pelvic lymphadenopathy with evidence of necrosis or abscess formation.

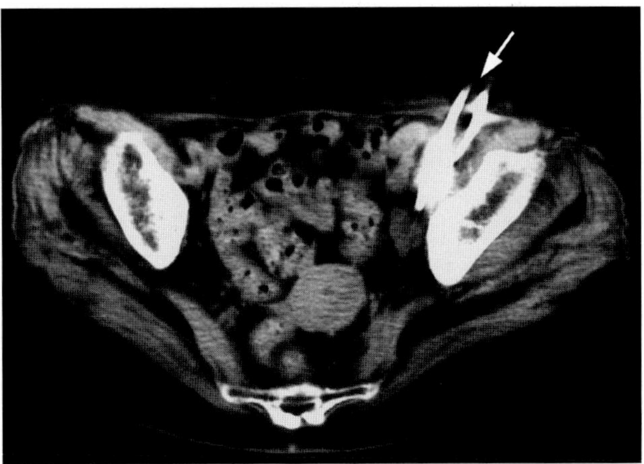

Figure 11. Axial CT image demonstrates a significant decrease in the size of the supraacetabular component of the abscess after 2 weeks of percutaneous drainage. Note the presence of two adjacent drainage tubes (arrow). (Compare to Figure 2.)

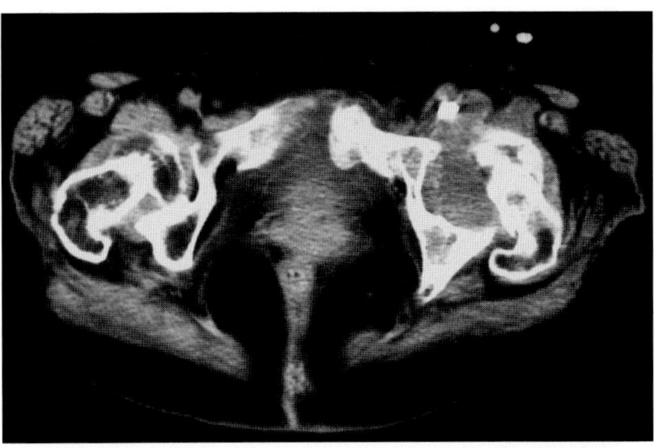

Figure 12. Axial CT image demonstrates increased left hip joint involvement by the abscess along with progressive femoral head destruction. (Compare to Figure 3.)

Selected Readings

Buxi TB, Doda SS, Mathur RK, et al. Computed tomography in spinal tuberculosis. Comput Med Imaging Graph 1991; 15:379–388.

Herranz AD, Moran APL, Lorena M, Rodriguez F, et al. [Left iliac psoas abscess in a patient treated for pulmonary tuberculosis]. Med Clin (Barc) 1995; 104:658–660.

Harrigan RA, Kauffman FH, Love MB. Tuberculous psoas abscess. J Emerg Med 1995; 13:493–498.

Perros P, Sim DW, MacIntyre D. Psoas abscess due to retroperitoneal tuberculous lymphadenopathy. Tubercle 1988; 69:299–301.

vanSonnenberg E, D'Agostino HB, Casola G, Halasz NA, Sanchez RB, Goodacre BW. Percutaneous abscess drainage: current concepts. Radiology 1991; 181:617–626.

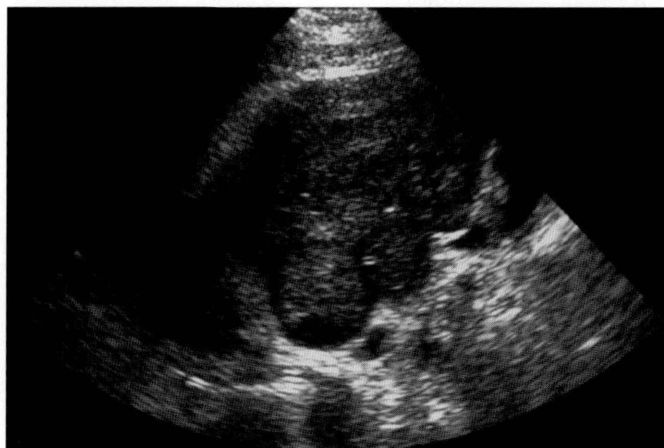

Figure 1. Transverse sonogram of the liver.

TEACHING FILE CASE 19

Richard D. Redvanly, M.D., and Ricardo Lencioni, M.D.

History

A 60-year-old man with a history of alcohol-related cirrhosis was hospitalized for hematemesis. Upper endoscopy revealed bleeding esophageal varices for which sclerotherapy was performed. Hematemesis continued despite sclerotherapy. Based on liver function tests, the patient's cirrhosis was classified as Childs class C. In addition, the serum alpha-fetoprotein was mildly elevated (36 μg/L; normal <15 μg/L). The patient underwent abdominal ultrasonography **(Fig. 1)**.

What is your diagnosis?

Radiographic Findings

The sonogram shows a cirrhotic liver with a 3-cm hepatic mass in the posterior segment of the right lobe **(Fig. 2)**.

Diagnoses

1. Childs class C cirrhosis.
2. Solitary hepatocellular carcinoma.

What treatment would you recommend?

Management

Because this patient had a small, solitary hepatocellular carcinoma (HCC) and severe underlying cirrhosis, he was treated with percutaneous ethanol ablation therapy (PEAT). Under CT guidance, an 18-gauge needle was placed into various sites in the tumor and a total of 35 mL absolute ethanol was injected in two separate sessions.

One month following PEAT, contrast-enhanced CT scanning demonstrated persistent nodular enhancement along the anterior aspect of the treated tumor. CT-directed biopsy confirmed the presence of viable tumor **(Fig. 3)**. Under sonographic guidance, 15 mL of ethanol was injected into the tumor **(Fig. 4)**. The patient has survived 12 months without tumor recurrence.

Discussion

This case demonstrates the advantages of PEAT, which include the ease of performance and the ability to re-treat residual or recurrent disease. Moreover, this case emphasizes the importance of close clinical and radiologic follow-up of patients with chronic liver disease. HCC has a high rate of local and distant recurrence. PEAT is a valuable treatment option in the patient with cirrhosis and a small HCC who is not a surgical candidate. PEAT has achieved good long-term survival rates in these cases, and is safe and relatively easy to perform. Additionally, because PEAT is a local treatment, minimal damage is inflicted on healthy liver parenchyma, and the procedure can be repeated if viable tumor persists or recurs.

Selected Readings

Livraghi T, Giorgio A, Marin G, et al. Hepatocellular carcinoma and cirrhosis in 746 patients: long-term results of percutaneous ethanol injection. Radiology 1995; 197:101–108.

Livraghi T, Solbiati L. Percutaneous ethanol injection in liver cancer: method and results. Semin Intervent Radiol 1993; 10:69–77.

Redvanly RD, Chezmar JL. Percutaneous ethanol ablation therapy of malignant hepatic tumors using CT guidance. Semin Intervent Radiol 1993; 10:82–87.

Shiina S, Niwa Y, Omata M. Percutaneous ethanol injection therapy for liver neoplasms. Semin Intervent Radiol 1993; 10:57–68.

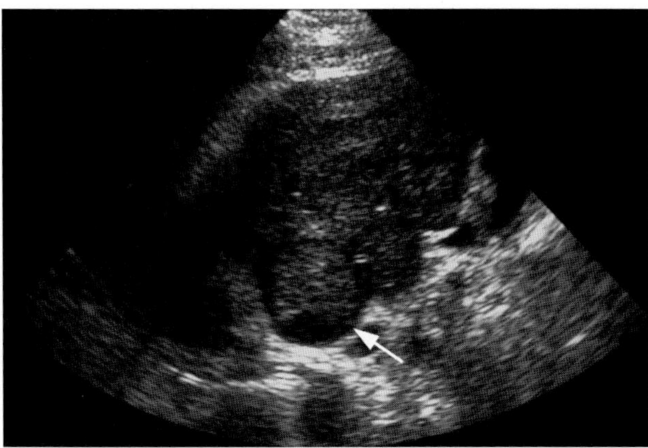

Figure 2. Sonogram demonstrates a focal isoechoic 3-cm mass (arrow) with a hypoechoic capsule in the posterior segment of the right lobe of the liver (segment 6).

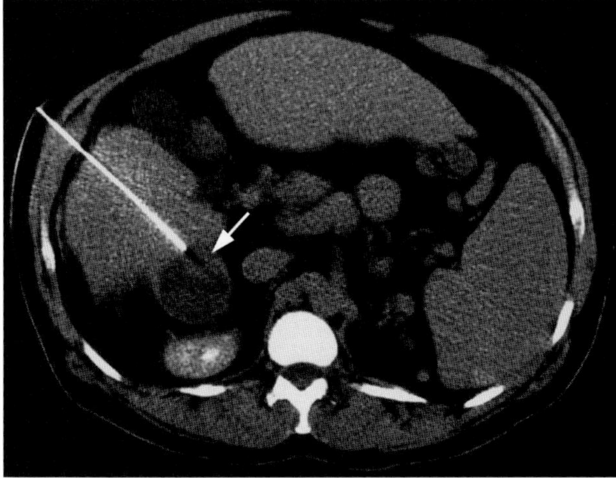

Figure 3. CT-directed biopsy 1 month after initial PEAT confirms the presence of viable tumor (arrow) at the periphery of the previously treated tumor.

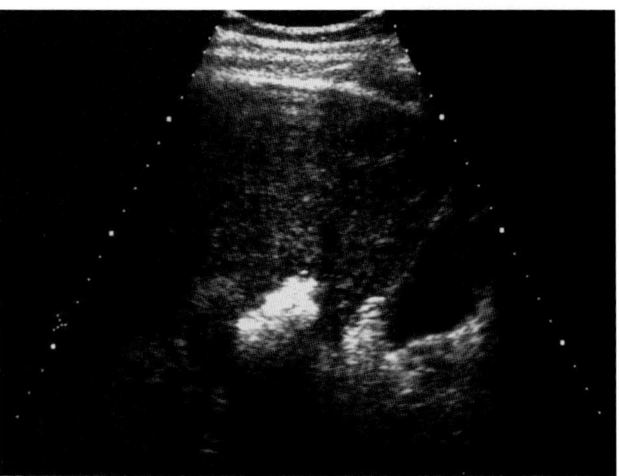

Figure 4. Sonography during PEAT shows a hyperechoic area which represents ethanol injected into viable tumor.

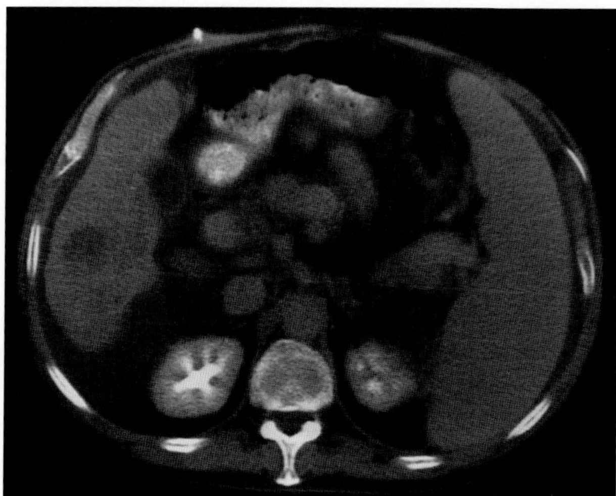

Figure 1. Contrast-enhanced CT scan through the liver.

TEACHING FILE CASE 20

Richard D. Redvanly, M.D., and Ricardo Lencioni, M.D.

History

A 45-year-old man with hepatitis C came to the hospital for evaluation of an elevated serum alpha-fetoprotein level. Laboratory tests revealed Childs class C cirrhosis. He underwent contrast-enhanced computed tomography (CT) scanning **(Fig. 1)**.

What is your diagnosis?

Radiographic Findings

The contrast-enhanced CT scan reveals a cirrhotic-appearing liver with a solitary 3-cm hypoattenuating mass in the anterior segment of the right lobe **(Fig. 2)**.

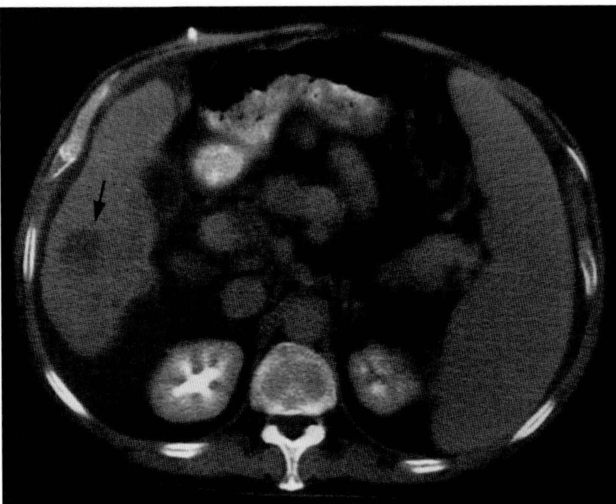

Figure 2. CT scan reveals a cirrhotic-appearing liver with a focal 3-cm hypoattenuating mass (arrow) in the anterior segment of the right lobe (segment 5).

Diagnoses

1. Childs class C cirrhosis.
2. Solitary hepatocellular carcinoma.

What treatment would you recommend?

Management

Because of the patient's cirrhosis, he was not an appropriate candidate for hepatic resection. However, because he had a solitary small hepatocellular carcinoma (HCC), he was a good candidate for percutaneous ethanol ablation therapy (PEAT). An 18-gauge needle was placed into various portions of the tumor and a total of 35 mL of ethanol was injected in two treatment sessions. Immediately following PEAT, a CT scan demonstrated the tumor to be completely hypodense **(Fig. 3)**. A follow-up CT scan obtained 1 month after PEAT revealed the lesion to be nonenhancing, suggesting adequate tumor ablation **(Fig. 4)**. The patient underwent orthotopic liver transplantation 3 months later (as treatment for cirrhosis and portal hypertension as well as for the HCC) and has survived 3 years without recurrence. Histopathological examination of the explanted liver revealed complete tumor necrosis.

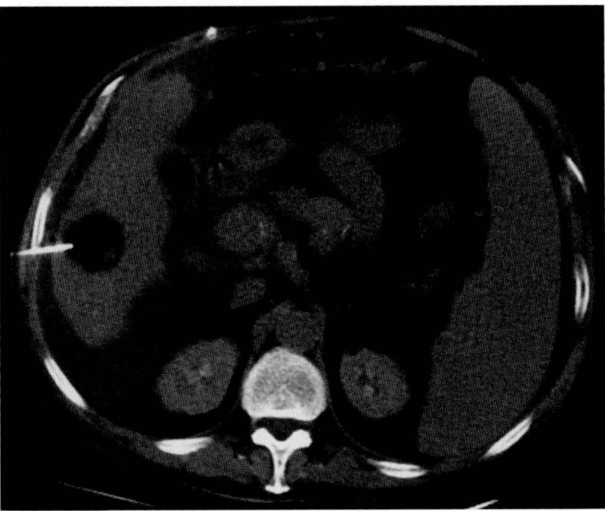

Figure 3. CT scan immediately following PEAT shows the tumor to be completely hypoattenuating, suggesting adequate tumor ablation.

Discussion

This case illustrates a potential role for PEAT as an effective adjunctive treatment option for patients who are poor candidates for surgical resection. Orthotopic liver transplantation provides an opportunity to remove the tumor as well as the cirrhotic liver. PEAT may be useful in patients with a small HCC as a means to prevent disease progression while awaiting liver transplantation.

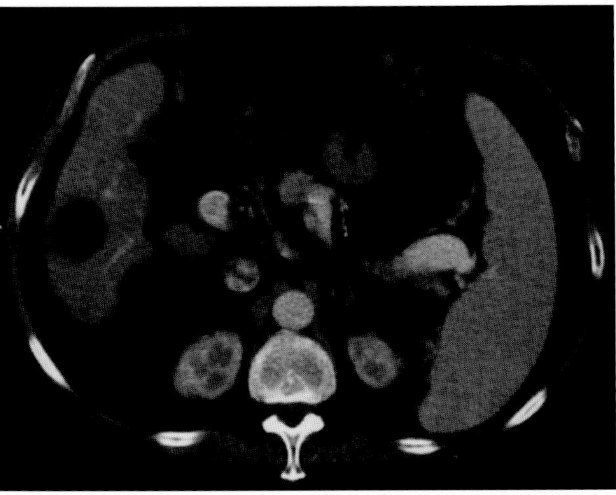

Figure 4. Follow-up contrast-enhanced CT scan 1 month after PEAT. The tumor is completely nonenhancing, consistent with tumor necrosis.

Selected Readings

Livraghi T, Giorgio A, Marin G, et al. Hepatocellular carcinoma and cirrhosis in 746 patients: long-term results of percutaneous ethanol injection. Radiology 1995; 197:101–108.

Livraghi T, Solbiati L. Percutaneous ethanol injection in liver cancer: method and results. Semin Intervent Radiol 1993; 10:69–77.

Redvanly RD, Chezmar JL. Percutaneous ethanol ablation therapy of malignant hepatic tumors using CT guidance. Semin Intervent Radiol 1993; 10:82–87.

Shiina S, Niwa Y, Omata M. Percutaneous ethanol injection therapy for liver neoplasms. Semin Intervent Radiol 1993; 10:57–68.

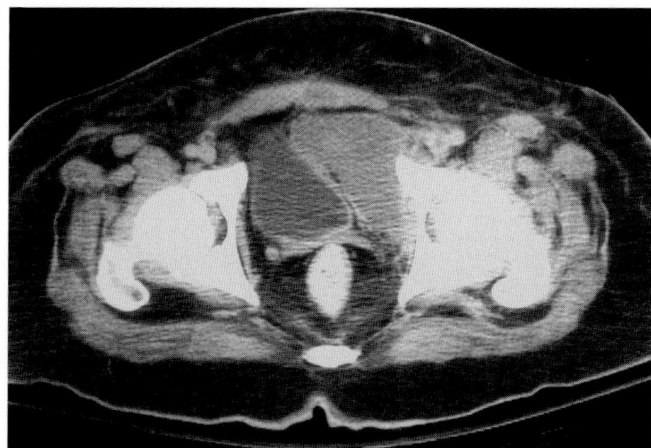

Figure 1. Abdominal CT scan.

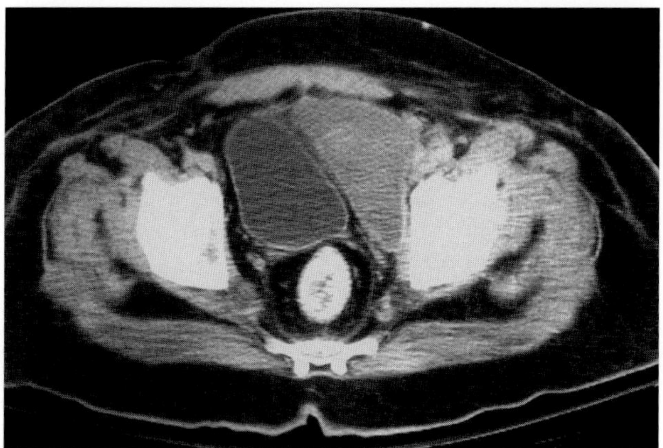

Figure 2. CT image superior to Figure 1.

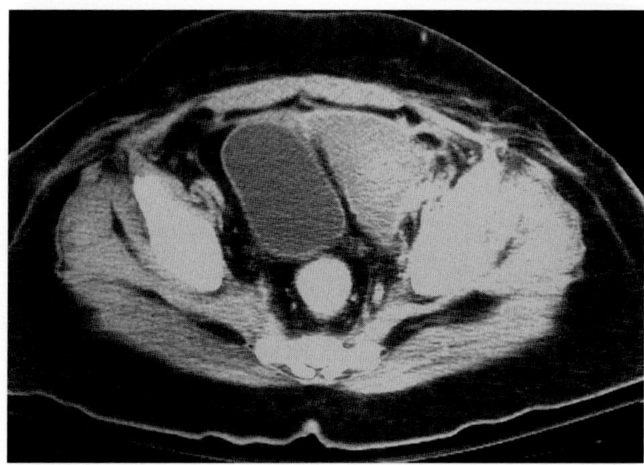

Figure 3. More superior image.

TEACHING FILE CASE 21

Lance Arnder, M.D., and Jeet Sandhu, M.D.

History

A 62-year-old man was struck by an automobile. He was found to have a pelvic hematoma but was clinically stable. Several days later, he developed fevers with positive blood cultures, and a computed tomography (CT) scan was obtained to exclude an abdominal abscess **(Figs. 1–3)**.

What is your diagnosis?

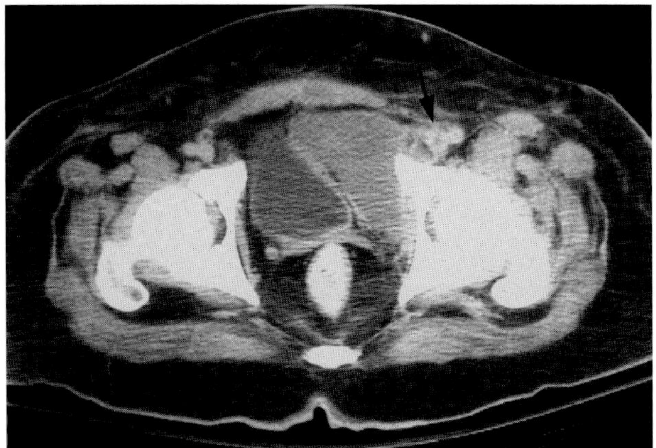
Figure 4. High-density collection compatible with a hematoma adjacent to the bladder. Note thrombus in the left common femoral vein (arrow).

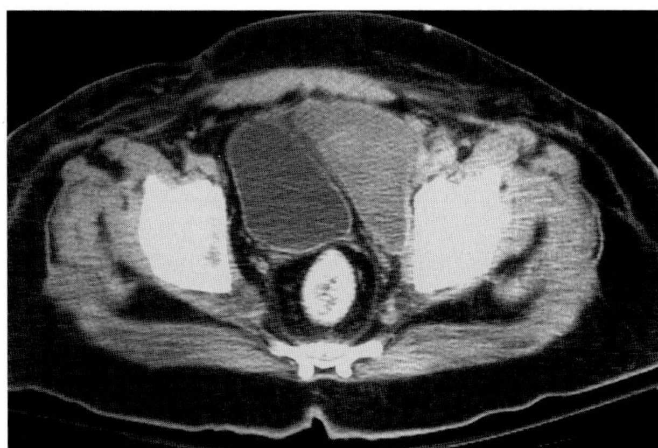
Figure 5. Image more cephalad to Figure 4.

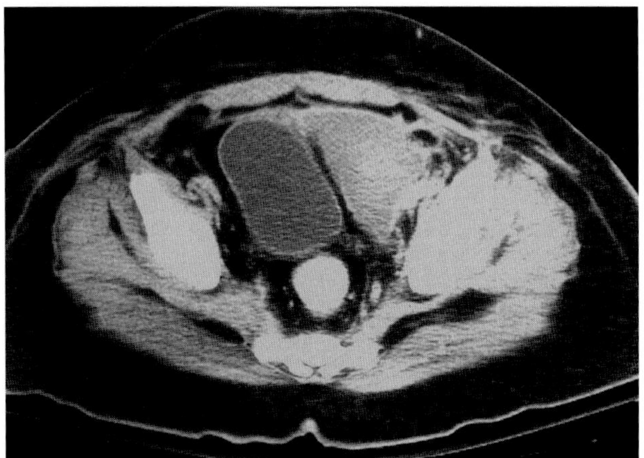
Figure 6. Cephalad extent of the hematoma.

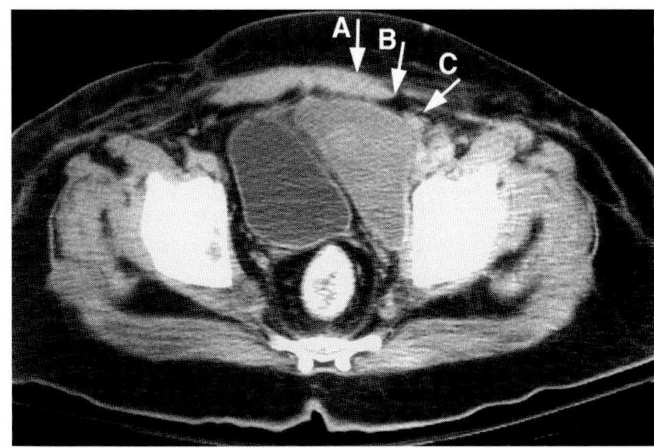

Figure 7. Which route would you choose to drain this hematoma: A, B, or C?

Radiographic Findings
The CT images demonstrate a complex fluid collection with an enhancing rim to the left of the urinary bladder and producing mass effect upon it **(Figs. 4–6)**. Given the patient's recent trauma and the high density of the collection, these findings most likely represent a pelvic hematoma. The enhancing rim around the collection is probably due to active reabsorption of the hematoma. Based on the patient's clinical symptoms, superinfection of the hematoma cannot be excluded. A left common femoral deep vein thrombosis was identified incidentally.

Diagnosis
Pelvic hematoma with possible superinfection.

Because infection of the hematoma could not be excluded, and given the ongoing sepsis, the clinical service deemed the patient a poor surgical risk and requested drainage of the collection.

Would you attempt percutaneous drainage and if so, which route would you choose **(Fig. 7)**?

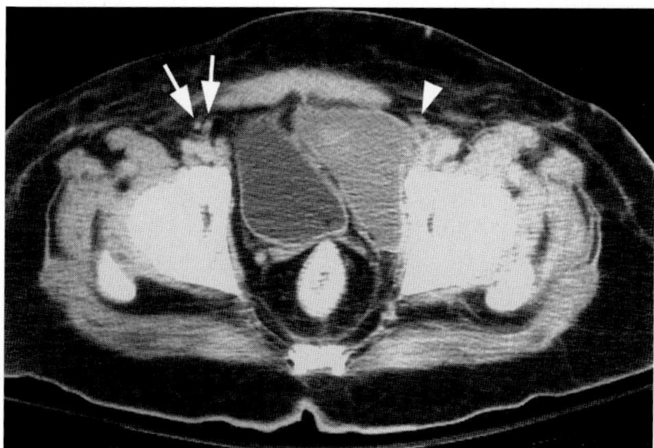

Figure 8. Inferior epigastric vessels on the left (arrowhead) overlie the hematoma, precluding the use of access route C. The right inferior epigastric artery and vein (arrows) are noted originating from the common femoral artery and vein.

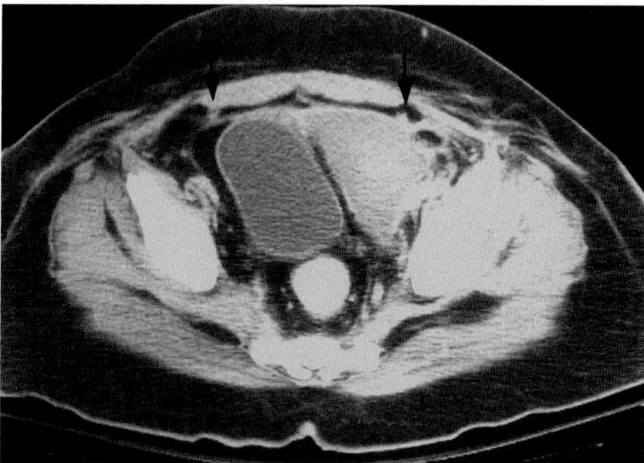

Figure 9. Inferior epigastric vessels (arrows) along the lateral edge of the rectus muscle.

Management

Percutaneous drainage from a transrectus abdominus approach (approach A) was performed, and old blood was obtained that yielded gram-positive cocci on culture. With continued drainage supplemented by local thrombolytic therapy in conjunction with intravenous antibiotics, the patient responded well and did not require surgery.

Discussion

Hematomas can be difficult to drain percutaneously because of their viscous, dense nature. Older hematomas that have liquefied may be easier to drain. Although hematomas can be difficult to drain, percutaneous drainage should be attempted in certain circumstances.

If the hematoma is infected, if the patient has bacteremia with no other source, or if the patient has severe pain or obstructive symptoms, drainage can be attempted. A large-bore catheter should be placed and as much of the liquefied component drained as possible. Urokinase in varying doses can be injected into the collection to facilitate further liquefaction of the hematoma. In patients with suspected superinfection of the hematoma, the catheter can be removed within 48 to 72 hours if cultures remain negative; this minimizes any chance of infecting the hematoma. If the patient does not meet any of the criteria for drainage, the hematoma should not be disturbed because most hematomas will resolve spontaneously over time.

In this case and in all cases where an anterior approach is used to drain a collection, the location of the epigastric vessels must be kept in mind. Because the inferior epigastric artery courses through the path of the most direct access to the collection (approach C) **(Fig. 8)**, placement of a drainage catheter along this course may result in significant bleeding. Approach B is along the edge of the rectus muscle, where the epigastric vessels lie **(Fig. 9)**. The inferior epigastric artery lies posterior to the lateral aspect of the rectus muscle at the superior aspect of the collection, and courses laterally over the collection to join the external iliac artery. A transrectus approach is the most direct approach that would also avoid the inferior epigastric artery.

The reason for avoiding the rectus muscles during percutaneous procedures is to avoid the epigastric vessels. Paradoxically, in this case the transrectus approach is the best approach for avoiding the epigastric vessels.

The inferior epigastric artery originates from the external iliac artery and travels superiorly and medially until it lies just posterior to the ipsilateral rectus muscle along the lateral edge **(Fig. 10)**. Lying just anterior to the parietal peritoneum, it then courses superiorly behind the ipsilateral rectus muscle to anastomose with the superior epigastric artery above the umbilicus. The superior epigastric artery is a continuation of the internal mammary artery beyond the origin of the musculophrenic artery.

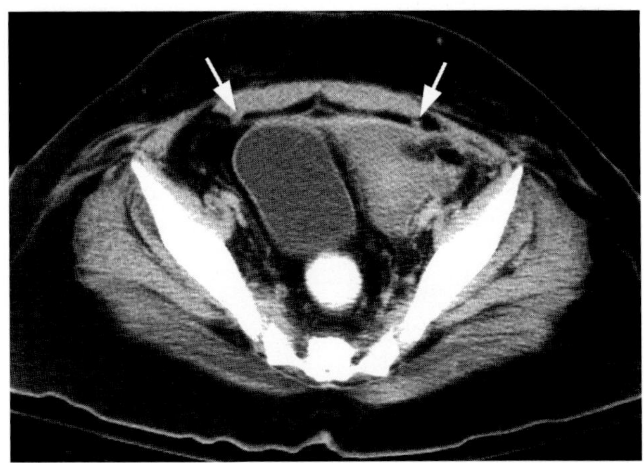

Figure 10. Normal inferior location of the inferior epigastric vessels immediately posterior to the lateral third of the rectus abdominus (arrows).

The course of the inferior epigastric artery is gently medial as it extends cranially so that inferiorly, it lies behind the lateral third of the ipsilateral rectus muscle, and more superiorly, it lies behind the middle third of the ipsilateral rectus muscle.

Major vascular complications involving the inferior epigastric, the superior epigastric, and the internal mammary arteries during percutaneous procedures are rare. However, a review of the literature reveals that major complications involving percutaneous damage to these vessels do occur. In one case, a patient expired secondary to injury of the inferior epigastric artery. The death was due at least in part to delayed recognition of the injury, which emphasizes the need for close postprocedure monitoring of the patient.

If possible, percutaneous puncture along the described courses of these arteries should be avoided. If this is not possible, consideration should be given to CT guidance. As with the epigastric vessels, which may be injured with anterior abdominal approaches, the internal mammary artery can be injured with parasternal biopsies or drainages. With respect to the internal mammary arteries, a puncture at least 2.5 cm lateral to the sternal border should avoid these vessels. Similarly, an immediate parasternal approach should also avoid these vessels, although CT guidance in this situation is recommended.

Selected Readings

Glassberg RM, Sussman SK. Life-threatening hemorrhage due to percutaneous transthoracic intervention: importance of the internal mammary artery. AJR 1990; 154:47–49.

Glassberg RM, Sussman SK, Glickstein MF. CT anatomy of the internal mammary vessels: importance in planning percutaneous transthoracic procedures. AJR 1990; 155:397–400.

Nordestgaard AG, Bodily KC, Osborne RW, Buttorff JD. Major vascular injuries during laparoscopic procedures. Am J Surg 1995; 169:543–545.

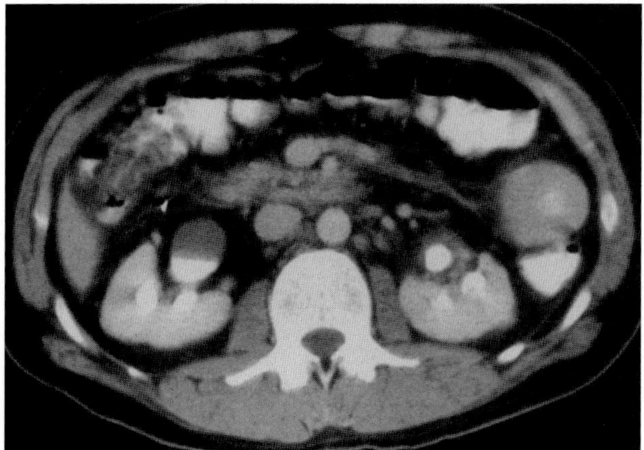

Figure 1. Abdominal CT scan.

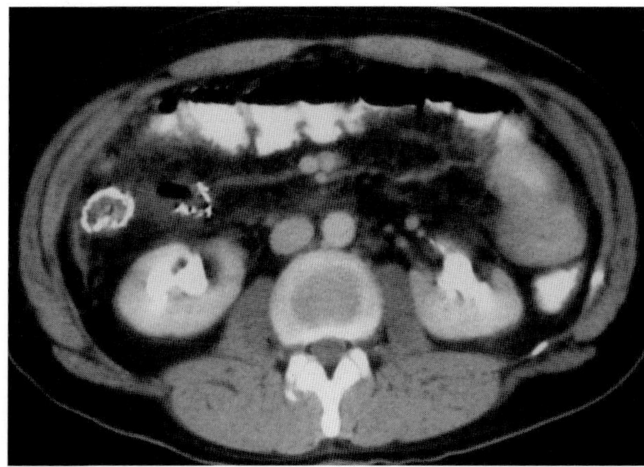

Figure 2. Abdominal CT scan.

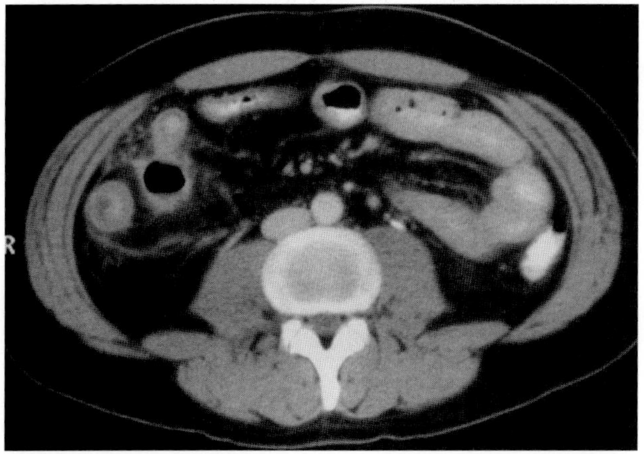

Figure 3. Abdominal CT scan.

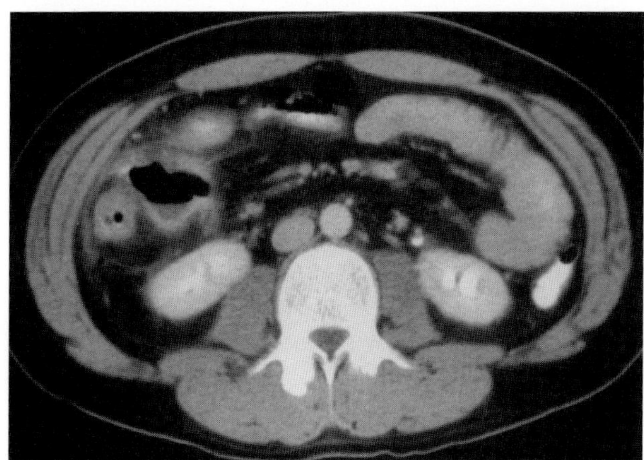

Figure 4. Abdominal CT scan.

TEACHING FILE CASE 22

Jeet Sandhu, M.D.

History

This 23-year-old man came to the hospital with fevers, diarrhea, abdominal pain, and a palpable abdominal mass. A computed tomography (CT) scan was obtained **(Figs. 1–4)**.

What is your diagnosis?

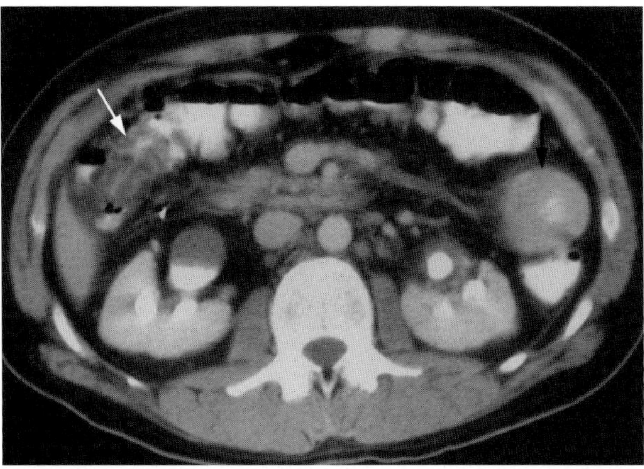

Figure 5. Wall thickening identified in the proximal transverse colon (white arrow) and a thickened loop of small bowel (black arrow).

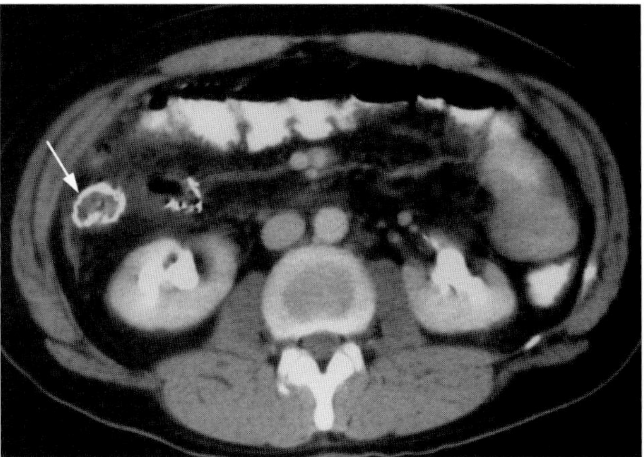

Figure 6. Anastomotic site from prior bowel resection (arrow).

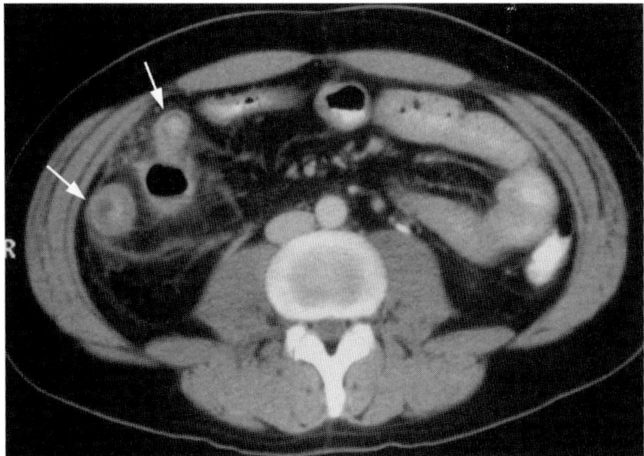

Figure 7. Loop of distal small bowel (arrows) with thickened bowel wall. An extraluminal air-filled cavity with surrounding infiltration of the fat and thickening of Gerota's fascia is present.

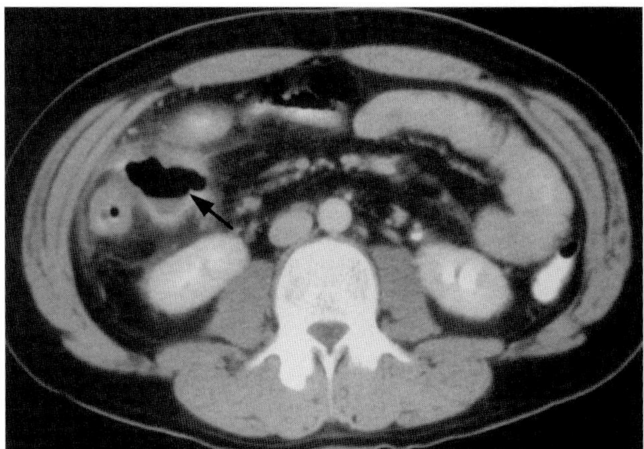

Figure 8. CT image inferior to Figure 7 demonstrates fluid in the cavity (arrow) with surrounding inflammation of the tissues. The cavity is suggestive of an abscess and, given the large amount of air in the cavity, a fistula should be suspected.

Radiographic Findings

Wall thickening of the colon and a small bowel loop are present **(Fig. 5)**. The patient has had prior surgical resection of a portion of his terminal ileum and colon for Crohn's disease with primary re-anastomosis **(Fig. 6)**. Two markedly thickened loops of ileum are present, with an adjacent air-filled extraluminal cavity surrounded by stranding and inflammatory changes in the fat which suggest an abscess **(Fig. 7)**. Although the air in the cavity could be from gas-producing organisms, it is much more likely to come from the bowel via a fistula to the abscess.

On a scan slightly inferior to the level of the prior scan, a small amount of fluid is present in the cavity and the inflammatory changes and bowel thickening are again identified **(Fig. 8)**. Even without the prior history of Crohn's disease, in a young patient with multiple areas of bowel abnormality with an associated abscess, the leading diagnosis should be Crohn's disease. However, the possibility of a lymphoma with perforation should also be considered.

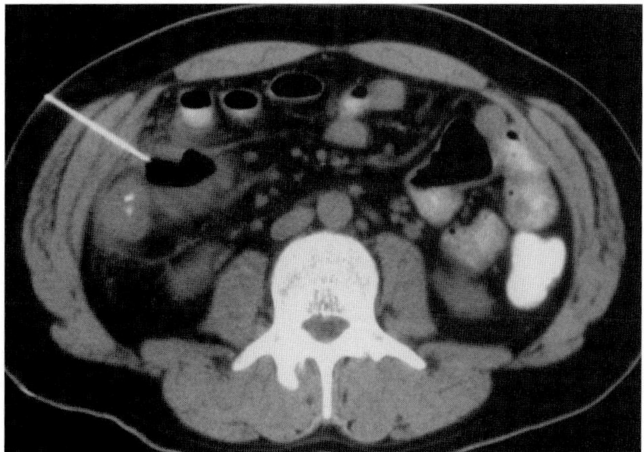

Figure 9. CT-guided drainage of the abscess with the needle tip in the collection.

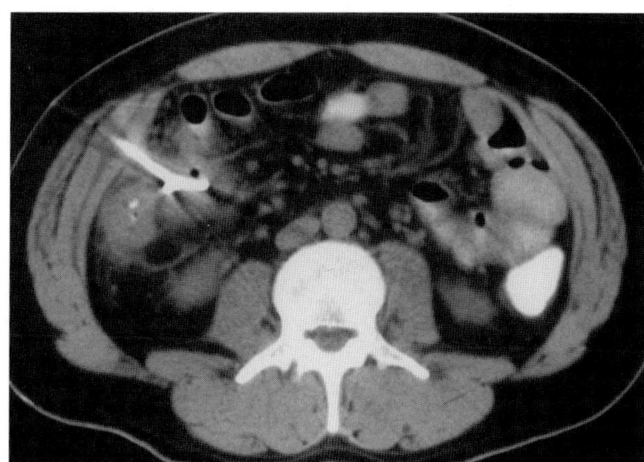

Figure 10. Placement of a Cope loop catheter for evacuation of the collection.

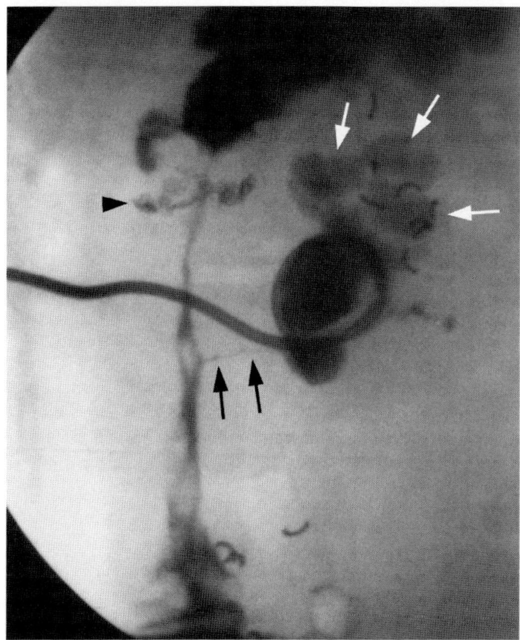

Figure 11. Initial tube check after catheter placement demonstrates a fistula (black arrows) originating from a markedly diseased ileal segment proximal to the prior ileocolic anastomosis (arrowhead). The cavity is the same size as the loop of the catheter. White arrows show renal calculi superior to the abscess cavity.

Diagnosis

Abdominal abscess with likely enteric fistula from Crohn's disease.

How would you manage this patient?

Management

Percutaneous drainage of the abdominal abscess was performed under CT guidance **(Fig. 9)**. Ten mL of purulent material was obtained and a catheter was left in the cavity **(Fig. 10)**. A follow-up tube check several days later demonstrated that the cavity was the same size as the Cope loop **(Fig. 11)**. However, a fistula to the ileum is now visible, with diffuse wall thickening of the bowel segment from which the fistula originated. The fistula is distant from the anastomotic site. Given the extensive bowel wall abnormalities, it was unlikely that prolonged tube drainage would allow closure of the fistula, but this was attempted anyway.

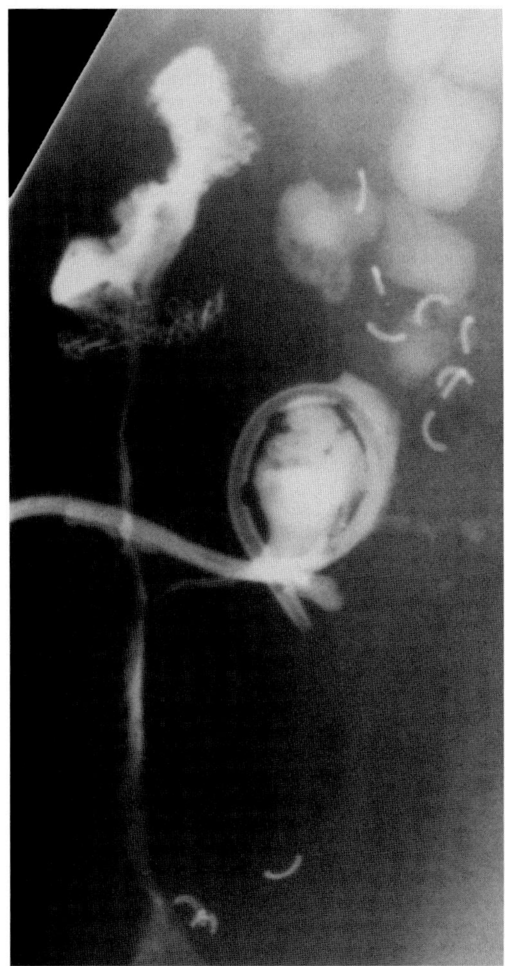

Figure 12. Tube check 2 months after initial drainage demonstrates a persistent fistula with persistent bowel thickening. Renal calculi are still seen superior and adjacent to the abscess cavity.

A repeat fistulogram in 2 months demonstrated a persistent fistula to the ileum; the appearance of the bowel was unchanged **(Fig. 12)**. At this time the patient underwent surgical resection of the diseased bowel.

Discussion

Fistulas may be found in 15% of all cases of abdominal abscess drainage. Fistulas can occur to the bowel, to the pancreatic duct or the biliary tree, to the urinary tract, or to the skin. Most fistulas occur postoperatively, with the majority of them occurring from leakage at the enteric anastomotic site. The etiologies of spontaneous fistulas include peptic ulcer disease, inflammatory bowel disease, diverticulitis, appendicitis, trauma, and malignancy with perforation.

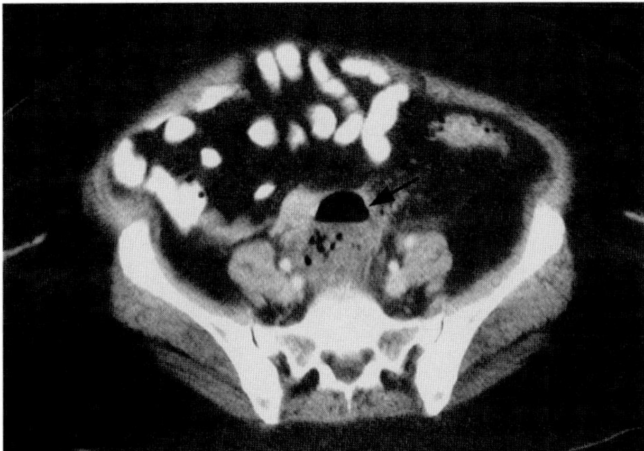

Figure 13. Sigmoid diverticular abscess with air in the collection suggestive of a fistula (arrow).

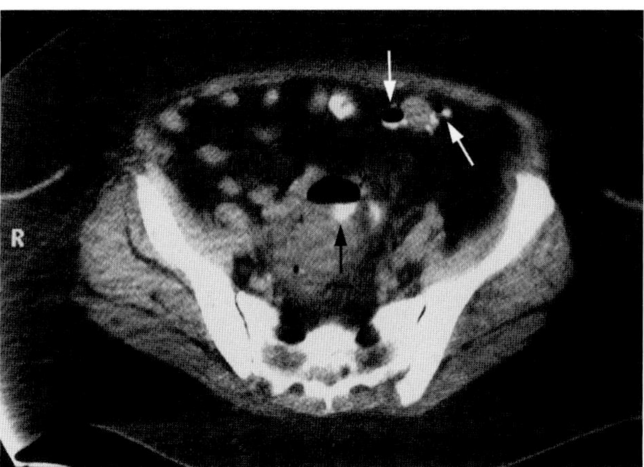

Figure 14. Delayed CT scan demonstrates extravasation of contrast material (black arrow) into the abscess collection. Multiple other diverticula from the proximal sigmoid colon are present (white arrows).

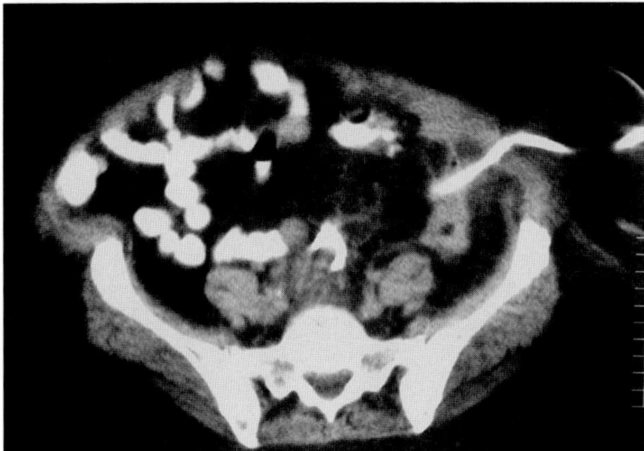

Figure 15. Placement of a catheter into the collection under CT guidance.

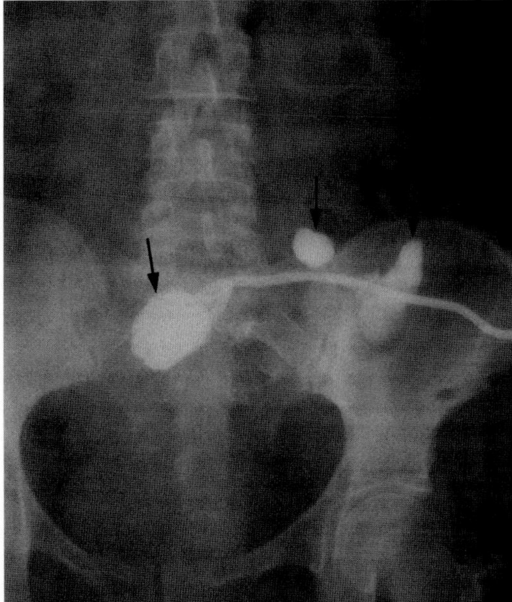

Figure 16. Tube injection 3 days after catheter placement shows filling of the sigmoid colon (arrows) from the abscess cavity. Over the course of 8 weeks of tube drainage, the fistula closed with no communication from the cavity to the bowel.

The success of nonoperative management in closing the fistula will depend on the etiology of the underlying fistula as well as the ability to divert the pancreatic, biliary, or enteric contents away from the site of the fistula. Overall success rates in fistula closure with percutaneous drainage alone are approximately 60%. There is no significant difference in closure of high-output fistulas (>200 mL per day) versus low-output fistulas. Fistulas secondary to diverticulitis or appendicitis have a near 100% closure rate with percutaneous drainage **(Figs. 13–16)**. Post-traumatic fistulas also close successfully with percutaneous drainage. Postoperative fistulas have a variable closure rate depending partly on the location within the bowel. Esophageal fistulas have a very high spontaneous closure rate with catheter drainage, while small bowel and colonic fistulas have a variable closure rate and may require prolonged drainage.

Fistulas caused by perforated malignancy have a very poor spontaneous closure rate with percutaneous drainage. Similarly, fistulas associated with Crohn's disease respond poorly to percutaneous drainage, in part due to the significant underlying intrinsic bowel disease associated with Crohn's disease.

Crohn's disease, also known as regional enteritis, regional ileitis, ileocolitis, or granulomatous ileocolitis, is an inflammatory condition of unknown etiology that results in necrotizing inflammation of the gastrointestinal tract anywhere from the mouth to the anus, although it is typically found in the ileum. Discontinuous involvement is a distinguishing feature of Crohn's disease; abnormal areas of bowel are separated by normal areas of uninvolved bowel. Necrotizing inflammation is the hallmark of Crohn's disease and results in mucosal linear ulcerations and distortion of mucosal folds that give a "cobblestone" appearance to the bowel.

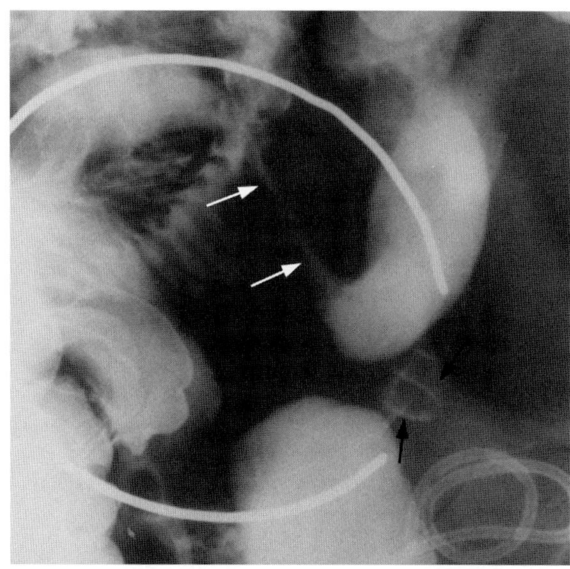

Figure 17. Deep penetrating ulcers (black arrows) with bowel wall thickening (white arrows) are characteristic of Crohn's disease.

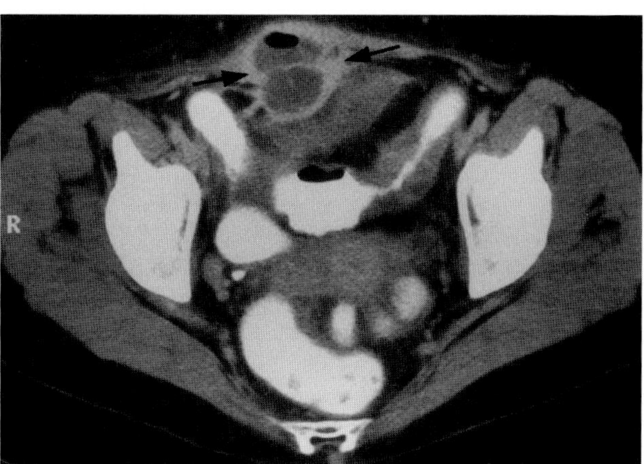

Figure 18. Small bowel wall thickening and luminal narrowing from the transmural inflammation associated with Crohn's disease. The patient also has an anterior abdominal wall abscess (arrows) due to perforation from another diseased bowel segment.

The etiology of Crohn's disease is unknown but it is believed to represent an autoimmune disorder, possibly due to an abnormal platelet activating factor coupled with failure of suppresser T-cells and abnormally active helper T-cells. As a result, there is an exaggerated immune response that triggers an activation of the inflammatory cascade with consequent ulceration and inflammation of the bowel wall. Certainly genetic, familial, and racial factors play a role in the development of Crohn's disease. It is much more common in Caucasian individuals, in developed countries, and in those individuals with a family history of Crohn's disease.

Although the etiology is unknown, the clinical scenario is relatively characteristic, with patients presenting with abdominal pain, diarrhea, and mild gastrointestinal bleeding. With chronic inflammation, patients may develop strictures within the bowel resulting in intestinal obstruction. As indicated earlier, Crohn's disease can affect any segment of the gastrointestinal tract, and skip areas are common. Because of the inflammation in the bowel wall, transmural involvement is relatively characteristic with associated deep fissures, ulcers, and narrowing of the bowel lumen due to the thickened bowel wall **(Fig. 17)**. On cross-sectional imaging, the thickened bowel wall and resultant narrowing of the lumen can be easily identified **(Fig. 18)**.

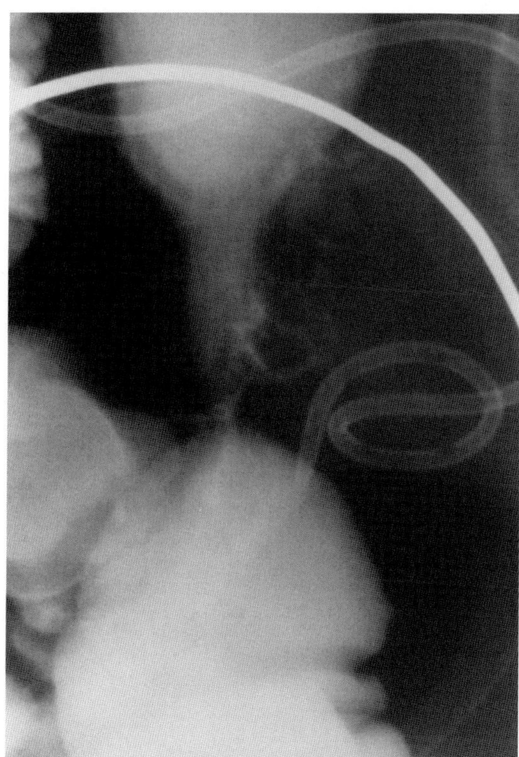

Figure 19. A spot image from a small bowel follow-through in a patient with Crohn's disease in whom an abscess had been drained. Narrowing of the lumen is present. The abscess site is near to the numerous deep ulcers in the diseased segment of the bowel.

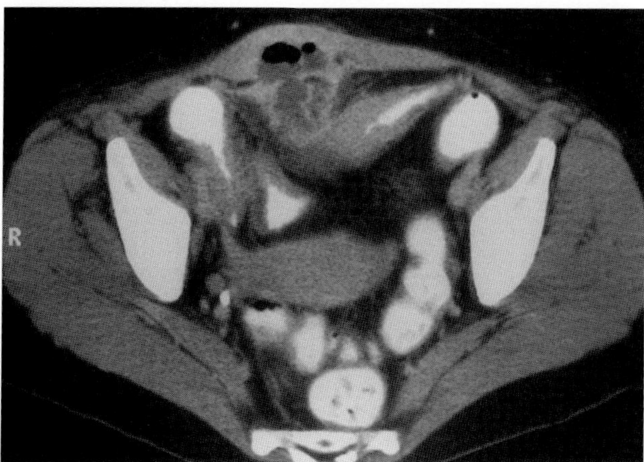

Figure 20. Abdominal wall abscess in a patient with Crohn's disease.

Because of this transmural inflammation, micro- or macroscopic perforation is relatively common and can result in abdominal abscesses **(Fig. 19)**. Fifteen to twenty-five percent of patients with Crohn's disease will develop an intraabdominal abscess at some point. Abscesses occur more frequently in patients with ileal or ileocolic involvement. In patients who present with fever and an abdominal mass, there should be a high suspicion for an abdominal abscess and a CT scan should be obtained **(Fig. 20)**.

For abscesses secondary to Crohn's disease, the traditional surgical dictum has been to incise and drain the abscess, then perform delayed bowel resection and anastomosis. However, up to 85% of surgically drained abscesses developed cutaneous fistulas that necessitated resection of the fistula in addition to the diseased bowel. However, numerous reports have now shown that percutaneous drainage of abscesses associated with Crohn's disease can be performed safely without the development of enterocutaneous fistulas or other complications. Draining the abscess and clearing the infected field permits a single-stage surgical resection with primary anastomosis rather than a two-stage operation. In addition, abscess drainage can be a temporizing measure, allowing the patient's nutritional and surgical status to improve, which minimizes the morbidity of the surgical intervention. If no fistula is demonstrated, percutaneous drainage of the abscess may be the definitive procedure which, in conjunction with medical therapy, may avoid surgery.

Fistulas to the bowel will be identified after percutaneous abscess drainage. This is not surprising given the transmural nature of the inflammation that induces the perforation, resulting in the abscess. The success rate of prolonged catheter drainage in allowing nonsurgical closure of enteric fistulas in patients with Crohn's disease is quite variable. In one report, almost 60% of patients had closure of their fistulas with prolonged catheter drainage.

Other reports have not been as encouraging, demonstrating closure of the fistulas in 0%–40% of cases. The ability to close the fistula may depend on the stage of the Crohn's disease. If the fistula originates from a strictured, fibrotic, thickened segment of the bowel as occurs in chronic end-stage Crohn's disease, it is unlikely that the fistula will close. When a fistula is discovered, a trial of prolonged catheter drainage to determine whether the fistula will close may be warranted; however, it should be kept in mind that the patient may still require surgical resection of the diseased bowel segment and associated fistula.

Selected Readings

Casola G, vanSonnenberg E, Neff CC, Saba RM, Withers C, Emarine C. Abscesses in Crohn's disease: percutaneous drainage. Radiology 1987; 163:19–22.

Kerlan RK, Jeffrey RB, Pogany AC, Ring EJ. Abdominal abscess with low-output fistula: successful percutaneous drainage. Radiology 1985; 155:73–75.

LaBerge JM, Kerlan RK, Gordon RL, Ring EJ. Nonoperative treatment of enteric fistulas: results in 53 patients. J Vasc Interv Radiol 1992; 3:353–357.

Lambiase RE, Cronan JJ, Dorfman GS, Poalella LP, Haas RA. Percutaneous drainage of abscesses in patients with Crohn's disease. AJR 150:1043–1045.

Safrit HD, Mauro MA, Jaques PF. Percutaneous abscess drainage in Crohn's disease. AJR 1987; 148:859–862.

Schuster MR, Crummy AB, Wojtowycz MM, McDermott JC. Abdominal abscesses associated with enteric fistulas: percutaneous management. J Vasc Interv Radiol 1992; 3:359–363.

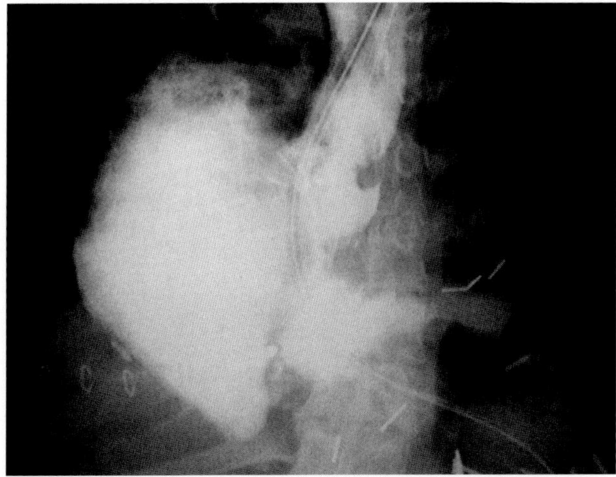

Figure 1. Radiograph of the lower chest following instillation of water-soluble contrast material through an indwelling nasoenteric tube.

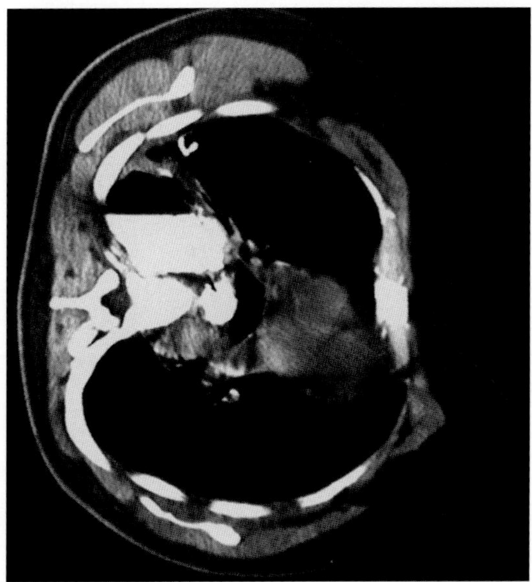

Figure 2. Thoracic CT scan with the patient in a left lateral decubitus position obtained after the gastrointestinal series.

TEACHING FILE CASE 23

Robert K. Kerlan, Jr., M.D., and Ernest J. Ring, M.D.

History

A 37-year-old man underwent a distal esophagectomy with transverse colon interposition for a benign stricture secondary to lye ingestion. Three days after surgery the patient developed chest pain and fever. An upper gastrointestinal series with water-soluble contrast material was performed **(Fig. 1)**, followed by thoracic computed tomography (CT) scanning **(Fig. 2)**.

What is your diagnosis?

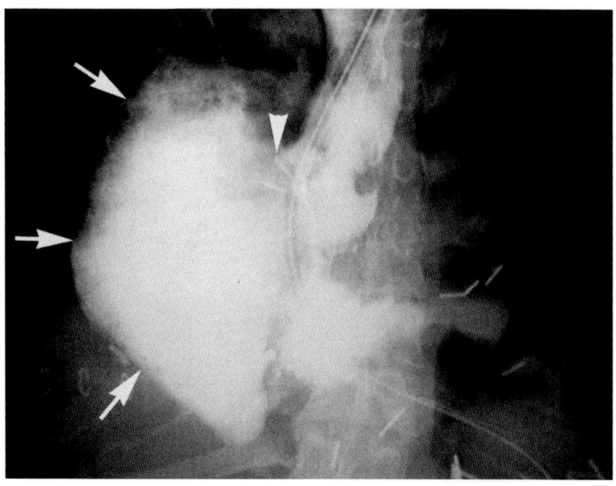

Figure 3. Massive leakage of contrast material (arrows) into the right thoracic cavity from the esophagus. The site of perforation (arrowhead) can be visualized in the anticipated position of the esophagocolonic anastomosis.

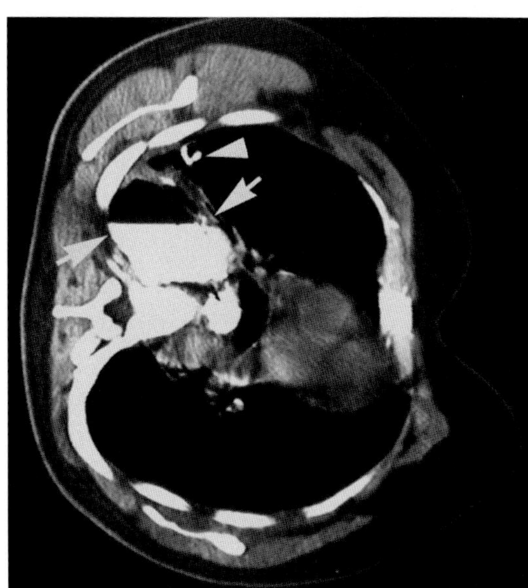

Figure 4. Thoracic CT scan depicts the anatomic position of the extravasated contrast material (arrows) in the posterior aspect of the right hemithorax. A surgically placed thoracostomy tube (arrowhead) can be seen anterior and lateral to the collection.

Radiographic Findings

The upper gastrointestinal series **(Fig. 3)** shows massive leakage of contrast material from the mid esophagus into the right thoracic cavity. A perforation is identified along the right lateral aspect of the mid esophagus, presumably at the site of the esophagocolonic anastomosis.

The thoracic CT scan **(Fig. 4)** confirms the leak into a cavity that contains both extravasated contrast material and air in the posterior aspect of the right hemithorax. The collection is adjacent to the colonic interposition immediately caudal to the anticipated position of the esophagocolonic anastomosis.

Diagnosis

Enteric perforation into the mediastinum and right pleural space most likely due to partial dehiscence of the esophagocolonic anastomosis.

How would you manage this patient?

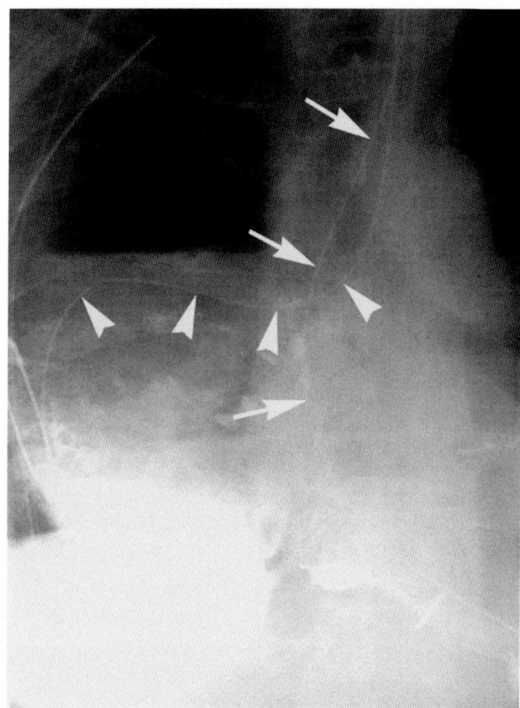

Figure 5. An 18-F Salem sump (arrowheads) has been advanced from the nose, through the esophageal perforation, and into the pleural fluid collection. An additional transnasal 16-F Salem sump (arrows) has been placed intraluminally across the anastomosis to diminish the amount of material leaking through the defect.

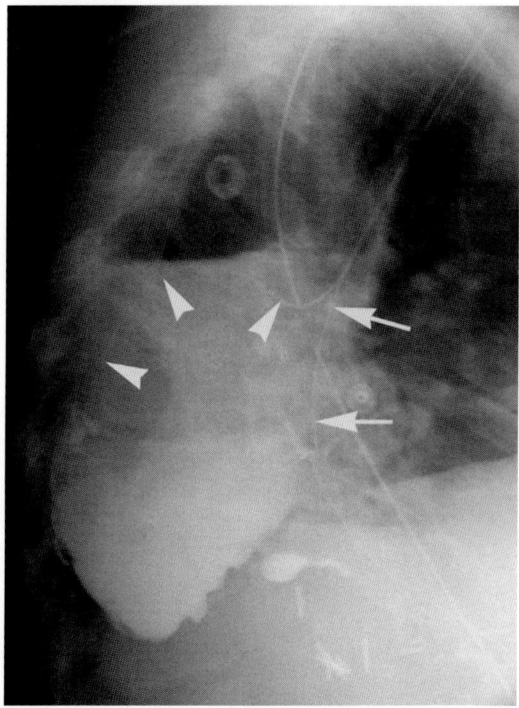

Figure 6. Lateral chest radiograph confirms the position of the transesophageal thoracic drainage tube (arrowheads) and naso-enteric sump (arrows). A surgically placed thoracostomy tube is also visible.

Management

Under fluoroscopic guidance, a selective catheter was manipulated through the esophageal perforation into the pleural collection. An exchange guide wire was placed and an 18-F Salem sump tube was advanced over the guide wire into the loculated pleural space. An additional sump tube was positioned within the esophageal lumen adjacent to the perforation spanning the esophagocolonic anastomosis **(Figs. 5, 6)**. Both tubes were placed to low-continuous wall suction. The pleural collection gradually collapsed into a mature fistulous track. After 4 weeks, the transesophageal tube was removed. After an additional week of naso-esophageal suction, the perforation healed and the patient was discharged home.

Discussion

Disruption of the enteric anastomosis with contamination of the mediastinum and pleural spaces is the most common cause of mortality following esophageal surgery. Though small leaks confined to the para-anastomotic area may be managed conservatively with naso-esophageal suction, larger defects usually require aggressive therapy.

When leaks are detected acutely, re-exploration with primary repair can be curative. However, most patients will have considerable contamination which precludes the creation of a fresh anastomosis. In these patients, surgery is directed at draining any associated abscesses and controlling the fistula. Percutaneous and transesophageal drainage can replace the more invasive open surgical procedure in this clinical setting.

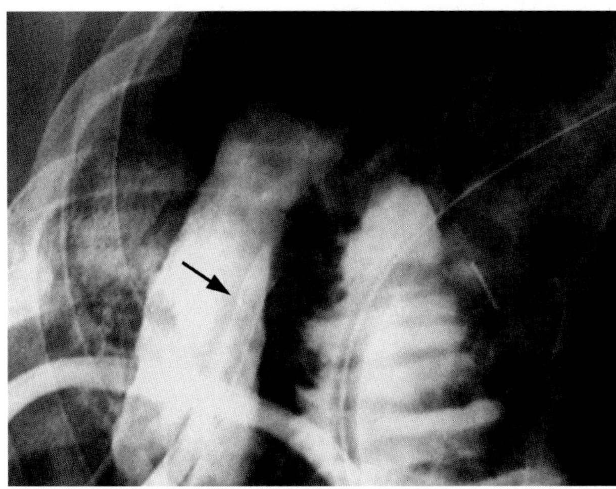

Figure 7. 24-F sump tube (arrow) placed percutaneously into the loculated right posterior pleural collection adjacent to the leaking esophagocolonic anastomosis.

Mediastinal and pleural collections can be approached through a direct percutaneous puncture **(Figs. 7, 8)**, if an appropriate window devoid of aerated lung and major vascular structures is present. However, mediastinal and pleural collections can also be evacuated through the site of perforation via the transnasal route. Catheter lengths in excess of 50 cm are often required to reach the collection from this approach. The transnasal route also has the advantage of partially obturating the hole, diminishing the amount of leakage from the esophagus into the mediastinum and pleural space.

Maroney et al reported successful percutaneous management in six of six patients with leaking esophageal anastomoses. Percutaneous drainage was used in three patients, and transesophageal drainage was used in three. All patients had a large-bore (18–20-F) sump drainage of the esophageal lumen adjacent to the dehiscence. Repeat sinograms were used to adjust the tube positions as needed until all associated cavities had healed sufficiently to allow tube withdrawal. The average length of therapy was 36 days.

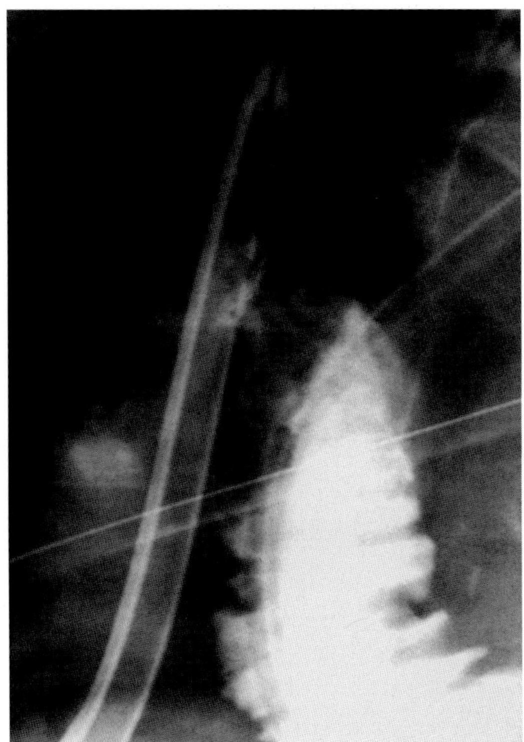

Figure 8. Same patient as in Figure 7. The side-holes of the drainage tube are positioned adjacent to the site of perforation and the cavity has been completely evacuated.

Selected Readings

Brewer LA, Carter R, Mulder GA, Stiles QR. Options in the management of perforations of the esophagus. Am J Surg 1986; 152:62–69.

Chang AE, Schwartz W, Ring EJ, et al. Transluminal catheter drainage of an esophageal disruption: an adjunct to nonoperative management. Surg Gastroenterol 1982; 1:135–138.

Maroney TP, Ring EJ, Gordon RL, Pellegrini CA. Role of interventional radiology in the management of major esophageal leaks. Radiology 1989; 170:1055–1057.

Vauthey JN, Lerut J, Laube M, Donati D, Gertsch P. Blunt oesophageal perforation: treatment with surgical exclusion and percutaneous drainage under computed tomographic guidance. Eur J Surg 1992; 158(9):509–510.

Wright CD, Mathisen DJ, Wain JC, Moncure AC, Hilgenberg AD, Grillo HC. Reinforced primary repair of thoracic esophageal perforation. Ann Thorac Surg 1995; 60(2):245–249.

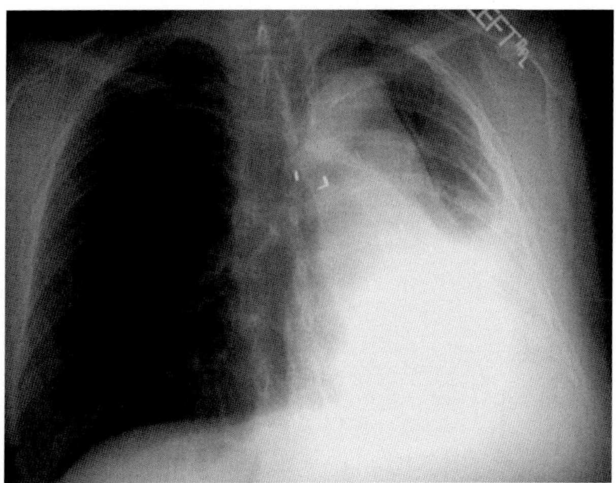

Figure 1. Chest radiograph.

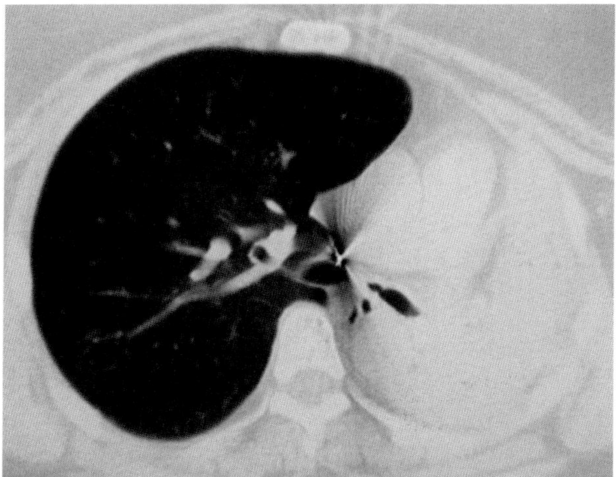

Figure 2. Axial CT image immediately caudal to the carina.

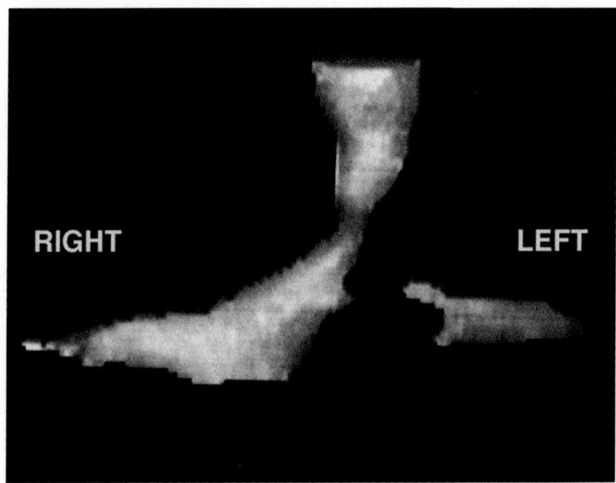

Figure 3. Three-dimensional reconstruction (shaded-surface display) of the tracheobronchial tree in the region of the carina.

TEACHING FILE CASE 24

Robert K. Kerlan, Jr., M.D., Roy L. Gordon, M.D., and Jeffrey A. Golden, M.D.

History

A 33-year-old woman with acquired immunodeficiency syndrome (AIDS) came to the hospital with a 6-month history of dyspnea. The patient's work-up included microbiologic analysis of the sputum, bronchoscopy, and mediastinoscopy. Imaging evaluation included a chest radiograph **(Fig. 1)** and thoracic computed tomography (CT) scanning **(Fig. 2)** with three-dimensional reconstruction of the proximal tracheobronchial tree **(Fig. 3)**.

What is your diagnosis?

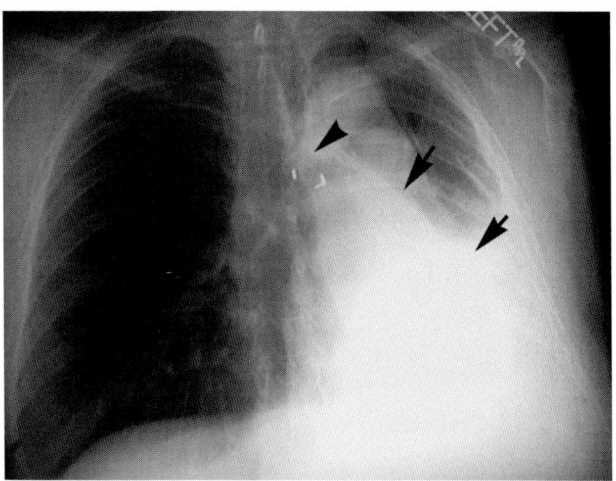

Figure 4. Chest radiograph reveals dense opacification (arrows) of the left lower lobe associated with significant volume loss. Surgical clips (arrowhead) from previous mediastinoscopy are visible.

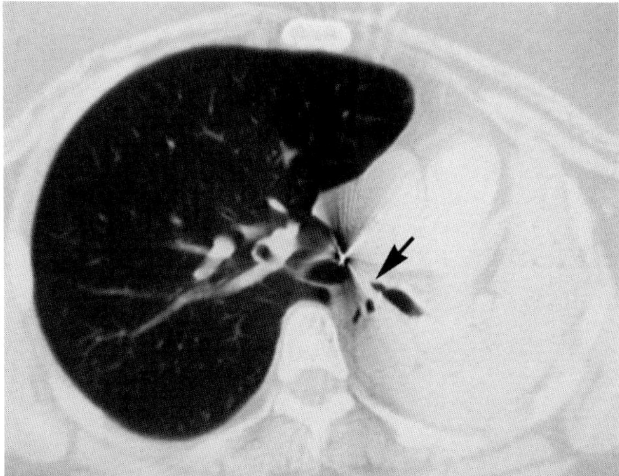

Figure 5. Thoracic CT scan reveals narrowing of the proximal left mainstem bronchus (arrow). Dense opacification of the left lower lobe is also evident.

Radiographic Findings

The chest radiograph **(Fig. 4)** reveals dense opacification of the left lower lobe with volume loss. The trachea and proximal bronchial structures are difficult to visualize on this image. However, the CT scan **(Fig. 5)** shows marked narrowing of the left mainstem bronchus as well as dense opacification at the left base. Other axial images showed narrowing of the distal trachea. The three-dimensional reconstruction **(Fig. 6)** shows the narrowing of the trachea and occlusion of the origin of the left mainstem bronchus. However, complete occlusion may not be present, as shaded-surface-display reconstructions may overestimate the degree of narrowing.

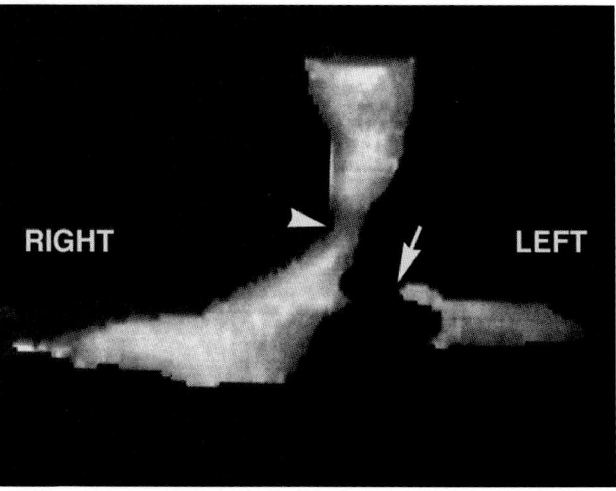

Figure 6. Three-dimensional reconstruction depicts narrowing of the distal trachea extending into the origin of the right mainstem bronchus (arrowhead). The proximal left mainstem bronchus appears to be occluded (arrow).

Diagnosis

Tracheobronchial stenosis.

How would you manage this patient?

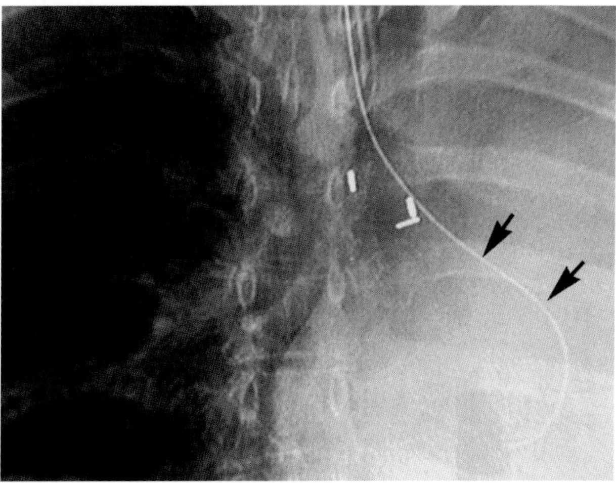

Figure 7. A guide wire (arrows) is advanced through the narrowing of the left mainstem and lower lobe bronchus.

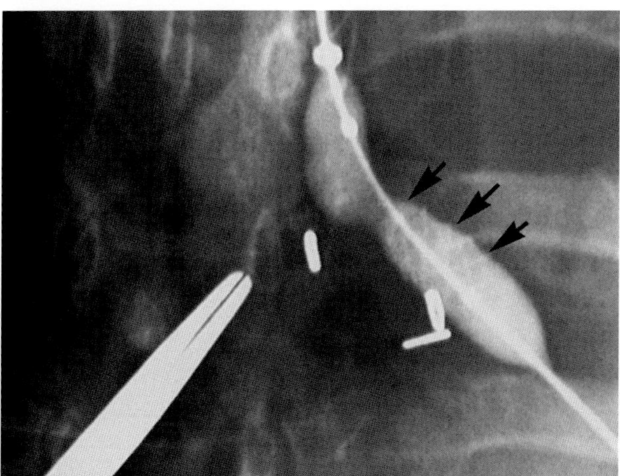

Figure 8. An 8-mm-diameter balloon is used to deploy the expandable stent (arrows).

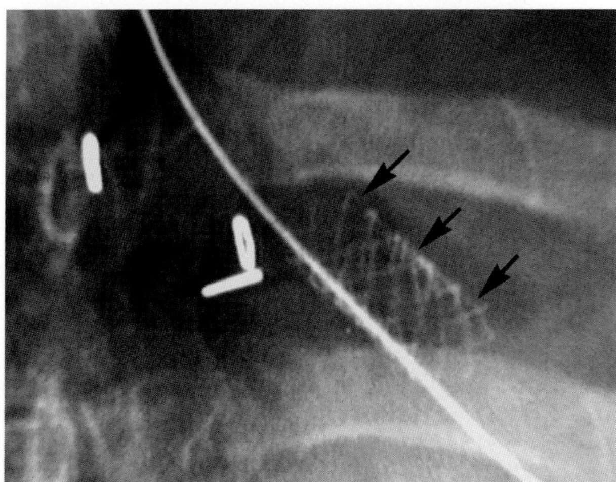

Figure 9. Palmaz stent deployed across the obstructing lesion (arrows).

Management

The appropriate management depends on the underlying cause of the obstruction. If AIDS-related lymphoma was responsible for the airway compression, chemotherapy and radiation may be the optimal treatment. If a specific infectious agent could be identified, culture-directed antibiotic therapy would be indicated. Unfortunately, neither a neoplasm nor a specific infectious agent could be identified by sputum analysis, bronchoscopy, or mediastinoscopy. It was therefore elected to treat the patient empirically with balloon dilation and stent placement.

The patient was given general anesthesia and both fluoroscopic and bronchoscopic guidance were used to advance a guide wire through the left mainstem bronchus into the conducting airways of the left lower lobe **(Fig. 7)**. A 90-cm-long 8-F sheath was shortened to approximately 50 cm and advanced over the wire beyond the obstructing lesion. A 20-mm-long Palmaz balloon expandable stent (Johnson & Johnson Interventional Systems, Warren, NJ) was mounted on an 8-mm balloon and advanced through the sheath into the appropriate position. The sheath was retracted and the balloon inflated with dilute contrast material **(Fig. 8)**, deploying the stent **(Fig. 9)**.

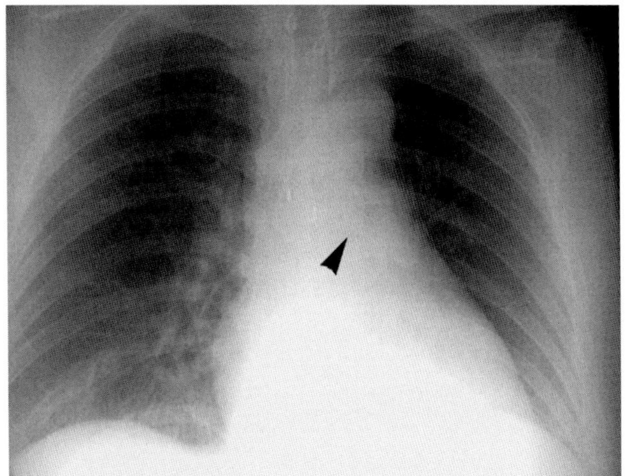

Figure 10. Chest radiograph shows improved aeration of the left lower lobe. The stent (arrowhead) is barely visible.

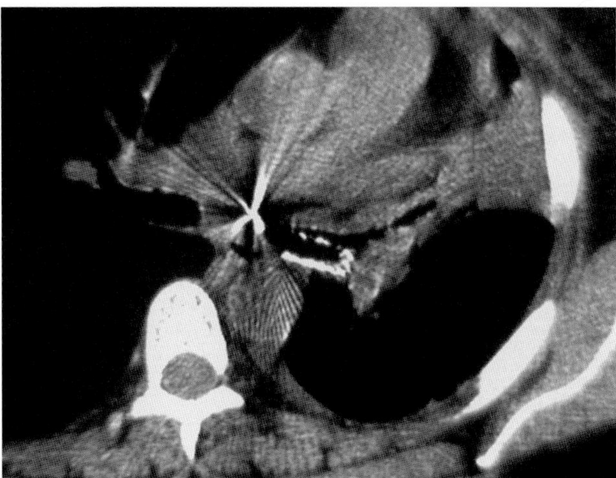

Figure 11. CT image immediately caudal to the carina shows dramatically improved caliber of the left mainstem bronchus and improved aeration of the left lower lobe.

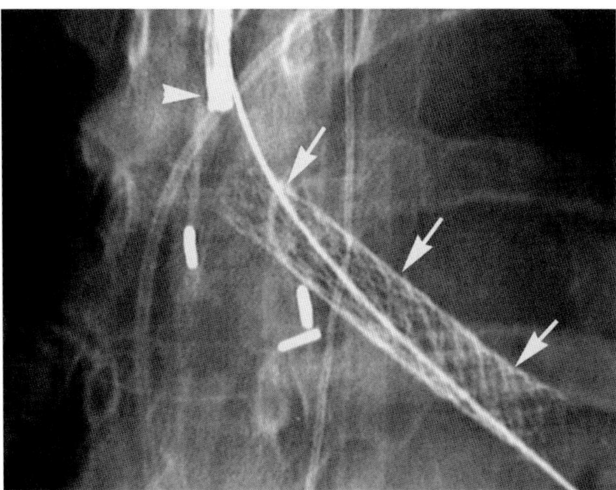

Figure 12. A Palmaz stent is placed coaxially into the left lower lobe bronchus (arrows), where a stent had been previously placed, extending the metallic bridge to the carina (arrowhead).

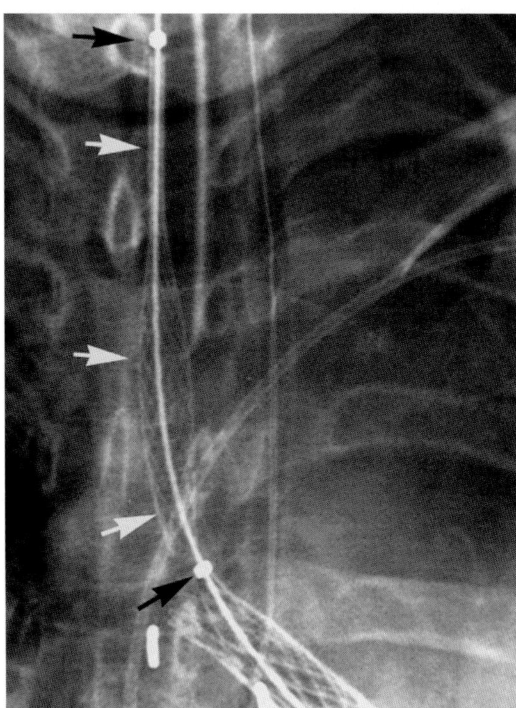

Figure 13. A self-expanding Wallstent (white arrows) is deployed under fluoroscopic guidance within the trachea. Close observation of the positioning markers (black arrows) is necessary for precise positioning and to avoid deployment within the endotracheal tube.

The procedure was terminated. A follow-up chest radiograph **(Fig. 10)** and thoracic CT scan **(Fig. 11)** confirmed improved diameter of the left mainstem bronchus and improved aeration of the left lower lobe.

The patient experienced symptomatic improvement but continued to have significant dyspnea on exertion. It was therefore elected to extend the left mainstem bronchial stent to the carina **(Fig. 12)** and stent the trachea **(Figs. 13–15)**. A 16-mm-diameter, 40-mm-long self-expandable Wallstent (Schneider, Minneapolis, MN) was placed in the trachea. After the stent was deployed, a 14-mm-diameter balloon **(Fig. 14)** was used to expand it. The patient subsequently had resolution of her dyspnea and progressive clearing of her left lower lobe consolidation **(Fig. 16)**.

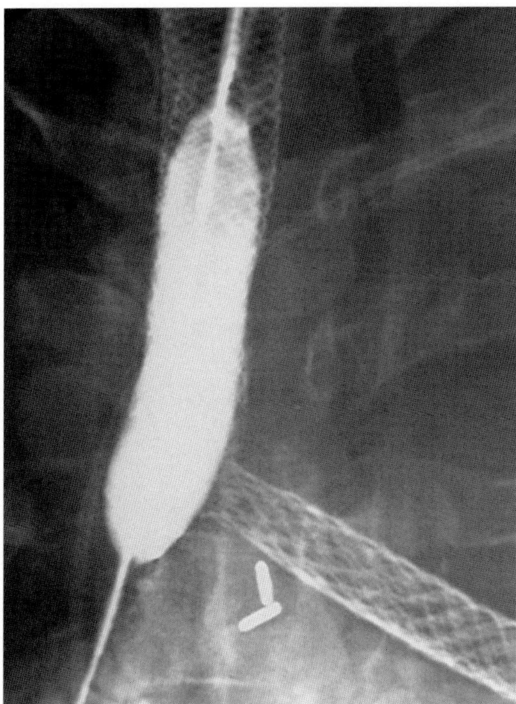

Figure 14. A 14-mm-diameter balloon is used to more fully expand the stent.

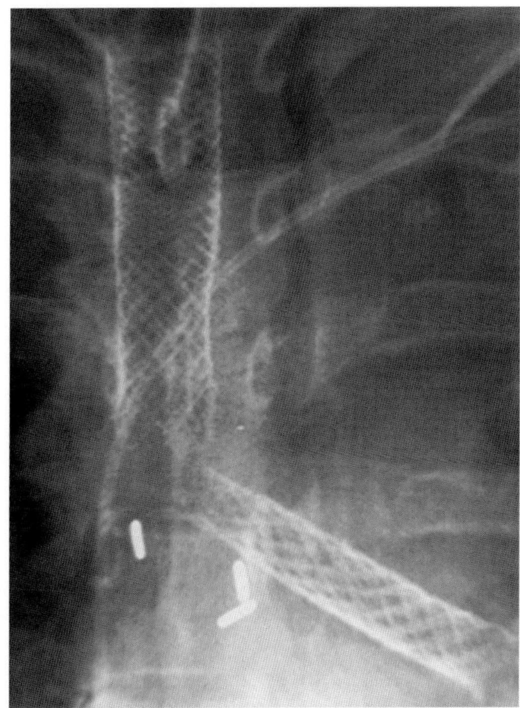

Figure 15. Completion image shows both the tracheal and left mainstem bronchial stents.

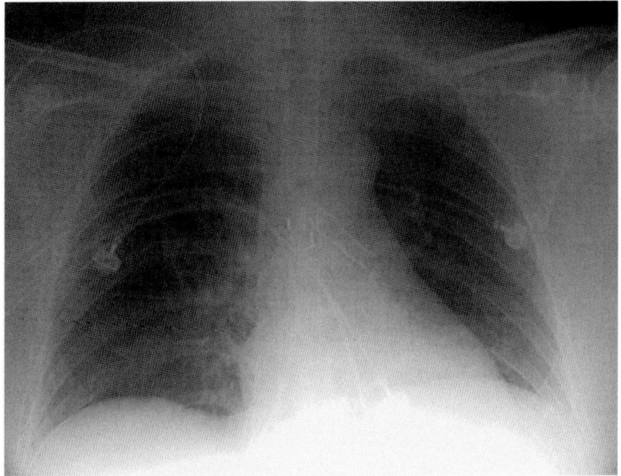

Figure 16. Chest radiograph obtained 2 months after stent placement shows complete resolution of the left lower lobe atelectasis.

Discussion

Metallic stents are being used with increasing frequency to manage obstruction of the major airways. The majority of patients reported have had stent placement for unresectable malignancy. Wilson et al reported symptomatic improvement in 77% of 56 patients with malignant tumor that could not be managed with radiotherapy, chemotherapy, or surgical resection. The mean survival time in this group of patients was 77 days.

Sonett et al reported a more diverse group of patients that included 23 patients with malignancy, 24 with stenoses following lung transplantation, and 10 with benign stenoses. In this latter group of patients (including four post-intubation, four inflammatory, one malacia, and one bronchial fistula), 80% experienced symptomatic relief. Silicone-coated stents were used, and the longest period of follow-up was 43 months.

Filler et al reported implantation of Palmaz stents in seven children, including three who had undergone repair of congenital tracheal stenosis and four with tracheo- or bronchomalacia. Three of the seven developed recurrent airway obstruction within 1 month. One child died at 1 year and the remaining three have done well, with a mean follow-up of 11 months.

Technical aspects of this procedure need refinement. Care must be taken not to cover branch airways, which can be difficult to visualize fluoroscopically. Moreover, the ideal stent has not been developed and it is unclear which of the commercially available stents are best suited for the tracheobronchial tree.

Tracheobronchial stents are tolerated surprisingly well. Coughing and irritation from stent placement is usually minimal. At follow-up bronchoscopy, noncovered stents may be incorporated and lined with a thin layer of connective tissue or neo-epithelium.

As the follow-up period for the numerous trials in progress increases, the role of stents in the major airways will become better defined. It is currently accepted as the treatment of choice for malignant tracheobronchial obstruction resistant to other forms of therapy. The role of stent placement in benign disease is less well defined but is generally warranted for diseases in which no other therapeutic alternatives are available.

Selected Readings

Filler RM, Forte V, Fraga JC, Matute J. The use of expandable metallic airway stents for tracheobronchial obstruction in children. J Ped Surg 1995; 30:1050–1055.

Sonett JR, Keenan RJ, Ferson PF, Griffith BP, Landreneau RJ. Endobronchial management of benign, malignant, and lung transplantation airways stenoses. Ann Thorac Surg 1995; 59:1417–1422.

Wilson GE, Walshaw MJ, Hind CR. Treatment of large airway obstruction in lung cancer using expandable metal stents inserted under direct vision via the fiberoptic bronchoscope. Thorax 1996; 51:248–252.

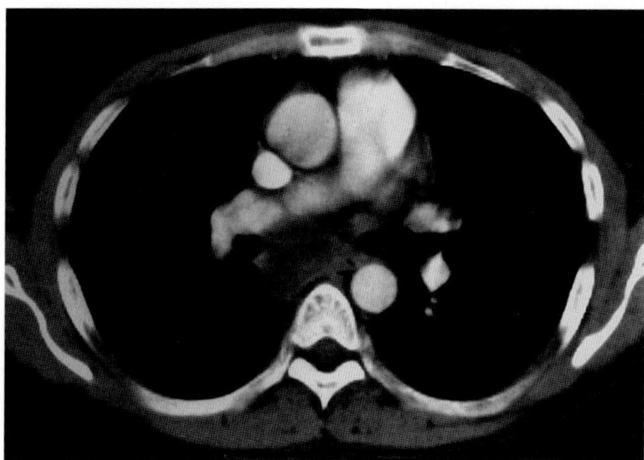

Figure 1. Contrast-enhanced CT scan of the chest.

TEACHING FILE CASE 25

Jeet Sandhu, M.D.

History

This is a 32-year-old patient with cystic fibrosis who underwent a double lung transplant two months earlier. The patient now returns with fever and an elevated white blood cell count. Blood cultures were positive for Pseudomonas. Because the patient had some chest discomfort, a computed tomography (CT) scan of the chest was obtained **(Fig. 1)**.

What is your diagnosis?

Radiographic Findings

A 5-cm-diameter low-density lesion is identified which extends from the subcarinal region to the inferior border of the left atrium **(Fig. 2)**. Given the patient's symptoms and blood cultures, the lesion is presumed to represent a mediastinal abscess.

How would you approach this lesion?

Management

The options for draining this abscess are relatively limited. Given the intimate relationship between this abscess and the esophagus, transesophageal drainage is theoretically possible. However, appropriate needle lengths are not available for endoscopic placement, and given the elasticity of the esophagus and the acute angles that would be required to puncture it, an endoscopically or sonographically guided transesophageal drainage would be technically difficult. Because the lesion is located immediately underneath the carina, transbronchial drainage with a Wang needle and/or endoscopy is another possible option. However, the presence of a drainage tube through the trachea and vocal cords would be uncomfortable for the patient.

Open surgical drainage could be performed. However, this is a significantly invasive procedure that entails significant morbidity in a patient who has had a recent operation. Because the surgeons were reluctant to operate on the patient again, percutaneous options were discussed.

The location of this abscess makes simple percutaneous drainage quite challenging. A catheter could be advanced through the lung parenchyma into the mediastinal abscess. However, because the patient had recently undergone lung transplantation and had already had numerous pneumothoraces, both the patient and referring clinicians were leery—and rightly so—of direct transparenchymal drainage with its risk of a significant pneumothorax. To avoid puncturing the lung parenchyma and perhaps inducing a pneumothorax, it was decided to attempt artificial widening of the mediastinum in order to create an extrapleural, extraparenchymal pathway for the drainage catheter.

The patient was placed in the prone position and appropriate skin markers were used to determine the puncture site **(Fig. 3)**. The lidocaine needle was then used to determine the appropriate position and approach angle. A 25-gauge spinal needle was then advanced and positioned with CT guidance such that it was in an extrapleural location immediately anterior to the costovertebral junction. At this point, 10 mL of lidocaine was injected into the extrapleural space **(Fig. 4)**. Significant lung parenchyma still remained between the abscess and the skin entry site.

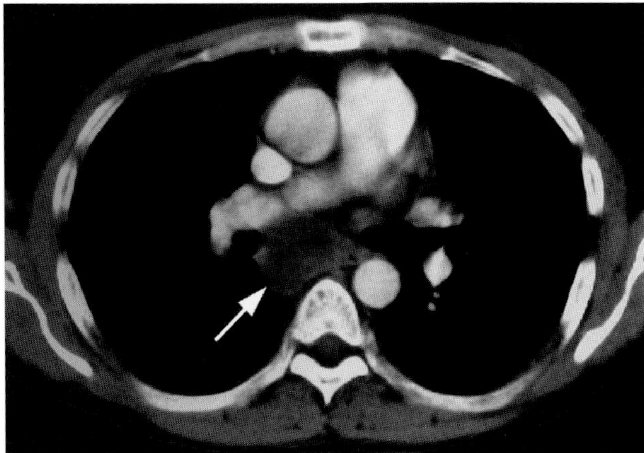

Figure 2. 5-cm-diameter fluid collection (arrow) in the azygoesophageal recess immediately adjacent to the esophagus and behind the right pulmonary artery.

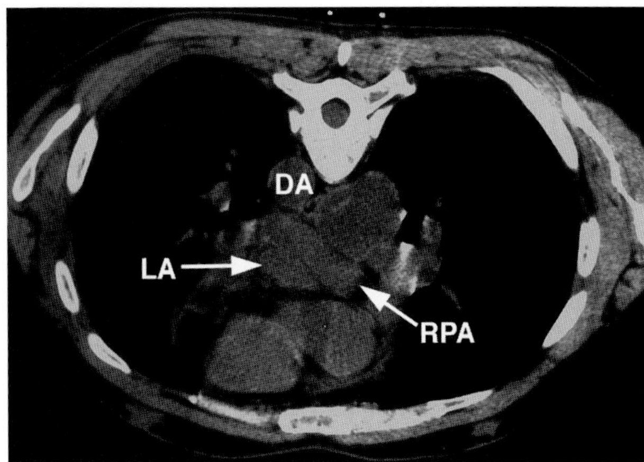

Figure 3. Noncontrast localizing prone CT scan for drainage of the mediastinal abscess. Air is noted in the esophagus. LA=left atrium; DA=descending thoracic aorta; RPA=right pulmonary artery.

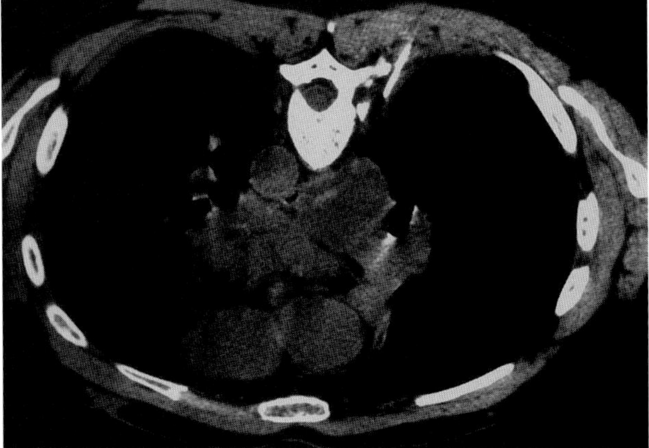

Figure 4. 25-gauge needle advanced into the extrapleural space immediately anterior to the costovertebral junction with injection of lidocaine to widen the extrapleural spaces.

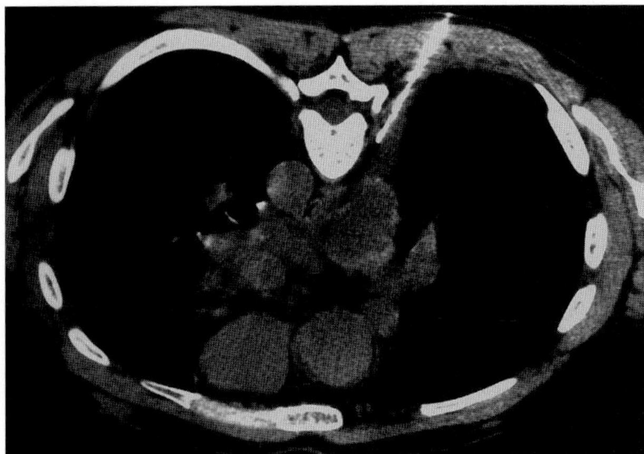

Figure 5. Advancement of a 25-gauge spinal needle with injection of 80 mL lidocaine and saline to displace the lung from the azygoesophageal recess. The lung has been pushed laterally so that lung tissue is no longer interposed between the needle trajectory and the abscess.

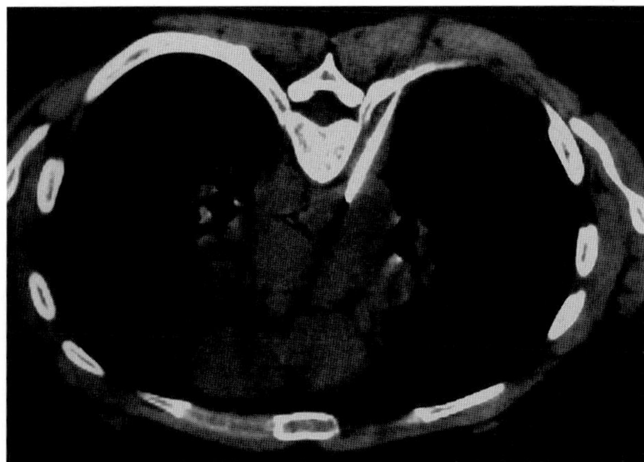

Figure 6. Advancement of an 18-gauge needle into the mediastinal abscess via the widened mediastinum.

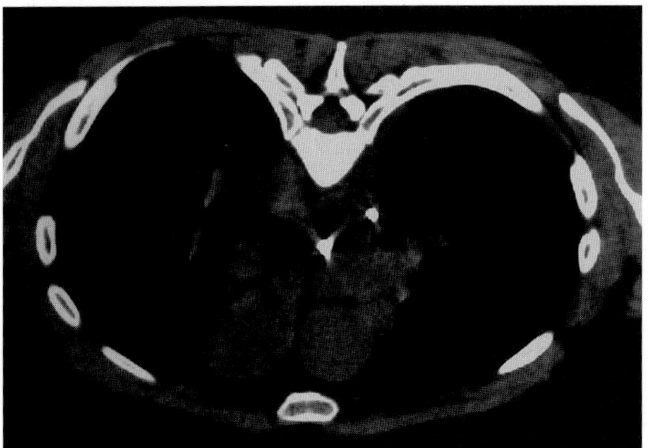

Figure 7. Cope loop drainage catheter in the abscess cavity.

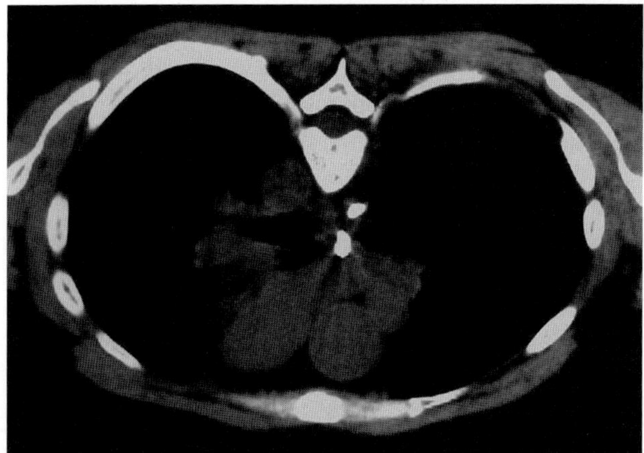

Figure 8. Decompressed abscess cavity after aspiration of abscess contents.

The 25-gauge spinal needle was advanced immediately anterolateral to the vertebral body and a total of 80 mL of sterile saline and lidocaine was injected to widen the mediastinum **(Fig. 5)**. Through the artificially widened mediastinum, an 18-gauge needle was advanced until the tip was in the mid portion of the mediastinal abscess **(Fig. 6)**. Several mL of purulent and gelatinous fluid was aspirated, confirming that the needle was located within the abscess cavity. With standard Seldinger technique, an 8-F locking Cope loop drainage catheter was inserted into the cavity **(Fig. 7)**. A total of 45 mL of gelatinous purulent material was drained from the abscess cavity which eventually grew a monoculture of Pseudomonas. Repeat CT scanning after aspiration of the material showed collapse of the cavity **(Fig. 8)**. Follow-up CT scanning and chest radiography showed no evidence of pneumothorax.

Discussion

Drainage of abscesses throughout the body is a well-established, safe, and effective technique. In certain locations, percutaneous access to the collection is limited by intervening vital structures. In this case, a significant amount of lung parenchyma lay between the skin entry site and the mediastinal abscess. Although a catheter can be inserted through the lung parenchyma, this route carries significant risks. Pneumothorax rates of 25%–40% have been documented for fine needle lung biopsies, and the incidence will certainly be greater with an 8-F drainage catheter. In addition to pneumothoraces, transparenchymal drainage can result in significant hemoptysis, air embolus, and seeding of the lung parenchyma with infectious material from the abscess. To prevent these complications, routes that go through the lung parenchyma should be avoided.

The technique of artificial mediastinal widening to create an extraparenchymal path for large-gauge cutting needle biopsies of mediastinal abnormalities has been well described. The same technique can be used to create an extraparenchymal path for the drainage catheter, as was done in this case, thereby minimizing the risk of pneumothorax. The use of this technique provides access to areas and lesions that have previously been difficult to approach for biopsy or drainage. The amount of saline required to create an adequate extrapleural pathway varies. Up to 180 mL of saline can be injected. Creation of the mediastinal widening may induce patient discomfort, so adequate sedation should be administered to ensure patient cooperation.

From a technical point of view, thin-section CT images should be obtained with the initial localizing scan because the extrapleural space anterior to the costovertebral junction, which is the target for initial needle placement, is relatively small. Thin-section images also aid in planning an adequate intercostal approach without volume averaging of the adjacent ribs.

Because aerated lung is avoided, the chances of inducing a pneumothorax are minimal, and the technique of artificial mediastinal widening should be considered for drainage of inaccessible mediastinal fluid collections.

Selected Readings

Günther RW. Percutaneous interventions in the thorax. J Vasc Interv Radiol 1992; 3:379–390.

Moulton JS. Artificial extrapleural window for mediastinal biopsy. J Vasc Interv Radiol 1993; 4:825–829.

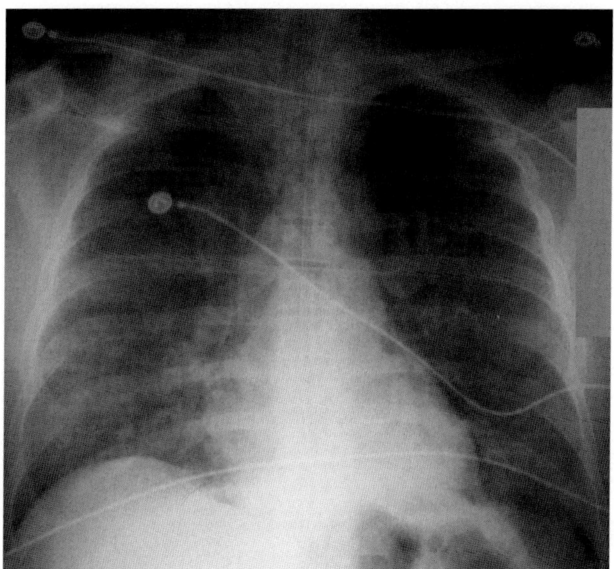

Figure 1. Initial chest radiograph.

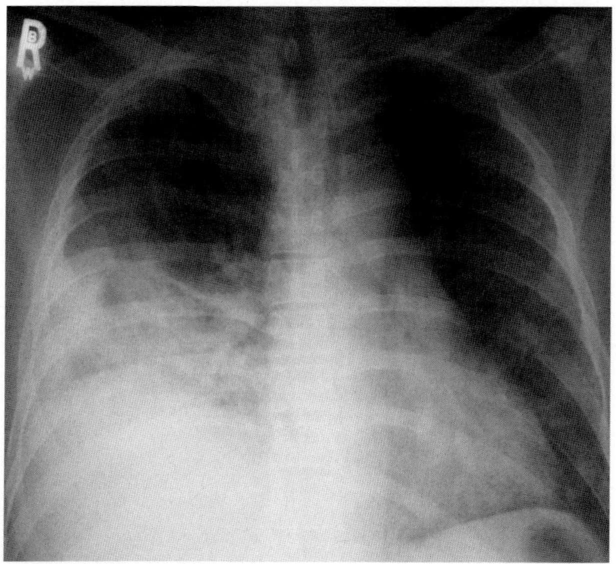

Figure 2. Chest radiograph 20 days later.

TEACHING FILE CASE 26

Scott R. Schultz, M.D., and
Jeffrey S. Klein, M.D.

History

A 36-year-old man came to the hospital with fever, malaise, cough, and shortness of breath. An initial chest radiograph revealed a diffuse multinodular parenchymal process. Initial sputum cultures were negative. Two days after admission, the patient's progressive shortness of breath developed into respiratory arrest requiring intubation **(Fig. 1)**. The patient's respiratory status gradually improved. On hospital day 20, a chest radiograph was obtained **(Fig. 2)**.

What is your diagnosis?

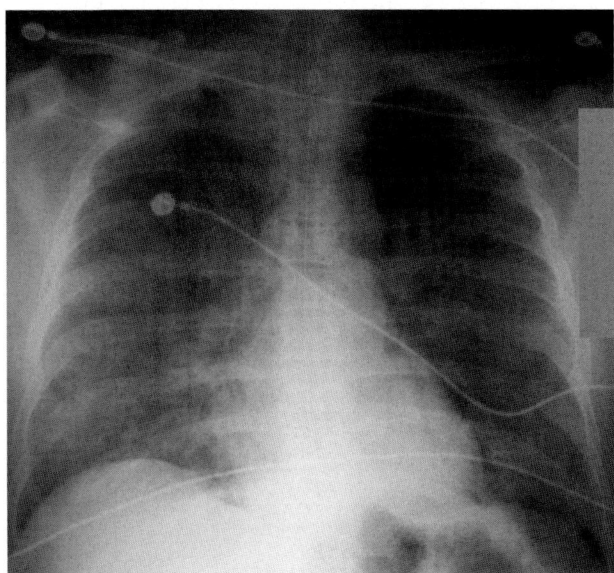

Figure 3. Initial chest radiograph shows infiltrations.

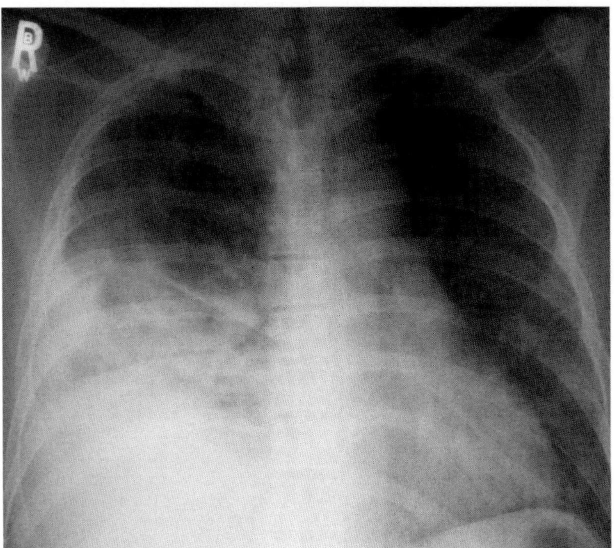

Figure 4. Chest radiograph 20 days later shows a right pleural fluid collection.

Radiographic Findings

The initial chest radiograph reveals a diffuse multinodular infiltrate, a pneumomediastinum, and the endotracheal and nasogastric tubes **(Fig. 3)**. The chest radiograph taken on hospital day 20 reveals some resolution of the bilateral nodular opacities with interval development of a moderately sized right pleural effusion and associated parenchymal opacity **(Fig. 4)**.

Diagnoses

1. Severe pneumonia resulting in acute respiratory distress syndrome.
2. Right-sided pleural fluid collection.

How would you manage this patient?

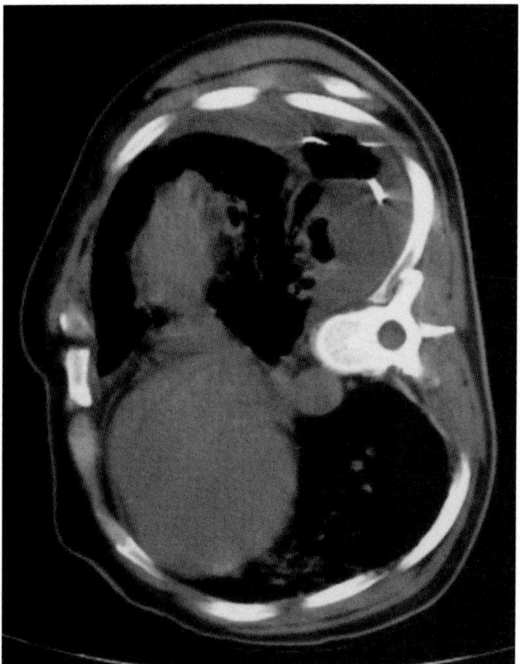

Figure 5. CT scan in a left lateral decubitus position demonstrates a loculated pleural fluid collection which was drained with a 10-F pigtail catheter.

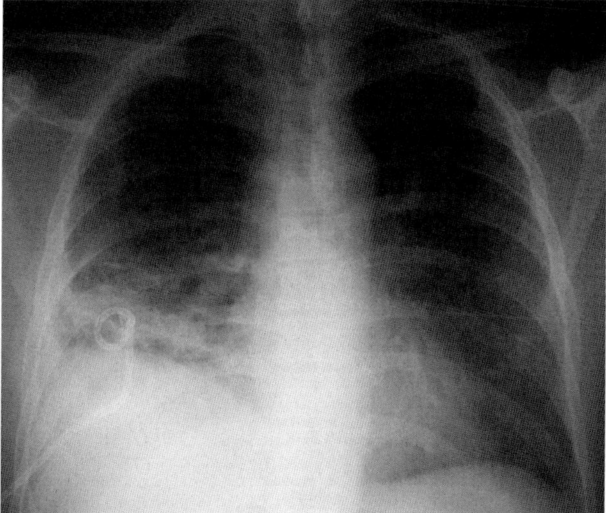

Figure 6. Chest radiograph 12 days after tube placement shows resolution of the pleural fluid collection.

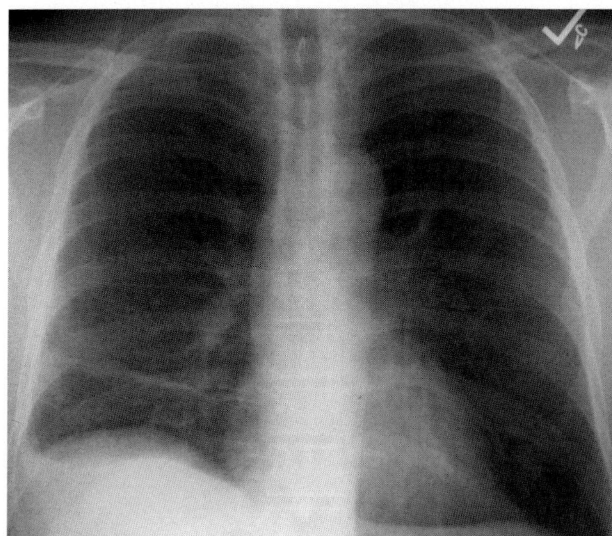

Figure 7. Follow-up chest radiograph 1 month after the acute event demonstrates some pleural scarring.

Management

A computed tomography (CT) scan of the chest obtained on hospital day 21 documented a loculated right pleural fluid collection in the right chest **(Fig. 5)**. Drainage of the collection was requested to improve the patient's ventilatory status as well as to exclude an empyema. This was drained percutaneously under CT guidance with a 10-F pigtail catheter. Twelve days later a chest radiograph revealed almost complete resolution of the fluid collection and the tube was removed **(Fig. 6)**.

The patient returned 1 month later for a follow-up chest radiograph which showed only some residual scarring at the right lung base **(Fig. 7)**.

Discussion

This is a case of a severe viral (varicella) pneumonia which progressed to acute respiratory distress syndrome and respiratory failure. The patient's course was complicated by the development of pneumomediastinum and a right-sided empyema. Empyemas most often develop as a consequence of pulmonary infections or secondary infection of a pre-existing hydro- or hemothorax. Parapneumonic effusions occur very frequently with pulmonary infections, as in this case, and they may become infected. Classically, empyemas are defined as having frankly purulent pleural fluid. However, it is now recognized that fluid collections with positive Gram stain or bacterial cultures should be classified as empyemas. Empyemas appear as loculated pleural fluid collections with the "split pleura sign." All frankly purulent material or material showing positive Gram stain on thoracentesis should be drained. Percutaneous drainage with 8–16-F pigtail catheters is the least invasive and a highly effective means of draining pleural fluid. In patients in whom percutaneous drainage is unsuccessful, surgical thoracotomy and debridement with pleural decortication may be required.

Parapneumonic pleural effusions develop in approximately 40% of patients with community-acquired pneumonia. Most of these parapneumonic effusions will resolve with antibiotic therapy alone. However, in some patients with a "complicated" parapneumonic effusion, antibiotic therapy alone is insufficient, and percutaneous drainage is required. These complicated parapneumonic effusions have exudative characteristics with a low pH, elevated lactate dehydrogenase, and low glucose. If these characteristics are found on diagnostic thoracentesis, percutaneous drainage should be considered.

Patients with a suspected loculated pleural collection (non-free flowing on decubitus films) should undergo CT scanning to further characterize its appearance and location. If a thick pleural peel is identified on the CT scan and the symptoms have been present for longer than 3 weeks, initial surgical drainage should be considered. If the diagnostic thoracentesis shows frank pus or positive Gram stain, the symptoms have been present less than 3 weeks, and a non-thickened pleural peel is seen, percutaneous drainage should be pursued. Percutaneous drainage can be performed with Seldinger or trocar techniques. After placement of the tube in the dependent portion of the collections and attachment of the tube to a Pleurevac (Deknatel, Inc., Fall River, MA), daily output should be recorded. Once the radiographs show resolution of the pleural fluid and the output is less than 10 mL per day, the catheter can be removed.

If drainage is inadequate, the catheter should be repositioned to ensure that it is in an optimal location to drain the fluid. If the fluid is particularly thick or viscous, a larger-bore tube may be used. Administration of urokinase through the catheter may aid in lysing the adhesions and septa, allowing more optimal flow of the fluid. Percutaneous drainage of parapneumonic effusions and empyemas has a success rate of 70%–90%, which compares very favorably to that of surgical large-bore tube drainage.

Selected Readings

Alfageme I, Munoz F, Pena N, Umbria S. Empyema of the thorax in adults: etiology, microbiologic findings, and management. Chest 1993; 103:839–843.

Klein JS, Schultz S, Heffner JE. Interventional radiology of the chest: image-guided percutaneous drainage of pleural effusions, lung abscess, and pneumothorax. AJR 1995; 164:581–588.

Merriam MA, Cronan JJ, Dorfman GS, Lambiase RE, Haas RA. Radiologically guided percutaneous catheter drainage of pleural fluid collections. AJR 1988; 151:1113–1116.

Silverman SG, Mueller PR, Saini S, et al. Thoracic empyema: management with image-guided catheter drainage. Radiology 1988; 169:5–9

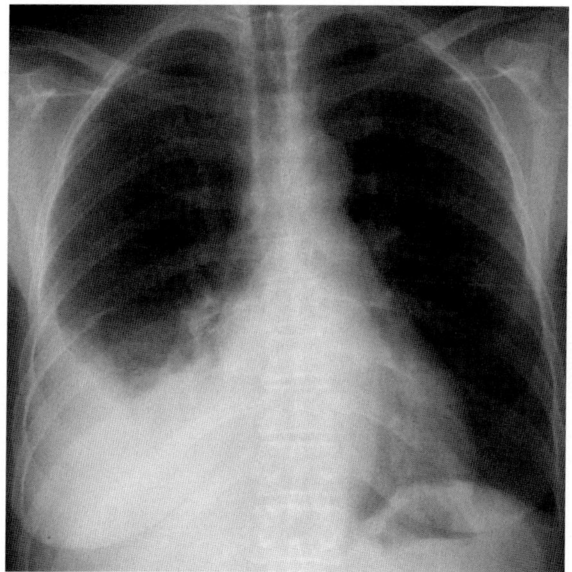
Figure 1. Initial chest radiograph.

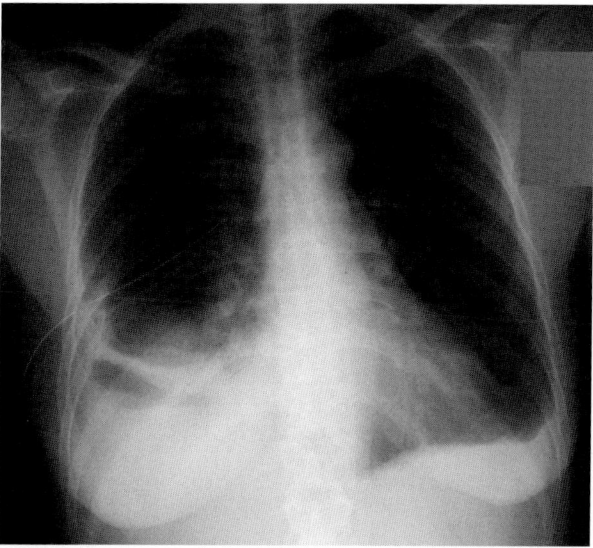
Figure 2. Follow-up chest radiograph after drainage from the surgical thoracostomy tube had diminished dramatically.

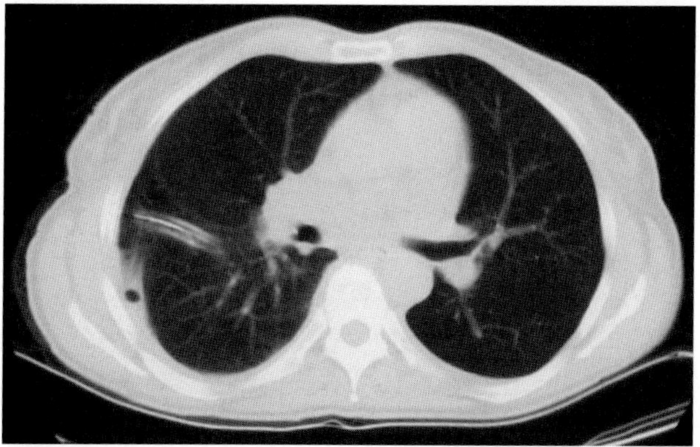
Figure 3. CT scan at the level of the chest tube tip.

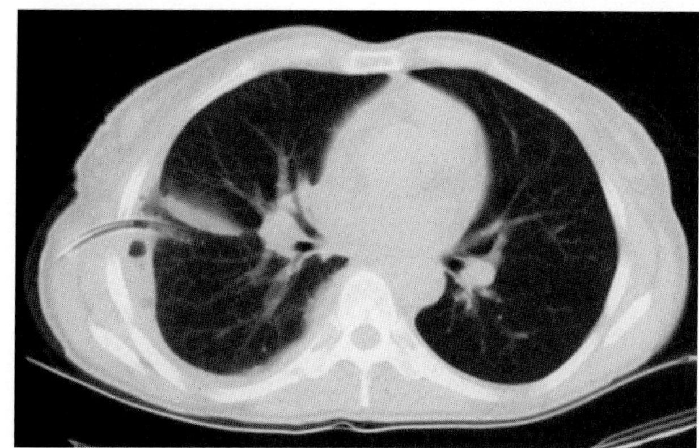
Figure 4. CT scan at a slightly lower level.

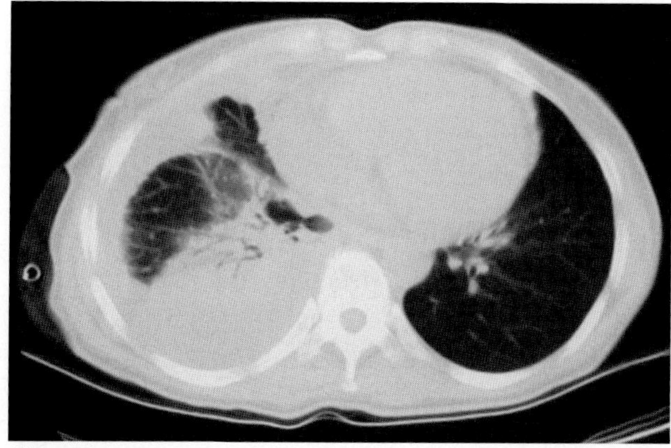
Figure 5. Lower image of the CT scan.

TEACHING FILE CASE 27

Scott R. Schultz, M.D., and
Jeffrey S. Klein, M.D.

History

A 53-year-old man came to the hospital with shortness of breath and fever. An initial chest radiograph revealed a large right-sided pleural effusion and marked right middle and lower lobe atelectasis **(Fig. 1)**. Because of this, a surgical chest tube was placed in the emergency room. Cultures revealed that the patient had a severe streptococcus pneumonia. On hospital day 3, the chest tube drainage stopped. A chest radiograph **(Fig. 2)** and a computed tomography (CT) scan of the chest **(Figs. 3–5)** were obtained.

What is your diagnosis?

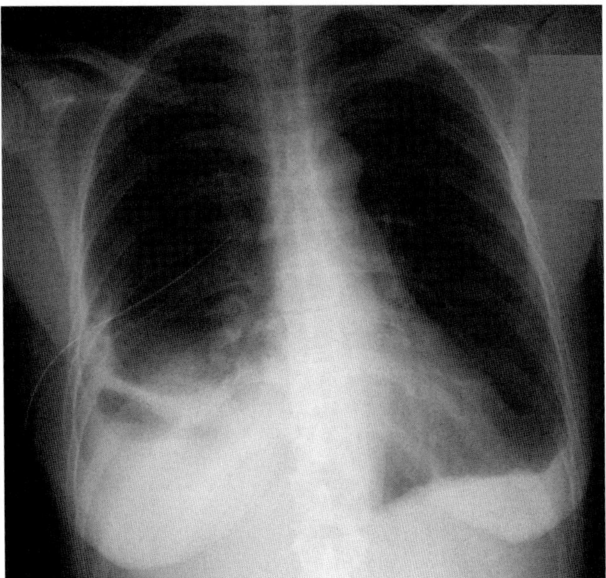

Figure 6. Right chest tube in place with residual pleural fluid most notable at the lung base.

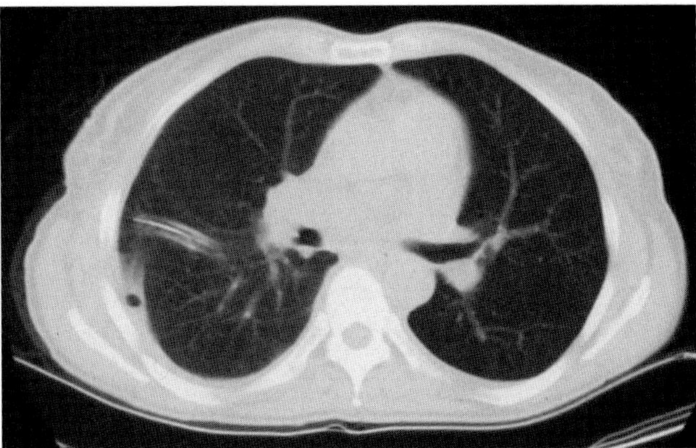

Figure 7. CT scan demonstrates the chest tube in the major fissure.

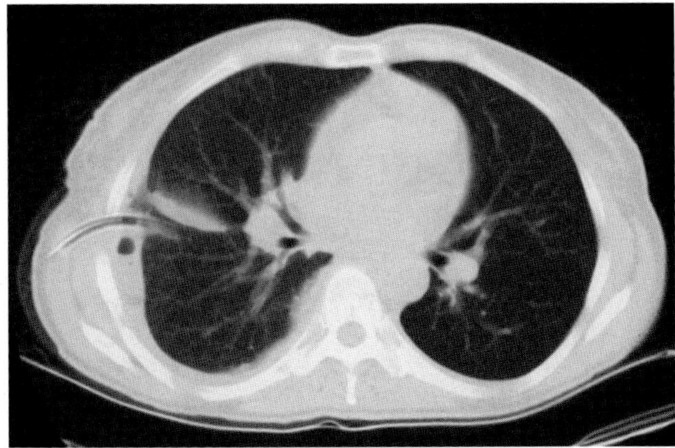

Figure 8. Lower image shows pleural fluid laterally with a loculated air collection.

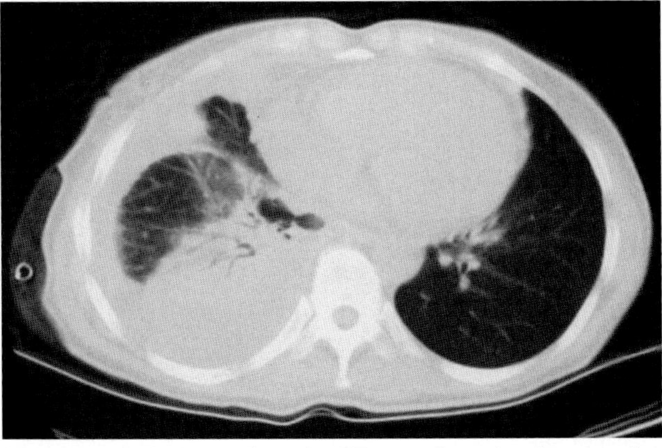

Figure 9. Inferior image from the CT scan shows basilar consolidation with air bronchograms and significant residual pleural fluid.

Radiographic Findings

The chest radiograph and CT scan reveal a loculated fluid collection in the right posterior basilar pleural space **(Figs. 6–9)**. The right-sided chest tube is within the major fissure.

Diagnoses

1. Streptococcal pneumonia.
2. Significant parapneumonic effusion.
3. Surgical chest tube within the major fissure.

How would you manage this patient?

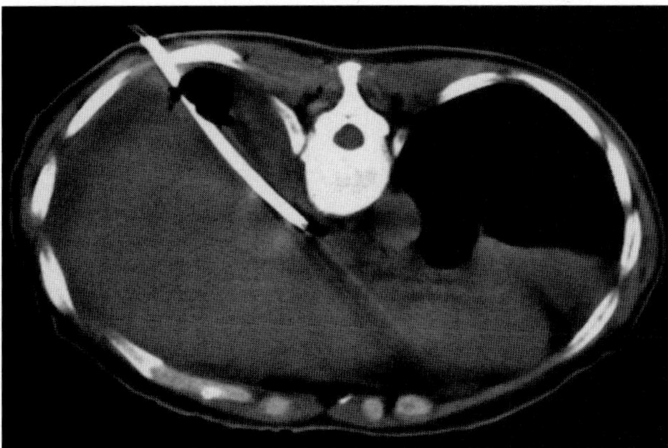

Figure 10. Percutaneous CT-guided placement of a drainage catheter into the posterior pleural fluid collection. The patient is in the prone position.

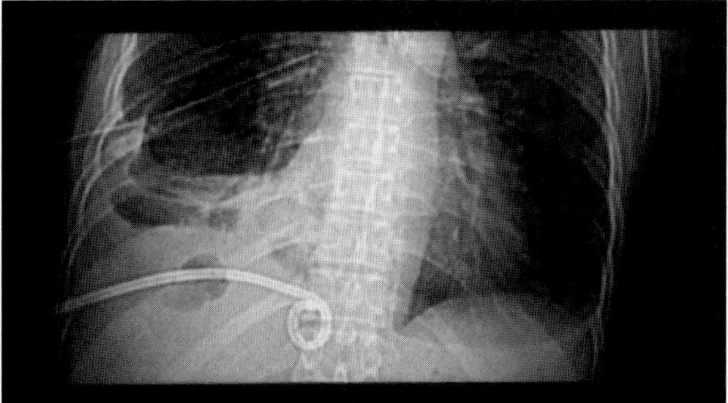

Figure 11. CT scan demonstrates the final position of the percutaneous catheter.

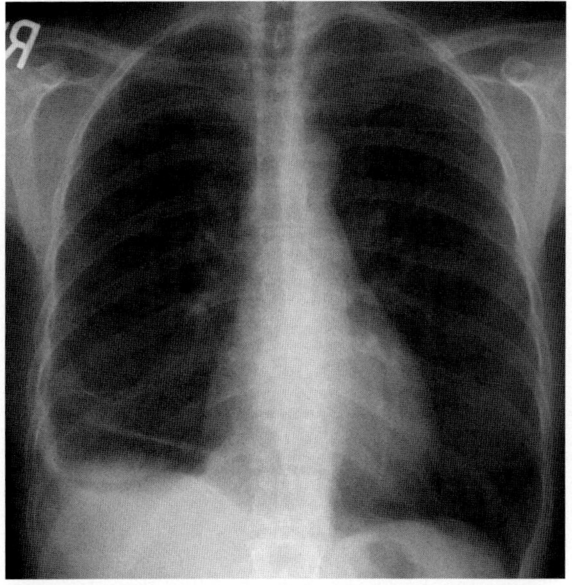

Figure 12. Follow-up chest radiograph 1 month later shows resolution of the fluid with only minimal scarring.

Management

Because the surgical tube was in the fissure and was therefore not draining the parapneumonic effusion, a percutaneous drain was placed under CT guidance **(Figs. 10, 11)**. The drain was left in place for several days and removed after the output fell to less than 10 mL per day. The patient was discharged from the hospital and returned 1 month later for a follow-up chest radiograph. At that time, there was no residual effusion and only minimal scarring **(Fig. 12)**.

Discussion

This case demonstrates a potential problem with blindly placed chest tubes: they can end up in the fissures as the lung re-expands. In a situation such as this, a percutaneous drain can easily be placed into the collection under imaging guidance, thus avoiding inadvertent placement into the fissure. The use of imaging, either CT or sonography, allows precise placement of the chest tube, especially into loculated collections.

Parapneumonic effusions may occur in up to 40% of cases of community-acquired pneumonia. Most parapneumonic effusions do not need to be drained percutaneously as they will resolve with appropriate antibiotic therapy alone. Occasionally, these parapneumonic effusions will evolve to empyemas. If the diagnostic thoracentesis yields grossly purulent material or fluid that shows organisms on Gram stain, percutaneous drainage should be performed. "Complicated" parapneumonic effusions, although not frankly infected, may also need to be drained; they will not resolve with antibiotic therapy alone and may progress to an organized stage that will eventually require surgical decortication. These complicated parapneumonic effusions will have exudative characteristics on the thoracentesis with a low pH, low glucose, and high lactate dehydrogenase. Regardless of the characteristic of the fluid, when the effusions are large and are causing respiratory compromise, they need to be drained.

Selected Readings

Klein JS, Schultz S, Heffner JE. Interventional radiology of the chest: image-guided percutaneous drainage of pleural effusions, lung abscess, and pneumothorax. AJR 1995; 164:581–588.

Light RW. Parapneumonic effusions and empyema. Clin Chest Med 1985; 6: 55–62.

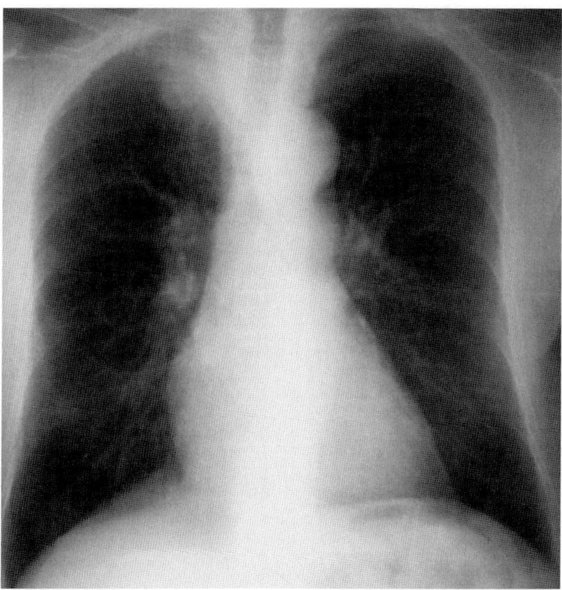

Figure 1. Chest radiograph.

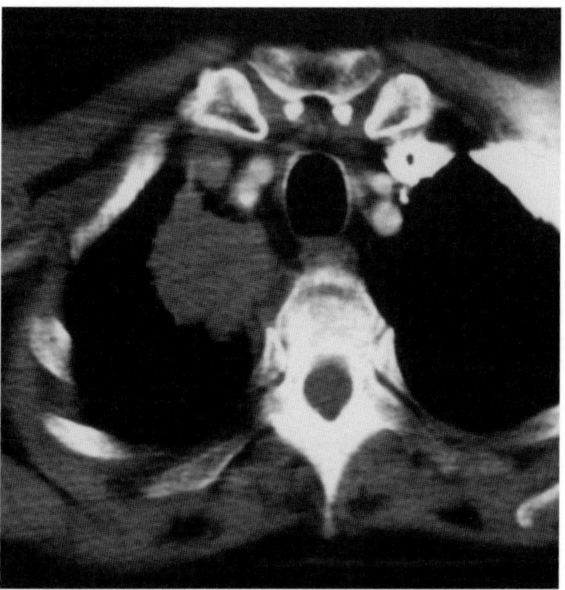

Figure 2. Contrast-enhanced CT scan of the chest.

TEACHING FILE CASE 28

Shelley R. Marder, M.D., and
Robert K. Kerlan, Jr., M.D.

History

A 75-year-old man with a significant smoking history came to the hospital with weight loss. A radiograph of the chest was obtained **(Fig. 1)**. Further evaluation included a contrast-enhanced thoracic computed tomography (CT) scan **(Fig. 2)**.

What is your diagnosis?

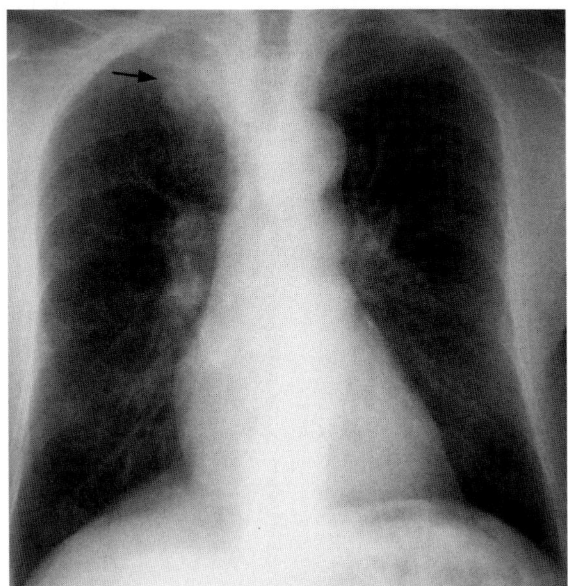

Figure 3. Chest radiograph demonstrates a right apical lung mass (arrow) abutting the mediastinum.

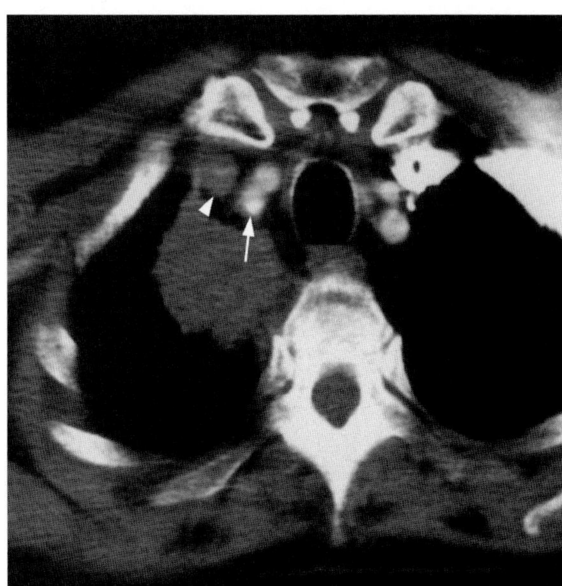

Figure 4. CT scan reveals an apical mass posterior to the subclavian artery (arrow) and innominate vein (arrowhead). The mass measures 4.5 cm and has spiculated margins.

Radiographic Findings

The chest radiograph reveals a right apical mass **(Fig. 3)**. No pleural effusion is identified. The CT scan demonstrates the mass to have spiculated margins. It measures approximately 4.5 cm in maximum dimension and is adjacent to the subclavian artery and superior mediastinum **(Fig. 4)**. There is no significant adenopathy. CT-guided biopsy was contemplated, but access was considered difficult because of the proximity of the mass to the brachiocephalic vessels and innominate vein. Furthermore, the clavicle appeared to obstruct the most direct path, and transgression of aerated lung would be necessary in order to approach the lesion.

Diagnosis

Right apical lung mass highly suspicious for malignancy.

What are the options for obtaining diagnostic tissue percutaneously?

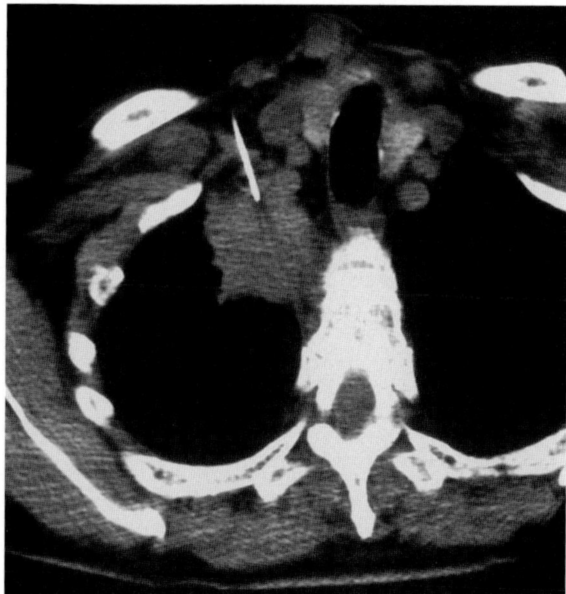

Figure 5. Westcott needle within the mass (mediastinal windows)—bone and vessels are no longer in the path.

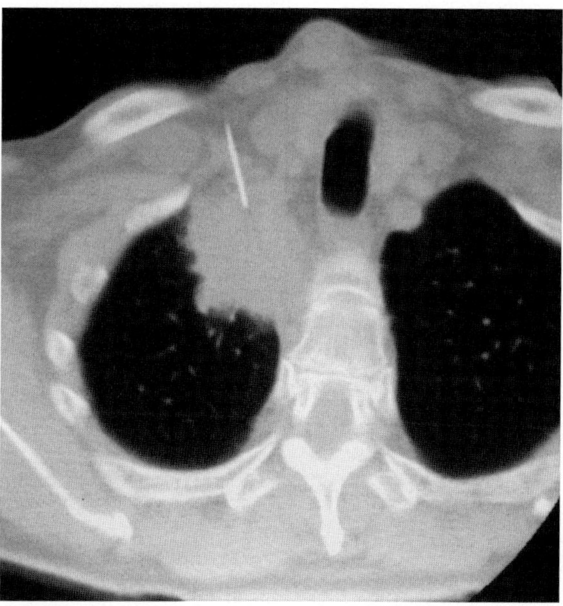

Figure 6. Needle within the mass (lung windows)—no aerated lung was traversed.

Management

Percutaneous CT-guided transthoracic fine-needle aspiration biopsy was undertaken with use of CT gantry angulation (approximately 30 degrees cranial to caudal). A path was visualized which avoided overlying bone **(Fig. 5)**, vascular structures, and aerated lung **(Fig. 6)**. The specimen was obtained with a 22-gauge Westcott needle and was provided to an on-site cytologist for immediate review following fixation in alcohol and toluidine blue staining. Malignant cells consistent with squamous cell carcinoma were identified.

Discussion

This case illustrates the utility of gantry angulation to provide a safer approach for biopsy of a lung lesion. Bone, blood vessels, and aerated lung were avoided, thereby reducing the risk of the procedure. The method was originally described for use in the abdomen to avoid traversing the left lobe of the liver when placing a transgastric drain into a pancreatic pseudocyst. It is probably applied most often in adrenal biopsy to prevent a transpleural path across the costophrenic sulcus. Other methods for angled CT approaches, including geometric calculation, triangulation, and stereotaxis are cumbersome. Furthermore, these methods do not permit direct visualization of the entire needle path and tip, which is one of the major advantages of CT guidance.

CT-guided aspiration/biopsy has been shown to have a high degree of accuracy (80%–90%). CT makes it possible to obtain tissue from lesions not well seen fluoroscopically and to avoid vital structures and aerated lung. Requirements include a skilled cytologist and a patient who can cooperate with breathing instructions. Although pneumothorax rates are higher with CT guidance (19%–47%) than with fluoroscopic technique (15%–27%), this may be attributable to the types of lesions attempted, with longer intraparenchymal paths requiring multiple passes, along with the delays in confirming needle tip position. Efforts to decrease the likelihood of pneumothorax include avoiding bullae and fissures, limiting the number of pleural crossings, and observing the patient after the procedure, with the patient in a reclined position with the biopsy site dependent.

Selected Readings

Austin JH, Cohen MB. Value of having a cytopathologist present during percutaneous fine-needle aspiration biopsy of lung: report of 55 cancer patients and meta-analysis of the literature. AJR 1993; 160:175–177.

Haramati LB, Austin JH. Complications after CT-guided needle biopsy through aerated versus nonaerated lung. Radiology 1991; 181:778.

Harter LP, Moss AA, Goldberg HI, Gross BH. CT-guided fine-needle aspirations for diagnosis of benign and malignant disease. AJR 1983; 140:363–367.

Hussain S. Gantry angulation in CT-guided percutaneous adrenal biopsy. AJR 1996; 166:537–539.

Moore EH, Shepard JA, McLoud TC, Templeton PA, Kosiuk JP. Positional precautions in needle aspiration lung biopsy. Radiology 1990; 175:733–735.

Onik G, Cosman ER, Wells TH Jr, et al. CT-guided aspirations for the body: comparison of hand guidance with stereotaxis. Radiology 1988; 166:389–394.

Perlmutt LM, Johnston WW, Dunnick NR. Percutaneous transthoracic needle aspiration: a review. AJR 1989; 152:451–455.

Picus D, Weyman PJ, Anderson DJ. Interventional computed tomography. In: Lee JKT, Sagel SS, Stanley RJ, eds. Computed body tomography with MRI correlation. 2nd edition. New York: Raven Press, 1989; 89–108.

vanSonnenberg E, Casola G, Ho M, et al. Difficult thoracic lesions: CT-guided biopsy experience in 150 cases. Radiology 1988; 167:457–461.

vanSonnenberg E, Lin AS, Deutsch AL, Mattrey RF. Percutaneous biopsy of difficult mediastinal, hilar, and pulmonary lesions by computed-tomographic guidance and a modified coaxial technique. Radiology 1983; 148:300–302.

vanSonnenberg E, Wittenberg J, Ferrucci JT, Mueller PR, Simeone JF. Triangulation method for percutaneous needle guidance: the angled approach to upper abdominal masses. AJR 1981; 137:757–761.

Yueh N, Halvorsen RA Jr, Letourneau JG, Crass JR. Gantry tilt technique for CT-guided biopsy and drainage. J Comput Assist Tomogr 1989; 13:182–184.

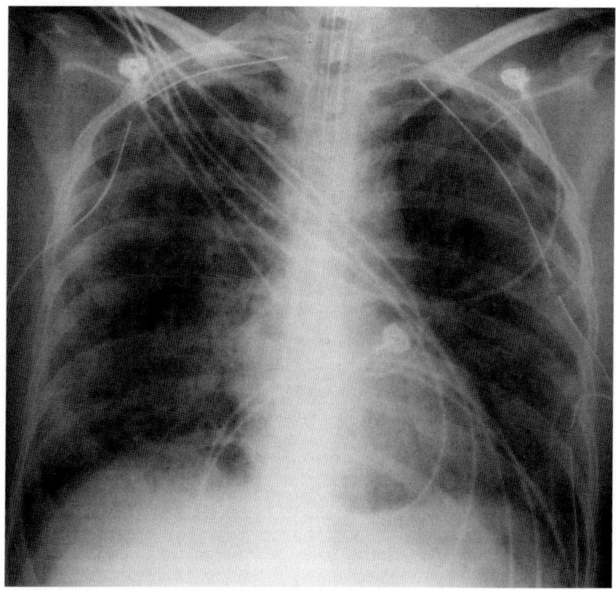

Figure 1. Initial chest radiograph.

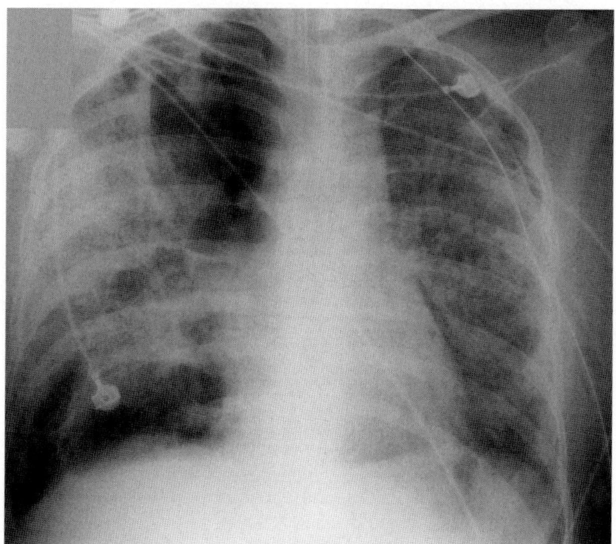

Figure 2. Chest radiograph after tube removal.

TEACHING FILE CASE 29

Vincent D. McCormick, M.D.

History

This 36-year-old patient admitted with pneumococcal pneumonia and sepsis developed acute respiratory distress syndrome (ARDS) and required mechanical ventilation for oxygenation. After the patient had been on mechanically assisted ventilation for several days, bilateral pneumothoraces developed which were treated with placement of large-bore chest tubes **(Fig. 1)**. Following removal of the right chest tube, a chest radiograph was obtained **(Fig. 2)**.

What is your diagnosis?

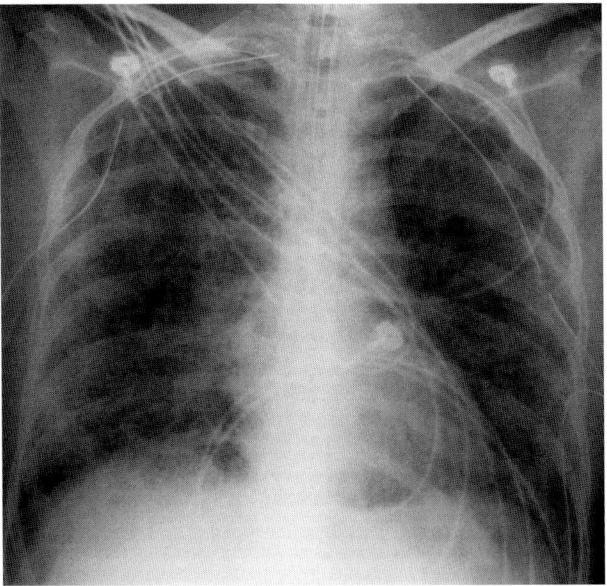

Figure 3. Endotracheal, feeding, and bilateral chest tubes are present. Diffuse, heterogeneous opacification of the lungs is consistent with the clinical diagnosis of ARDS.

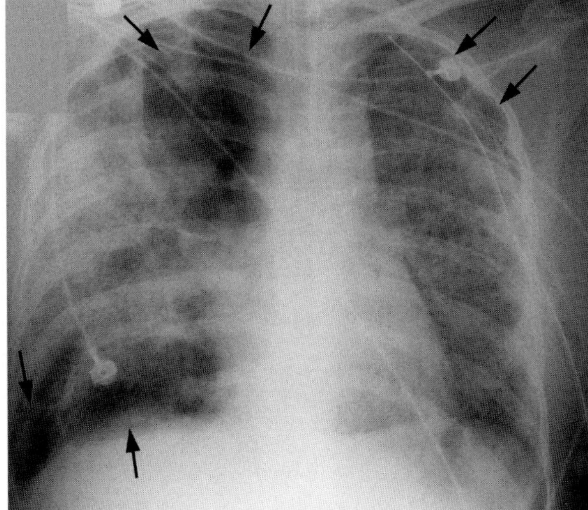

Figure 4. Following removal of the right chest tube, right apical and right basilar pneumothoraces developed, and a left upper pneumothorax is also apparent (arrows).

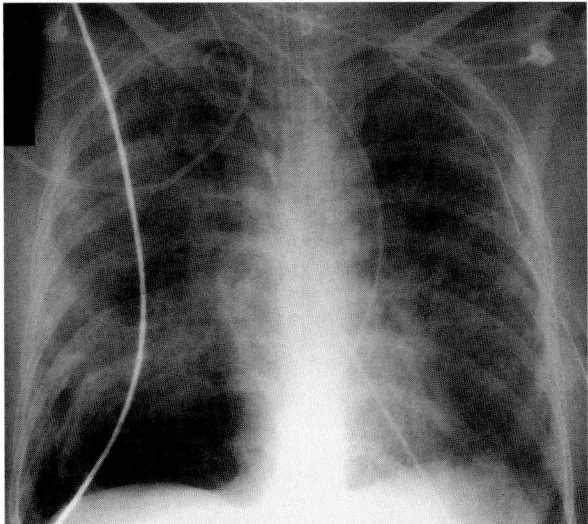

Figure 5. After placement of a right chest tube, the apical collection has resolved but the right basilar pneumothorax displays increasing evidence of tension.

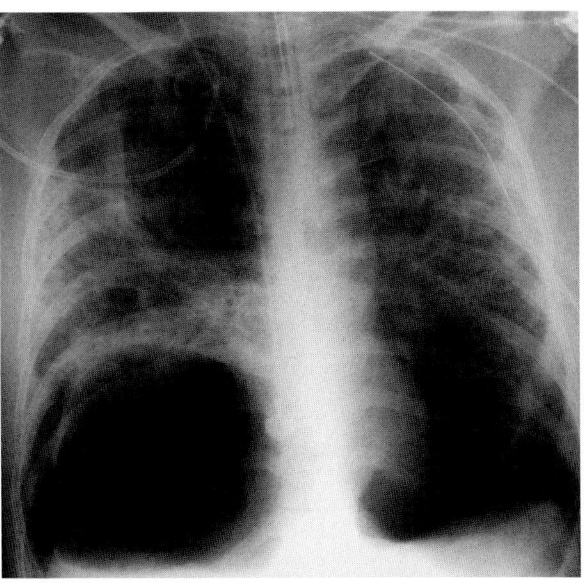

Figure 6. Bibasilar tension pneumothoraces are now present.

Radiographic Findings

The initial chest radiograph demonstrates diffuse bilateral parenchymal opacities consistent with the clinical diagnosis of ARDS **(Fig. 3)**. An endotracheal tube and bilateral chest tubes are present. The chest radiograph obtained following removal of the right chest tube shows the development of right apical and basilar and left upper pneumothoraces **(Fig. 4)**.

Diagnosis

Multiple bilateral tension pneumothoraces.

How would you manage this patient?

Management

In the interventional suite, a 14-F pigtail catheter was placed into the apical pneumothorax under fluoroscopic control. Bibasilar tension pneumothoraces developed over the next 3 days **(Figs. 5, 6)** and a computed tomography (CT) scan demonstrated the extent of the bibasilar collections and confirmed the persistence of a large right apical pneumothorax **(Figs. 7, 8)**.

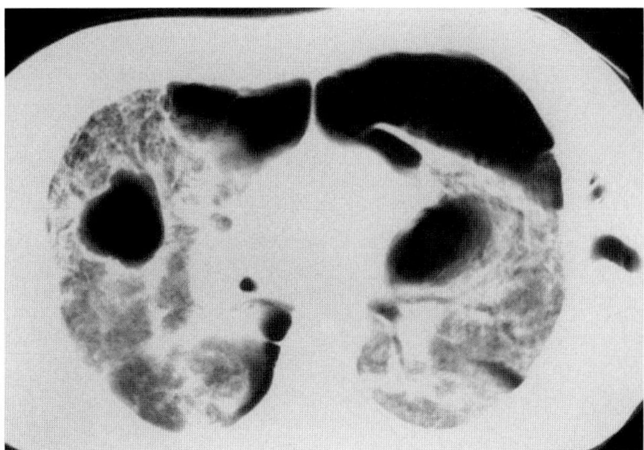

Figure 7. CT scan confirms the presence of large bibasilar tension pneumothoraces and their superior extension to the mid thorax.

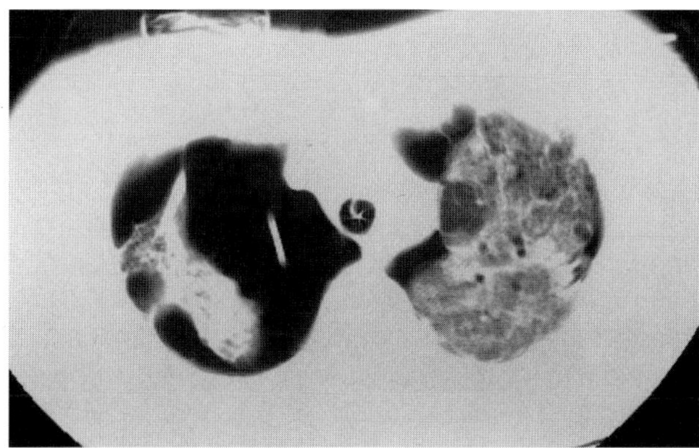

Figure 8. The right apical collection is considerably larger than suspected based on the chest radiograph.

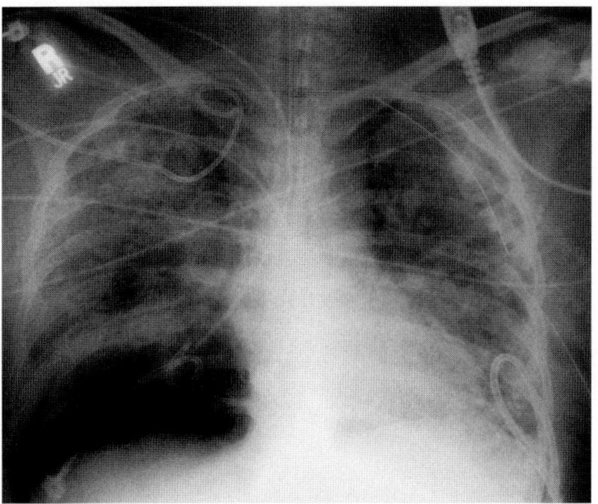

Figure 9. Following placement of bibasilar tubes, the left basilar collection has been evacuated while the right basilar collection has decreased in size and exhibits diminished signs of tension.

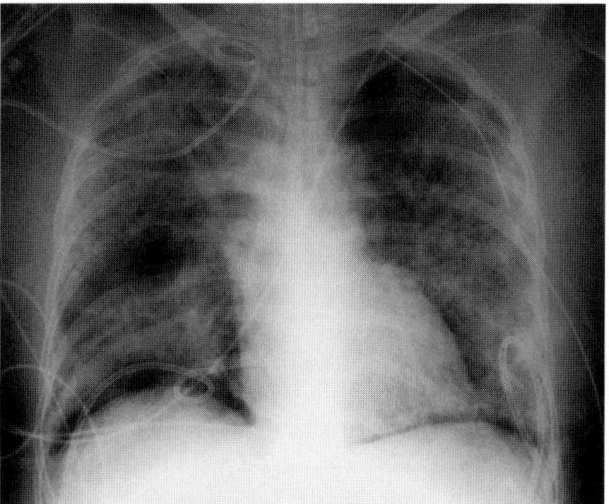

Figure 10. Small, residual bibasilar pneumothoraces are visible. The left apical pneumothorax is unchanged.

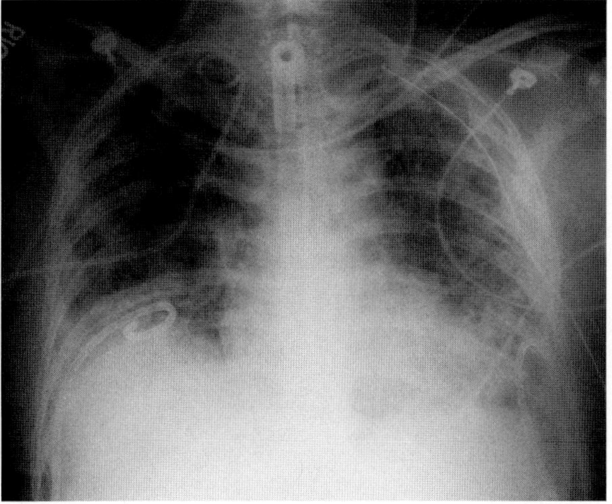

Figure 11. The pneumothoraces are no longer present.

The bibasilar pneumothoraces were managed with bilateral pigtail catheters positioned under fluoroscopic guidance **(Fig. 9)**. Three days later, a chest radiograph demonstrated almost complete evacuation of the pneumothoraces **(Fig. 10)**, and a week later they were no longer apparent **(Fig. 11)**.

Discussion

Critically ill patients requiring mechanical ventilation in the setting of severe parenchymal lung disease are prone to develop pneumothoraces, which can be life-threatening. A cascade of events in barotrauma (pulmonary injury and air leak due to mechanical ventilation) begins with alveolar wall rupture producing interstitial emphysema which tracks to the mediastinum, often resulting in pneumomediastinum and/or pneumothorax. Stiffened lung parenchyma and/or adhesions in patients with pneumonia, ARDS, and severe interstitial disease may prevent the collapse of involved lung segments when a pneumothorax occurs. In these circumstances, even a small pneumothorax may be under tension and the usual signs of tension may not be apparent on chest radiography.

Of special note, pneumothoraces in patients on mechanically assisted ventilation almost always progress to tension, in up to 96% of cases in one reported series. Because loculated pneumothoraces are not easily treated with blind surgical techniques, imaging-guided placement of drainage catheters is the procedure of choice in these situations.

Pneumothorax drainage can be performed with fluoroscopically guided trocar technique or Seldinger technique to position 8–10-F catheters. Use of larger chest tubes (16 F) obviates the kinking or clogging which may occur with smaller-caliber tubes.

CT scanning may be necessary to confirm the presence of a pneumothorax that is suspected but not definitively demonstrated on an anteroposterior supine chest radiograph. Similarly, CT scanning may be crucial to proper positioning of a drainage catheter into a small loculated collection.

Complete re-expansion of a pneumothorax in these patients may not be apparent on chest radiographs or CT scans for several days after chest tube placement. Additionally, significant clinical improvement does not always follow evacuation of tension pneumothoraces in these cases, probably because of the severity of the underlying lung disease. However, catheter placement for tension pneumothorax evacuation stabilizes these patients and slows or halts the deterioration of gas exchange, which accounts for significant morbidity and mortality. As noted in this case, multiple tubes may be required for the multiple loculated pneumothoraces. Treatment of such air collections should be pursued aggressively to improve the clinical situation as much as possible because there may be no other recourse in these patients.

Selected Readings

Boland CW, Lee MJ, Sutcliffe, NP, Mueller PR. Loculated pneumothoraces in patients with acute respiratory disease treated with mechanical ventilation: preliminary observations after image-guided drainage. J Vasc Interv Radiol 1996; 7:247–252.

Klein JS, Schultz S. Interventional chest radiology. Curr Probl Diagn Radiol 1992; 21:219–277.

Steier M, Ching N, Roberts EB, Nealon TF. Pneumothorax complicating continuous ventilatory support. J Thorac Cardiovasc Surg 1974; 67:17–23.

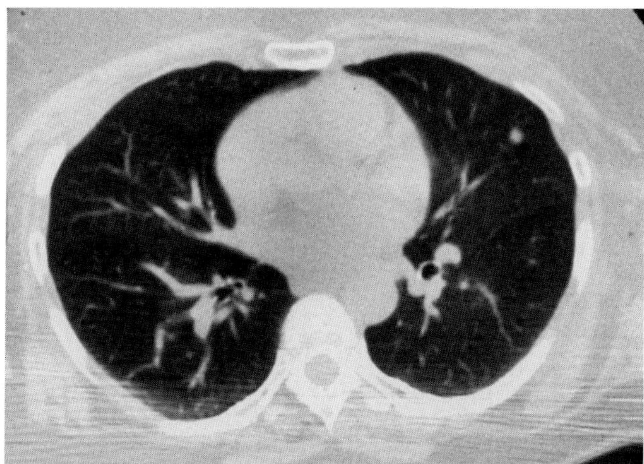

Figure 1. CT scan in a patient with a new lung nodule.

TEACHING CASE FILE 30

Ana M. Salazar, M.D., and
Rosita M. Shah, M.D.

History

A 64-year-old smoker was found to have a new small lingular nodule on a routine chest radiograph. A computed tomography (CT) scan was obtained **(Fig. 1)**.

What is your diagnosis?

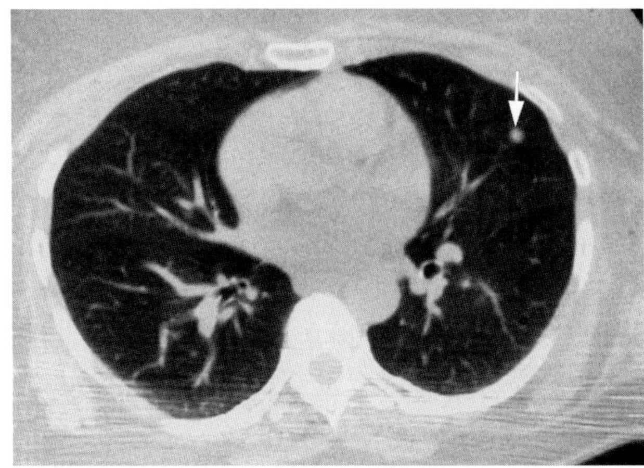

Figure 2. CT scan shows an 8-mm peripheral nodule (arrow).

Radiographic Findings

An 8-mm noncalcified nodule is present **(Fig. 2)**. Given the fact that this is a new nodule in a patient with a history of smoking, and no known tumor is present elsewhere, it must be assumed that this is a primary pulmonary neoplasm.

Diagnosis

Lingular nodule, probably a primary neoplasm.

How would you manage this patient?

Management

Fine needle aspiration (FNA) is possible, but the subcentimeter size of the lesion precluded FNA in this case because a negative biopsy would not provide a high level of confidence that the lesion is benign. The patient was referred for thoracoscopic excision of the nodule.

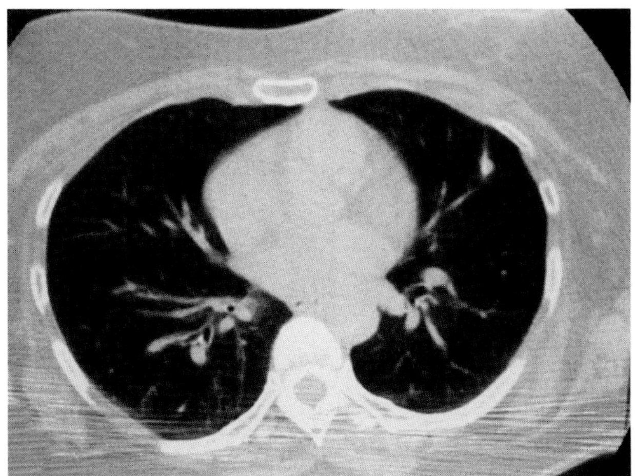

Figure 3. Needle localization.

The small size and the location deep to the pleura may make this nodule difficult to localize at thoraco-scopy because it could neither be palpated nor visualized. Preoperative wire localization is necessary in this case and was performed from an anterior approach. **Figure 3** shows the position of the introducer and stylet. The introducer needle is optimally placed through the nodule and slightly distal to it. The localizing wire was placed through the needle **(Fig. 4)**. The wire must remain unanchored on the chest wall to allow movement with respiration. Anchoring the wire will cause it to dislodge. At surgery the nodule was found to be a peripheral carcinoid.

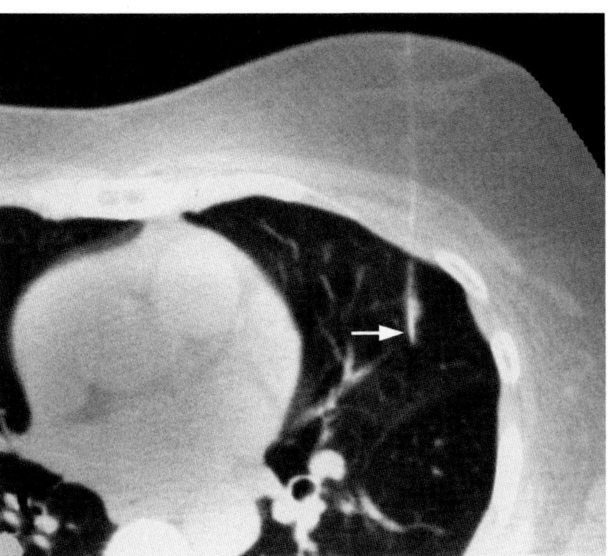

Figure 4. Localizing wire placement (arrow).

Selected Readings

Mack MJ, Gordon MJ, Postma TW, et al. Percutaneous localization of pulmonary nodules for thoracoscopic lung resection. Ann Thorac Surg 1992; 53:1123–1124.

Shah RM, Spirn PW, Salazar AM, et al. Localization of peripheral pulmonary nodules for thoracoscopic excision: value of CT-guided wire placement. AJR 1993; 161:279–283.

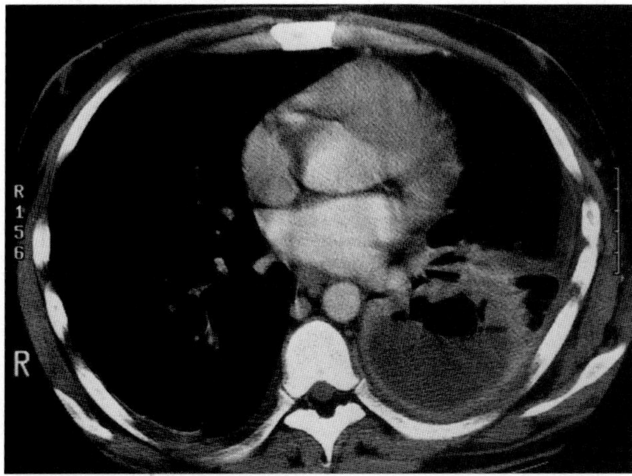

Figure 1. CT scan of the chest.

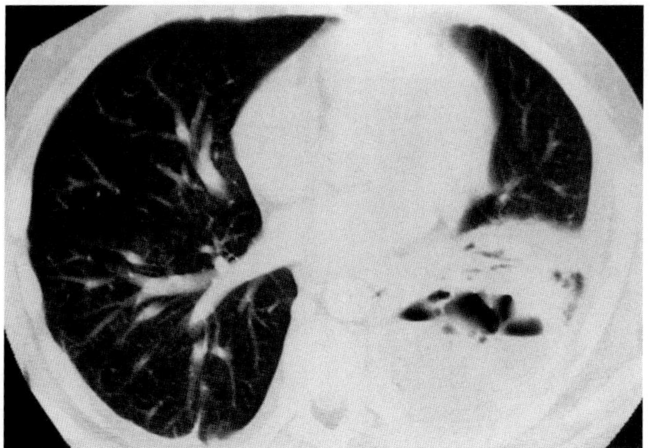
Figure 2. CT scan of the chest.

TEACHING FILE CASE 31

James F. Gruden, M.D.

History

A 43-year-old man with a history of intravenous drug use came to the emergency department complaining of several days of high fever, chills, left pleuritic chest pain, and a productive cough. A chest radiograph (not shown) demonstrated consolidation in the superior segment of the left lower lobe with a small pleural effusion blunting the costophrenic angle. Sputum Gram stain was nondiagnostic.

The patient was admitted to the hospital for broad-spectrum intravenous antibiotic therapy, but on the fourth hospital day he still had fevers to 39 degrees C. A repeat chest radiograph (not shown) showed progression of pleuroparenchymal abnormalities on the left. A computed tomography (CT) scan was obtained **(Figs. 1, 2)**.

What is your diagnosis?

Radiographic Findings

A large fluid collection is present in the posterior left mid lung zone **(Fig. 3)**. Lung windows confirm the presence of scattered air-fluid levels with evident septations **(Fig. 4)**. The collection is fairly round and forms acute angles with the adjacent lung parenchyma. The anterior and lateral walls are thick and irregular. Adjacent compressive atelectasis is present in the posterior subsegment of the left upper lobe.

The collection is consistent with a lung abscess given its round shape (acute angles formed with the lung) and areas of wall thickening. The location (superior segment of the lower lobe) is also typical and is often related to aspiration. The posterior smooth pleural enhancement, however, can cause this to be mistaken for a pleural collection and possible empyema.

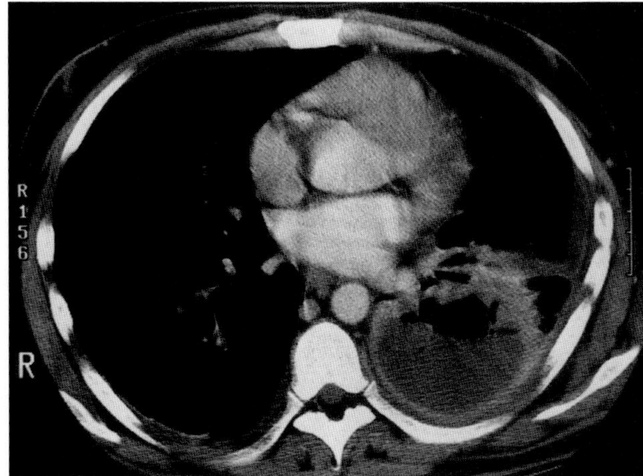

Figure 3. Fluid collection in the left posterior chest has imaging characteristics of a lung abscess. Note the thick, irregular anterior and lateral walls, the acute angles formed with the lung, and compressive atelectasis in the adjacent upper lobe.

Diagnoses

1. Lung abscess, superior segment of the right lower lobe.
2. Compressive atelectasis, left upper lobe.

Management

The CT scan was interpreted as an air-containing empyema and a surgical consult was obtained. A left chest tube was placed at the bedside by the surgical resident in an effort to achieve pleural drainage, and gross pus was drained from the tube. The Gram stain showed polymicrobial infection with mixed anaerobic and aerobic organisms.

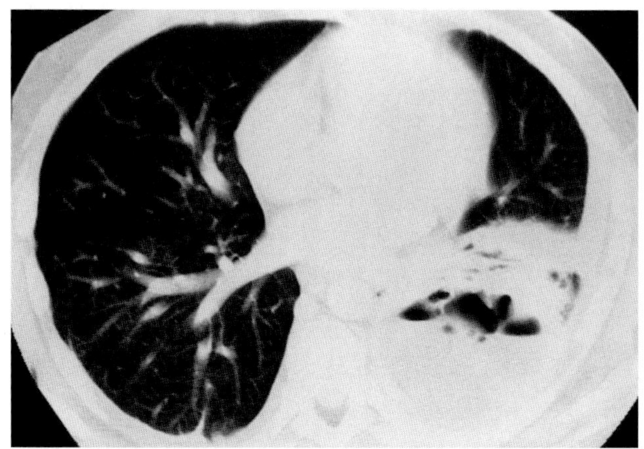

Figure 4. Lung windows confirm the presence of several air-fluid levels in the thick-walled abscess along with multiple small septations.

Several days later, the patient remained febrile, and the chest tube output, initially minimal, had ceased altogether. A CT scan obtained to assess the adequacy of "pleural drainage" shows that the chest tube has retracted into the left pleural space **(Fig. 5)**. The large collection seen earlier is smaller, but it is still present anterior to the tube and contains a persistent air-fluid level, which was confirmed on lung windows. This parenchymal abscess is thick-walled and round.

A pleural collection is now present on the left. It has a typical crescentic shape and also contains foci of air (confirmed on lung windows). This new collection forms obtuse angles with the adjacent lung and does not have the irregular wall thickening evident in most lung abscesses.

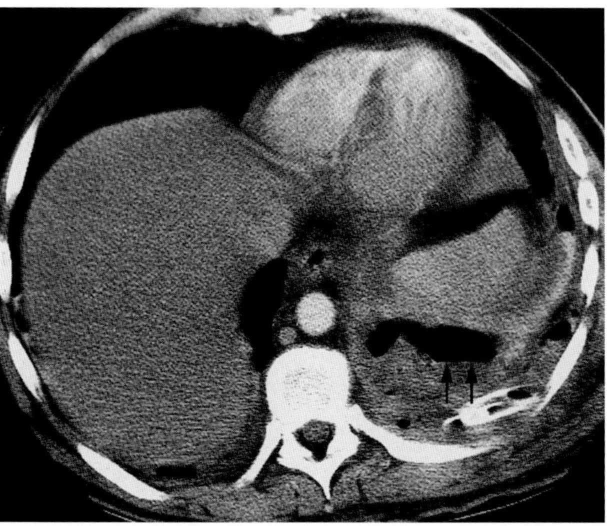

Figure 5. Chest tube in the pleural space with a new pleural collection; the lung abscess is still present anteriorly but has been decompressed, presumably into the pleural space, and contains a persistent air-fluid level (arrows).

Because the patient was still symptomatic and there was no output from the chest tube, the Interventional Radiology service was asked to place percutaneous pigtail catheters in order to optimize drainage of the parenchymal and pleural collections. With use of CT guidance to select the optimal location for the tube (using metallic letters on the skin surface), a 16-F catheter was placed with Seldinger technique. Thick pus emanated immediately from the drainage catheter, so attempts were made to aspirate as much material as possible while the patient was in the CT suite. With use of a syringe connected to the pigtail catheter, approximately 50 mL of purulent material was aspirated.

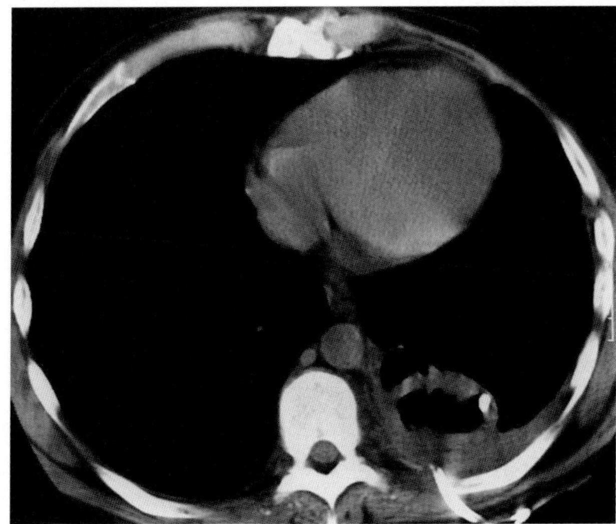

Figure 6. Pigtail catheter coiled in the abscess space (now continuous with the pleural space because of the presence of a bronchopleural fistula).

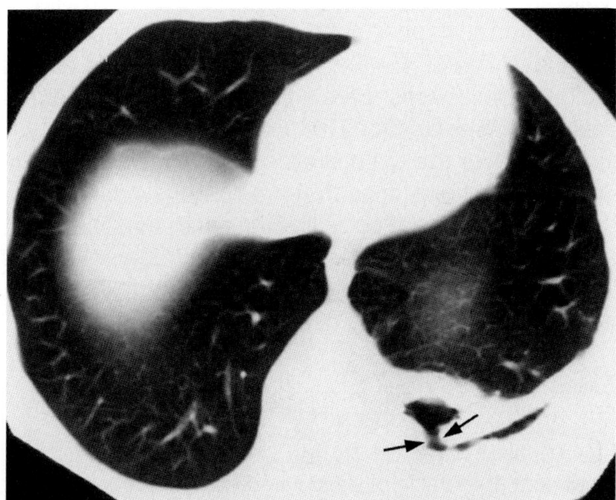

Figure 7. Inferiorly, the site of the bronchopleural fistula is identified (arrows); air is noted in the pleural space posteriorly and in the abscess cavity anteriorly.

A postprocedural CT scan showed the catheter coiled in the parenchymal abscess cavity **(Fig. 6)**, and a more inferior image **(Fig. 7)** showed direct communication between the parenchymal and pleural collections, forming a bronchopleural fistula. Because of the generous communication between the two spaces, it was decided to leave the catheter in the abscess instead of placing an additional catheter in the pleural space.

Urokinase (Abbott Laboratories) mixed with normal saline was then administered through the catheter, and the tube was clamped for 2 hours. Several hundred mL of material drained out when the tube was unclamped. The procedure was repeated the following day with similar results.

On the third day after pigtail catheter placement the patient was afebrile, and the pigtail catheter had no output. A repeat CT scan (not shown) showed resolution of the parenchymal and pleural fluid, with only a thick-walled air-containing cavity in the left lower lobe. The tube was removed, and the patient had an uneventful recovery.

The final diagnosis was lung abscess presumably related to aspiration, complicated by empyema, probably iatrogenic.

Discussion

This case illustrates several important points. First, distinguishing between a lung abscess and an empyema is important but can be difficult; abscesses typically respond to intravenous antibiotics, although clinical improvement can be quite slow. Empyemas require tube drainage. In patients who require tube drainage, imaging-guided placement of relatively small-bore tubes should be performed. Given the fact that this lung abscess abutted the pleural space and there was no intervening aerated lung, percutaneous imaging-guided tube placement could have been performed easily.

Second, although empyema may have complicated the clinical course without intervention, the blind placement of a surgical chest tube probably played a role in creating the bronchopleural fistula by spilling infected material from the pus-filled abscess into the pleural space. This thick material was difficult to drain with the tube. In general, lung abscesses are better treated medically, but imaging-guided catheter placement should be considered when intervention is required. Although pigtail catheter placement in a lung abscess can occasionally result in bronchopleural fistula formation, the chances are much lower than with large-bore tube placement. Small catheter placement, if feasible, can be a much better alternative than open thoracostomy.

The third important point illustrated by this case is the technique for management of pleural collections. In general, parapneumonic effusions respond to medical therapy; empyemas require tube drainage. Pleural fluid analysis is usually performed to assess the type of fluid present (not done in this case because of the presence of gross pus). Light's criteria are used to make this distinction: gross pus, positive Gram stain, pH below 7.0, or glucose level below 40 mg/dL define empyema and are indications for drainage. However, in an unstable patient or when respiratory function is compromised, drainage may be indicated regardless of the characteristics of the fluid. Late empyemas, with significant parietal pleural thickening (over 5 mm) or a "honeycomb" appearance on ultrasound, often do not respond to percutaneous drainage and require open thoracotomy.

Imaging-guided tube thoracostomy is preferable to surgical tube placement for several reasons: 1) patient comfort; 2) the ability to place the tube into the largest portion of the collection using CT or ultrasound guidance, thus avoiding tube malposition; 3) the low complication rate of pigtail catheter placement compared to blind surgical tube placement; and 4) the ability to administer thrombolytic therapy through the catheter as needed. In addition, multiple catheters can be placed, if needed, and individual catheter position can be altered. The success rate of imaging-guided percutaneous catheter placement in the treatment of empyema is 70%–80%.

The role of urokinase in the treatment of empyemas is not at all clear. Although thrombolytic therapy has been reported to result in increased tube drainage and to cause no significant untoward effects, no consistent protocol for urokinase administration exists. It is not clear whether frequent administration of small amounts (50,000–100,00 IU) is more efficacious than large boluses (250,000 IU). In addition, various researchers in this area have clamped the tube for different lengths of time: for 1 to 3 hours or even overnight. No controlled study has been performed comparing urokinase with the administration of saline alone, and it is not known whether beneficial effects derive from thrombolytic therapy or mechanical irrigation. Lastly, some authors connect catheters to negative pressure, while others employ only gravity drainage.

Urokinase converts plasminogen to its active form (plasmin), which breaks down fibrin and theoretically lyses small adhesions within the pleural space that limit drainage. Again, this is theoretical; attempts to measure fibrin split products in pleural fluid before and after urokinase therapy have yielded inconclusive results. Whatever the mechanism, and despite the lack of uniform controlled clinical trials, urokinase now has a role in the treatment of pleural collections that are not satisfactorily drained by pigtail catheter placement and tube irrigation alone.

It is important to treat empyemas similar to infected collections elsewhere in the body. As much material as possible should be aspirated and drained at the time of initial tube placement. Tube irrigation with 10–20 mL of sterile saline should be done two or three times per day, and the tube should be connected to low suction (-20 cm H_2O). With this protocol, most empyemas can be drained without supplemental thrombolytic therapy. In cases in which the catheter(s) is (are) positioned adequately but drainage is suboptimal, catheter patency should first be confirmed. If the catheter is patent, repeat imaging (chest radiography or CT scanning) is indicated to evaluate the collection.

Collections which persist despite the presence of a patent, correctly positioned catheter may respond to urokinase. Again, the exact dose and timing of administration varies. Tubes are clamped from 1 to 12 hours. Despite these variations in the treatment protocol, success rates are quite similar, consistently exceeding 80% even in collections that are obviously difficult to drain. No significant complications with urokinase administration have been reported with the doses used in the pleural space. Monitoring of serum fibrinogen or degradation products is not required.

Selected Readings

Lee KS, Im JG, Kim YH, Hwang SH, Bae WK, Lee BH. Treatment of thoracic multiloculated empyemas with intracavitary urokinase. Radiology 1991; 179:771–775.

Light RW. Parapneumonic effusions and empyema. Clin Chest Med 1985; 6:55–62.

Moulton JS, Moore PT, Mencini RA. Treatment of loculated pleural effusions with transcatheter intracavitary urokinase. AJR 1989; 153:941–945.

Park CS, Chung WM, Lim MK, Cho CH, Suh CH, Chung WK. Transcatheter instillation of urokinase into a loculated pleural effusion: analysis of treatment effect. AJR 1996; 167:649–652.

Ryan JM, Boland GW, Lee MJ, Mueller PR. Intracavitary urokinase therapy as an adjunct to percutaneous drainage in a patient with a multiloculated empyema. AJR 1996; 167:643–647.

vanSonnenberg E, Nakamoto SK, Mueller PR, et al. CT- and sonographic-guided catheter drainage of empyemas after chest-tube failure. Radiology 1984; 151:349–353.

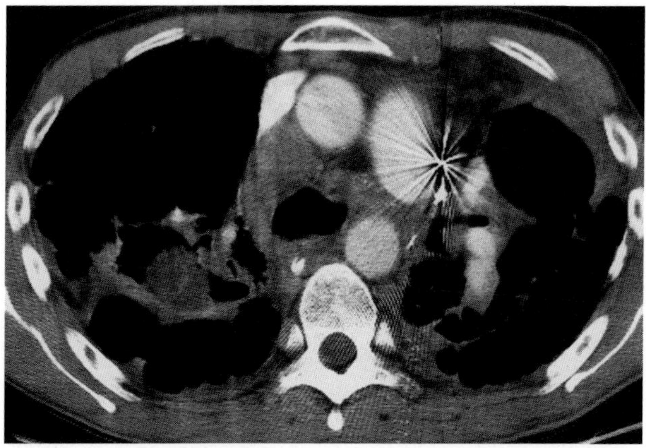

Figure 1. Soft-tissue windows from a CT scan in a patient with massive hemoptysis.

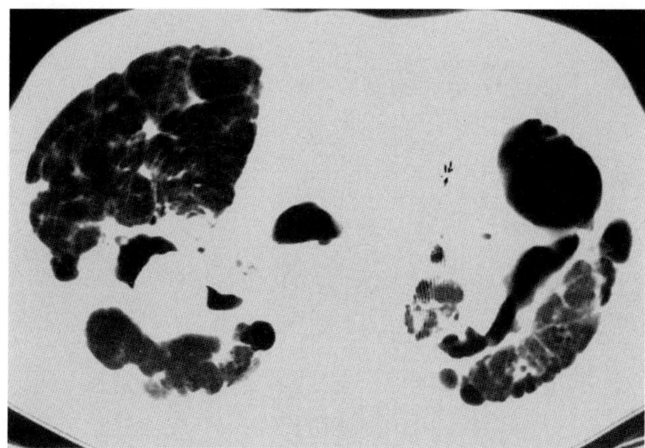

Figure 2. Lung windows of the section shown in Figure 1.

TEACHING FILE CASE 32

James F. Gruden, M.D.

History

A 38-year-old man with a long history of sarcoidosis came to the emergency department with massive hemoptysis (several cups of bright red blood within the previous hour). While in the emergency room, he had recurrent, massive, bright red hemoptysis and was admitted to the hospital. A computed tomography (CT) scan of the chest was obtained **(Figs. 1, 2)**.

What is your diagnosis?

Radiographic Findings

The CT scan shows low-attenuation, rounded, dependent intracavitary soft tissue in the right upper lobe **(Fig. 3)**. Bulky retrocaval paratracheal and precarinal adenopathy is evident. Surgical clips are the residua of remote mediastinoscopy. Note the subtle air-fluid level in the right mainstem bronchus **(Fig. 4)**.

Bilateral parahilar parenchymal consolidation is present, associated with architectural distortion and multiple bilateral peripheral cystic or cavitary areas. The main pulmonary artery is also enlarged.

Diagnoses

1. Mycetoma, right upper lobe.
2. Blood within the right mainstem bronchus.
3. End-stage lung disease secondary to sarcoidosis.
3. Secondary pulmonary arterial hypertension.

What should be done next?

Management

Fiberoptic bronchoscopy was performed to confirm the CT findings and to definitively localize the bleeding site. Bright red blood filled the right mainstem bronchus and brisk bleeding during the procedure precluded further assessment of the right bronchial tree. No blood was present on the left. The patient became hemodynamically unstable and was intubated (selective left mainstem) and transferred to the intensive care unit.

The patient was not a candidate for surgery, so emergent selective bronchial artery embolization was requested. The cavitary lesion in the right upper lobe was supplied by numerous tortuous and enlarged bronchial vessels (not shown) originating from a combined intercostal/bronchial artery trunk. The bronchial artery was embolized with particulate Ivalon (Unipoint, High Point, NC) until feeding vessels could no longer be identified at angiography and no forward flow in the bronchial artery was present.

Several hours after the embolization, massive hemoptysis recurred and continued intermittently for the next several days. What do you have to offer at this point?

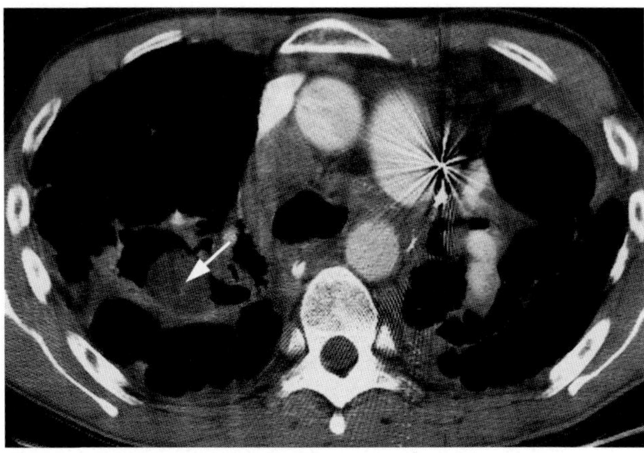

Figure 3. Mycetoma (arrow) in the right upper lobe cavity and extensive mediastinal adenopathy.

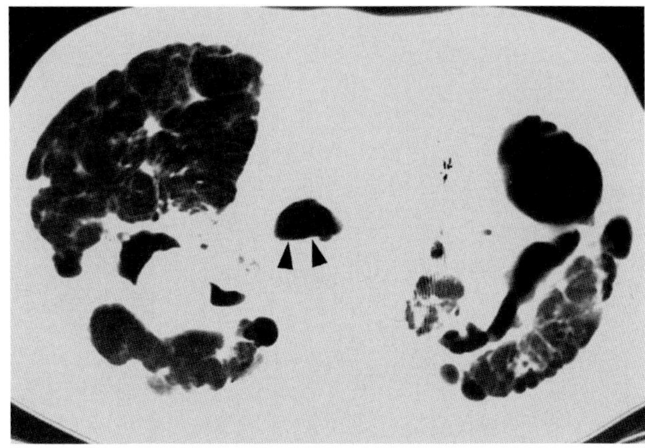

Figure 4. Lung windows show bilateral parenchymal fibrosis and cavitary disease consistent with sarcoidosis. Blood-fluid level is seen in the right mainstem bronchus (arrowheads).

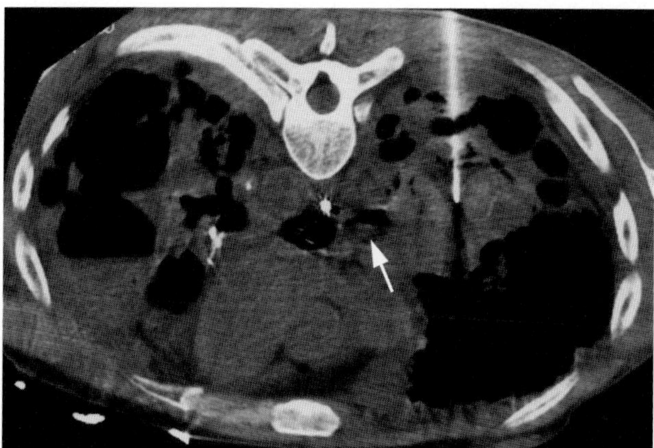

Figure 5. Percutaneous needle positioned in the cavity, with the gelatin-amphotericin mixture in the cavity and some of the mixture in the right mainstem bronchus (arrow).

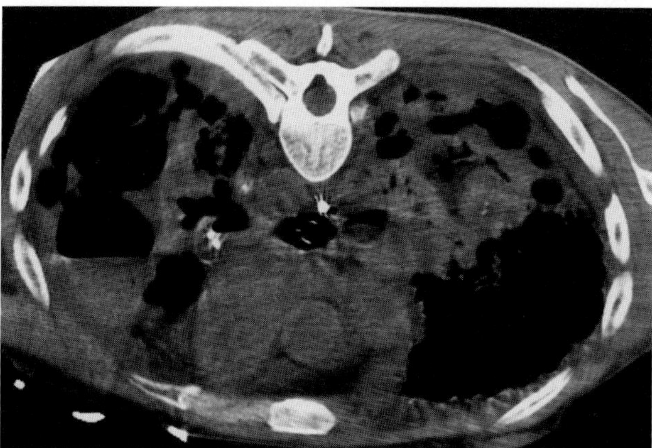

Figure 6. After needle removal, gelatin material remains in the cavity and bronchus. The left mainstem bronchus is selectively intubated.

The patient was scheduled for percutaneous intracavitary therapy. The intubated patient was placed in the prone position on the CT gantry, and the cavity containing the mycetoma was entered percutaneously with an 18-gauge needle. A solution of 50 mg amphotericin B in 10 mL sterile dextrose and water was administered through the needle; this solution was emitted immediately through the tracheostomy tube. Postprocedural CT images (not shown) demonstrated no retained solution within the cavity.

In an effort to facilitate retention of the amphotericin B mixture within the cavity, a gelatin-based solution was prepared according to a protocol previously described by Munk. Six grams of oxoid standard laboratory gelatin was dissolved in 8.5 mL sterile water in a hot water bath at 40 degrees C to which 50 mg amphotericin was then added. The solution was drawn up in a heated syringe (40 degrees C) immediately prior to instillation and the syringe attached directly to the 18-gauge needle. The gelatin solution was administered rapidly because it solidifies at room temperature and is semisolid at body temperature.

The postinjection prone CT scan **(Fig. 5)** shows the suspension within the cavity. The needle was removed, and the therapeutic gelatin mixture remained within the cavity **(Fig. 6)**.

The patient remained in the intensive care unit and had no further hemoptysis; however, he suffered cardiopulmonary arrest on day 21 of his hospitalization and could not be resuscitated.

Discussion

Fungal superinfection of pre-existing cystic or cavitary lung lesions is most commonly due to *Aspergillus* species; these aspergillomas are complicated at some point by hemoptysis in the majority of cases, which can be massive (>300 mL in 24 hours). Although surgical resection is the treatment of choice, many patients are not surgical candidates because of underlying cardiopulmonary disease and/or unstable hemodynamics at the time of active hemoptysis.

Bronchial artery embolization is often helpful in the immediate control of hemoptysis, but it cannot offer definitive therapy for the underlying mycetoma. In addition, hemoptysis recurs in nearly one quarter of all patients within 6 months. This recurrent bleeding may result from capillary oozing within the inner wall of the superinfected cystic or cavitary parenchymal lesion in conjunction with parasitization of collateral vessels over time.

Intracavitary therapy is effective in the immediate control of hemoptysis in nearly all patients, and partial or complete resolution of the mycetoma is noted at follow-up in the majority of patients. While some investigators have advocated daily administration of liquid solutions through an indwelling pigtail catheter placed in the cavity or via repeated cavity punctures at various intervals, the administration of amphotericin in a solid mixture (such as gelatin in this case) permits single-session therapy.

The mechanism by which intracavitary therapy produces beneficial effects is probably related to the sclerosing properties of ampho-tericin, although in the long term, local antifungal action is probably important as well. In patients who benefit from solution-based therapy, mechanical irrigation may also contribute to partial or complete resolution of the mycetoma. On an acute basis, however, hemoptysis is controlled because of obliteration of the bleeding small vessels in the cavity wall regardless of the solid or liquid nature of the agent.

The optimal dose of amphotericin has not been defined for either short-term control of hemoptysis or long-term resolution of the mycetoma. However, 50 mg seems to be adequate based on available reports; if hemoptysis recurs, administration can be repeated.

Complications of intracavitary therapy are uncommon. Pneumothorax is rare because of common pleural adhesions or fibrothorax related to the underlying disease process (usually tuberculosis or sarcoidosis). Hemoptysis during the procedure can occur because of the hypervascularity present in and around the parenchymal lesion and pleura, particularly if a guide wire is used prior to pigtail catheter insertion for daily solution-based therapy. This is another advantage of single-session treatment with gelatin or glycerin-based amphotericin.

The roles of bronchial artery embolization and intracavitary therapy are evolving, and patients with life-threatening hemoptysis secondary to an intracavitary mycetoma may benefit from both. However, it is prudent to attempt intracavitary treatment of the mycetoma first; it is faster, simpler, and has high immediate and long-term success rates.

Selected Readings

Giron JM, Poey CG, Fajadet PP, et al. Inoperable pulmonary aspergilloma: percutaneous CT-guided injection with glycerin and ampho-tericin B paste in 15 cases. Radiology 1993; 188:825–827.

Lee KS, Kim HT, Kim YH, Choe KO. Treatment of hemoptysis in patients with cavitary aspergilloma of the lung: value of percutaneous instillation of amphotericin B. AJR 1993; 161:727–731.

Munk PL, Vellet AD, Rankin RN, Müller NL, Ahmad D. Intracavitary aspergilloma: transthoracic percutaneous injection of amphotericin gelatin solution. Radiology 1993; 188:821–823.

Uflacker R, Kaemmerer A, Picon PD, et al. Bronchial artery embolization in the management of hemoptysis: technical aspects and long-term results. Radiology 1985; 157:637–644.

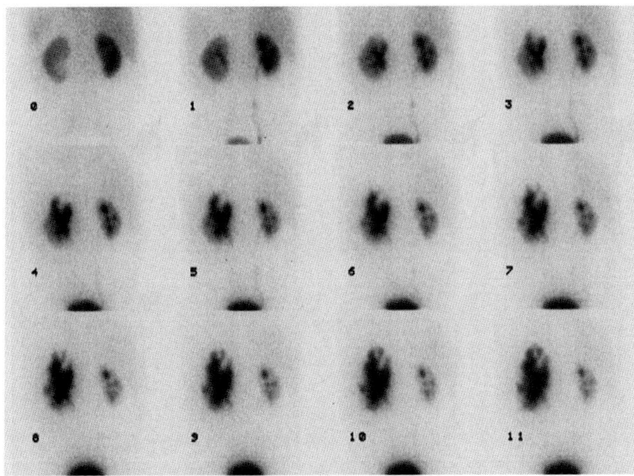

Figure 1. Excretory phase of a technetium-99m MAG-3 radionuclide renal scan (posterior view).

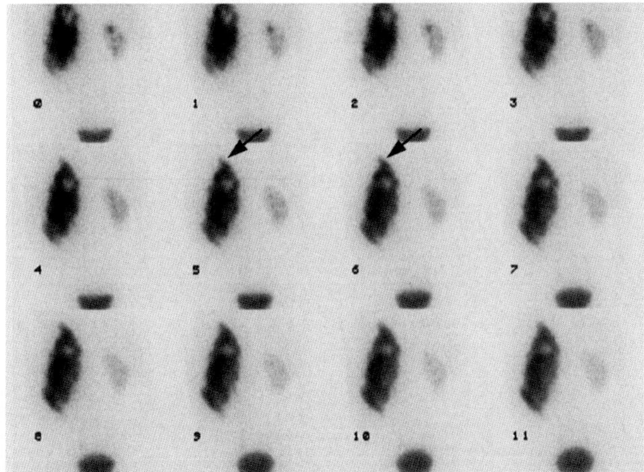

Figure 2. Renal scan after the administration of Lasix (posterior view).

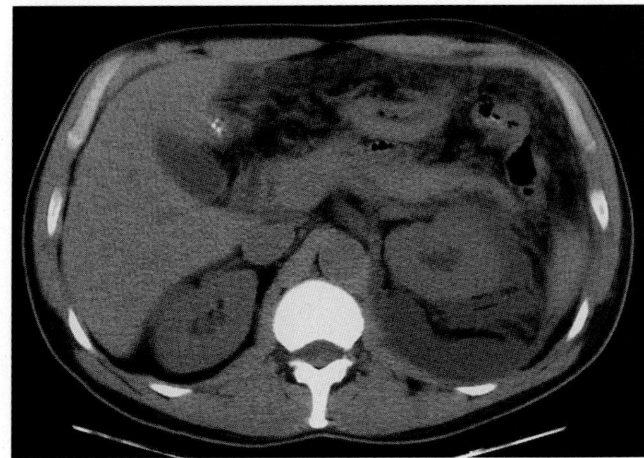

Figure 3. CT scan of the kidneys.

TEACHING FILE CASE 33

Phillip Kohanski, M.D.

History

The patient is a 50-year-old man who was seen by a gastroenterologist for a complaint of postprandial abdominal pain. A malignant gastric mass was detected at upper endoscopy. A nuclear medicine Lasix renal scan was performed because of worsening renal function **(Figs. 1, 2)**. Following the renal scan, a computed tomography (CT) scan of the abdomen was obtained **(Fig. 3)**.

What is your diagnosis?

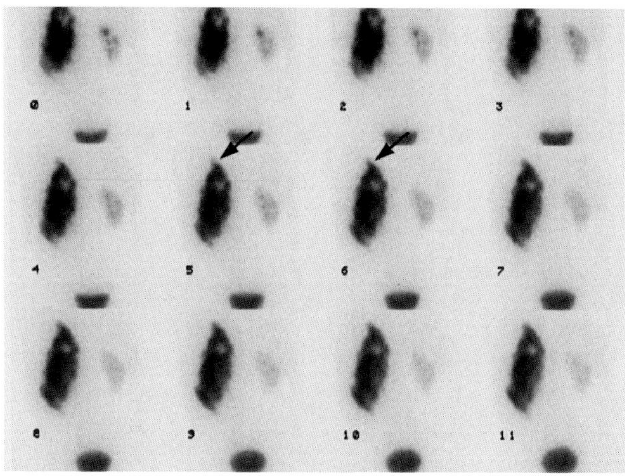

Figure 4. Renal scan after administration of Lasix. Arrows point to urine extravasation (posterior view).

Radiographic Findings

The nuclear medicine study demonstrates extravasation of urine from the left renal collecting system **(Fig. 4)**. The CT scan demonstrates left ureteral obstruction. Urinoma formation and inflammatory changes are also evident in the perirenal tissues **(Fig. 5)**.

Diagnosis

Left ureteral obstruction due to gastric mass metastasis to the retroperitoneum with urine extravasation and urinoma formation.

How would you treat this patient?

Management

When the urinoma was demonstrated on the CT scan, the referring physician requested urinoma drainage and placement of a nephrostomy catheter into the renal collecting system. The patient was placed in the prone position and a localizing grid was taped to his skin. A CT slice was obtained to delineate the relationship of the skin markers to the urinoma **(Fig. 6)**.

Depth and angle measurements were made from the CT slice. The patient was prepared and draped and given local anesthesia. The anesthesia needle was retained in its position as a guide, and a CT slice was taken through the needle **(Fig. 7)**.

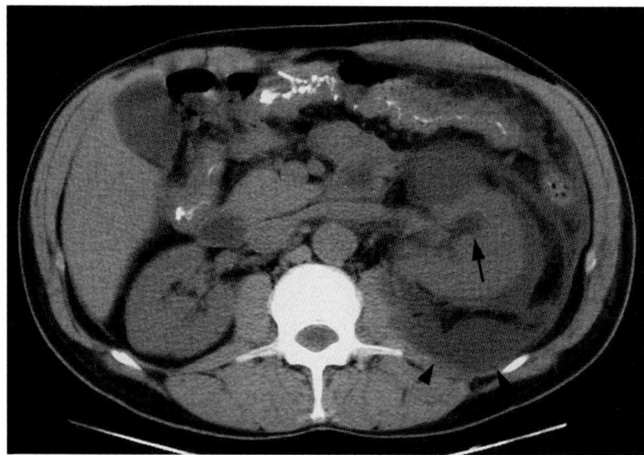

Figure 5. CT scan shows a dilated left renal collecting system (arrow) and a urinoma surrounding the left kidney (arrowhead).

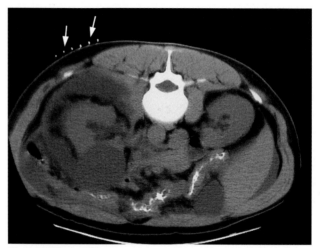

Figure 6. Prone CT scan with a marking grid in place (arrows).

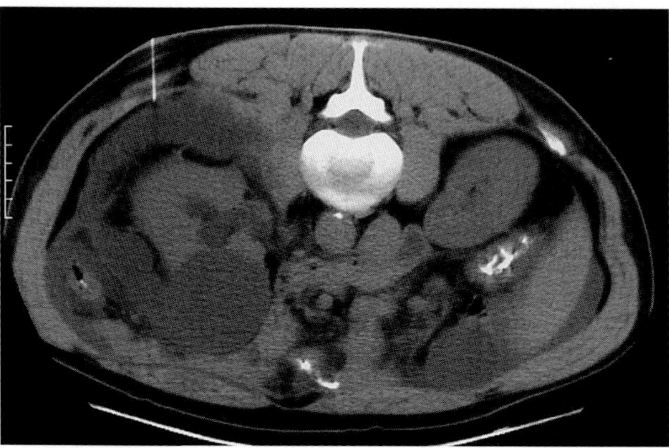

Figure 7. Prone CT slice through the needle used to administer local anesthesia.

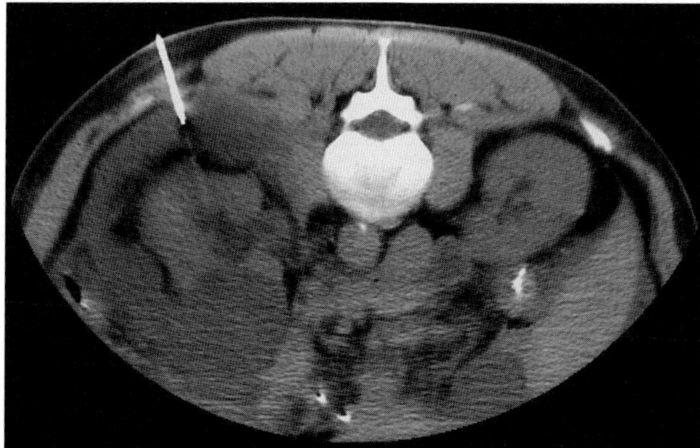

Figure 8. Prone CT scan with the all-purpose drain inserted using trocar technique.

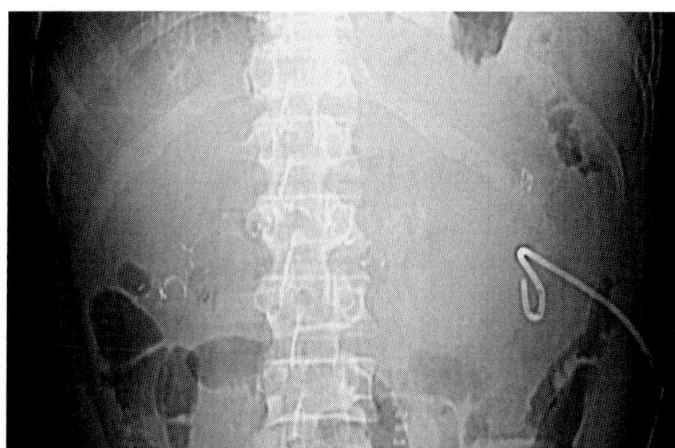

Figure 9. Supine orientation CT scout scan with the all-purpose drain deployed in the left flank.

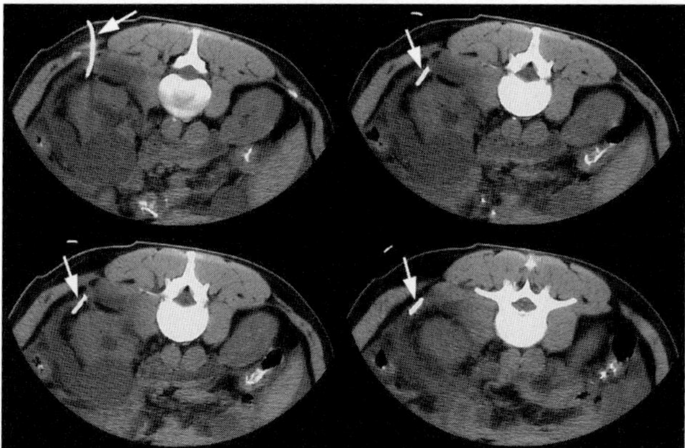

Figure 10. Prone CT scan through the urinoma with the all-purpose drain (arrows) in place.

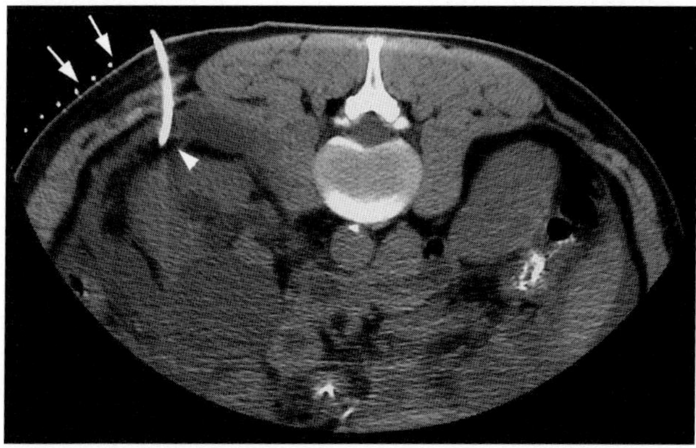

Figure 11. Prone CT scan with the marking grid (arrows) in place. Note the all-purpose drain (arrowhead).

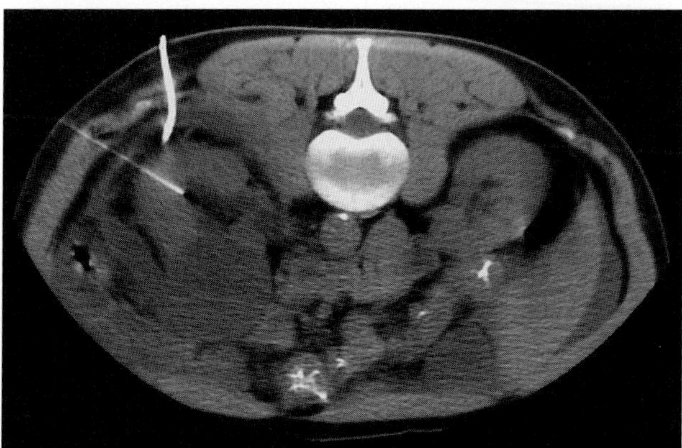

Figure 12. Prone CT scan with a 22-gauge needle in the renal calyx.

An all-purpose drain was placed with use of trocar technique **(Fig. 8)**. The catheter was placed over a trocar into the edge of the urinoma. The trocar was then removed. The position of the catheter was verified by aspirating urine. Once it was confirmed that the catheter tip was in the urine collection, the trocar was partially replaced (with the utmost care to ensure the trocar did not perforate or lacerate the catheter), and the catheter was fed off of the trocar into the fluid collection. A scout CT image and several CT slices through the region of the drain were obtained **(Figs. 9, 10)**. The catheter was sutured in place and connected to a drainage bag.

The skin grid was replaced and a CT slice was made through the kidney **(Fig. 11)**. The angle and depth from the skin marker to a renal calyx were measured from the CT monitor. A 22-gauge needle was inserted into the collecting system and urine aspirated. A small amount of air was injected to serve as contrast material. A CT slice through the needle was obtained **(Fig. 12)**.

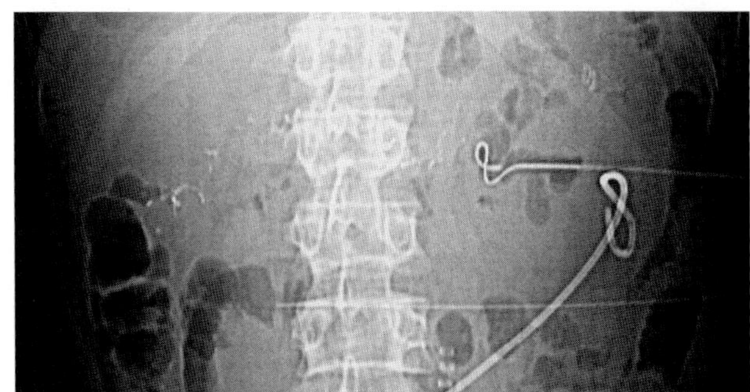

Figure 13. Supine orientation CT scout scan with an 0.018-inch wire in the left collecting system.

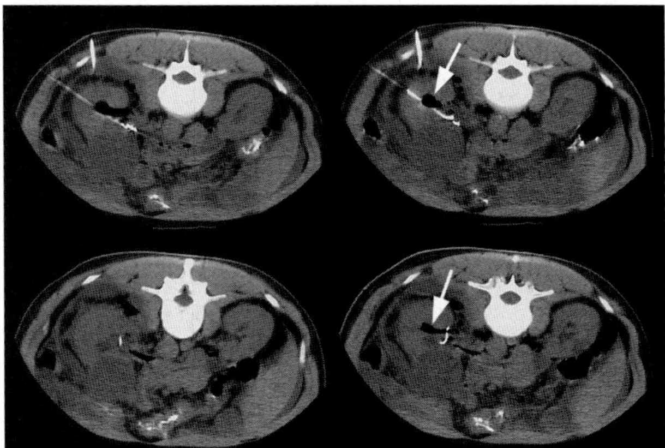

Figure 14. Prone CT scans through an 0.018-inch wire. Note the air introduced into the renal collecting system as contrast material (arrows).

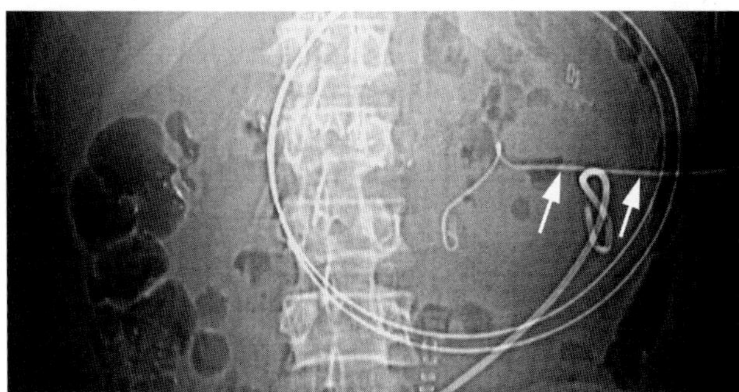

Figure 15. Supine orientation CT scout scan confirms that the sheath (arrows) and the 0.035-inch wire are in the left collecting system.

An 0.018-inch guide wire was advanced into the renal collecting system. A scout CT scan was obtained **(Fig. 13)**, and several CT slices were also made to confirm that the wire was within the collecting system **(Fig. 14)**. A measurement was obtained from these slices to determine the depth for subsequent placement of the sheath dilator.

The sheath dilator was placed over the 0.018-inch guide wire, and the dilator and 0.018-inch wire were removed. A floppy-tipped 0.035-inch guide wire was then advanced through the sheath. A CT scout scan and several CT slices were obtained to ensure that the wire remained within the collecting system **(Fig. 15)**. The nephrostomy tube was then advanced over the 0.035-inch guide wire, and another CT scout scan was obtained **(Fig. 16)**.

The catheter was then locked by pulling the drawstring and suturing the catheter to the skin. The patient was transferred to a fluoroscopy room, where a nephrostogram was obtained **(Fig. 17)**. This demonstrated narrowing and irregularity in the mid ureter and complete obstruction to the distal ureter.

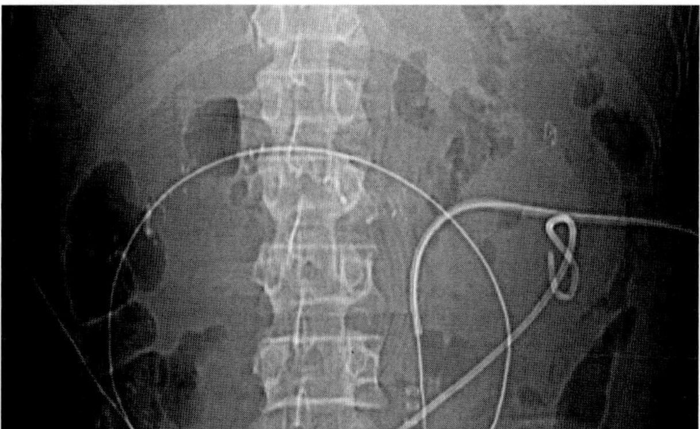

Figure 16. Supine orientation CT scout scan confirms the position of the nephrostomy catheter in the proximal ureter.

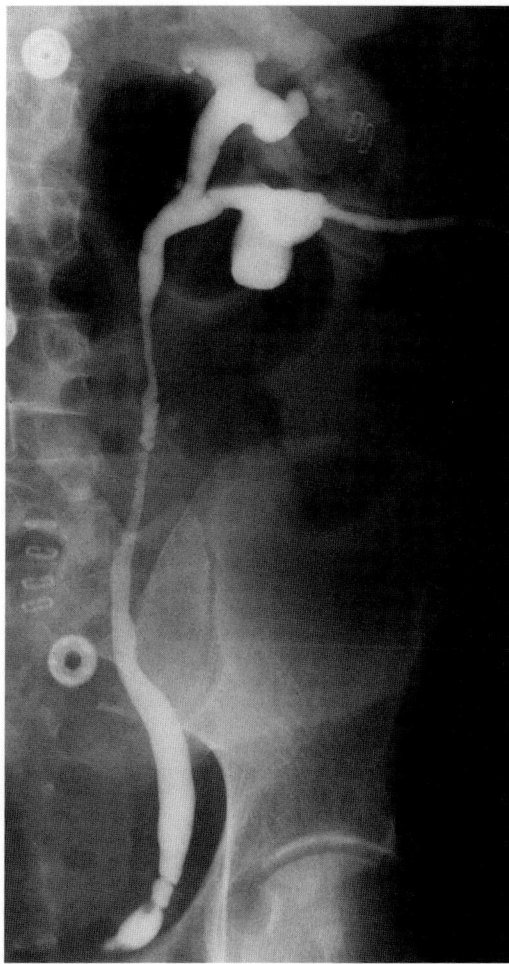

Figure 17. Follow-up supine nephrostogram shows good catheter position.

Discussion

This case demonstrates the management of a completely obstructed urinary system by extrinsic tumor with leakage of urine, probably from a ruptured renal calyx. It also demonstrates CT-guided external drainage of a nondistended urinary system. Additional modalities that can be used for drainage of a nondilated urinary system include ultrasound, fluoroscopy, and endoscopy.

Urine in the retroperitoneum causes lipolysis of the retroperitoneal fat, with a resultant fibrotic reaction. This can progress to cause a ureteral stricture and complete occlusion of the ureter with subsequent loss of function in the affected kidney. Urinomas should be drained either percutaneously or surgically and the cause of the urine leak addressed. Most urinomas form secondary to ureteral obstruction with subsequent rupture of a calyceal fornix. Often, as in this case, once the urinary system is decompressed and the urinoma aspirated, the urothelium will heal and spontaneously seal the forniceal tear.

Urinomas also form as the result of urinary tract trauma. Usually for a ureteral transection a stent can be placed, either percutaneously from the kidney in an antegrade fashion or endoscopically in a retrograde direction, resulting in adequate healing. Urinomas caused by direct renal trauma often need to be treated surgically. Urinomas that result from renal transplantation are often treated with catheter drainage with or without percutaneous drainage and stent placement. Most urinary drainage procedures are performed under fluoroscopic guidance. The nondilated renal collecting system presents greater technical difficulty. In this case, CT guidance was used because simultaneous percutaneous nephrostomy (in a minimally dilated system) and urinoma drainage were desired.

Selected Readings

Clayman RV, Kavoussi LR. Endosurgical techniques for the diagnosis and treatment of noncalculous disease of the ureter and kidney. In: Walsh PS, Vaughan ED, eds. Campbell's urology. 6th edition. Philadelphia: W.B. Saunders Company, 1992.

Coleman CC. Antegrade pyelography and percutaneous nephrostomy. In: Kadir S, ed. Current practice of interventional radiology. St. Louis: Mosby Year Book, 1991.

Lang EK, Glorioso L. Management of urinomas by percutaneous drainage procedures. Radiol Clin North Am 1986; 24:551–559.

Yoder IC, Papanicolaou N, Pfister RC. Percutaneous approach to the renal transplant. In: Kadir S, ed. Current practice of interventional radiology. St. Louis: Mosby Year Book, 1991.

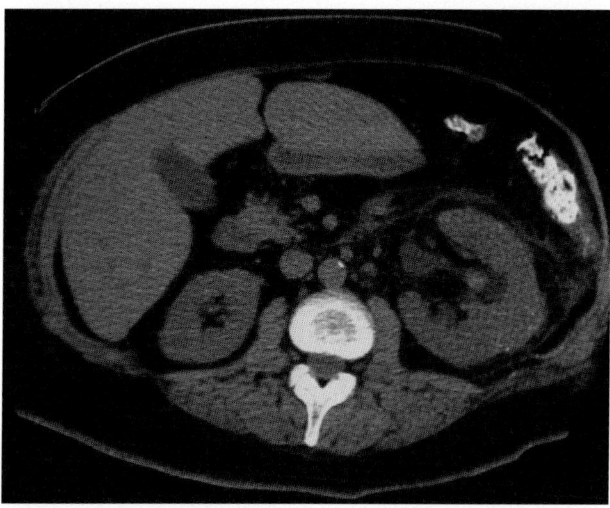

Figure 1. Supine noncontrast CT scan through the interpolar region of the left kidney.

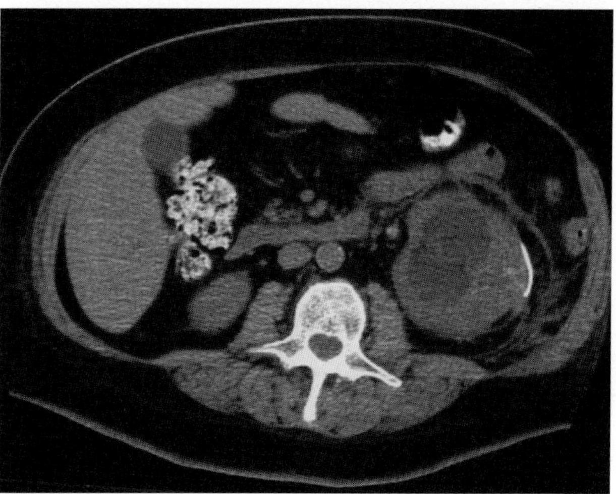

Figure 2. Noncontrast CT scan through the lower pole of the left kidney.

TEACHING FILE CASE 34

Allen J. Meglin, M.D., Paul R. Cazier, M.D., and Charles E. Swallow, M.D.

History

A 58-year-old woman was sent from an outside institution with sepsis and pyonephrosis following an unsuccessful attempt at percutaneous drainage of a partially obstructed left lower pole renal collecting system. A noncontrast computed tomography (CT) scan of the left kidney and perinephric tissues was obtained **(Figs. 1, 2)**.

What is your diagnosis?

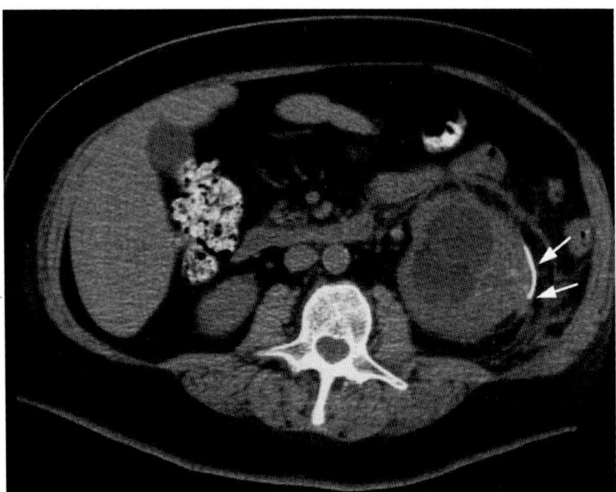

Figure 3. Noncontrast CT scan shows a retained wire fragment (arrows).

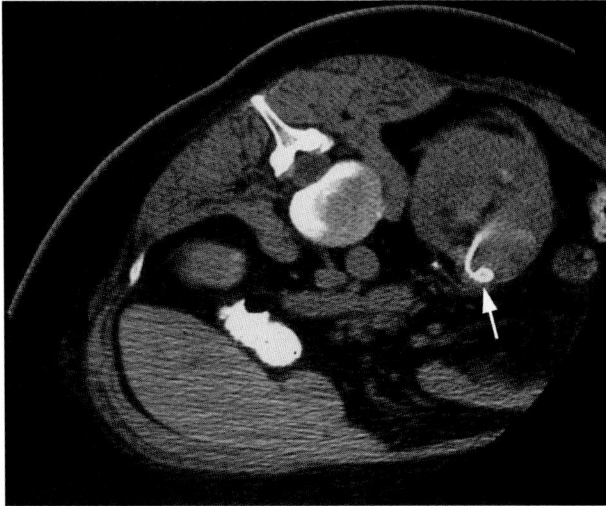

Figure 4. Prone noncontrast CT scan shows a wire coiled anteriorly in the renal parenchyma instead of the collecting system (arrow) during the initial percutaneous nephrostomy drainage.

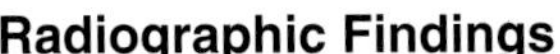

Radiographic Findings

The CT scan shows a metallic density adjacent to but not in the left kidney **(Fig. 3)**. Apparently, a short segment of 0.035-inch metallic guide wire was inadvertently sheared off during the previous attempt at CT-guided renal drainage **(Figs. 4–6)**. The retained foreign body is located outside the renal capsule but inside Gerota's fascia. The CT scan of the initial drainage procedure shows that the nephrostomy tube was not in the collecting system at the time of the initial drainage, and it is likely that attempts to reposition the tube resulted in wire fracture **(Fig. 7)**. The sheared segment of wire was withdrawn out of the kidney when the malpositioned tube was removed. The wire did not come all the way out of the patient, but was trapped by Gerota's fascia. Inflammatory changes suggesting infection can be seen in the perinephric space on a subsequent CT scan, and the heterogeneous area of low attenuation in the lower pole of the left kidney represents focal pyelonephritis **(Fig. 8)**.

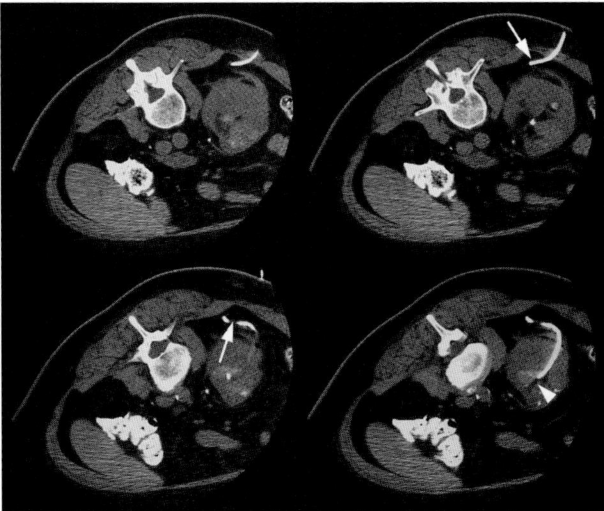

Figure 5. Prone noncontrast CT scan shows a catheter coiled outside the renal parenchyma (arrow) with the tip of the catheter in the renal parenchyma (arrowhead).

A ureteral stent was subsequently placed endoscopically from the urinary bladder into the upper pole of the left kidney. The lower pole collecting system remained filled with pus as it was partially obstructed by a poorly visualized calculus **(Figs. 9, 10)**. Imaging from the endoscopic procedure (unavailable) revealed that only a small amount of contrast material could flow past the stone into the infected lower pole.

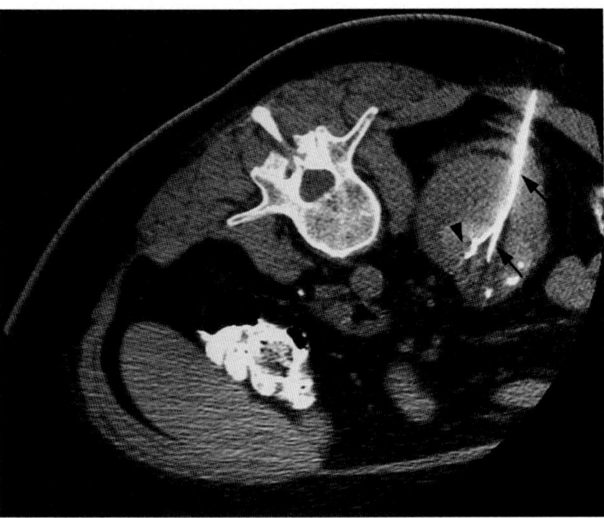

Figure 6. Prone noncontrast CT scan shows a metal stiffening cannula and catheter (arrow) replaced over the wire (arrowhead) in an attempt to reaccess the collecting system.

Diagnoses

1. Focal pyelonephritis of the lower pole of the left kidney with an isolated, obstructed, and infected lower pole collecting system.
2. Retained perinephric foreign body.

What are your management options?

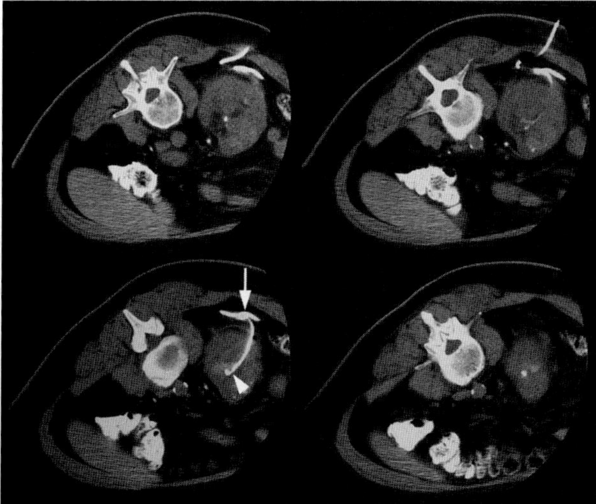

Figure 7. Prone noncontrast CT scan shows a catheter (arrow) and the sheared-off wire segment (arrowhead) still in the renal parenchyma after catheter repositioning.

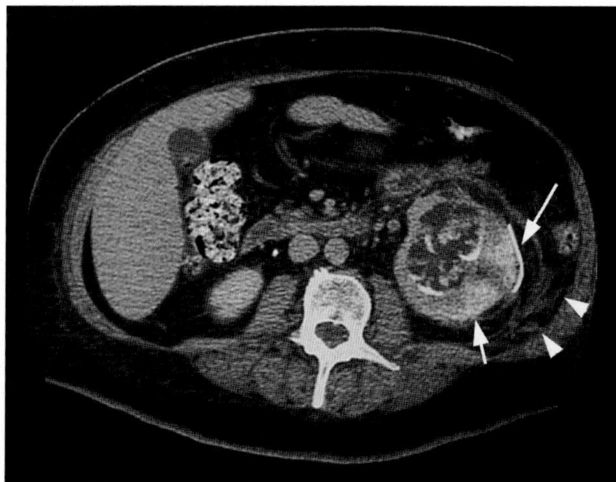

Figure 8. Supine contrast-enhanced CT scan shows the wire segment (long arrow), inflammatory changes (arrowheads), and focal pyelonephritis (short arrow).

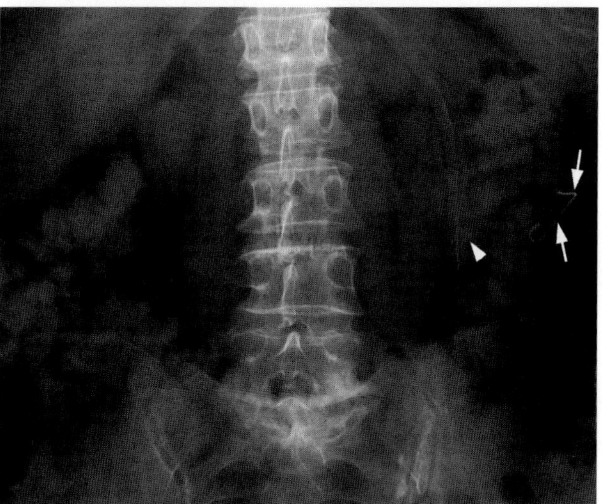

Figure 9. Plain film shows the lower pole (arrowhead) and the retained foreign body (arrows).

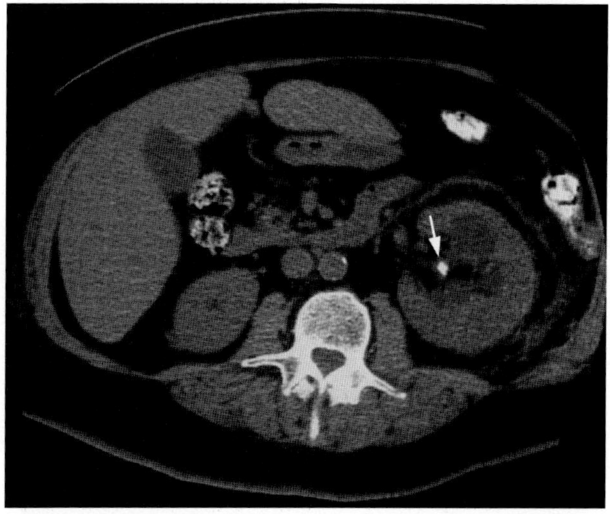

Figure 10. Noncontrast CT scan shows a lower pole collecting system calculus (arrow).

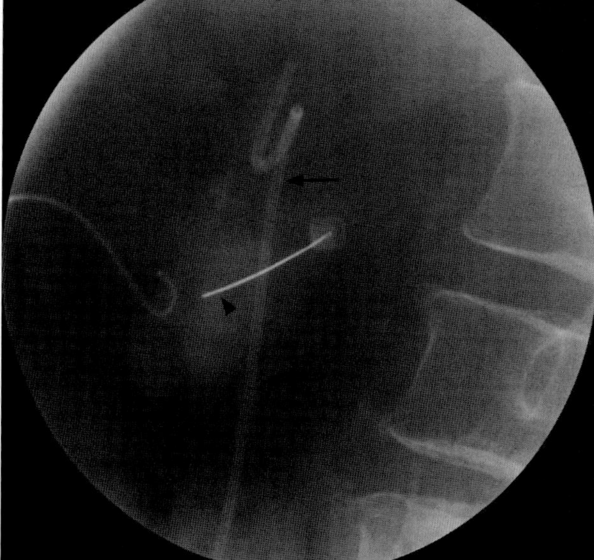

Figure 11. Prone fluoroscopic spot image shows faint opacification of the lower pole, a double-J ureteral stent (arrows), and the retained foreign body. The needle is directed (arrowhead) into the lower pole collecting system for routine PCN.

Management

The infected, partially obstructed lower pole collecting system was decompressed with routine fluoroscopically guided percutaneous nephrostomy (PCN) tube placement **(Fig. 11)**. The lower pole calyx calculus was not removed at the time of initial decompression because it could not be visualized fluoroscopically. It was removed with use of a ureteroscope after the patient had been stabilized.

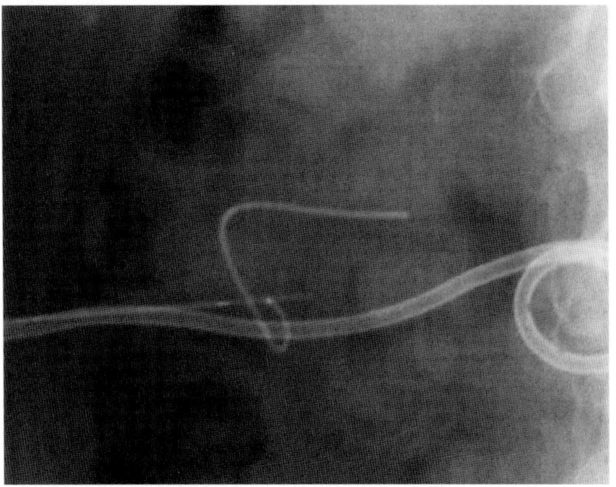

Figure 12. A percutaneous nephrostomy tube has been placed into the isolated lower pole. A Chiba needle has now been placed adjacent to the foreign body.

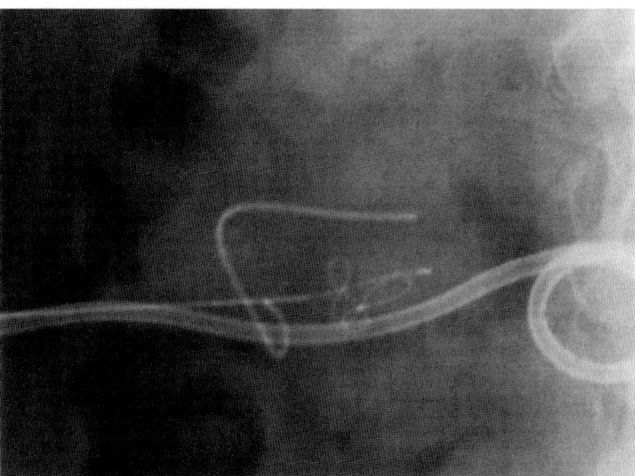

Figure 13. Platinum-tipped wire coiled just past the foreign body.

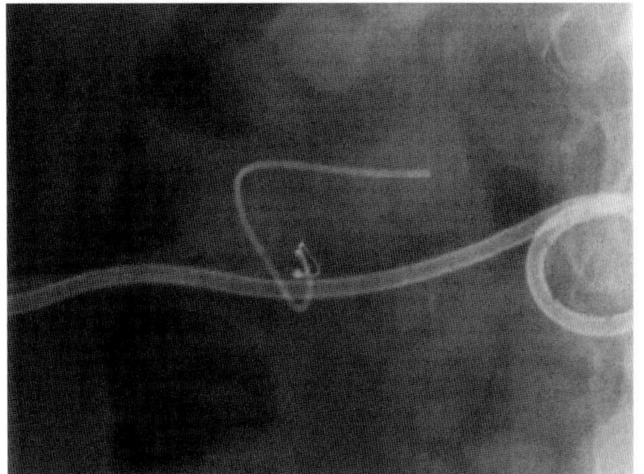

Figure 14. Snare around the foreign body.

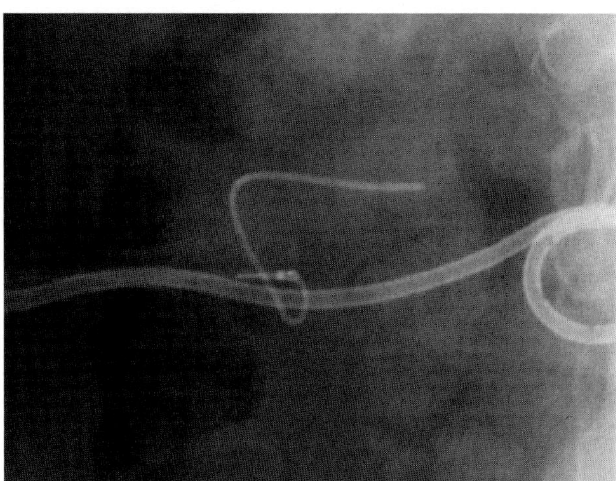

Figure 15. Snare secured around the foreign body.

The wire fragment was assumed to be infected, so percutaneous removal of the foreign body was undertaken immediately after the nephrostomy tube drainage. Through the same skin incision and needle track used for the PCN, a 22-gauge Chiba needle, an 0.018-inch wire, and then a sheath were placed adjacent to the foreign body. The needle tip position was confirmed by touching the wire fragment with the needle tip **(Fig. 12)**. A platinum-tipped wire was then coiled just past the foreign body **(Fig. 13)**. The needle was then exchanged for a sheath. With the sheath positioned just a few millimeters from the wire, a 5-mm snare was placed through the sheath around the foreign body **(Fig. 14)**. Once the foreign body was secured within the snare, the end of the wire was pulled through the 6.3-F sheath and out of the patient **(Figs. 15–19)**.

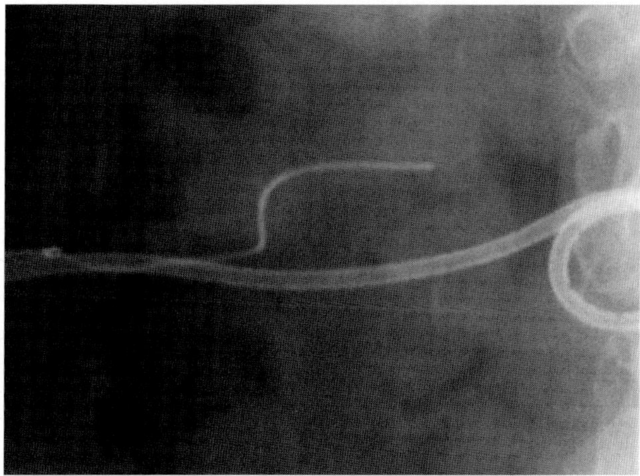

Figure 16. The snare is retracted, pulling the foreign body out through the percutaneous track.

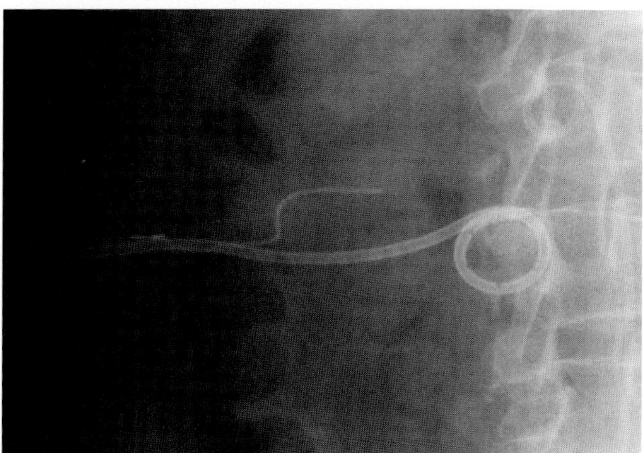

Figure 17. Foreign body exiting the track. The PCN drains the lower pole.

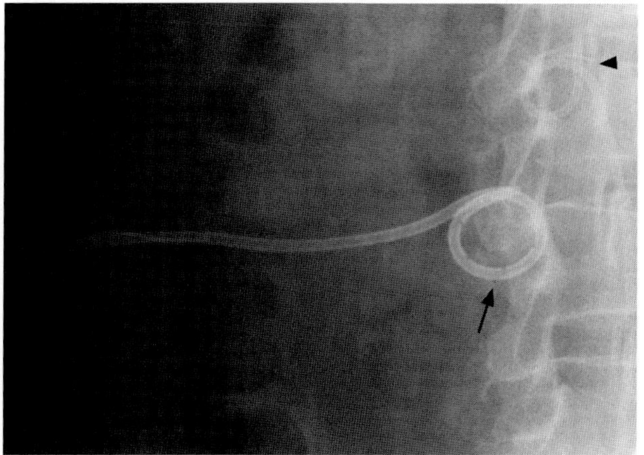

Figure 18. Foreign body removed. PCN in the lower pole (arrow). Ureteral catheter in the upper pole (arrowhead).

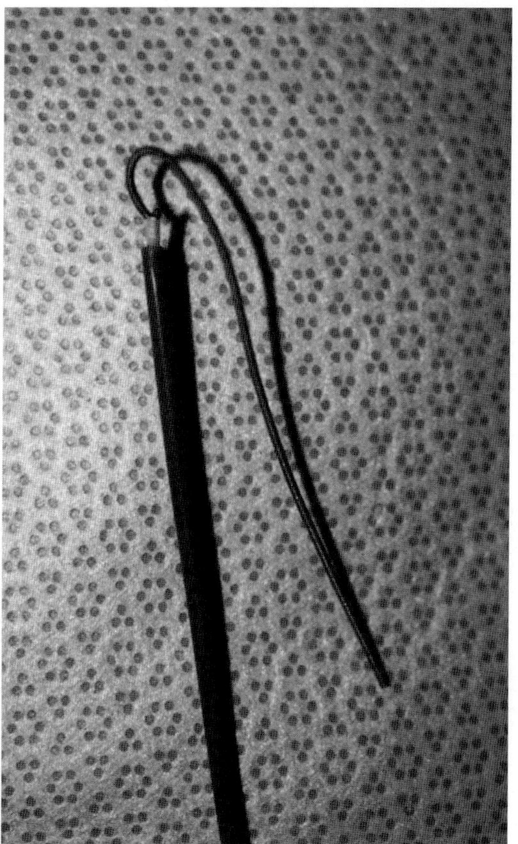

Figure 19. Foreign body in the snare and sheath.

Discussion

Percutaneous nephrostomy for decompression of an obstructed or infected renal pelvis is a standard technique. Percutaneous foreign body removal can be performed with use of many of the same techniques required for percutaneous nephrostomy and stone extraction. As with stone extraction, it is critical to select a safe access site so as to avoid traversing the pleural space, bowel, liver, or spleen. Three-dimensional localization of the object may be facilitated with use of C-arm fluoroscopy, which allows the operator to pass the needle directly down onto the foreign body by passing it parallel to the x-ray beam. After the needle has been advanced onto the target, an over-the-wire exchange for the appropriate sized dilator, sheath, snare, or basket can be made to extract the soft tissue or nonvascular foreign body.

In this case, the wire fragment was considered an infected foreign body. Percutaneous drainage of the lower pole pyonephrosis and removal of the foreign body obviated the need for surgical intervention. With a single procedure, all of the early, infectious complications of prior unsuccessful percutaneous nephrostomy were treated. This permitted delayed, elective removal of the partially obstructing lower pole calculus. Early treatment of the serious infectious process was essential to the successful outcome of this case.

Selected Readings

Egglin TK, Dickey KW, Rosenblatt M, Pollak JS. Retrieval of intravascular foreign bodies: experience in 32 cases. AJR 1995; 164:1259–1264.

Kadir S, ed. Current practice of interventional radiology. St. Louis: Mosby Year Book, 1991.

Nazarian GK, Myers TV, Bjarnason H, Stackhouse DJ, Dietz CA, Hunter DW. Applications of the Amplatz snare device during interventional radiologic procedures. AJR 1995; 165:673–678.

Nosher JL, Seigel R. Percutaneous retrieval of nonvascular foreign bodies. Radiology 1993; 187:649–651.

Pollack HM, Banner MP. Percutaneous extraction of upper urinary tract calculi. Urol Radiol 1984; 6(2):124–137.

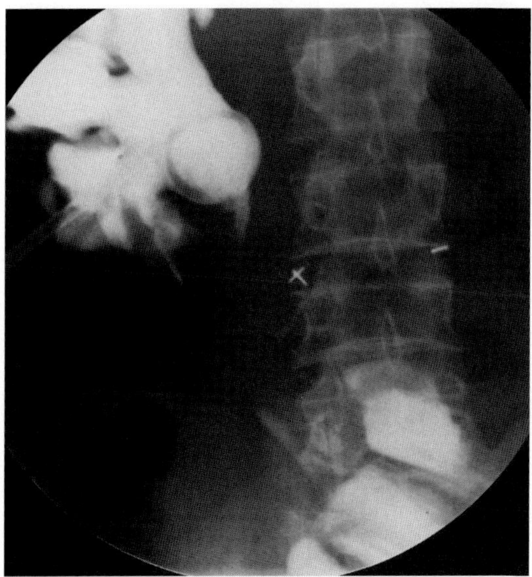

Figure 1. Nephrostogram following injection of contrast material via the nephrostomy catheter.

TEACHING FILE CASE 35

Adam B. Winick, M.D.

History

A 25-year-old man came to the hospital with left flank pain and a complicated past medical history. He had a rhabdomyosarcoma of the bladder at the age of five. He underwent radiation therapy, chemotherapy, and cystoprostatectomy with creation of an ileal loop conduit. Three months prior to this presentation, his ileal conduit was revised for recurrent bouts of infection and stenosis of the left ureteroileal anastomosis. At the time of the revision, the distal half of the left ureter was stenotic with only the proximal 5 cm of the ureter remaining viable. The revision had been performed because the ureteroileal anastomosis had been balloon dilated and a stent placed at another institution with unsatisfactory clinical results.

During this admission, a left percutaneous nephrostomy catheter was placed and injection of the catheter was performed **(Fig. 1)**.

What is your diagnosis?

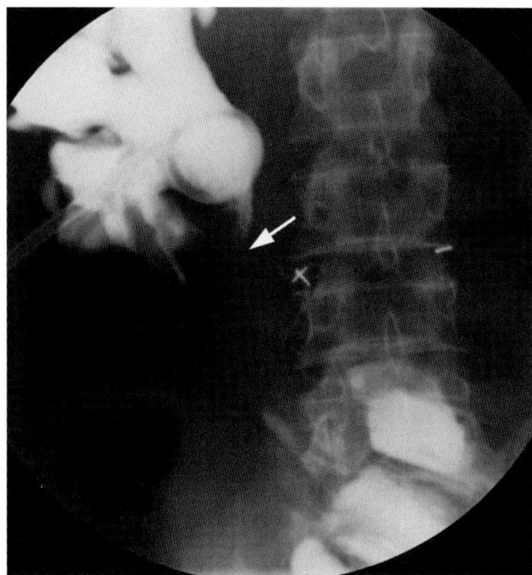

Figure 2. Nephrostogram shows ureteropelvic junction obstruction (arrow).

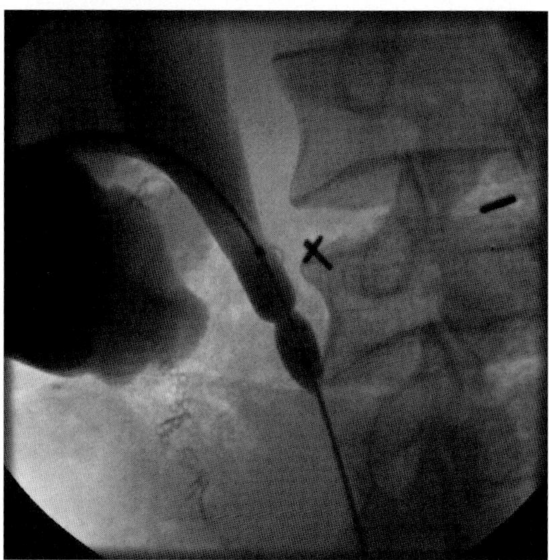

Figure 3. Percutaneously placed balloon catheter across the stenosis. The balloon waist demonstrates the site of ureteral stenosis.

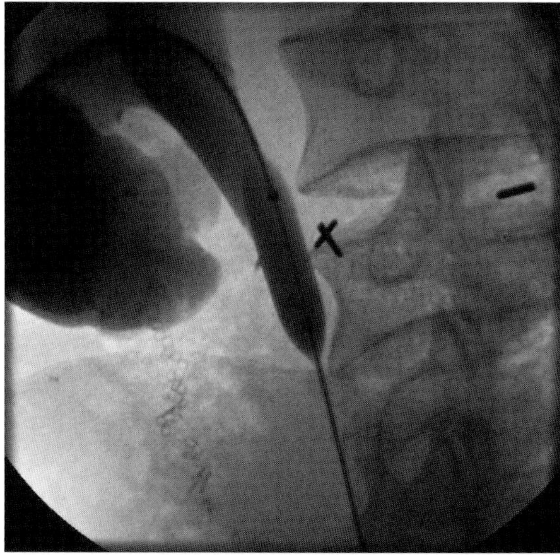

Figure 4. The balloon catheter has been fully expanded, and the waist is now effaced.

Radiographic Findings
Contrast material injection with the patient in the prone position reveals marked hydronephrosis with complete occlusion of the left ureter at the uretero-pelvic junction **(Fig. 2)**.

Diagnosis
Benign postoperative ureteral stricture.

How would you manage this patient?

Management
The stricture was crossed and the patient underwent ureteroplasty with a 6-mm balloon. Effacement of the balloon waist was subsequently noted **(Figs. 3, 4)**. A 12-F nephroureteral stent was placed with the tip coiled in the neobladder **(Fig. 5)**. The stent was left in place for 3 weeks, at which time the patient returned for a Whitaker test **(see Tutorial 20: Urodynamic Measurement: The Whitaker Test)**. An unusually large amount of infusate fluid was necessary during the Whitaker test because of the increased capacity of the collecting system. The pressure gradient from the renal pelvis to the ileal loop conduit exceeded 20 cm H_2O; therefore, the patient failed the Whitaker test. At no point during the test did contrast material flow distally into the neobladder.

The stricture was crossed again and ureteroplasty was repeated with an 8-mm balloon. The balloon waist was effaced at 7 atmospheres of pressure. A 14-F nephroureteral stent was placed for long-term stent placement.

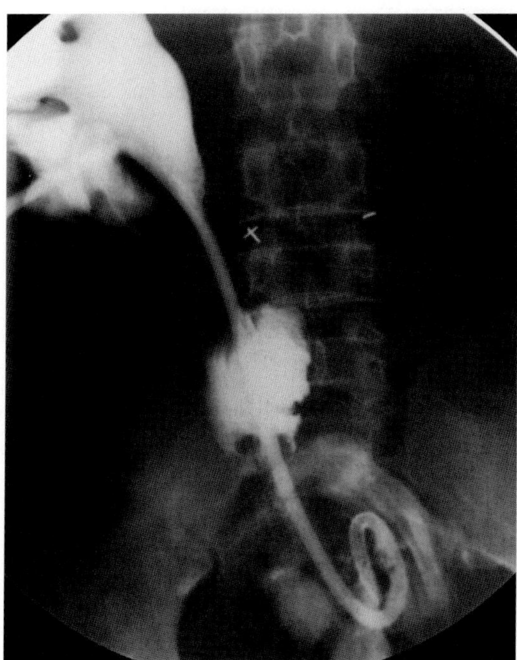

Figure 5. Nephrostogram with the nephroureterostomy catheter in place.

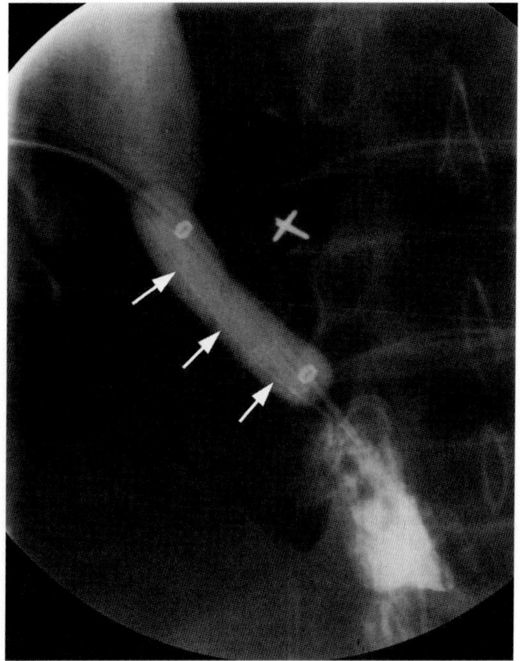

Figure 6. Repeat balloon angioplasty. Arrows show the laterally located electrocautery wire coursing along the angioplasty balloon.

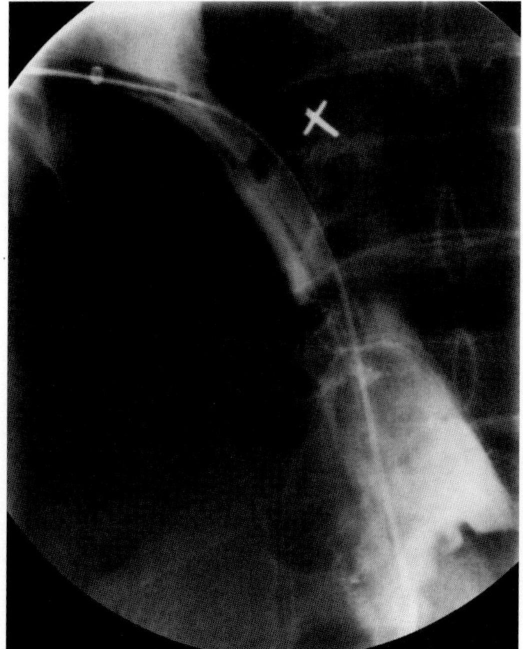

Figure 7. Nephrostogram shows no evidence of urine extravasation at the ureteroplasty site.

The patient returned 8 weeks later for a repeat Whitaker test. The pressure gradient was greater than 20 cm H_2O after infusion of 150 mL of contrast material. Therefore, a percutaneous endopyelotomy was performed with a balloon/cauterizing catheter in a combined procedure with a urologist. The catheter had a standard balloon at the end, with a thin wire alongside the balloon which was connected to a power pack. The wire was placed laterally to avoid incising the inferior vena cava **(Fig. 6)**. Three short bursts of electricity were passed through the wire to incise the ureter in the area of the stricture. Afterwards, the balloon was left inflated for 10 minutes. Injection of contrast material after the balloon was deflated showed a patent ureter with contrast material flowing into the bladder and no extravasation **(Fig. 7)**. The 14-F nephroureteral stent was replaced for further stent placement.

A repeat nephrostogram obtained through the nephroureteral stent 7 weeks after the incision of the ureter showed no extravasation. The stent was exchanged for a regular nephrostomy tube placed above the stricture and capped for a clinical trial of 1 week. The patient developed left flank pain and fever 2 days later, indicating failure of the clinical trial. The ureter then had to be reaccessed, which was very difficult even with an 0.016-inch wire.

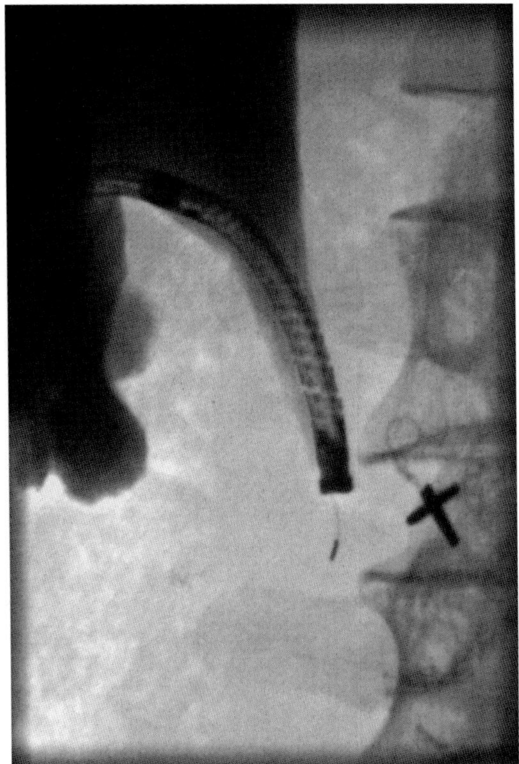

Figure 8. Fluoroscopic spot image shows the nephroscope directed down the ureter.

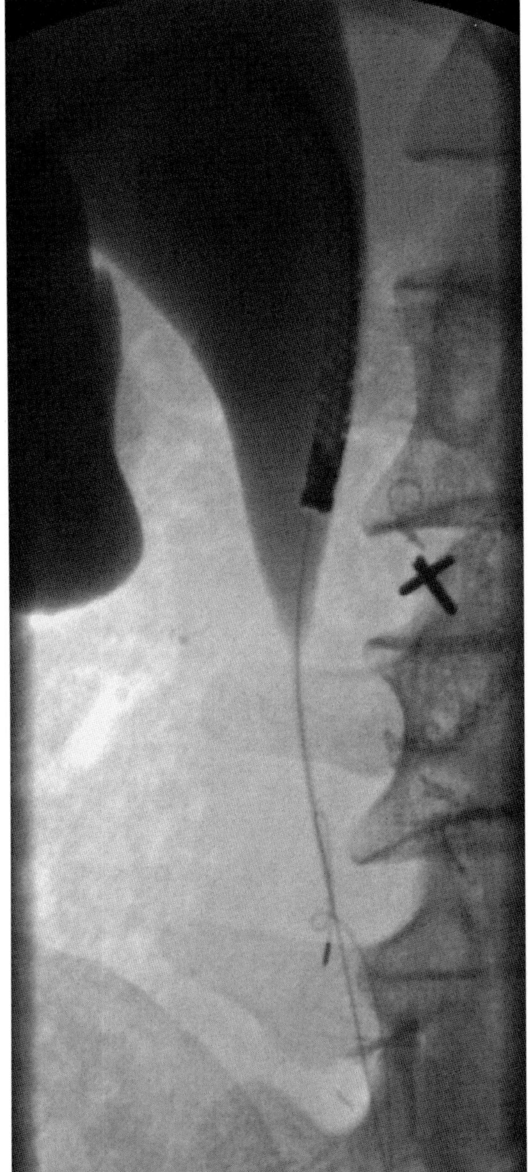

Figure 9. Under nephroscopic guidance, an 0.016-inch wire is passed across the ureteral stricture.

A 9-F ureteroscope was required to find the ureteral orifice in order to cannulate it with an 0.016-inch wire **(Figs. 8, 9)**. Following catheter and guide wire exchanges, an 8-mm x 4-cm high-pressure balloon was used to dilate the stenotic segment of the ureter **(Figs. 10, 11)**. An 8-mm x 2-cm Wallstent (Schneider, Minneapolis, MN) was then deployed across the stenosis **(Figs. 12, 13)**. The distal end of the stent did not cross into the neobladder.

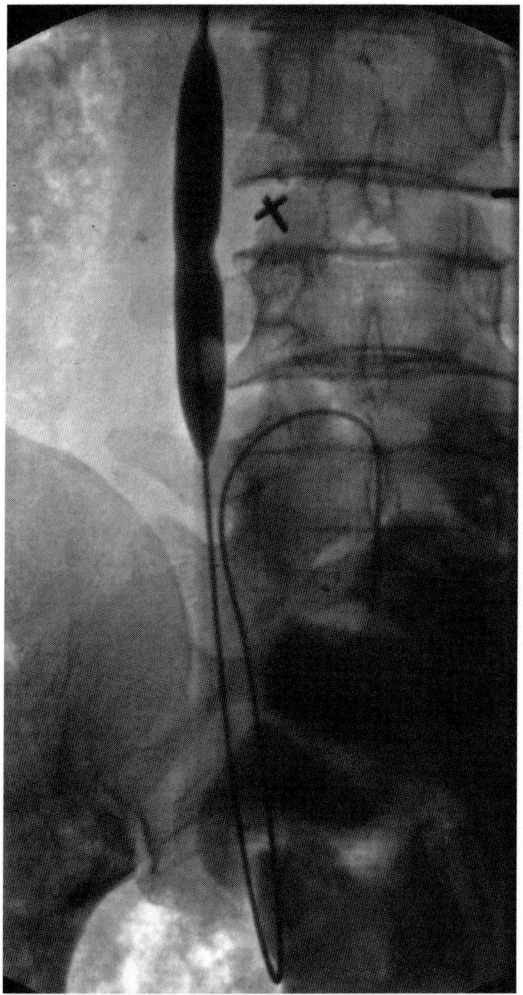

Figure 10. High-pressure angioplasty balloon being used to dilate the ureteral stricture.

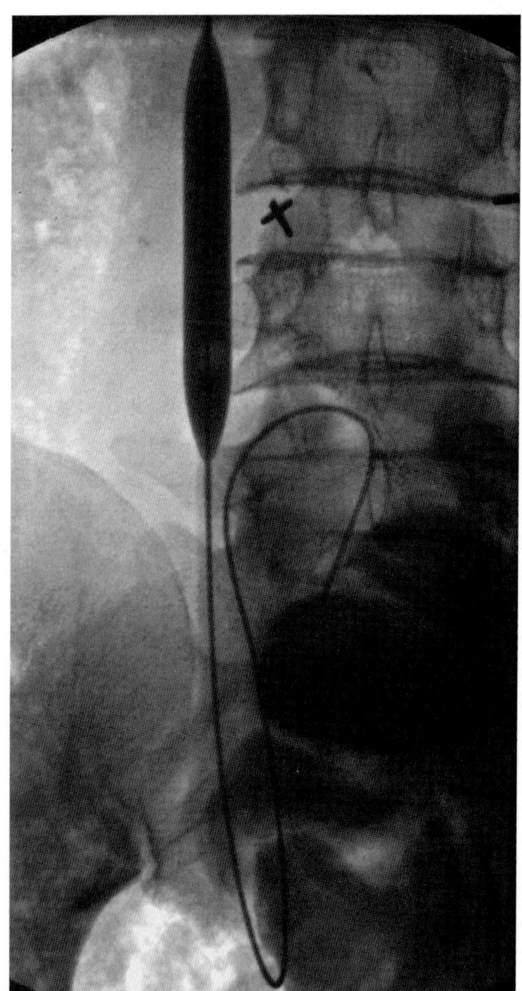

Figure 11. The waist on the angioplasty balloon is effaced, indicating a successful ureteroplasty.

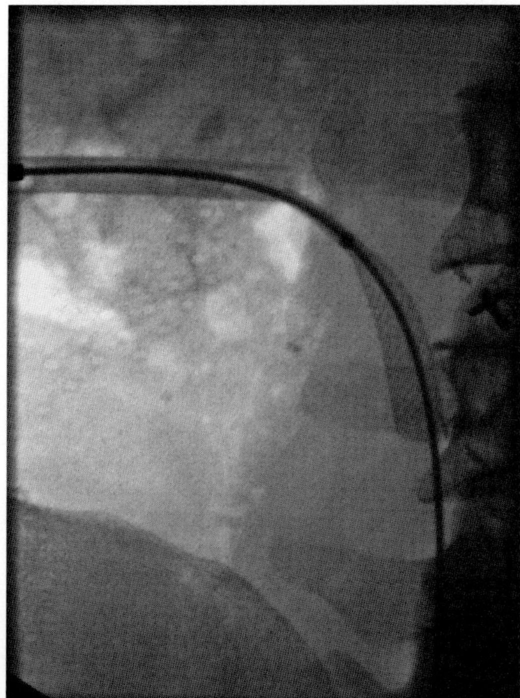

Figure 12. Wallstent being deployed across the ureteral stricture.

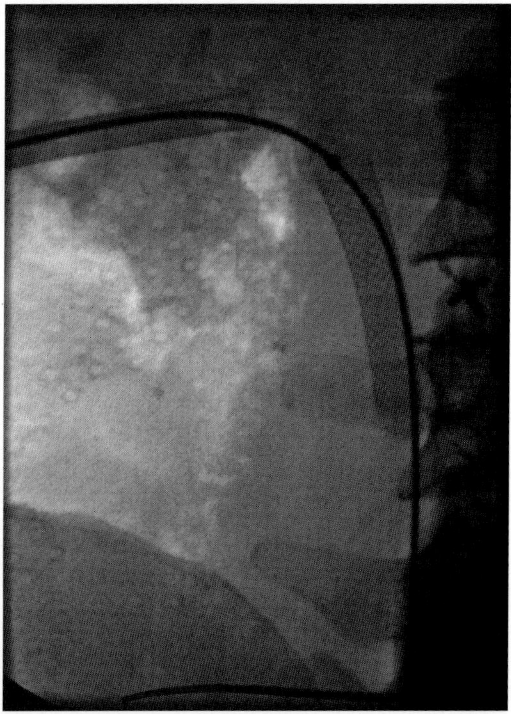

Figure 13. Wallstent fully deployed.

After stent deployment, there was good flow of contrast material into the neobladder **(Fig. 14)**. The nephrostomy tube was replaced and capped. Unfortunately, the patient returned 5 days later with flank pain and fever. A nephrostogram revealed complete occlusion of the ureteral Wallstent. The patient required a nephrectomy because of the continued difficulty with the ureteral stricture. At pathologic examination, no tumor was seen.

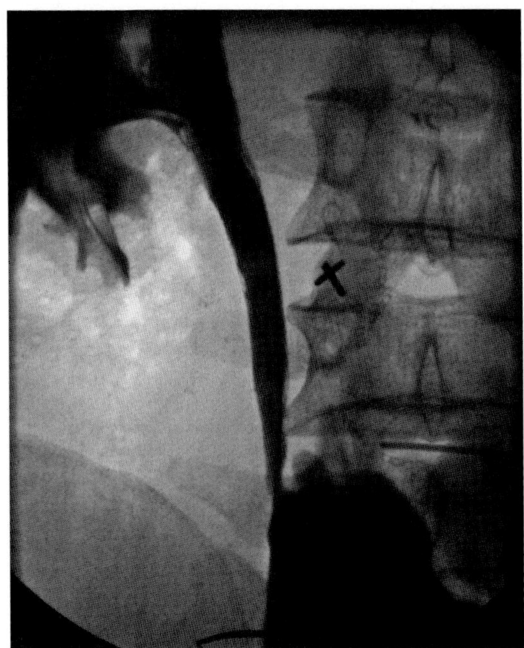

Figure 14. Nephrostogram shows a widely patent ureter and the Wallstent.

Discussion

Benign strictures of the ureter may result from multiple etiologies including postoperative changes related to ischemia, radiation therapy, endourologic manipulation, inflammatory conditions such as tuberculosis, or periureteral fibrosis from retroperitoneal fibrosis. It can be difficult to maintain patency of a surgically created ureteroenteric anastomosis if a stricture develops. Long-term results following dilation of ureteral strictures have not yielded high 1-year success rates. For example, only a 16% 1-year patency rate was found by Shapiro et al, and 70% of the patients studied developed recurrent strictures within 6 months.

The use of metallic stents has not been shown to aid in maintaining patency following ureteral dilation. Stent placement was performed in this case as a last resort to try to salvage the otherwise functional kidney. In a study by Pollak et al, only one ureteral stent out of six (17%) was patent at 11-month follow-up. The other five stents had occluded between 1 and 11 months. On pathologic evaluation of the stents, the occlusions were due to ingrowth of hyperplastic uroepithelium and granulation tissue. Although the size of this series is small, the low patency rates are problematic.

The use of electroincision combined with balloon dilation may be the treatment of choice in the future, following further study with larger numbers of patients. Kramolowsky et al report a success rate of 71% in seven strictures, with an average follow-up of 16 months. Cornud et al have a 66% success rate, with a 6-month follow-up.

The current consensus recommendation is to avoid placing ureteric metallic stents for benign disease. If a stricture is resistant to balloon dilation with catheter placement to prevent fibrosis, the next step is either surgical revision or surgery and prolonged catheter stent placement with repeat dilations as necessary. Electroincision of ureteral strictures may be the best option in the future, but further investigation is warranted before the procedure becomes accepted for widespread applications.

Selected Readings

Beckman CF, Roth RA, Bihrle W III. Dilatation of benign ureteral strictures. Radiology 1989: 172:437–441.

Cornud F, Mendelsberg M, Chretien Y, et al. Fluoroscopically guided percutaneous transrenal electroincision of uretero-intestinal anastomotic strictures. J Urol 1992; 147:578–581.

Kramolowsky EV, Clayman RV, Weyman PJ. Management of ureterointestinal anastomotic strictures: comparison of open surgical and endourological repair. J Urol 1988; 139:1195–1198.

Kwak S, Leef JA, Rosenblum JD. Percutaneous balloon catheter dilatation of benign ureteral strictures: effect of multiple dilatation procedures on long-term patency. AJR 1995; 165:97–100.

Pollak JS, Rosenblatt MM, Egglin TK, Dickey KW, Glickman M. Treatment of ureteral obstructions with the Wallstent endoprosthesis: preliminary results. J Vasc Interv Radiol 1995; 6:417–425.

Shapiro MJ, Banner MP, Amendola MA, Gordon RL, Pollak HM, Wein AJ. Balloon catheter dilation of ureteroenteric strictures: long-term results. Radiology 1988: 168:385–387.

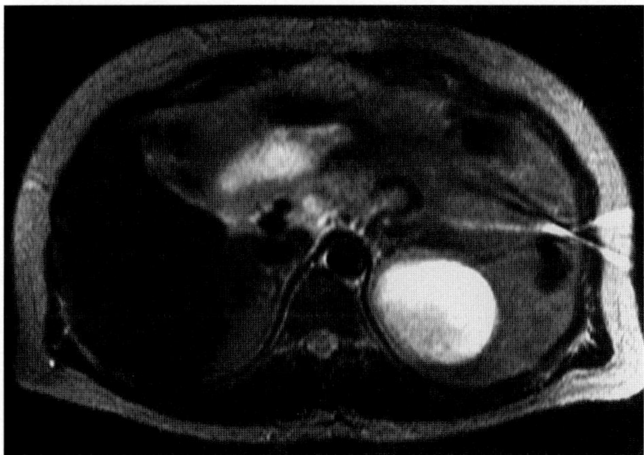

Figure 1. T2-weighted MR image through the upper pole of the left kidney.

TEACHING FILE CASE 36

Mark L. Lukens, M.D.

History

A 39-year-old man came to the hospital with a 3-month history of left flank pain. Physical examination suggested a musculoskeletal origin for the flank pain. Urine and serologic analyses were normal. Magnetic resonance (MR) imaging of the abdomen was performed to evaluate the paraspinal muscles **(Fig. 1)**.

What is your diagnosis?

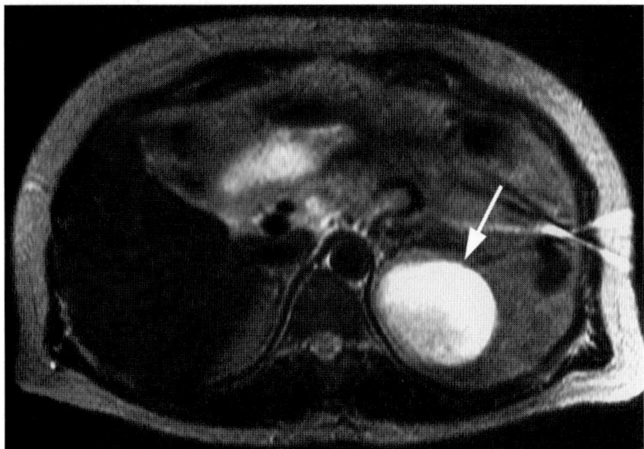

Figure 2. T2-weighted MR image shows a rounded hyperintense structure arising from the upper pole of the left kidney (arrow).

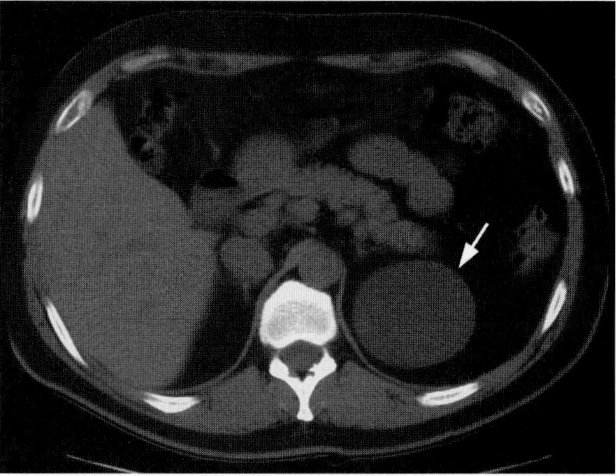

Figure 3. Noncontrast CT scan of the abdomen shows a rounded, low-density structure arising from the upper pole of the left kidney consistent with a simple cyst (arrow). Hounsfield measurements (not shown) within the collection were 15, consistent with fluid.

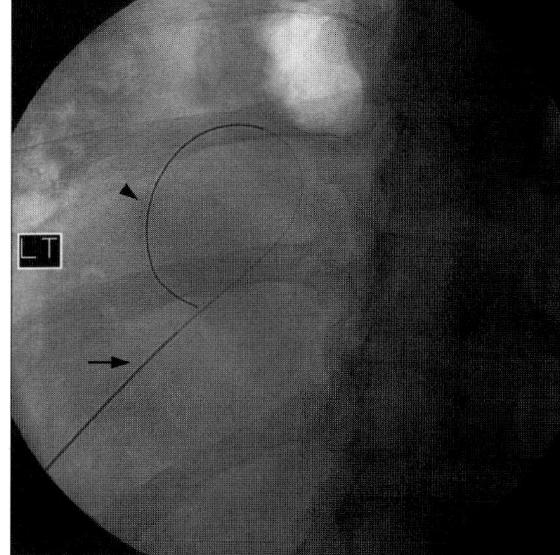

Figure 4. Digital spot radiograph shows a 21-gauge needle (arrow) placed within the cyst and an 0.018-inch wire (arrowhead) coiled within the cyst cavity.

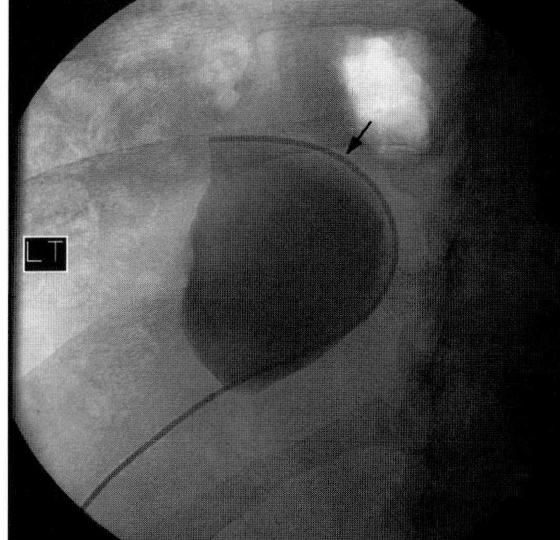

Figure 5. 6-F dilator system (arrow) within the cyst, with a small amount of contrast material injected into the cyst.

Radiographic Findings

The MR image showed no musculoskeletal abnormality, but a large, rounded fluid collection arising from the upper pole of the left kidney was identified **(Fig. 2)**.

Diagnosis

Large simple cyst within the upper pole of the left kidney.

Management

Following MR imaging, an abdominal spiral computed tomography (CT) scan was obtained which confirmed the findings in the left kidney **(Fig. 3)**. Given the patient's history of left flank pain, palliative cyst puncture and drainage were performed. Under sonographic guidance, a 21-gauge needle, an 0.018-inch guide wire, and a 6-F dilator system were placed into the cyst and their positions confirmed fluoroscopically **(Figs. 4, 5)**. Thirty-five mL of straw-colored fluid was withdrawn from the cyst and sent for cytology and laboratory evaluation.

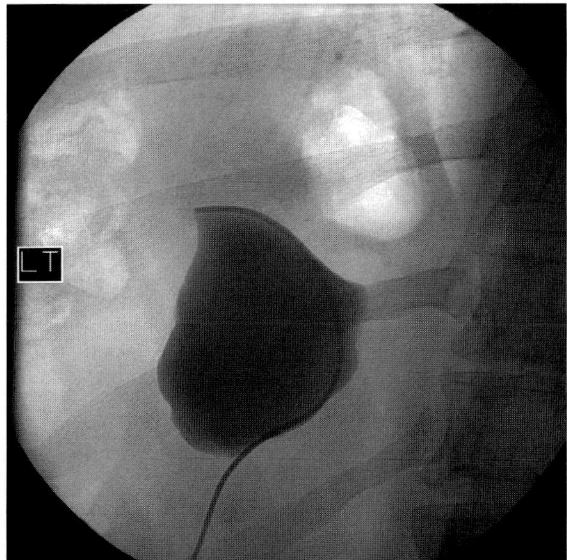

Figure 6. Cystogram with full-strength contrast material shows smooth walls and no communication with the collecting system.

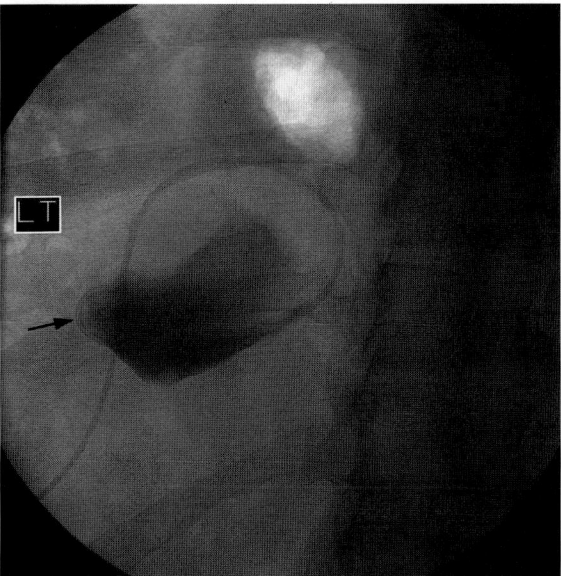

Figure 7. 6-F pigtail catheter within the cyst during aspiration (arrow).

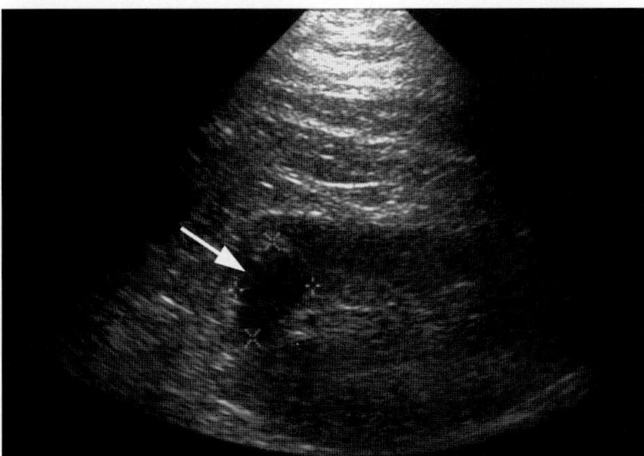

Figure 8. Sonogram shows the small 1.5-cm x 1-cm residual cyst cavity (arrow).

Contrast material was injected to delineate the walls of the cyst cavity **(Fig. 6)**. A 6-F pigtail catheter was placed to ensure complete evacuation of the cyst cavity **(Fig. 7)**. Sclerotherapy of the cyst was declined by both the patient and the referring clinician. The flank pain resolved quickly after the cyst drainage. Follow-up sonography the next day showed only a small residual cyst **(Fig. 8)**. The patient remained asymptomatic at 1-year follow-up.

Discussion

With the advent of sonography and CT scanning as noninvasive techniques for diagnosing renal cysts, percutaneous renal cyst puncture is rarely used as a diagnostic modality. CT scanning and sonography can diagnose benign cysts with a high degree of accuracy. The current diagnostic indications for renal cyst puncture include evaluation of an indeterminate mass, inconclusive or conflicting sonographic and CT findings, and unexplained hematuria or fever with an apparent simple cyst. Therapeutic cyst puncture is performed to relieve obstruction of the renal collecting system, in cases of renin-dependent hypertension and nonspecific abdominal pain.

Access to the cyst can be guided by sonography, CT, or fluoroscopy. Following drainage, the fluid is sent for laboratory studies to include cytology, culture, and analysis of lactate dehydrogenase, protein, and fat content. Elevated fat content is characteristic of neoplasm, and increased protein may be due to tumor or inflammation. Contrast material and air can then be injected to delineate the cyst wall. Smooth, round contours are consistent with a simple cyst, and nodular or irregular walls raise the suspicion of a neoplasm or a mass of inflammatory nature. Therapeutic cyst puncture can be followed by sclerosis, because the cyst recurs after simple aspiration in 30%–78% percent of cases.

Sclerosis is performed following placement of a pigtail catheter into the cyst. Once the cyst fluid has been aspirated, absolute ethanol (approximately 25% of the cyst volume) is instilled. The patient is placed in the prone, supine, and both decubitus positions for 5 minutes each, after which the ethanol and catheter are removed. Major complications are rare (1.4%) but include perirenal hemorrhage, pneumothorax, arteriovenous fistula, infection, urinoma, and bowel injury. Minor complications (10%) include hematuria, fever, pain, and contrast material extravasation. Sclerosis, although used infrequently, can be diagnostic, palliative, and therapeutic, thereby sparing the patient an open surgical procedure.

Selected Readings

Bean WJ. Renal cysts: treatment with alcohol. Radiology 1981; 138:329–331.

Bosniak MA. The current radiological approach to renal cysts. Radiology 1986; 158:1–10.

Lang EK. Renal cyst puncture and aspiration: a survey of complications. AJR 1977; 128:723–727.

Lang EK, Johnson B, Chance HL, et al. Assessment of avascular renal mass lesions: the use of nephrotomography, arteriography, cyst puncture, double contrast study and histochemical and histopathologic examination of the aspirate. South Med J 1972; 65:1–10.

McClennan BL, Stanley RJ, Melson GL, Levitt RG, Sagel SS. CT of the renal cyst: is cyst aspiration necessary? AJR 1979; 133:671–675.

Pollack HM, Banner MP, Arger PH, Peters J, Mulhern CB Jr, Coleman BG. The accuracy of gray-scale renal ultrasonography in differentiating cystic neoplasms from benign cysts. Radiology 1982; 143:741–745.

Sandler CM, Houston GK, Hall JT, Morettin LB. Guided cyst puncture and aspiration. Radiol Clin North Am 1986; 24:527–537.

Stevenson JJ, Sherwood T. Conservative management of renal masses. Br J Urol 1971; 43:646–647.

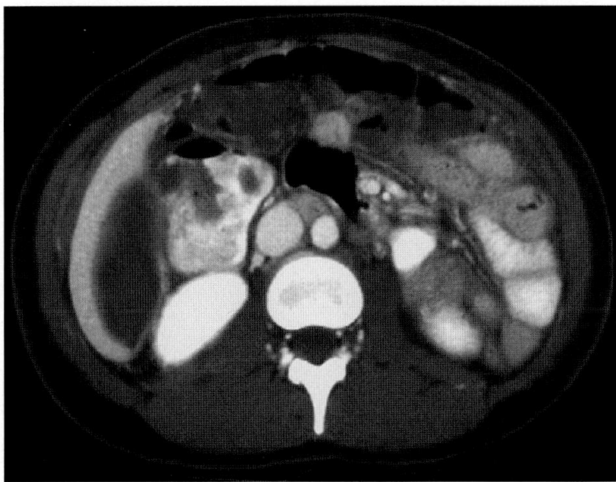

Figure 1. Contrast-enhanced spiral CT scan of the abdomen and pelvis.

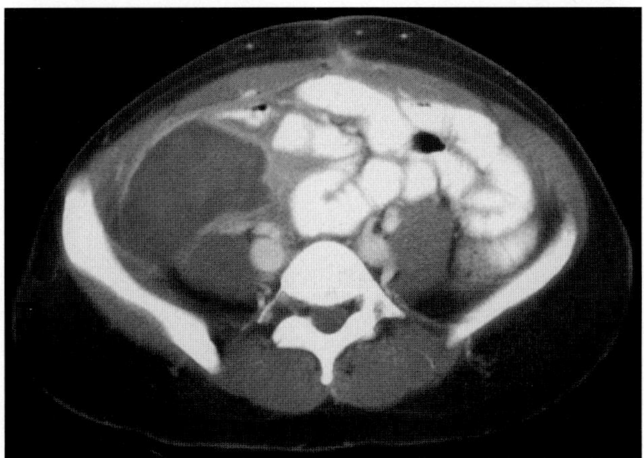

Figure 2. Contrast-enhanced spiral CT scan of the abdomen and pelvis.

TEACHING FILE CASE 37

Mark L. Lukens, M.D., and
Daniel Boyle, M.D.

History

A 30-year-old woman with a history of endometriosis underwent resection of an endometrioma and ileocecectomy with primary ileocolic reanastomosis. Fourteen days after the surgery, she came to the hospital with an elevated white blood cell count of 14,000, a fever of 101 degrees F, and right lower quadrant tenderness. A spiral computed tomography (CT) scan of the abdomen and pelvis was obtained with oral and intravenous contrast material **(Figs. 1, 2)**.

What is your diagnosis?

Radiographic Findings

The CT scan showed a well-defined, low-density collection extending from the inferior margin of the right lobe of the liver to the right iliac fossa **(Fig. 3)**. Regions of increased density are noted within the collection **(Fig. 4)**. The fluid collection extended to the ileocolic anastomotic suture line **(Fig. 5)**.

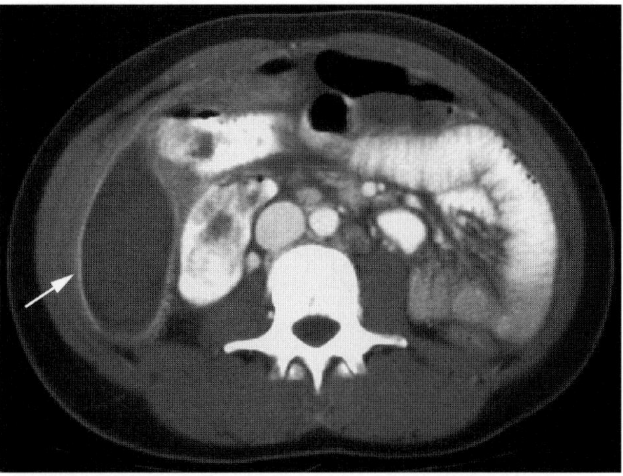

Figure 3. CT image shows a low-density fluid collection along the right paracolic gutter. Note the thickened enhancing ring surrounding the collection (arrow).

Preliminary Diagnosis

Complex fluid collection near the ileocolic anastomosis.

Management

The differential diagnosis includes abscess, postoperative hematoma, seroma, complicated urinoma, lymphocele, and tubo-ovarian abscess. In light of the patient's leukocytosis and fever, an abscess was considered the most likely diagnosis and percutaneous drainage was requested. Intravenous antibiotics were also initiated. Before drainage, a sonogram showed a complex fluid collection with considerable echogenic material **(Fig. 6)**. A 21-gauge needle and an 0.018-inch wire were placed into the fluid collection under sonographic guidance and the wire position was confirmed fluoroscopically **(Figs. 7, 8)**. A 10-F all-purpose drain was placed, and 80 mL of loose thrombus and blood was withdrawn.

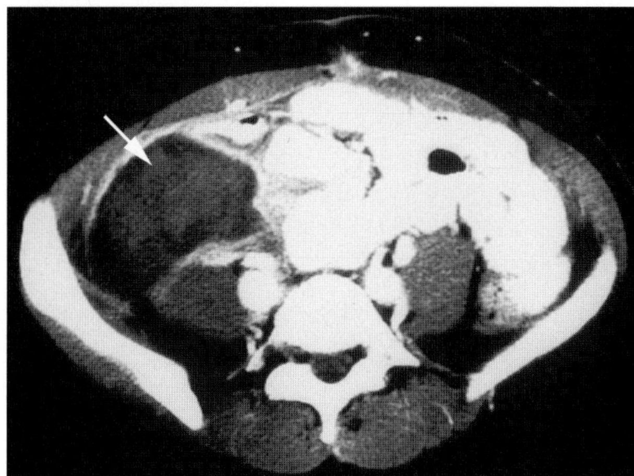

Figure 4. CT image with narrow contrast levels shows increased density within the fluid collection (arrow).

The drainage fluid was sent for laboratory evaluation and subsequent cultures grew *Escherichia coli*. The catheter was attached to a suction grenade for 3 days, during which time a small amount (~20 mL) of dark blood was drained each day. To encourage drainage and resolution of the hematoma, it was decided to instill 250,000 units of urokinase diluted in 40 mL of normal saline into the cavity. Lavage of the cavity was performed in the angiographic suite with two aliquots of 20 mL each. The urokinase was left in the cavity for 20 minutes and vigorous flushing was performed to better distribute the urokinase throughout the collection.

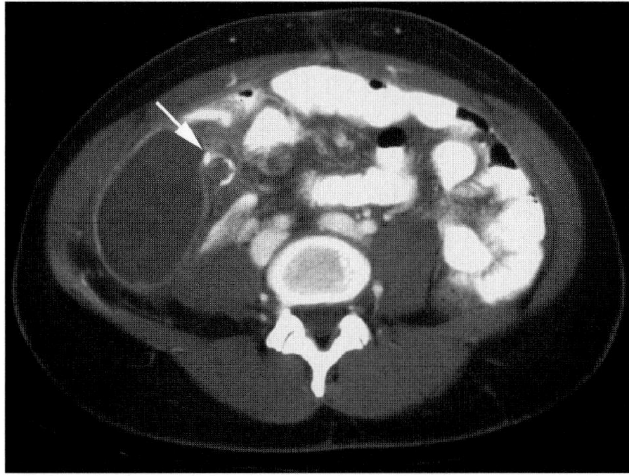

Figure 5. Arrow shows the close relationship of the fluid collection to the anastomotic suture line.

A sinogram performed prior to the urokinase instillation showed irregular internal borders of the cavity **(Fig. 9)**. After urokinase treatment, approximately 80 mL of dark blood and loose thrombus was withdrawn and the borders of the cavity became considerably smoother **(Fig. 10)**. Follow-up CT scanning showed significant resolution of the hematoma with only a minimal residual collection **(Fig. 11)**.

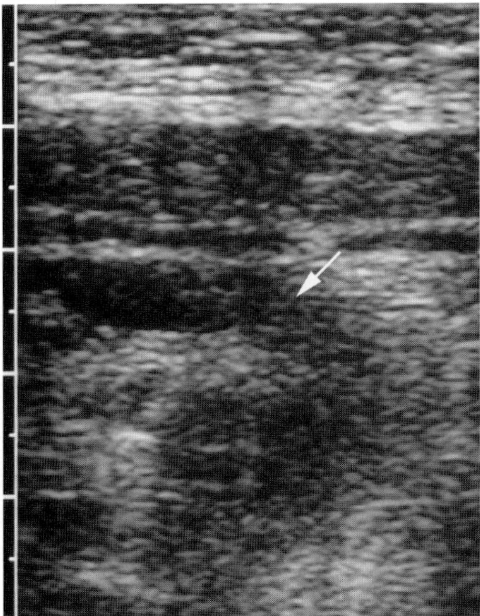

Figure 6. Sonogram obtained before drainage shows a complex fluid collection in the right lower quadrant (arrow).

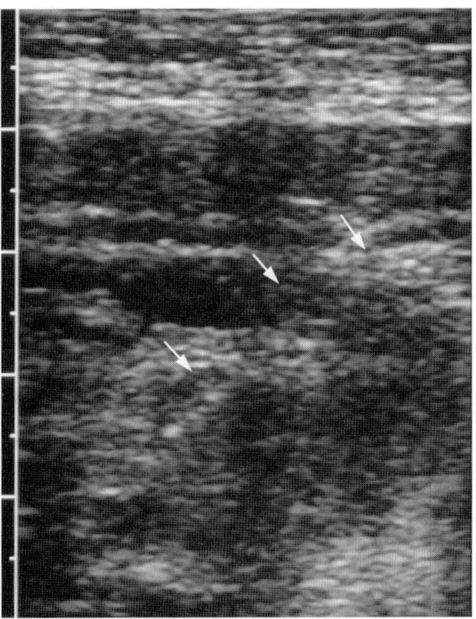

Figure 7. Arrows show the 21-gauge needle placed in the collection under sonographic guidance.

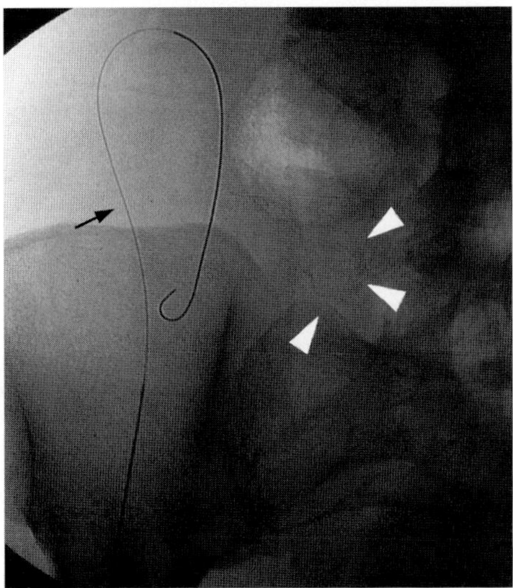

Figure 8. Digital spot radiograph shows the needle and wire within the cavity (arrow). Arrowheads show the proximity of the anastomotic sutures.

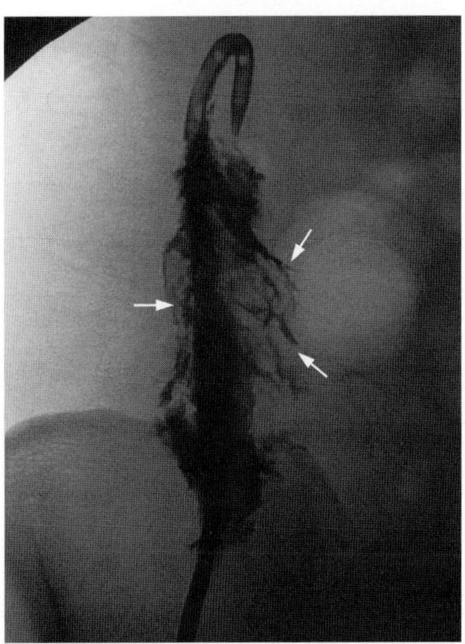

Figure 9. Sinogram shows irregular internal borders (arrows).

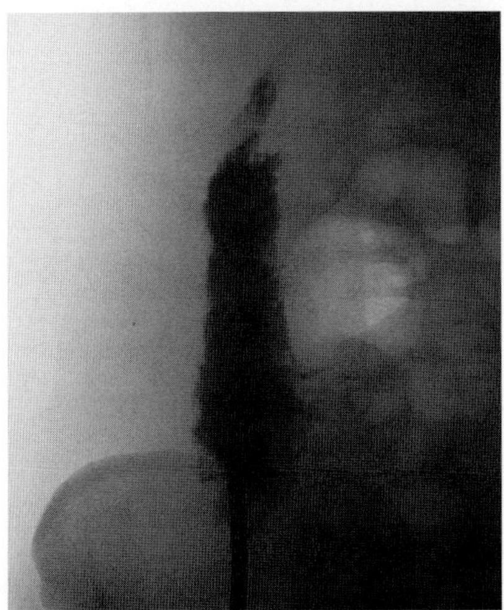

Figure 10. Post-urokinase sinogram shows smoother internal borders.

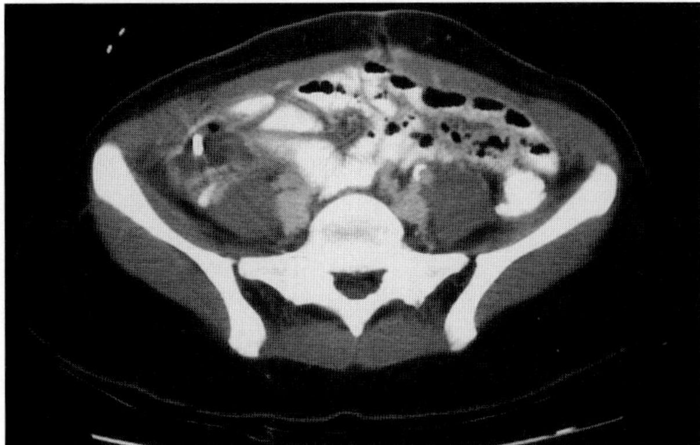

Figure 11. Repeat CT scan after initial urokinase therapy shows reduction in the size of the fluid collection.

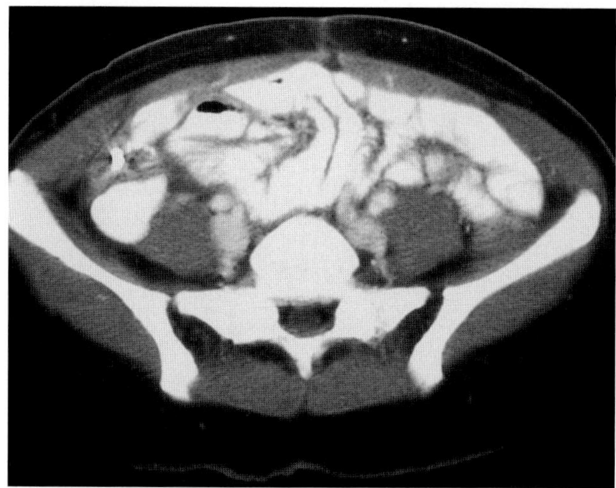

Figure 12. CT scan obtained after the second round of urokinase therapy shows resolution of the hematoma.

Additional urokinase therapy was initiated after 7 days of drainage. Another CT scan showed resolution of the hematoma. The catheter was removed 12 days after the initial drainage **(Fig. 12)**.

Final Diagnosis

Infected postoperative hematoma.

Discussion

Postoperative hematomas are difficult to drain because of their increased viscosity and possible superimposed infection. More expedient drainage can be achieved with larger caliber drains. Because of their tenacious nature, a method was sought for better drainage of organized hematomas. Working from the experience with fibrinolytic instillation in empyemas and abscesses, Vogelzang et al have proposed using urokinase for extravascular hematomas. Urokinase activates the conversion of plasminogen to plasmin, which then degrades the fibrin, leading to thrombolysis and, in theory, easier drainage.

Recent work has shown that intracavitary urokinase causes no significant change in serologic values and no significant increase in the rate of hemorrhagic complications. With these results, urokinase should be considered as adjunctive therapy in percutaneous abscess and hematoma drainage.

Selected Readings

Bergh NP, Ekroth R, Larsson S, Nagy P. Intrapleural streptokinase in the treatment of haemothorax and empyema. Scand J Thorac Cardiovasc Surg 1977; 11:265–268.

Berglin E, Ekroth R, Teger-Nilsson AC, William-Olsson G. Intrapleural instillation of streptokinase: effects on systemic fibrinolysis. Thorac Cardiovasc Surg 1981; 29:124–126.

Griebling TL, Chang PJ, Loening SA, Williams RD. Percutaneous thrombolysis of an infected retroperitoneal hematoma with urokinase. J Urol 1995; 154:1477.

Lahorra JM, Haaga JR, Stellato T, Flanigan T, Graham R. Safety of intracavitary urokinase with percutaneous abscess drainage. AJR 1993; 160:171–174.

Moulton JS, Moore PT, Mencini RA. Treatment of loculated pleural effusions with transcatheter intracavitary urokinase. AJR 1989; 153:941–945.

Park JK, Kraus FC, Haaga JR. Fluid flow during percutaneous drainage procedures: an in vitro study of the effects of fluid viscosity, catheter size, and adjunctive urokinase. AJR 1993; 160:165–169.

Saldinger E, Bookstein JJ. Mechanisms of fibrinolysis: native and exogenous systems. Semin Intervent Radiol 1985; 2:321–330.

Tillet WS, Sherry S, Read CT. The use of streptokinase-streptodornase in the treatment of chronic empyema. J Thorac Surg 1951; 21:325–341.

Vogelzang RL, Tobin RS, Burstein S, Anschuetz SL, Marzano M, Kozlowski JM. Transcatheter intracavitary fibrinolysis of infected extravascular hematomas. AJR 1987; 148:378–380.

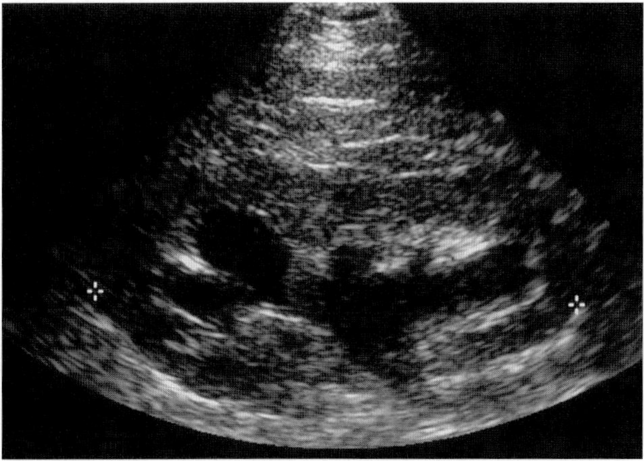

Figure 1. Left renal sonogram, longitudinal image.

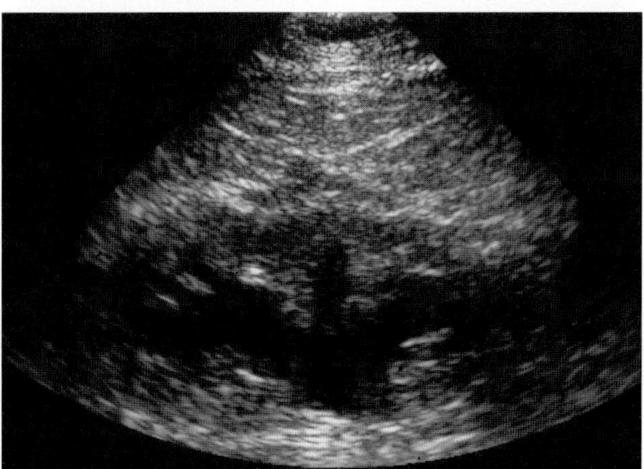

Figure 2. Right renal sonogram, longitudinal image.

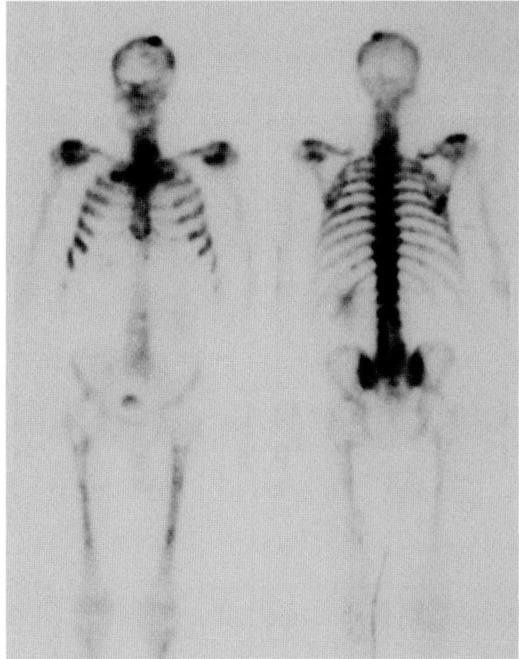

Figure 3. Whole body bone scan.

TEACHING FILE CASE 38

Ellen M. Chung, M.D.

History

An 81-year-old man with known metastatic prostate cancer developed worsening of his previously stable chronic renal insufficiency. A renal ultrasound examination was performed to evaluate the kidneys and renal collecting systems **(Figs. 1, 2)**. The patient had also recently undergone a bone scan for follow-up of skeletal metastases **(Fig. 3)**.

What is your diagnosis?

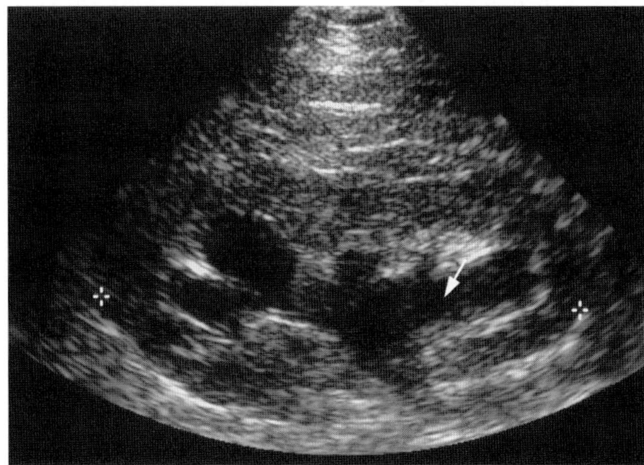

Figure 4. Left renal sonogram shows a dilated pyelocaliceal system (arrow).

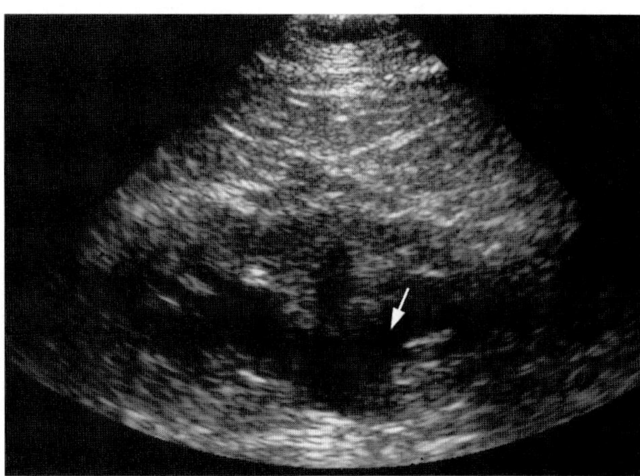

Figure 5. Right renal sonogram also shows a dilated collecting system (arrow).

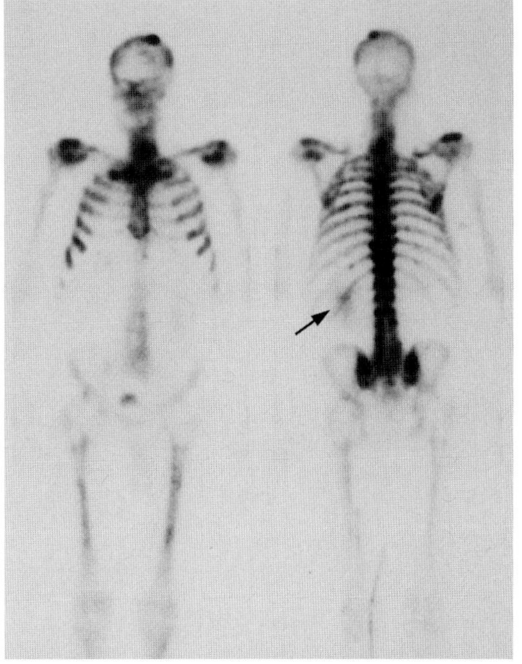

Figure 6. The bone scan demonstrates normal left renal activity (arrow), which is absent on the right. Also shown is increased uptake in the skull, due to recent scalp biopsy, and in the right sacroiliac joint, due to a metastasis.

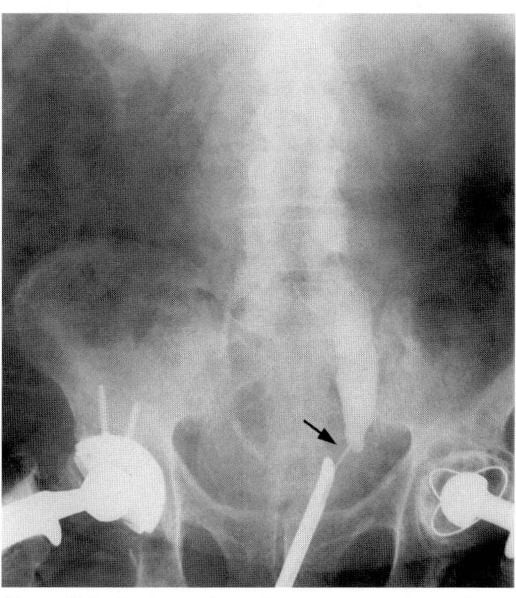

Figure 7. Left retrograde ureterogram reveals a column of contrast material terminating at the site of obstruction near the left ureterovesical junction (arrows).

Radiographic Findings

The sonogram showed bilateral hydronephrosis **(Figs. 4, 5)**. The bone scan demonstrated absent renal activity on the right and normal renal activity on the left **(Fig. 6)**. A cystoscopic left retrograde ureterogram shows dilatation of the proximal left ureter and obstruction of the left ureter near the ureterovesical junction **(Fig. 7)**.

Diagnosis

Bilateral ureteral obstruction due to metastatic prostate cancer.

What treatment can you offer?

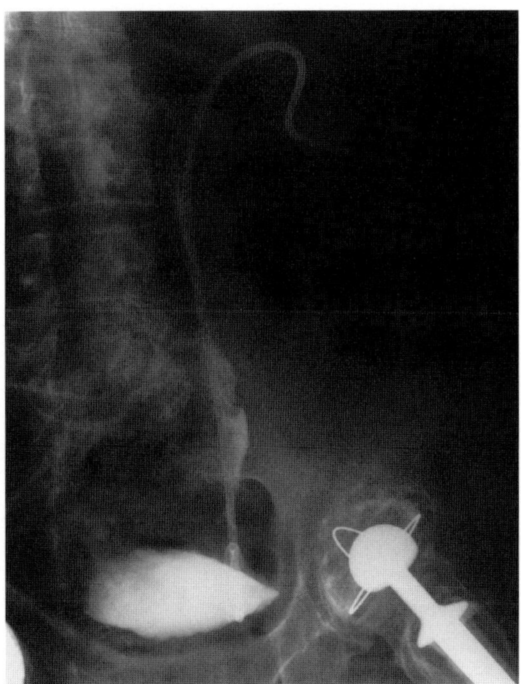

Figure 8. Radiograph demonstrates placement of a left externalized nephroureterostomy tube.

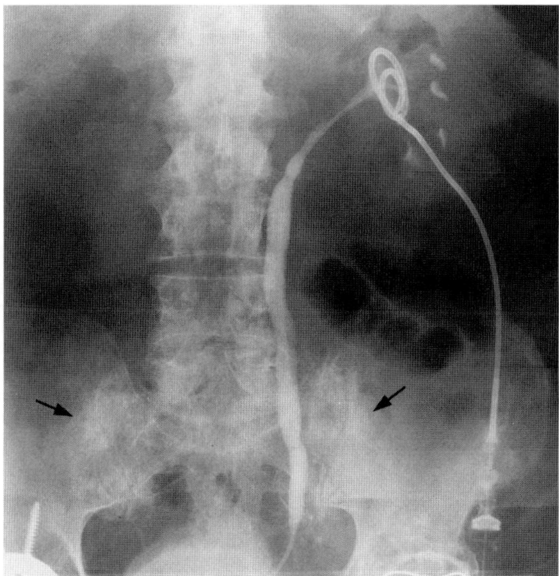

Figure 9. Radiograph after instillation of contrast material into the renal pelvis via the nephrostomy tube shows the antegrade double-pigtail ureteral stent in the ureter and the nephrostomy tube coiled in the left renal pelvis. Arrows show sclerotic metastases.

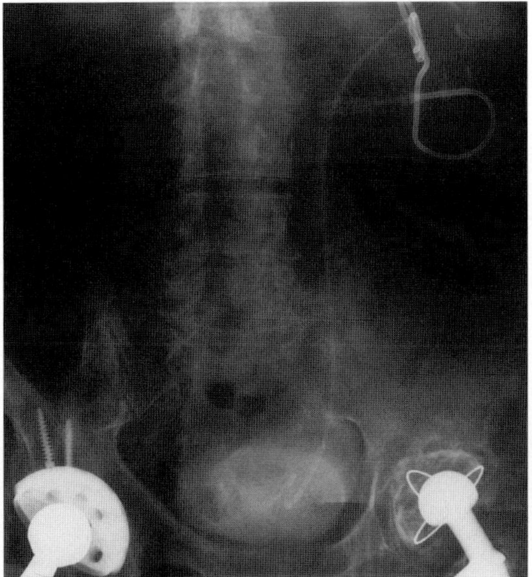

Figure 10. Radiograph shows that contrast material has drained into the bladder via the antegrade double-pigtail ureteral stent.

Management

At cystoscopy, a wire could not be passed in retrograde fashion into either ureter. Given the lack of excretion of technetium-99m by the right kidney and the patient's poor overall prognosis, palliative drainage of the left kidney was performed by placing a percutaneous nephrostomy tube **(Fig. 8)**. In an effort to improve the patient's quality of life, an internal double-J ureteral stent was placed via the percutaneous nephrostomy track **(Figs. 9, 10)**. A nephrostomy tube was left in place after the stent was placed to maintain temporary external access to the collecting system. It was removed after patency of the ureteral catheter was confirmed.

Discussion

Ureteral stent placement was initially developed for the treatment of ureteral injuries or for patients undergoing ureteral surgery; however, ureteral stents are now frequently used to relieve ureteral obstruction due to benign or malignant neoplasms. Malignant ureteral obstruction has, at least in the past, carried an ominous prognosis, and the benefit of tube drainage has come under a great deal of scrutiny.

In the case of newly diagnosed primary tumor the benefit is clear, as some lasting response to antitumor therapy is expected. Furthermore, urinary diversion is expected to improve or preserve renal function, which may allow use of some aggressive chemotherapeutic regimens that would otherwise be contraindicated in the face of renal insufficiency or obstruction.

The benefit of urinary diversion is less clear in the case of metastatic or recurrent abdominopelvic malignancy. In such cases, patient selection is particularly important. Of course, when therapy is palliative, each decision should be made on an individual basis, in concert with the primary physician, the patient's family, and, particularly, the patient. Factors to be considered are functional status, overall life expectancy, and the availability of some treatment for the tumor.

The preferred method of urinary diversion for such patients is retrograde placement of a ureteral stent via cystoscopy, as no external tube is needed. In some cases this procedure is technically impossible due to the bulk of the tumor. A percutaneous antegrade approach can then be taken. This method involves placement of a percutaneous nephrostomy, followed by placement of a ureteral stent via the nephrostomy, then removal of the nephrostomy tube. If the patient has an adequate life expectancy, the ureteral stent should be changed every 6 months.

In most instances, bilateral diversion has no benefit to renal function over unilateral drainage. Bilateral percutaneous nephrostomy tubes may make it difficult for the patient to lie fully supine. For these reasons, the kidney with the most residual function is selected for initial drainage.

Selected Readings

Chapman ME, Reid JH. Use of percutaneous nephrostomy in malignant ureteric obstruction. Br J Radiol 1991; 64:318–320.

Kadir S, ed. Current practice of interventional radiology. St. Louis: Mosby Year Book, 1991.

Keidan RD, Greenberg RE, Hoffman JP, Weese JL. Is percutaneous nephrostomy for hydronephrosis appropriate in patients with advanced cancer? Am J Surg 1988; 156:206–208.

Mitty HA, Train JS, Dan SJ. Placement of ureteral stents by antegrade and retrograde techniques. Radiol Clin North Am 1986; 24:587–600.

Watkinson AF, A'Hern RP, Jones A, King DM, Moskovic EC. The role of percutaneous nephrostomy in malignant urinary tract obstruction. Clin Radiol 1993; 47:32–35.

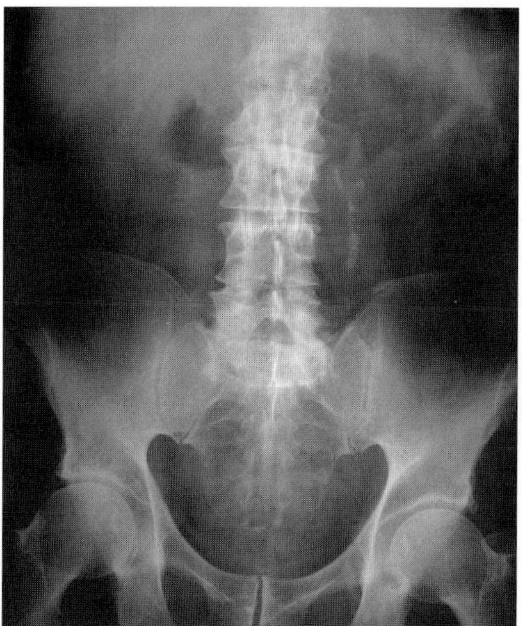

Figure 1. Supine abdominal radiograph.

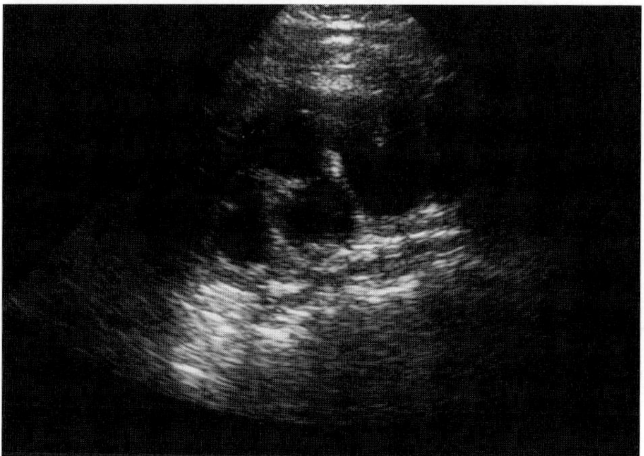

Figure 2. Longitudinal sonogram of the left kidney.

TEACHING FILE CASE 39

Robert D. Lyon, M.D.

History

A 78-year-old man came to the hospital with fever and left flank pain 2 weeks after extracorporeal shock wave lithotripsy (ESWL). A supine radiograph of the abdomen was obtained in the emergency department **(Fig. 1)**. An abdominal ultrasound examination was then performed **(Fig. 2)**.

What is your diagnosis?

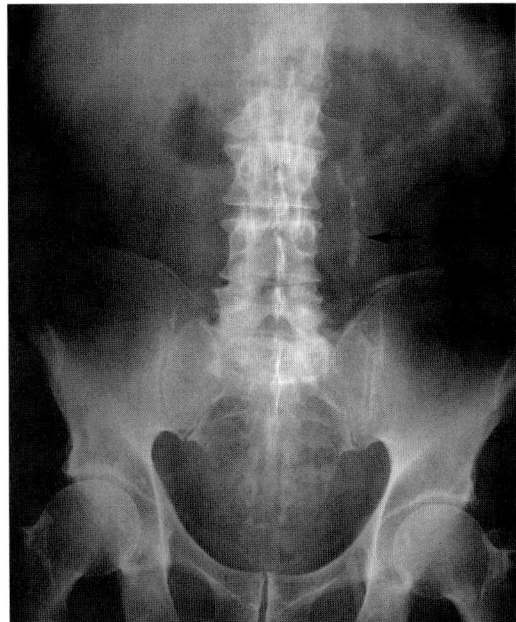
Figure 3. Abdominal radiograph shows a 4-cm-long row of ureteral calculi (arrow).

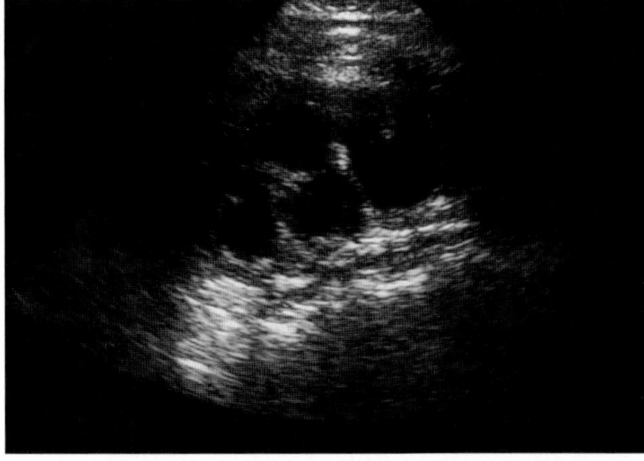
Figure 4. Sonogram of the left kidney shows hydronephrosis and hydroureter proximal to the obstructive ureteral calculi.

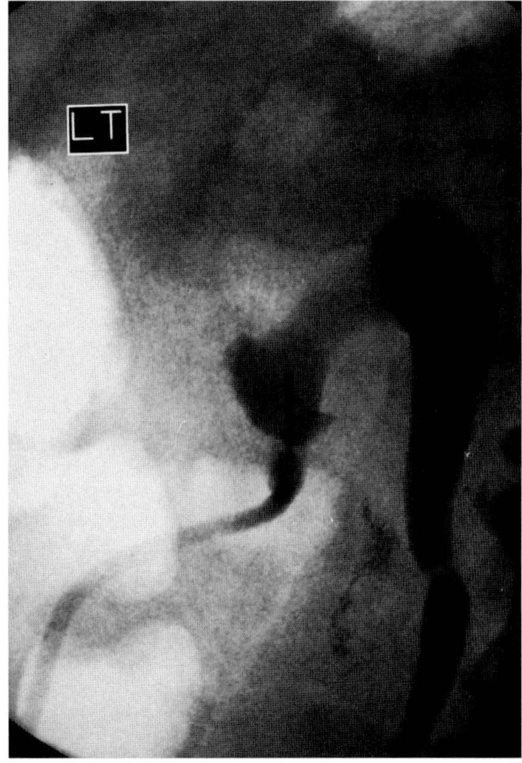

Figure 5. Spot radiograph shows needle placement into an anterior renal calyx.

Radiographic Findings

The abdominal radiograph showed a 4-cm length of retained ureteral stone fragments ("steinstrasse") **(Fig. 3)** obstructing the left ureter. The ultrasound examination **(Fig. 4)** showed hydronephrosis and proximal hydroureter.

Diagnosis

Retained ureteral stone fragments following extracorporeal shock wave lithotripsy.

What treatment would you recommend?

Management

Percutaneous nephrostomy with use of a two-needle technique was performed to decompress the urinary system. **Figure 5** shows the first needle in an anterior calyx that is filled with contrast material. Iodinated contrast material is denser than urine and settles in the dependent, anterior portion of the renal collecting system. **Figure 6** shows the second needle in an air-filled posterior calyx. Urine cultures and Gram stains were obtained prior to contrast material injection to help guide subsequent antibiotic therapy.

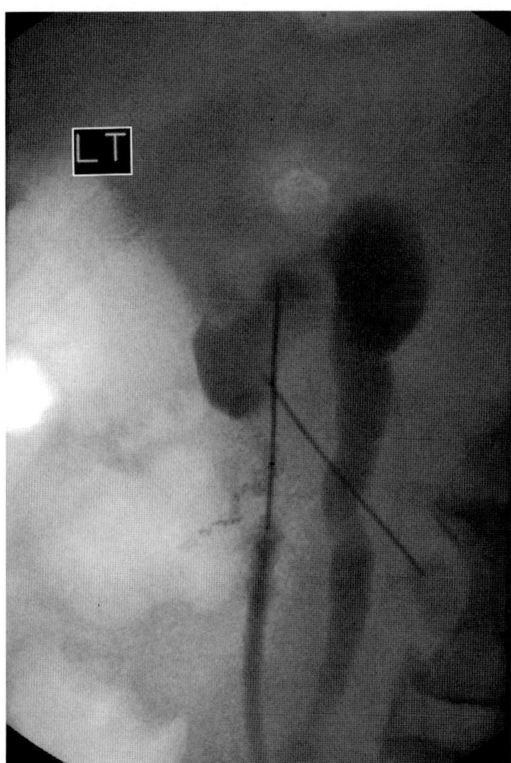

Figure 6. Spot radiograph shows air and a second needle in the nondependent, posterior calyx.

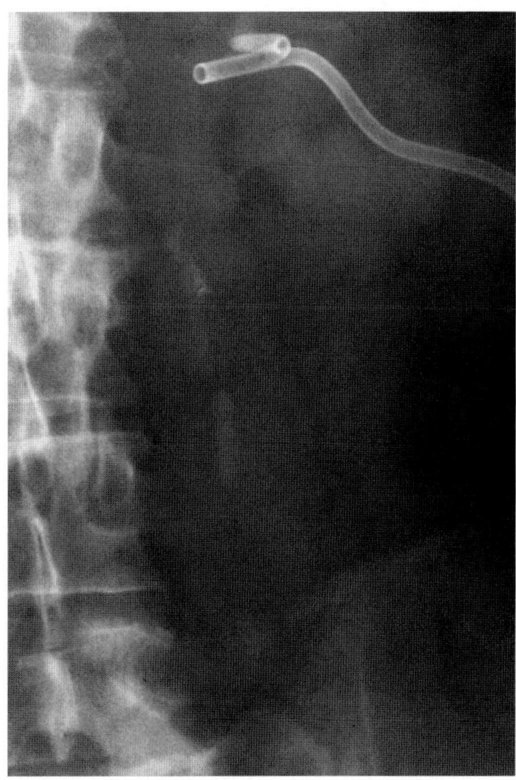

Figure 7. 8-F nephrostomy catheter in the renal pelvis.

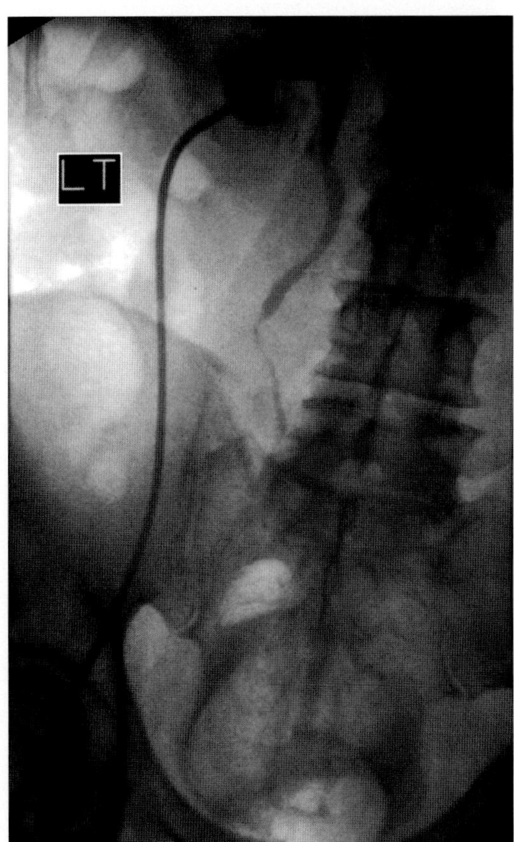

Figure 8. Antegrade pyelogram shows complete ureteral obstruction by the steinstrasse.

An 8-F self-locking nephrostomy catheter was placed into the left renal pelvis **(Fig. 7)**. The patient was admitted to the hospital, and antibiotic therapy was begun. An antegrade pyelogram was obtained the next day and showed significant ureteral obstruction at the level of the retained stones **(Fig. 8)**. The nephrostomy catheter was therefore left to external drainage. The patient ultimately required ureteral lithotripsy to fragment the most caudal stone. This allowed the smaller, more proximal stones to pass spontaneously.

Discussion

ESWL is a highly effective technique for treating most urinary tract calculi. Retained stones are a significant complication, however, that may necessitate percutaneous intervention to treat incipient urinary tract obstruction. Some patients with retained stones will do well with observation alone, as smaller (less then one-half cm) fragments may pass spontaneously. Patients with symptoms of ureteral colic and fever require percutaneous nephrostomy (PCN) to relieve symptoms and prevent life-threatening sepsis.

PCN and subsequent nephroureteral stent placement permit spontaneous passage of ureteral stones by relieving ureteral spasm. In most cases, however, ureteral obstruction requires further intervention with percutaneous stone extraction using stone basket and flushing techniques, repeat ESWL, or endoscopic lithotripsy. Surgical stone removal is rarely required.

Selected Readings

Dretler SP. Management of "steinstrasse." Endourology 1986; 1:1.

Gillenwater JY. Extracorporeal shock wave lithotripsy for the treatment of urinary calculi. In: Gillenwater JY, Graybeck JT, Howards SS, Duckett JW. Adult and pediatric urology. 3rd edition. St. Louis: Mosby Year Book, 1996; 913–930.

Tegtmeyer CJ, Kellum CD, Jenkins A, et al. Extracorporeal shock wave lithotripsy: interventional radiologic solutions to associated problems. Radiology 1986; 161:587–592.

Weinerth JL, Flatt JA, Carson CC. Lessons learned in patients with large steinstrasse. J Urol 1989; 142:1425–1427.

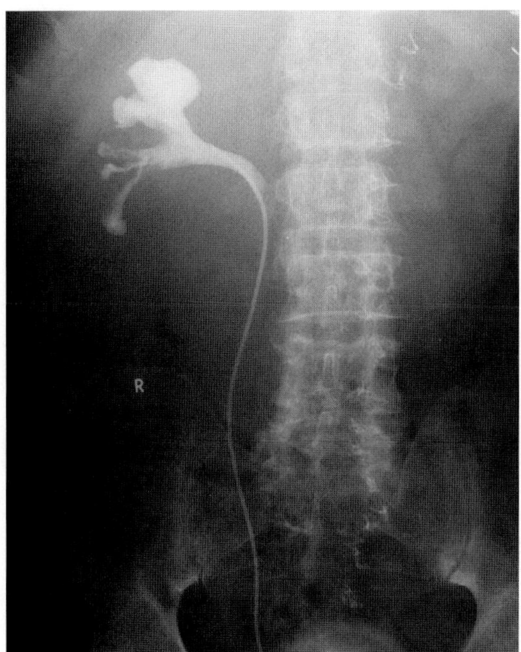

Figure 1. Right retrograde ureterogram.

TEACHING FILE CASE 40

Steven D. Stowell, M.D.

History

A 66-year-old man came to the hospital with weight loss and gross hematuria. An intravenous urogram was obtained, which revealed a distorted intrarenal collecting system. A retrograde ureterogram was also obtained **(Fig. 1)**.

What is your diagnosis?

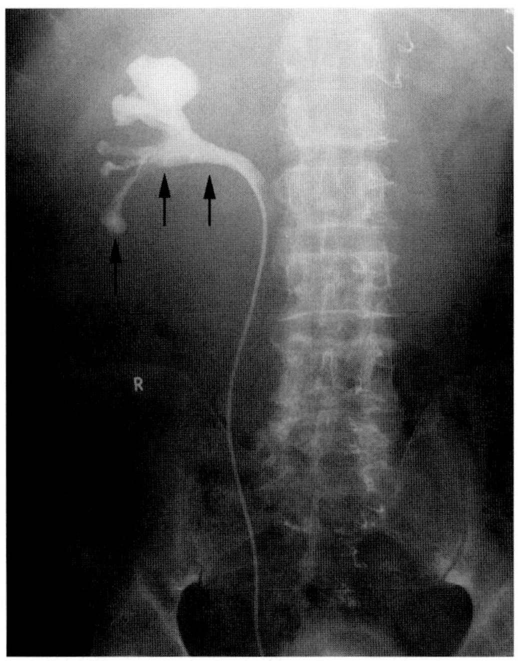

Figure 2. Right retrograde ureterogram reveals marked irregularity of the lower intrarenal collecting system mucosa (arrows).

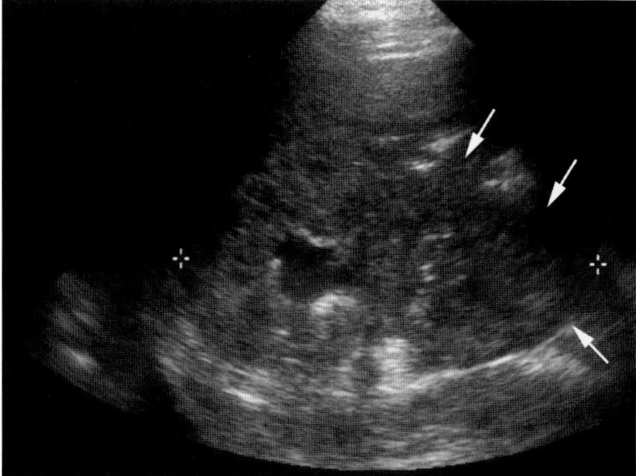

Figure 3. Sonogram of the right kidney. The lower pole of the kidney is replaced by a heterogeneous mass (arrows).

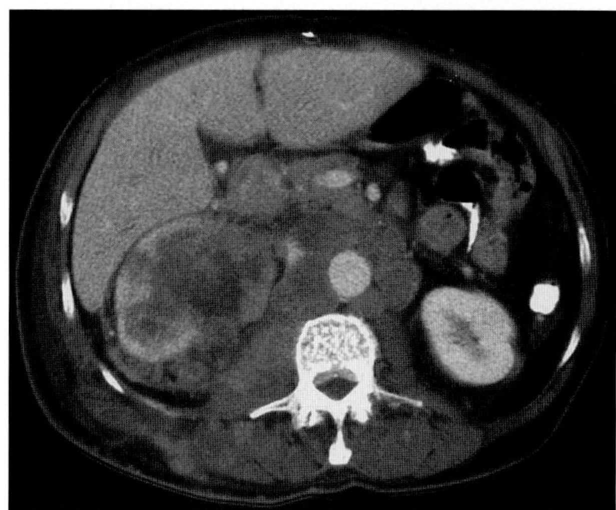

Figure 4. CT scan of the abdomen reveals a large mass of the right kidney. Marked periaortocaval and renal hilar lymphadenopathy are present.

Radiographic Findings

The retrograde ureterogram showed marked irregularity of the right renal collecting system **(Fig. 2)**. An ultrasound examination was performed to further define the etiology of the patient's hematuria. The ultrasound revealed a large mass involving the right kidney **(Fig. 3)**. A computed tomography (CT) scan revealed a large exophytic heterogeneous mass with regional lymph node involvement **(Fig. 4)**. Subsequent nuclear scintigraphy revealed 7% function in the right kidney **(Fig. 5)**. An arteriogram of the right kidney showed multiple vessels that had an irregular course and contour, and pooling of contrast material in the lower pole **(Fig. 6)**. These findings were indicative of tumor neovascularity, which was thought to be the source of the patient's hematuria. Several lumbar vessels showed similar findings **(Figs. 7, 8)**.

Diagnosis

Hematuria secondary to renal cell carcinoma.

How would you manage this patient?

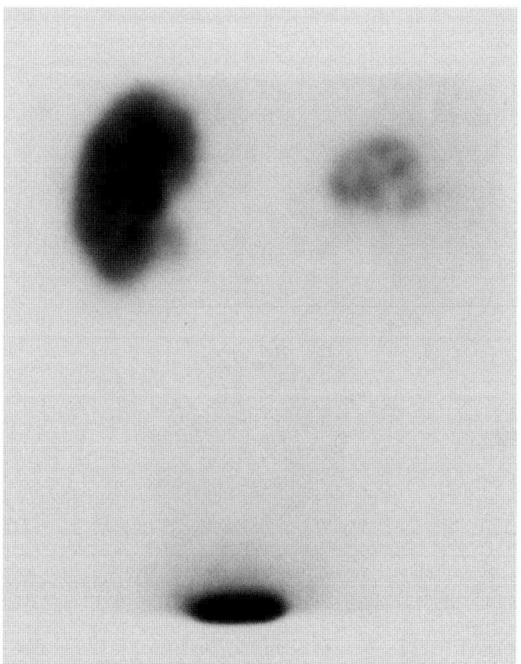

Figure 5. Technetium-99m MAG-3 study shows minimal uptake of the radiotracer in the upper pole of the right kidney, revealing 7% function.

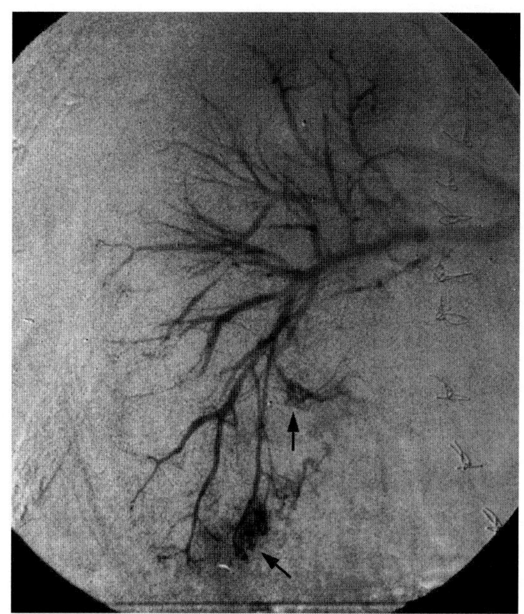

Figure 6. Right renal arteriogram. The lower pole shows multiple vessels with abnormal courses and irregular contours. Pooling of contrast material in the lower pole of the right kidney is seen (arrows).

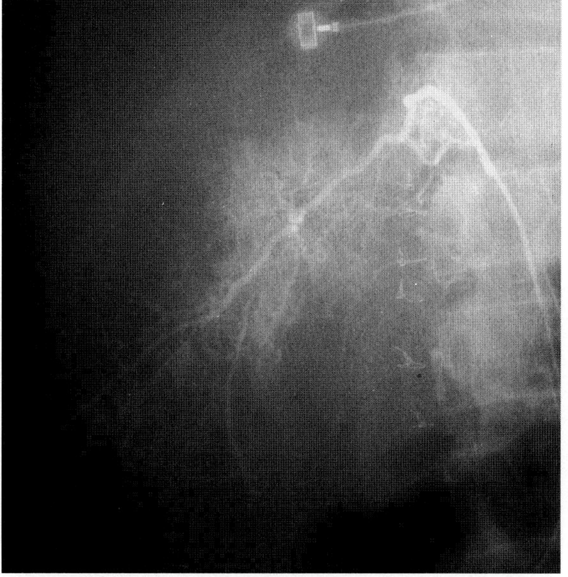

Figure 7. Arteriogram of a right L1 vessel shows irregular vessels representing tumor vascularity.

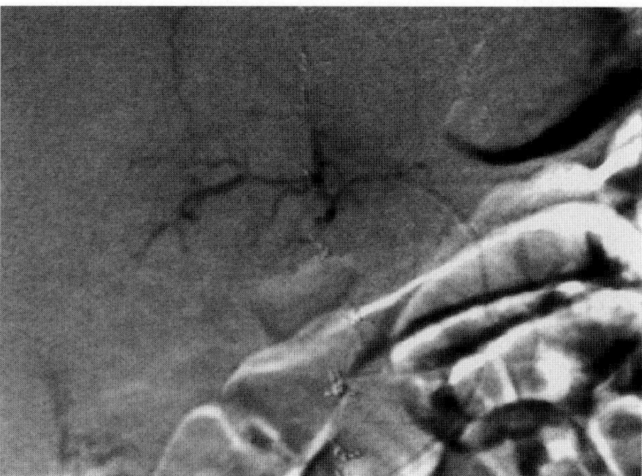

Figure 8. Arteriogram of a right L2 vessel shows irregular vessels representing tumor vascularity.

Management

Because the right kidney showed minimal function on scintigraphy, it was decided to embolize the kidney and tumor to palliate the hematuria. The renal artery was selected with a 5-F cobra catheter, and the kidney was embolized with polyvinyl alcohol particles in a 50-50 mixture of saline and contrast material. Follow-up images showed no hypervascular tumor stain **(Fig. 9)**. The patient still had hematuria 24 hours later, so repeat arteriography was performed. The arteriogram revealed a small lumbar vessel with mild vascular irregularity and pooling of a small amount of contrast material, indicating extravasation from the tumor **(Fig. 10)**. The vessel was subsequently embolized.

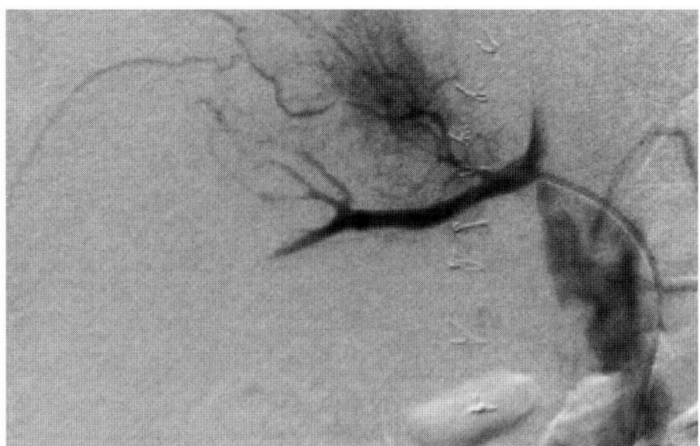

Figure 9. Postembolization arteriogram of the right kidney with markedly decreased vascularity. Compare to Figure 6.

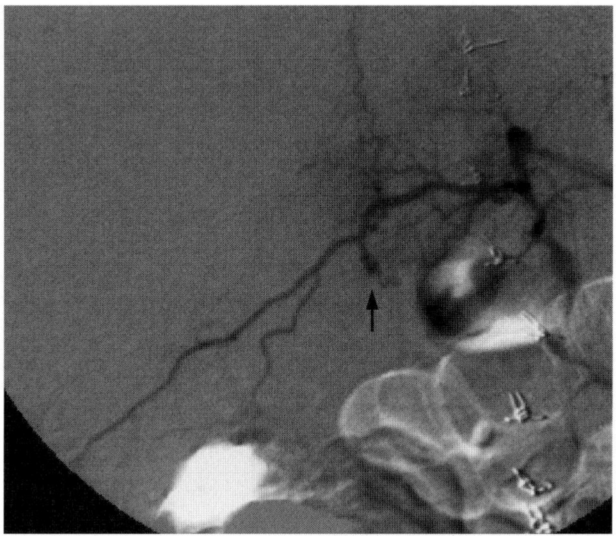

Figure 10. Right L3 arteriogram with irregular vessels. Pooling of contrast material (arrow) represents extravasation from the tumor.

Discussion

Embolization to control hematuria is the preferred treatment for unresectable renal tumors. As shown in this case, the tumor may recruit vessels from outside the kidney. Partial embolization of the kidney may be performed if preservation of the uninvolved renal tissue eliminates the need for dialysis. Total renal ablation was performed in this case due to massive tumor involvement and minimal renal function, and because it was thought that embolization posed a much lesser risk than surgical nephrectomy. Polyvinyl alcohol was chosen as the embolic agent because it causes distal, permanent occlusion. Ethanol can also be used as an embolic agent, but this is often very painful both at the time of the procedure and afterwards. Care must be taken when embolizing renal tumors; the embolic agent can spill into the aorta or flow through arteriovenous fistulas of the tumor. Additionally, when large tissue masses are embolized, the patient is likely to experience postembolization syndrome, with local pain, elevated white blood count, fever, and possible soft-tissue gas. This is often treated effectively with antibiotics and anti-inflammatory and analgesic agents.

Selected Readings

Kadir S, ed. Current practice of interventional radiology. St. Louis: Mosby Year Book, 1991.

Keller FS, Rösch J, Baur GM, Taylor LM, Dotter CT, Porter JM. Percutaneous angiographic embolization: a procedure of increasing usefulness: review of a decade of experience. Am J Surg 1981; 142:5–13.

Wojtowycz M. Handbook of interventional radiology and angiography. 2nd edition. St. Louis: Mosby Year Book, 1995.

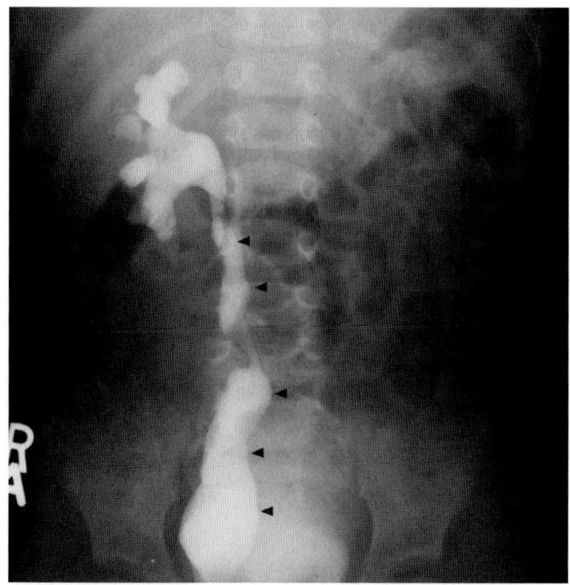

Figure 1. Intravenous urogram shows a markedly dilated right ureter (arrowheads).

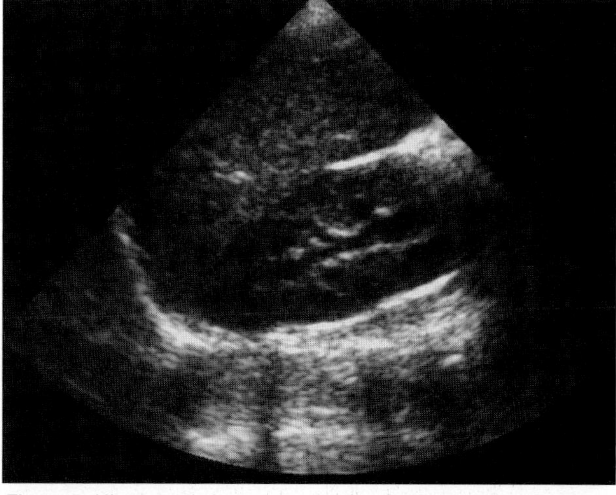

Figure 2. Ultrasound shows very mild hydronephrosis of the right kidney.

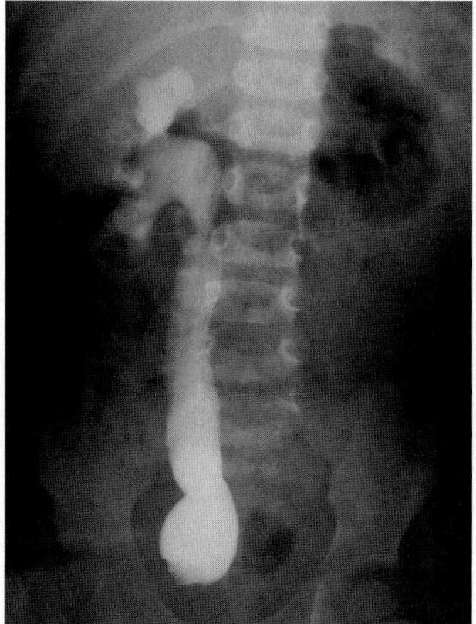

Figure 3. Postoperative intravenous urogram at 10 minutes.

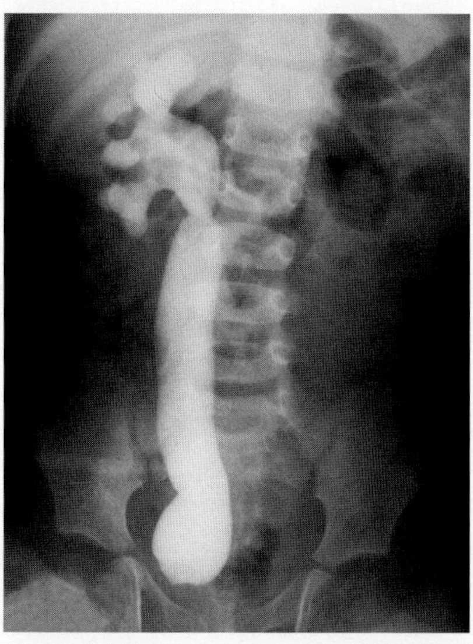

Figure 4. Intravenous urogram at 20 minutes.

TEACHING FILE CASE 41

Steven D. Stowell, M.D.

History

A 2-year-old boy was brought to the hospital with fever, chills, and pyuria. An intravenous urogram revealed slight right pyelocaliectasis and marked right ureterectasis. The left kidney was not seen **(Fig. 1)**. A voiding cystourethrogram showed grade 4 reflux on the right and a short, blind-ending left ureter. An ultrasound study revealed mild right hydronephrosis and nonvisualization of the left kidney **(Fig. 2)**. A technetium-99m dimercaptosuccinic acid scan confirmed the absence of the left kidney. There was cortical scarring of the right kidney.

A ureterocystostomy of the distal right ureter was performed for repair of primary megaureter by surgically tapering the distal ureter and creating an oblique tunnel through the bladder wall in order to minimize the reflux of urine. A double-J stent was placed from the renal pelvis into the bladder during surgery. After the stent was removed, the patient could not void spontaneously, and an intravenous urogram was obtained **(Figs. 3, 4)**.

What is your diagnosis?

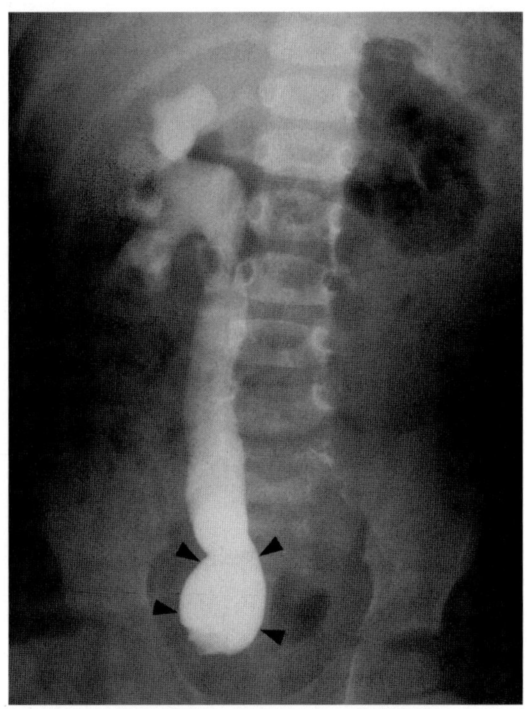

Figure 5. Postoperative intravenous urogram at 10 minutes shows persistent marked dilatation of the right ureter (arrowheads).

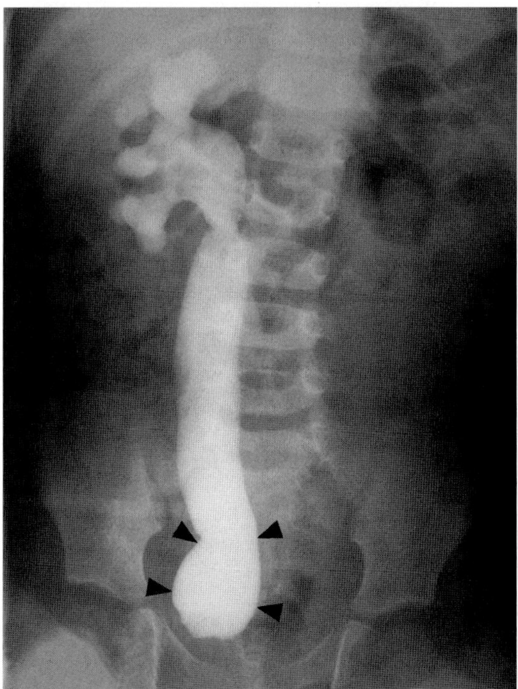

Figure 6. An intravenous urogram at 20 minutes shows marked pyelocaliectasis and ureterectasis. No change is noted from the urogram at 10 minutes. The arrowheads point to the aperistaltic distal ureteral segment.

Radiographic Findings

The postoperative intravenous urogram revealed marked pyelocaliectasis and ureterectasis persisting at 10 and 20 minutes without flow into the bladder. A segment of the distal ureter is aperistaltic **(Figs. 5, 6)**.

Diagnosis

Postoperative physiologic ureteral obstruction with an aperistaltic distal ureteral segment.

What treatment would you recommend?

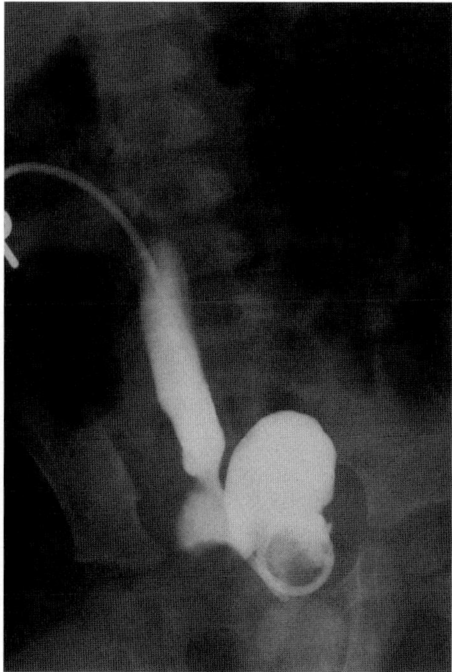

Figure 7. Nephroureterostomy tube with the loop of the tube in the bladder. Contrast material flows through the tube, opacifying both the ureter and the bladder.

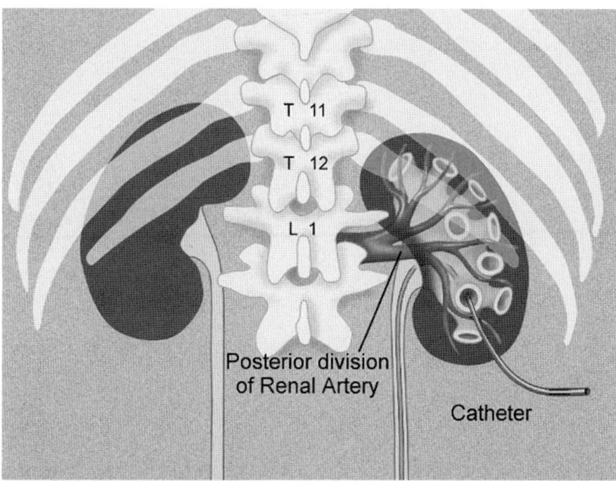

Figure 8. Optimal approach to the renal collecting system with respect to renal arterial anatomy.

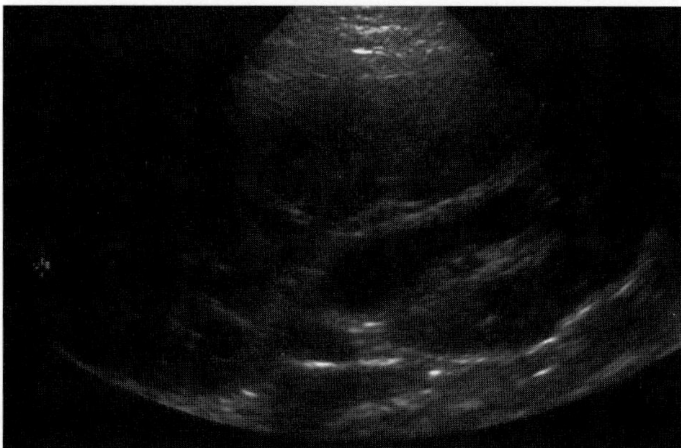

Figure 9. Ultrasound 2 years after surgery reveals mild pyelocaliectasis with normal renal parenchyma.

Management

The patient was referred for percutaneous nephrostomy (PCN) to drain the physiologically obstructed renal collecting system. An 8-F nephroureterostomy tube was created by modifying a PCN tube by making multiple proximal side-holes. The tube was placed via a posterior lower pole calyx **(Fig. 7)**. The nephroureterostomy tube allowed urine to bypass the aperistaltic ureteral segment and flow into the bladder. Spontaneous voiding confirmed good function of the tube.

Discussion

Percutaneous nephrostomy is commonly used for decompression of obstructed upper urinary tracts. A posterior lower pole calyx is the preferred access site because it minimizes the risk of pneumothorax by permitting entry below the twelfth rib. Also, most kidneys have a dominant anterior blood supply with the posterior blood supply passing beneath the lower pole infundibulum. Therefore, the posterolateral kidney is a watershed zone, and puncture in this area minimizes bleeding **(Fig. 8)**. This approach also allows a single smooth curve of the tube from the skin into the ureter.

While meant to be a temporary palliative measure, some patients may develop irreversible strictures or have malignant obstruction and may require permanent indwelling percutaneous nephrostomy catheters, necessitating tube changes every 4 to 6 weeks due to catheter encrustation. This patient had significant perioperative edema at the neoureterostomy site which caused the acute obstruction. The patient, however, was able to have his tube removed after 1 month with good results. An ultrasound examination 2 years later revealed mild pyelocaliectasis with normal renal parenchyma **(Fig. 9)**.

Selected Readings

Castaneda-Zuniga WR, et al. Percutaneous radiologic techniques. In: Castaneda-Zuniga WR, Tadavarthy SM, eds. Interventional radiology. 2nd edition. Baltimore: Williams and Wilkins, 1992.

Gillenwater J, Grayhack J, Howards S, Duckett J. Adult and pediatric urology. 2nd edition. St. Louis: Mosby Year Book, 1991.

Kadir S, ed. Current practice of interventional radiology. St. Louis: Mosby Year Book, 1991.

Wojtowycz M. Handbook of interventional radiology and angiography. 2nd edition. St. Louis: Mosby Year Book, 1995.

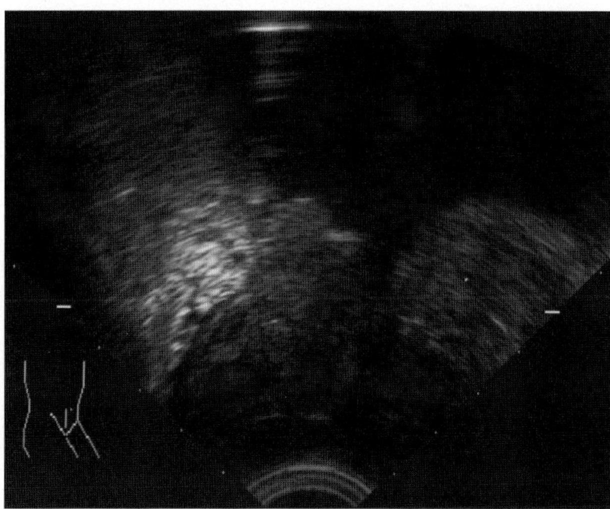

Figure 1. Transrectal prostatic ultrasound.

TEACHING FILE CASE 42

Kevin L. Quinn, M.D.

History

A 98-year-old man with a history of benign prostatic hypertrophy (BPH) and frequent voiding was referred to interventional radiology. The patient was not a candidate for transurethral resection of the prostate (TURP) and had failed to respond to medical therapy. Long-term Foley catheter placement was an unacceptable option due to a history of repeated, forcible Foley catheter removal by the patient. Prior to any therapy, a transrectal ultrasound (TRUS) examination was performed **(Fig. 1)**.

What is your diagnosis?

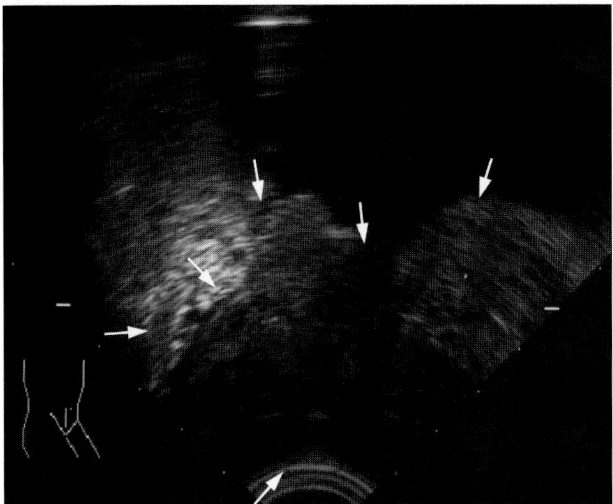

Figure 2. Transrectal prostatic ultrasound demonstrates an enlarged prostate extending into the bladder (arrows) with compression of the urethral opening at the bladder neck.

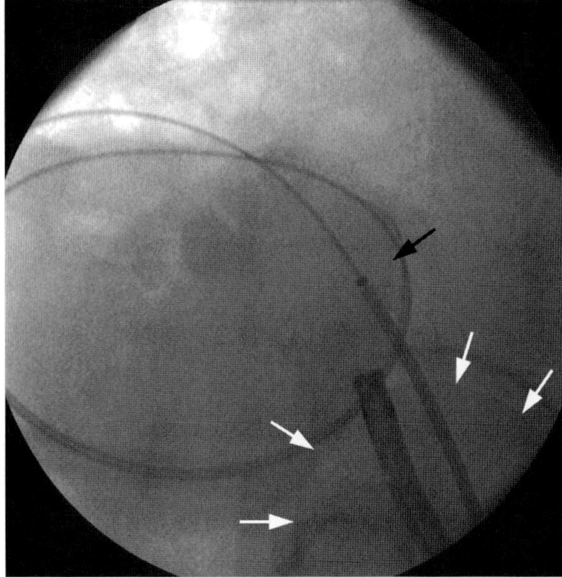

Figure 3. Lateral radiograph shows that the position of the distal end of the Wallstent (black arrow) at the urethral opening in the bladder is confirmed with use of the cystoscope. White arrows outline the femoral head.

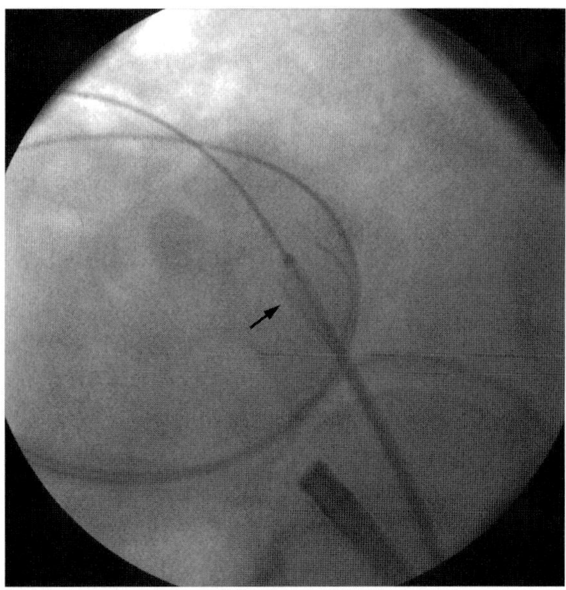

Figure 4. Lateral radiograph shows that the cystoscope is withdrawn and the stent is partially deployed (arrow).

Radiographic Findings

TRUS demonstrated an enlarged prostate with a prominent intravesicular component and significant post-void residual **(Fig. 2)**.

Diagnosis

Marked benign prostatic hypertrophy with urinary retention.

What palliative treatment would you recommend?

Management

This patient presented a difficult clinical problem because traditional conservative care had been unsuccessful and he was not a suitable surgical candidate. Permanent internal stent placement offered a potential solution. A hydrophilic guide wire was introduced into the bladder via the urethra, and a flexible cystoscope was advanced in tandem with the wire to the prostate under mucosal anesthesia. The distance from the bladder neck to the urogenital diaphragm was measured at 6 cm. A 10-mm x 68-mm Wallstent (Schneider, Minneapolis, MN) was introduced over the wire and the distal end placed at the urethral orifice using direct cystoscopic visualization **(Fig. 3)**. The scope was then withdrawn and the stent deployed **(Fig. 4)**.

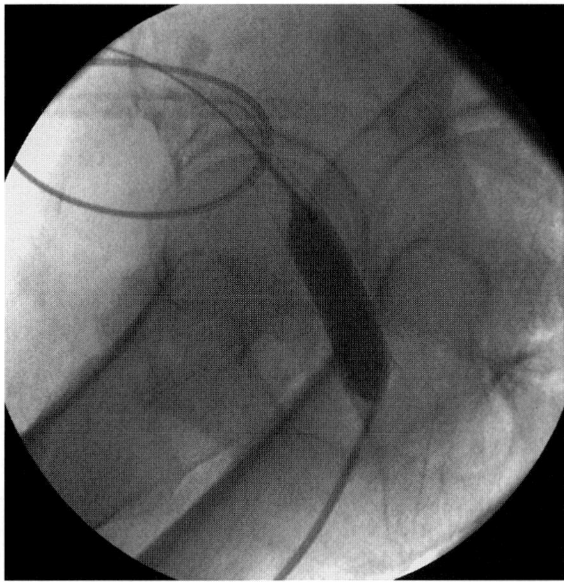

Figure 5. Lateral radiograph shows the stent embedded with an angioplasty balloon.

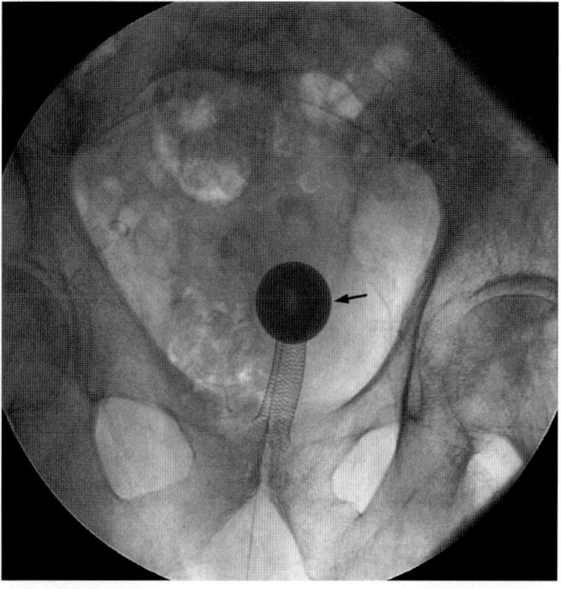

Figure 6. Anteroposterior view of the stent in the prostatic urethra with the Foley catheter. The Foley balloon is inflated (arrow).

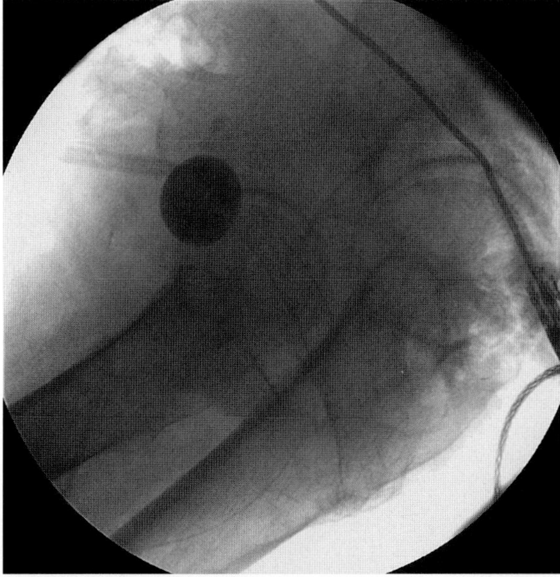

Figure 7. Lateral view of the stent.

A 14-mm x 4-cm angioplasty balloon was then used to embed the stent into the prostatic urothelium **(Fig. 5)**. A Foley catheter was left in place for 24 hours **(Figs. 6, 7)**, although postprocedural bleeding was minimal. After the procedure, the patient experienced occasional incontinence which gradually diminished over the ensuing 9 months follow-up. The patient remained otherwise asymptomatic, and there was no infection or reobstruction during that time.

Discussion

The standard surgical management of BPH has included TURP or open prostatectomy. Patients who are not candidates for prostatic surgery may respond to medical treatment or may require chronic drainage with a Foley catheter or suprapubic cystostomy. Several permanently implanted metal stents, including the Urolume Wallstent (Schneider), ProstaCoil (Angiomed/Bard, Germany), and Memotherm (Instent Inc, Minneapolis, MN) have recently been tested in clinical trials on this group of patients. The Urolume Wallstent has recently received Food and Drug Administration approval for human use as an effective and safe treatment in properly selected men who are otherwise healthy. Reported complications from permanent metal stent placement of the urethra have included malpositioning, intractable detrusor instability, stent encrustation, stent migration, severe prostatic urethral epithelial hyperplasia, and epididymitis.

In this case, TRUS as well as direct visualization with the cystoscope were used to ensure that the stent did not project beyond the prostate into the bladder lumen. It was thought that this stent placement would minimize stent encrustation and detrusor instability. Overexpansion of the 10-mm-diameter stent with a 14-mm balloon was also intended to minimize encrustation by embedding the stent well into the urothelium.

Selected Readings

Kletscher BA, Oesterling JE. Prostatic stents: current perspectives for the management of benign prostatic hyperplasia. Urol Clin North Am 1995; 22(2):423–430.

Oesterling JE, Kaplan SA, Epstein HB, Defalco AJ, Reddy PK, Chancellor MB. The North American experience with the UroLume endoprosthesis as a treatment for benign prostatic hyperplasia: long-term results. Urology 1994; 44(3):353–362.

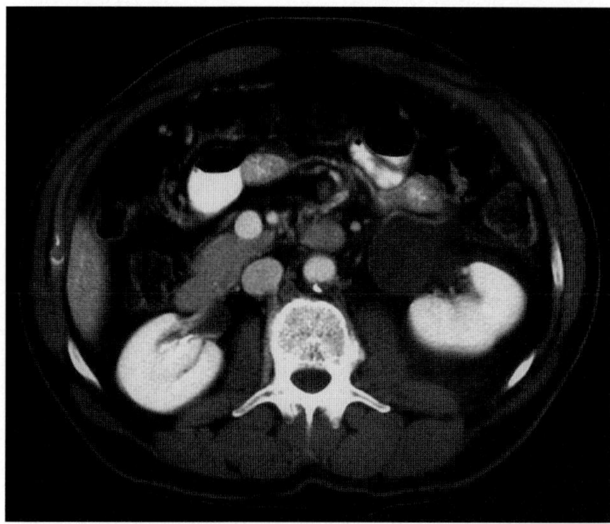

Figure 1. Axial cut from the initial contrast-enhanced abdominal/ pelvic CT scan.

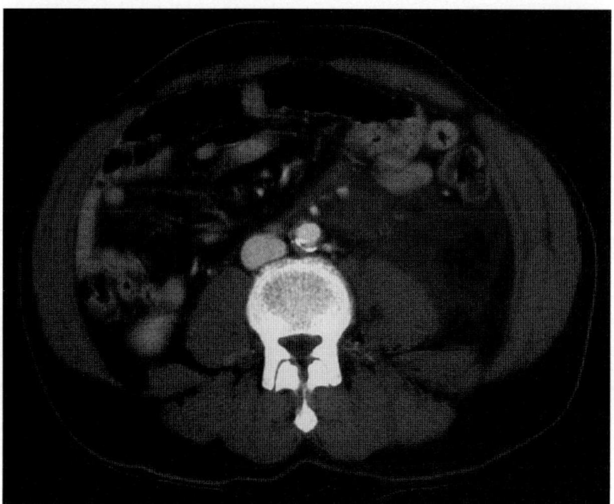

Figure 2. A more caudal image from the same scan.

TEACHING FILE CASE 43

Ellen Chung, M.D., Allen J. Meglin, M.D., and Aaron L. Stack, M.D.

History

A 52-year-old man underwent a percutaneous discectomy at the L4-L5 level from a left flank approach. There were no immediate surgical complications, but the patient experienced increasing left flank pain postoperatively. A computed tomography (CT) scan was obtained **(Figs. 1, 2)**.

What is your diagnosis?

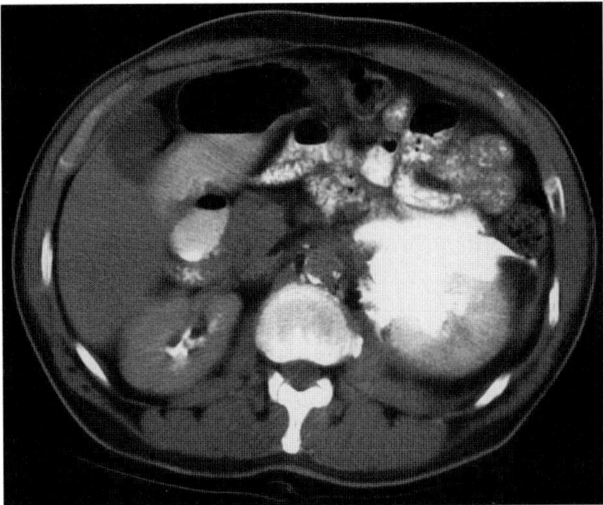

Figure 3. Axial image from the delayed CT scan.

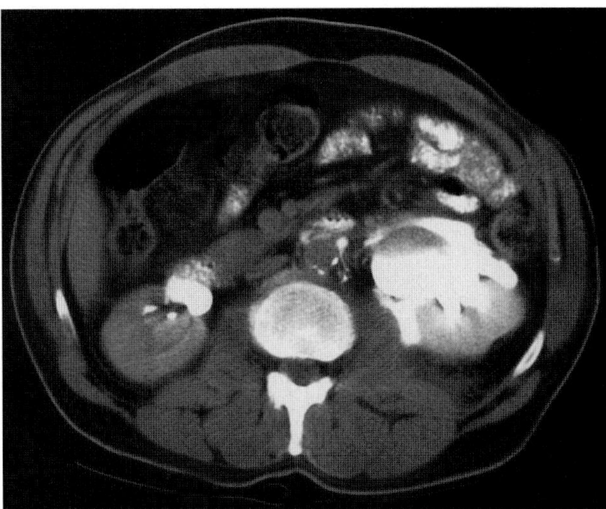

Figure 4. More caudal axial image from the same delayed scan.

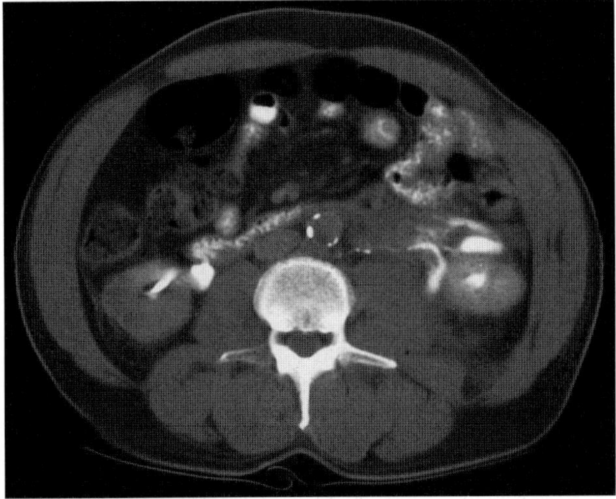

Figure 5. Still more caudal axial image from the delayed scan.

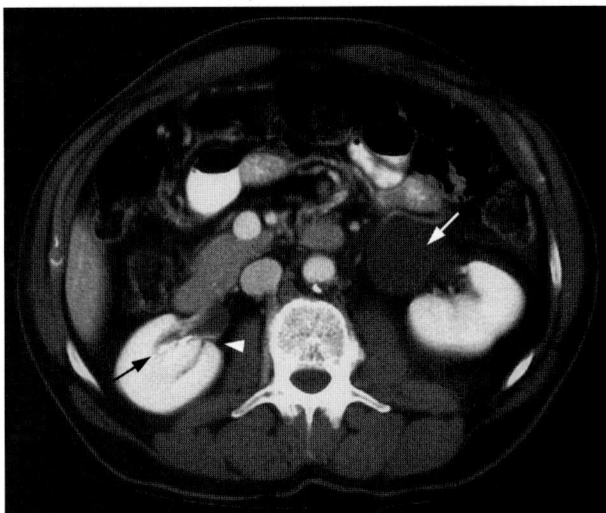

Figure 6. Axial image from the initial contrast-enhanced CT scan shows a normal left nephrogram but no contrast material in the dilated left renal pelvis (white arrow). Compare the normal right side with contrast material in the calyces (black arrow) and nondilated ureter (arrowhead).

A delayed CT scan was also obtained several hours later without the use of additional contrast material **(Figs. 3–5)**.

What is your diagnosis now?

Radiographic Findings

The initial CT scan shows a left nephrogram, but there was no contrast material within the dilated left renal pelvis **(Fig. 6)**. Compare the normal right side, which demonstrates contrast in the calyces and ureter. Additionally, there is an abnormal fluid collection in the left retroperitoneum **(Fig. 7)**.

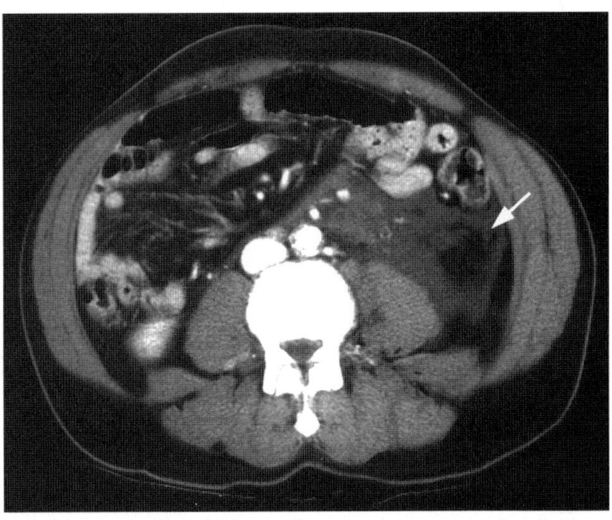

Figure 7. A more caudal image from same scan reveals a fluid collection in the left retroperitoneum (arrow).

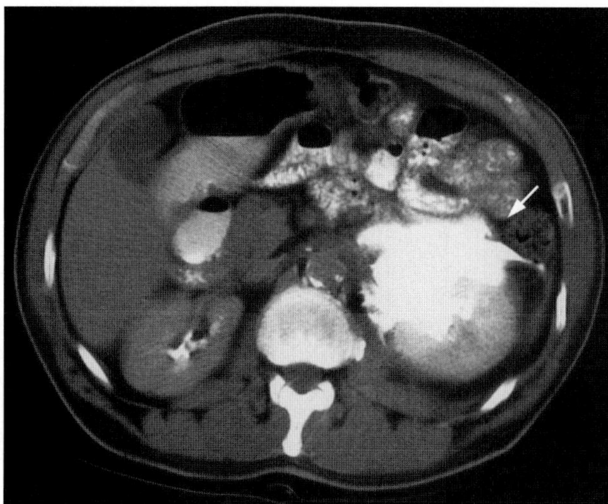

Figure 8. Axial image from the delayed CT scan demonstrates extravasation of contrast material into the retroperitoneal space (arrow).

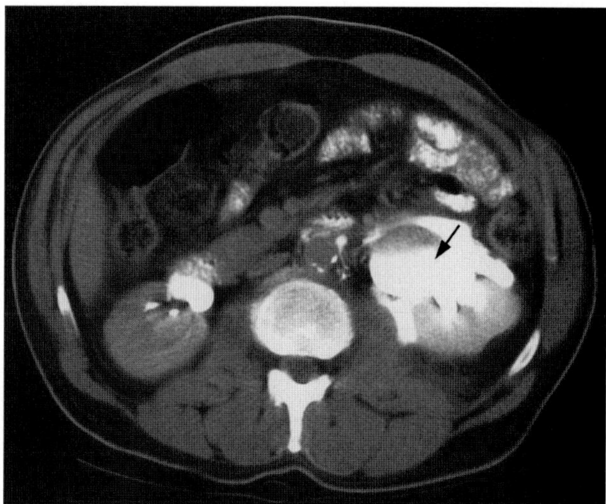

Figure 9. A more caudal image from the same scan shows delayed excretion of contrast material into the left renal calyces and into the dilated left renal pelvis (arrow).

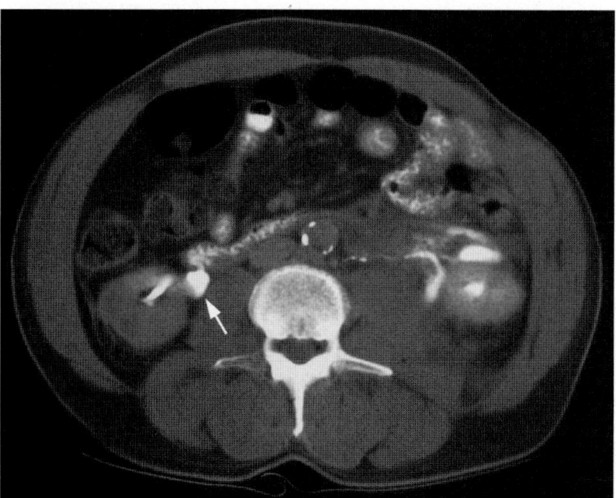

Figure 10. Axial image caudal to the L4-L5 level shows contrast material in the right ureter (arrow) but no contrast-filled left ureter.

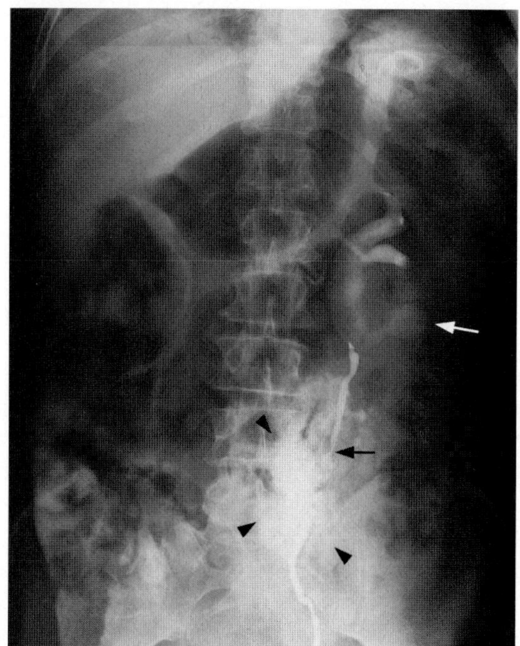

Figure 11. Retrograde ureterogram shows disruption of the contrast-filled ureter at the L4-L5 level (black arrow), and adjacent extensive extravasation of contrast material (arrowheads). Note also the distended left renal pelvis and lower pole calyx (white arrow).

The delayed CT scan reveals extensive extravasation of contrast material in the left retroperitoneal space **(Fig. 8)** and delayed filling of the dilated left renal pelvis with contrast material **(Fig. 9)**; however, no contrast-filled ureter is seen on the left caudal to the L4-L5 level **(Fig. 10)**.

A retrograde ureterogram performed via cystoscopy showed disruption of the left ureter with extravasation of contrast material into surrounding tissues **(Fig. 11)**. Multiple cystoscopic attempts to cross the disruption with a wire were unsuccessful.

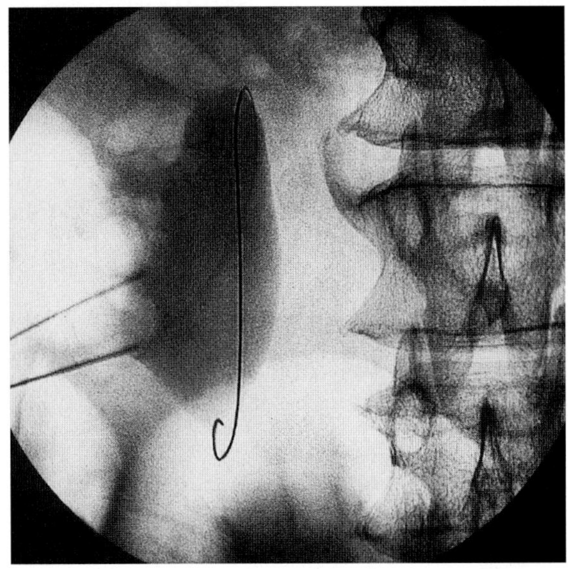

Figure 12. Prone digital image demonstrates the needle and fine wire access into the left renal pelvis.

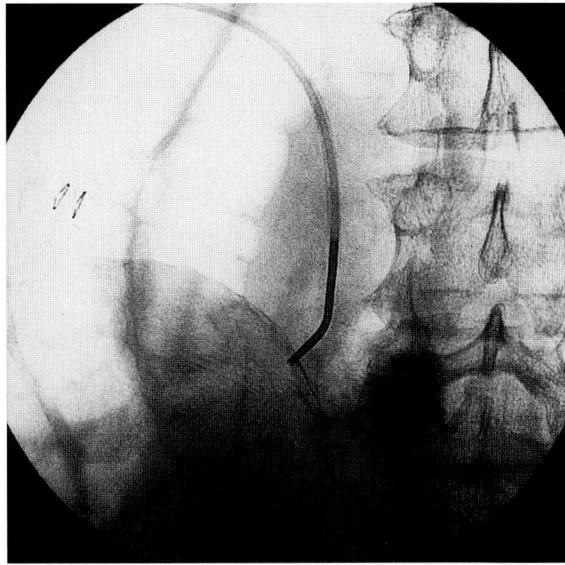

Figure 13. Digital image shows the curved catheter within the sheath traversing the ureter.

Diagnosis

Nearly complete ureteral transection due to inadvertent injury at the time of percutaneous discectomy.

What treatment can you offer?

Management

The renal pelvis was accessed with use of a 21-gauge needle and an 0.018-inch wire **(Fig. 12)**. A sheath-dilator set was then inserted, allowing placement of a thicker wire, over which an anchoring sheath was deployed into a lower pole calyx to provide stable access to the renal pelvis. A gently curved 5-F catheter was then threaded through the sheath **(Fig. 13)** and contrast material was injected directly into the distal ureter **(Fig. 14)**.

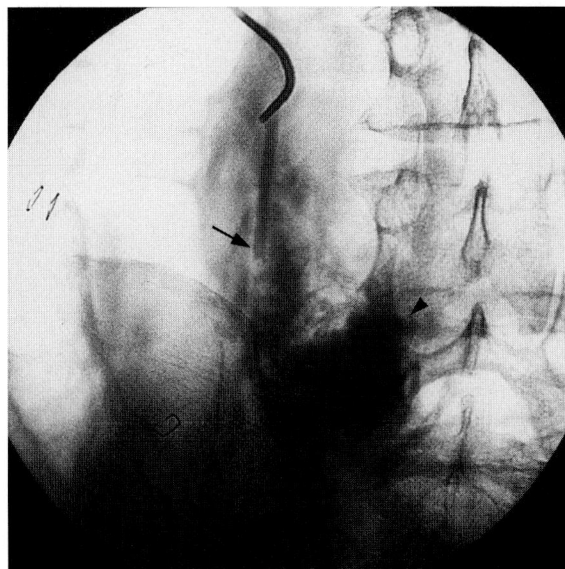

Figure 14. Injection of contrast material through the catheter in the left ureter shows abrupt cut-off of the contrast column (arrow) and extravasation (arrowhead) at the L4-L5 level.

Roadmapping was used to visualize both the ureter and the wire. The nearly completely transected ureter was then crossed with an 0.035-inch hydrophilic-coated, highly torquable wire. The wire and catheter were then passed through the distal ureter and into the urinary bladder **(Fig. 15)**. The wire was exchanged for a stiff wire, providing secure access to the bladder.

An 8-F nephroureterostomy tube was placed with the tip in the bladder, the side-holes in the renal pelvis, and the proximal end extending through the skin in the flank **(Figs. 16–18)**. The tube was left to external drainage for 4 days and then capped, providing internal drainage only.

What would be your next plan of action?

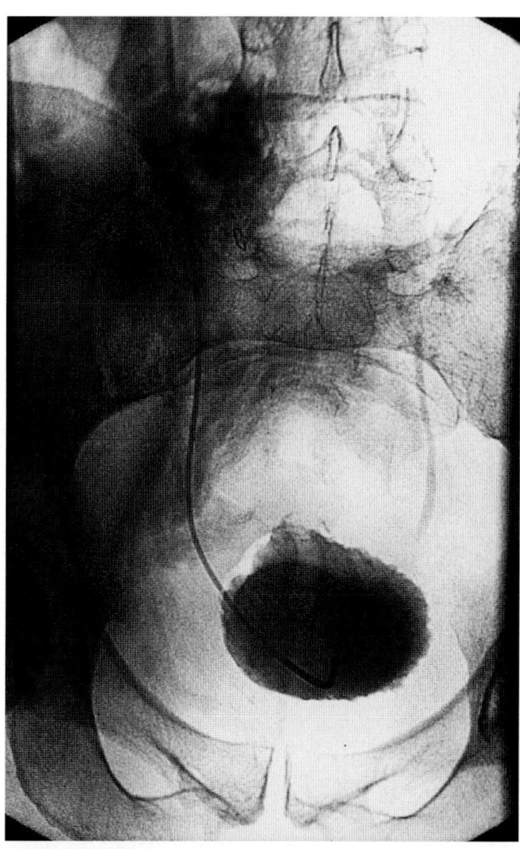

Figure 15. Prone digital image shows the curved catheter and wire positioned across the ureteral tear with their distal tips in the contrast-filled bladder.

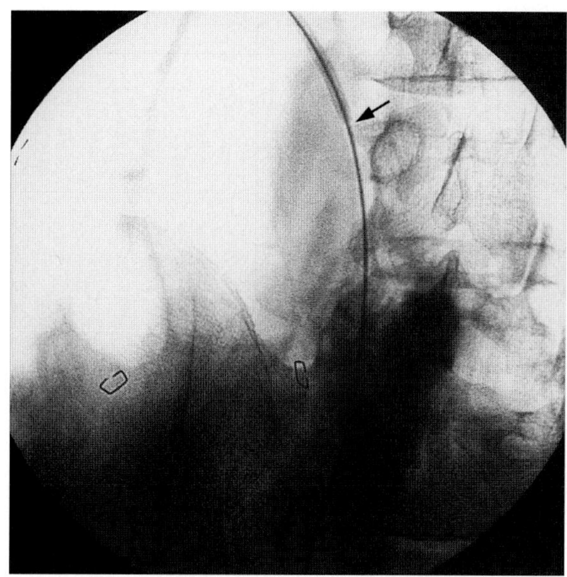

Figure 16. Prone digital image shows the nephroureteral tube (arrow) being advanced along the stiff wire through the ureter.

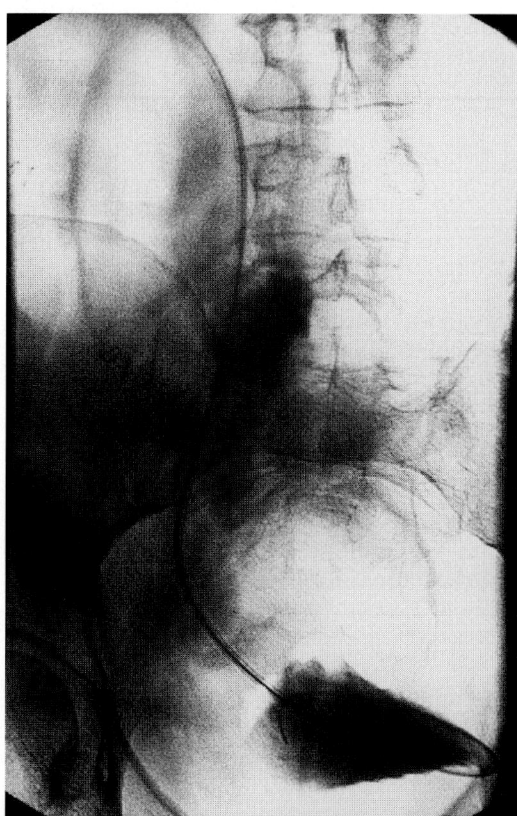

Figure 17. Prone digital image shows the nephroureteral tube being advanced along the stiff wire through the ureter.

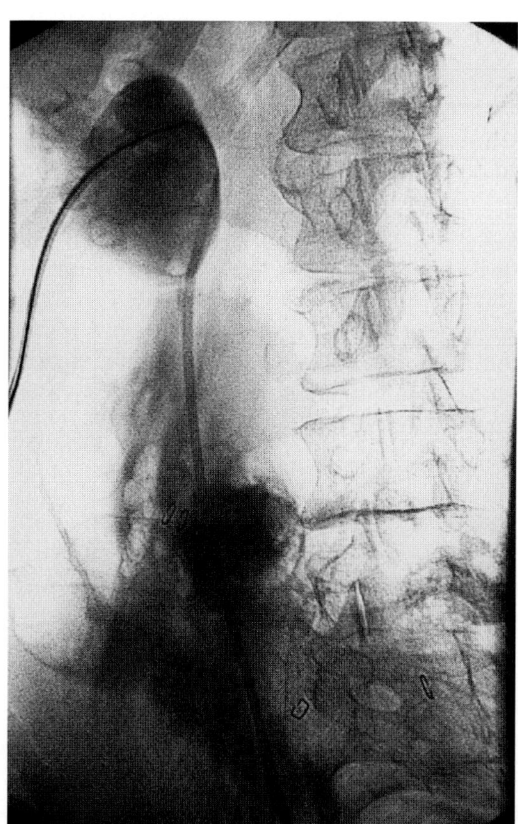

Figure 18. Prone digital image demonstrates withdrawal of the stiff wire from the tube.

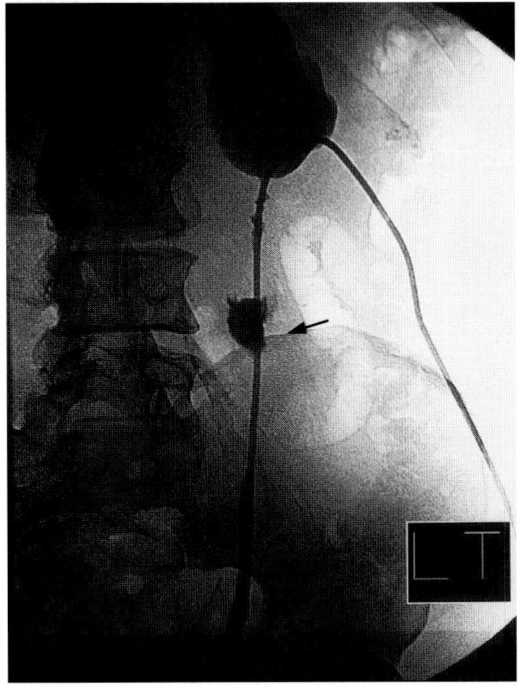

Figure 19. Nephrostogram performed 4 weeks after the injury demonstrates a less extensive focus of extravasation (arrow).

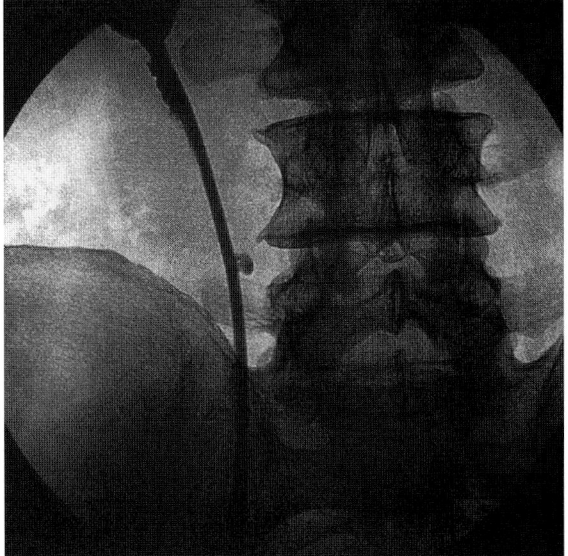

Figure 20. Nephrostogram performed 6 weeks after the injury reveals minimal extravasation of contrast material.

Four weeks later the nephroureterostomy tube was injected with contrast material. A much smaller but still significant area of extravasation was demonstrated at the site of injury **(Fig. 19)**, so the nephroureterostomy tube was left in place.

Six weeks after the injury, injection of the tube revealed only a minimal focus of extravasation **(Fig. 20)**. At this time a wire was passed through the tube into the bladder and the tube was removed. A double-J internal ureteral stent was then advanced over the wire and into the ureter. A week later the nephrostomy tube was removed **(Fig. 21)**, leaving the patient with no external tube. The ureteral stent was later removed via cystoscopy when there was no further extravasation of contrast material from the ureter.

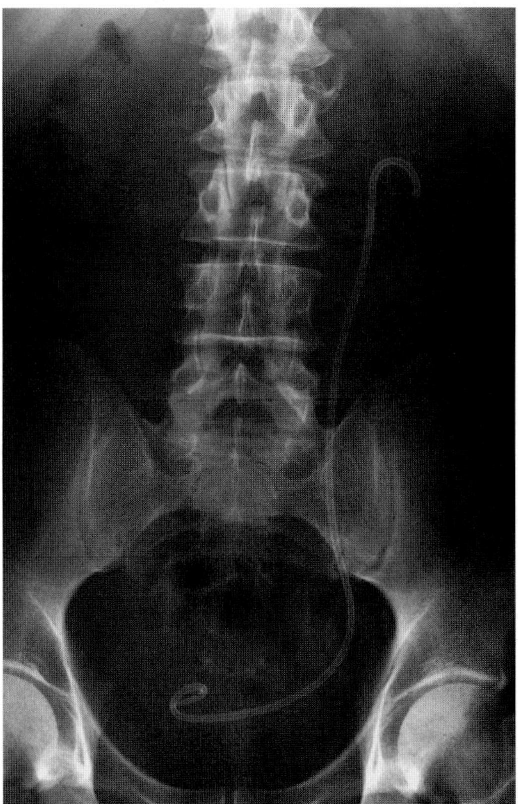

Figure 21. Supine radiograph demonstrates the internal double-J ureteral stent following removal of the external drainage tube.

Discussion

Ureteral injury is more commonly caused by penetrating wounds (especially gunshot wounds) rather than blunt trauma. An important cause of ureteral injury is iatrogenic trauma, particularly during gynecologic surgery. Ureteral trauma, unfortunately, is difficult to diagnose acutely, and delay in diagnosis occurs in approximately one third of trauma cases. This is thought to be due to associated life-threatening injuries and the low index of suspicion. More than 90% of ureteral injuries are associated with injuries of other organ systems and these are often serious, because the mechanism required to produce a ureteral injury is either a gunshot or stab wound or severe blunt trauma.

Signs and symptoms are often absent or nonspecific. Hematuria is only present in two thirds of patients, and is usually microscopic. Furthermore, preoperative radiologic studies often fail to demonstrate ureteral injuries. CT scanning and intravenous pyelography each prospectively demonstrate only approximately one third of such injuries. Suggestive findings include adjacent lumbar vertebral body injuries, ureteral deviation or dilatation, bladder displacement, and nonvisualization of the contrast-filled ureter below the level of the disruption. Delayed images are helpful in demonstrating extravasation of contrast material but are not routinely obtained in the trauma setting.

For ureteral injury or surgery, the stent is important for two reasons. First, it provides urinary diversion, preventing the formation of urinomas which cause periureteral scarring, stricture, and fistula formation. Second, the stent provides a mold or scaffold for ureteral epithelialization, making stricture formation less likely.

Encrustation with salts may occur with stents placed for long periods and may cause occlusion of the stent. Encrustation can be prevented by keeping the urine dilute and promptly treating urinary infections, particularly those caused by urea-splitting organisms. Patency of the stent can be assessed by cystography or duplex sonography. A functioning stent is expected to freely reflux on cystography, and absence of free reflux is an indication for stent exchange.

The duration of ureteral stent placement depends on the indication. If placed for malignant obstruction, the stent remains for the duration of the illness, usually the rest of the patient's life. It should be exchanged every 6 months via a retrograde approach. If placed for ureteral trauma, duration depends on the severity of the injury. As a guideline, if the ureter was not disrupted but merely manipulated, causing edema, then 3–5 days of stent placement is adequate. For a routine surgical anastomosis, 10–15 days is adequate, but twice that period should be considered if the anastomosis is at risk. A stent placed across a leak should be left in place for 35–45 days.

Selected Readings

Campbell EW Jr, Filderman PS, Jacobs SC. Ureteral injury due to blunt and penetrating trauma. Urology 1992; 40:216–220.

Faubert C, Caspar W. Lumbar percutaneous discectomy: initial experience in 28 cases. Neuroradiology 1991; 33:407–410.

Guerriero WG. Ureteral injury. Urol Clin North Am 1989; 16:237–248.

Kadir S, ed. Current practice of interventional radiology. St. Louis: Mosby Year Book, 1991.

Lang EK, Glorioso L III. Management of urinomas by percutaneous drainage procedures. Radiol Clin North Am 1986; 24:551–559.

Maroon JC, Onik G, Sternau L. Percutaneous automated discectomy: a new approach to lumbar surgery. Clin Orthop 1989; 238:64–70.

Mitty HA, Train JS, Dan SJ. Placement of ureteral stents by antegrade and retrograde techniques. Radiol Clin North Am 1986; 24:587–600.

Platt JF, Ellis JH, Rubin JM. Assessment of internal ureteral stent patency in patients with pyelocaliectasis: value of renal duplex sonography. AJR 1993; 161:87–90.

Townsend M, DeFalco AJ. Absence of ureteral opacification below ureteral disruption: a sentinel CT finding. AJR 1995; 164:253–254.

Uflacker R, Wholey M. Interventional radiology. New York: McGraw-Hill, Inc., 1991; 501–535.

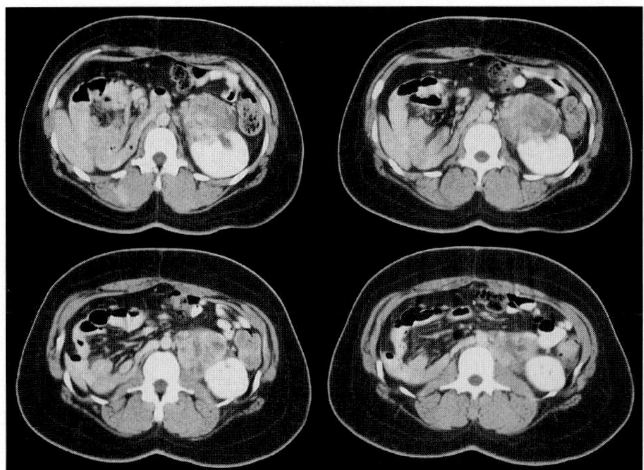

Figure 1. Contrast-enhanced CT scan.

TEACHING FILE CASE 44

Hector Ferral, M.D., and
Michael Wholey, M.D.

History

The patient is a 30-year-old woman with a history of retroperitoneal sarcoma who had previously undergone resection of the right kidney secondary to tumor invasion. She came to the hospital with severe back pain, malaise, and declining renal function as shown by elevated creatinine (5.0 mg/dL) and decreased urinary output. A computed tomography (CT) scan was obtained **(Fig. 1)**.

What is your diagnosis?

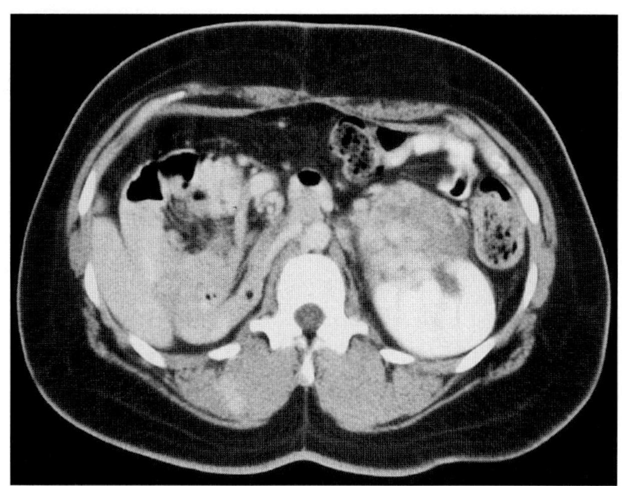

Figure 2. Selected image from Figure 1. The CT scan shows minimal hydronephrosis of the left kidney and a large mass compressing the collecting system and ureter.

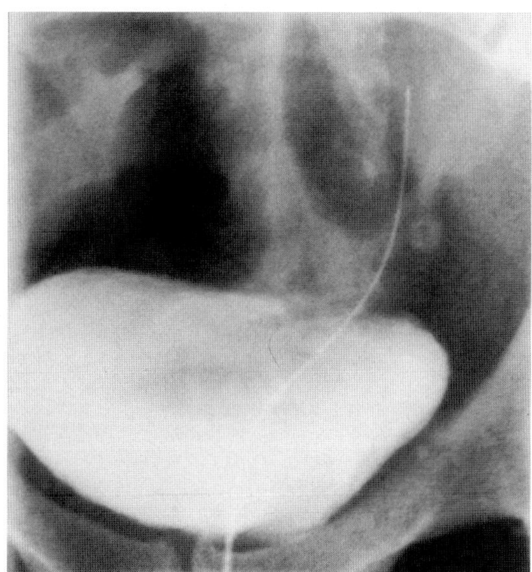

Figure 3. Fluoroscopic image shows a catheter and wire entering the left ureter.

Radiographic Findings

A CT scan showed a large heterogeneous mass in the anterior pararenal space. The mass displaces the kidney posterolaterally and compresses the renal pelvis. Despite ureteral obstruction, only minimal hydronephrosis is present, due to compression of the renal pelvis by the mass **(Fig. 2)**. An ultrasound (not available) showed segmental dilatation of the left collecting system with compression of the renal pelvis by tumor.

Diagnosis

Extrinsic compression of the left renal pelvis by recurrent tumor with minimal dilatation of the collecting system.

Management

Retrograde catheterization of the left ureter for double-J stent placement was attempted by the urologists without success. Percutaneous nephrostomy tube placement was then requested to decompress the obstructed left collecting system. However, the collecting system could not be opacified secondary to tumor compression, and percutaneous nephrostomy tube placement was not attempted.

The patient was subsequently placed in a supine position and a Council-tip catheter was inserted into the bladder. The catheter was then removed over a guide wire. With use of a 5-F JB1 catheter and a Glidewire (Terumo, Medi-Tech, Natick, MA), retrograde catheterization of the ureter was performed under fluoroscopic guidance only. The bladder was approximately three quarters full when the ureter was selected **(Fig. 3)**.

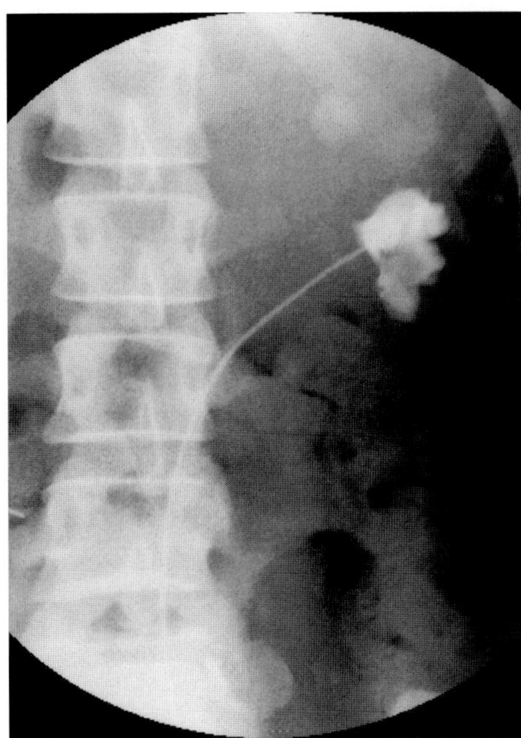

Figure 4. Fluoroscopic image shows the diagnostic catheter in the renal pelvis.

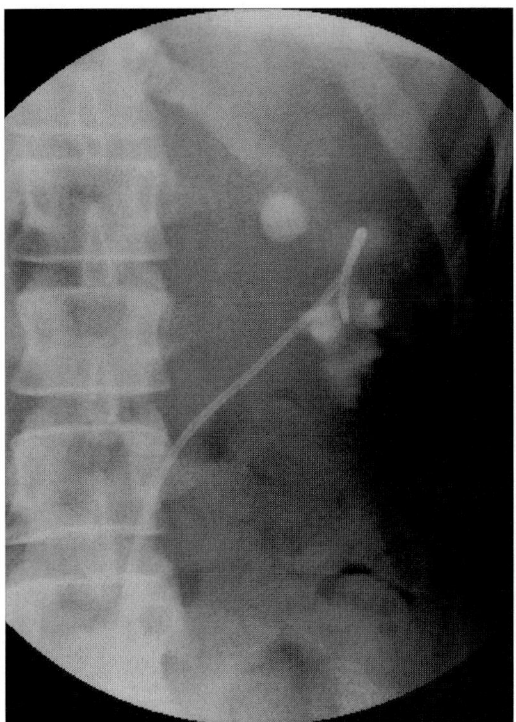

Figure 5. Fluoroscopic image of the renal pelvis shows that the diagnostic catheter has been exchanged for a double-J catheter.

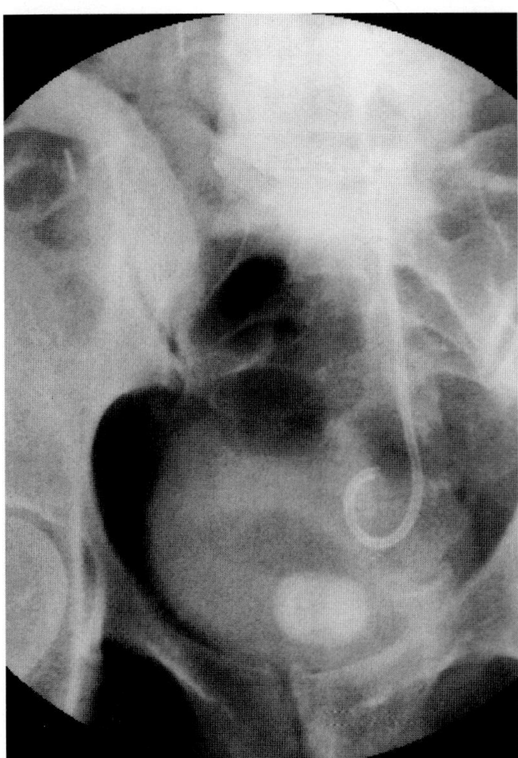

Figure 6. Fluoroscopic image of the double-J catheter in the bladder.

Once the ureter was selected, the catheter and wire were carefully advanced up the ureter and into the renal pelvis **(Fig. 4)**. Contrast material was injected to confirm catheter position within the renal pelvis **(Fig. 5)**. The Glidewire was exchanged for an 0.035-inch Amplatz Super Stiff guide wire (Medi-Tech). An 8-F, 24-cm double-J catheter was advanced over the guide wire. Adequate position of the double-J catheter was confirmed and the catheter was deployed with use of the usual technique **(Fig. 6)**.

Discussion

Fluoroscopically directed retrograde catheter placement into the distal ureter without cystoscopic assistance is a relatively new technique described by Babel and Winterkorn. Retrograde catheterization of the ureter was attempted in this case because of difficulty placing a percutaneous nephrostomy tube secondary to the massive renal pelvis compression induced by the tumor. This is a safe technique with minimal risk or discomfort to the patient.

The ureter is catheterized under fluoroscopic guidance without the use of cystoscopic visualization by probing the expected location of the ureteral orifice along the posterior lateral bladder wall near the bladder trigone. Once the catheter engages the ureteral orifice (with use of standard vessel selection probing techniques), a Glidewire can be used to gently probe the distal ureter. Microadvancement of the catheter followed by injection of contrast material can be done to confirm catheter placement in the ureter and not the bladder wall. Once the catheter is clearly in the ureter, routine catheter and wire techniques can be used to gain access to the renal pelvis.

This technique may be useful in similar cases where percutaneous nephrostomy tube placement for collecting system decompression is difficult or contraindicated due to coagulopathy or other concomitant medical problems. The use of a Glidewire and angiographic catheter greatly helps to negotiate the stenotic or tortuous areas of the ureter.

Selected Reading

Babel SG, Winterkorn KG. Retrograde catheterization of the ureter without cystoscopic assistance: preliminary experience. Radiology 1993; 187:547–549.

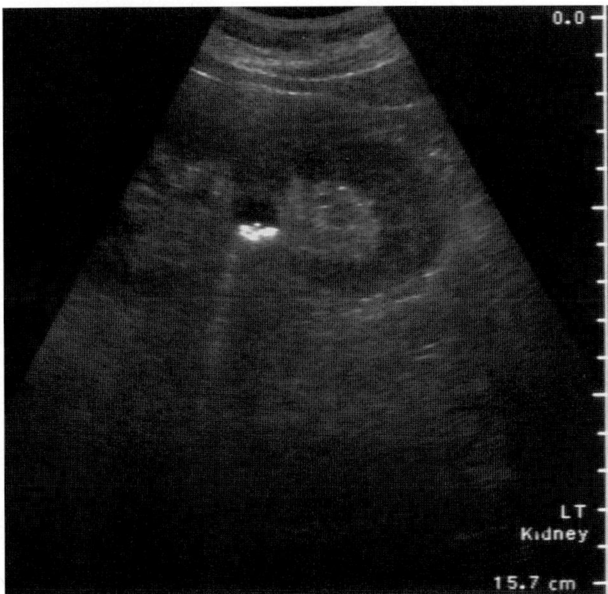

Figure 1. Longitudinal sonogram of the left kidney.

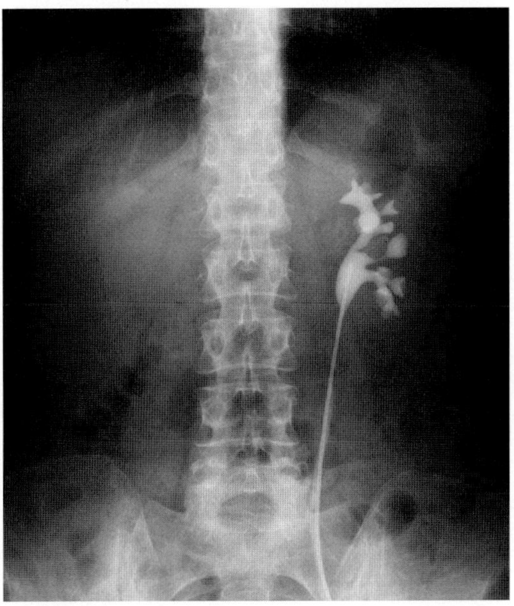
Figure 2. Retrograde ureterogram of the left kidney, at contrast run-in.

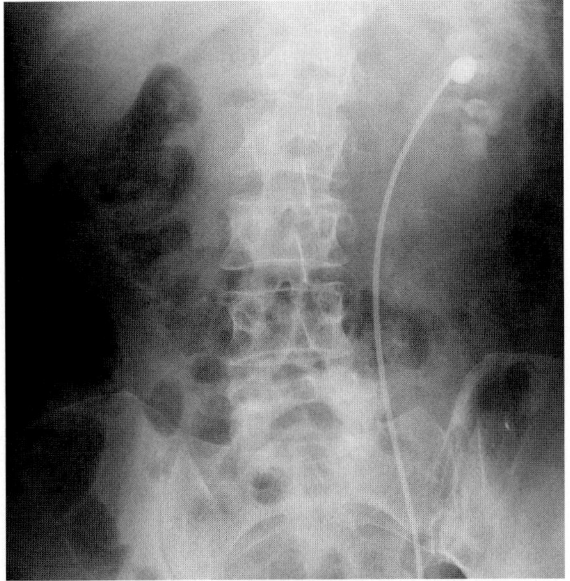
Figure 3. Retrograde ureterogram, after contrast material has drained from the collecting system.

TEACHING FILE CASE 45

Allen J. Meglin, M.D., Stephen J. Brown, M.D., and Ellen M. Chung, M.D.

History

A 52-year-old woman with a neurogenic bladder and a history of multiple upper urinary tract infections and calculi came to the hospital with a 1-day history of flank pain and fever. A sonogram was obtained **(Fig. 1)**. The patient then underwent retrograde ureterography **(Figs. 2, 3)**.

What is your diagnosis?

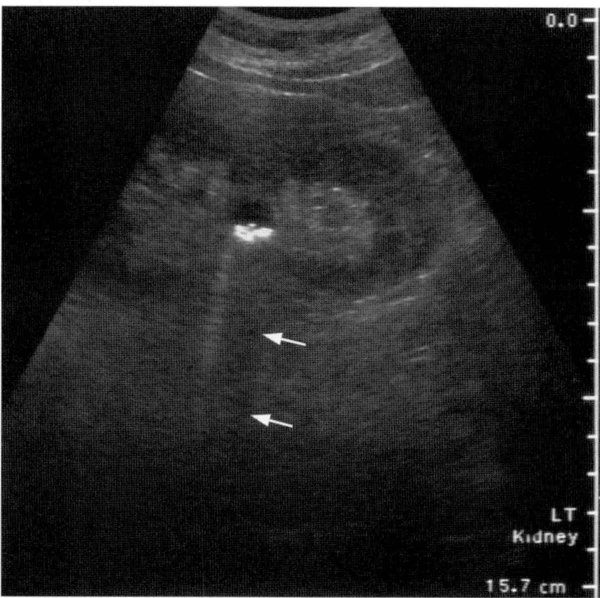

Figure 4. Ultrasound shows an echogenic focus with posterior shadowing (arrows).

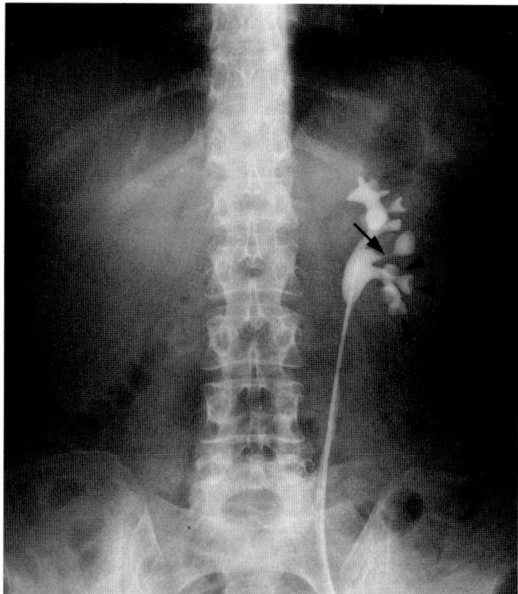

Figure 5. Retrograde ureterogram shows contrast material filling the interpolar calyx with narrowed infundibulum (arrow). Note the three minor calyces in the lower pole (arrowheads).

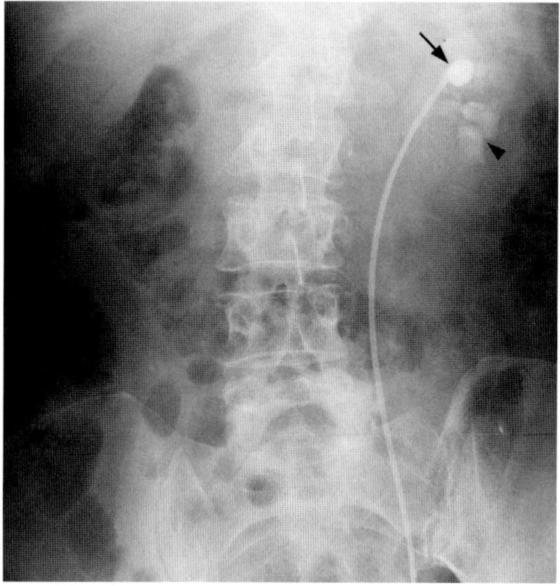

Figure 6. Delayed image shows retention of contrast material in the three lower pole minor calyces (arrowhead). There is now filling of an interpolar diverticulum (arrow). No calculi are seen.

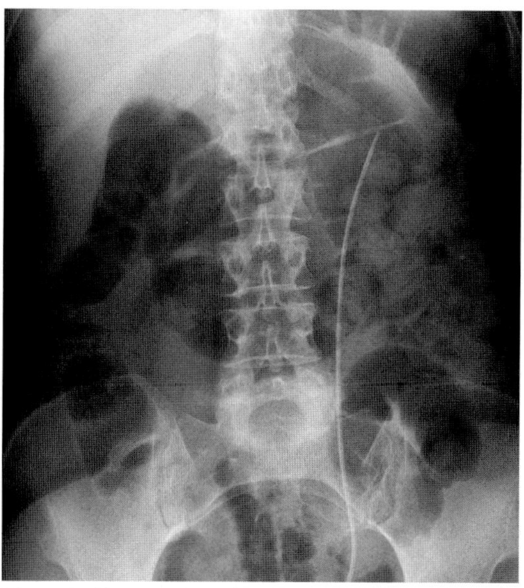

Figure 7. Retrograde catheter placed.

Radiographic Findings

The sonogram shows stones in the interpolar region of the left kidney **(Fig. 4)**. The calculi were small and radiolucent and therefore not evident on the subsequent retrograde ureterogram (RU). Early and late RU images show filling of the calyces, with retention of contrast material in a calyceal diverticulum **(Figs. 5, 6)**.

Diagnosis

Left interpolar region calyceal diverticulum containing radiolucent calculi.

How would you manage this patient?

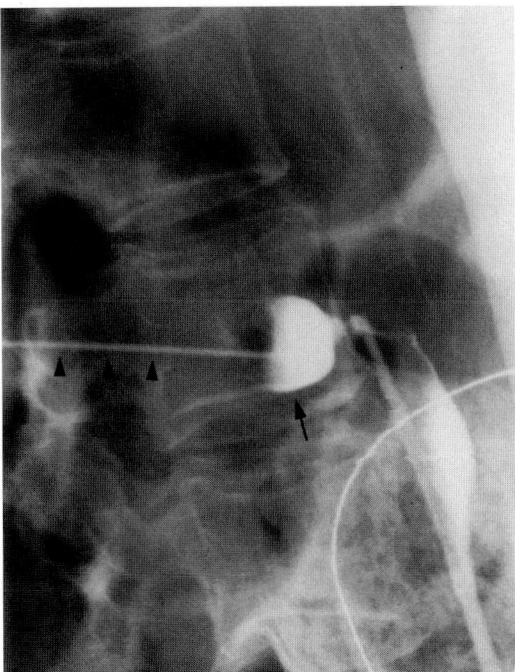

Figure 8. Lateral view with the patient in the prone position. Air and contrast material in the renal pelvis. A needle (arrowheads) was placed from the posterior aspect of the patient into the calyceal diverticulum (arrow).

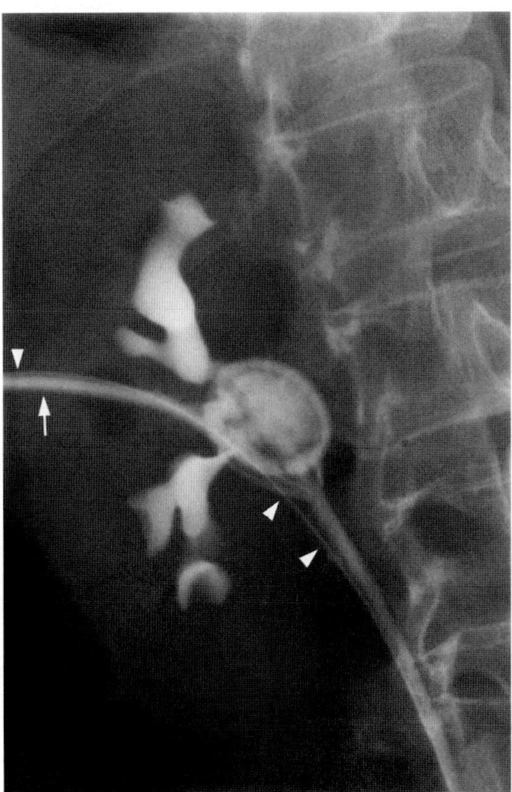

Figure 9. Guide wire (arrowheads) and catheter (arrow) placed through the neck of the diverticulum into the renal pelvis.

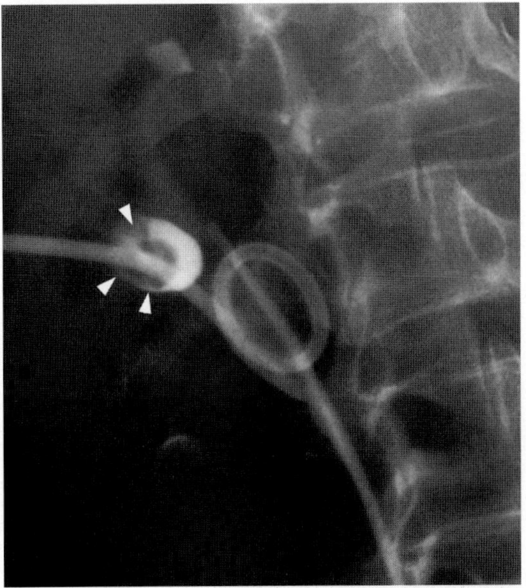

Figure 10. Stones (arrowheads) appear as filling defects in the contrast material in the diverticulum, posterior to the drainage catheter.

Management

Two attempts at extracorporeal shock wave lithotripsy (ESWL) were unsuccessful. Flexible ureteroscopy was unsuccessful in gaining access to the diverticulum. The patient underwent percutaneous nephrostomy after retrograde placement of a ureteral catheter **(Fig. 7)**. Air and contrast material were injected into the renal pelvis from a ureteral catheter, and a 21-gauge diamond-tipped needle was used to directly access the diverticulum under fluoroscopic guidance **(Fig. 8)**. A guide wire and an 8-F catheter were placed through the diverticulum into the renal pelvis **(Fig. 9)**. A completion radiograph showed contrast material and a filling defect (the stones) in the diverticulum **(Fig. 10)**.

Discussion

Percutaneous nephrostomy was performed with the goal of externalizing the diverticulum or reconnecting it sufficiently to the renal pelvis. The diverticulum was accessed directly in this case. Percutaneous nephrostomy to decompress the collecting system and allow for resolution of infection can be safely performed on an outpatient basis. Once this is accomplished, subsequent nephrolithotomy for larger stones or simple percutaneous extraction of small stones with or without diverticular ablation can be undertaken.

This case demonstrates stones in a calyceal diverticulum in a patient with a neurogenic bladder and a 1-day history of fever. Calyceal diverticula are partially excluded from the collecting system. The stone is a foreign body that may be seeded with bacteria and must be removed. ESWL is the treatment of choice for small uncomplicated stones. However, while it may be successful in fragmenting the stone, ESWL may not reduce the particle size sufficiently to allow the particle to pass through the narrow neck of the diverticulum, and stone reformation may occur. Flexible ureteroscopy with basket removal of stones less than 5 mm in diameter is an attractive approach, but this was not technically possible in this patient because of the diverticular stenosis which prevented retrograde access to the stones. If the stones were larger, ESWL may also have been an attractive option.

After the patient had been allowed to defervesce, the stones were removed via the percutaneous nephrostomy track with use of standard basket extraction techniques. Lithotripsy was not required because the stones were small and easily fragmented with basket techniques.

Selected Readings

Bellman GC, Silverstein JI, Blickensderfer S, Smith AD. Technique and follow-up of percutaneous management of calyceal diverticula. Urology 1993; 42:21–25.

Carr LK, Honey J, Jewett MA, Ibanez D, Ryan M, Bombardier C. New stone formation: a comparison of extracorporeal shock wave lithotripsy and percutaneous nephrolithotomy. J Urol 1996; 155:1565–1567.

Dretler SP. A new useful endourologic classification of calyceal diverticula. (Abstr). J Endourol 1992; (Suppl) 6:F–17.

Gray RR, So CB, McLoughlin RF, Pugash RA, Saliken JC, Macklin NI. Outpatient percutaneous nephrostomy. Radiology 1996; 198:85-88.

LeRoy AJ. Diagnosis and treatment of nephrolithiasis: current perspectives. AJR 1994; 163:1309–1313.

Sun BY, Lee YH, Jiaan BP, Chen KK, Chang LS, Chen KT. Recurrence rate and risk factors for urinary calculi after extracorporeal shock wave lithotripsy. J Urol 1996; 156:903–906.

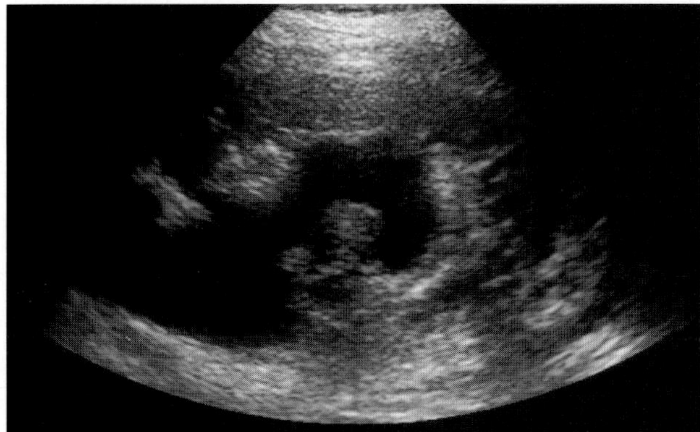

Figure 1. Longitudinal sonogram of the left kidney.

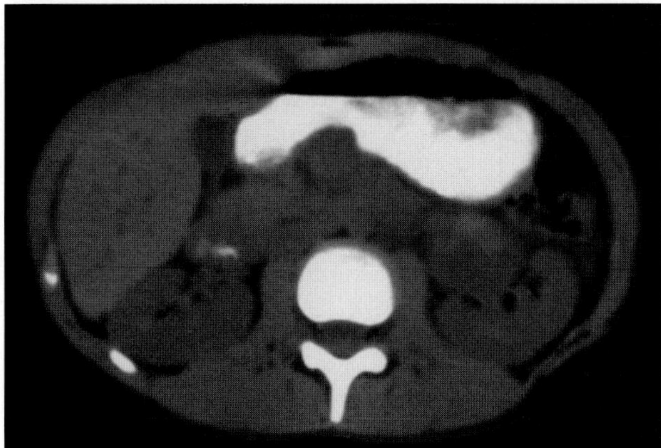

Figure 2. Noncontrast renal CT scan.

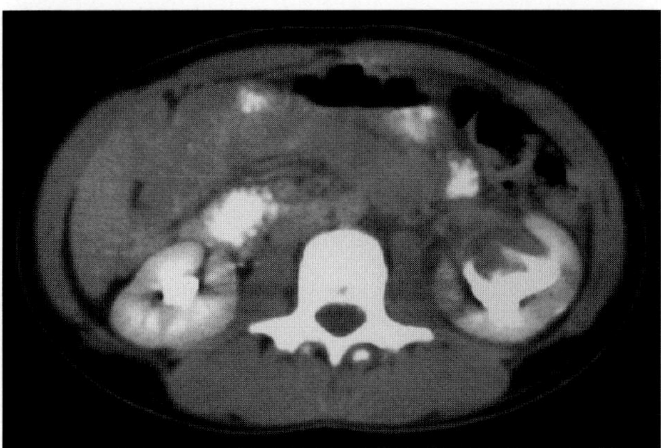

Figure 3. Contrast-enhanced renal CT scan.

TEACHING FILE CASE 46

Joseph A. Ronsivalle, D.O., and Dennis S. Peppas, M.D.

History

A 13-year-old girl with known asymptomatic left ureteropelvic junction (UPJ) obstruction came to the hospital with complaints of severe left flank pain after experiencing mild trauma. The pain was sudden in onset and was worsening progressively. Renal sonography **(Fig. 1)** and computed tomography (CT) scanning were performed **(Figs. 2, 3)**.

What is your diagnosis?

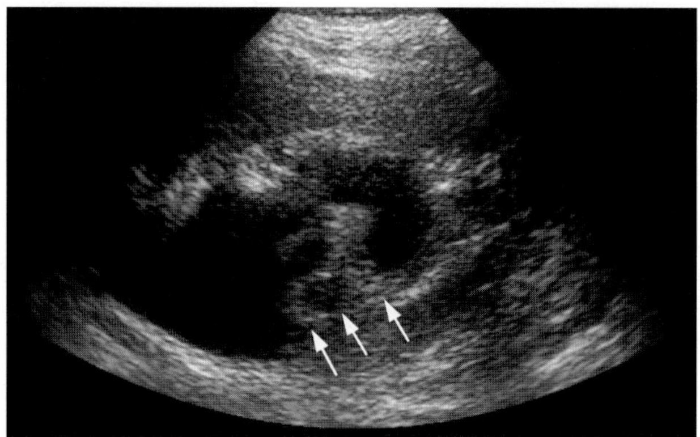

Figure 4. Longitudinal sonogram of the left kidney shows hydronephrosis. There is echogenic material within the collecting system (arrows).

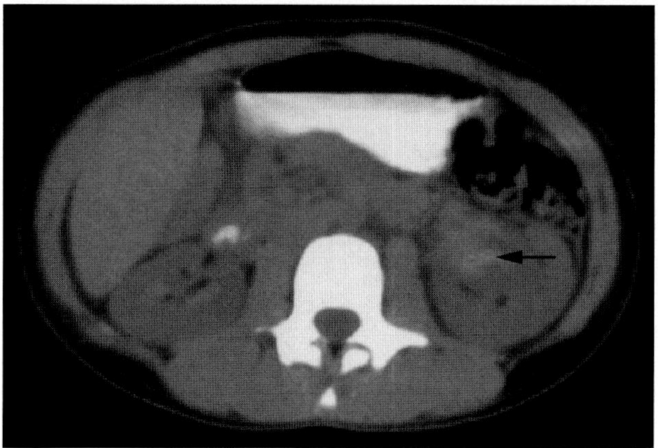

Figure 5. Noncontrast CT scan shows dilatation of the left collecting system and relatively hyperdense acute clot in the renal pelvis (arrow).

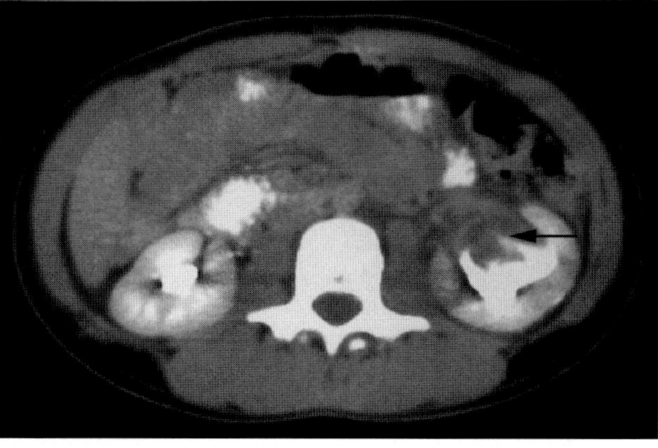

Figure 6. Contrast-enhanced CT scan shows a central filling defect in the renal pelvis due to the blood clot (arrow).

Radiographic Findings

The sonogram **(Fig. 4)** demonstrates a dilated left intrarenal collecting system with a central area of increased echoes within the renal pelvis. The noncontrast computed tomography scan **(Fig. 5)** similarly demonstrates a dilated intrarenal collecting system on the left with areas of increased attenuation centrally within the renal pelvis. The clot is acute and therefore relatively hyperdense with respect to urine in the collecting system. The contrast-enhanced scan **(Fig. 6)** demonstrates an opacified left intrarenal collecting system with a central filling defect within the renal pelvis.

Diagnoses

1. Thrombus within the left renal pelvis completely obstructing a pre-existing partial UPJ obstruction.
2. Rule out left UPJ disruption.

How would you manage this patient?

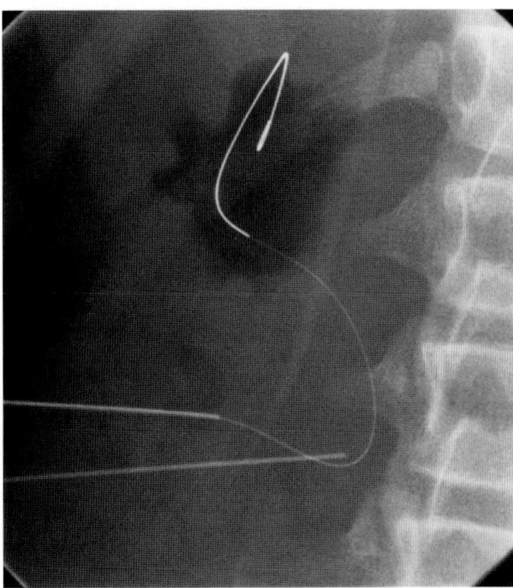

Figure 7. Fluoroscopic spot image shows two needles and a guide wire within the collecting system.

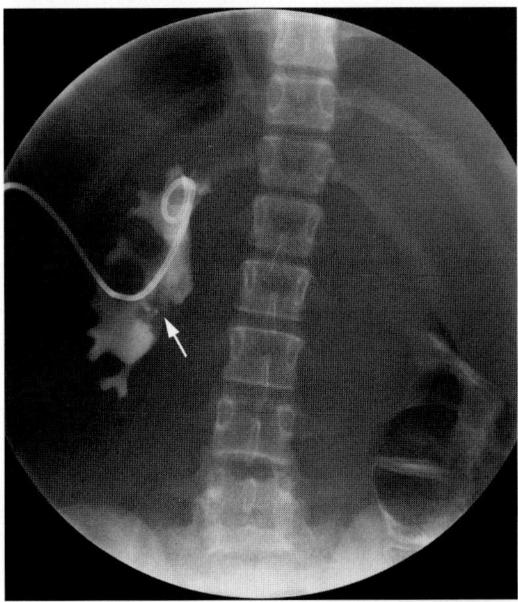

Figure 8. Fluoroscopic spot image after placement of nephrostomy catheter and instillation of contrast material. Arrow shows filling defect representing thrombus within the collecting system.

Management

The patient complained of progressive flank pain. A partial or complete avulsion in the area of the left UPJ could not be excluded on the basis of the CT scan alone. A Lasix renogram was obtained, again demonstrating UPJ obstruction but no definite urine leak. Given the acute setting with increasing clinical suspicion of urinary extravasation, a percutaneous nephrostomy tube was placed.

The percutaneous nephrostomy was performed using a double access technique. With the patient in the prone position, a 22-gauge Chiba needle was inserted into the renal pelvis and a small amount (1–3 mL) of room air was injected to fill the posterior nondependent calyces. A second 21-gauge needle was then inserted into a posterior inferior calyx **(Fig. 7)**. This track was subsequently dilated and a 10-F nephrostomy catheter was placed **(Fig. 8)**. The patient experienced immediate relief of pain after decompression of the collecting system. The nephrostomy tube was left in place for 3 months to allow sufficient time for inflammation and scarring to resolve.

A preoperative nephrostogram revealed marked left hydronephrosis, without passage of contrast material into the left ureter **(Fig. 9)**. The patient then underwent successful open pyeloplasty. At the time of pyeloplasty, she was noted to have a high ureteral insertion into her left renal pelvis and a crossing lower pole renal vessel, both of which contributed to obstruction at the UPJ. In addition, there was a significant amount of perirenal scarring, consistent with probable leakage of urine at the time of injury, despite the lack of definite extravasation on the imaging studies. On postoperative Lasix renography, there was no evidence of obstruction, with a post-Lasix half-life of 6 minutes.

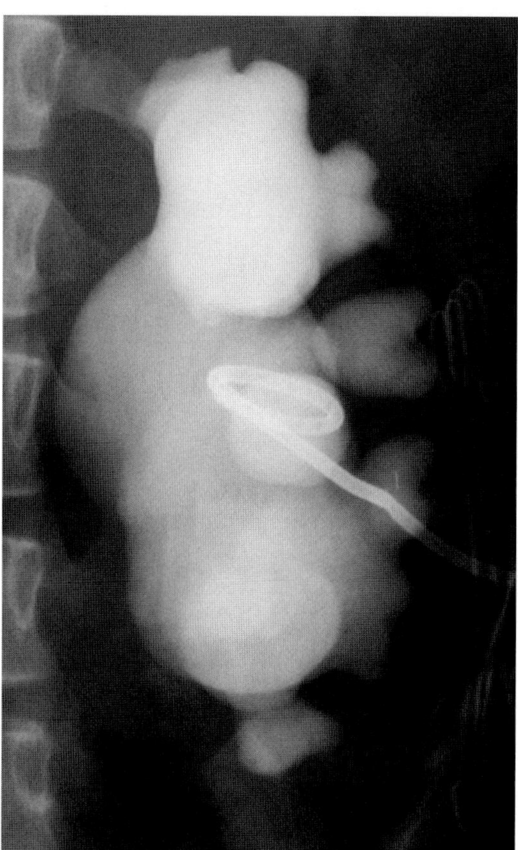

Figure 9. Delayed image from a preoperative antegrade nephrostogram demonstrates persistent hydronephrosis and no passage of contrast material into the left ureter.

Discussion

Hemorrhage after minor trauma is commonly seen in patients with congenital ureteropelvic junction obstruction. Most often the presenting symptoms are pain and hematuria. This patient experienced minor trauma and subsequently had severe left flank pain. Thrombus within the renal pelvis was diagnosed using multiple modalities including ultrasound and CT. The high density on CT scanning confirmed the acute nature of the clot. A relatively large-caliber nephrostomy tube was used to decrease the likelihood of the tube becoming obstructed by blood products. After decompression of the thrombus-filled collecting system with percutaneous nephrostomy there was immediate relief of symptoms. The definitive solution was surgical repair of the UPJ obstruction, which was subsequently performed.

UPJ obstruction is most often diagnosed perinatally during the evaluation of antenatal hydronephrosis. Since prenatal ultrasonography is not performed universally, a percentage of patients with UPJ obstruction will grow and thrive and perhaps never come to medical attention. Some patients are seen during late adolescence and adulthood for acute flank pain during times of increased urine output. The presentation of a UPJ obstruction following blunt abdominal trauma is a rare entity. Disruption of the UPJ is also an extremely rare event, with an acute deceleration/acceleration almost always being the mechanism of injury. Young people are the most common subset of the population to experience a disruption, representing over 50% of cases.

Additionally, although room air was safely used to visualize the collecting system in this case, the risk of air embolus suggests that CO_2 may be a better agent.

Selected Readings

Boone TB, Gilling PJ, Husmann DA. Ureteropelvic junction disruption following blunt abdominal trauma. J Urol 1993; 150:33–36.

Novik AC, Stremm SB. Surgery of the kidney. In: Walsh PC, Retik AB, Stamey TA, Vaughn ED, eds. Campbell's urology. 6th edition. Philadelphia: W.B. Saunders Company, 1992.

Palmer JM, Drago JR. Ureteral avulsion from non-penetrating trauma. J Urol 1981; 125:108–111.

Pfister RC, Yoder IC. Intrinsic diseases of the ureter. In: Taveras JM, Ferrucci JT, eds. Radiology: diagnosis, imaging, intervention. Philadelphia: J.B. Lippincott Company, 1986.

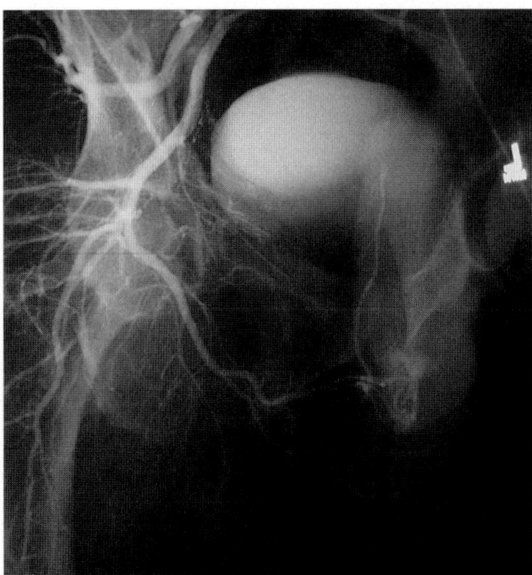

Figure 1. Selective right internal iliac arteriogram with use of nonionic contrast material.

TEACHING FILE CASE 47

Mark L. Lukens, M.D., and Allen J. Meglin, M.D.

History

A 35-year-old active duty soldier came to the hospital 7 weeks after sustaining straddle-type blunt trauma to the perineum from a fall in his jeep. Shortly after the injury he noticed partial tumescence and curvature of the penis to the left. Corporal aspiration and injection of epinephrine were performed and resulted in transient, 30-minute penile detumescence. Subsequent erections were persistent and not fully rigid. Penile arterial blood gas measurements had a high oxygen concentration, suggesting a "high-flow" or arterial abnormality. The patient was then referred for pelvic arteriography **(Fig. 1)**.

What is your diagnosis?

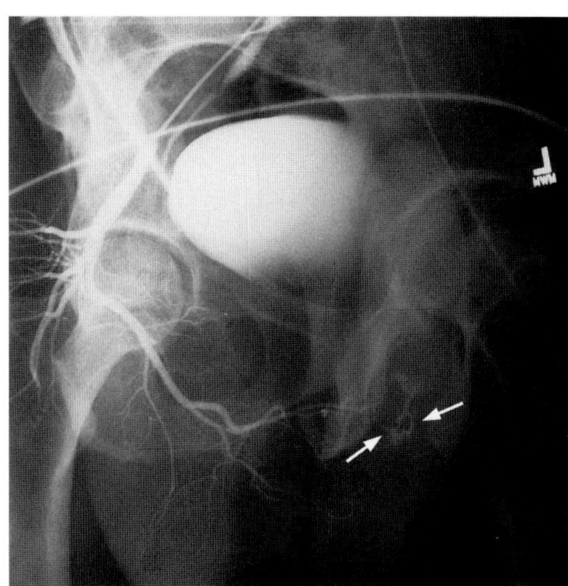

Figure 2. Arrows show filling of emissary veins and corpus cavernosum early in the arterial phase of internal iliac arteriography.

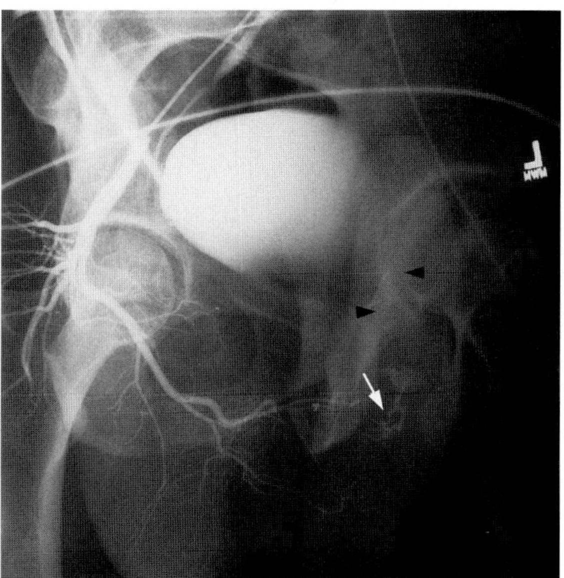

Figure 3. Arrow shows arteriovenous fistula of the right bulbourethral artery. The dorsal penile artery does not fill, secondary to shunting through the arteriovenous fistula (arrowheads).

Radiographic Findings

From a left (contralateral) common femoral approach, selective internal iliac arteriography was performed. There was evidence of filling of the right corpus cavernosum from the right bulbourethral artery **(Figs. 2, 3)**.

Diagnosis

Post-traumatic arteriovenous fistula of the right bulbourethral artery to the corpus cavernosum.

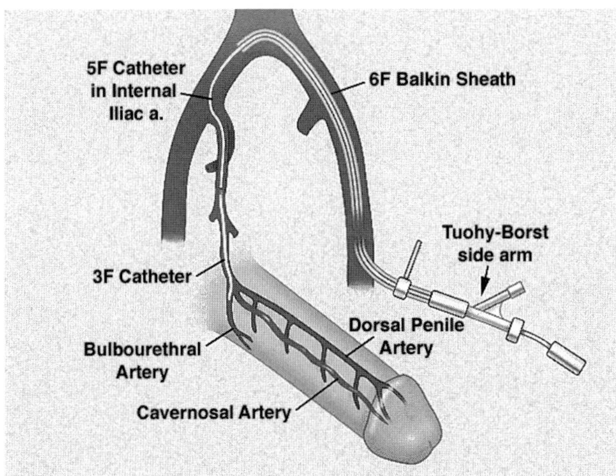

Figure 4. Triaxial system for embolization of the bulbourethral artery.

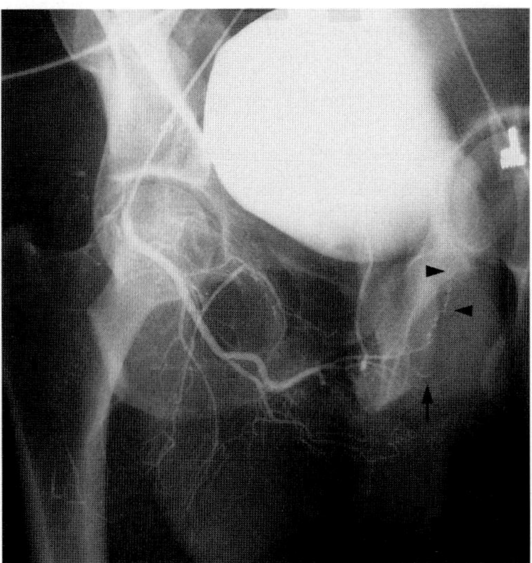

Figure 5. Postembolization arteriogram shows no evidence of persistent arteriovenous fistula. Arrow shows the area of prior fistula. Note the patent distal dorsal penile artery (arrowheads).

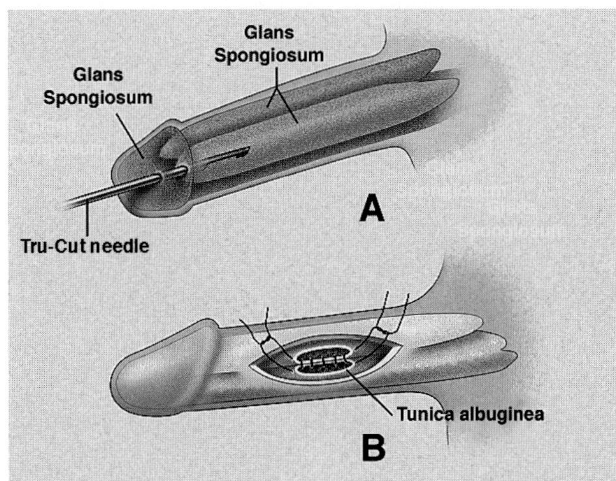

Figure 6. A. Tru-Cut needle being used to create a surgical shunt from the glans spongiosum to the corpus cavernosum. B. Creation of a surgical shunt from the cavernosum to the spongiosum in the shaft of the penis.

Management

Following identification of the arteriovenous fistula, a triaxial system consisting of a Balkin sheath (Cook, Bloomington, IN), a 5-F straight catheter, and a 3-F microcatheter was used to gain access to the internal pudendal artery from the contralateral groin. Distal vessel selection was performed by advancing the 3-F catheter directly into the right bulbourethral artery **(Fig. 4)**. Gelfoam slurry (Upjohn, Kalamazoo, MI) was then used to embolize the artery. Follow-up arteriography showed a normal dorsal penile artery and disappearance of the arteriovenous fistula. There was no evidence of emissary vein or corporal filling **(Fig. 5)**. There was significant detumescence after embolotherapy without subsequent loss of the ability to achieve an erection.

Discussion

Priapism is defined as prolonged, painful erection unrelated to sexual stimulation. Priapism is idiopathic in up to 50% of cases and is usually related to venous outflow obstruction. Other causes include sickle cell disease and traumatic and iatrogenic injury.

Rarely, priapism is caused by increased arterial blood flow. Initial treatment consists of spinal anesthesia followed by aspiration and irrigation of the corpus cavernosum. If these measures are unsuccessful, surgical shunting can be performed for venous outflow abnormalities **(Fig. 6)**.

In the past, high-flow priapism was treated by ligation of one or both internal pudendal arteries. Although successful, this treatment was associated with impotence and gangrene.

Recently, transcatheter techniques aimed at reducing the arterial blood flow have been utilized to treat high-flow priapism with good results. Occlusion should be temporary to afford both healing of the abnormality and recanalization to preserve potency. Gelfoam was used in this case to temporarily decrease flow through the arteriovenous fistula. As a temporary agent, it allows return of normal flow to the penis within 5 to 7 days. Early, accurate diagnosis of high-flow priapism can obviate the need for a surgical shunt and may result in complete healing without penile damage.

Selected Readings

Cosgrove MD, LaRocque MA. Shunt surgery for priapism: review of results. Urology 1974; 4:1–5.

Crummy AB, Ishizuka H, Madsen PO. Post-traumatic priapism: successful treatment with autologous clot embolization. AJR 1979; 133:329–330.

LaRocque MA, Cosgrove MD. Priapism: a review of 46 cases. J Urol 1974; 112:770–773.

Ji MX, He NS, Wang P, Chen G. Use of selective embolization of the bilateral cavernous arteries for post-traumatic arterial priapism. J Urol 1994; 151:1641–1642.

Puppo P, Belgrano E, Germinale F, Bottino P, Giuliani L. Angiographic treatment of high-flow priapism. Eur Urol 1985; 11:397–400.

Ravi R, Baijal SS, Roy S. Embolotherapy of priapism. Arch Esp Urol 1992; 45:587–588.

Walker TG, Grant PW, Goldstein I, Krane RJ, Greenfield AJ. "High-flow" priapism: treatment with superselective transcatheter embolization. Radiology 1990; 174:1053–1054.

Wasmer JM, Carrion HM, Mekras G, Politano VA. Evaluation and treatment of priapism. J Urol 1981; 125:204–207.

Wear JB Jr, Crummy AB, Munson BO. A new approach to the treatment of priapism. J Urol 1977; 117:252–254.

Winter CC. Cure of idiopathic priapism: new procedure for creating fistula between glans penis and corpora cavernosa. Urology 1976; 8:389–391.

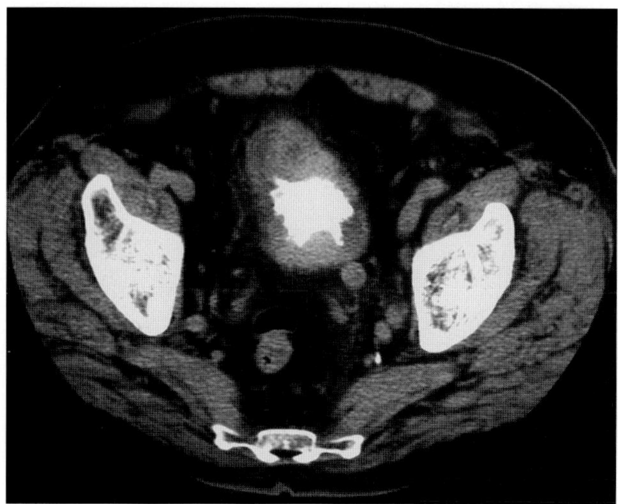

Figure 1. Contrast-enhanced computed tomography (CT) scan of the pelvis, at the level of the urinary bladder.

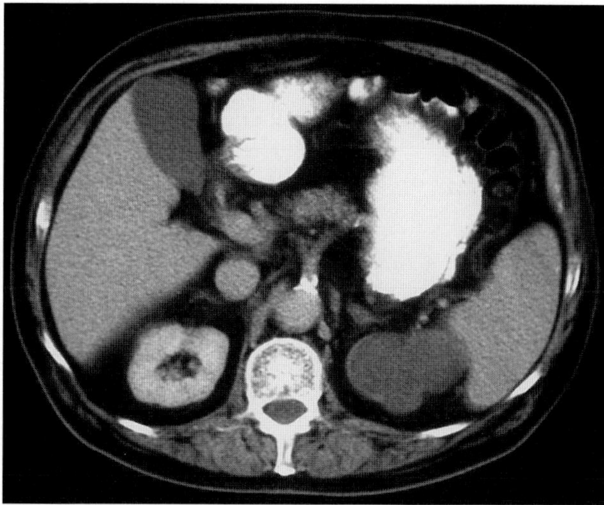

Figure 2. Noncontrast CT scan through the kidneys.

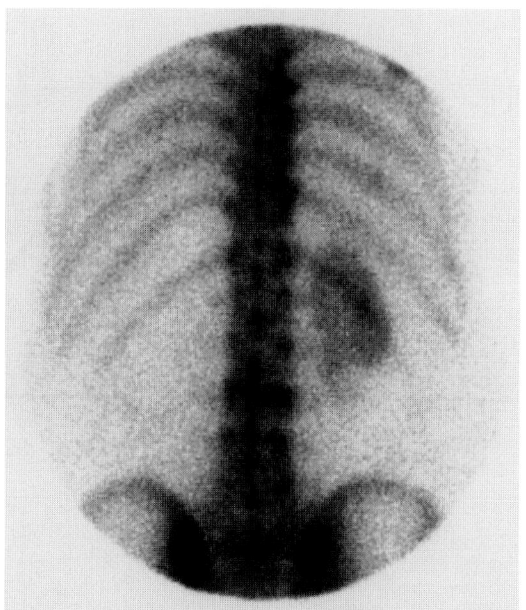

Figure 3. Posterior image from a bone scan.

TEACHING FILE CASE 48

Robert T. Andrews, M.D.

History

A 68-year-old man was referred by his urologist with a complaint of intractable bladder pain, which was exacerbated by even minimal bladder filling. The presence of urine, and even the balloon of a Foley catheter, were unbearable to the patient. Other medical problems included severe angina, a left ventricular ejection fraction of 40%, and a large aortic aneurysm. The patient underwent noncontrast and contrast-enhanced (CT) computed tomography scans of the abdomen and pelvis **(Figs. 1, 2)**, as well as a bone scan **(Fig. 3)**.

What is your diagnosis?

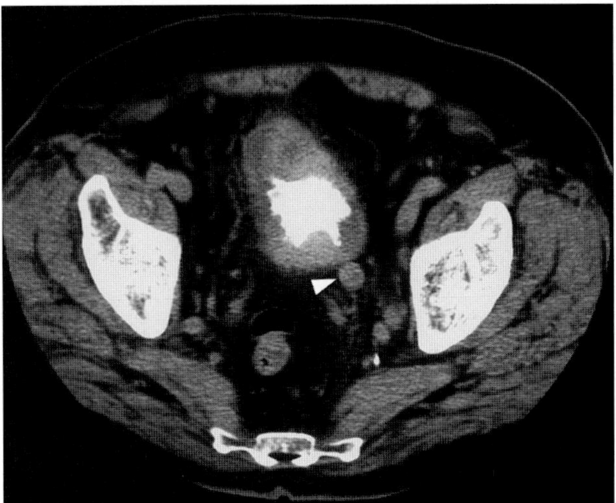

Figure 4. CT scan shows that the bladder wall is thickened and irregular. The perivesical fat is infiltrated, and pathologic retrovesical dilatation of the ureter is present (arrowhead).

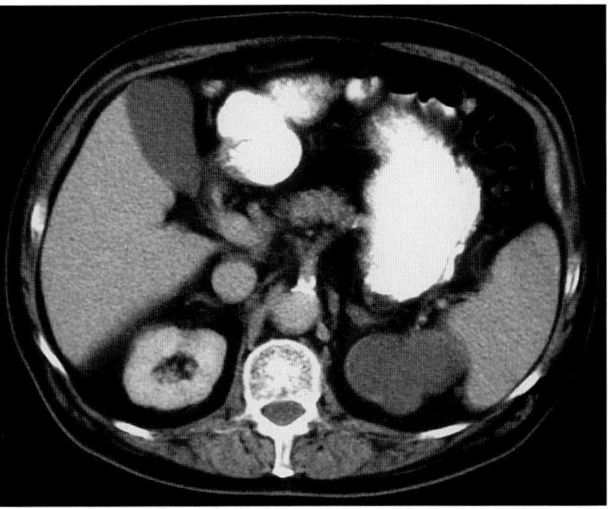

Figure 5. Grade 4 hydronephrosis on the left, with a normal right kidney. An infrarenal abdominal aortic aneurysm was present but is not shown.

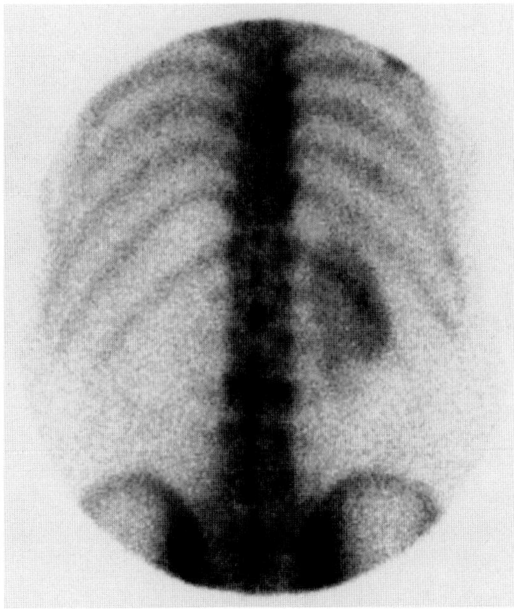

Figure 6. Posterior image from the bone scan shows no function of the left kidney. There is normal function on the right.

Radiographic Findings

The CT images show a thickened, highly irregular bladder wall, with infiltration of the adjacent fat **(Fig. 4)**. The left ureter is markedly dilated, and there is grade 4 hydronephrosis of the left kidney **(Fig. 5)**. The right kidney is normal. A single image from the bone scan shows a functional right kidney but no function in the left kidney **(Fig. 6)**.

Diagnoses

1. Stage D transitional cell carcinoma of the bladder.
2. End stage obstructive uropathy on the left.
3. Significant cardiovascular disease, which increases the risk of standard surgical urinary diversion.

What treatment would you recommend?

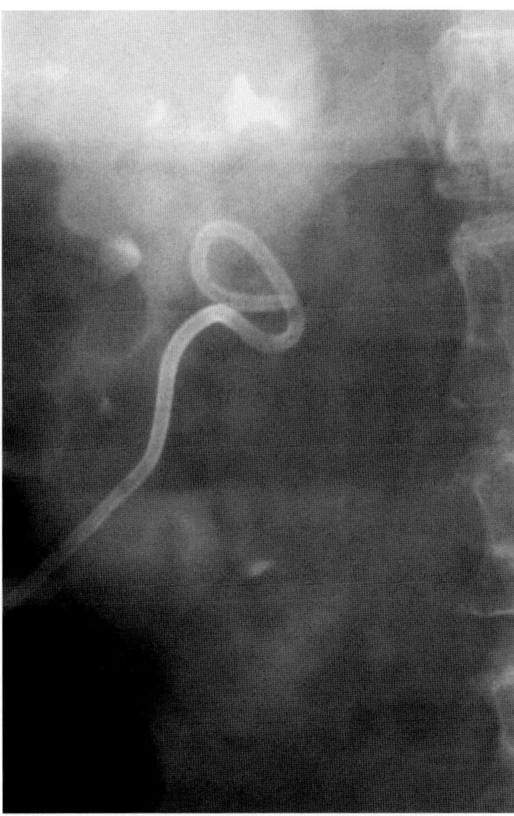

Figure 7. Supine image shows a percutaneous nephrostomy catheter in place in the right kidney.

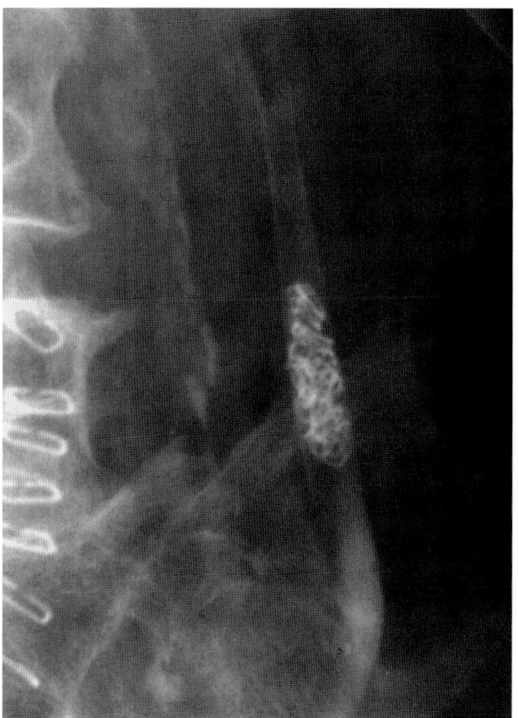

Figure 8. Prone image of the right kidney shows embolization of the distal right ureter with use of a biliary Wallstent and Gianturco coils.

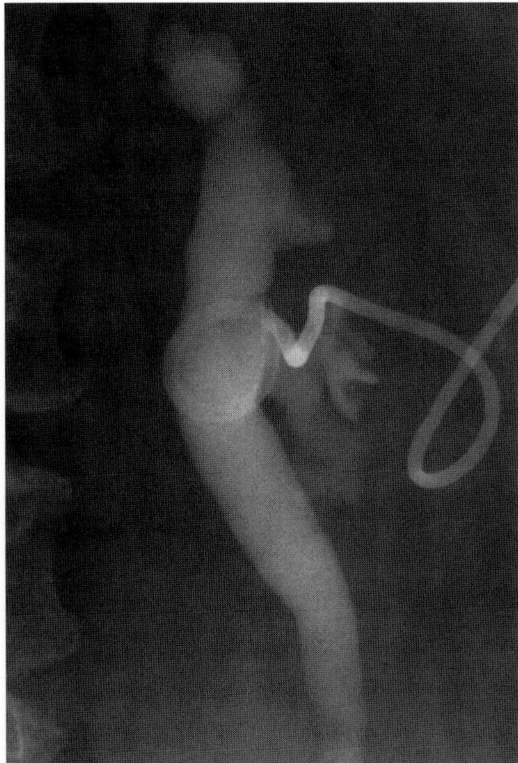

Figure 9. Prone nephrostogram shows right hydroureteronephrosis due to distal occlusion.

Management

The left kidney was not contributing to urine formation, so it did not require decompression. A percutaneous nephrostomy catheter was placed in the right renal collecting system **(Fig. 7)**. The right ureter was then occluded at the sacral promontory with use of a 6-mm x 40-mm biliary Wallstent (Schneider, Minneapolis, MN) and 16 complex helical coils (Cook, Bloomington, IN) **(Figs. 8, 9)**. Over the subsequent week, the urine output from the patient's Foley catheter dropped precipitously, with a concomitant increase in output from his nephrostomy. The Foley catheter was removed 1 week after the procedure, and the patient's pain abated. He did not have any further urine output from his urethra. The patient died of pneumonia 6 months later, and did not undergo further imaging prior to his death.

Discussion

Permanent urinary diversion is indicated in patients who have advanced pelvic pathology that causes obstructive uropathy, fistula formation, or pain. In patients who cannot tolerate surgical diversion, the minimally invasive percutaneous approach described here may be appropriate. The procedure can be performed unilaterally or bilaterally. Embolization coils and metallic stents both alone and together have been shown to cause significant ureteral wall thickening and stricture formation, with resultant ureteral occlusion.

Permanent ureteral occlusion, while a desirable goal, can be difficult to achieve. Self-expanding metallic stents alone may not occlude the ureter and they carry the risk of both migration and erosion through the ureter. Coils alone may not completely occlude the ureter, and in cases of ureteral leak, may permit enough urine to flow through the leak to maintain its patency. It appears that a combination of these agents may be effective by reducing the impact of their individual disadvantages. Other embolic methods, such as alcohol ablation, tissue glues, and detachable balloons and hydrogel may also be effective in permanent ureteral occlusion.

Selected Readings

Bing KT, Hicks ME, Figenshau RS, et al. Percutaneous ureteral occlusion with use of Gianturco coils and gelatin sponge. Part I. Swine model. J Vasc Interv Radiol 1992; 3(2):313–317.

Bing KT, Hicks ME, Picus D, Darcy MD. Percutaneous ureteral occlusion with use of Gianturco coils and gelatin sponge. Part II. Clinical experience. J Vasc Interv Radiol 1992; 3(2):319–321.

Gaylord GM, Johnsrude IS. Transrenal ureteral occlusion with Gianturco coils and gelatin sponge. Radiology 1989; 172:1047–1048.

Gunther R, Klose KJ, Alken P, Bohl J. Transrenal ureteral occlusion using a detachable balloon. Urol Radiol 1984; 6:210–214.

Gunther R, Marberger M, Klose KJ. Transrenal ureteral embolization. Radiology 1979; 132:317–319.

Millward SF, Thijssen AM, Marriner JR, Moors DE, Mai KT. Effect of a metallic balloon expanded stent on normal rabbit ureter. J Vasc Interv Radiol 1991; 2:557–560.

Wright KC, Dobben RL, Magal C, Ogawa K, Wallace S, Gianturco C. Occlusive effect of metallic stents on canine ureters. Cardiovasc Intervent Radiol 1993; 16(4):230–234.

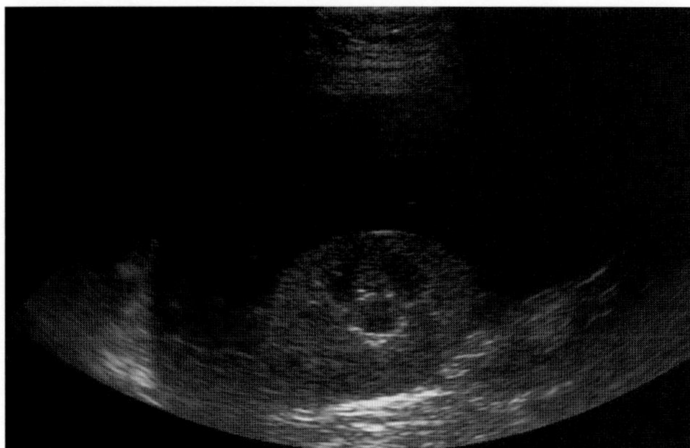

Figure 1. Transverse sonogram of the left iliac fossa.

TEACHING FILE CASE 49

Joseph A. Ronsivalle, D.O.

History

The patient is a 60-year-old man who came to the hospital with pelvic discomfort 2 weeks after receiving a cadaveric renal transplant for end stage renal disease and hypertension. An ultrasound examination of the renal transplant was performed **(Fig. 1)**.

What is your diagnosis?

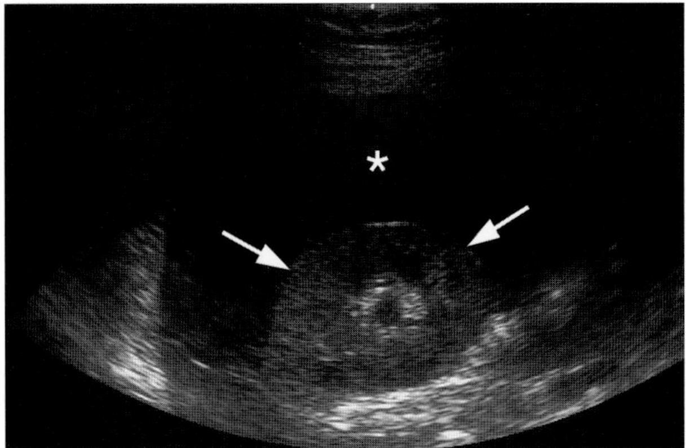
Figure 2. Sonogram reveals an anechoic fluid collection (asterisk) next to the renal transplant (arrows).

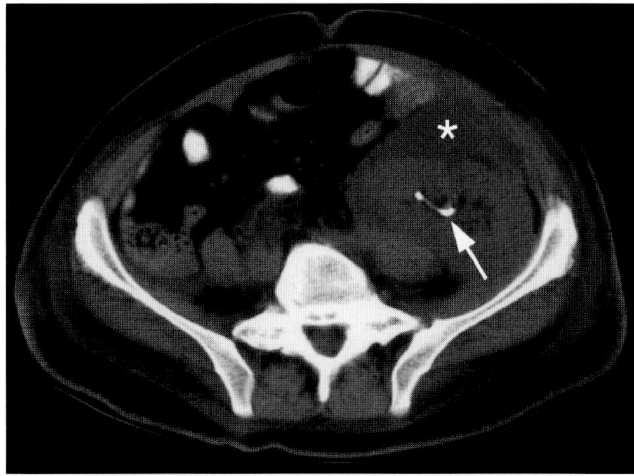
Figure 3. Noncontrast CT scan of the pelvis demonstrates a perinephric fluid collection (asterisk). A stent is present in the collecting system (arrow).

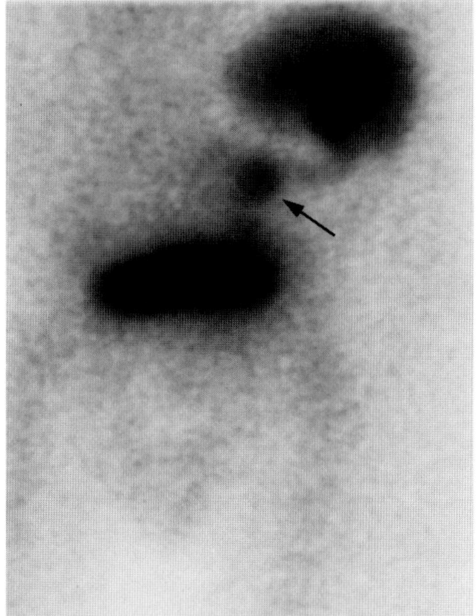
Figure 4. 12-minute image from a renal transplant scintigram demonstrates a focal accumulation of increased radiopharmaceutical activity at the mid portion of the ureter (arrow).

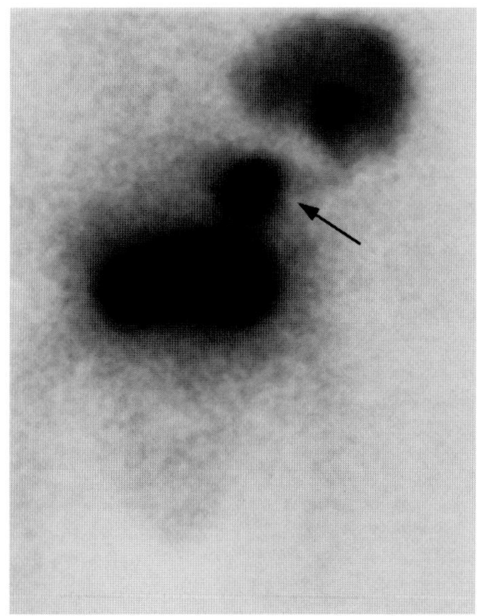
Figure 5. 32-minute image from a renal transplant scintigram demonstrates further accumulation of radiopharmaceutical activity at the mid portion of the ureter (arrow).

Radiographic Findings

The sonogram demonstrates a large, predominantly anechoic fluid collection adjacent to the transplanted kidney within the left iliac fossa **(Fig. 2)**. A noncontrast computed tomography (CT) examination demonstrated a crescentic fluid collection surrounding the transplanted kidney, and a stent in the collecting system **(Fig. 3)**. Renal scintigraphy demonstrated extravasation of the radiopharmaceutical **(Figs. 4, 5)**. Delayed scintigraphic images correlated with the CT findings **(Fig. 6)**.

What is your diagnosis now?

Diagnosis

Peritransplant urinoma secondary to breakdown of the ureteroureterostomy anastomosis.

How would you manage this patient?

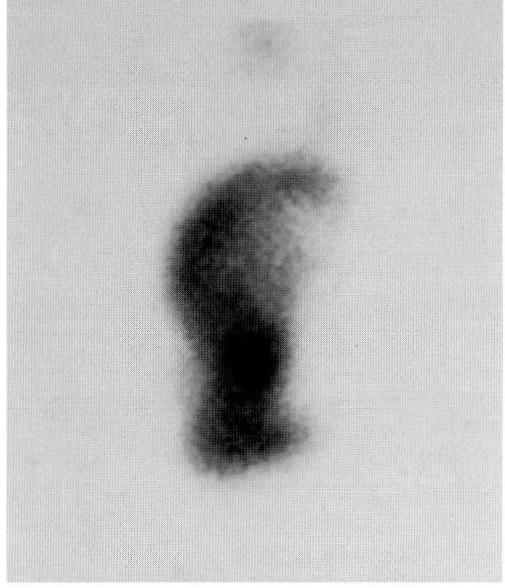
Figure 6. Four-hour delayed image demonstrates a crescentic collection of radiopharmaceutical that correlates with the CT findings.

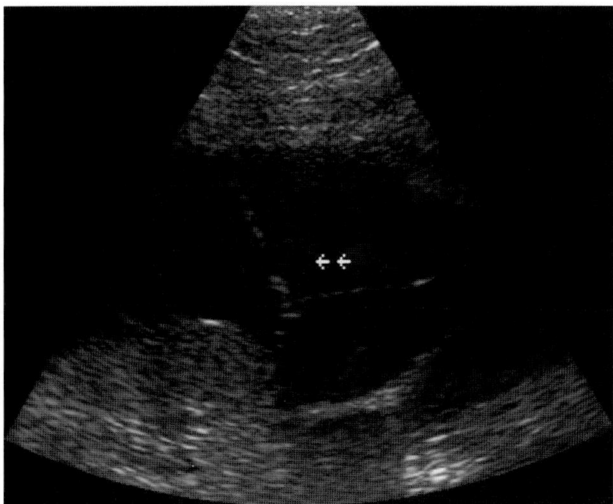

Figure 7. Transverse sonographic image demonstrates an echogenic needle within the fluid collection (arrows).

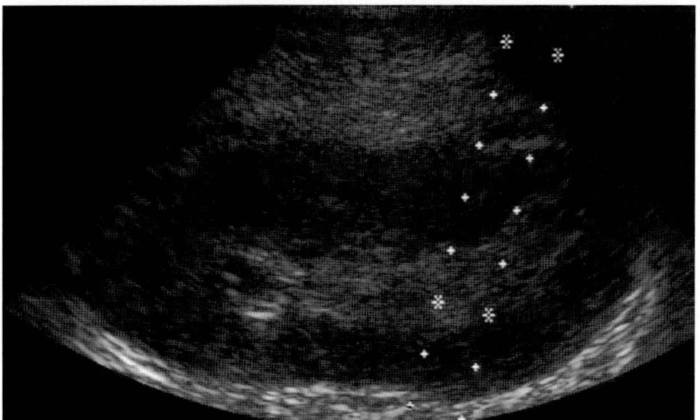

Figure 9. A needle guide is used to direct the puncture.

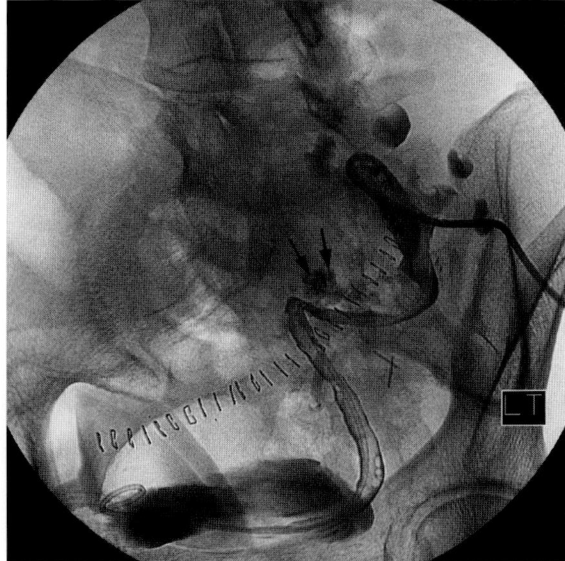

Figure 11. Anteroposterior image from a nephrostogram demonstrates the nephrostomy catheter within the contrast-filled collecting system. There is a focal collection of contrast material outside of the ureter at the site of the leak (arrows).

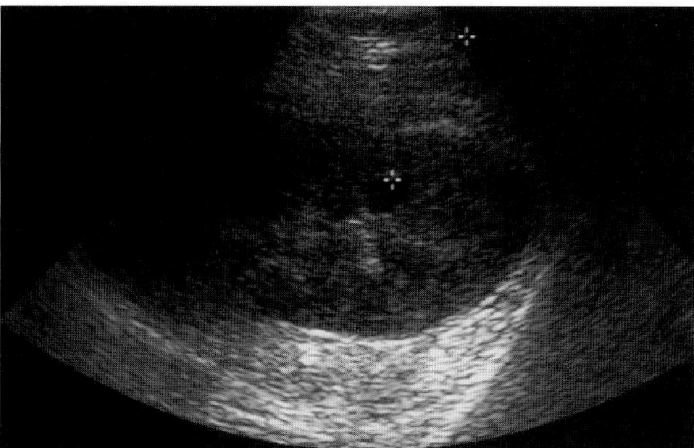

Figure 8. Longitudinal sonogram demonstrates the approach to the collecting system of the transplant kidney.

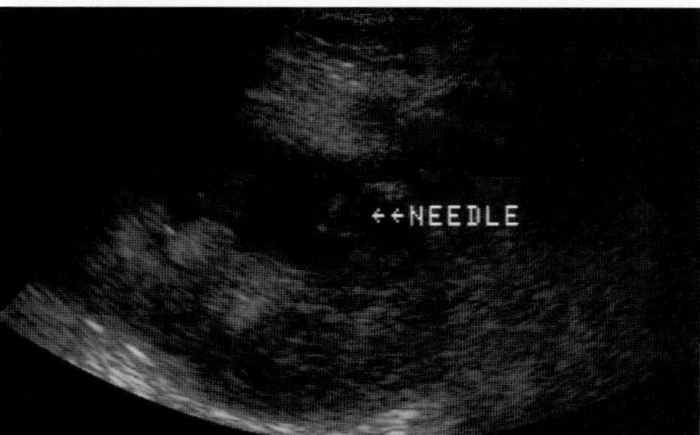

Figure 10. The needle tip is seen within the collecting system.

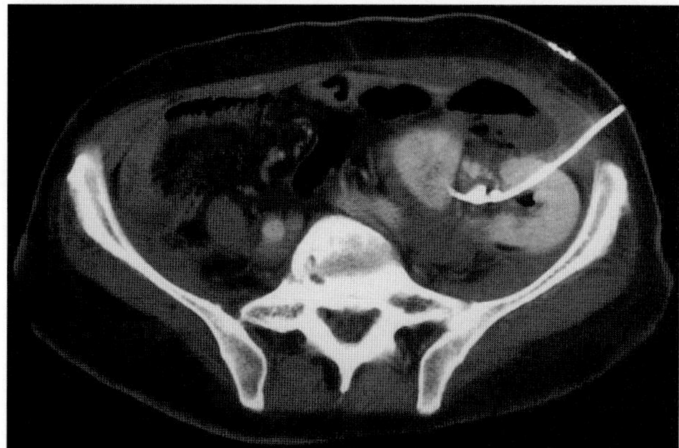

Figure 12. Contrast-enhanced CT image demonstrates the percutaneously placed nephrostomy catheter within the collecting system of the transplant kidney.

Management

Ultrasound guidance was used for diagnostic percutaneous aspiration of the fluid **(Fig. 7)**. Laboratory analysis of the aspirated fluid revealed a creatinine of 12.6 mg/dL. No organisms were seen on Gram stain, and cultures were negative. These findings confirmed that the fluid collection represented an uncomplicated urinoma. The patient was managed with prolonged ureteral stent placement in the hope that the ureteral leak would close spontaneously. Subsequent sonography and CT scanning revealed persistence of the perinephric fluid collection. It was therefore decided that total ureteral diversion was warranted. A percutaneous nephrostomy tube was placed under ultrasound guidance **(Figs. 8–11)**. Follow-up CT scanning revealed good position of the nephrostomy tube and ureteral stent **(Fig. 12)**.

Discussion

Peritransplant fluid collections are common, occurring in up to 50% of renal transplant patients. Although the etiology of the fluid collection may be suggested by the complexity of the fluid, the time at which the fluid appears, or the size of the collection, imaging findings are often nonspecific and the etiology remains unknown. Because management of the collection depends on the etiology of the fluid (ie, surgical management of a urinoma versus conservative management of a seroma), diagnostic percutaneous aspiration of the fluid can help guide the appropriate therapy.

Although the ureteral stent was not completely occluded in this case, urine following a less resistant path continued leaking from the anastomosis. The etiology of the leak was likely secondary to ischemia of the native and/or donor segments of the ureter at the surgical anastomosis. Percutaneous rather than surgical diversion was chosen in this patient because it posed less of a risk to the transplant kidney while diverting urine away from the leaking anastomosis.

Percutaneous intervention of renal allografts poses challenges not encountered in the native kidney. The transverse orientation of the kidney, the ventral location of the renal arteries and veins, and the potential for traversing intervening structures create a narrow window of opportunity for percutaneous access to the kidney. CT or sonographic guidance may assist in overcoming these anatomic challenges unique to the renal allograft. Often, cross-sectional imaging coupled with fluoroscopic imaging provides the safest access to the transplanted kidney.

Selected Readings

Hunter DW, Castaneda-Zuniga WR, Coleman CC, Herrera M, Amplatz K. Percutaneous techniques in the management of urological complications in renal transplant patients. Radiology 1983; 148:407–412.

Letourneau JG, Day DL, Feinberg SB. Ultrasound and computed tomographic evaluation of renal transplantation. Radiol Clin North Am 1987; 25:267–279.

Tublin ME, Dodd GD. Sonography of renal transplantation. Radiol Clin North Am 1995; 33:447–459.

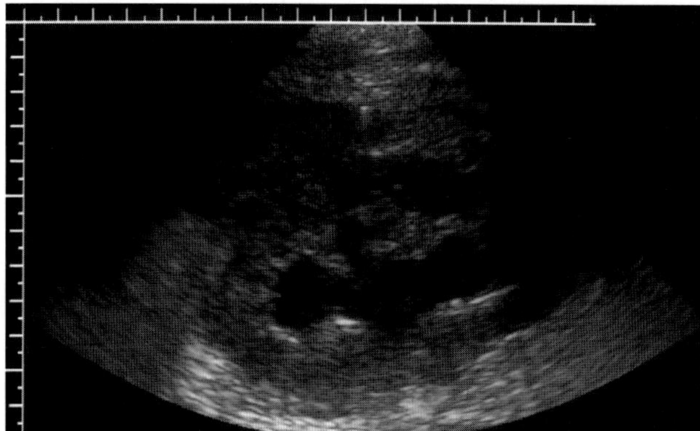

Figure 1. Left renal sonogram, longitudinal image.

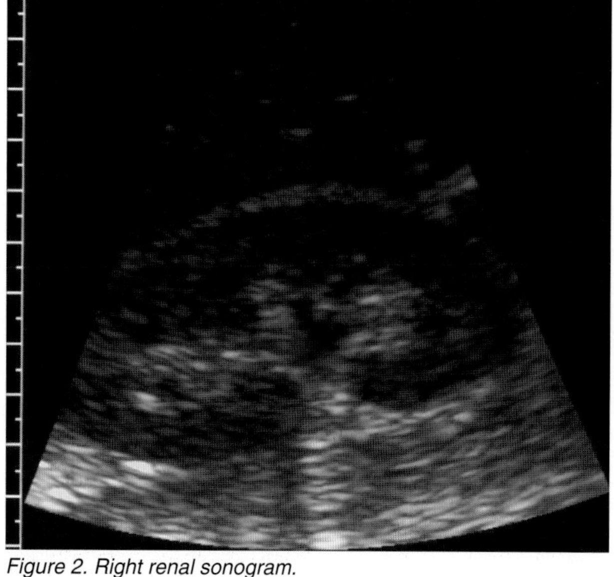

Figure 2. Right renal sonogram.

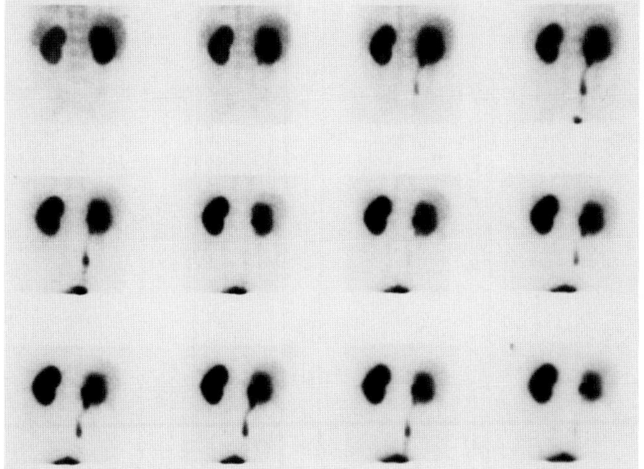

Figure 3. Nuclear renogram prior to administration of Lasix.

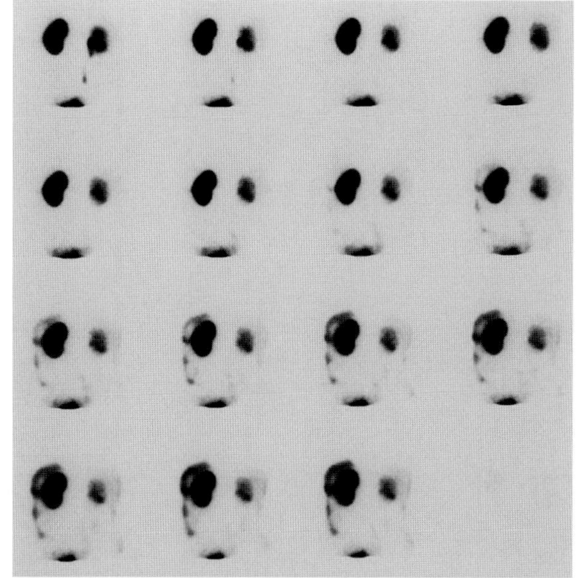

Figure 4. Nuclear renogram, post Lasix.

TEACHING FILE CASE 50

Ellen M. Chung, M.D.

History

A 65-year-old man with a remote history of radical cystectomy, Bricker loop formation for urinary diversion, and pelvic irradiation for bladder cancer was referred 2 days after a low anterior resection for rectal cancer with a rising serum creatinine. A renal ultrasound examination was performed **(Figs. 1, 2)**. Based upon the ultrasound results, a nuclear medicine Lasix renogram was obtained **(Figs. 3, 4)**.

What is your diagnosis?

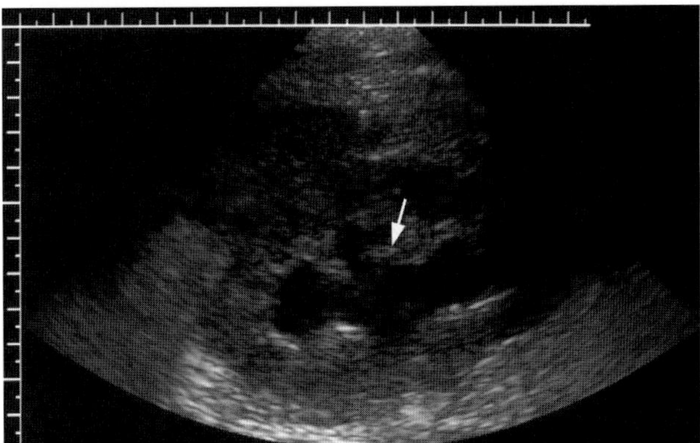

Figure 5. Left renal sonogram shows a dilated collecting system (arrow).

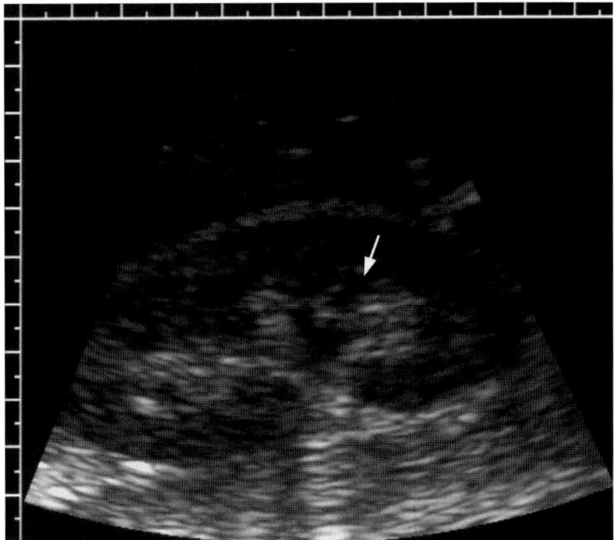

Figure 6. Right renal sonogram with minimal pyelocaliectasis (arrow).

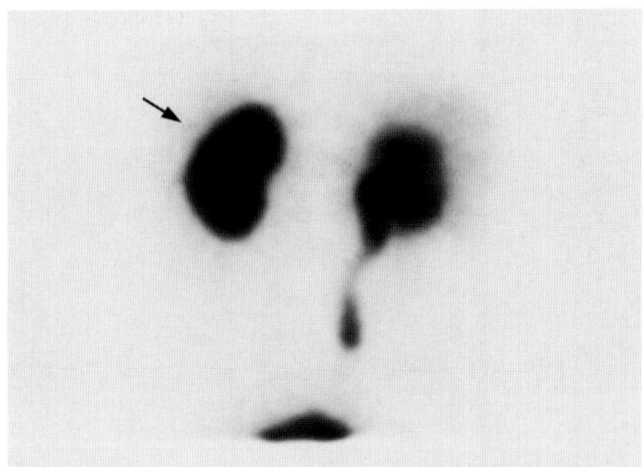

Figure 7. Pre-Lasix nuclear renogram. The left kidney (arrow) exhibits delayed excretion of the radiopharmaceutical compared with the right.

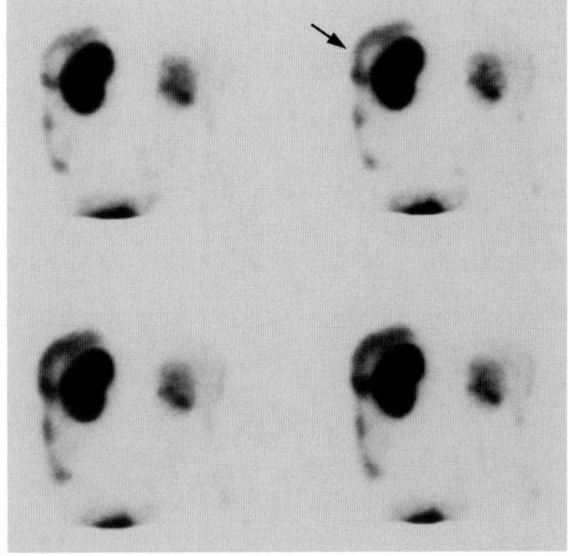

Figure 8. Post-Lasix nuclear renogram shows extravasation in the left renal fossa (arrow).

Radiographic Findings

Moderate pyelocaliectasis was seen on the left **(Fig. 5)** with only mild dilatation of the collecting system noted on the right **(Fig. 6)**.

The nuclear renogram showed diminished extraction and excretion of the radiopharmaceutical by the left kidney **(Fig. 7)**, which contributed only 28% of the total renal function. Furthermore, after the administration of Lasix, extravasation was seen in the left renal fossa **(Fig. 8)**. Review of the images on computed cine loop revealed that the leak originated from the region of the distal left ureter.

A left antegrade (transrenal) pyeloureterogram **(Fig. 9)** was obtained to further evaluate the nature of the injury and to determine if percutaneous treatment was possible. The ureterogram showed persistent abrupt cut-off of the contrast column in the left ureter, consistent with complete ureteral ligation. Therefore, it was inferred that the leak originated either at the distal left ureteral stump or the uretero-enterostomy junction.

Diagnosis

Inadvertent left ureteral ligation.

What treatment can you offer now?

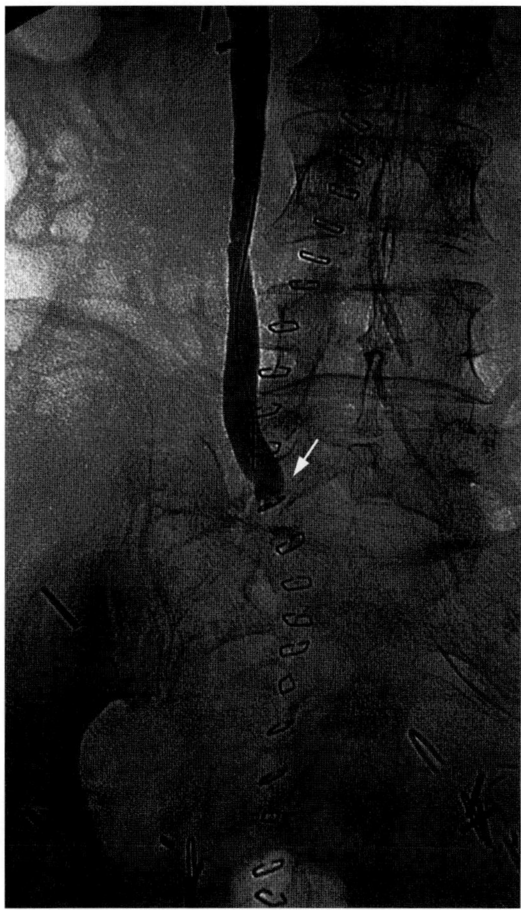

Figure 9. Left antegrade ureterogram with the patient in the prone position. The distal portion of the antegrade ureterogram (right) demonstrates abrupt cut-off of the contrast column in the mid left ureter (arrow).

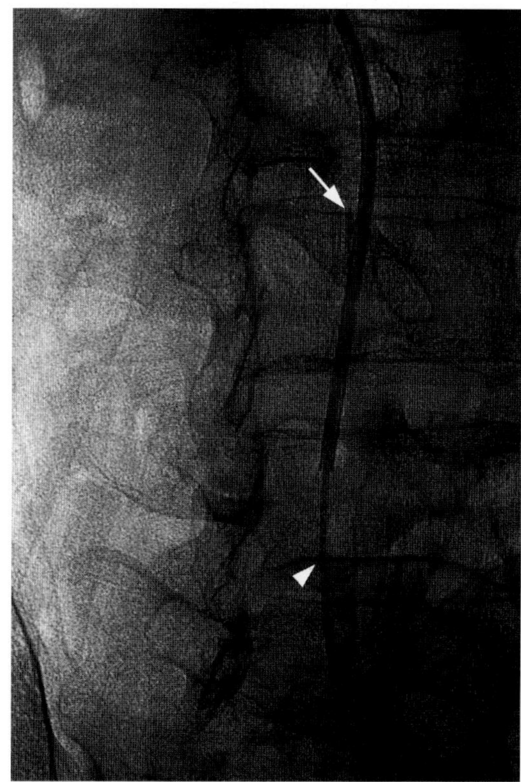

Figure 10. Digital image shows the nephrostomy tube (arrow) with the 5-F catheter (arrowhead) passing through it to the site where the left ureter is ligated.

Management

If the ureter were lacerated with the cut ends remaining in close proximity or partial continuity, the gap could have been crossed with a wire and a ureteral stent could have been placed via the antegrade approach. In this case, however, surgical reanastomosis was necessary to repair the complete ureteral ligation.

The surgeon anticipated that localization of the ureter in the surgical field would be difficult because of the patient's prior surgery and radiation therapy, so preoperative placement of a stent in the proximal ureteral stump was requested. The surgeon also wanted a nephrostomy tube left in place for drainage proximal to the new anastomosis. These aims were both accomplished with use of a straight drain and a smaller coaxial 5-F catheter through the drainage tube. The distal tip of the drainage tube was left in the renal pelvis. The tip of the 5-F catheter was advanced to the site of the obstruction so it could be palpated at surgery to locate the proximal ureter **(Fig. 10)**. At the conclusion of surgery, the 5-F catheter was removed, leaving the straight nephrostomy tube in place.

At surgery the left ureter was found to be ligated twice and cut between the sutures, as it had been mistaken for a blood vessel. Surprisingly, the *right* ureter was found to be lacerated, and direct examination revealed urine freely spilling from it. Thus, it was the *right* ureter, rather than the left, that was the source of the extravasated urine. Because of the surgically altered anatomy, the ureteral leak allowed urine to track along the left ureter and collect in the left renal fossa. A new Bricker loop was created with reimplantation of both repaired ureters into this new enterostomy.

Discussion

Bilateral ureteral injuries are rare; however, they are seen in cases of iatrogenic ureteral injury. Unfortunately, iatrogenic ureteral injury is most often diagnosed postoperatively. Delay in recognizing the ureteral injury increases the associated morbidity from 10% to 40%. Complications include urinoma, abscess, fistula, and stricture formation. Hematuria is often absent. Making the diagnosis is easier when there is obstruction, but with a normally functioning contralateral kidney, even complete obstruction can go unrecognized.

With standard operative technique, the incidence of ureteral injury in uncomplicated abdominal hysterectomy is still 0.9%, which has been unchanged for decades. Ureteral injury also occurs in nongynecologic surgery, particularly in pelvic surgery. The incidence is increased in cancer surgery because of tumor encasement and displacement of the ureters.

Despite its common use as a screening examination, ultrasound is not as sensitive in detecting ureteral injury as intravenous urography. Therefore, a normal ultrasound examination does not exclude the diagnosis of ureteral disruption, and further work-up should be pursued.

Selected Readings

Campbell EW Jr, Filderman PS, Jacobs SC. Ureteral injury due to blunt and penetrating trauma. Urology 1992; 40:216–220.

Guerriero WG. Ureteral injury. Urol Clin North Am 1989; 16:237–248.

Kadir S, ed. Current practice of interventional radiology. St. Louis: Mosby Year Book, 1991.

Mitty HA, Train JS, Dan SJ. Placement of ureteral stents by antegrade and retrograde techniques. Radiol Clin North Am 1986; 24:587–600.

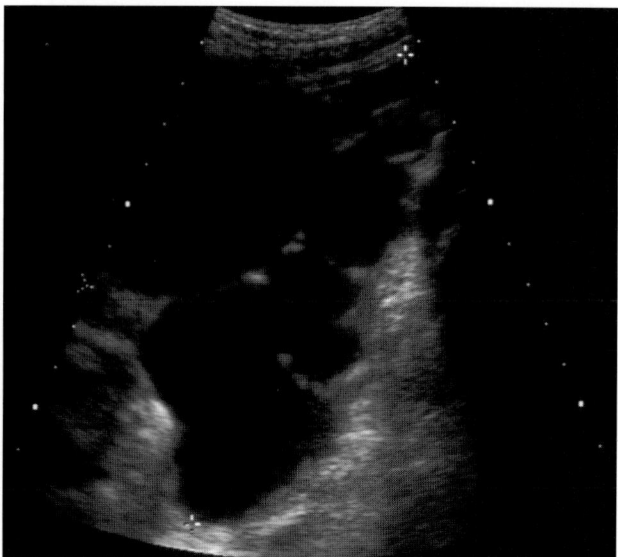

Figure 1. Longitudinal sonogram of the left kidney.

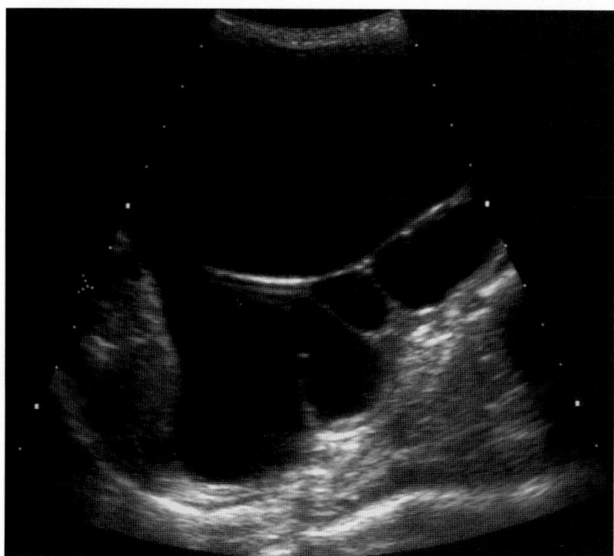

Figure 2. Transverse sonogram of the left kidney.

TEACHING FILE CASE 51

John D. Statler, M.D.

History

A 6-month-old otherwise asymptomatic boy was brought to the hospital after his parents detected a large, firm left flank mass. An ultrasound examination was performed **(Figs. 1, 2)**.

What is your diagnosis?

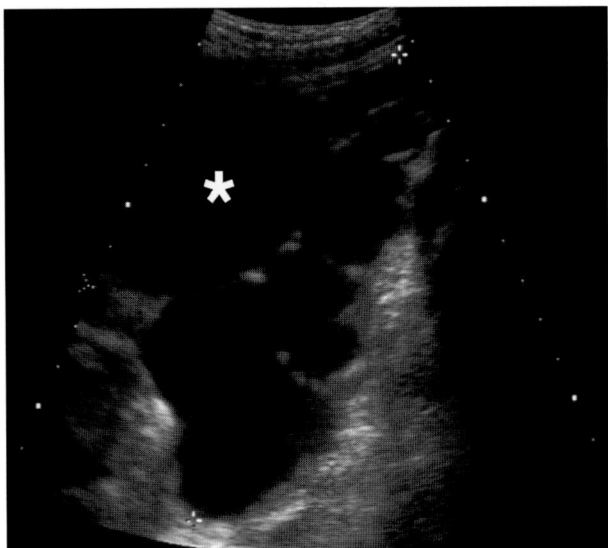

Figure 3. Sonogram shows marked hydronephrosis, confirmed by communication between the renal pelvis and the calyces (asterisk).

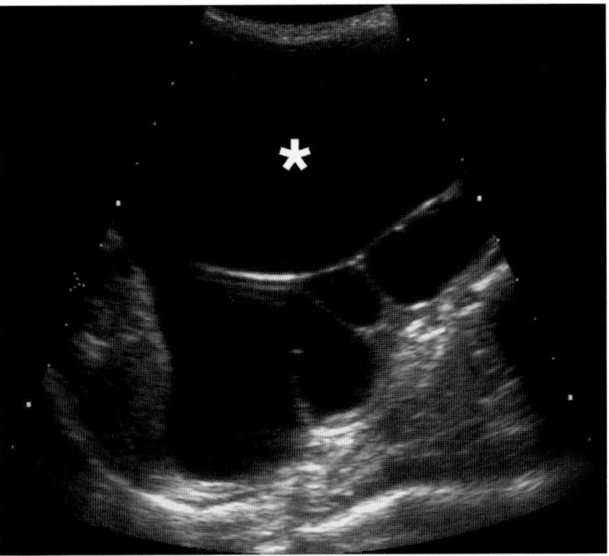

Figure 4. Communication between the pelvis (asterisk) and the calyces is again seen on the transverse sonogram.

Radiographic Findings

Severe hydronephrosis with little remaining renal parenchyma was noted in the left renal fossa **(Figs. 3, 4)**. It was unclear if these findings were due to ureteropelvic junction (UPJ) obstruction or vesicoureteral reflux. An intravenous pyelogram (IVP) was obtained **(Fig. 5)**.

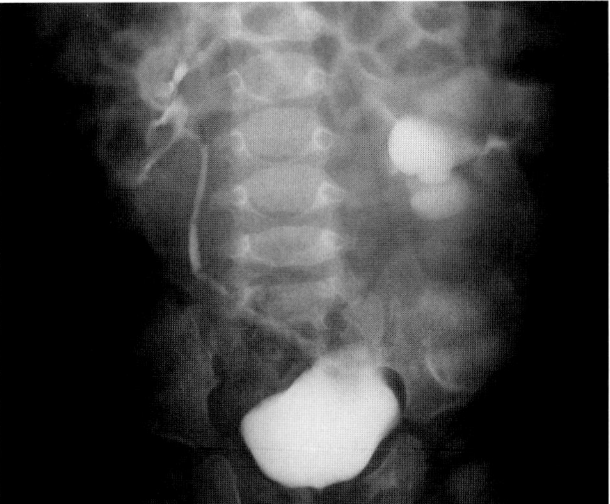

Figure 5. IVP shows delayed filling of a dilated left renal pelvis, and a normal right kidney and collecting system.

Now what is your diagnosis?

The IVP showed delayed filling of a dilated left renal pelvis with a normal right collecting system. No contrast material was seen distal to the left ureteropelvic junction on delayed images. A nuclear renal scan with technetium-99m MAG-3 revealed a dilated left renal collecting system and a minimal rim of functional renal cortex **(Fig. 6)**. Split renal function was 42% on the left and 58% on the right. Voiding cystourethrography was not performed.

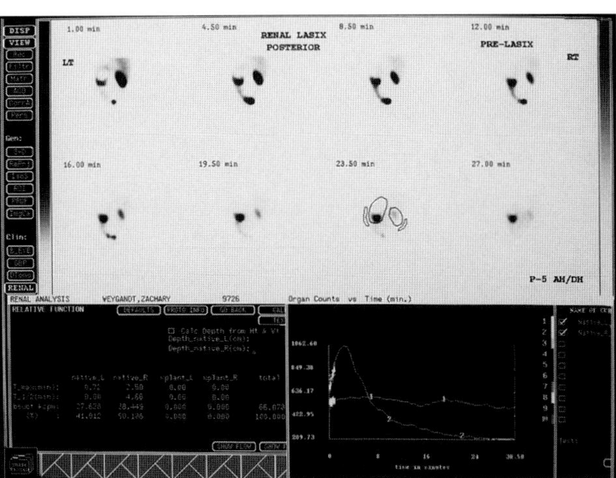

Figure 6. Technetium-99m MAG-3 scan shows a dilated left collecting system with 42% of the total renal function occurring on the left.

Diagnosis

Left ureteropelvic junction obstruction.

How would you manage this patient?

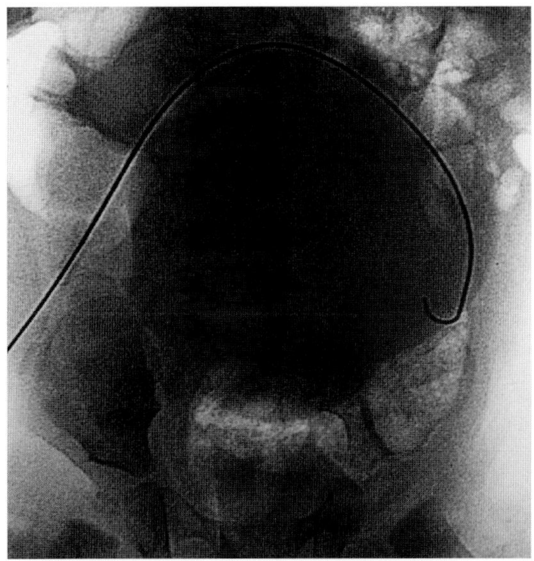

Figure 7. At percutaneous nephrostomy, the guide wire outlines the extent of renal pelvic dilatation.

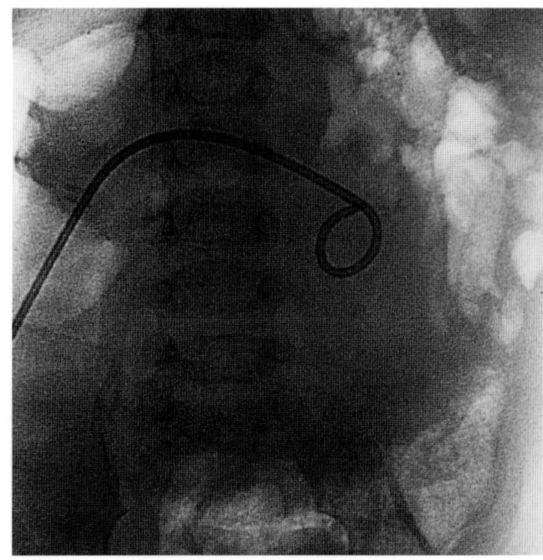

Figure 8. Pediatric nephrostomy tube in place.

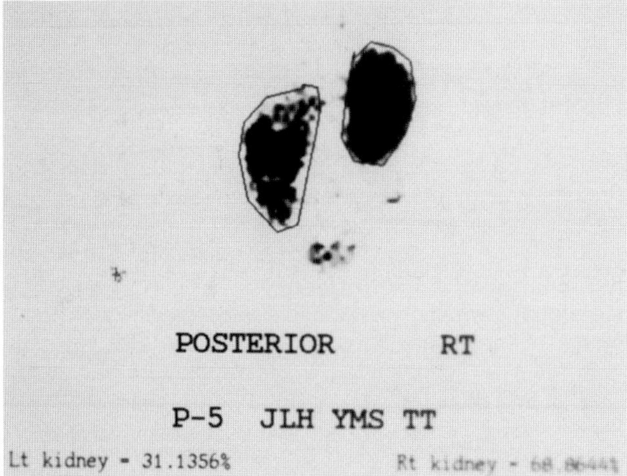

Figure 9. Technetium-99m DMSA scan after percutaneous nephrostomy, before pyeloplasty.

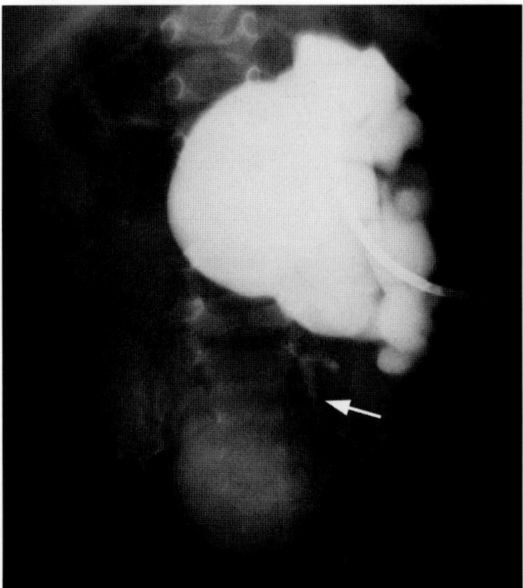

Figure 10. Nephrostogram demonstrates an enlarged left renal pelvis and distorted calyces, but the distal left ureter is normal (arrow).

Management

The right kidney was normal, and despite the UPJ obstruction, the imaging studies suggested a salvageable left kidney. To preserve cortical function, a left percutaneous nephrostomy was performed. With the patient in the prone position, the left renal pelvis was accessed with use of a 21-gauge needle and an 0.018-inch wire. The wire was noted to coil in the enlarged renal pelvis **(Fig. 7)**. A sheath was placed and contrast material was injected to confirm the correct position. The track was subsequently dilated to 6 F, and a 6-F pediatric pigtail nephrostomy catheter was placed **(Fig. 8)**.

Two months later the patient underwent a technetium-99m dimercaptosuccinic acid (DMSA) nuclear renal scan to assess the cortical response to decompression. The function on the left had decreased from 42% to 31%, suggesting that treatment with percutaneous nephrostomy alone was inadequate **(Fig. 9)**. The patient, therefore, underwent dismembered pyeloplasty. A repeat nephrostogram showed a dilated pelvis with distorted calyces but a normal-appearing left ureter **(Fig. 10)**.

Discussion

The differential diagnosis for neonatal flank mass includes UPJ obstruction, hydronephrosis, multicystic dysplastic kidney, and cystic nephroma. UPJ obstruction is the most common cause of childhood urinary tract obstruction and is the result of abnormal development of the ureter at or near the UPJ. Histologically, disordered smooth muscle and connective tissue result in luminal narrowing. Approximately one third of UPJ obstructions are associated with abnormal vessels crossing the lower pole.

Some authors think that UPJ obstruction results from a physiologic abnormality rather than an anatomic obstruction. The normal peristaltic mechanism of the renal pelvis is altered, resulting in a physiologic obstruction to urine egress. This mechanism is supported by the finding of pinhole patency of the UPJ at surgery. In this case, however, true anatomic obstruction existed.

Treatment options are based on functional scintigraphic evaluation. When kidneys demonstrate no parenchymal function, nephrectomy is indicated. If the obstructed kidney contributes at least 15% of the total renal function it may be considered salvageable. Kidneys with severe hydronephrosis and preserved function are best treated with pyeloplasty or endopyelotomy. Percutaneous nephrostomy can be a temporizing measure that preserves function and allows decompression of the dilated collecting system before pyeloplasty or endopyelotomy. Selected patients with hydronephrosis and more than 40% split renal function can be effectively treated with percutaneous nephrostomy alone.

Ransley et al have shown that over 70% of patients with good cortical function require percutaneous nephrostomy with no further surgical intervention. If corrected by 1 year of age, many kidneys with UPJ obstruction show improved function. Percutaneous nephrostomy is performed for congenital UPJ obstruction to relieve obstruction and azotemia prior to surgery, to demonstrate recoverable renal function, and to drain pyonephrosis. Complications of percutaneous nephrostomy include hemorrhage, infection, perirenal fluid collection, and injury to adjacent organs. The major contraindications to percutaneous nephrostomy in UPJ obstruction are coagulopathy or a nonsalvageable kidney.

Selected Readings

Irving HC, Arthur RJ, Thomas DF. Percutaneous nephrostomy in pediatrics. Clin Radiol 1987; 38:245–248.

Karlin G, Badlani G, Smith AD. Percutaneous pyeloplasty (endopyelotomy) for congenital ureteropelvic junction obstruction. Urology 1992; 39:533–537.

Koff SA, Hayden LJ, Cirulli C, Shore R. Pathophysiology of ureteropelvic junction obstruction: experimental and clinical observations. J Urol 1986; 136:336–338.

O'Brien WM, Matsumoto AH, Grant EG, Gibbons MD. Percutaneous nephrostomy in infants. Urology 1990; 36:269–272.

Owen RJ, Lamont AC, Brookes J. Early management and postnatal investigation of prenatally diagnosed hydronephrosis. Clin Radiol 1996; 51:173–176.

Peters CA. Urinary tract obstruction in children. J Urol 1995; 39:1874–1884.

Putman CE, Ravin CE. Textbook of diagnostic imaging. 2nd edition. Philadelphia: W.B. Saunders Company, 1994; 1070–1075.

Ransley PG, Dhillon HK, Gordon I, Duffy PG, Dillon MJ, Barratt TM. The postnatal management of hydronephrosis diagnosed by prenatal ultrasound. J Urol 1990; 144:584–587.

Silverman FN, Kuhn JP. Caffey's pediatric x-ray diagnosis: an integrated imaging approach. 9th edition. St. Louis: Mosby Year Book, 1993; 2110–2113.

Endnote

Case courtesy of Dennis S. Peppas, M.D.

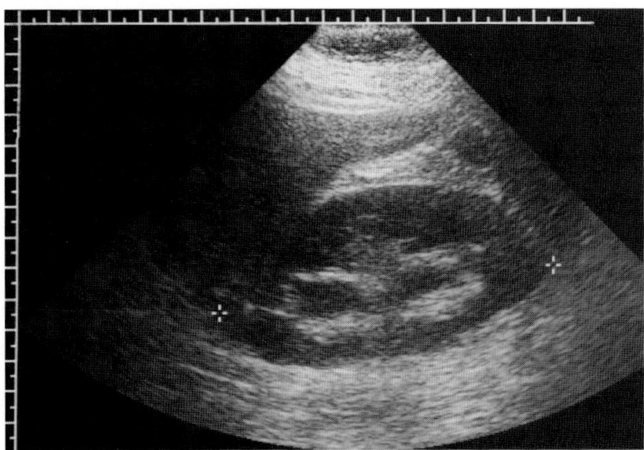

Figure 1. Longitudinal sonogram of the right kidney.

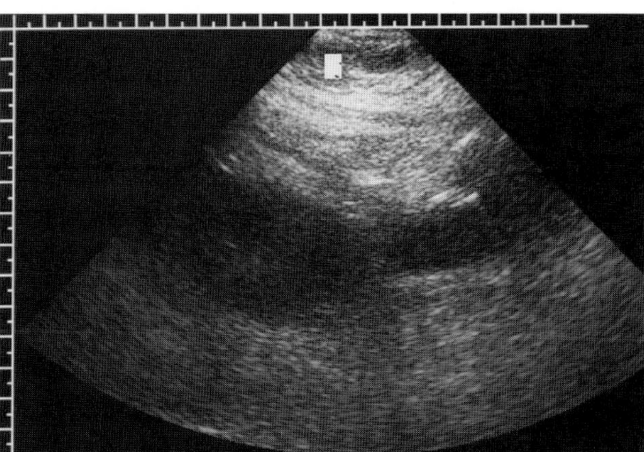

Figure 2. Longitudinal sonogram of the proximal ureter.

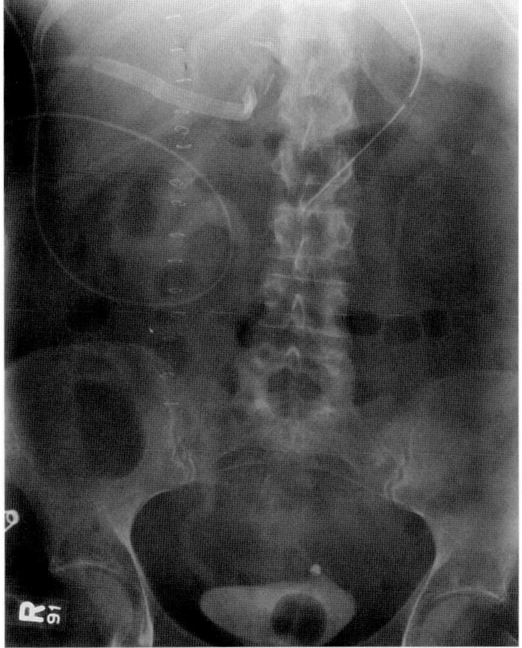

Figure 3. Twenty-minute film from an IVP. Note the skin staples over the right abdomen from a recent cholecystectomy prior to admission.

TEACHING FILE CASE 52

Daniel Boyle, M.D., Allen J. Meglin, M.D., and Mark L. Lukens, M.D.

History

A 59-year-old woman came to the hospital with nausea, vomiting, dysuria, and right flank pain. On initial evaluation she was febrile, hypotensive, and had an elevated white blood cell count. Urine and blood cultures grew *E. coli.* A renal sonogram **(Figs. 1, 2)** and intravenous pyeloureterogram (IVP) **(Fig. 3)** were obtained.

What is your diagnosis?

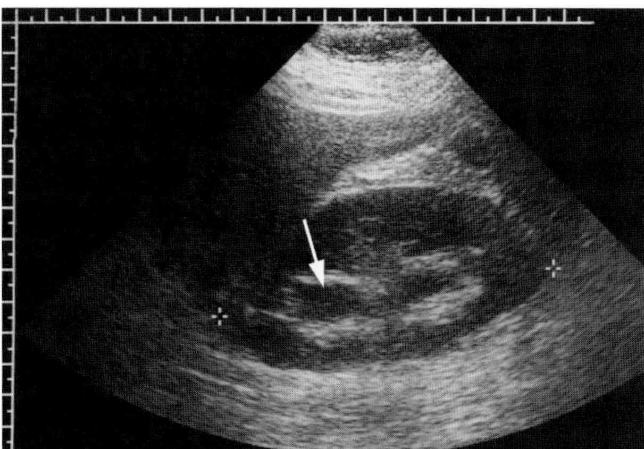

Figure 4. Longitudinal sonographic image of the right kidney demonstrates moderate hydronephrosis (arrow) and ureteral dilatation.

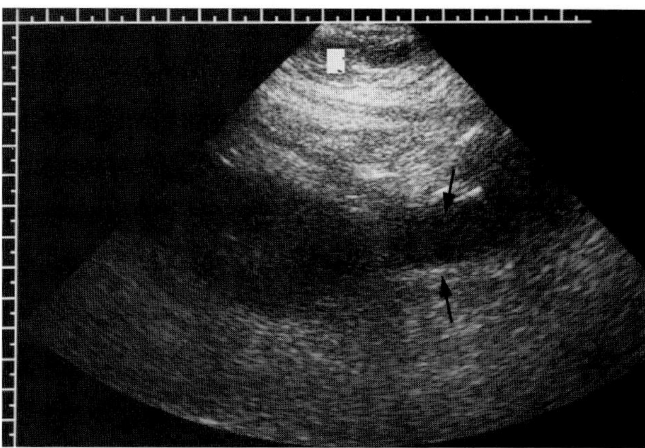

Figure 5. Longitudinal sonographic image of the proximal ureter demonstrates moderate ureteral dilatation (arrows).

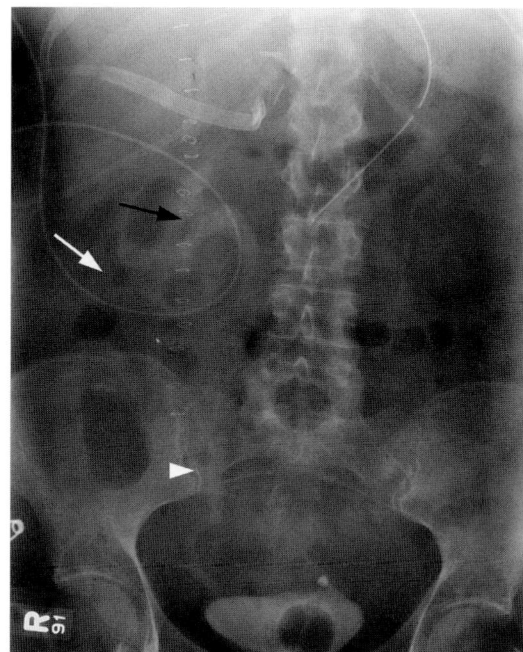

Figure 6. Twenty-minute film from an IVP shows moderate hydroureteronephrosis (black arrow) with ureteral ectasia (arrowhead). Note the position of the colon (white arrow).

Radiographic Findings

The sonogram demonstrates moderate right hydronephrosis and a dilated proximal ureter **(Figs. 4, 5)**. The IVP reveals moderate right hydroureteronephrosis with ureteral ectasia extending to the ureterovesical junction **(Fig. 6)**.

Diagnosis

Urosepsis secondary to an obstructed right renal collecting system.

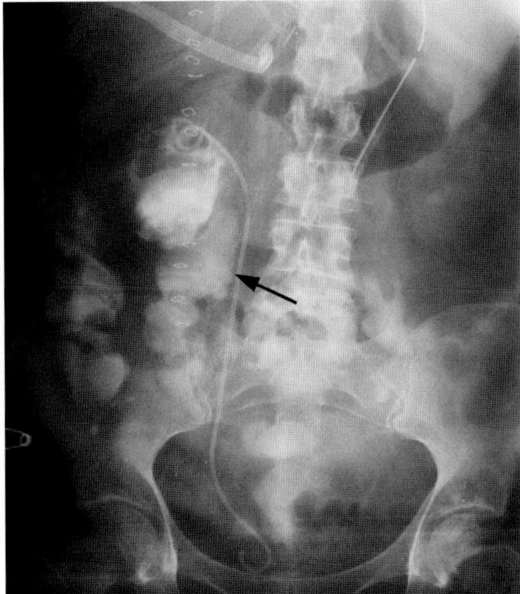

Figure 7. Abdominal film obtained immediately after retrograde ureteral stent placement demonstrates marked extravasation of contrast material into the colon (arrow).

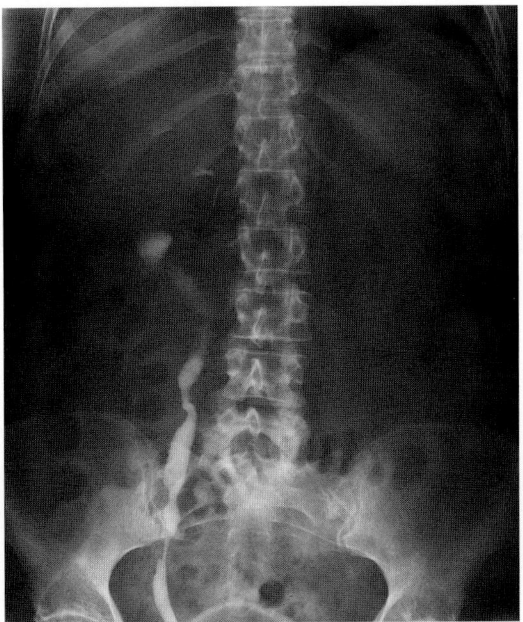

Figure 8. Three-week follow-up retrograde pyelo-ureterogram shows resolution of the pyelocolofistula with no extravasation of contrast material.

Management

The urologist was unable to place a retrograde ureteral stent due to ureteral ectasia. Interventional Radiology then attempted percutaneous nephrostomy (PCN), which was also unsuccessful. Subsequent retrograde ureteral stent placement was ultimately successful, and a stone was removed from the ureterovesical junction during the procedure. A pyelocolofistula was noted at the site of the unsuccessful nephrostomy and manifested as extravasation of contrast material into the colon **(Fig. 7)**. The patient's colonic perforation was treated conservatively with intravenous antibiotics and urinary decompression. The patient improved clinically and the ureteral stent was removed after 3 weeks. A follow-up retrograde pyeloureterogram **(Fig. 8)** demonstrated no evidence of obstruction or persistence of the pyelocolofistula.

Discussion

Colonic perforation is an uncommon complication of PCN, with an incidence of 0.2%. The risk of colonic perforation can be minimized with optimal needle and catheter positioning. This can be accomplished by imaging the renal collecting system in multiple fluoroscopic projections prior to passing the needle through the skin. At our institution, we try to create an "elevator shaft of opportunity" from the renal calyx to the proposed skin entry site. Careful evaluation of the proposed needle track with fluoroscopy, sonography, or computed tomography (CT) scanning can be done to ensure that no intervening structures are present in the "elevator shaft."

A posterolateral approach to the kidney is preferred, using the posterior axillary line as a reference for the location of the skin incision. The ideal renal collecting system entry site is in the middle or inferior pole, passing through the Brödel avascular plane and entering a posterior calyx end on. This approach avoids the larger renal vessels which usually lie along the anterior and posterior surface of the calyces.

Sonography can also be used, either alone or in conjunction with fluoroscopy, to direct needle placement. This helps to avoid the colon or adjacent organs. However, the value of sonography is limited in obese patients or where there is no dilated collecting system.

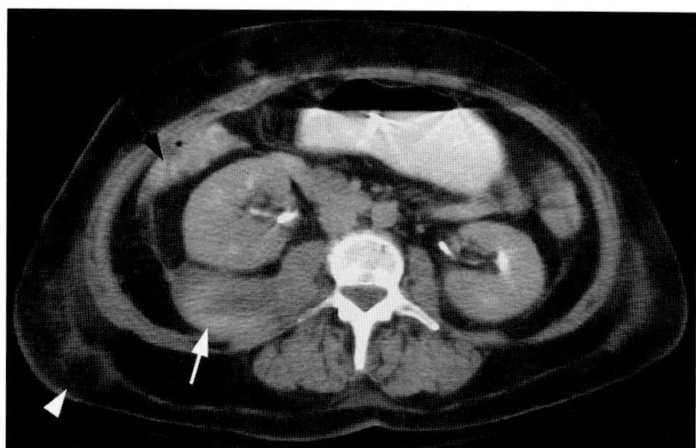

Figure 9. CT scan of the abdomen reveals a right perinephric hematoma (white arrow). Note the lateral position of the colon (black arrow) and the adjacent soft-tissue changes from the attempted nephrostomy (arrowhead).

The colon is a lateral structure in relation to the kidney and lies in the posterior pararenal space. Certain patients may be more vulnerable to colonic injury during PCN access. An increased risk exists in patients with an air-distended colon or an unusually posterior colon which may even be retrorenal in location. The risk of colonic injury tends to be higher in patients who have had an ileal-jejunal bypass procedure for obesity because the colon is more distended with fluid. Thin patients appear to be at a slightly higher risk of colonic perforation. Too lateral a puncture site also increases the chance of colonic injury. Colonic perforation is more common in the small percentage of patients who have mobile kidneys. CT scanning may be a useful guide in these cases or where there is a history of altered anatomy or previous surgery **(Fig. 9)**. Colonic perforation usually becomes evident in the immediate postprocedure period. Most colonic injuries are extraperitoneal and will heal with conservative treatment without developing a fistula, abscess, or peritonitis. Intraperitoneal injury usually necessitates open repair to prevent peritonitis.

In addition to the colonic perforation, a second complication of PCN occurred in this case. **Figure 9** shows that a perinephric hematoma is present. The colon was not malpositioned in this case and the complications of bleeding and bowel injury likely resulted from too lateral a puncture site. A small renal branch artery was probably lacerated, causing retroperitoneal hemorrhage. This occurred as the needle was advanced through a laterally located portion of the kidney, away from the avascular plane of Brödel.

Severe bleeding occurs in fewer than 3% of percutaneous renal procedures. Most bleeding complications are associated with the initial puncture or repeated punctures. Management may consist of observation, embolization, or nephrectomy. Delayed bleeding can also result from renal artery pseudoaneurysm or arteriovenous fistula formation, which occur in fewer than 1% of PCN cases.

Selected Readings

Leroy AJ, Williams HJ, Bender CE, Segura JW, Patterson DE, Benson RC. Colon perforation following percutaneous nephrostomy and renal calculus removal. Radiology 1985; 155:83–85.

Morse RM, Spirnak JP, Resnick MI. Iatrogenic colon and rectal injuries associated with urological intervention: report of 14 patients. J Urol 1988, 140:101–103.

Smith AD. Controversies in endourology. Philadelphia: W.B. Saunders Company, 1995; 179–181.

Vallancien G, Capdeville R, Veillon B, Charton M, Brisset JM. Colonic perforation during percutaneous nephrolithotomy. J Urol 1985; 134:1185–1187.

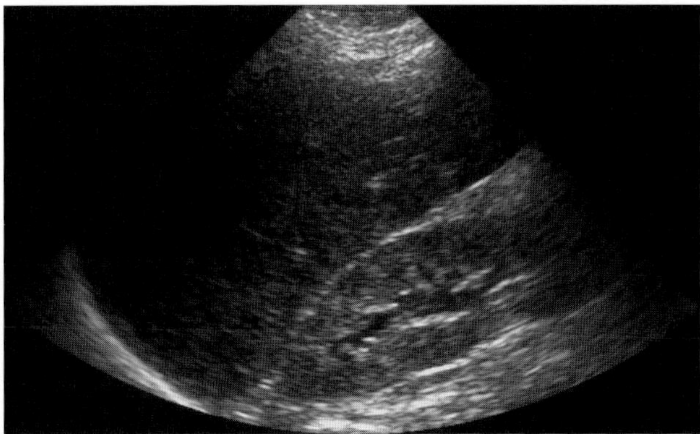

Figure 1. Sonogram of the right kidney.

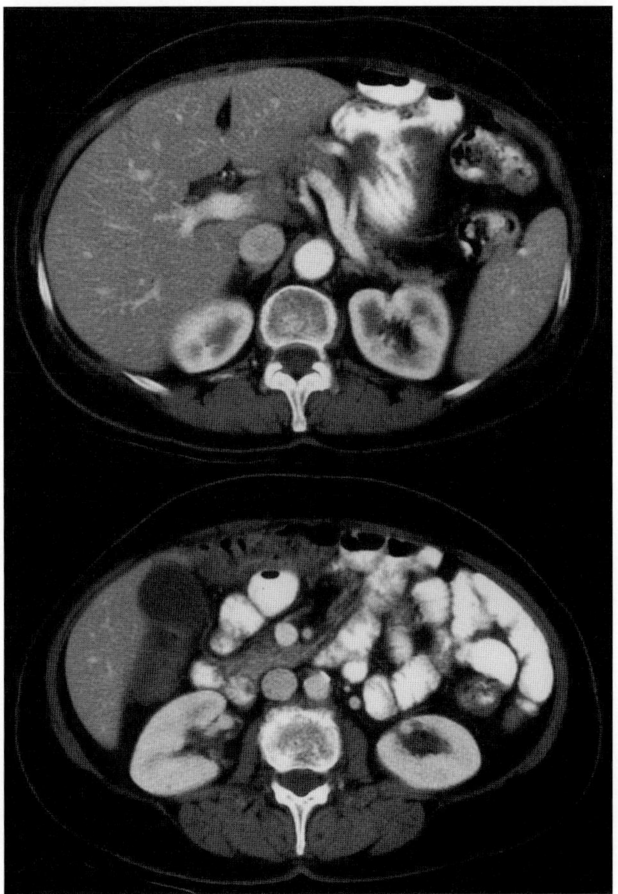

Figure 2. Representative sections from a renal CT scan.

TEACHING FILE CASE 53

William H. Marshall, M.D., and Allen J. Meglin, M.D.

History

A 34-year-old man underwent a left orchiectomy 14 years ago for nonseminomatous testicular cancer. After the orchiectomy, he was treated with a testosterone patch for 2 years. He now comes to the hospital with a right testicular mass. Before a second orchiectomy was undertaken, routine preoperative urinalysis demonstrated marked proteinuria. Renal sonography **(Fig. 1)** and computed tomography (CT) scanning **(Fig. 2)** were performed.

What is your diagnosis?

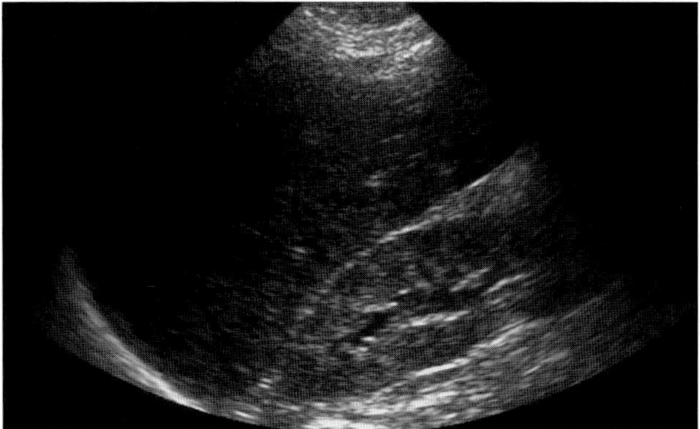

Figure 3. Renal sonogram demonstrates minimally increased echotexture with no evidence of mass lesion or hydronephrosis.

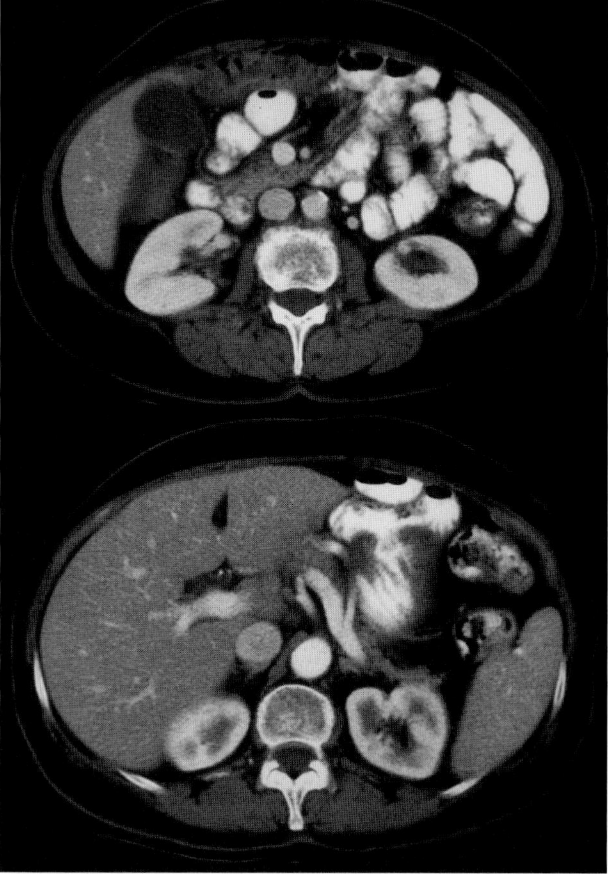

Figure 4. CT scan reveals symmetric uptake of contrast material without mass lesion or retroperitoneal adenopathy.

Radiographic Findings

The sonogram demonstrates minimally increased cortical echogenicity consistent with medical renal disease **(Fig. 3)**. No evidence of a renal mass, perinephric adenopathy, or hydronephrosis is seen. Doppler evaluation of the renal vasculature demonstrates normal arterial and venous anatomy. The CT scan reveals bilateral symmetric nephrograms without mass or significant retroperitoneal adenopathy **(Fig. 4)**.

Diagnosis

Unexplained proteinuria.

How would you manage this patient?

Management

The imaging studies did not explain the proteinuria, so a percutaneous renal biopsy was performed, after confirming that the patient's coagulation parameters were normal. Real-time sonography was used to localize the kidney and to provide continuous needle guidance **(Fig. 5)**. The lower pole of the kidney was localized to avoid the large vessels of the renal sinus. A spring-loaded biopsy gun was placed through a needle guide attached to the transducer, and the needle tip was followed sonographically to the point of renal cortex entry. Three cores of renal parenchyma were obtained and confirmed as diagnostically adequate by immediate gross examination.

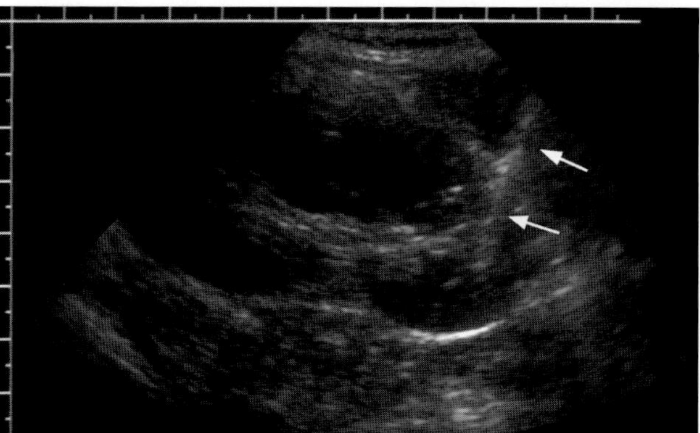

Figure 5. Ultrasound of the percutaneous biopsy shows the needle (arrows) entering the lower pole of the renal parenchyma.

Discussion

Percutaneous renal biopsy is a valuable tool for diagnosis, management, and prognosis of renal diseases in both native and transplanted kidneys. The diagnostic information it provides is critical in directing disease-specific management. The procedure was introduced in 1951 by Iverson and Brun and later popularized and standardized by Kark and Muehrcke. Several methods of kidney localization and biopsy guidance have been used over the past four decades, including radiography, radionuclide imaging, fluoroscopy with or without intravenous pyelography, and CT imaging. Real-time ultrasound is used for both localization and continuous observation of the kidney and biopsy device during the biopsy procedure.

For several reasons, sonographic guidance is gaining favor among physicians who perform renal biopsy. It carries with it a low risk of complications, it is easy to use, and more physicians are becoming comfortable using it. Presently, over 95% of sonographically directed biopsies yield a diagnosis, with a risk of life-threatening complications lower than 0.5%.

Continuous ultrasound guidance is reported in several studies to provide improved safety when compared with other modalities. Marwah et al reported that out of 394 patients who underwent percutaneous biopsy with use of ultrasound, 6.6% experienced minor and major complications. The minor complications were gross hematuria and/or self-limited subcapsular or perinephric hematoma. The major complications included hemorrhage requiring transfusion of blood products or resulting in hemodynamic instability, acute renal obstruction or failure, septicemia, and death. Another series of 200 renal biopsies reported an 8.1% minor complication rate and a 5.6% major complication rate.

Renal biopsy equipment has also advanced, with an evolution from manual aspiration to the manual needle and, most recently, to the automated spring-loaded device. The newer equipment facilitates needle mechanics for those less experienced in the biopsy technique, reduces the actual time that the biopsy needle is within the kidney, and requires less dexterity for tissue procurement. A review by Ballal et al of 107 renal biopsies performed with use of an 18-gauge automated spring-loaded "gun" type device revealed a 4.7% incidence of minor complications and no major complications.

An analysis of the risk factors associated with the two available needle types (14-gauge Franklin-Silverman needle and the 18-gauge automated core biopsy needle) found overall complication rates of 16.0% and 10.5%, respectively, and clinically significant complication rates of 6.5% and 2.5%, respectively. Because they yield adequate tissue samples, have low complication rates, and are easy to handle, spring-loaded "gun" devices seem to be the instruments of choice for performing percutaneous renal biopsy. In a review of 544 renal biopsies by Mendelssohn et al, a mean of 12.04 glomeruli were obtained for analysis, with a 96.9% pathologic diagnosis rate.

Conclusion

Although renal biopsies can be performed with use of surface landmarks or fluoroscopic or CT guidance, sonography has proven to be safe and effective, and is emerging as the modality of choice for performing renal biopsies. It also has great utility in the obese patient with high-riding kidneys who would otherwise be at great risk of life-threatening complications.

Selected Readings

Ballal SH, Nayak R, Dhanraj P, Kocher P, Bastani B. Percutaneous renal biopsy: a single center experience with automated spring-loaded biopsy gun type device. Clin Nephrol 1995; 44:274–275.

Birnholz JC, Kasinath BS, Corwin HL. An improved technique for ultrasound-guided percutaneous renal biopsy. Kidney Int 1985; 27:80–82.

Burstein DM, Schwartz MM, Korbet SM. Percutaneous renal biopsy with the use of real-time ultrasound. Am J Nephrol 1991; 11:195–200.

Corwin HL, Schwartz MM, Lewis EJ. The importance of sample size in the interpretation of renal biopsy. Am J Nephrol 1988; 8:85–89.

Fraser IR, Fairley KF. Renal biopsy as an outpatient procedure. Am J Kidney Dis 1995; 25:876–878.

Gibba A, Borella T, Michelone G, Dionisio P, Caramello E, Bajardi P. Percutaneous renal biopsy utilizing ultrasonic guidance and a semi-automated device. Urology 1994; 43:541–543.

Kadir S, ed. Current practice of interventional radiology. St. Louis: Mosby Year Book, 1991.

Kolb LG, Velosa JA, Bergstralh EJ, Offord KP. Percutaneous renal allograft biopsy: a comparison of two needle types and analysis of risk factors. Transplantation 1994; 1742–1746.

Marwah DS, Korbet SM. Timing of complications in percutaneous renal biopsy: what is the optimal period of observation? Am J Kidney Dis 1996; 28:47–52.

Mendelssohn FC, Cole EH. Outcomes of percutaneous kidney biopsy, including those of solitary native kidneys. Am J Kidney Dis 1995; 26:580–585.

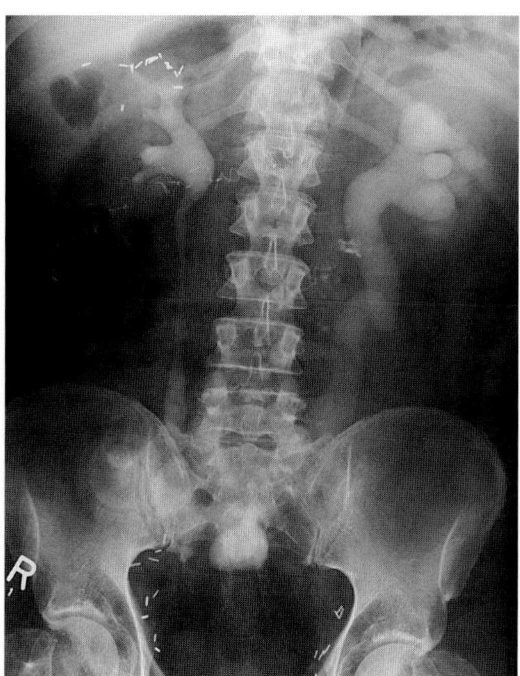

Figure 1. IVP performed after Bricker loop ileal diversion and revision.

TEACHING FILE CASE 54

Dean E. Baird, M.D.

History

A 58-year-old man underwent a cystoprostatectomy and Bricker ileal diversion for transitional cell carcinoma of the bladder. A revision of the ileal diversion was performed 4 years later to treat left ureteral obstruction. A technetium-99m MAG-3 renal scan performed 7 years after the revision showed a decrease in left renal function from 47% to 37% differential perfusion compared with a renal scan performed 2 years earlier. An intravenous pyelogram (IVP) was obtained **(Fig. 1)**.

What is your diagnosis?

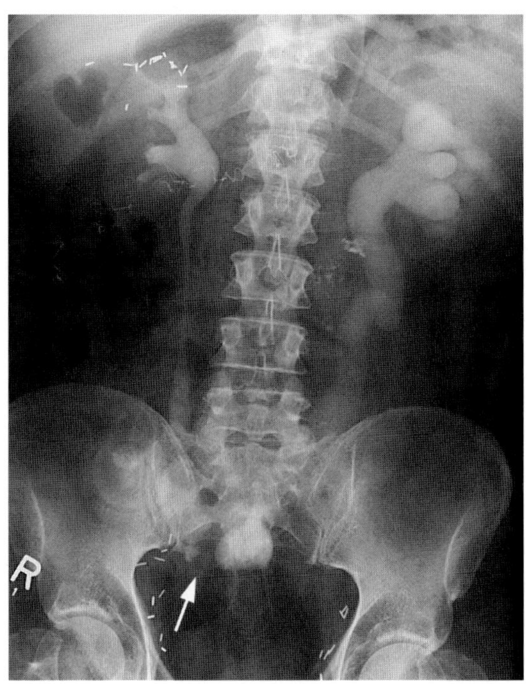

Figure 2. IVP shows the site of ureteral obstruction (arrow).

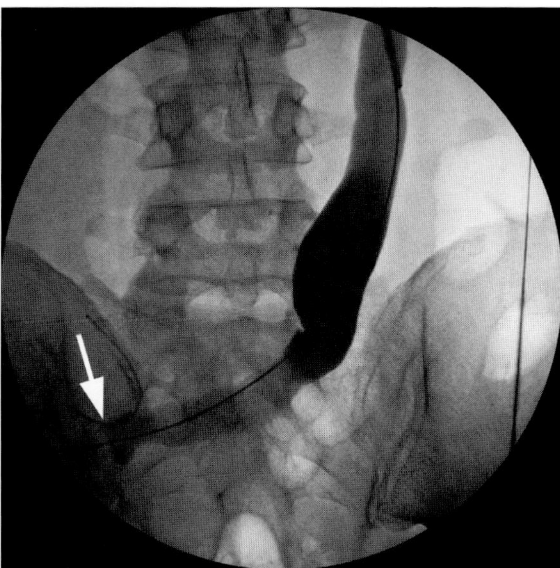

Figure 3. Antegrade left nephrostogram demonstrates ureteral obstruction at the level of the anastomosis with the ileal loop (arrow).

Radiographic Findings

The IVP showed obstruction of the left collecting system at the level of the ureteral anastomosis with the ileal loop **(Fig. 2)**. An antegrade left nephrostogram obtained after percutaneous nephrostomy shows complete obstruction of the distal left ureter at the level of insertion with the ileal conduit **(Fig. 3)**. Despite vigorous hand injection, no contrast material entered the conduit from the left ureter.

What is your diagnosis now?

Diagnosis

Distal left ureteral anastomotic stricture resulting in left ureteral obstruction and interval diminished left renal function.

What treatment would you recommend?

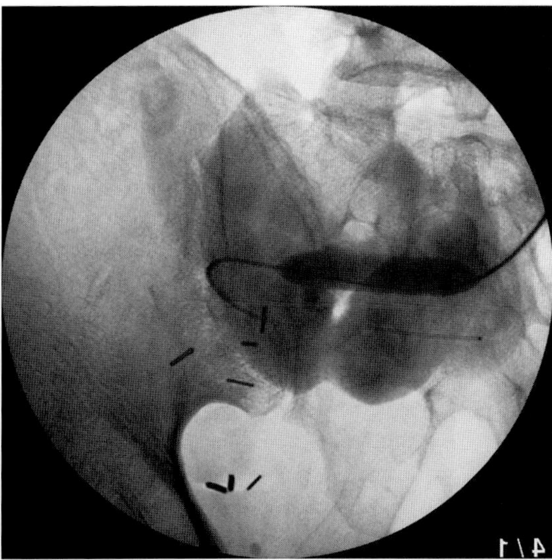

Figure 4. Inflated balloon catheter across the ureteral stenosis site.

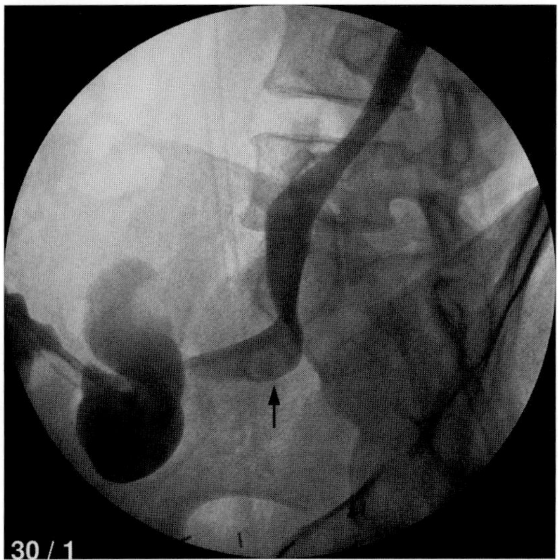

Figure 5. Antegrade left nephrostogram demonstrates a distal ureteral ovoid filling defect (arrow).

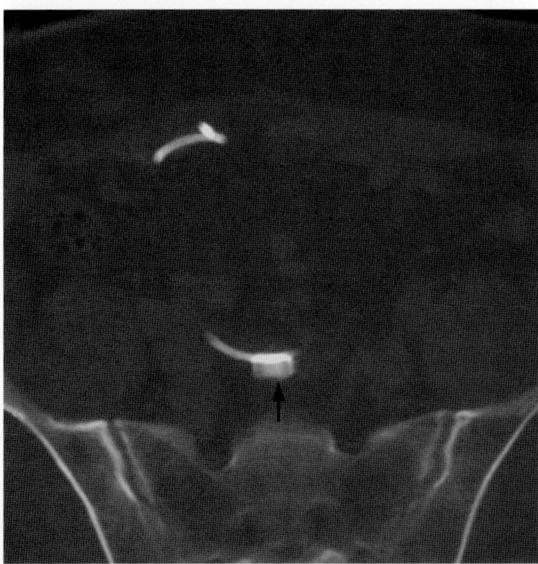

Figure 6. CT scan demonstrates a distal left ureteral stone (arrow) and a ureteral stent.

Management

The left ureteral anastomotic stricture was dilated from an antegrade approach. Under fluoroscopic guidance, the stricture was crossed with an 0.035-inch hydrophilic guide wire. After the wire was advanced into the ileal conduit, a 5-F, 65-cm straight catheter was placed and the wire exchanged for an 0.035-inch wire. After removal of the straight catheter, an 8-mm x 3-cm percutaneous angioplasty balloon catheter was placed across the stenosis and inflated until no waist could be seen on fluoroscopy **(Fig. 4)**. The subsequent contrast study showed free flow of contrast material through the anastomosis into the ileal conduit without evidence of extravasation. An 8-F double-J Strecker stent was then placed, and a 10-F back-up nephrostomy catheter was placed into the renal pelvis.

An antegrade nephrostogram performed 2 weeks later revealed an ovoid filling defect at the distal left ureter **(Fig. 5)**, consistent with a radiolucent ureteral calculus. This finding was confirmed on a computed tomography (CT) scan performed on the same day **(Fig. 6)**. The calculus was later fragmented and removed by ureteroscopy.

Discussion

This case demonstrates the utility of percutaneous balloon catheter dilatation in the management of benign ureteral strictures in postoperative patients. Benign ureteral strictures occur in 7%–10% of ureteroenteric anastomosis patients and can be complicated by urinary tract stones, pyelonephritis, and urinary sepsis. Surgical revision is technically difficult because of postoperative fibrous adhesions and any adjuvant radiation therapy. Successful balloon dilatation of ureteral strictures is achieved in nearly all patients. However, ureteral patency more than 6 months after the procedure is seen in only 18%–50% of patients. The prime determinants of success include chronicity of the stricture, length of the stricture, and stricture etiology.

Strictures of longer duration are less amenable to successful dilatation, which indicates the need for catheter dilatation as soon as possible. After ureteroplasty, stents are placed in all ureters for 4–8 weeks to maintain ureteral patency. This procedure can also be used in post-renal transplantation strictures as an alternative to surgical revision in a significant percentage of patients. Recent alternative therapies include combined balloon dilatation with electrosurgical incision. These alternative measures will further reduce the need for open surgical intervention of ureteroenteric anastomotic strictures.

Selected Readings

Beckmann CF, Roth R, Bihrle W. Dilation of benign ureteral strictures. Radiology 1989; 172:437–441.

Kim JC, Banner MP, Ramchandani P, Grossman RA, Pollack HM. Balloon dilation of ureteral strictures after renal transplantation. Radiology 1993; 186:717–722.

Kwak S, Leef JA, Rosenblum JD. Percutaneous balloon catheter dilatation of benign ureteral strictures: effect of multiple dilatation procedures on long-term patency. AJR 1995; 165:97–100.

Razvi HA, Martin TV, Sosa RE, Vaughan ED. Endourologic management of complications of urinary intestinal diversions. In: AUA Update Series, Lesson 22, Volume XV, 1996.

Shapiro MJ, Banner MP, Amendola MA, Gordon RL, Pollack HM, Wein AJ. Balloon catheter dilatation of ureteroenteric strictures: long-term results. Radiology 1988; 168:385–387.

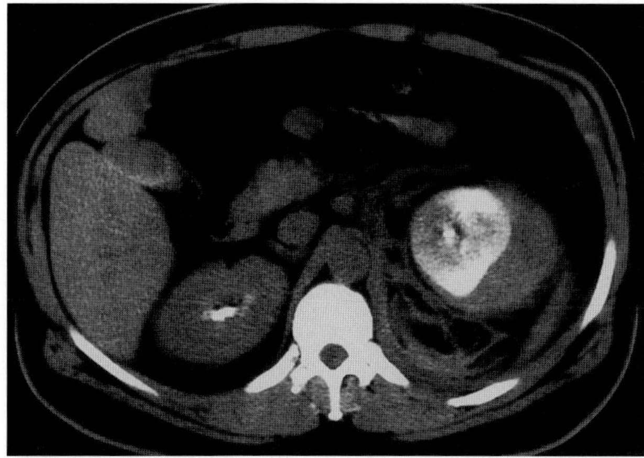

Figure 1. Delayed contrast-enhanced CT scan of the upper portions of the kidneys.

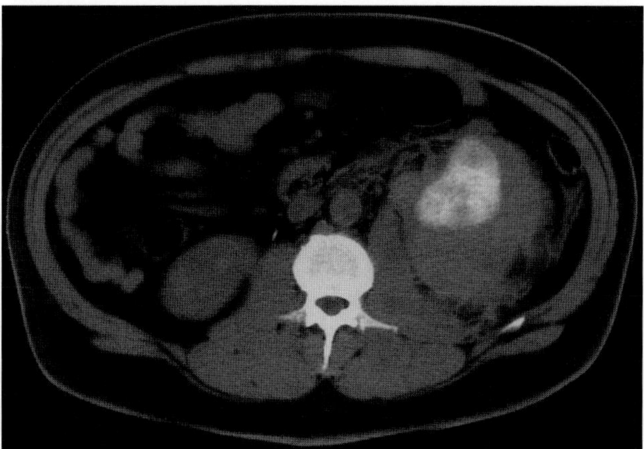

Figure 2. Delayed contrast-enhanced CT scan of the lower portions of the kidneys.

TEACHING FILE CASE 55

Jeet Sandhu, M.D.

History

The patient is a 32-year-old man who experienced the sudden onset of left flank pain after a wrestling match. A computed tomography (CT) scan was obtained 4 hours after the administration of contrast material **(Figs. 1, 2)**.

What is your diagnosis?

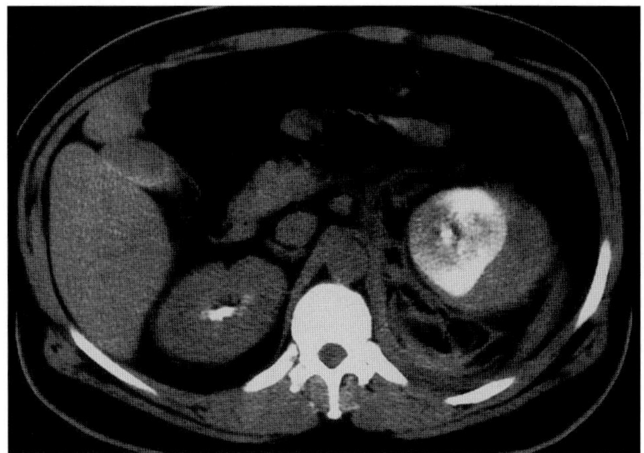

Figure 3. Delayed contrast-enhanced CT scan shows a persistently dense nephrogram of the left kidney with a subcapsular hematoma.

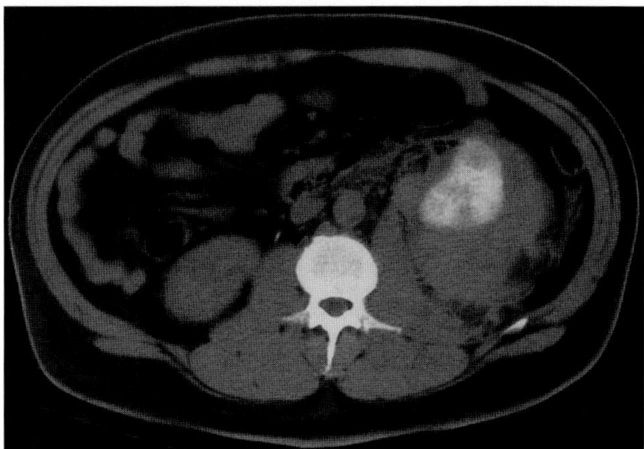

Figure 4. Inferior CT scan shows the inferior extension of the subcapsular component of the hematoma as well as a posterior pararenal hematoma with compression of the psoas muscle.

Radiographic Findings

The left kidney is compressed by a subcapsular hematoma **(Fig. 3)**. Significant impairment of left kidney function is evidenced by a persistently dense nephrogram. No renal parenchymal contrast material is identified in the right kidney; all of the contrast material has been excreted into the collecting system.

The uniformly high density of the subcapsular hematoma suggests that this is an acute, fresh hematoma. The more inferior CT image also demonstrates both the subcapsular component of the hematoma as well as a posterior pararenal hematoma compressing the left psoas muscle **(Fig. 4)**. Differential enhancement of the kidneys is again noted.

Diagnosis

Acute Page kidney phenomenon from a subcapsular hematoma compressing the renal parenchyma.

How would you manage this patient?

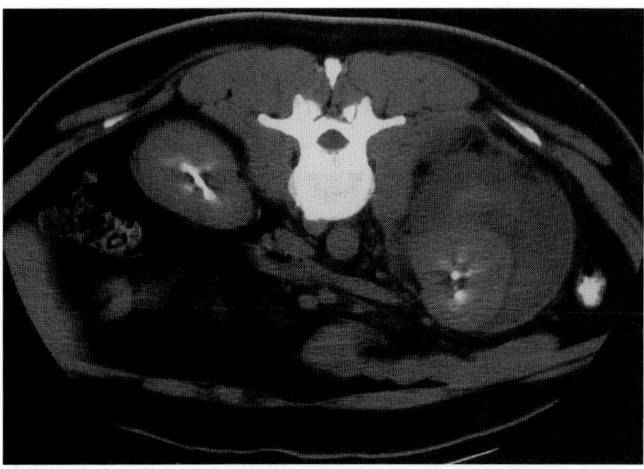

Figure 5. Prone CT scan obtained 3 weeks after the initial evaluation shows a persistent subcapsular hematoma.

Management

Because of the persistently dense nephrogram, a renal ultrasound examination was performed to exclude left renal vein thrombosis. The left renal vein was normal on both ultrasound and catheter-based contrast venography. Although the patient had been in a wrestling match, the trauma to his flank seemed insufficient to produce these findings. When patients have renal or pararenal hematomas after minimal trauma, a causative etiology to the underlying hemorrhage, which often turns out to be a tumor, should be sought. Although no tumor or mass was identified in the left kidney on the CT scan, the patient underwent renal arteriography to evaluate for an occult tumor. The left renal arteriogram was also normal, with no evidence of abnormal vascularity. After the initial evaluation and work-up, it was decided to follow the patient conservatively to see whether the hematoma would resolve spontaneously.

Three weeks after the initial CT scan was obtained, the patient had a technetium-99m diethylenetetramine pentaacetic acid (DTPA) renal scan which showed reduced function of the left kidney. A repeat CT scan showed persistent subcapsular hematoma **(Fig. 5)**. Compared to the initial CT scan, the hematoma was not as uniformly dense, suggesting that some interval liquefaction and lysis of the hematoma had taken place. The hematoma was clearly subcapsular in location, because Gerota's fascia could be identified separate from the margin of the hematoma. Although the patient was not hypertensive, his left renal function was significantly impaired.

How would you manage this patient now?

Because of the decreased left renal function quantified by the nuclear medicine study, it was decided that the hematoma needed to be evacuated. The options were to drain it surgically or percutaneously.

Because of the lower morbidity associated with percutaneous intervention and the technical accessibility of the hematoma, percutaneous drainage was attempted. Under CT guidance a needle was advanced into the hematoma from a posterolateral approach **(Fig. 6)**. Standard Seldinger technique was used to advance a wire into the collection **(Fig. 7)**, then a 16-F drainage catheter was advanced over the wire into the subcapsular hematoma **(Figs. 8, 9)**. Approximately 100 mL of old blood was obtained. The catheter was removed a week later after follow-up CT scanning showed no significant residual subcapsular hematoma. Follow-up CT scanning at 3 months also showed no significant residual hematoma **(Fig. 10)**, and a nuclear medicine renal study at that time demonstrated equivalent normal function of the kidneys.

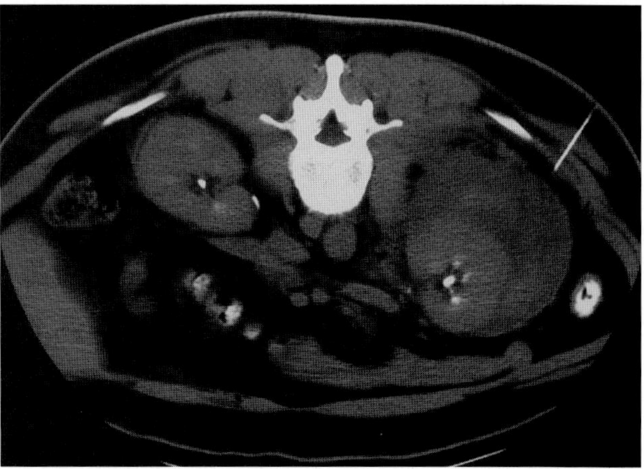

Figure 6. A needle is advanced into the subcapsular hematoma under CT guidance.

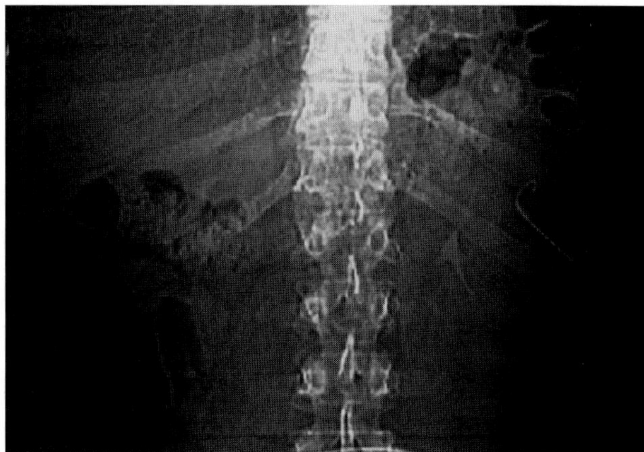

Figure 7. Wire in the subcapsular hematoma.

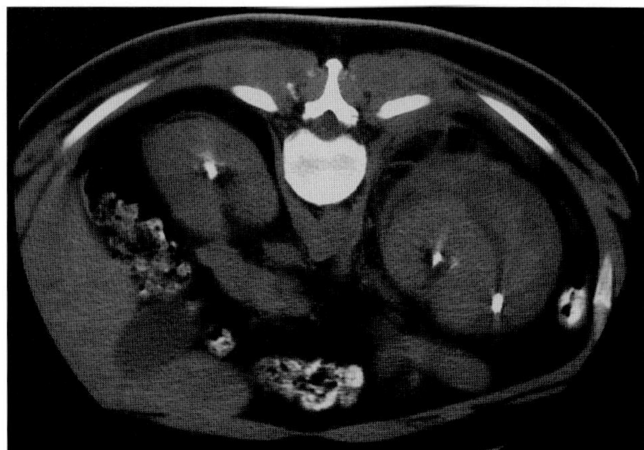

Figure 8. Prone CT scan shows the drain in the subcapsular hematoma.

Discussion

The Page kidney phenomenon is caused by the accumulation of blood in the perirenal or subcapsular space which results in compression of the renal parenchyma and consequent renal ischemia. The renal capsule is a very tough, confining structure with little space between the kidney and capsule. Collections of blood or fluid in this location exert significant pressure on the renal parenchyma, which causes compression of the kidney. Because of the compression, intrarenal pressures increase, producing an apparent decrease in the glomerular filtration rate which the kidney interprets as resulting from decreased blood flow. In response to this perceived renal ischemia, the renin-angiotensin system is activated and hypertension results.

The most common etiology of a Page kidney is flank trauma that causes a subcapsular or perirenal hematoma. Although football is most commonly implicated, almost any contact sport can result in this syndrome. Subcapsular bleeding after a renal biopsy or surgical intervention can also lead to the Page kidney phenomenon. In 10% of cases, no known antecedent event explains the hematoma. If left untreated, the hematoma compresses the renal parenchyma, as in this case, and induces ischemic hypertension and/or deterioration in renal function.

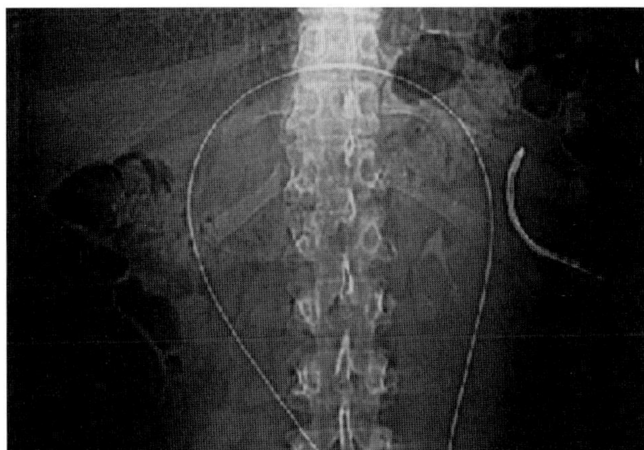

Figure 9. Drain in the subcapsular hematoma.

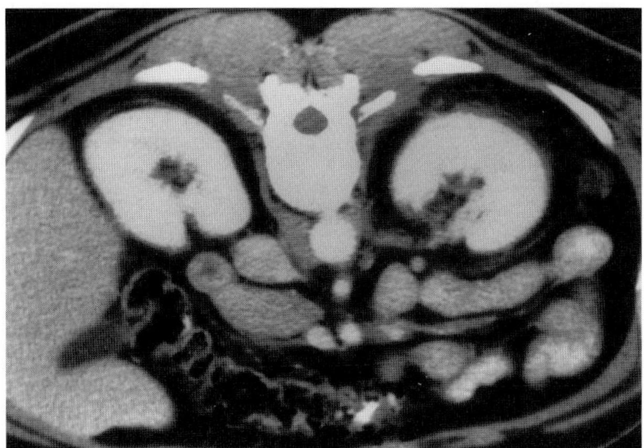

Figure 10. Follow-up CT scan at 3 months shows resolution of the subcapsular and posterior pararenal hematomas.

Over time the hematoma may be converted to a thick, fibrous capsule which causes continued compression of the kidney. This continued compression, now by the capsule itself, sustains the activation of the renin-angiotensin system. This explains why many patients present with hypertension long after the initial event. If discovered in the acute phase, the hematoma should be evacuated before it can convert into a fibrous capsule. In the absence of a fibrous capsule, percutaneous drainage will likely evacuate the majority of the hematoma. However, if a fibrous capsule is present, surgical therapy will be required. This capsule is best identified with CT or magnetic resonance imaging.

In general, asymptomatic hematomas will resorb spontaneously. Percutaneous drainage should be considered for all symptomatic hematomas. If the hematoma becomes infected, it should be drained. Symptomatic hematomas that produce significant pain or compress surrounding structures should also be drained. Hematomas are much more difficult to drain percutaneously than simple fluid collections because of the numerous septations, the viscosity of the blood, and organization of the clot. However, percutaneous drainage of hematomas may preclude the need for more invasive and morbid surgical evacuation. In this case, numerous dense areas which were suggestive of more organized thrombus were identified within the hematoma even 3 weeks after the initial event. Fortunately, simple catheter drainage with a large-bore tube sufficed.

The object of drainage is to drain as much of the liquefied component as possible. Mechanical destruction of the septations or fragmentation of organized thrombus with a guide wire or basket may improve drainage. The instillation of thrombolytic agents such as urokinase may also further liquefy the hematoma, permitting more successful percutaneous drainage.

In an acute hematoma causing a Page kidney phenomenon, percutaneous drainage should be considered as an alternative to surgical evacuation. It is important to drain the hematoma before a thick capsule develops.

Selected Readings

Aragona F, Artibani W, Calabro A, Villi G, Cisternino A, Ostardo E. Page kidney: a curable form of arterial hypertension. Case report and review of the literature. Urol Int 1991; 46:203–207.

Dempsey J, Gavant ML, Cowles SJ, Gaber AO. Acute Page kidney phenomenon: a cause of reversible renal allograft failure. South Med J 1993; 86:574–577.

McCune TR, Stone WJ, Breyer JA. Page kidney: case report and review of the literature. Am J Kidney Dis 1991; 18:593–599.

Mita K, Kobukata Y. Conservative management of nontraumatic subcapsular renal hematoma: a case report. Int J Urol 1994; 1:181–182

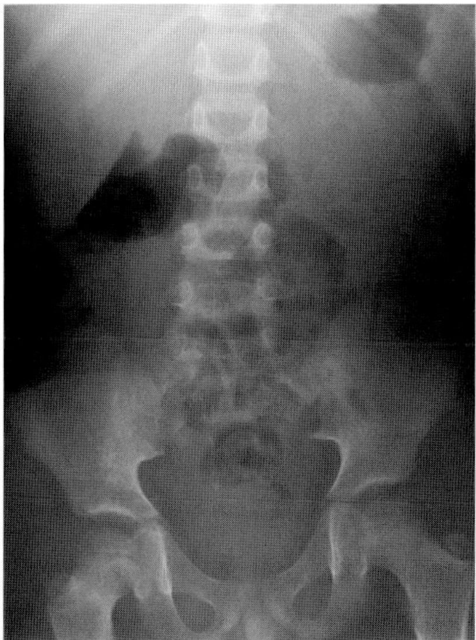
Figure 1. Scout film.

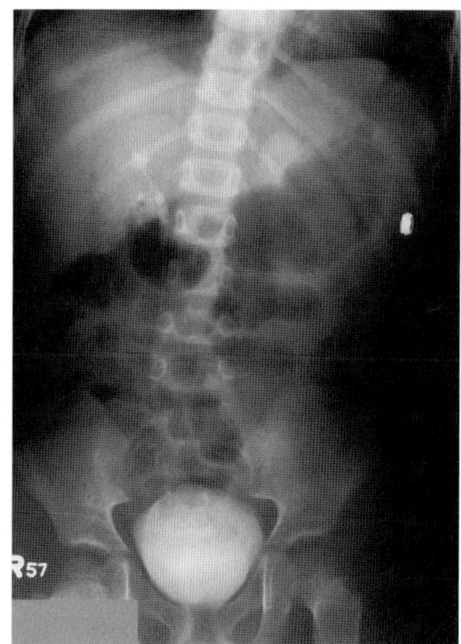

Figure 2. Excretory urogram 15 minutes after injection.

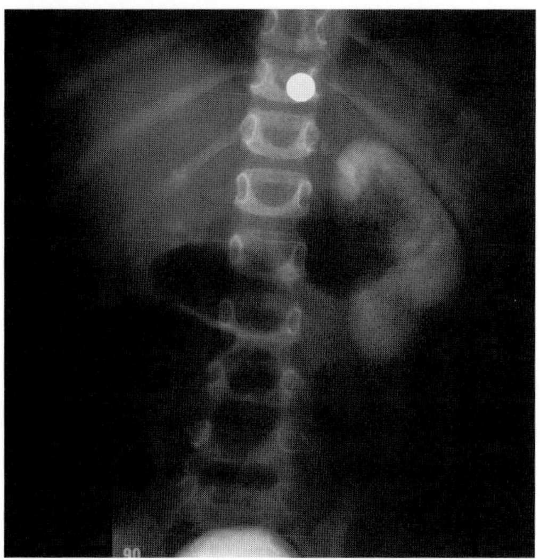
Figure 3. Film at 4 hours, 45 minutes after injection.

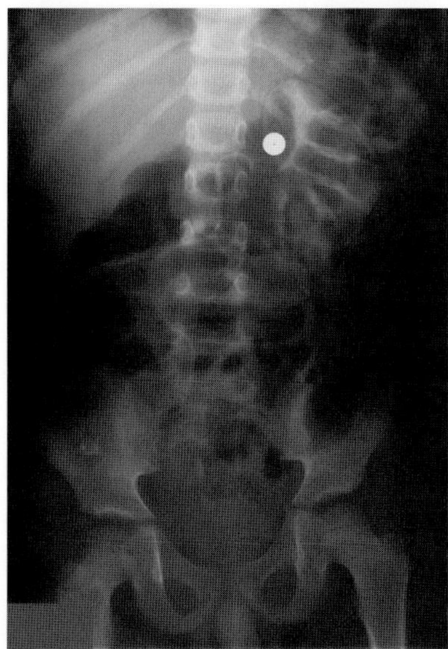
Figure 4. Delayed film at 15 hours.

TEACHING FILE CASE 56

Michelle Neuder, M.D., and Anthony C. Venbrux, M.D.

History

A 6-year-old boy was admitted to the hospital with left-sided abdominal pain that developed acutely and continued to worsen progressively over a 24-hour period. This was accompanied by a decreased appetite and level of activity. There had been no previous urinary tract infection, hematuria, trauma, or fever. The past medical history was significant for asthma, for which the patient was being treated with prednisone.

On admission, the child was afebrile and exhibited mild left upper quadrant and costovertebral angle tenderness on physical examination. No palpable masses were noted. The remainder of the physical examination was unremarkable.

Serum chemistries were within normal limits except for a bicarbonate of 19 and an anion gap of 21. The complete blood count was also within normal limits. On urinalysis, the urine was hazy with a pH of 7.5 and a small amount of ketones. Microscopically, 0–1 red blood cells per high-powered field (hpf), occasional white blood cells per hpf, and a few bacteria per hpf were seen. No casts or crystals were present. Urine culture was negative.

The patient's family history is significant for the child's father having a history of gout. After an ultrasound examination documented left-sided hydronephrosis (not shown), an excretory urogram was obtained **(Figs. 1–4)**.

What is your diagnosis?

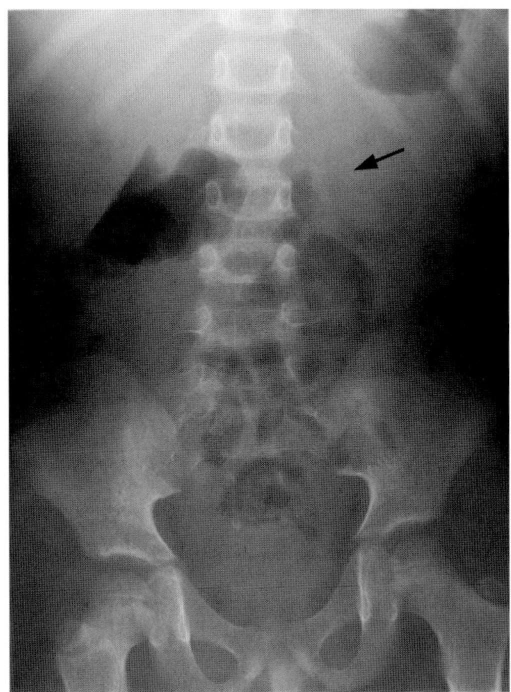

Figure 5. Scout film shows a faint calcific density over the left renal outline (arrow).

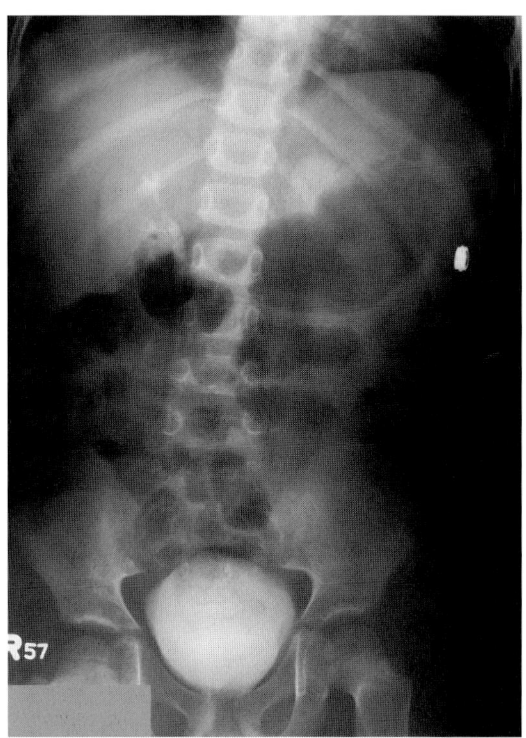

Figure 6. Excretory urogram 15 minutes after injection.

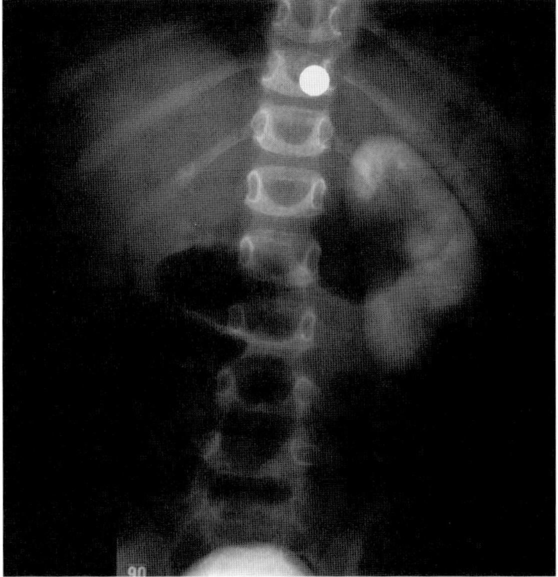

Figure 7. Delayed excretion of contrast material on the left at 4 hours, 45 minutes after injection.

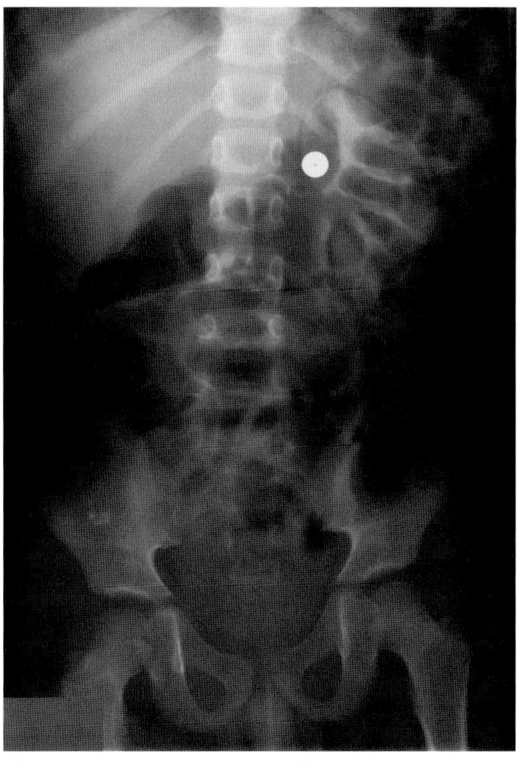

Figure 8. Distal ureter does not fill on follow-up film 15 hours after injection. This indicates obstruction.

Radiographic Findings

The scout film shows a faint calcific density over the left renal outline **(Fig. 5)** which did not correspond with the kidney based on oblique views (not shown). The excretory urogram confirms left-sided ureteral obstruction **(Figs. 6, 7)** with no observed filling of the distal left ureter on an abdominal follow-up film 15 hours later **(Fig. 8)**. The right renal collecting system and ureter cleared normally.

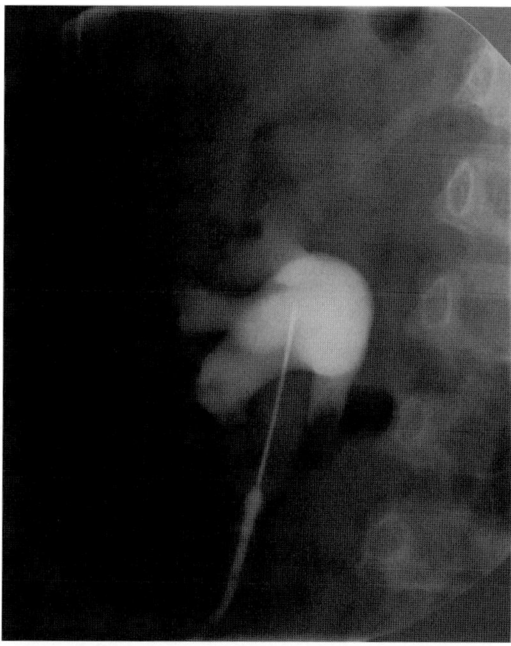

Figure 9. Anteroposterior spot film from a left antegrade nephrostogram performed with a "skinny" needle. The patient is prone.

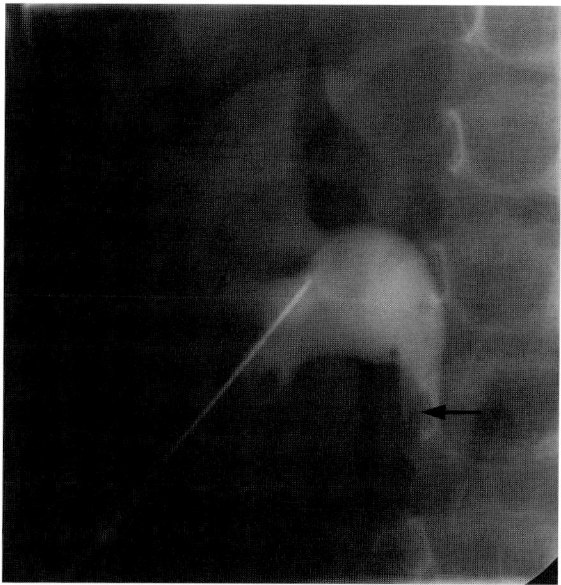

Figure 10. With the patient in the prone position, antegrade pyelogram shows complete obstruction of the left ureter at the level of the UPJ. Arrow shows a filling defect at the UPJ.

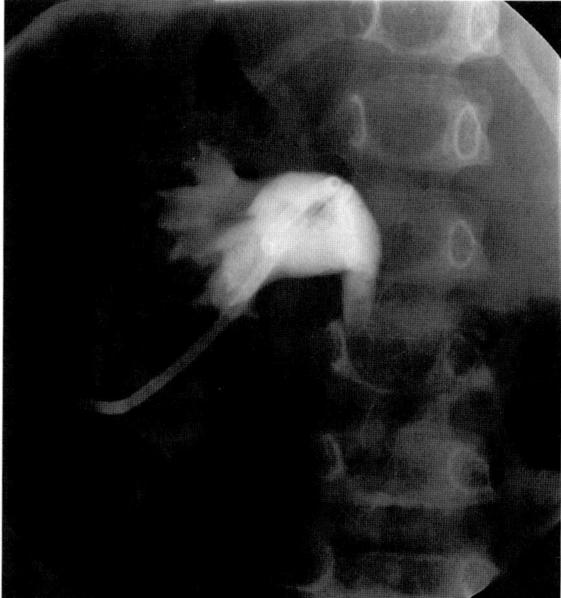

Figure 11. Prone nephrostogram shows the percutaneous nephrostomy tube in place. Again, no contrast material gets past the UPJ obstruction.

A left percutaneous antegrade pyeloureterogram obtained under ultrasound and fluoroscopic guidance demonstrates a filling defect at the uretero-pelvic junction (UPJ) that measures approximately 1 cm x 1.5 cm without evidence of calcification **(Figs. 9, 10)**. The ureter just distal to the UPJ was not visualized. The left renal pelvis and calyces were mildly dilated. The left kidney contour was normal.

Diagnosis

Radiolucent uric acid stone.

The differential diagnosis includes a blood clot or a primary obstructing lesion such as a malignant mass; however, this latter possibility is highly unlikely given the patient's age, clinical examination, and laboratory results.

How would you manage this patient?

Management

The patient was treated by urinary tract decompression and urine diversion with an 8-F nephrostomy tube placed percutaneously into the left renal pelvis **(Fig. 11)**. One day after nephrostomy tube placement, serum uric acid measurement revealed hyperuricemia (uric acid, 6.9 mg/dL; normal 2.0–5.5 mg/dL). Throughout the following week, urine pH ranged from 6.0 to 7.5.

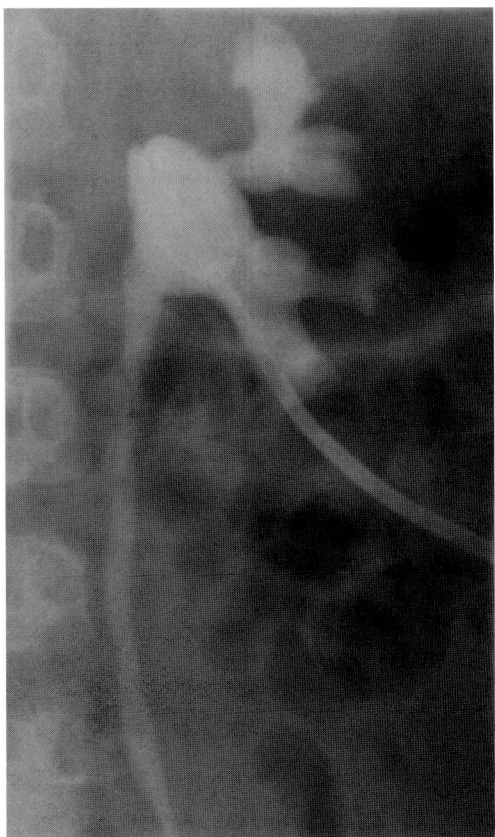

Figure 12. Coned-down supine antegrade nephrostogram after the UPJ stone had passed shows ureteral irregularity around the site of prior obstruction and a normal distal ureter.

A repeat nephrostogram 3 days after nephrostomy tube placement demonstrated a patent left ureter and only mild irregularity at the site of the prior filling defect **(Figs. 12, 13)**. The patient's serum uric acid levels slowly declined to normal over several days.

The left nephrostomy tube was capped to allow internal drainage. The child did well afterwards and remained asymptomatic. The final nephrostogram (not shown) demonstrated free flow beyond the site of focal narrowing. The pediatric urologist thought that the child had spontaneously passed the stone. Although the patient's urine was filtered, the stone was not recovered and therefore stone composition could not be analyzed.

Serum and urine chemistries, as well as urine microscopy, were followed up at 2 weeks, 3 months, and 9 months after discharge. An excretory urogram obtained at 9 months follow-up demonstrated an unobstructed urinary collecting system bilaterally **(Fig. 14)**. The proximal left ureter showed evidence of a mild focal narrowing which was thought to be a small stricture. No evidence of urinary obstruction was seen distal to this site. The patient has remained asymptomatic at 4 years follow-up.

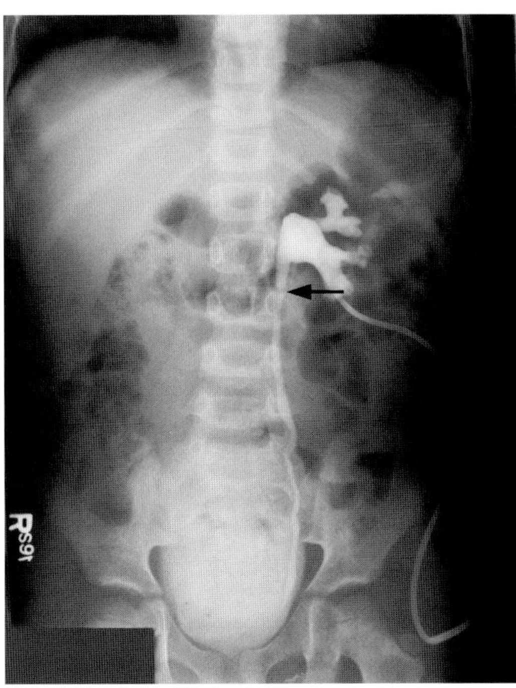

Figure 13. Repeat nephrostogram 3 days after nephrostomy tube placement. Arrow shows that the site of prior UPJ obstruction is now near normal, with only mild mucosal irregularity.

Discussion

Pediatric urolithiasis, a relatively rare phenomenon in the United States, is a complication of many different disorders. Most children with urolithiasis present with renal or ureteral calculi, often associated with a pre-existing condition such as a congenital anomaly, metabolic abnormality, or a history of trauma with prolonged immobilization. Urolithiasis may also be associated with chronic and recurrent urinary tract infections. Spontaneous stone passage may occur in about 40% of patients (as in this patient) while an additional 40% or more may require surgery or extracorporeal shock wave lithotripsy (ESWL). The mean age of presentation in the United States ranges between 8 and 12 years.

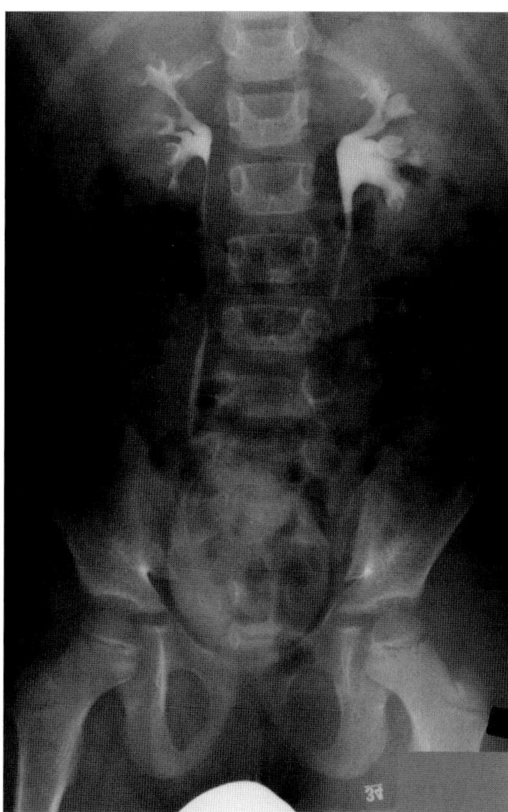

Figure 14. Supine urogram 9 months later is normal.

The predominant etiology of stone formation in children in the United States is metabolic (53% of all patients), secondary to an increased excretion of solutes or a decreased excretion of solubilizing substances. Disorders of metabolism resulting in an increased excretion of solutes include idiopathic hypercalciuria (33%–50% of patients), hyperparathyroidism, distal renal tubular acidosis, primary oxaluria, cystinuria, gout, and Lesch-Nyhan syndrome. Those disorders characterized by a decreased excretion of solubilizing substances involve decreased excretion of citrate, magnesium, and pyrophosphate. The congenital anomalies most often encountered in children (20%–44%) are UPJ obstruction and vesicoureteral reflux.

In younger children and infants, diagnosis of calculi is difficult, with pain or gross or microscopic hematuria being the most commonly encountered presentation. Abdominal pain is typically diffuse, occurring in 40% to 75% of patients, while 25% to 40% will present with hematuria. A third subset of patients, usually girls under 5 years old, will have symptoms of a urinary tract infection (10%–30%). Recurrent urinary tract infections, persistent gross hematuria not associated with glomerulonephritis, and recurrent severe abdominal pain implicate urolithiasis as a likely etiology.

Age of onset, family history, fluid intake, diet, and drug history are important additional factors to consider in making the diagnosis of urolithiasis. Urinalysis, urine culture, serum electrolytes (including calcium, phosphorus, uric acid), and a 24-hour urine collection to measure volume, calcium, oxalate, uric acid, citrate, cystine, phosphate, and creatinine should be performed. Intravenous pyelography should also be performed to define subtle anatomic anomalies and to identify renal scarring.

The surgical management of urolithiasis in children has changed dramatically in the last 15 years. Open surgery has largely been superceded by ESWL, improved percutaneous techniques, and the availability of smaller, more flexible ureteroscopes for extraction of mid and lower ureteral stones. Open surgery has been used mainly to manage urolithiasis in children who have a congenital obstruction, such as UPJ obstruction, or in patients with severe orthopedic deformities that preclude the use of endourologic procedures and ESWL.

Percutaneous management is very effective in the symptomatic patient with urolithiasis. Percutaneous nephrostomy has been performed successfully in children for the treatment of upper tract pathology. The most common indication for percutaneous catheter placement is temporary decompression of the obstructed kidney. Percutaneous nephrostomy has been used successfully in other percutaneous manipulations including extraction of renal calculi, incision of a UPJ obstruction, and dilation and stent placement to treat ureteral strictures. These techniques should not be used in patients with bleeding diatheses (ie, a coagulopathy that cannot be corrected). Potential complications of interventional therapy include bleeding, sepsis, and tube dislodgement. Patients may be discharged with nephrostomy catheters in place, with tube changes performed on an outpatient basis every 2 to 3 months.

ESWL has demonstrated a high degree of safety, at least in the short term, in the treatment of upper tract stones smaller than 2.0 cm in diameter, although some initial degree of measurable renal damage is associated with stone destruction. There are also long-term effects on both renal and bone growth that have yet to be defined. Large stones or staghorn calculi cannot be removed by ESWL alone. Such stones require percutaneous access, tract dilation, and debulking with use of ultrasonic and/or electrohydraulic lithotripsy first, followed by ESWL.

Selected Readings

Cohen TD, Ehreth J, Kin LR, Preminger GM. Pediatric urolithiasis: medical and surgical management. Urology 1996; 47:292–303.

Faerber GJ, Bloom DA. Pediatric endourology. In: Gillenwater JY, Grayback SS, Howards JW, Duckett JW. Adult and pediatric urology. St. Louis: Mosby Year Book, 1996; 2739–2758.

Harmon EP, Neal DE, Thomas R. Pediatric urolithiasis: review of research and current management. Pediatr Nephrol 1994; 8:508–512.

Segura JW. Role of percutaneous procedures in the management of renal calculi. Urol Clin North Am 1990; 17:207–216.

Stanley P, Diament MJ. Pediatric percutaneous nephrostomy: experience with 50 patients. J Urol 1986; 135:1223–1226.

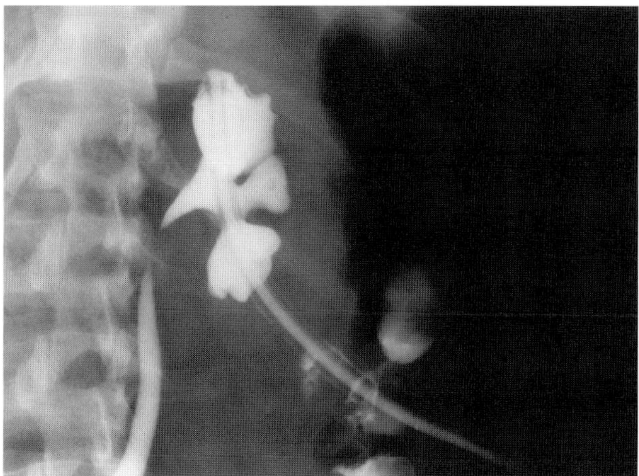

Figure 1. Nephrostogram in a patient after nephrolithotomy.

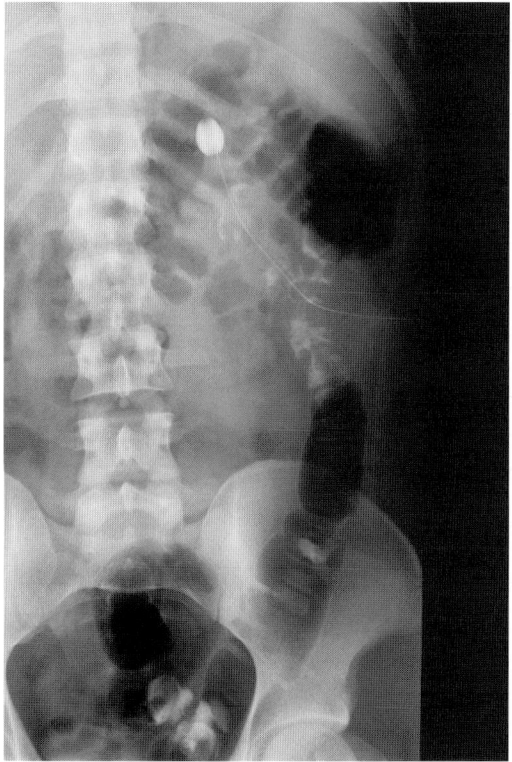

Figure 2. Full abdominal film.

TEACHING FILE CASE 57

Lance Arnder, M.D., and
Jeet Sandhu, M.D.

History

A 30-year-old patient underwent percutaneous nephrolithotomy. The nephrostomy was performed by the urologic service, but the patient is referred to the interventional suite for a tube check to exclude residual stones and evaluate drainage **(Figs. 1, 2)**.

What is your diagnosis?

Radiographic Findings

The nephrostogram demonstrates contrast material within a dilated left renal collecting system and ureter **(Fig. 3)**. Contrast material is also seen tracking around the tube and into the descending colon. This was not seen on the scout film. A less coned-in view demonstrates contrast material within the descending and sigmoid colon as well as thickened colonic folds in the region of the proximal descending colon **(Fig. 4)**.

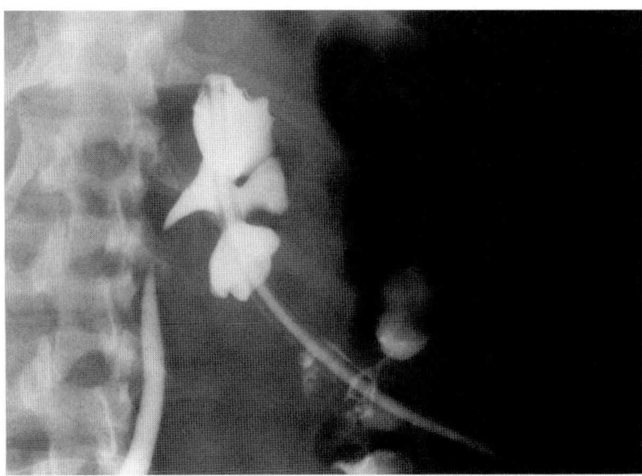

Figure 3. Nephrostogram shows no residual stones with brisk flow of contrast material down the ureter. Contrast material tracks back along the nephrostomy catheter and enters the colon. (The filling defect in the mid pole calyx is an air bubble).

Diagnosis

Colonic perforation by the percutaneous nephrostomy tube.

How would you manage this patient?

Management

Because the nephrostomy tube had been in place for less than 48 hours, it was decided to simply remove the tube and treat the patient with antibiotics. The patient did well and had no untoward sequelae.

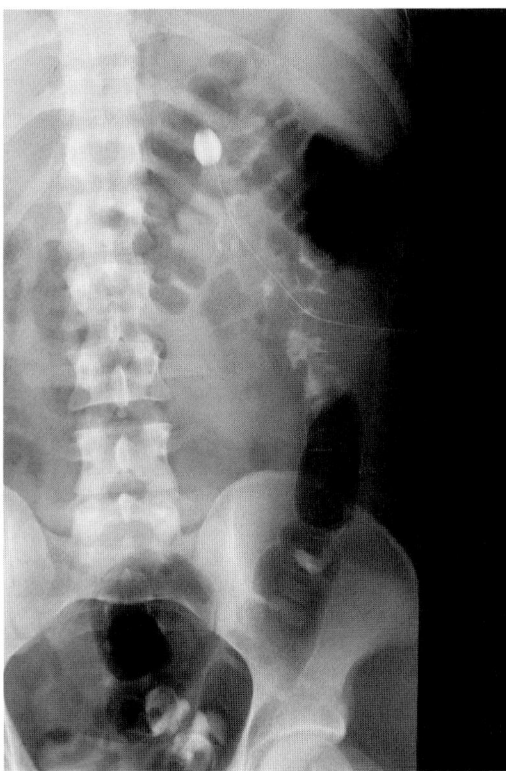

Figure 4. Abdominal radiograph shows contrast material in the colon from the colonic perforation with thickening of the colonic folds in the area of injury.

Discussion

Percutaneous nephrostomy tube placement is a safe and effective procedure that is successful in 98% of cases. The mortality rate is 0.2% and the incidence of major complications—those requiring a specific treatment to correct the complication or those that require extending the patient's hospital stay—is 4%. The complications associated with percutaneous nephrostomy tube placement can be divided into three categories: vascular, infectious, and catheter-related.

Vascular Complications

Vascular complications include arteriovenous fistula formation, pseudoaneurysm formation, and more commonly, hemorrhage. These complications are minimized when a posterolateral approach is used with entry into a calyx along or nearly along the mid-coronal plane of the kidney (the "bloodless" plane of Brödel).

Entering the posterior calyx minimizes the amount of renal parenchyma traversed and allows access to the collecting system as far from the larger renal and segmental vessels as possible. Any hemorrhage from the traversed renal parenchyma will be tamponaded to some extent by the nephrostomy catheter. The risk of vascular injury is greater with an anterior calyx because more parenchyma is traversed and the larger segmental vessels are located anteriorly.

Infectious Complications
Although vascular complications can and do occur, the most common major and minor complications of the procedure are infectious: perirenal abscess and sepsis, respectively. Because the factors leading to urinary tract infection—obstruction, stasis, or renal calculi—are the same ones that create the need for the nephrostomy, the use of periprocedural antibio-tics has been recommended for all patients undergoing this procedure, especially those at high risk for infection. High-risk patients are defined as those with infected urine documented by urinalysis or culture, those with a urinary ostomy, and in particular, those with struvite stones. The use of prophylactic antibio-tics has been shown to reduce the incidence of septic complications from 50% to 9% in this high-risk group.

Although ultrasound can suggest the presence of pyonephrosis, any patient with an unexplained fever and hydronephrosis, even if totally clear fluid is evident on the sonogram, should be presumed to have infected urine and given prophylactic antibio-tics. To avoid sepsis, postprocedure nephrostograms should be delayed until the infection has been treated adequately.

Catheter-Related Complications
Most catheter-related complications result from misplacement of the catheter into or through an organ, viscus, or pleural space. Direct placement into the renal pelvis can even occur. Perforation of the colon occurs in approximately 0.2% of cases and most often occurs in patients whose colons are abnormally high and posterior in position. At least a portion of the colon extends behind the medial two thirds of the kidney in 4.7% of prone patients. This statistic is the most important because patients most often lie prone during the procedure. Since the normal angle of entry used for nephrostomies is within 30 degrees of a true dorsal approach, this angle should prevent entry into colon that does not extend beyond the lateral third of the kidney. In this case, the entry site was too lateral, which resulted in the colonic injury.

Colonic Position
The retrorenal colon is more common in men than in women, and in older than in younger individuals. This is especially true on the right. It is interesting to note that while colonic extension behind the kidney is more common on the left, significant extension or extension behind the medial two thirds of the kidney is more common on the right. In either side it was only present at the level of the lower renal pole in one study. Based on this information, a true dorsal approach through a superior or mid pole posterior calyx is the safest approach with respect to the colon.

Of course, this consideration must be balanced against placement through the paraspinal muscles and the desirability of an approach along the plane of Brödel. In most patients, an approach into a lower pole calyx is chosen because the approach to the mid and upper pole calyces lies in an axial plane superior to the inferior border of the 12th rib.

The risk of traversing the pleural space increases when an approach superior to the 12th rib is chosen. In one study, all patients with significant retrorenal colon had extensively distended bowel. Attention should be directed to the bowel gas under fluoroscopy before choosing an approach. The use of ultrasound guidance will also minimize any chances of colonic injury as it allows the operator to easily identify and avoid the bowel.

Management of Colonic Perforation

It is important to recognize early that colonic perforation has occurred. This reduces the amount of time in which a colorenal fistula can mature and hastens the institution of appropriate management.

If the tube has been in place for only a short period of time and the pressure within the colonic lumen is not elevated, conservative management with antibiotic therapy after removal of the tube is appropriate. If recognition of the colonic injury is delayed, the nephrostomy catheter should still be removed from the kidney; it can be reinserted from an alternative route if needed. The original nephrostomy catheter should be left in the colon to decompress it. If after a few days a sinogram demonstrates no colorenal fistula, the catheter can be removed from the colon. A CT examination can be performed to evaluate for any abscess formation that might require drainage. If any increased luminal pressure is evident within the affected colon, the colon should be decompressed.

Fortunately, colonic perforation from nephrostomy placement is a rare event that is seldom life-threatening. Despite dilation of the track to a significant size (30 F), this complication can usually be managed conservatively and its incidence minimized by adhering to proper technique when inserting the initial nephrostomy catheter.

Selected Readings

Cochran ST, Barbaric ZL, Lee JJ, Kashfian P. Percutaneous nephrostomy tube placement: an outpatient procedure? Radiology 1991; 179:843–847.

Ferral H, Stackhouse DJ, Bjarnason H, Hunter DW, Castaneda-Zuniga WR. Complications of percutaneous nephrostomy tube placement. Semin Intervent Radiol 1994; 11:198–206.

Hopper KD, Sherman JL, Luethke JM, Ghaed N. The retrorenal colon in the supine and prone patient. Radiology 1987; 162:443–446.

Lang EK. Percutaneous nephrostolithotomy and lithotripsy: a multi-institutional survey of complications. Radiology 1987; 162:25–30.

LeRoy AJ, Williams HJ, Bender CE, Segura JW, Patterson DE, Benson RC. Colon perforation following percutaneous nephrostomy and renal calculus removal. Radiology 1985; 155:83–85.

Stables DP. Percutaneous nephrostomy: techniques, indications, and results. Urol Clin North Am 1982; 9:15–29.

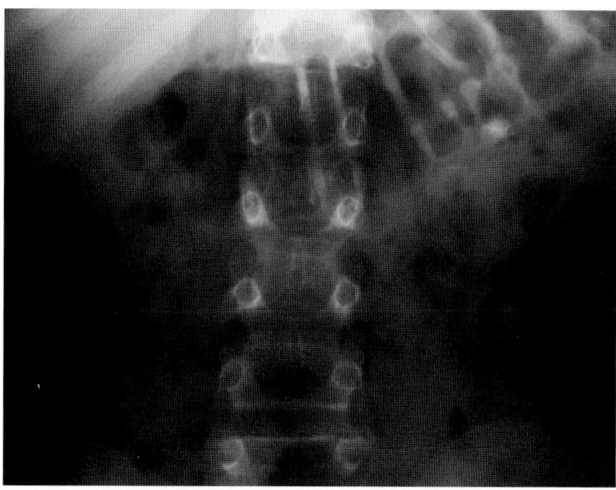

Figure 1. Scout film of an intravenous pyelogram.

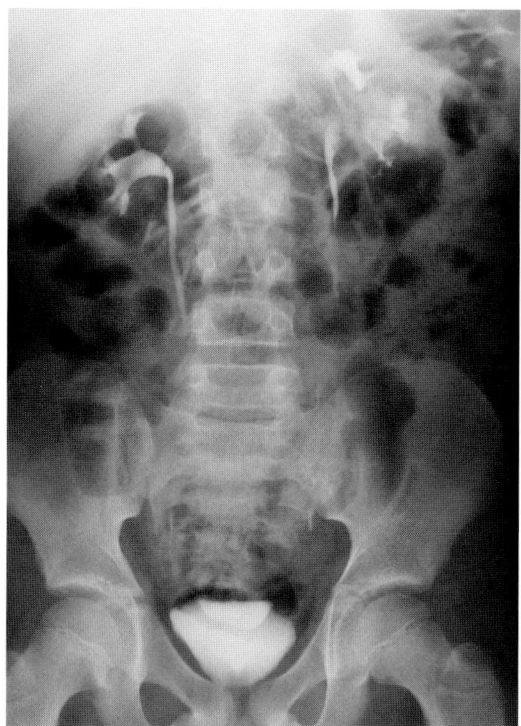

Figure 2. Radiograph obtained 5 minutes after injection of intravenous contrast material.

TEACHING CASE FILE 58

Dennis S. Peppas, M.D., and Ellen M. Chung, M.D.

History

A 10-year-old boy is being evaluated for microscopic hematuria with an intravenous pyelogram (IVP) **(Figs. 1, 2)**.

What is your diagnosis?

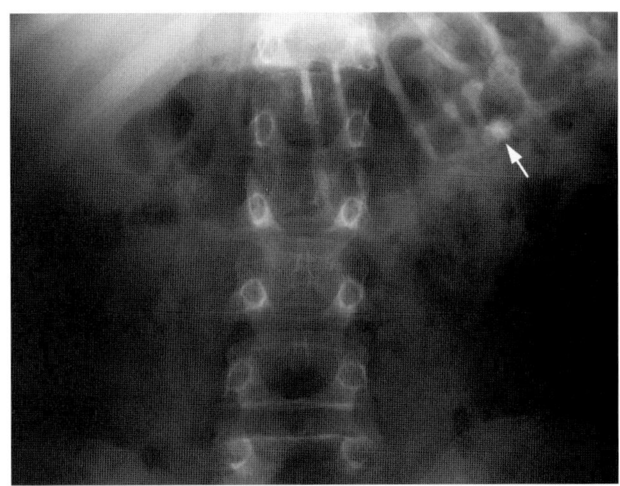

Figure 3. Scout film of an IVP demonstrates a radiopacity overlying the left renal outline (arrow).

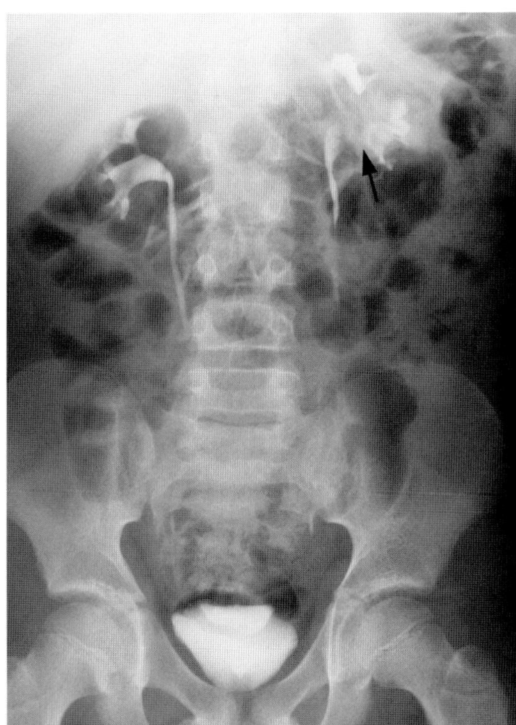

Figure 4. Film obtained 5 minutes after injection of intravenous contrast material demonstrates a filling defect within the left renal pelvis (arrow) due to the dense calculus seen on the scout film.

Radiographic Findings

The IVP demonstrates a 1.2 x 0.9-cm radiopacity overlying the left renal pelvis on the scout film **(Fig. 3)** which corresponds to a filling defect on the film obtained 5 minutes after injection of intravenous contrast material **(Fig. 4)**. There is no evidence of urinary obstruction (eg, ureteropelvic junction or ureterovesical junction obstruction), or medical renal disease.

Diagnosis

Renal calculus.

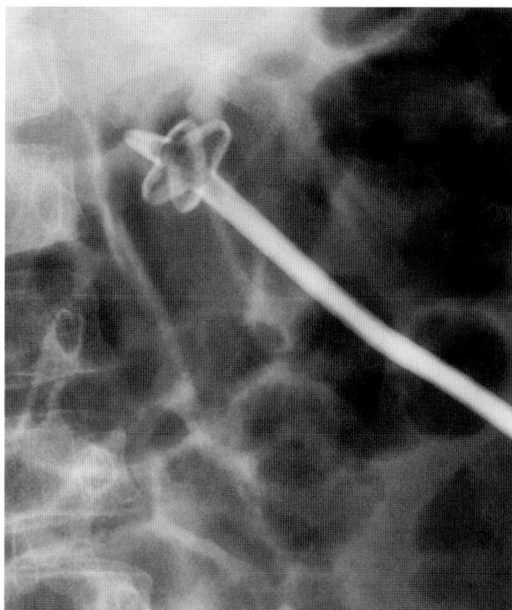

Figure 5. Radiograph obtained following nephrostolithotomy shows a percutaneous nephrostomy tube in the collecting system. There are no retained stone fragments.

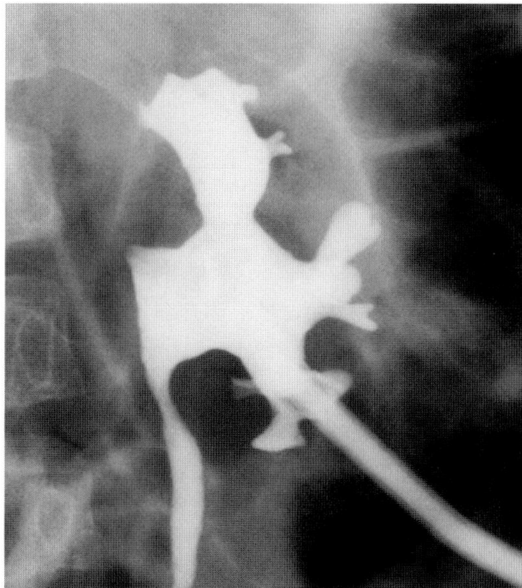

Figure 6. Antegrade nephrostogram performed prior to removal of the nephrostomy tube shows good flow of contrast material through the ureteropelvic junction.

Management

The child underwent two sessions of extracorporeal shock wave lithotripsy (ESWL). Both ESWL treatments failed to disrupt or fragment the stone. Further treatment options presented to the parent included open pyelolithotomy and percutaneous nephrolithotomy (PCNL). The parent opted for PCNL, which was performed without complication. The coned-down view of the left kidney from the postoperative kidneys, ureters, bladder study **(Fig. 5)** and antegrade nephrostogram **(Fig. 6)** failed to reveal any retained stone fragments or extravasation of contrast material to suggest disruption of the collecting system.

Discussion

It is estimated that the pediatric population accounts for less than 1% of the total number of patients who present with calculus disease of the urinary tract. The etiology of calculi in this patient population is usually a metabolic disorder (eg, renal tubular acidosis, hyperparathyroidism, etc) or recurrent urinary tract infection with vesicoureteral reflux. PCNL is a safe and effective method of treating urinary calculi. In over 500 cases of percutaneous nephrostolithotomy, Lee et al were able to achieve acceptable stone-free rates with a minimum of postoperative morbidity.

Selected Readings

Hulbert JC, Reddy PK, Gonzalez R, et al. Percutaneous nephrostolithotomy: an alternative approach to the management of pediatric calculus disease. Pediatrics 76(4):610–612.

Lee WJ, Smith AD, Cubelli V, Vernace FM. Percutaneous nephrolithotomy: analysis of 500 consecutive cases. Urol Radiol 1986; 8(2):61–66.

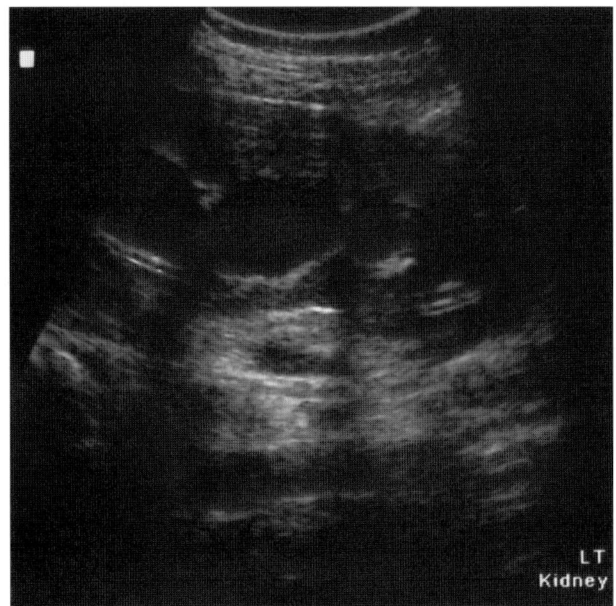

Figure 1. Ultrasound with full bladder.

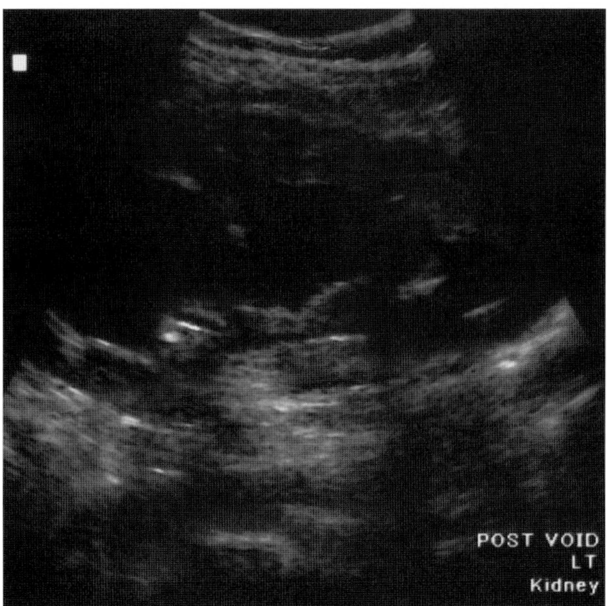

Figure 2. Left renal sonogram after voiding.

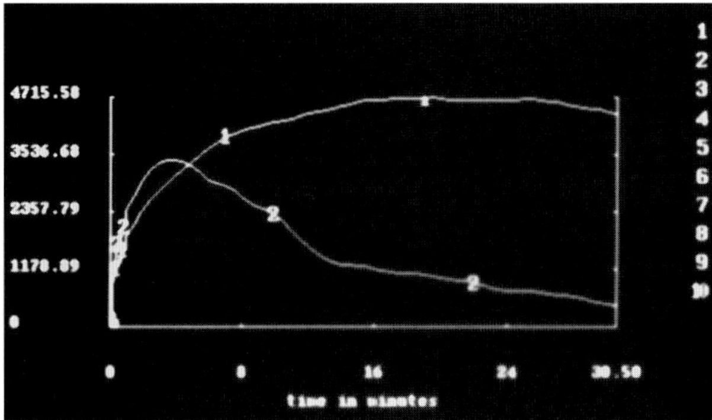

Figure 3. Lasix renogram.

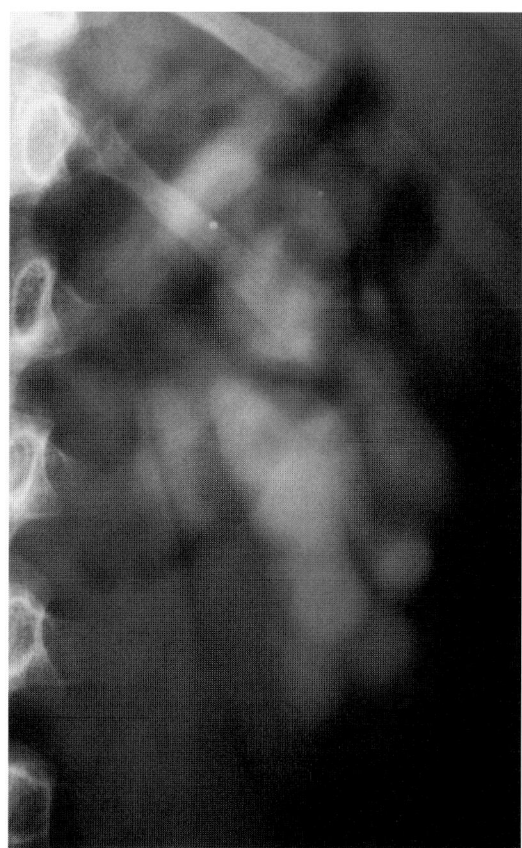

Figure 4. 6-minute film from an IVP.

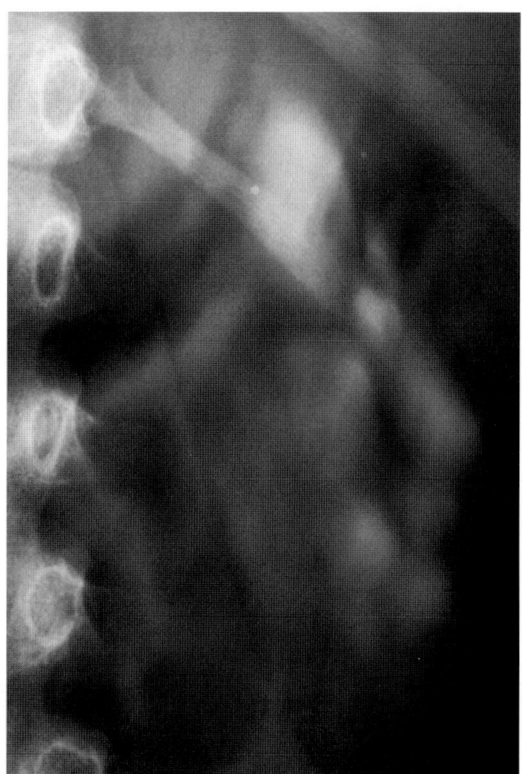

Figure 5. IVP following the administration of Lasix.

TEACHING FILE CASE 59

Dennis S. Peppas, M.D., and Ellen M. Chung, M.D.

History

An 8-year-old girl is being evaluated for a urinary tract infection with a voiding cystourethrogram (VCUG) and ultrasound **(Figs. 1, 2)**. Based on the results of these studies a Lasix renogram was obtained **(Fig. 3)**. She was followed with serial renal and bladder ultrasound examinations and Lasix renal scans which showed no significant changes from her original studies. In order to obtain an anatomic as well as physiologic evaluation, an intravenous pyelogram (IVP) with Lasix was obtained **(Figs. 4, 5)**.

What is your diagnosis?

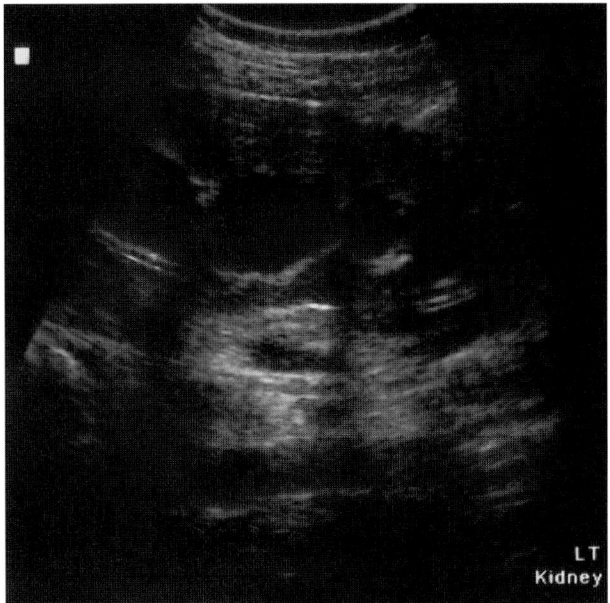

Figure 6. Longitudinal view of the left kidney demonstrates moderate caliectasis, with relative preservation of the renal cortex.

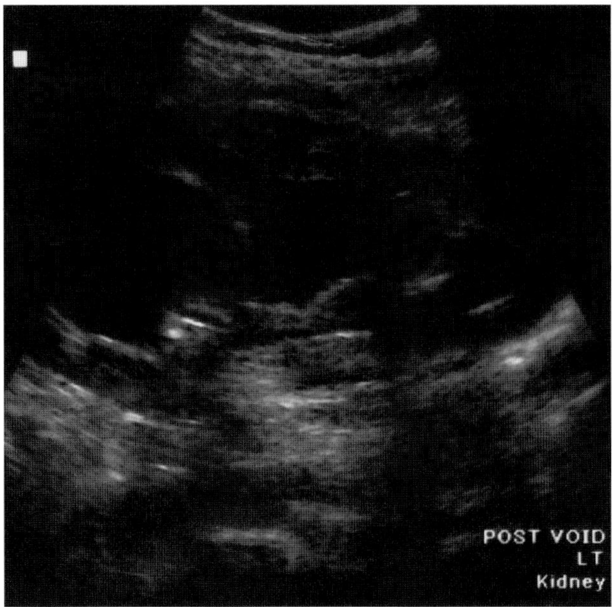

Figure 7. Post-void longitudinal view of the left kidney demonstrates persistent caliectasis, unchanged from the pre-void state.

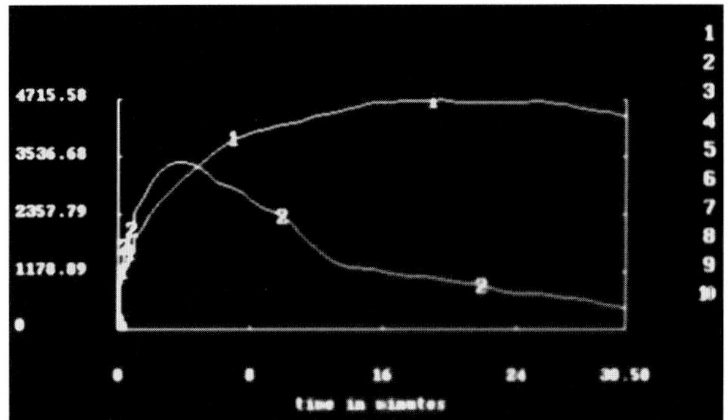

Figure 8. Renogram curves, post Lasix, demonstrate a prolonged half-life consistent with obstruction.

Radiographic Findings

The VCUG is normal with no reflux **(Fig. 6)**. The sonogram demonstrates hydronephrosis without hydroureter or renal cortical thinning **(Fig. 7)**. The Lasix renogram demonstrates an elevated half-life in the obstructed range, but function between the left and right kidney is equivalent **(Fig. 8)**. The IVP reveals persistent left hydronephrosis without visualization of the ipsilateral ureter throughout the course of the study **(Figs. 9, 10)**.

Diagnosis

Left ureteropelvic junction obstruction.

Management

In an older child with ureteropelvic junction (UPJ) obstruction, observation is not an acceptable alternative. Therefore, the alternatives for treatment discussed with this family included the standard open pyeloplasty and endopyelotomy. The parents opted for endopyelotomy.

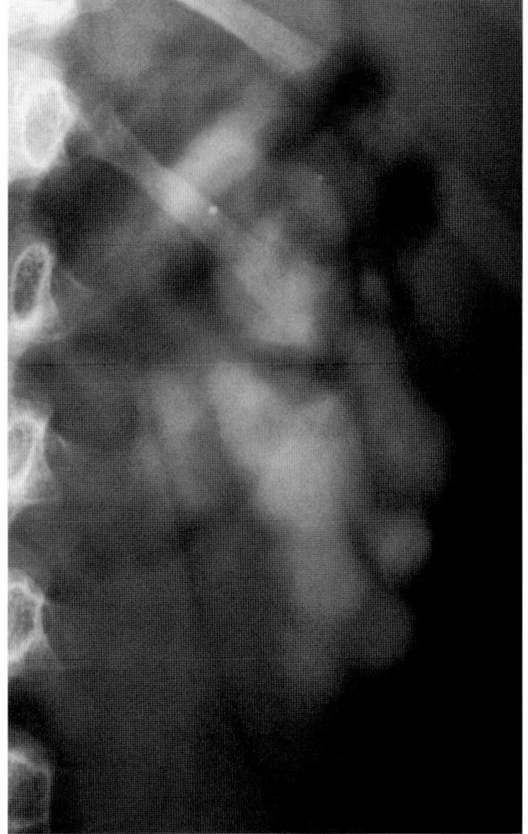

Figure 9. 6-minute film from an IVP with Lasix demonstrates delayed filling of the left renal collecting system.

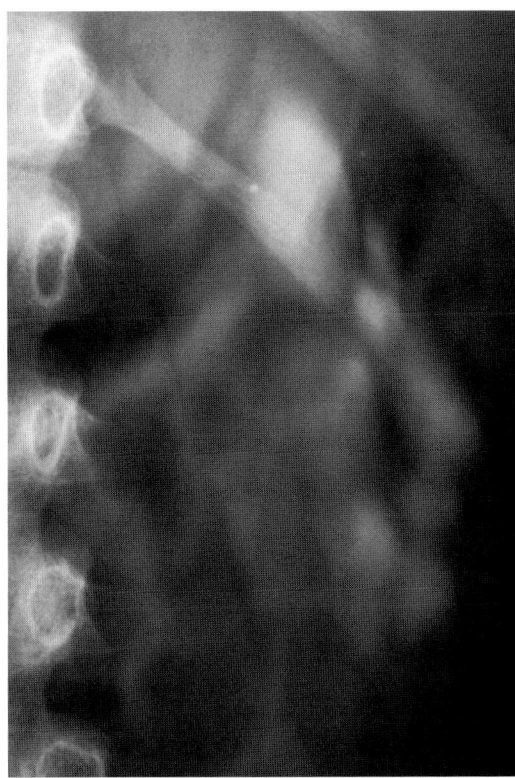

Figure 10. Following administration of Lasix there is no passage of contrast material through the left UPJ, confirming once again the diagnosis of left UPJ obstruction.

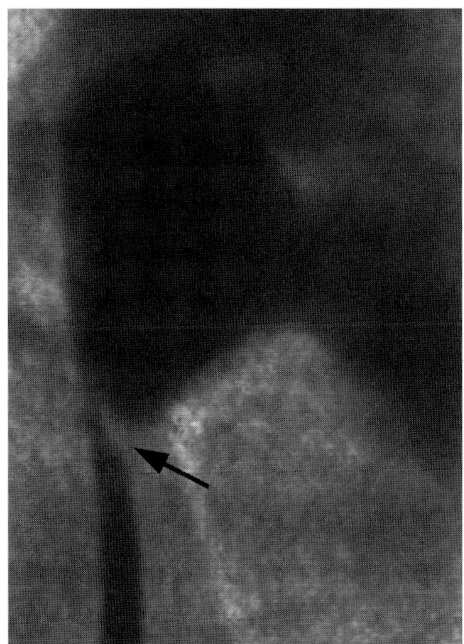

Figure 11. The initial phase of an endopyelotomy procedure is to obtain a retrograde pyeloureterogram. This demonstrates narrowing in the region of the left UPJ (arrow).

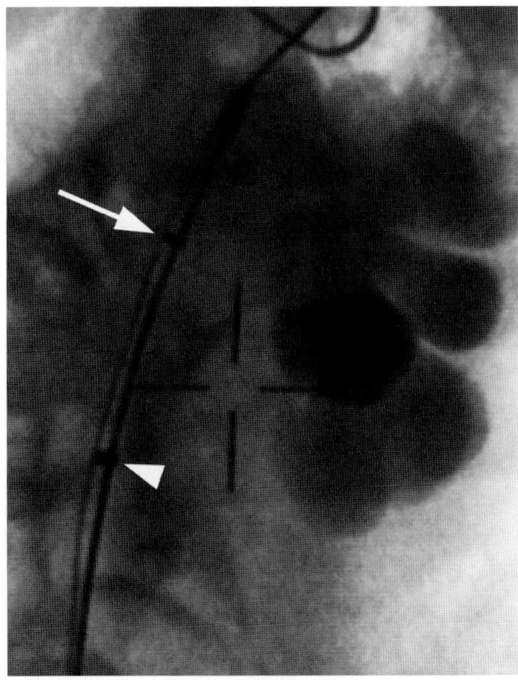

Figure 12. The Accusize catheter is placed through the area of the left UPJ. The distal (arrow) and proximal (arrowhead) dots are maneuvered to either side of the obstruction prior to inflation of the balloon.

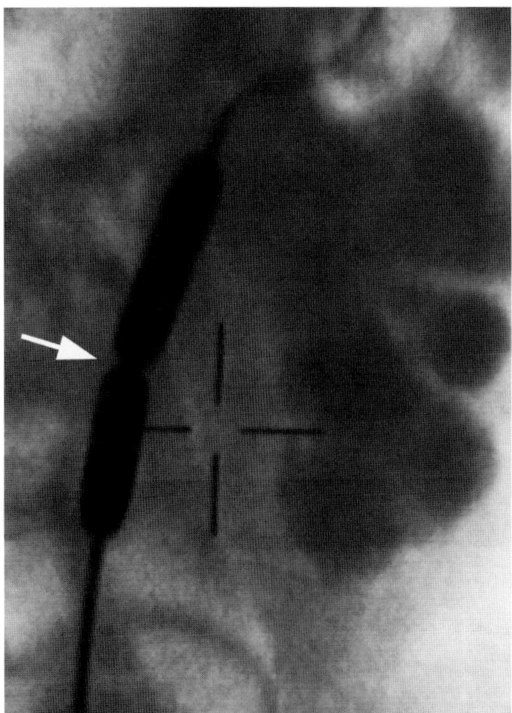

Figure 13. The balloon is inflated and demonstrates a "waist" (arrow) at the level of the UPJ obstruction.

An Accusize catheter was placed through a cystoscope into the area of the obstruction **(Figs. 11, 12)**. Once appropriate placement had been achieved, the balloon portion of the catheter was inflated, ensuring that the electrosurgical wire element was securely applied to (unopposed to) the area of obstruction **(Fig. 13)**.

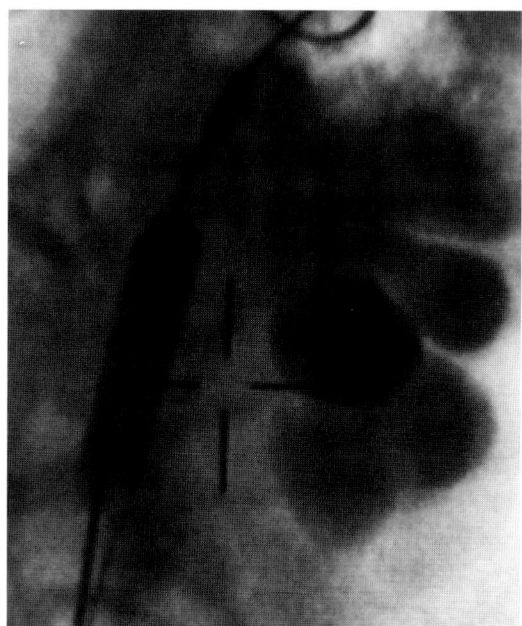

Figure 14. The cautery unit is then activated and the Accusize wire incises the left UPJ, with loss of the "waist" seen in Figure 13.

The electrosurgical unit was then engaged, incising the narrowed UPJ **(Fig. 14)**. A repeat retrograde ureteropyelogram was then obtained to confirm extravasation of contrast material **(Fig. 15)**. A stent was then placed and the procedure terminated. Following stent removal, a repeat Lasix renogram was obtained which demonstrated no evidence of obstruction, with a half-life of 3.7 minutes.

In the younger patient, endopyelotomy is not the treatment of choice, as the endoscopic equipment and supplies needed to perform such a procedure are not readily available in the appropriate sizes. However, this child was large enough that the procedure could be performed with the use of adult-sized materials. She is currently doing well and has no evidence of recurrent obstruction.

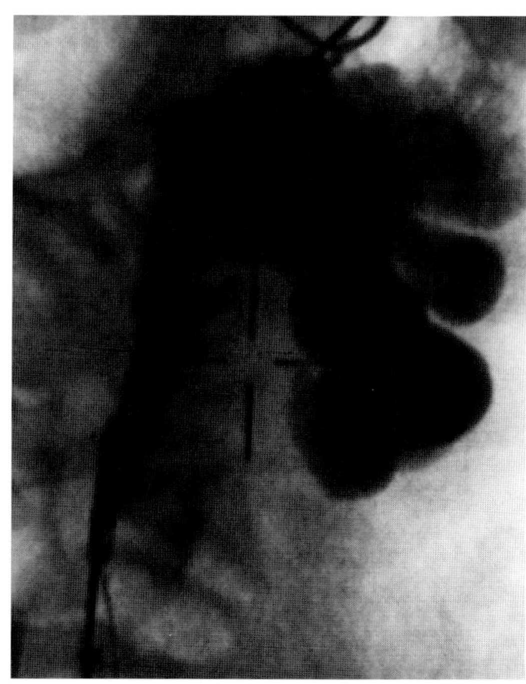

Figure 15. A repeat retrograde ureteropyelogram demonstrates some mild extravasation of contrast material, confirming that the UPJ was incised.

Selected Readings

Brooks JD, Kavoussi LR, Preminger GM, Schuessler WW, Moore RG. Comparison of open and endourologic approaches to the obstructed ureteropelvic junction. Urology 1995; 46(6):791–795.

Clayman RV, Basler JW, Kavoussi L, Picus DD. Ureteronephroscopic endopyelotomy. J Urol 1990; 144:246–252.

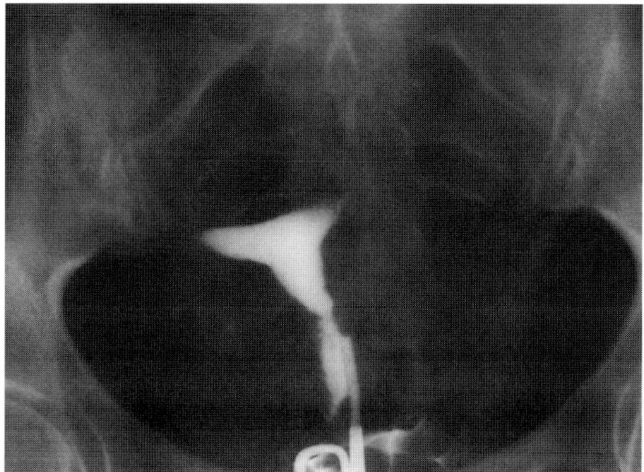
Figure 1. HSG.

TEACHING FILE CASE 60

Mark L. Lukens, M.D., and
John F. Cardella, M.D.

History

The patient is a 28-year-old woman with a 2-year history of infertility (unsuccessful egg fertilization despite unprotected intercourse). Sperm analysis of the spouse has shown normal numbers and forms of spermatozoa. Medical therapy has been unsuccessful. A hysterosalpingogram (HSG) was obtained with use of water-soluble contrast material via a transvaginal cannula with a rubber acorn tip and cervical traction provided by a tenaculum **(Fig. 1)**.

What is your diagnosis?

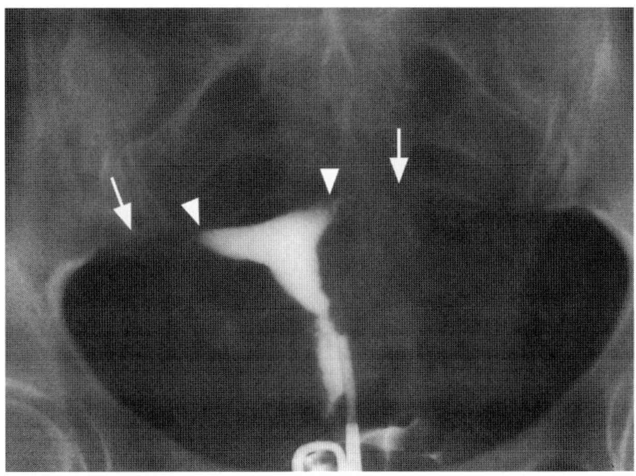

Figure 2. Direct hysterosalpingography shows nonvisualization of the fallopian tubes bilaterally. The uterine contour is smooth. The endocervical canal is patent. Note the rounded contours of the cornua bilaterally (arrowheads). Arrows show the expected location of the fallopian tubes.

Radiographic Findings

The HSG shows bilateral non-visualization of the fallopian tubes **(Fig. 2)**. The uterine cavity is smooth in contour without evidence of mass effect or filling defect. The cervical canal is patent without irregularity. There is spilling of contrast material into the vagina due to an incomplete seal at the external os.

Preliminary Diagnosis

Bilateral nonvisualization of the fallopian tubes.

What treatment would you suggest?

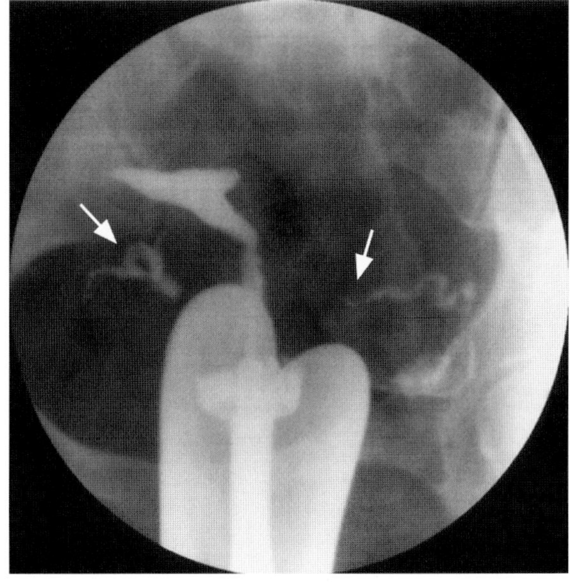

Figure 3. Hysterosalpingography with use of a Hysterocath shows patent fallopian tubes bilaterally (arrows).

Management

One possible treatment would be surgical reconstruction and recanalization of the fallopian tubes. Instead the patient was referred for direct salpingography and possible fallopian tube dilation. Repeat dedicated hysterosalpingography was performed with use of a vacuum Hysterocath (Cook, Bloomington, IN). Periprocedural doxycycline was given for 5 days surrounding the procedure. The final hysterosalpingogram shows patency of both fallopian tubes with peritoneal spilling of contrast material **(Fig. 3)**.

Diagnosis

False positive hysterosalpingogram due to poor filling.

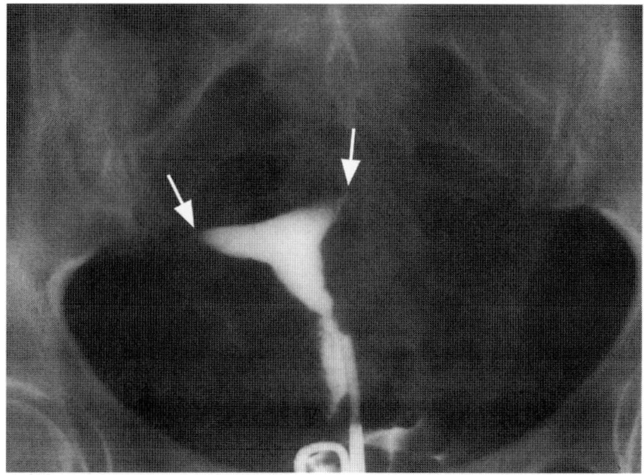

Figure 4. Note again the rounded contours of the cornua bilaterally suggesting inadequate filling of the uterine cavity (arrows).

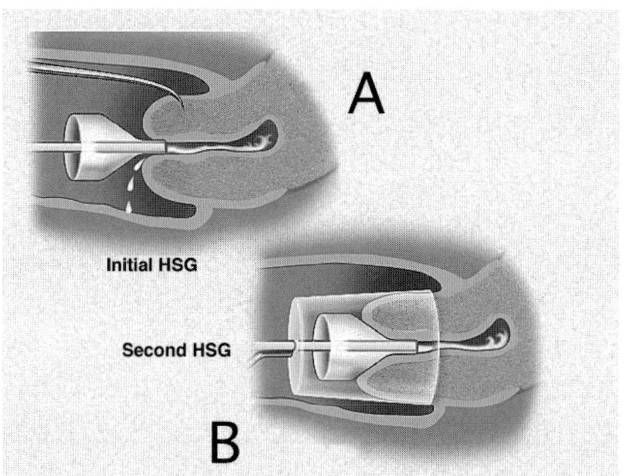

Figure 5. A. The lack of a watertight seal enables contrast material to leak from the external cervical os. B. A watertight seal allows the needed pressure for full opacification of the uterine cavity and fallopian tubes.

Discussion

In general, hysterosalpingography is performed in the follicular phase of the menstrual cycle, typically around the 10th day of the cycle. This case demonstrates the utility and importance of adequate preliminary hysterosalpingography. The initial HSG was obtained with use of a diagnostic catheter rather than a catheter system designed specifically for hysterosalpingography. False positive HSGs are not uncommon with conventional hysterosalpingography, and direct salpingography may be required for accurate diagnosis. A rounded cornua without evidence of tubal filling suggests insufficient instillation of contrast material **(Fig. 4)**.

Adequate pressure needed for good hysterosalpingography cannot be achieved without a watertight seal at the cervical os. Proper cannulation and seal at the cervical os are shown in **Figure 5**. The vacuum seal at the cervix also enables easy sterile catheterization of the uterus and fallopian tubes. Additionally, traction can be placed on the cervix to better delineate the uterine body anatomy.

Selected Readings

Hunt RB. Hysterosalpingography: techniques and interpretation. Chicago: Year Book Medical Publishers, 1990.

Thurmond AS, Novy M, Uchida BT, Rösch J. Fallopian tube obstruction: selective salpingography and recanalization. Work in progress. Radiology 1987; 163:511–514.

Thurmond AS, Uchida BT, Rösch J. Device for hysterosalpingography and fallopian tube catheterization. Radiology 1990; 174:571–572.

Yoder IC. Hysterosalpingography and pelvic ultrasound: imaging in infertility and gynecology. Boston: Little, Brown and Company, 1988.

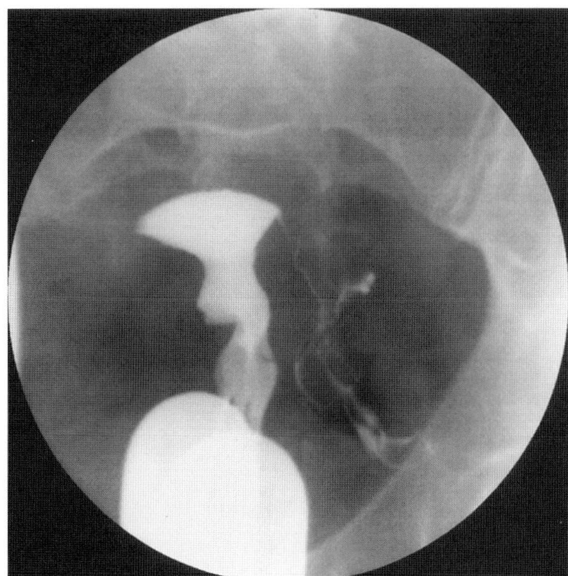

Figure 1. HSG.

TEACHING FILE CASE 61

Mark L. Lukens, M.D., and
John F. Cardella, M.D.

History

The patient is a 32-year-old woman who has been unable to conceive over the past 2 years despite unprotected intercourse. She has no prior history of pelvic inflammatory disease, tubal ligation, or known congenital anomaly. A hysterosalpingogram (HSG) was obtained **(Fig. 1)**.

What is your diagnosis?

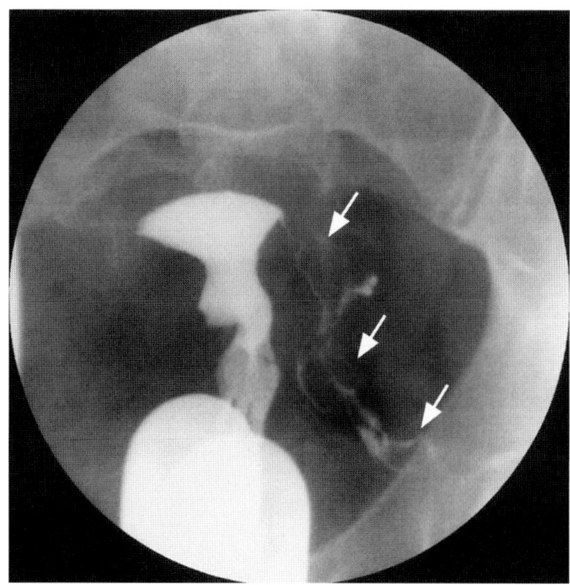

Figure 2. Hysterosalpingography shows a normal endocervical canal and smooth uterine contour. The left fallopian tube is patent and shows peritoneal spilling of contrast material (arrows).

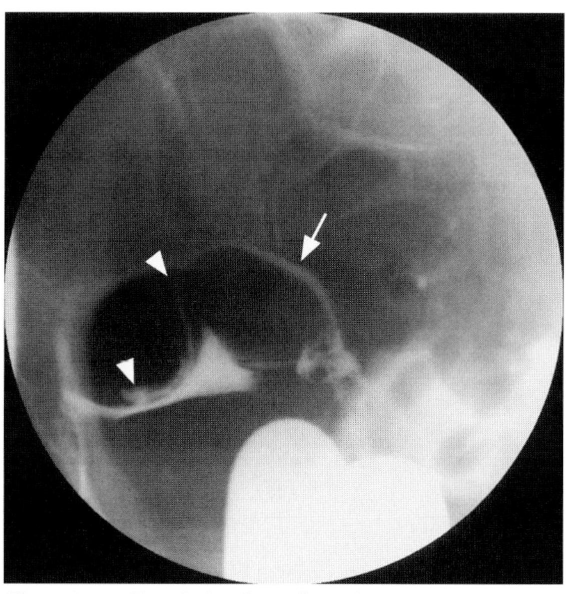

Figure 3. 5.5-F angled catheter (arrow) seated in the right fallopian tubal ostium during direct salpingography. Note the thin, patent fallopian tube with peritoneal spilling of contrast material on the right (arrowheads).

Radiographic Findings

The HSG performed with water-soluble contrast material shows a normal uterine contour and a patent left fallopian tube with peritoneal spilling. The right fallopian tube is not visualized **(Fig. 2)**.

Diagnoses

1. Patent left fallopian tube.
2. Occluded right fallopian tube at the cornual level.

What treatment would you recommend?

Management

Following the initial HSG, an 0.035-inch J-tipped guide wire was advanced into the uterine cavity toward the right uterine cornu. A 5.5-F angled catheter was then advanced into the cornu and direct salpingography was performed. Gentle injections of contrast material cleared the tube and showed peritoneal spilling **(Fig. 3)**. Follow-up hysterosalpingography performed with a vacuum cup Hysterocath (Cook, Bloomington, IN) shows a patent right fallopian tube **(Fig. 4)**.

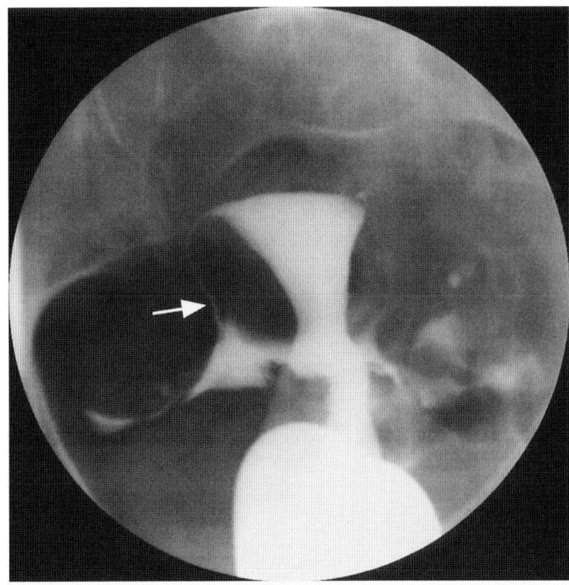

Figure 4. Follow-up HSG shows a patent right fallopian tube with spilling of contrast material into the peritoneal cavity (arrow).

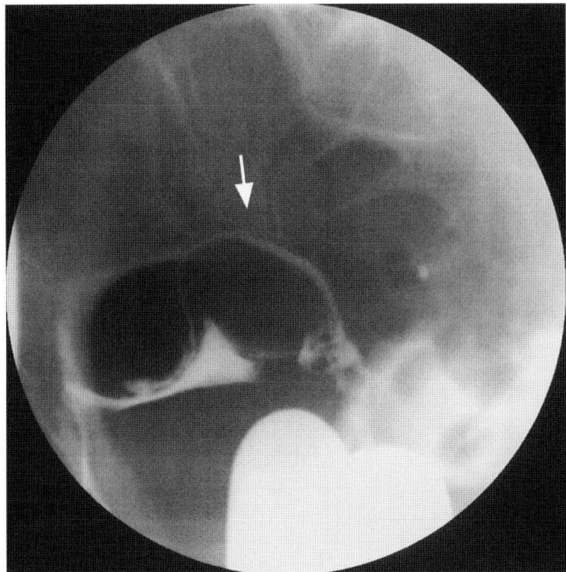

Figure 5. Note the position of the angled catheter in the cornua of the fallopian tube (arrow).

Discussion

This case shows the value of direct selective salpingography. Gentle direct injection of contrast material into the uterine cornua will often clear the cellular debris that causes proximal tubal occlusion. It is important that the catheter be placed directly into the ostium of the fallopian tube to avoid myometrial injection, which is painful to the patient **(Fig. 5)**. If the tube is incompletely visualized, then the patient can proceed to fallopian tube recanalization.

Selected Readings

Rösch J, Thurmond AS, Uchida BT, Sovak M. Selective transcervical fallopian tube catheterization: technique update. Radiology 1988; 168:1–5.

Thurmond AS. Selective salpingography and fallopian tube recanalization. AJR 1991; 156:33–38.

Thurmond AS, Novy M, Uchida BT, Rösch J. Fallopian tube obstruction: selective salpingography and recanalization. Work in progress. Radiology 1987; 163:511–514.

Thurmond AS, Rösch J. Fallopian tubes: improved technique for catheterization. Radiology 1990; 174:572–573.

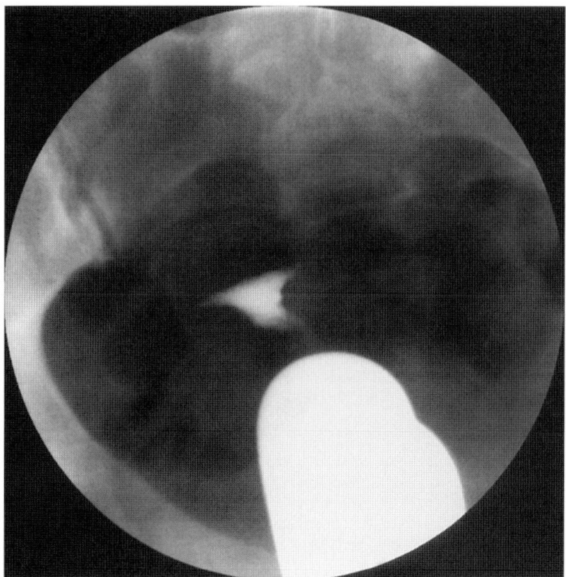

Figure 1. HSG.

TEACHING FILE CASE 62

Mark L. Lukens, M.D., and
John F. Cardella, M.D.

History

The patient is a 30-year-old woman who has been unable to conceive over the past 2 years despite unprotected intercourse. No history of prior surgery or pelvic inflammatory disease was elicited. A hysterosalpingogram (HSG) was obtained **(Fig. 1)**.

What is your diagnosis?

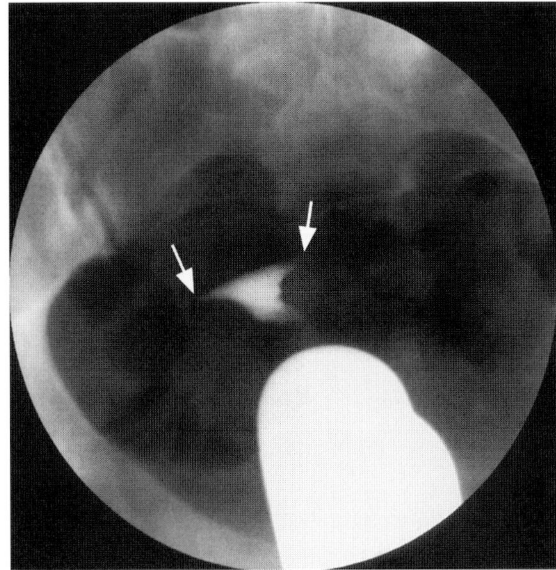
Figure 2. Initial hysterosalpingography shows a small uterine cavity without evidence of mass or mucosal abnormality. There is proximal occlusion of the fallopian tubes bilaterally (arrows).

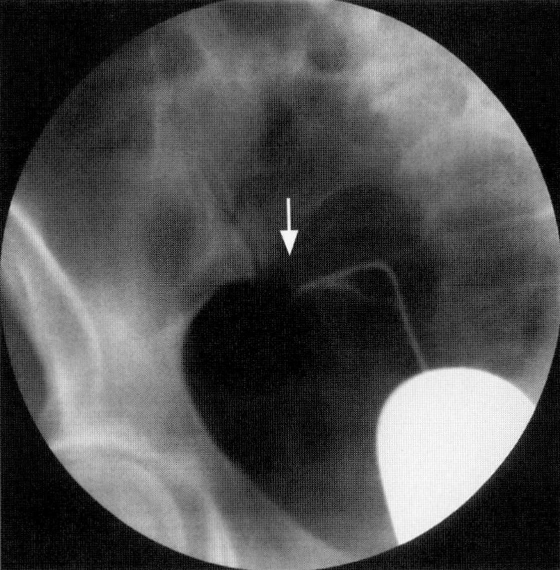
Figure 3. Direct salpingography with a 5.5-F catheter in the right uterine cornua shows persistent proximal occlusion (arrow).

Radiographic Findings

The initial HSG shows bilateral tubal occlusion **(Fig. 2)**. Direct salpingography with use of water-soluble contrast material and a 5.5-F angled catheter in the right fallopian tube ostium shows persistent occlusion proximally **(Fig. 3)**. Direct salpingography on the left shows an irregular, dilated, and occluded fallopian tube **(Figs. 4, 5)**.

Diagnoses

1. Proximal occlusion of thc right fallopian tube with nonvisualization distally.
2. Dilated and occluded distal left fallopian tube, with questionable hydrosalpinx.

How would you manage this patient?

Management

Following direct salpingography, coaxial fallopian tube dilation was performed with use of a 3-F straight catheter and an 0.018-inch platinum-tipped guide wire advanced via the 5.5-F angled catheter. The 3-F catheter was initially placed in the proximal tube and the wire was gently advanced through the point of obstruction **(Fig. 6)**. The catheter was then advanced over the wire to further dilate the fallopian tube. Follow-up salpingography through the 3-F catheter initially in the mid tube, then at the uterine cornu showed patency of the fallopian tube with free peritoneal spilling **(Fig. 7)**. Attempts to dilate the left tube were unsuccessful because the wire would not pass through the irregular and dilated mid portion of the tube **(Fig. 8)**.

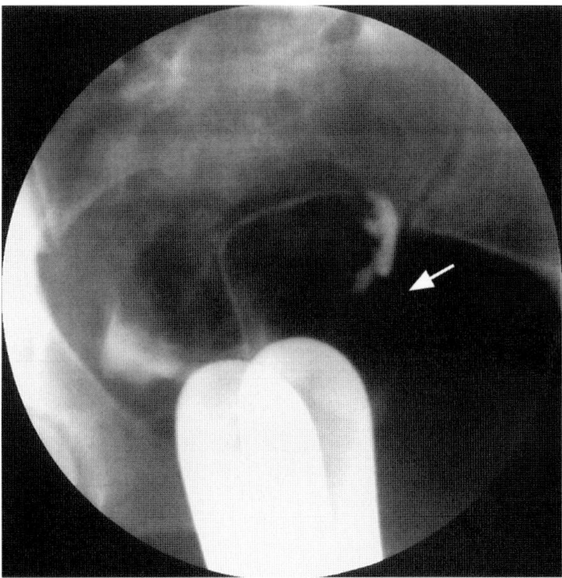
Figure 4. Direct salpingography with a 5.5-F angled catheter in the left uterine cornua shows an irregular, dilated tube with mid tubal occlusion (arrow).

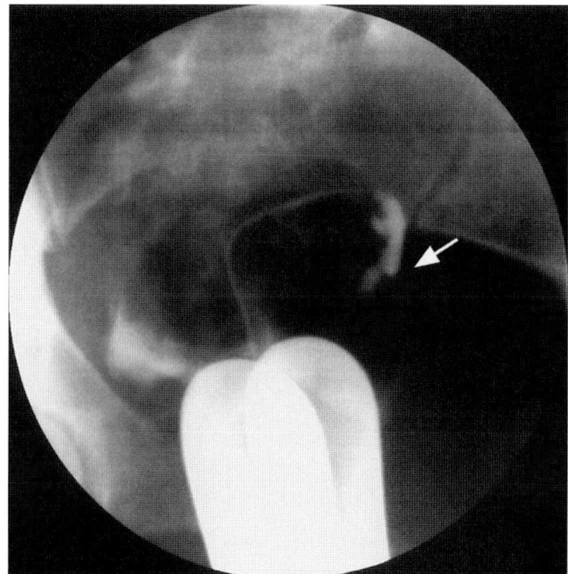

Figure 5. Arrow shows a focally dilated segment of the left fallopian tube.

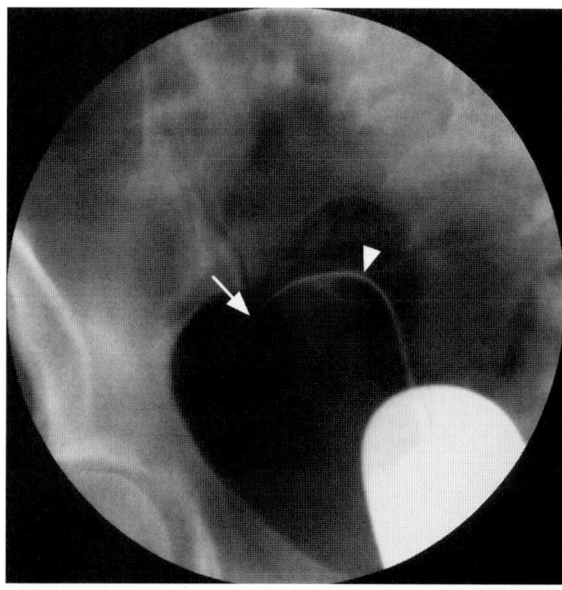

Figure 6. Fallopian tube recanalization with an 0.018-inch wire (arrow) in the right mid tube via a 3-F catheter (arrowhead).

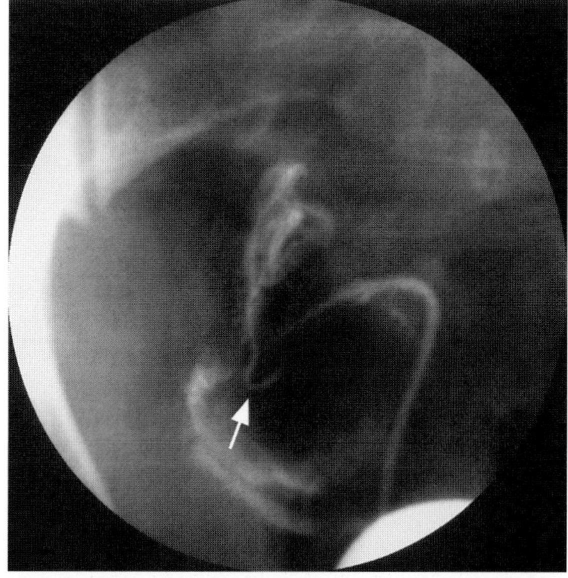

Figure 7. Follow-up salpingography through the 3-F catheter in the mid tube shows a recanalized patent fallopian tube with peritoneal spilling on the right (arrow).

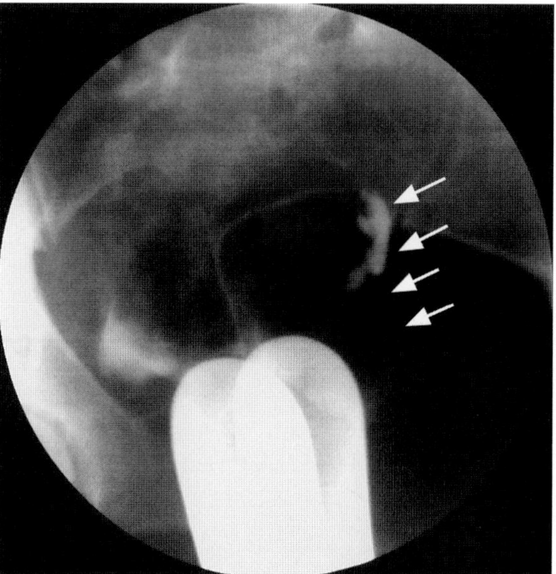

Figure 8. Arrows show the focally obstructed tube. Multiple guide wires failed to pass this obstruction.

Discussion

This case shows that tubal dilation with a 3-F catheter and an 0.018-inch wire can clear a tube that remains obstructed after selective salpingography. The technical success rate is 70%–80%, with pregnancy rates as high as 37%. Complications such as perforation of the fallopian tube occur in approximately 5%–10% of cases. Perforation usually occurs in patients with pre-existing conditions such as salpingitis isthmica nodosa or previous tubal surgery. Hysterosalpingography with fallopian tube dilation is now supported by the American Fertility Society for the treatment of infertile women prior to microsurgery or in vitro fertilization.

Selected Readings

Hovsepian DM, Bonn J, Eschelman DJ, Shapiro MJ, Sullivan KL, Gardiner GA Jr. Fallopian tube recanalization in an unrestricted patient population. Radiology 1994; 190:137–140.

Rösch J, Thurmond AS, Uchida BT, Sovak M. Selective transcervical fallopian tube catheterization: technique update. Radiology 1988; 168:1–5.

Thurmond AS. Pregnancies after selective salpingography and tubal recanalization. Radiology 1994; 190:11–13.

Thurmond AS. Selective salpingography and fallopian tube recanalization. AJR 1991; 156:33–38.

Thurmond AS, Novy M, Uchida BT, Rösch J. Fallopian tube obstruction: selective salpingography and recanalization. Work in progress. Radiology 1987; 163:511–514.

Thurmond AS, Rösch J. Fallopian tubes: improved technique for catheterization. Radiology 1990; 174:572–573.

Thurmond AS, Rösch J. Nonsurgical fallopian tube recanalization for treatment of infertility. Radiology 1990; 174:371–374.

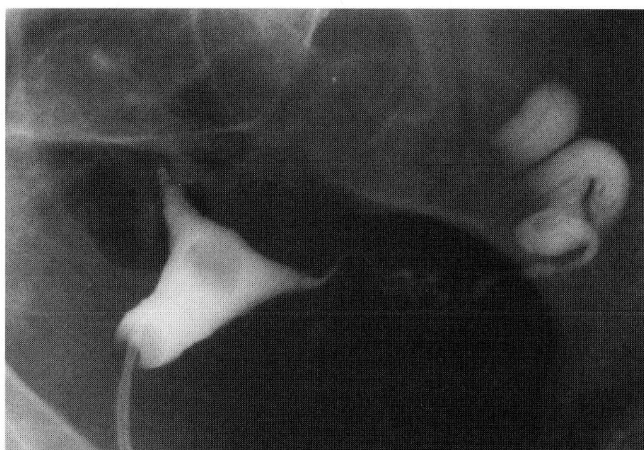

Figure 1. Oblique hysterosalpingogram.

TEACHING FILE CASE 63

Vincent D. McCormick, M.D.

History

This 35-year-old woman with a previous history of pelvic inflammatory disease (PID) is being evaluated for infertility. **Figure 1** is an oblique film from a hysterosalpingogram obtained after the injection of 7 mL of contrast material.

What is your diagnosis?

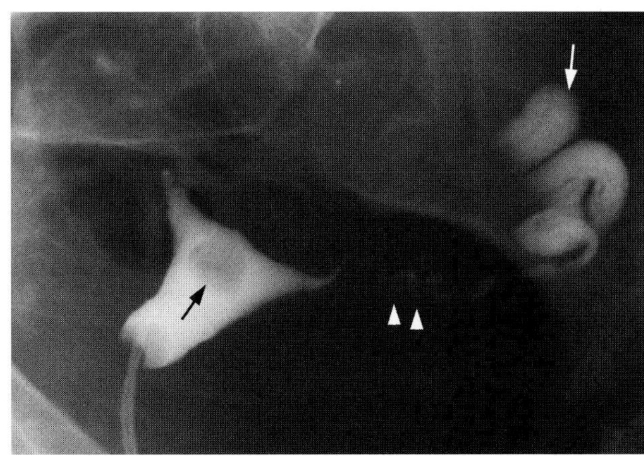

Figure 2. Hysterosalpingogram shows collections of contrast material resembling diverticula in the left tube (arrowheads) with hydrosalpinx (white arrow). An endometrial cavity filling defect is also present (black arrow).

Radiographic Findings

Diverticular-like collections of contrast material arise from the mid-isthmic portion of the left tube, associated with hydrosalpinx and obstruction of the ampullary segment **(Fig. 2)**. A 13-mm filling defect in the endometrial cavity, non-filling of the right tube, and a linear lucency crossing the left cornu are also apparent.

Diagnoses

1. Salpingitis isthmica nodosa with hydrosalpinx.
2. Uterine myoma.
3. Cornual ring.

What treatment would you recommend?

Discussion

The typical appearance and site of salpingitis isthmica nodosa (SIN) are illustrated by this case. SIN is often associated with PID with or without hydrosalpinx, and is complicated by ectopic pregnancy in up to 10% of cases. Resection of the segment of the tube involved with SIN can be undertaken. In the current case, repair of the fimbriated portion of the tube with tubal reimplantation or anastomosis would be necessary as well. Treatment of proximal tubal obstruction with transcervical recanalization techniques has a reported success rate of 80%–90%. However, tubal recanalization cannot be used where there is ampullary obstruction, as in this case. Endovaginal sonography confirmed that the uterine filling defect represented a submucosal myoma. The lucency in the left cornu is a normal variant.

Selected Readings

Creasy JL, Clark RL, Cuttino JT, Groff TR. Salpingitis isthmica nodosa: radiologic and clinical correlates. Radiology 1985; 154:597–600.

Hovsepian DM, Bonn J, Eschelman DJ, et al. Fallopian tube recanalization in an unrestricted patient population. Radiology 1994; 190:137–140.

Thurmond AS. Fallopian tube recanalization. Semin Intervent Radiol 1992; 9:73–79.

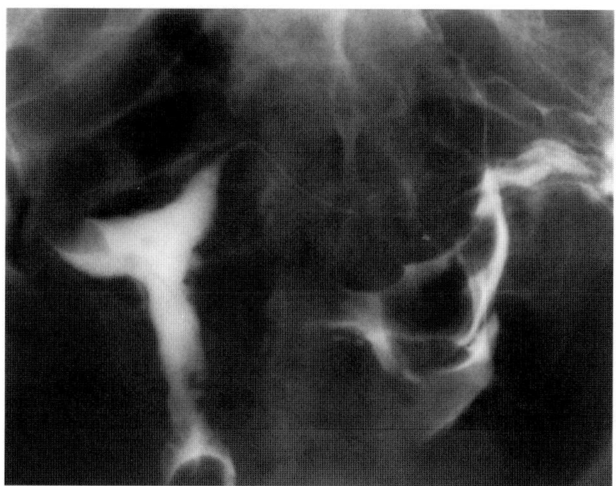

Figure 1. Hysterosalpingogram.

TEACHING FILE CASE 64

Vincent D. McCormick, M.D.

History

The patient is a 40-year-old woman who is being evaluated for menorrhagia. An enlarged uterus was noted on physical examination. The patient underwent a post partum dilation and curettage (D&C) years ago. Hysterosalpingography was performed **(Fig. 1)**.

What is your diagnosis?

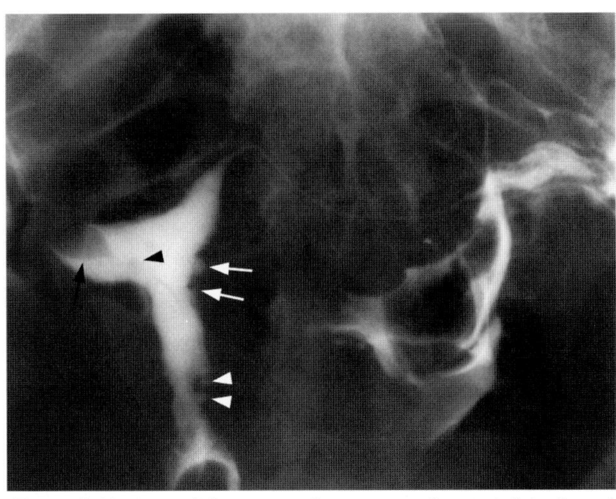

Figure 2. Hysterosalpingogram shows narrowing and distortion of the lower uterine segment (white arrowheads). Note small cavities along the left side of the uterine body (white arrows), and filling defects are present within the endometrial cavity (black arrowhead). The right tube does not fill due to a cornual filling defect (black arrow).

Radiographic Findings

On the hysterosalpingogram, irregular filling defects cause narrowing and distortion of the lower uterine segment **(Fig. 2)**. Small cavities arise from the left side of the body of the uterus, and small polypoid/linear filling defects are evident within the endometrial cavity. Free spillage of contrast material from the left tube indicates patency. A sharply marginated filling defect in the right cornu is associated with nonfilling of the right tube.

Diagnoses

1. Synechiae.
2. Adenomyosis.
3. Cornual polyp.

Discussion

The irregular filling defects and distortion of the lower uterine segment are characteristic of synechiae, which almost always occur with a history of post partum D&C. The smaller polypoid lesions could be due to endometrial polyps or synechiae, whereas the linear defect is probably another adhesion. The uterine body cavities represent adenomyosis, and the cornual lesion is an endometrial polyp obstructing the fallopian tube.

Adenomyosis may be focal or, more commonly, diffuse. If it is associated with severe, increasing dysmenorrhea and menorrhagia, the definitive therapy is hysterectomy. Magnetic resonance (MR) imaging is the modality of choice for evaluation of adenomyosis because neither hysterosalpingography nor sonography can accurately detect or characterize this disease. Patients hoping to retain reproductive capability should undergo MR examination to determine whether the disease is focal or diffuse. In the case of focal disease, excision of an encapsulated adenomyoma may be a therapeutic option.

Selected Readings

Krysiewicz S. Infertility in women: diagnostic evaluation with hysterosalpingography and other imaging techniques. AJR 1992; 159:253–261.

Williams TJ. Endometriosis. In: Thompson JD, Rock JA. Te Linde's operative gynecology. Philadelphia: J.B. Lippincott Company, 1992; 463–466.

Yoder IC, Hall DA. Hysterosalpingography in the 1990s. AJR 1991; 157:675–683.

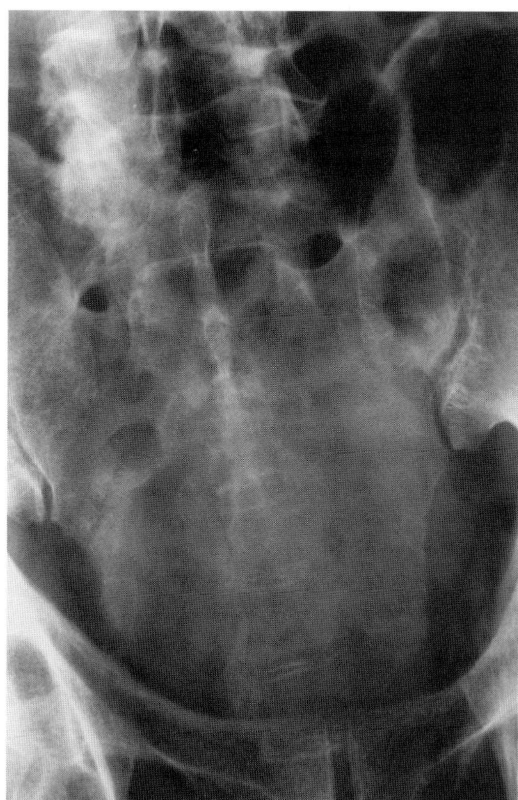

Figure 1. Frontal radiograph of the sacrum.

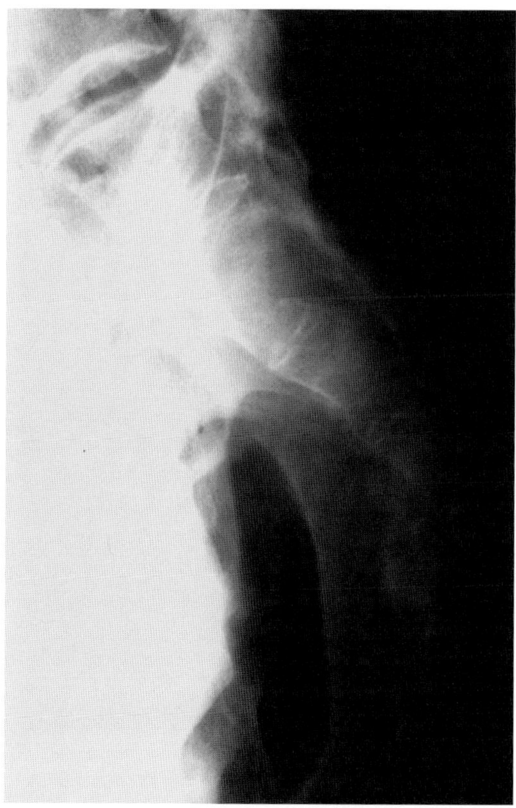

Figure 2. Lateral radiograph of the sacrum.

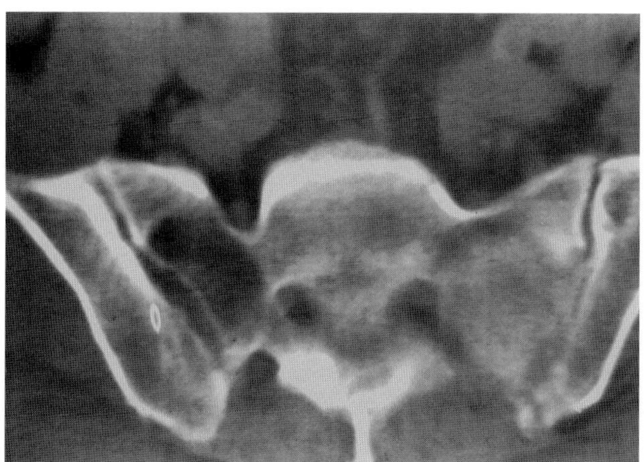

Figure 3. CT scan of the sacrum.

TEACHING FILE CASE 65

William Clark, M.D., and
Georges Y. El-Khoury, M.D.

History

A 73-year-old man came to the hospital with pain in the left hip and buttock. The buttock pain had been present for 12 months, was not constant, and was absent at night. It radiated into the left hip. He also had a 6-month history of constipation. The physical examination revealed point tenderness over the sacrum. The rectal examination was normal, with a firm but symmetric prostate gland. There were no other physical findings. Radiographs **(Figs. 1, 2)** and a computed tomography (CT) scan **(Fig. 3)** of the sacrum were obtained.

What is your diagnosis?

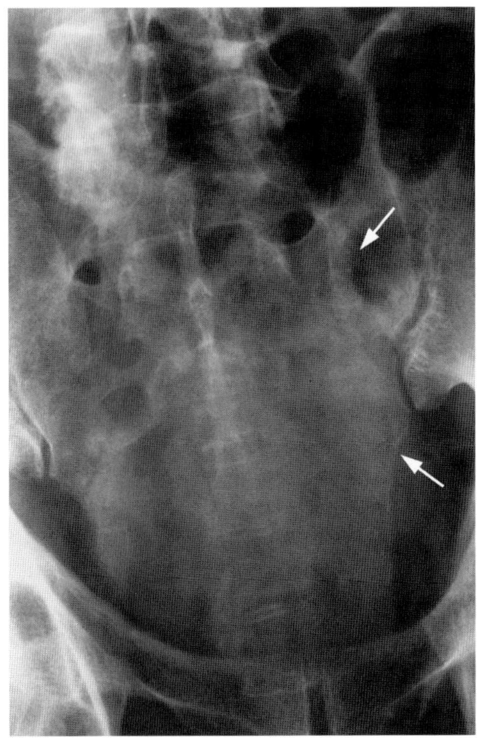

Figure 4. Frontal radiograph of the sacrum shows increased density diffusely over the left side of the sacrum (arrows).

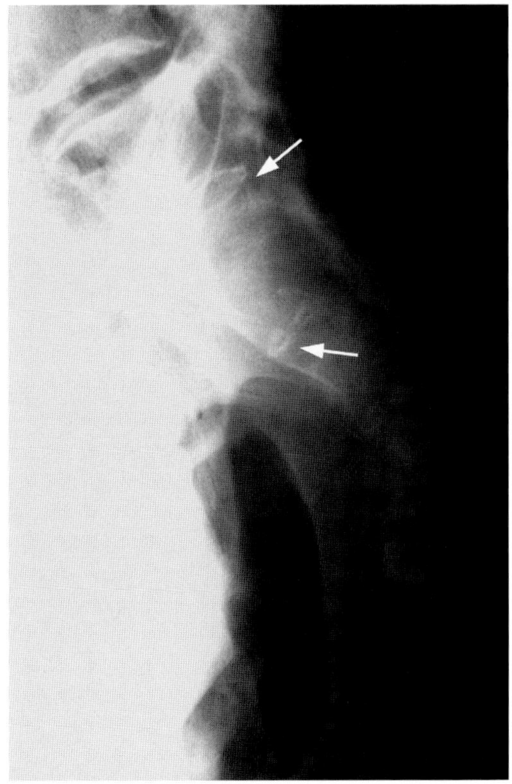

Figure 5. Lateral radiograph of the sacrum demonstrates sclerosis of the anterior portion of the sacrum (arrows).

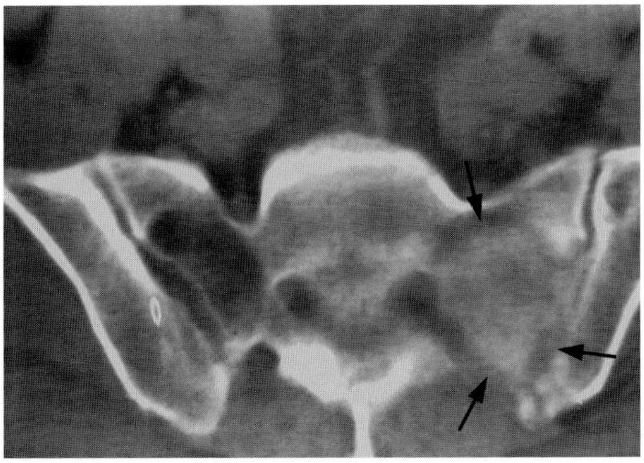

Figure 6. Selected transaxial CT image through the sacrum confirms irregular mottled increased density of the left side of the sacrum (arrows), especially when compared to the right side.

Radiographic Findings

The frontal radiograph of the sacrum demonstrates increased density of the left side of the sacrum from S3 to S5 **(Fig. 4)**. The arcuate lines show loss of clarity at S3 on the left. The lateral film shows increased sclerosis in the anterior portion of the sacrum **(Fig. 5)**. The CT scan confirmed the ill-defined sclerosis of the left side of the sacrum **(Fig. 6)**. A bone scan (not shown) demonstrated increased radioisotope uptake in the sacrum but no other focal bony abnormality.

Initial Diagnosis

Sclerotic bone lesion.

What is your differential diagnosis? What is your recommendation for further investigation?

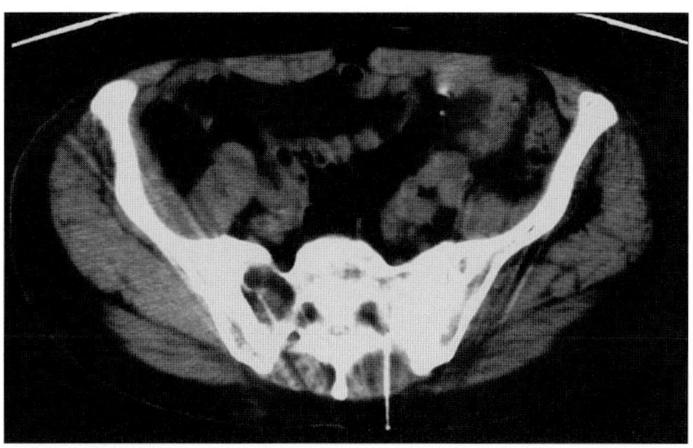

Figure 7. Fine needle aspiration of the sacrum.

Management

Tissue for cytology was obtained by CT-guided fine needle aspiration **(Fig. 7)**. Three passes were made with a 22-gauge spinal needle. In each case the needle penetrated the posterior cortex of the sacrum in the region of the abnormality. Cytology demonstrated adenocarcinoma, with cells staining positive with prostatic antibodies. Further clinical evaluation showed that the serum alkaline phosphatase was 353 IU/L (normal range: 30–115 IU) and prostatic specific antigen was 426 ng/mL (normal: <4). These values further suggested that the prostate was the primary site of the metastatic lesion in the sacrum.

Final Diagnosis

Carcinoma of the prostate gland with metastasis to the sacrum.

Discussion

Differential diagnosis of a solitary sclerotic lesion of the sacrum should include metastasis, infection, healing fracture, primary bone sarcoma, chordoma, lymphoma, and benign tumor such as osteoblastoma. In a 73-year-old man, a sclerotic metastasis is statistically the most likely cause and this is most commonly prostatic in nature.

In this case, an adequate sample for cytology was obtained with fine needle aspiration. A cytopathologist should always be on site to evaluate the adequacy of a tissue sample. Were the fine needle unable to traverse the sclerotic cortex of the sacrum, a trephine needle would have been necessary. Care must be exercised to avoid the sacral nerve roots when a larger-bore needle is used.

Selected Readings

El-Khoury GY, Terepka RH, Mickelson MR, Rainville KL, Zaleski MS. Fine-needle aspiration biopsy of bone. J Bone Joint Surg Am 1983; 65:522–525.

Logan PM, Connell DG, O'Connell JX, Munk PL, Janzen DL. Image-guided percutaneous biopsy of musculoskeletal tumors: an algorithm for selection of specific biopsy techniques. AJR 1996; 166:137–141.

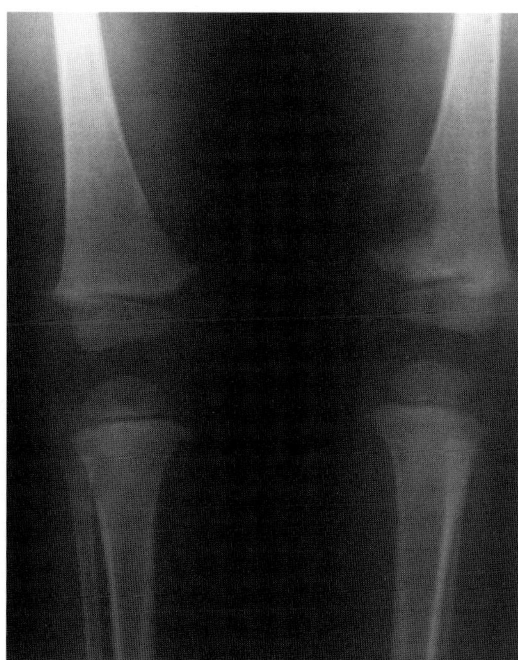

Figure 1. Frontal radiograph of the knees.

TEACHING FILE CASE 66

William Clark, M.D., and
Georges Y. El-Khoury, M.D.

History

A 15-month-old boy was brought to the hospital because he awoke refusing to walk or bear weight on his right leg. The child had been active the previous day. The parents had also described a 1-week history of poor appetite and nocturnal restlessness and a 24-hour history of fever. On examination the patient was irritable but consolable. He had a temperature of 39.4 degrees and a pulse rate of 200/minute. He had tenderness to palpation over the medial aspect of the distal left femur, and this area felt somewhat fuller than the corresponding contralateral region. No other clinical findings were noted. A radiograph of the knees was obtained **(Fig. 1)**.

What is your diagnosis?

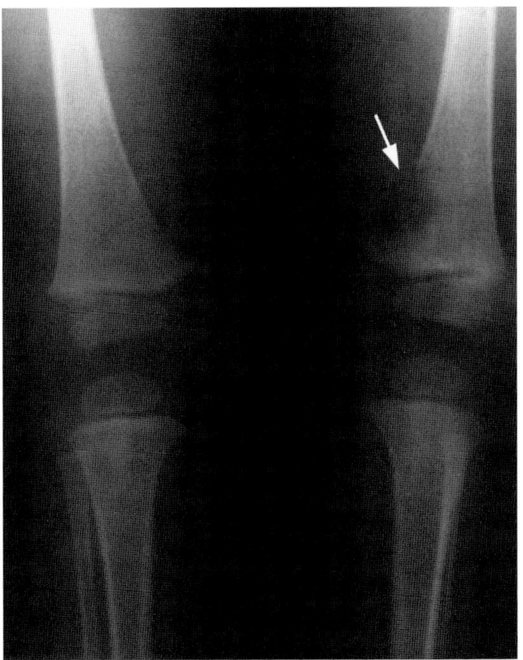

Figure 2. Frontal radiograph of the knees shows a lytic lesion of the left femur (arrow).

Radiographic Findings

The radiograph of the left femur **(Fig. 2)** revealed a 3-cm lytic lesion in the medial aspect of the left distal femoral metaphysis. The margins of the lesion were nongeographic but reasonably well defined. The cortex was destroyed, with minimal periosteal reaction. No conspicuous soft-tissue mass was evident. A skeletal survey and radioisotope bone scan did not show any other lesions.

What is your differential diagnosis and further plan of investigation?

Differential Diagnosis

Differential diagnosis in this age group includes:
1. Eosinophilic granuloma.
2. Round-cell tumor—neuroblastoma, lymphoma, rhabdomyosarcoma, Ewing's sarcoma.
3. Aneurysmal bone cyst.
4. Osteomyelitis.

Bone Biopsy

The patient was sedated with chloral hydrate. Fine needle aspiration biopsy was performed under fluoroscopic guidance **(Fig. 3)**. Four passes were made with a 22-gauge needle—three for cytology and one for bacteriology. The biopsy was easy to perform from a technical standpoint because of the cortical destruction.

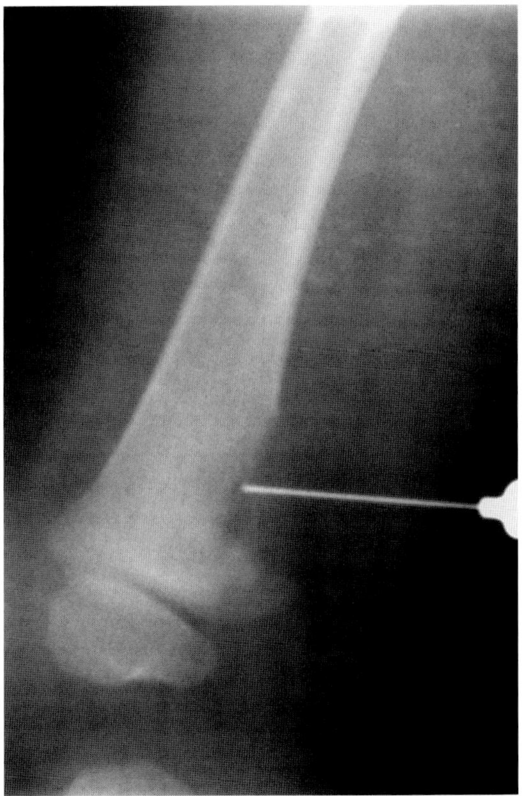

Figure 3. Fine needle aspiration of the distal femoral lesion.

Cytology

The cells had a round, monocytoid appearance suggesting the differential diagnosis of a small round-cell malignancy. Immunohistochemistry suggested a neural phenotype (neuroblastoma), although the diagnosis was not considered certain. Urine catecholamines were grossly elevated. A computed tomography scan of the abdomen revealed a 6-cm left suprarenal mass which on open biopsy was a neuroblastoma, thus confirming the diagnosis of metastatic neuroblastoma in the leg.

Selected Readings

El–Khoury GY, Terepka RH, Mickelson MR, Rainville KL, Zaleski MS. Fine-needle aspiration biopsy of bone. J Bone Joint Surg Am 1983; 65:522–525.

Logan PM, Connell DG, O'Connell JX, Munk PL, Janzen DL. Image-guided percutaneous biopsy of musculoskeletal tumors: an algorithm for selection of specific biopsy techniques. AJR 1996; 166:137–141.

CME QUIZZES

Tutorial 1: Overview of Biopsy Technique and Biopsy Needles

1. True or false? In the patient with normal anticoagulation status, no difference in bleeding rates is seen with 18–22-gauge aspiration needles.

2. True or false? Platelet inhibitors do not influence the bleeding rates after biopsy.

3. True or false? A single forward thrust is used to obtain tissue with cutting needles such as the Menghini.

4. The type of needle used for a biopsy depends on:
   a. patient cooperation
   b. location of the lesion
   c. vascularity of the lesion
   d. the clinical question to be answered
   e. all of the above

5. True or false? More tissue is obtained with a 22-gauge Chiba needle with a 25-degree bevel than a 22-gauge Chiba needle with a 45-degree bevel.

Tutorial 2: Ultrasound in Interventional Radiology: Applications and Techniques

1. Percutaneous interventional procedures which are amenable to real-time ultrasound guidance include:
   a. breast cyst aspiration
   b. peripheral venous access
   c. cholecystostomy tube placement
   d. fine needle aspiration biopsy of a liver mass
   e. all of the above

2. True or False? Fluoroscopic or CT guidance is preferred over ultrasound guidance for percutaneous aspiration or drainage when bone, gas-filled bowel, or aerated lung overlie the target lesion.

3. Compared to the free-hand technique, use of the needle guide attachment for ultrasound-guided procedures offers the following advantages:
   a. the needle is introduced in a single prescribed, predetermined pathway
   b. it can be easier to perform and therefore preferred when operators are less familiar with the use of ultrasound
   c. it provides greater flexibility and options for needle approaches and a wider range of accessible targets
   d. a and b
   e. all of the above

4. True or False? In general, a sector array ultrasound transducer is preferred for guiding needle procedures in superficial soft tissues and a linear array transducer is preferred for guiding deep intraabdominal procedures.

5. Maneuvers which can improve needle visibility on the ultrasound screen include:
   a. aligning the transducer with the needle to ensure that the needle shaft lies within the narrow sound beam emitted by the transducer
   b. moving the transducer toward the needle entry site so that the angle between the needle shaft and the insonant sound beam approaches zero degrees
   c. increasing the overall gain and number of focal zone settings
   d. a and b
   e. all of the above

Tutorial 3: Percutaneous Liver Biopsy

1. The following are advantages of CT-guided biopsy (True or False):
   a. it has minimal operator dependence
   b. it is a real-time procedure
   c. some lesions may be seen only by CT
   d. it is ideal for lesions high in the liver
   e. it is quicker to perform than ultrasound-guided liver biopsy

2. All of the following are relative contraindications to ultrasound-guided liver biopsy except:
   a. ascites
   b. PT >15 sec
   c. PTT >45 sec
   d. hemangioma at the liver surface
   e. platelets <50,000

3. An abdominal CT scan of a patient shows a small lesion near a vessel in the liver parenchyma seen only after contrast enhancement. The patient had a normal abdominal sonogram 3 days earlier. If the lesion is to be biopsied, the next best step is
   a. biopsy the approximate area of the lesion under CT guidance
   b. laparoscopy
   c. repeat sonography with direct reference to the CT films to visualize and then biopsy the lesion
   d. fluoroscopic biopsy after injection of contrast into the hepatic artery
   e. none of the above

4. The safest approach in any imaging-guided liver biopsy is:
   a. high intercostal
   b. low intercostal
   c. anterior
   d. posterior
   e. subcostal

5. Which of the following is the most common serious complication of imaging-guided liver biopsy?
   a. hemoperitoneum
   b. pain
   c. pneumothorax
   d. hemobilia
   e. tumor seeding of the biopsy track

6. The following steps need to be taken to optimize the image on sonography before starting the biopsy except:
   a. the highest frequency suitable transducer should be used
   b. the depth should be decreased so that it is just enough to show the far edge of the lesion
   c. the gain should be adjusted to show the lesion well
   d. the focal zone should be set at the far edge of the lesion
   e. the PRF of the color Doppler should be adjusted to show flow

7. To minimize complications when performing ultrasound-guided liver lesion biopsy with an 18-gauge core biopsy gun, the following conditions must be met except:
   a. there should be no blood vessel in the biopsy path as shown by color Doppler
   b. there should be at least 2.5 cm distance between the final position of the needle tip and a large vessel or liver capsule distal to it
   c. the lesion should not be hypervascular
   d. normal liver should not be present between the liver capsule and the lesion if at all possible
   e. the coagulation parameters should be reviewed and if abnormal, corrected before undertaking the biopsy

8. After an imaging-guided liver biopsy:
   a. all patients should be admitted to the hospital for 24-hour observation
   b. the patient should be discharged immediately if no complications are observed
   c. hemobilia is the most common complication
   d. the patient should have nothing by mouth for 4 hours
   e. vital signs should be monitored for 4 hours

9. Regarding CT-guided liver biopsy:
   a. a localizing grid is only used for small lesions
   b. "homemade" localizing grids have poor performance compared to commercially available grids
   c. lesions high in the liver are more easily targeted by tilting the gantry
   d. biopsies are performed only with the patient supine
   e. this is the best way of avoiding the pleural space

10. Regarding ultrasound-guided liver biopsies:
    a. in-and-out movements of the needle are helpful for localizing the needle tip
    b. it is difficult to avoid major vessels
    c. color Doppler of the intended track is only performed if there is a large vessel crossing the track
    d. the complication rate is higher than with CT-guided biopsy
    e. the needle track cannot be visualized immediately after the biopsy

Tutorial 4: Pancreatic Biopsy

1. True or False? Pancreatic biospies should always be performed with CT guidance.

2. All of the following are limitations of using CT guidance for pancreatic biopsies except:
   a. limited angulation capabilities
   b. inability to monitor needle advancement
   c. limited gantry aperture in certain patients
   d. inability to visualize surrounding structures well
   e. more time-consuming than US-guided procedures

3. True or False? US guidance for pancreatic biopsy is less sensitive and less accurate than CT guidance.

4. True or False? Pancreatic biopsy is limited to excluding neoplasms of the pancreas.

5. True or False? Percutaneous biopsies of pancreatic allografts should not be performed.

6. True or False? Use of a needle guide as opposed to freehand sonographic biopsy allows the operator to predetermine the needle path.

7. Overall complication rates for pancreatic biopsy are:
   a. 0.01%
   b. 0.1%
   c. 0.5%
   d. 1.0%
   e. 5.0%

8. True or False? Most structures surrounding the pancreas can be safely traversed with small-guage aspiration needles.

9. True or False? Detachable hub core biopsy needles should not be used during CT-guided biopsies.

10. True or False? It is advantageous to have the cytopathologist in attendance during pancreatic biopsies.

Tutorial 5: Adrenal Biopsy

1. Adrenal lesions can be noted in what percentage of abdominal CT scans obtained for various indications?

a. 0.5%
b. 1%
c. 3%
d. 5%
e. 10%

2. Which criteria have been used in the attempt to distinguish benign from malignant adrenal lesions?

a. lesion size
b. lesion stability over time
c. CT attenuation values
d. chemical shift MR imaging
e. all of the above

3. Adrenal masses greater than what size should be considered suspicious for malignancy?

a. 5 mm
b. 1 cm
c. 2 cm
d. 3 cm
e. 5 cm

4. True or False? The principal indication for needle biopsy of the adrenal gland is to determine the nature of the adrenal lesion in patients with potentially curable extra-adrenal malignancy.

5. True or False? Adrenal biopsies cannot be performed with ultrasound guidance.

6. The direct translumbar approach for biopsy of adrenal masses with CT guidance is limited by which anatomic approach?

a. paraspinal muscles which may cause significant pain when transgressed
b. transgression of the diaphragm which makes needle positioning difficult
c. needle path through the kidney which may result in hemorrhage
d. posterior costophrenic sulcus which may contain lung, resulting in a pneumothorax if transgressed
e. interposed vascular structures such as the aorta or inferior vena cava which may result in significant hemorrhage if punctured

7. True or False? The angled translumbar approach to the adrenal gland with CT biopsy usually can avoid the lung and diaphragm.

8. True or False? Needle biopsy of adrenal lesions shows an accuracy of approximately 90% with a specificity for metastatic disease approaching 100%.

9. True or False? Anterior or lateral biopsies from a transhepatic, transgastric, and transsplenic route can be used and are not associated with higher complication rates when compared to posterior angled approaches.

10. True or False? The overall rate of major complications with adrenal biopsy is 4%–5%.

1. For deep, centrally located abscesses which imaging modality is recommended for access guidance?
   a. fluoroscopy
   b. computed tomography
   c. sonography
   d. use of anatomic landmarks

2. Drainage catheter removal criteria include:
   a. patient clinically well
   b. no residual cavity on tube check
   c. tube output <20 mL/day
   d. a and b
   e. all of the above

3. The use of multiple catheters may be necessary for:
   a. thick fluid collections
   b. multilocular collections
   c. unilocular collections
   d. a and b
   e. all of the above

4. Collections with enteric fistulas characteristically have:
   a. low drainage output, for shorter duration
   b. high drainage output, for longer duration
   c. complete resolution following initial drainage

5. The most common cause of enteric fistulas is:
   a. inflammatory conditions
   b. postoperative anastomotic breakdown
   c. malignancy
   d. drainage catheter placement

6. Which of the following is incorrect concerning catheter placement for drainage?
   a. the catheter should be placed through an uninvolved organ to help tamponade potential bleeding
   b. transgression of the pleura should be avoided
   c. CT or US should be used to aid in procedural planning

7. What percentage of abdominal abscesses are successfully treated percutaneously?
   a. 0%–30%
   b. 30%–60%
   c. 70%–100%

8. Recommendations for preprocedure preparation for patients undergoing percutaneous catheter placement include:
   a. appropriate preprocedure imaging
   b. obtaining informed consent
   c. correcting significant coagulopathy
   d. all of the above

9. Good percutaneous drainage success rates should be expected for:
   a. complex, multilocular collections
   b. phlegmonous collections
   c. unilocular collections
   d. intraloop collections

10. Sump catheters are advantageous when:
    a. abscess fluid is thin
    b. the use of suction devices is anticipated
    c. the fluid is not infected
    d. a long access route is planned

1. The leading cause of hepatic abscess worldwide is:
   a. amebiasis
   b. echinococcal disease
   c. pyogenic abscess
   d. penetrating trauma

2. Which of the following can lead to pyogenic abscesses?
   a. biliary obstruction
   b. intraabdominal infection
   c. penetrating trauma
   d. indwelling hepatic arterial pumps
   e. all are correct

3. True or false? Cryptogenic pyogenic liver abscesses (where no identifiable source of the infection can be determined) are common.

4. Air in a liver abscess commonly suggests:
   a. presence of gas-forming organisms
   b. fistula to the bowel
   c. fistula to the lung
   d. prior aspiration or drainage

5. A 6-cm complex multiseptated liver abscess should be treated in which fashion?
   a. simple needle aspiration
   b. aspiration and lavage through a catheter with removal of the catheter after lavage
   c. placement of an indwelling catheter until the cavity has resolved
   d. antibiotic therapy without drainage

6. True or false? For a liver abscess secondary to biliary obstruction, decompression of the biliary system is not required.

7. True or false? When draining a liver abscess, it is important to try to traverse some normal liver parenchyma before entering the abscess.

8. True or false? Multiseptated liver abscesses require a catheter in each of the loculations.

9. When draining liver abscesses, what is the success rate in treating, temporizing, or palliating the patient?
   a. 50%–60%
   b. 65%–70%
   c. 70%–80%
   d. 80%–85%
   e. 90%–95%

10. Failure of percutaneous drainage of liver abscesses may be due to:
   a. inadequate drainage
   b. persistent fistula
   c. infected tumor
   d. infected hematoma
   e. all of the above

Tutorial 8: Drainage of Deep Pelvic Abscesse IncludingTransgluteal, Transrectal, and Transvaginal Approaches

1. True or False? The majority of pelvic abscess are postoperative in nature.

2. True or False? Although a pelvic fluid collection appears simple on the CT scan, the US can demonstrate multiple septations in the collection.

3. True or False? One should not drain complex multiloculated pelvic abscesses.

4. True or False? If possible, one should always perform an endocavitary drainage of a pelvic abscess.

5. True or False? Which does not influence the route and guidance choice in pelvic abscess drainage?
    a. location of the abscess
    b. intervening structures in the planned path
    c. age of the patient
    d. surgical back-up
    e. size of the abscess

6. True or False? Fistulas are often demonstrated during the procedural sinogram.

7. True or False? When performing a transgluteal drainage, one should stay below the piriformis and as close to the ischial spine as possible.

8. True or False? A significant number of patients may have persistent pain after a transgluteal drainage.

9. True or False? Sonography allows one to perform an endoluminal drainage without visualizing the abscess bulging into the rectum or vagina.

10. True or False? Simple transrectal needle aspiration and lavage of the abscess cavity has no role in the management of pelvic abscesses.

11. True or False? One should not perform a transrectal drainage because of the risk of causing superinfection of the abscess is too great and one risks creating a chronic colonic fistula.

1. Disadvantages of imaging pancreatitis with contrast-enhanced CT include which of the following?
    a. poor delineation of fluid collections
    b. inability to detect hemorrhagic complications
    c. potential exacerbation of pancreatitis
    d. inability to detect signs of pancreatic necrosis
    e. inability to plan routes of percutaneous drainage

2. Common clinical signs and laboratory features of pancreatitis include all of the following *except*:
    a. fever
    b. nausea and vomiting
    c. bradycardia
    d. abdominal pain
    e. elevated serum lipase

3. Etiologic factors associated with pancreatitis include all of the following *except*:
    a. cirrhosis
    b. performance of ERCP
    c. alcohol abuse
    d. gallstones
    e. infectious agents

4. Principles of tube management following drainage of fluid collections associated with pancreatitis include all of the following *except*:
    a. use of large-bore tubes for thick collections
    b. frequent catheter flushing and irrigation
    c. imaging by CT or sinograms when drainage changes abruptly in volume or character
    d. irrigation of the catheter with octreotide
    e. placement of additional tubes for multilocular or poorly drained collections

5. Factors entering into the decision whether to drain a collection associated with pancreatitis include which of the following:
    a. demonstration of pancreatic necrosis on contrast-enhanced CT scanning
    b. results of needle aspiration of the collection
    c. natural history of acute pancreatic fluid collections
    d. natural history of pseudocysts
    e. all of the above

6. Which of the following is *not* true regarding pancreatic pseudocysts?
    a. pseudocysts have a well-defined wall
    b. pseudocysts may resolve spontaneously
    c. pseudocysts may bleed
    d. pseudocysts typically develop within a few days after the onset of acute pancreatitis
    e. all of the above

7. Which of the following is least likely to be effectively treated by percutaneous drainage?
    a. pancreatic abscess
    b. infected pancreatic necrosis
    c. acute pancreatic fluid collection
    d. pancreatic pseudocysts
    e. postoperative pancreatic abscesses

8. Factors adversely affecting the closure of pancreatic fistulas include all of the following except:
    a. malnutrition
    b. obstruction of the pancreatic duct between the duodenum and a drained collection
    c. administration of total parenteral nutrition
    d. high-dose steroid therapy
    e. persistent infection or inflammation

9. Which of the following imaging studies is incorrectly matched with its advantages in the setting of acute severe pancreatitis:
    a. ERCP—assessment of pancreatic ductal integrity
    b. arteriography—demonstration of pseudoaneurysms
    c. ultrasonography—demonstration of gallstones
    d. ultrasonography—good definition of the presence and extent of acute pancreatic fluid collections
    e. ultrasonography—ability to effectively guide percutaneous drainage

10. Which of the following is false regarding vascular complications of pancreatitis?
    a. they are often life-threatening
    b. extrahepatic portal hypertension is one example
    c. common sites of pseudoaneurysm include the splenic artery and its branches
    d. arteriography is the method of choice for diagnosis of suspected arterial complications
    e. surgical therapy is almost invariably necessary for their treatment

Tutorial 10: Percutaneous Ethanol Ablation Therapy of Hepatocellular Carcinoma

1. Aggressive screening programs in patients with cirrhosis have improved detection of hepatocellular carcinoma. Approximately what percentage of patients with cirrhosis and hepatocellular carcinoma are candidates for hepatic resection?

   a. 5%
   b. 10%
   c. 30%
   d. 75%
   e. 90%

2. Advantages of percutaneous ethanol ablation therapy include all of the following except:

   a. it is safe
   b. it is relatively inexpensive
   c. it causes relatively minimal damage to nontumorous hepatic parenchyma
   d. it cannot be repeated on recurrent or residual disease

3. Important factors that determine whether a tumor will be ablated successfully include:

   a. tumor size
   b. internal characteristics of the tumor
   c. needle placement
   d. volume of injected ethanol
   e. all of the above

4. The optimal patient for PEAT of HCC is one with:

   a. a solitary, small ($\leq$3 cm) tumor
   b. multiple small hepatocellular carcinomas
   c. a small hepatocellular carcinoma with vascular invasion
   d. none of the above

5. Following PEAT, CT findings suggestive of persistent or locally recurrent viable tumor include:

   a. a completely nonenhancing lesion
   b. nodular foci of contrast enhancement
   c. areas of calcification
   d. air present within the treated lesion

6. Which one (or more) of the following suggest(s) the presence of viable tumor foci with MR imaging:

   a. areas of high signal intensity within the treated lesion on T2-weighted images
   b. the entire lesion is of low signal intensity on T2 weighted images
   c. central heterogeneous enhancement on dynamic gadolinium-enhanced T1-weighted images
   d. no enhancement on dynamic gadolinium-enhanced T1-weighted images

7. Important factors that influence long-term survival rates in patients with HCC treated by PEAT are:

   a. number of lesions
   b. tumor size
   c. severity of underlying cirrhosis
   d. presence of vascular invasion
   e. all of the above

8. Following tumor ablation, pain and fever frequently occur and are related to the following:

   a. volume of injected ethanol
   b. level of serum AFP
   c. presence of ascites
   d. peritoneal reflux of ethanol back along the needle track

9. Peritoneal reflux along the needle track is related to all of the following except:

   a. size of the needle
   b. tumor location
   c. length of the needle
   d. presence of ascites
   e. the rate of injection

10. Which of the following are true regarding HCC recurrence following PEAT?

   a. the tumor never recurs
   b. local tumor recurrence is approximately 15%–20% at five years
   c. most recurrent lesions are distinct new tumors in portions of the untreated liver
   d. the tumor always recurs locally
   e. overall 5-year tumor recurrence rate is 20%

Tutorial 11: Radiographically Guided Percutaneous Gastrostomy and Gastrojejunostomy

1. The most common indication for enteric tube placement is?
   a. gastric decompression
   b. feeding
   c. other

2. Which of the following patients would benefit from a gastrostomy or gastrojejunostomy tube for feeding?
   a. patient with esophageal cancer
   b. patient with short gut syndrome
   c. patient with distal small bowel obstruction

3. Which of the following is not an absolute contraindication to placement of either a gastrostomy or gastrojejunostomy tube?
   a. portal hypertension with gastric varices
   b. gastric Carcinomatosis
   c. coagulopathy
   d. extensive abdominal burns

4. All of the following are considered relative contraindications to placement of either a gastrostomy or gastrojejunostomy tube except?
   a. prior gastric surgery
   b. gastric outlet obstruction
   c. ascites
   d. esophageal Cancer

5. Which of the following items should be performed prior to placement of either a gastrostomy or gastrojejunostomy tube?
   a. obtain short history and physical examination
   b. maintain patients NPO for 12 to 24 hours prior to the procedure
   c. check laboratory findings with special attention to PT, PTT, and platelets
   d. place NG tube/catheter
   e. All of the above

6. Which of the following medications can be used to assist in insufflating the stomach?
   a. Versed (midazolam)
   b. Sublimaze (fentanyl citrate)
   c. glucagon
   d. morphine

7. The performance of a gastropexy provides the following advantages:
   a. it firmly attaches the stomach to the anterior abdominal wall
   b. it reduces the risk of peritonitis if the there is early dislodgement of the tube
   c. it prevents the stomach from being pushed away as dilators, wires, and sheaths are advanced into the stomach
   d. all of the above

8. True or False? Directing the needle toward the antrum of the stomach can facilitate placement of gastrojejunostomy.

9. Gastrojejunostomies are preferred over gastrostomy placement in the following situations?
   a. patients who are prone to aspirate
   b. patients with a partial duodenal obstruction
   c. patients with esophageal obstructions
   d. a and b
   e. a and c

10. The distal tip of a jejunostomy tube or gastrojejunostomy tube should be placed:
   a. slightly distal to the pylorus
   b. in the third portion of the duodenum
   c. beyond the ligament of Treitz
   d. none of the above

11. Postprocedure orders should include the following:
   a. limited use of the gastric port for medications and feedings during the first 24 hours
   b. administration of medications through the jejunal port only
   c. monitor patient for signs of peritonitis
   d. none of the above

12. Which of the following are potential procedural complications of gastrostomy and gastrojejunostomy placement?
   a. bleeding
   b. peritonitis
   c. aspiration
   d. perforation of the colon
   e. vasovagal reactions
   f. all of the above

13. Which of the following are postprocedure complications?
   a. wound and stomal infections
   b. tube dislodgement
   c. clogging the tube lumen
   d. all of the above

14. Radiographically guided percutaneous gastrostomy and gastrojejunostomy are associated with?
   a. Low complication rates
   b. Decreased costs when compared to surgically placed tubes
   c. High success rates in placement
   d. All of the above

Tutorial 12: Direct Percutaneous Jejunostomy

1. Indications for percutaneous jejunostomy include:
   a. previous gastric surgery
   b. chronic aspiration
   c. abnormal stomach position
   d. recurrent inadvertent tube dislodgement
   e. all of the above

2. Contraindications to DPJ include:
   a. underlying malignancy
   b. history of recurrent aspiration
   c. underlying coagulopathy
   d. prior gastrostomy tube

3. Gastrograffin is given 12 hours prior to the DPJ procedure in order to opacify:
   a. the stomach
   b. the jejunum
   c. the colon
   d. none of the above

4. When entering the jejunum, the needle is kept perpendicular to the skin in order to avoid the:
   a. stomach
   b. mesenteric vessels
   c. transverse colon
   d. none of the above

5. The skin puncture is made lateral to the midline but within the rectus abdominis muscle to avoid the:
   a. superior epigastric vessels
   b. liver
   c. spleen
   d. transverse colon

1. Which of the following is NOT true about TNAB?
   a. it can be used to diagnose both benign and malignant disease
   b. lesions only 1 cm or larger can be biopsied reliably
   c. TNAB can be performed in an outpatient setting
   d. fluoroscopy and CT are the most common methods of guiding TNAB

2. Which of the following is NOT true about fluoroscopically guided TNAB?
   a. most lesions visible on a chest radiograph can be biopsied under fluoroscopic guidance
   b. some lesions seen on a chest radiograph may not be visible on fluoroscopy
   c. a lesion must be visible on both posteroanterior and lateral chest radiographs to be amenable to fluoroscopic biopsy
   d. pre-biopsy fluoroscopy can be performed to confirm visibility of the lesion on fluoroscopy

3. Which of the following is NOT true about biopsy planning?
   a. the shortest distance between the skin and the lesion is usually taken
   b. some biopsies require that multiple pleural surfaces be crossed
   c. a lateral approach is sometimes preferred
   d. the needle should never cross an interlobar fissure

4. Which of the following is NOT true about fluoroscopically guided biopsies?
   a. ribs overlying the lesion prohibit performance of TNAB
   b. angled fluoroscopy can be used to check the depth of the needle
   c. movement of the needle opposite of the lung indicates that it is in the intercostal muscle
   d. the choice of biopsy needle is a matter of personal preference

5. Which of the following is NOT true about TNAB sampling?
   a. sampling the margins of the lesion is often better than sampling the central portion of the lesion
   b. resistance is always felt when the biopsy needle hits the lesion
   c. tilting the biopsy needle in different directions while sampling will increase the amount of sample obtained
   d. coaxial needle systems have the advantage of allowing multiple samples to be obtained

6. Which of the following is NOT true about CT-guided TNAB?
   a. the tip of the biopsy needle may produce a shadowing artifact
   b. body position may be important in finding a suitable biopsy approach
   c. CT level and width should be adjusted as needed
   d. ribs overlying the lesion prevent CT-guided biopsies from being performed

7. Which of the following is NOT true about TNAB sampling?
   a. injection of saline into an area of suspected infection probably decreases the chance of identifying the organism
   b. the presence of a cytologist during the TNAB increases the yield of the procedure
   c. many different types of studies may be performed on TNAB samples
   d. the wall of an abscess should be biopsied prior to aspirating the contents of the abscess

8. Which of the following is NOT true concerning post-biopsy care?
   a. patients can be discharged immediately following completion of the biopsy
   b. the patient should lie flat with the biopsy side dependent for 1 hour following completion of the biopsy
   c. if aerated lung was not traversed by the biopsy needle, the observation period can be abbreviated
   d. patients can ambulate during most of the observation period

9. The most common complication encountered following TNAB is:
   a. pulmonary contusion
   b infection
   c. pneumothorax
   d. seeding of the needle track with tumor

10. The injection of saline and anesthetic solution is useful in aiding the biopsy of:
   a. lung nodule
   b. posterior mediastinal adenopathy
   c. pleural lesions
   d. never of use

Tutorial 14: Evaluation and Treatment of Pneumothorax

1. True or False? Spontaneous pneumothoraces are often caused by rupture of subpleural blebs.

2. True or False? A small, stable pneumothorax after transthoracic lung biopsy is an indication for chest tube placement.

3. True or False? A patient with a 10% pneumothorax and dyspnea does not require treatment of the pneumothorax.

4. True or False? Drainage of pneumothoraces via small-bore chest tubes (6–8 F) is successful in over 90% of cases.

5. True or False? When a chest tube is placed for pneumothorax, the chest tube should be placed on the waterseal and evaluated for an air leak before the tube is removed.

1. Procedures amenable to video-assisted thoracoscopic surgical resection include:
   a. pleural staging and sclerosis
   b. lung biopsy
   c. resection of pulmonary nodules
   d. all of the above

2. Regarding resection of pulmonary nodules by VATS, all of the following are true except:
   a. VATS may be the first step in the diagnosis of a 7-mm pulmonary nodule
   b. only nodules >1.5 cm are amenable to VATS
   c. VATS may be considered for treatment of bronchogenic carcinoma in some patients
   d. VATS has a role in treating limited metastases

3. The resection of limited metastases is indicated in certain malignancies except:
   a. malignant melanoma
   b. seminoma
   c. thyroid carcinoma
   d. colon carcinoma

4. Which of the following statements is false?
   a. nodules deeper than 3–4 cm from the pleura may not be amenable to thoracoscopic resection
   b. the presence of a nodule 2 cm from the pleura with coexisting pulmonary disease may make thoracoscopic resection difficult, and preoperative localization in this setting is recommended
   c. a pneumothorax that occurs during the localization procedure should always be re-expanded prior to surgery
   d. nodules on the pleural surface or immediately subpleural are usually accessible to thoracoscopic resection without the need for preoperative localization

5. Preoperative localization of pulmonary nodules should be considered if:
   a. multiple lesions are present
   b. there is extensive interstitial fibrosis
   c. the nodule is in a posterobasal location
   d. the nodule is deep to the pleura
   e. all of the above

6. Regarding preoperative localization methods, which of the following statements is true?
   a. methylene blue dye is always used in combination with hookwire placement
   b. hookwire placement is always used in combination with instillation of methylene blue dye
   c. the optimal hookwire for pulmonary localizations lacks flexibility
   d. multiple types of hookwires have been used successfully

7. Regarding the localization procedure, which of the following statements is false?
   a. the introducer is used with a stylet in it until it is exchanged for the wire in order to maintain a "closed system"
   b. the operator should plan a route for the wire that minimizes the amount of lung that will need to be resected
   c. the hookwire should optimally be within 2 cm of the nodule
   d. the localization procedure should immediately precede surgery

8. Regarding the localization procedure, which of the following statements is true?
   a. a transfissural course is not prohibitive to localization and VATS resection
   b. positioning of the wire shaft beyond a 5-mm radius prevents successful resection
   c. patients should always be positioned supine during the localization procedure
   d. the external portion of the hookwire must be safely secured at the skin surface following the localization procedure

9. Reported complications of preoperative localization for VATS include:
   a. pleuritic pain
   b. hemorrhage
   c. pneumothorax
   d. all of the above

10. Which of the following statements is false?
   a. wire dislodgement can be followed by successful resection
   b. pneumothorax prevents the induction of anesthesia
   c. prolonged delays increase the risk of wire dislodgement
   d. prolonged delays may make localization with methylene blue dye alone difficult

1. Imaging-guided percutaneous drainage has proven most effective in which of the following stages of parapneumonic effusions?
   - a. exudative
   - b. fibrinopurulent
   - c. organized

2. The approximate dose of intrapleural urokinase for fibrinolysis of complex effusions is:
   - a. 10,000–20,000 IU
   - b. 50,000–100,000 IU
   - c. 500,000–750,000 IU

3. Reasons for failure of imaging-guided empyema drainage include all of the following except:
   - a. viscous fluid
   - b. catheter malfunction
   - c. aerobic infection
   - d. thick pleural peel

4. Agents successfully used for the sclerosis of malignant pleural effusions include all of the following except:
   - a. erythromycin
   - b. bleomycin
   - c. doxycycline
   - d. talc

5. Sclerosis of a malignant effusion is best performed when tube output has diminished to:
   - a. <100 mL/day
   - b. <250 mL/day
   - c. <500 mL/day
   - d. once catheter drainage has been established

6. Failure of drainage and sclerosis of a malignant effusion may be due to:
   - a. size of the effusion
   - b. duration of the effusion
   - c. size of the drainage tube/catheter
   - d. presence of an endobronchial lesion

7. Methods of managing hepatic hydrothorax include all of the following except:
   - a. diuresis
   - b. serial thoracenteses
   - c. tube drainage and sclerosis
   - d. thoracoscopic repair of diaphragmatic communications

8. The single factor most closely associated with an increased incidence of complications from imaging-guided catheter drainage of lung abscess is:
   - a. size of the abscess
   - b. size of the catheter
   - c. duration of the symptoms
   - d. traversal of normal lung between the pleural surface and the abscess

9. The most common indication for pericardial drainage is:
   - a. uremic pericarditis
   - b. post-pericardiotomy syndrome
   - c. lupus pericarditis
   - d. pericardial tamponade

10. Mediastinal bronchogenic cysts may produce symptoms by compression of all of the following structures except:
    - a. superior vena cava
    - b. left atrium
    - c. tracheobronchial tree
    - d. esophagus

Tutorial 17: Tracheal and Esophageal Stent Placement

1. Tracheobronchial stents can be used in all of the following situations except:
   a. malignant obstruction
   b. post lung transplant stenosis
   c. post tracheostomy stenosis
   d. tracheomalacia
   e. bronchial avulsion

2. True or false? Self-expanding stents must be used for tracheobronchial stenting.

3. When using conventional silicone stents to treat tracheobronchial stenoses, their greatest disadvantage is:
   a. rigid nature
   b. poor external diameter to internal diameter ratio
   c. large delivery systems
   d. traumatic placement
   e. prone to migration in short stenoses

4. The most likely etiology for stenoses in lung transplant patients is:
   a. poor surgical technique
   b. ischemia
   c. foreign body reaction
   d. rejection
   e. infection

5. For high tracheal lesions, the stent should be placed at least ____ below the vocal cords.
   a. 1 cm
   b. 2 cm
   c. 3 cm
   d. 4 cm
   e. 5 cm

6. After stent placement, improvement in the respiratory status of the treated patient can be expected in what percentage of cases?
   a. 50%
   b. 60%
   c. 70%
   d. 80%
   e. 90%

7. True or false? Patients with grade 1 and higher dysphagia should be treated with esophageal stent placement.

8. Patients with ERF:
   a. have a 6-month life expectancy
   b. can not be treated with a covered stent
   c. have recurrent episodes of aspiration and infection
   d. usually develop it as a consequence of infection, especially tuberculosis
   e. respond better to covered stenting if the ERF is not associated with an esophageal stricture

9. With the techniques currently available, the best treatment for inoperable malignant esophageal obstruction is:
   a. surgical bypass
   b. bouginage
   c. endoscopic laser therapy
   d. plastic esophageal endoprosthesis
   e. esophageal metallic stents

10. True or false? Substantial chest pain may occur after the placement of esophageal stents.

11. When using metallic stents to relieve malignant esophageal obstruction:
   a. there is a near 100% technical success rate
   b. relief of the dysphagia is seen in 95% of patients
   c. continued dysphagia is usually due to an achalasia-like syndrome produced by the tumor
   d. upper gastrointestinal bleeding can occur after stent placement and is usually related to the underlying tumor
   e. all of the above

Tutorial 18: Diagnostic Imaging of Urinary Tract Obstruction

1. Chronic renal obstruction is characterized by all of the following except:
   a. dilatation of the collecting system
   b. decreased renal blood flow
   c. increased pelvic pressure
   d. decreased glomerular filtration rate
   e. loss of parenchyma

2. On urography, an increasingly dense nephrogram is seen with all of the following except:
   a. acute ureteral obstruction
   b. chronic ureteral obstruction
   c. systemic hypotension
   d. acute tubular blockade (eg, lysis syndrome)
   e. renal vein thrombosis

3. All of the following are possible sonographic findings of ureteral obstruction except:
   a. dilatation of the collecting system
   b. thinning of renal parenchyma
   c. absence of ureteral jets
   d. increased frequency of ureteral jets
   e. increased resistive index

4. Computed tomography is highly effective in all of the following roles in evaluation of suspected urinary tract obstruction except:
   a. detection of obstruction
   b. identification of the level of obstruction
   c. identification of the cause of obstruction
   d. diagnosing or excluding ureteral calculus in the setting of acute pain
   e. determining salvageability of the kidney

5. Advantages of nuclear imaging in suspected obstruction include all of the following except:
   a. high accuracy no matter how poorly the kidney functions
   b. good reproducibility from exam to exam
   c. assessment of functional significance
   d. ability to assess salvageability
   e. ability to diagnose low-grade obstruction

Tutorial 19: Percutaneous Nephrostomy

1. All of the following are contraindications to PCN except:
    - a. coagulopathy
    - b. urinary tract infection
    - c. untreated pyonephrosis
    - d. solitary pelvic kidney surrounded by bowel

2. All of the following are potential complications of PCN except:
    - a. pneumothorax
    - b. renal hemorrhage
    - c. colonic perforation
    - d. biliary sepsis

3. All of the following are potential indications for PCN except:
    - a. hydronephrosis
    - b. obstructing ureteral calculus
    - c. extrarenal pelvis
    - d. antegrade nephrostogram

4. True or False? Use of an intercostal access site to the kidney requires that the hemidiaphragm be crossed.

5. What percentage of kidneys have larger, predominately laterally directed posterior renal calyces?

6. What percentage of kidneys have smaller, predominately posteriorly directed posterior renal calyces?

7. All of the following require percutaneous nephrostomy for subsequent interventions except:
    - a. complete staghorn calculus
    - b. hormone-refractory prostate cancer with obstructive uropathy
    - c. UPJ obstruction with equivocal renal scan

8. When air is injected into the renal pelvis with the patient in the prone position, the first calyx to fill with air is which of the following:
    - a. interpolar region, anterior calyx
    - b. interpolar region, posterior calyx
    - c. upper pole, posterior calyx
    - d. lower pole, posterior calyx

9. All of the following imaging modalities can be used to guide percutaneous nephrostomy except:
    - a. fluoroscopy
    - b. CT
    - c. sonography
    - d. nuclear medicine

10. The vascular plane of Brödel is defined by:
    - a. the watershed zone between anterior and posterior renal artery divisions
    - b. the preferred renal parenchymal access track
    - c. parallel to the posterior renal calyx
    - d. all of the above

1. Which of the following would be interpreted as a normal Whitaker test? (Upper tract pressure/Bladder pressure)
   a. 18 cm H_2O/4 cm H_2O
   b. 28 cm H_2O/19 cm H_2O
   c. 31 cm H_2O/22 cm H_2O
   d. a and b
   e. b and c

2. A falsely normal Whitaker test might be seen with:
   a. neurogenic bladder
   b. failure to drain the urinary bladder between measurements
   c. failure to completely fill a massively dilated collecting system
   d. continuous infusion technique through an 8-F nephrostomy catheter
   e. b and c

3. A falsely positive Whitaker test might be seen with:
   a. neurogenic bladder
   b. failure to drain the urinary bladder between measurements
   c. failure to completely fill a massively dilated collecting system
   d. continuous infusion technique through an 8-F nephrostomy catheter
   e. a and d

4. Which situation would *most* indicate the need for a Whitaker test?
   a. urinary tract infection and hydronephrosis in a male child
   b. asymptomatic hydronephrosis in a patient with previous stone disease
   c. flank pain and a normal ultrasound in a patient following ureteral reimplantation
   d. hydronephrotic lower moiety of a duplicated system in an adult
   e. none of the above are appropriate

5. Which of the following is an endpoint for the Whitaker test?
   a. upper tract pressure of 28 cm H_2O with a bladder pressure of 10 cm H_2O
   b. visualization of reflux into the contralateral ureter
   c. visualization of a high-grade ureteral stricture
   d. visualization of pyelotubular backflow
   e. all of the above

6. Contraindications to a Whitaker test include:
   a. cystectomy with ileal conduit
   b. horseshoe kidney
   c. fever of unknown origin
   d. opening upper tract pressure of 22 cm H_2O
   e. all of the above

7. In a woman with cervical cancer, a rising creatinine, and a normal renal ultrasound, a Whitaker test:
   a. is unnecessary because the upper tracts are not obstructed
   b. is contraindicated by the presence of tumor
   c. is unnecessary if an antegrade nephrostogram shows communication with the bladder
   d. may demonstrate the need for percutaneous urinary drainage
   e. a and c

8. In the evaluation of hydronephrosis, a normal Whitaker test:
   a. excludes significant ureterovesical stenosis
   b. excludes significant vesicoureteral reflux
   c. excludes intrinsic renal disease
   d. excludes neurogenic bladder
   e. none of the above

9. Which of the following is *not* a cause of nondilated urinary tract obstruction?
   a. acute renal failure
   b. chronic renal failure
   c. retroperitoneal fibrosis
   d. hypovolemia
   e. none of the above

10. Which of the following is *not* a potential cause of nonobstructed hydronephrosis?
   a. vesicoureteral reflux
   b. transitional cell carcinoma
   c. hyperglycemia
   d. previous urolithiasis
   e. none of the above

Tutorial 21: Percutaneous Ureteral Stents

1. Indications for ureteral stent placement include all of the following except:
   a. endometriosis
   b. hemorrhagic cystitis
   c. ureteroenteric fistula
   d. traumatic ureteral leak
   e. preoperative stent placement prior to ESWL

2. Transplant ureteral obstruction can be caused by:
   a. ischemia
   b. stricture at the ureteroneocystostomy
   c. blood clot
   d. rejection
   e. all of the above

More than one answer may be correct:

3. Methods of double-J stent insertion include:
   a. CT-guided percutaneous antegrade placement
   b. fluoroscopically guided retrograde insertion
   c. fluoroscopically guided percutaneous antegrade placement
   d. CT-guided retrograde insertion
   e. cystoscopically guided retrograde placement

4. True or False? Silicone stents are less prone to encrustation then hydrophilically coated stents.

5. True or False? Metallic Wallstents are unequivocally superior to plastic stents.

6. True or False? Polyurethane stents are more easily inserted than Silastic stents.

7. True or False? Urinomas are a cause of ureteral obstruction in renal transplants.

9. Signs of renovascular injury from percutaneous ureteral stent placement include:
   a. pulsatile bleeding from the percutaneous track
   b. unremitting hematuria
   c. significant drop in hematocrit
   d. a and c
   e. a, b, and c

8. Malpositioned double-J stents:
   a. can be repositioned with a loop snare
   b. must always be removed cystoscopically
   c. usually result from maldeployment of the proximal loop
   d. a and c
   e. a, b, and c

9. Nephroureteral stents:
   a. can be changed percutaneously over a wire
   b. do not require periodic changing
   c. are usually used only in renal transplants
   d. a and c
   e. a, b, and c

10. Nephroureteral stents
   a. can be changed percutaneously over a wire
   b. do not require periodic changing
   c. are usually used only in renal transplants
   d. a and c
   e. a, b, and c

1. The use of ESWL is limited in all of the following except:
   a. large-burden upper tract stone disease
   b. infected stones
   c. inferior calyceal stones
   d. calyceal diverticular stones
   e. thin patients

2. Percutaneous nephrostomy tubes are placed for all of the following except:
   a. obstructive nephropathy
   b. pyonephrosis
   c. renal collecting system stones
   d. ureteropelvic junction obstruction
   e. exsanguinating renal hemorrhage

3. Which of the following are indications for percutaneous interventions?
1. stones larger than 2.5 cm in diameter
2. lower pole stones
3. ESWL failures
4. patients with morbid obesity
   a. 1 only
   b. 1 and 3
   c. 2 and 4
   d. 4 only
   e. all of the above

4. Which of the following are contraindications to percutaneous intervention?
   a. coagulopathy
   b. untreated urinary tract infection
   c morbid obesity
   d. all of the above
   e. none of the above

5. All of the following should be used to avoid pressure sores during PCN under general anesthesia except:
   a. chest support with rolled towels
   b. padding of the medial and lateral humeral condyles
   c. extension of the elbows and shoulders beyond 90 degrees
   d. padding of the knee caps
   e. none of the above

6. The stone-free rates following PNL depend upon the size, location, and anatomic complexity of the stone.

7. For optimal renal pelvic stones, PNL can have stone-free rates up to 95%.

8. PNL routinely has stone-free rates of greater that 85% for staghorn calculi.

9. Punctures lateral to the axillary line have a lower rate of colonic perforation when percutaneous nephrostomy is performed.

10. The most disastrous ramification of percutaneous nephrostomy/nephrostolithotomy is renal vascular pedicle injury.

Tutorial 23: Renal Embolization

1. Embolotherapy of the kidney can be employed as a:
   - a. definitive treatment
   - b. palliative treatment
   - c. surgical adjunct
   - d. all of the above

2. Proximal placement of embolic agents in the renal artery should be avoided prior to nephrectomy because:
   - a. it has a low likelihood of success
   - b. the embolic agent can be dislodged during surgery
   - c. it can interfere with the process of tumor removal
   - d. it can cause postembolization syndrome

3. The postembolization syndrome is:
   - a. not self-limited
   - b. often fatal
   - c. difficult to distinguish from infection
   - d. not accompanied by development of soft tissue gas

4. Prior to renal embolization the contralateral kidney should be assessed for:
   - a. renal artery stenosis
   - b. presence of tumor involvement
   - c. presence of normal function
   - d. all the above

5. All of the following are true of preoperative renal embolization except:
   - a. it increases perirenal edema, making separations of fascial planes more difficult
   - b. it can decrease the amount of operative blood loss
   - c. it may stimulate an antigenic response
   - d. it may improve postoperative survival
   - e. it is indicated in cases of emphysematous pyelonephritis

Tutorial 24: Hysterosalpingography

1. What are the indications for hysterosalpingography?

2. Contraindications to HSG include...

3. What are the causes of non-filling of the fallopian tubes? What measures can be taken to opacify non-filled tubes?

4. Several diagnostic possibilities must be considered when a prominent concavity of the uterine fundal contour is encountered. Name them.

5. What is the clinical significance of a hysterographic diagnosis of SIN?

6. Discuss the differential diagnosis of filling defects in the endometrial cavity.

7. Which HSG features differentiate bicornuate uterus from septate uterus?

8. When should supplemental imaging with sonography or MR be used in the evaluation of uterine anomalies?

9. Name the pathologic conditions which cause tubal obstruction and the usual site of involvement for each.

10. List the types of uterine myomas. Which are detectable by HSG and why?

Tutorial 25: Fallopian Tube Recanalization

1. True or False? Fallopian tube recanalization is best suited for proximal tubal occlusions.

2. True or False? Tubal spasm can mimic tubal occlusion.

3. True or False? If the occlusion is more than 2 cm from the ostium of the fallopian tube, a stiffer guide wire should be used to traverse the occlusion.

4. True or False? Fallopian tube perforation occurs in 10% of attempted fallopian tube recanalizations.

5. True or False? Visualization of pelvic veins is an indicator of perforation.

6. True or False? If perforation occurs, no special monitoring or treatment is required.

7. True or False? Fallopian tube recanalization has an 80%–85% success rate in re-establishing proximal tubal patency.

8. True or False? After fallopian tube recanalization, two thirds of the patients will have normal-appearing tubes.

9. True or False? The presence of hydrosalpinx or peritubular adhesions does not increase the risk of tubal pregnancy after recanalization of the fallopian tube.

10. True or False? Fallopian tube catheterization/recanalization is not a treatment for infertility.

Tutorial 26: Percutaneous Bone Biopsies

1. True or False? The transpedicular approach is more likely to injure the spinal nerve than the posterolateral approach in biopsy of the lumbar vertebral body.

2. True or False? The posterolateral approach provides access to a smaller portion of the vertebral body than the transpedicular approach in biopsy of the lumbar spine.

3. True or False? The transcostovertebral approach to thoracic spine biopsy has a high risk of pneumothorax.

4. True or False? Paralysis of the laryngeal nerve is a rare complication of cervical spine biopsy.

5. True or False? Transpedicular biopsies often require a “bone cutting” needle.

Tutorial 27: Musculoskeletal Spinal Intervention

1. True or False? Epidural steroid injections usually give relief within 24 hours if they are to be effective.

2. True or False? Facet injections cannot be successfully accomplished unless the joint line is visible fluoroscopically.

3. True or False? Sacral nerve block is usually performed with the patient lying prone.

4. True or False? The essential information from diskography is obtained from the CT diskogram.

5. True or False? The SI joint is most easily punctured by a posteromedial starting point, aiming at the inferior 1 cm of the joint.

INDEX

Tutorials

Teaching File Cases